Volume 2

The Knee

VOLUME 2

The Knee

W. NORMAN SCOTT, M.D.
Director
Insall Scott Kelly Institute
Beth Israel Hospital, North Division
New York, New York

With 1174 illustrations

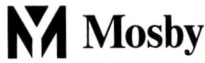 Mosby

St. Louis Baltimore Boston Chicago London Madrid Philadelphia Sydney Toronto

Publisher: George Stamathis
Editor: Robert Hurley
Associate Developmental Editor: Karyn Fell Taeyaerts
Project Manager: Nancy C. Baker
Project Supervisor: Carol A. Reynolds
Senior Production Editor: Jerry Schwartz
Proofroom Manager: Barbara M. Kelly
Designer: Carol A. Reynolds
Manufacturing Supervisor: Betty Richmond

Copyright © 1994 by Mosby–Year Book, Inc.

All rights reserved. No part of this publication may be reproduced, stored in a retrieval system, or transmitted, in any form or by any means, electronic, mechanical, photocopying, recording, or otherwise, without prior written permission from the publisher.

Permission to photocopy or reproduce solely for internal or personal use is permitted for libraries or other users registered with the Copyright Clearance Center, provided that the base fee of $4.00 per chapter plus $.10 per page is paid directly to the Copyright Clearance Center, 27 Congress Street, Salem, MA 01970. This consent does not extend to other kinds of copying, such as copying for general distribution, for advertising or promotional purposes, for creating new collected works, or for resale.

Printed in the United States of America.
Composition by Clarinda
Printing/binding by Maple-Vail

Mosby–Year Book, Inc.
11830 Westline Industrial Drive
St. Louis, Missouri 63146

Library of Congress Cataloging-in-Publication Data

The Knee / [edited by] W. Norman Scott.
    p. cm.
   Includes bibliographical references and index.
   ISBN 0-8016-6613-9
   1. Knee—Surgery. 2. Knee—Wounds and injuries. 3. Knee—Abnormalities. 4. Knee—Diseases I. Scott, W. Norman.
    [DNLM: 1. Knee—surgery. 2. Knee Joint—surgery. 3. Knee Injuries—rehabilitation. 4. Knee Prosthesis. 5. Arthroscopy. WE 870 K672 1993]
   RD561.K57   1993
   617.5′82—dc20   93-32910
   DNLM/DLC   CIP
   for Library of Congress

1 2 3 4 5 6 7 8 9 0 98 97 96 95 94

To our children, Eric, William, and Kelly

Careers and parenthood evolve through the daily challenges of intertwined failures and success which are responsive only to hard work, perseverance, and dedication to the distant and often elusive goal of personal happiness.

We dedicate this book to you, hoping both that your children give you as much happiness as you've afforded us, and that you pursue your careers with an unrelenting enthusiasm.

Contributors

Steven Albert, M.D.
Clinical Assistant Professor of Radiology
Cornell University Medical Center
Attending Radiologist
New York Hospital
New York, New York

Michael Alexiades, M.D.
Assistant Professor of Orthopaedic Surgery
Cornell University Medical College
Assistant Attending Orthopedic Surgeon
Hospital for Special Surgery
Lenox Hill Hospital
New York, New York

José A. Alicea, M.D.
Chief Resident, Department of Orthopaedics
Robert Wood Johnson University Hospital
University of Medicine and Dentistry of New Jersey
New Brunswick, New Jersey

Linda Altizer, R.N., M.S.N., O.N.C., C.E.N.
Nurse Manager, Staff Development
Washington County Hospital
Hagerstown, Maryland

Allen F. Anderson, M.D.
Clinical Instructor
Vanderbilt University
Director
Lipscomb Foundation for Education and Research
Nashville, Tennessee

James R. Andrews, M.D.
Medical Director
American Sports Medicine Institute
Clinical Professor of Orthopedics and Sports Medicine
University of Virginia Medical School
Orthopaedic Surgeon
Alabama Sports Medicine and Orthopaedic Center
Healthsouth Medical Center
Birmingham, Alabama

Steven Paul Arnoczky, D.V.M.
Wade O. Brinker Endowed Professor of Surgery
Director
Laboratory for Comparative Orthopaedic Research
College of Veterinary Medicine
Michigan State University
East Lansing, Michigan

Bernard R. Bach, Jr., M.D.
Associate Professor, Department of Orthopaedic Surgery
Director, Sports Medicine
Rush-Presbyterian-St. Luke's Medical Center
Chicago, Illinois

C. Lowry Barnes, M.D.
Assistant Clinical Professor, Department of Orthopaedic Surgery
University of Arkansas for Medical Sciences
Orthopaedic Specialists P.A.
Little Rock, Arkansas

James H. Beaty, M.D.
Associate Professor
University of Tennessee
The Campbell Clinic
Chief of Surgery
Le Bonheur Children's Medical Center
Memphis, Tennessee

Jeffrey R. Bechler, M.D.
Champion Orthopaedics
San Diego, California

Lee H. Bender, M.S., R.N., C.N.A.A.
Director, Patient Care Services
Shriners Hospitals for Crippled Children
Greenville, South Carolina

Jack M. Bert, M.D., F.A.C.S.
Clinical Professor
University of Minnesota School of Medicine
President
St. Paul Bone & Joint Specialists
St. Joseph's Hospital
St. Paul, Minnesota

Robert E. Booth, Jr., M.D.
Professor and Vice Chairman
Department of Orthopaedic Surgery
Jefferson Medical College
Thomas Jefferson University
Co-chief, Orthopaedic Surgery
Pennsylvania Hospital
Philadelphia, Pennsylvania

Robert W. Bucholz, M.D.
Professor and Chairman, Department of Orthopaedic Surgery
University of Texas Southwestern Medical School
Dallas, Texas

Frederick F. Buechel, M.D.
Clinical Professor of Orthopaedic Surgery
New Jersey Medical School
University of Medicine and Dentistry of New Jersey
Chief, Total Joint Reconstructive and Arthritis Surgery Services
Chairman, Department of Orthopaedics & Fractures
New Jersey Orthopaedic Hospital
Orange, New Jersey

David D. Bullek, M.D.
Fellow
Insall Scott Kelly Institute for Orthopaedics and Sports Medicine
Beth Israel Medical Center
New York, New York

Robert T. Burks, M.D.
Assistant Professor of Orthopaedic Surgery
University of Utah
Salt Lake City, Utah

Roger B. Butorac, F.R.A.C.S. (ORTHO)
Visiting Orthopaedic Surgeon
Launceston General Hospital
Launceston, Australia

Sturla Terrence Canale, M.D.
Professor, Department of Orthopaedics
University of Tennessee and The Campbell Clinic
Memphis, Tennessee
Chief of Pediatric Orthopaedics and Active Staff
Baptist Memorial Hospitals
The Regional Medical Center
Le Bonheur Children's Hospital
Memphis, Tennessee

W. Dilworth Cannon, Jr., M.D.
Professor of Clinical Orthopaedic Surgery
Director of Sports Medicine
University of California, San Francisco
San Francisco, California

Samuel W. Capra, Jr., M.D.
Tahoe Forest Hospital
Trucker, California

Susan M. Craig, M.D.
Assistant Professor of Surgery
Mt. Sinai School of Medicine
Assistant Attending Surgeon
Mt. Sinai Hospital
Beth Israel Medical Center, North Division
New York, New York

Robert D. D'Ambrosia, M.D.
Professor and Chairman, Department of Orthopaedic Surgery
Louisiana State University School of Medicine
New Orleans, Louisiana

Francis G. D'Ambrosio, M.D.
Clinical Instructor
Attending Orthopaedic Surgeon
Rancho Los Amigos Medical Center
Downey, California

Lawrence P. Davis, M.D.
Associate Professor, Department of Radiology
Wayne State University School of Medicine
Attending Physician, Department of Radiology
Harper Hospital
Detroit, Michigan

Jeffrey V. DeLuca, M.D.
Assistant Attending
Norwalk Hospital
Norwalk, Connecticut

Douglas A. Dennis, M.D.
Assistant Clinical Professor
University of Colorado Health Sciences Center
Attending Orthopaedic Surgeon
University Hospital
St. Joseph Hospital
P/SL Denver
Rose Medical Center
Children's Hospital
Vencor Hospital
Denver, Colorado

Lawrence D. Dorr, M.D.
Director & Professor, Department of Orthopaedic Surgery
University of Southern California Center for Arthritis and Joint Implant Surgery
Professor of Orthopaedic Surgery
USC University Hospital
Los Angeles, California

Scott F. Dye, M.D.
Assistant Clinical Professor of Orthopaedic Surgery
University of California, San Francisco
Chief of Orthopaedics
Davies Medical Center
Mount Zion Medical Center
California Pacific Medical Center
San Francisco, California

Robert W. Eberle
Research Coordinator
The Grant Orthopaedic Institute
Grant Medical Center
Columbus, Ohio

Gregory C. Fanelli, M.D.
Chief of Sports Medicine and Associate
Department of Orthopaedic Surgery
Geisinger Clinic
Geisinger Medical Center
Danville, Pennsylvania

Philip M. Faris, M.D.
Orthopaedic Surgeon
Kendrick Memorial Hospital
St. Frances Hospital
Mooresville, Indiana

Stephen V. Fealy, B.A.
Medical Student
Columbia University College of Physicians and Surgeons
New York, New York

Robert H. Fitzgerald Jr., M.D.
Professor and Chairman
Wayne State University School of Medicine
Chairman, Department of Orthopaedic Surgery
Detroit Medical Center
Detroit, Michigan

William F. Flynn, Jr., M.D.
Fellow, Joint Reconstruction
The Hospital for Special Surgery
New York, New York

Peter J. Fowler, M.D., F.R.C.S.(C)
Professor of Orthopaedic Surgery
Head, Section of Sports Medicine
University of Western Ontario
Orthopaedic Surgeon
University Hospital
London, Ontario

Andrew G. Franks, Jr., M.D., F.A.C.P.
Clinical Associate Professor
New York University Medical Center
Attending Rheumatologist
Hospital for Joint Diseases
Lenox Hill Hospital
New York, New York

Marc J. Friedman, M.D.
Assistant Clinical Professor, Division of Orthopaedics
University of California, Los Angeles School of Medicine
Southern California Orthopaedic Institute
Van Nuys, California

Freddie H. Fu, M.D.
Blue Cross of Western Pennsylvania
Professor, Orthopaedic Surgery
Chief, Division of Sports Medicine
Vice Chairman, Clinical Department of Orthopedic Surgery
University of Pittsburgh School of Medicine
Pittsburgh, Pennsylvania

John P. Fulkerson, M.D.
Professor
University of Connecticut School of Medicine
Farmington, Connecticut

Charles A. Gatto, M.D.
Resident, Orthopaedic Surgery
Albany Medical College
Albany Medical Center Hospital
Albany, New York

Matthew B. Gavin, M.D.
Orthopaedic Surgeon
National Hospital for Orthopaedics and Rehabilitation
Northern Virginia Hospital
Arlington, Virginia
Mount Vernon Hospital
Alexandria, Virginia

Bernard Ghelman, M.D.
Associate Professor of Radiology
Cornell University Medical College
Attending Radiologist
The Hospital for Special Surgery
New York Hospital
New York, New York

Mary Ann Gibney, R.N., M.P.H.
The Hospital for Special Surgery
New York, New York

Jonathan L. Glashow, M.D.
Adjunct Attending Physician
Lenox Hill Hospital
New York, New York

Victor M. Goldberg, M.D.
Charles H. Herndon Professor
Case Western Reserve University
Chairman, Department of Orthopaedics
University Hospitals of Cleveland
Cleveland, Ohio

John Goodfellow, M.S., F.R.C.S.
Honorary Consultant Surgeon
Nuffield Orthopaedic Centre
Oxford, United Kingdom

Robert S. Gotlin, D.O.
Instructor, Physical Medicine and Rehabilitation
Mount Sinai School of Medicine
Physician-in-Charge, Orthopaedic and Sports Section
Department of Physical Medicine and Rehabilitation
Beth Israel Medical Center
New York, New York

Mark A. Greenfield, D.O.
Fellow
Insall Scott Kelly Institute for Orthopaedics and Sports Medicine
New York, New York
Steingard Orthopaedics and Sports Medicine
Phoenix, Arizona

Alison B. Haimes, M.D.
Clinical Assistant Professor of Radiology
Cornell University Medical Center
Adjunct Clinical Assistant Attending
New York Hospital
Memorial Sloan Kettering Cancer Center
New York, New York

Gregory T. Hardin, M.D.
Fellow, Sports Medicine Section
Rush-Presbyterian-St. Lukes Medical Center
Chicago, Illinois

Mark L. Harlow, M.D.
Attending Orthopaedic Surgeon
Rapid City Region Hospital
Rapid City, South Dakota

John H. Healey, M.D.
Associate Professor of Orthopaedic Surgery
Cornell University Medical College
Chief of Orthopaedic Surgery
Memorial Sloan Kettering Cancer Center
New York, New York

William L. Healy, M.D.
Chairman, Department of Orthopaedic Surgery
Lahey Clinic
Burlington, Massachusetts

Robert C. Hendler, M.D.
Director
Mid-Hudson Orthopedic and Sports Medicine, P.C.
Attending Orthopaedic Surgeon
Arden Hill Hospital
Goshen, New York

Jacqueline C. Hodge, M.D.
Instructor, Musculoskeletal Radiology
Washington University Medical Center
The Mallinckrodt Institute of Radiology
St. Louis, Missouri

Aaron A. Hofmann, M.D.
Professor
University of Utah School of Medicine
University of Utah Medical Center
Salt Lake City, Utah

Timothy M. Hosea, M.D.
Clinical Assistant Professor of Orthopaedic Surgery
Robert Wood Johnson Medical School
University of Medicine and Dentistry of New Jersey
Attending Surgeon
Robert Wood Johnson University Hospital,
St. Peter's Medical Center
New Brunswick, New Jersey

Gordon Huie
Mount Sinai School of Medicine
Supervising Physician Assistant
Insall Scott Kelly Institute for Orthopaedics and Sports Medicine
Beth Israel Medical Center, North Division
New York, New York

John N. Insall, M.D.
Director
Insall Scott Kelly Institute for Orthopaedics and Sports Medicine
Attending Orthopaedic Surgeon
Beth Israel Medical Center, North Division
New York, New York

Glen E. Johnson, M.D.
Associate Clinical Professor
Washington University School of Medicine
Missouri Baptist Hospital, St. Louis, Missouri
St. Joseph Hospital, St. Charles, Missouri
Barnes Hospital, St. Peters, Missouri

Robert J. Johnson, M.D.
Professor of Orthopaedic Surgery
University of Vermont
Attending in Orthopaedic Surgery
Medical Center Hospital of Vermont
Burlington, Vermont

Stuart D. Katchis, M.D.
Fellow, Department of Sports Medicine
The Cleveland Clinic Foundation
Cleveland, Ohio

Richard Katz, M.D.
Clinical Assistant Professor of Radiology
Cornell University Medical Center
Attending Radiologist
New York Hospital
New York, New York

Anne M. Kelly, M.D.
Orthopaedic Resident
George Washington University
George Washington University Hospital
Washington, District of Columbia

Michael A. Kelly, M.D.
Director
Insall Scott Kelly Institute for Orthopaedics and Sports Medicine
Beth Israel Medical Center, North Division
New York, New York

Matthew J. Kraay, B.S., M.S., M.D.
Assistant Professor of Orthopaedic Surgery
Case Western Reserve University
Attending Surgeon
University Hospitals of Cleveland
Cleveland, Ohio

Laurie Lewis, M.D.
Directors, Pain Service
Beth Israel Hospital, North Division
New York, New York

A. Brant Lipscomb, Jr., M.D.
Clinical Assistant Professor of Orthopaedics
Vanderbilt University
Nashville, Tennessee

Adolph V. Lombardi, Jr., M.D., F.A.C.S.
Clinical Assistant Professor
Department of Surgery
Division of Orthopaedics
Department of Biomedical Engineering
Ohio State University Hospitals
Director
Research of Grant Orthopaedic Institute
Grant Medical Center
Columbus, Ohio

Stephen J. Lombardo, M.D.
Associate Clinical Professor of Orthopaedic Surgery
University of Southern California Medical Center
Associate
Kerlan-Jobe Orthopaedic Clinic
Inglewood, California

Paul A. Lotke, M.D.
Professor of Orthopaedic Surgery
University of Pennsylvania School of Medicine
Chief of Implant Service
Delaware County Memorial Hospital
Drexel Hill, Pennsylvania

Michael G. Maday, M.D.
Former Fellow in Sports Medicine
University of Pittsburgh
Midland Orthopaedic Associates
Section of Orthopaedic Surgery
Mercy Hospital & Medical Center
Chicago, Illinois

James H. Maguire, M.D.
Associate Professor of Medicine
Harvard Medical School
Physician and Clinical Director
Infectious Disease Division
Brigham and Women's Hospital
Boston, Massachusetts

Mehrdad M. Malek, M.D., F.A.C.S.
Associate Professor
Howard University
Director, Washington Orthopaedic and Knee Clinic, Inc.
Oxon Hill, Maryland

Thomas H. Mallory, M.D., F.A.C.S.
Graduate Faculty of Biomedical Engineering
Clinical Assistant Professor of Orthopaedic Surgery
Ohio State University Hospitals
Chairman
Grant Orthopaedic Institute
Chairman of Section, Joint Implant Surgery
Grant Medical Center
Columbus, Ohio

Marilyn J. Manco-Johnson, M.D.
Associate Professor, Department of Pediatrics
University of Colorado Health Sciences Center
University Hospital
The Children's Hospital
Denver, Colorado

Michael A. Masini, M.D.
St. Vincent's Medical Center
The Toledo Hospital
Toledo, Ohio

Henry Masur, M.D.
Chief, Critical Care Medicine
Clinical Center, National Institutes of Health
Clinical Professor of Medicine
George Washington University Medical Center
Washington, D.C.

Alan C. Merchant, M.D.
Clinical Professor of Orthopaedic Surgery
Stanford University School of Medicine
Active Staff, Orthopaedics
El Camino Hospital
Mountain View, California

Lyle J. Micheli, M.D.
Associate Clinical Professor, Orthopaedic Surgery
Harvard Medical Center
Director, Division of Sports Medicine
The Children's Hospital
Boston, Massachusetts

Richard P. Mikosz, Ph.D.
Assistant Professor
Rush Medical College
Assistant Scientist
Rush-Presbyterian-St. Luke's Medical Center
Chicago, Illinois

Drew V. Miller, M.D.
St. Joseph's Hospital
Northside Hospital
Atlanta, Georgia

Craig G. Mohler, M.D.
Clinical Instructor
Rush Medical College
Joint Replacement Fellow
Rush-Presbyterian-St. Luke's Medical Center
Chicago, Illinois

Ryuji Nagamine, M.D.
Chief, Department of Orthopaedic Surgery
JR Kyushu Hospital
Kitakyushu-city Fukuoka, Japan

Claude E. Nichols, III, M.D.
Assistant Professor/Coordinator, Orthopaedic Surgery Residency Program
University of Vermont College of Medicine
Medical Center Hospital of Vermont, Burlington, Vermont
Fanny Allen Hospital of Vermont, Colchester, Vermont

Stephen J. O'Brien, M.D.
The Hospital for Special Surgery
New York, New York

John O'Connor, B.E., M.A., Ph.D.
Research Director
Oxford Orthopaedic Engineering Centre
University Lecturer
University of Oxford
Fellow, St. Peter's College
Oxford, United Kingdom

Lonnie E. Paulos, M.D.
Medical Director,
Orthopaedic Biomechanics Institute
Co-Director
The Orthopedic Specialty Hospital
Salt Lake City, Utah

Glenn B. Perry, M.D.
Orthopaedic Surgeon
Carolinas Medical Center
Presbyterian-Orthopaedic Hospital
University Memorial Hospital
Mercy Hospital
Charlotte, North Carolina

William R. Post, M.D.
Assistant Professor, Section of Sports Medicine
Department of Orthopaedics
West Virginia University
Morgantown, West Virginia

Chitranjan S. Ranawat, M.D.
Professor of Orthopaedic Surgery
Cornell University Medical College
New York Hospital
Director, Surgical Arthritis Service
Attending Physician
Hospital for Special Surgery
New York, New York

James A. Rand, M.D.
Professor of Orthopaedic Surgery
Mayo Medical School
Mayo Clinic Scottsdale
Scottsdale, Arizona

Bart P. Rask, M.D.
Fellow in Sports Medicine
The Children's Hospital
Harvard Medical School
Boston, Massachusetts

Bruce Reider, M.D.
Associate Professor of Surgery
University of Chicago Pritzker School of Medicine
Director of Sports Medicine
University of Chicago Hospitals
Chicago, Illinois

John P. Reilly, M.D.
Attending Surgeon
Staten Island University Hospital
Adjunct Attending Department of Orthopedic Surgery
Lenox Hill Hospital
Assistant Attending Department of Orthopedic Surgery
Beth Israel Medical Center, North Division
New York, New York

Arthur C. Rettig, M.D.
Associate Clinical Professor
Indiana University School of Medicine
Methodist Sports Medicine Center
Indianapolis, Indiana

Kayvon S. Riggi, M.D.
Senior Resident
Mayo Clinic, Rochester, Minnesota
Sports Medicine Fellow
Orthopedic Surgery and Athletic Medicine
University of Texas Health Science Center
San Antonio, Texas

Clare M. Rimnac, Ph.D.
Associate Professor
Cornell University Medical College
Associate Scientist
The Hospital for Special Surgery
New York, New York

William G. Rodkey, D.V.M.
Diplomate
American College of Veterinary Surgeons
Director, Research and Education
Steadman Sports Medicine Foundation
Director, Scientific Affairs
ReGen Biologics
Vail, Colorado

Aaron G. Rosenberg, M.D.
Associate Professor
Rush Medical College
Attending Surgeon
Rush-Presbyterian-St. Luke's Medical Center
Chicago, Illinois

Richard A. Rubinstein Jr, M.D.
Assistant Professor of Orthopaedic Surgery
Oregon Health Sciences University
Active Staff, Orthopaedic Surgery
Providence Medical Center
Portland, Oregon

Anthony J. Saraniti, M.S., P.T.
Director,
Eastside Sports Physical Therapy Center
Westside Sports Physical Therapy Center
New York, New York

Robert R. Scheinberg, M.D.
Dallas, Texas

Morton Schneider, M.D.
Lenox Hill Hospital
New York, New York

Richard D. Scott, M.D.
Associate Clinical Professor of Orthopaedic Surgery,
Harvard Medical School
Surgeon, Brigham and Women's Hospital
New England Baptist Hospital
Boston, Massachusetts

Giles R. Scuderi, M.D.
Attending Orthopedic Surgeon
Insall Scott Kelly Institute for Orthopaedics & Sports Medicine
Attending Orthopedic Surgeon
Beth Israel Medical Center, North Division
New York, New York

Thomas P. Sculco, M.D.
Clinical Professor, Orthopaedic Surgery
Cornell University Medical College
Director, Orthopaedic Surgery
The Hospital for Special Surgery
New York, New York

Dana G. Seltzer, M.D.
Chief of Sports Medicine and Shoulder Surgery
Phoenix Orthopaedic Residency Program
Maricopa Medical Center
Phoenix, Arizona

John H. Serocki, M.D.
Scripps Hospital
San Diego, California

K. Donald Shelbourne, M.D.
Assistant Clinical Professor
Indiana University School of Medicine
Methodist Sports Medicine Center
Indianapolis, Indiana

John M. Siliski, M.D.
Assistant Professor
Harvard Medical School

Chief, Reconstructive Knee Unit
Massachusetts General Hospital
Boston, Massachusetts

Stephen R. Soffer, M.D.
Co-Director
Eastern Sports Medicine and Orthopedic Institute
Orthopaedic Surgeon
Reading Hospital
West Reading, Pennsylvania

Moshe Solomonow, Ph.D
Professor and Director of Bioengineering
Department of Orthopaedic Surgery
Louisiana State University Medical Center
Director, Paraplegic Locomotion Program
Rehabilitation Institute of New Orleans
New Orleans, Louisiana

Norman F. Sprague, III, M.D.
Assistant Clinical Professor
University of California, Los Angeles School of Medicine
St. John's Hospital
Santa Monica, California

J. Richard Steadman, M.D.
Clinical Professor
University of Texas Southwestern Medical School, Dallas, Texas
Chairman of Medical Group and Chief Surgeon, United States Ski Team
Orthopaedic Surgeon
Steadman Hawkins Clinic
Vail, Colorado

Steven H. Stern, M.D.
Assistant Professor, Department of Orthopaedic Surgery
Northwestern University Medical School
Active Attending Orthopaedic Surgeon
Northwestern Memorial Hospital
Chicago, Illinois

Dania A. Sweitzer, P.T.
Director
Pleasantville Physical Therapy and Sports Care P.C.
Pleasantville, New York

Ronald W. Sweitzer, M.S. P.T.
Director
Pleasantville Physical Therapy and Sports Care, P.C.
Pleasantville, New York

David Templeman, M.D.
Assistant Professor, Department of Orthopaedic Surgery
University of Minnesota
Staff
Hennepin County Medical Center
Minneapolis, Minnesota

Richard M. Terek, M.D.
Assistant Professor, Department of Orthopaedics
Brown University
Surgeon
Rhode Island Hospital
Roger Williams Medical Center
Providence, Rhode Island

Thomas S. Thornhill, M.D.
Asociate Clinical Professor of Orthopaedics
Harvard Medical School
Brigham and Women's Hospital
New England Baptist Hospital
Boston, Massachusetts

Brad S. Tolin, M.D.
Clinical Assistant Professor of Orthopaedic Surgery
University of Texas Health Center at San Antonio
San Antonio, Texas

Alfred J. Tria, Jr., M.D.
Associate Clinical Professor of Orthopaedics
Robert Wood Johnson University Medical School
New Brunswick, New Jersey

Mary Ann Underhill, M.S., R.N., O.N.C.
Adjunct Assistant Professor
Indiana University School of Nursing
Clinical Nurse Specialist, Orthopaedics
Community Hospitals Indianapolis
Indianapolis, Indiana

Vincent J. Vigorita, M.D.
Associate Professor of Pathology
State University Health Science Center
Medical Director
Lutheran Medical Center
Brooklyn, New York

Kelly G. Vince, M.D., F.R.C.S.(C.)
Assistant Clinical Professor, Department of Surgery
University of California-Irvine College of Medicine
Senior Orthopaedic Surgeon
Centinela Hospital Medical Center, Inglewood, California
Consultant, Arthritis Service
Rancho Los Amigos Medical Center, Downey, California
Associate Orthopaedic Surgeon
Kerlan-Jobe Orthopaedic Clinic, Inglewood, California

Virginia D. Wade, M.D.
Attending Anesthesiologist
Beth Israel Medical Center, North Division
New York, New York

William C. Warner, Jr., M.D.
Assistant Professor, Department of Orthopaedic Surgery
University of Tennessee
The Campbell Clinic
Staff Physician
LeBonheur Children's Hospital
Memphis, Tennessee

Leo A. Whiteside, M.D.
Research Assistant Professor of Surgery
Department of Orthopaedic Surgery
Washington University
Chief of Orthopaedic Surgery
Director, Biomechanical Research Laboratory
DePaul Health Center
St. Louis, Missouri

Jerome D. Wiedel, M.D.
Professor & Chairman, Department of Orthopaedics
University of Colorado Health Sciences Center
University Hospital
Denver, Colorado

Richard M. Wilk, M.D.
Attending Surgeon, Department of Orthopaedic Surgery
Lahey Clinic
Burlington, Massachusetts

Steve A. Wilson, M.D.
Fellow, Sports Medicine
Beth Israel Medical Center, North Division
New York, New York

Timothy M. Wright, M.D.
Professor
Cornell University Medical College
Director, Department of Biomechanics
The Hospital for Special Surgery
New York, New York

S. Steven Yang, M.D., M.P.H.
Chief Resident, Orthopaedic Surgery
Lenox Hill Hospital
New York, New York

FOREWORD

The compilation of this book is indeed a gigantic effort and easily shows it in the end product. Dr. Scott has brought together a group of authors at various stages of their careers who have managed to produce an extremely comprehensive volume that covers every aspect of understanding and management of knee problems, from basic science through medical and surgical treatment and rehabilitation. This monumental task has produced a reference volume that will be indispensable to students and practitioners.

In their professional lives most knee surgeons emphasize either reconstructive surgery for arthritis or ligament reconstruction and arthroscopy for athletic injuries and their sequelae. Dr. Scott is the unusual individual who has extensive experience in not only reconstructive surgery such as arthroplasty, but also athletic injuries, ligament surgery, and arthroscopy. It is these talents that have enabled him to assemble such a comprehensive text.

In the past 30 years I have watched orthopaedic surgery move on a course of increasing subspecialization. This trend has resulted in the proliferation and growth of subspecialty societies, an increasing percentage of graduating residents taking fellowships for a variety of reasons, and tremendous technological advancement, and has culminated in the issue of Certificates of Added Qualification. However, with our current interest in health care reform and our movement toward managed care and possibly managed competition, it is likely that this trend toward subspecialization will at least lessen and perhaps reverse itself. The organization of this text and the information in it is most appropriate for subspecialist and generalist alike.

Those of us who have been involved in the growth of knee surgery in the last 2 decades frequently wonder if newer procedures are being overutilized. The growth of technology, competition, and marketing are certainly factors that tend to foster this overutilization. It is through familiarity with the information in a text such as *The Knee* that these factors can be put in perspective to the benefit of both the patient with knee problems and his surgeon.

John B. McGinty, M.D.
Charleston, South Carolina

PREFACE

When asked to develop a text on the knee about 10 years ago, I was both intrigued and overwhelmed by the project. From a practical viewpoint, it appeared that it would be best to publish several books on specific topics of particular interest to the knee student and subsequently combine them into an overall textbook. I did, indeed, publish three other books, *Total Knee Revision Arthroplasty, Arthroscopy of the Knee, and Ligament and Extensor Mechanism Injuries of the Knee.* The unbelievable progress in all aspects of the diagnosis and treatment of knee pathology, however, rendered many of the previous chapters obsolete. In fact, this explosion of scientific knowledge has necessitated expansion of the sections with more contributions to keep the information current.

This two-volume text, inclusive of 84 chapters, is a true mosaic of the various disciplines that overlap in the treatment of knee disorders. In the medical environment of the nineties, "gatekeepers," internists, nurses, physical therapists, physicians' assistants, bioengineers, radiologists, rheumatologists, anesthesiologists, physiatrists, and pediatricians are all involved to varying degrees in dealing with the symptomatic knee. The contributors are thus representative of this multi-disciplinary approach, hopefully appealing to a correspondingly wide spectrum of readers.

This book has been organized into 17 sections (parts) which include basic science and the diagnosis and treatment of specific knee injuries. There is some overlap which is purposeful, because many knee injuries often cannot be so easily partitioned. In Part I, the anatomy has been presented from a combined histological, gross, arthroscopic, radiologic, and clinical perspective. It is our aspiration that this functional approach will better integrate with the knee physiology, biomechanics, and imaging sections (Part II and III). While many physicians do not treat the pediatric patient, an understanding of both congenital anomalies and the pediatric knee (Part IV) is essential in caring for the adolescent athlete.

Similarly, there are many specific medical aspects with which the treating knee physician has to be familiar. Part V contains these topics: anesthesia, rheumatological aspects of knee disorders, hemophiliac arthropathy, HIV and its relationship to knee disorders, and reflex sympathetic dystrophy.

The "patella," or more accurately, the extensor mechanism, remains an enigma from the pediatric to the geriatric knee, and thus six chapters are devoted exclusively to this topic (Part VI). Part VII is an arthroscopic section which focuses on the history of arthroscopic equipment, setup, and a more detailed arthroscopic anatomy. Similarly, Part VIII focuses on the arthroscopic treatment of cartilage and synovial disorders. Parts IX, X, XI, and XII include 21 chapters discussing ligament pathology. This abundance of information is reflective of the controversy which still surrounds these seemingly more frequent injuries. On the contrary, Part XIII only contains two chapters on rather infrequent dislocations of the tibiofemoral and tibiofibular articulations.

The classic surgical approaches to the arthritic knee, osteotomy, knee replacement, and revision arthroplasty are discussed thoroughly in Parts XIV and XV. The various nonsurgical and operative complications can be devastating, and thus, these appropriate chapters are essential to the total knee student.

Fractures and tumors about the knee are more often treated by different subspecialists, but in view of a recent attempt to deemphasize the specialist, we thought it appropriate to include a summary of treatment modalities. It should be noted that for the first time, to the best of our knowledge, we have integrated the nursing and rehabilitation chapters in the specific parts rather that isolate them. It seems that this approach is both essential and reflective of better patient care.

As we look to the future, it might be an "unreachable goal" to outdo the last 20 years. In this interval, technology allowed us to diagnose the "internal derangement" with more accuracy, minimize the indications for arthrotomy for any type of cartilage and ligament surgery, and expand the indications for knee arthroplasty. As we accumulate the "hard" data and "soft" outcome study information in the next 5 years, we will all be challenged to pursue scientific excellence in an atmosphere of cost containment. While this is a discouraging interval for the medical community, history suggests that our resourcefulness will prevail and the goal of improving our patient's lives will not be lost. On behalf of all the contributors to this textbook, I hope we have presented a thorough and sometimes provocative text to stimulate and encourage all the professionals involved in the understanding and treatment of knee disorders.

W. Norman Scott, M.D.

ACKNOWLEDGMENT

Publishing a textbook is tremendous and often overwhelming detail work. It requires tireless and conscientious devotion. Since such patience is not necessarily my strongest suit, I've had to rely on Denise Henock and Gordon Huie to make this happen. To both of you, thanks for a tremendous effort.

Contents

Volume 2

Foreword   xv

Preface   xvii

PART XI: SURGICAL MANAGEMENT OF CRUCIATE AND COLLATERAL LIGAMENT INJURIES

41 / **Indications and a Surgical Philosophy for Managing Anterior Cruciate Ligament Disruption**   747
Jonathan Glashow and W. Norman Scott

42 / **Arthroscopic Anterior Cruciate Ligament Reconstruction Utilizing Patellar Tendon**   757
Bruce Reider

43 / **Iliotibial Myofascial Transfer**   773
W. Norman Scott and Gordon Huie

44 / **Intraarticular and Extraarticular Anterior Cruciate Ligament Reconstruction**   791
Mehrdad M. Malek, Gregory C. Fanelli, Jeffrey V. DeLuca

45 / **Intraarticular Semitendinosus Anterior Cruciate Ligament Reconstruction**   813
Robert C. Hendler

46 / **Anterior Cruciate Ligament Reconstruction With the Kennedy Ligament Augmentation Device**   829
Peter J. Fowler and Samuel W. Capra, Jr.

47 / **Artificial Cruciate Ligament Reconstruction**   839
Brad S. Tolin and Marc J. Friedman

48 / **Allografts in Knee Ligament Surgery**   865
Dana G. Seltzer and Stephen J. Lombardo

49 / **Posterior Cruciate Reconstruction With Bone-Patellar Tendon-Bone Autografts**   895
James R. Andrews and Stephen R. Soffer

50 / **Posterior Cruciate Ligament Reconstruction With Semitendinosus and Gracilis Tendons**   913
A. Brant Lipscomb, Jr. and Allen F. Anderson

PART XII: REHABILITATION, BRACING, AND NURSING CARE FOR CARTILAGE AND LIGAMENTOUS INJURIES

51 / **Rehabilitation of Cartilage Lesions**   921
Ronald W. Sweitzer, Dania A. Sweitzer, Anthony J. Saraniti

52 / **Knee Rehabilitation After Knee Ligament Injury or Surgery**   943
Lonnie E. Paulos

53 / **Knee Braces for Athletic Injuries**   957
Gregory T. Hardin and Bernard R. Bach, Jr.

54 / **Nursing Care of the Patient With a Ligament Injury**   983
Linda L. Altizer

PART XIII: KNEE DISLOCATION

55 / **Traumatic Dislocation of the Knee**   999
John M. Siliski

56 / **Dislocation of the Proximal Tibiofibular Joint**   1009
Stuart D. Katchis and W. Norman Scott

PART XIV: OSTEOTOMY AND PRIMARY TOTAL KNEE REPLACEMENT

57 / **Osteotomy in Treatment of the Arthritic Knee**   1019
William L. Healy and Richard M Wilk

58 / **Evolution of Total Knee Arthroplasty**   1045
Kelly G. Vince

59 / **Biomechanical Aspects of Knee Replacement Designs**   1079
Leo A. Whiteside and Ryuji Nagamine

60 / **Unicompartmental Knee Replacement** 1097
C. Lowry Barnes and Richard D. Scott

61 / **Cementless Total Knee Arthroplasty** 1105
Matthew J. Kraay and Victor M. Goldberg

62 / **Posterior Cruciate Ligament-Retaining Total Knee Arthroplasty** 1117
Kayvon S. Riggi and James A. Rand

63 / **The Role of Congruent Meniscal Bearings in Knee Arthroplasty** 1143
John Goodfellow and John O'Connor

64 / **Meniscal Bearing Knee Replacement: Development, Long-Term Results, and Future Technology** 1157
Frederick F. Buechel

65 / **Cruciate-Substituting Knee Arthroplasty** 1179
Steven H. Stern and John N. Insall

66 / **Ligament Releases in the Arthritic Knee** 1199
Francis G. D'Ambrosio and W. Norman Scott

67 / **Transfusion Considerations in Total Knee Arthroplasty** 1211
Phillip M. Faris

68 / **Thrombophlebitis in Knee Arthroplasty** 1217
Paul A. Lotke

69 / **Nursing Care of a Patient Having a Total Knee Arthroplasty** 1227
Mary Ann Underhill

PART XV: REVISION TOTAL KNEE REPLACEMENT

70 / **Mechanisms of Failure of Total Knee Arthroplasty** 1239
Lawrence D. Dorr and John H. Serocki

71 / **Retrieval Analysis of Knee Replacements** 1251
Clare M. Rimnac and Timothy M. Wright

72 / **Infected Total Knee Arthroplasty** 1261
Michael A. Masini, James H. Maguire, Thomas S. Thornhill

73 / **Sort Tissue Considerations in the Failed Total Knee Arthroplasty** 1279
Susan M. Craig

74 / **Principles of Planning and Prosthetic Selection for Revision Total Knee Replacement** 1297
Chitranjan S. Ranwat and William F. Flynn, Jr.

75 / **Constrained Knee Arthroplasty** 1305
Adolph V. Lombardi, Jr., Thomas H. Mallory, Robert W. Eberle

76 / **Patellar Complications in Total Knee Arthroplasty** 1325
Robert E. Booth, Jr.

77 / **Bone Grafting in Total Knee Arthroplasty** 1353
Thomas P. Sculco

78 / **Arthrodesis and Resection Arthroplasty for the Failed Total Knee Replacement** 1345
Douglas A. Dennis

PART XVI: FRACTURES ABOUT THE KNEE

79 / **Supracondylar and Intercondylar Distal Femoral Fractures** 1357
David Templeman

80 / **Tibial Plateau Fractures** 1369
John P. Reilly

81 / **Fractures of the Patella** 1393
Robert R. Scheinberg and Robert W. Bucholz

82 / **Periprosthetic Fractures** 1405
Mark L. Harlow and Aaron A. Hofmann

PART XVII: TUMORS ABOUT THE KNEE

83 / **Tumor and Tumor-Like Lesions of the Knee** 1421
Vincent J. Vigorita, Charles Gatto, Bernard Ghelman

84 / **Management of Bone and Soft Tissue Tumors About the Knee** 1441
John H. Healey and Richard M. Terek

Index xxv

Contents

Volume 1

Foreword xv

Preface xvii

PART I: EMBRYOLOGY, ANATOMY AND SURGICAL APPROACHES TO THE KNEE

1 / **Embryology of the Knee** 3
Timothy M. Hosea, Alfred J. Tria, Jr., Jeffrey R. Bechler

2 / **Anatomy** 15
Steve A. Wilson, Vincent J. Vigorita, W. Norman Scott

3 / **Surgical Approaches to the Knee** 55
Giles R. Scuderi

PART II: KNEE PHYSIOLOGY AND BIOMECHANICS

4 / **Basic Knee Biomechanics** 75
Aaron Rosenberg, Richard P. Mikosz, Craig G. Mohler

5 / **Gait Analysis and Its Relationship to Knee Function** 95
Aaron Rosenberg, Craig G. Mohler, Richard P. Mikosz

6 / **Neural Reflex Arcs and Muscle Control of Knee Stability and Motion** 107
Moshe Solomonow and Robert D. D'Ambrosia

PART III: IMAGING

7 / **Standard Radiologic Analysis of the Normal and Abnormal Knee** 123
Jacqueline C. Hodge and Bernard Ghelman

8 / **Magnetic Resonance Imaging of the Knee** 159
Steven Albert, Richard Katz, Morton Schneider, Alison B. Haimes

9 / **Nuclear Scans** 195
Robert H. Fitzgerald, Jr. and Lawrence P. Davis

PART IV: CONGENITAL DEFORMITIES AND THE PEDIATRIC KNEE

10 / **Congenital Deformities of the Knee** 209
William C. Warner, Jr., Sturla Terrence Canale, James H. Beaty

11 / **The Pediatric Knee** 229
Bart P. Rask and Lyle J. Micheli

12 / **Nursing Care of the Pediatric Patient With a Knee Disorder** 277
Lee H. Bender

PART V: ANESTHETIC AND SELECTED MEDICAL CONSIDERATIONS

13 / **Anesthetic Considerations for Knee Surgery** 299
Virginia D. Wade

14 / **Rheumatologic Aspects of Knee Disorders** 315
Andrew G. Franks, Jr.

15 / **Hemophilia and Knee Arthropathy** 331
Jerome D. Wiedel and Marilyn Manco-Johnson

16 / **Pathophysiology of HIV Infection and Its Relationship to Knee Disorders** 347
Lauren Wood and Henry Masur

17 / **Reflex Sympathetic Dystrophy** 365
Michael A. Kelly, Robert S. Gotlin, Laurie Lewis

PART VI: PATELLAR AND EXTENSOR MECHANISM DISORDERS

18 / **Functional Anatomy and Biomechanics of the Patellofemoral Joint** 381
Scott F. Dye

19 / **Patellofemoral Pain** 391
Mark A. Greenfield and W. Norman Scott

20 / **Extensor Mechanism Injuries: Classification and Diagnosis** 403
Alan C. Merchant

21 / **Nonoperative Treatment of Patellofemoral Pain** 415
David D. Bullek and Michael A. Kelly

22 / **Surgery of the Patellofemoral Joint: Indications, Effects, Results, and Recommendations** 441
William R. Post and John P. Fulkerson

23 / **Quadriceps and Patellar Tendon Disruptions** 469
Giles R. Scuderi

PART VII: ARTHROSCOPY: HISTORY, EQUIPMENT, APPROACHES, AND SURGERY OF THE KNEE JOINT

24 / **Arthroscopy: Past, Present, and Future** 481
Glenn B. Perry and David D. Bullek

25 / **Arthroscopic Equipment and Surgical Approaches** 487
Alfred J. Tria, Jr., Timothy M. Hosea, Jose A. Alicea

26 / **Arthroscopic Survey of the Knee Joint** 497
W. Dilworth Cannon, Jr.

27 / **Arthroscopic Laser Surgery** 515
Drew V. Miller, Stephen J. O'Brien, Stephen V. Fealy, Mary Ann Gibney, Anne M. Kelly

PART VIII: ARTHROSCOPIC SURGERY FOR CARTILAGE AND SYNOVIAL LESIONS

28 / **Arthroscopic Meniscal Resection** 527
Norman F. Sprague, III

29 / **Arthroscopic Meniscal Repair** 559
Michael G. Maday and Freddie H. Fu

30 / **Meniscal Allograft Replacement** 573
William G. Rodkey and J. Richard Steadman

31 / **Arthroscopic Treatment of Degenerative Arthritis of the Knee** 583
Jack M. Bert

32 / **Injuries and Diseases of Articular Surfaces of the Knee** 597
Robert T. Burks and Roger B. Butorac

33 / **Synovectomy of the Knee** 621
Matthew B. Gavin and W. Norman Scott

PART IX: DIAGNOSIS AND PRINCIPLES OF MANAGEMENT OF LIGAMENT INJURIES

34 / **History of Surgical Treatment of Knee Ligament Injuries** 637
S. Steven Yang and Michael Alexiades

35 / **Physiologic Principles of Ligament Injuries and Healing** 645
Steven Paul Arnoczky

36 / **Clinical Diagnosis and Classification of Ligament Injuries** 657
Alfred J. Tria, Jr., Timothy M. Hosea, Jose A. Alicea

37 / **Knee Laxity Testing Devices** 673
Bernard R. Bach, Jr.

PART X: NONOPERATIVE MANAGEMENT OF LIGAMENTOUS INJURIES

38 / **Medial and Lateral Ligament Injuries of the Knee** 703
Arthur C. Rettig and Richard A. Rubinstein, Jr.

39 / **Anterior Cruciate Ligament Injuries** 723
Claude Nichols and Robert J. Johnson

40 / **Posterior Cruciate Ligament Injuries** 737
K. Donald Shelbourne and Glen E. Johnson

Index xxv

Part XI

Surgical Management of Cruciate and Collateral Ligament Injuries

41
Indications and a Surgical Philosophy for Managing Anterior Cruciate Ligament Disruption

JONATHAN GLASHOW, M.D.
W. NORMAN SCOTT, M.D.

Operative repair
Intraarticular reconstruction
   Graft strength considerations
   Graft vascularity
   Isometric considerations

Types of grafts
   Autografts
   Allografts
   Prosthetic ligaments
Summary

Although credit for discovery of the anterior cruciate ligament (ACL) has been attributed to Galen in 170 A.D., it was not until 1850 that Stark recorded disruption of the ACL as a pathologic entity.[30] The surgical approach to this injury began in 1895 when Robson repaired a ruptured ACL.[29] There was a quiescent period, however, until the 1930s when extraarticular repairs were popularized.[6] Around 1936 intraarticular procedures, and specifically the use of the patellar tendon as a cruciate substitute, was recommended by Campbell.[10] In the 1950s O'Donoghue[54] recognized these injuries in intercollegiate athletes and utilized a surgical approach to return the athletes to their preinjury level of sports participation. The 1960s and 1970s were dominated by combinations of extraarticular and intraarticular procedures as espoused by Jones, Slocum, Larsen, and many others.[61] The most striking aspect of this era was the attempt to elucidate the diagnosis of a torn ACL by physical examination and develop an understanding of the natural history of an incompetent ACL.[1, 3, 5] Subsequently, numerous stability tests were described. While no test was pathognomonically unequivocal, a heightened awareness for diagnosing the injury was achieved. Surgically, intra- and extraarticular procedures were often combined to compensate for the ruptured ligament.

In the late 1980s arthroscopic procedures for reconstruction of the ACL resulted in less morbidity for the patients, more exacting placement of reconstructed ligaments, and the use of allografts and synthetic ligaments in addition to various autografts. Advances in data retrieval have allowed a more scientific approach in assessing reconstruction procedures of the ACL.[9] There is concern, however, that because of the improvements in surgical techniques, surgeons might misinterpret the natural history of a torn ACL that is still being unraveled. In developing a philosophy for the surgical treatment of the torn ACL, we cannot emphasize enough that not all patients must undergo reconstruction of an incompetent ACL.

The surgical treatment for a complete tear of the ACL must take into consideration the age, sex, lifestyle, and concomitant knee injuries. As we develop and challenge existing concepts, it is probably safe to say at the time of this writing that approximately one third of the patients who sustain a complete tear of the ACL, and who are treated nonoperatively, will be able to return to their previous level of functional sports participation with constant rehabilitation and appropriate bracing.[12, 20, 24, 37, 47] It is important to remember, whether one has a nonsurgical or surgical approach to a patient with a ruptured ACL, that normalcy has not been achieved, even in successful results. Return to functional preinjury levels is the desired goal since we have no way of thoroughly reconstructing a normal ACL. The ideal candidate for a reconstruction of the ACL is the younger athlete who is going to participate on an interscholastic, perhaps intercollegiate, and possibly professional level of sports requiring cutting, twisting, and jumping activities. These demands certainly stress the knee and logic dictates that this patient has less likelihood of overcoming a loss of one of the four major ligaments in the knee. While several studies strongly suggest that concomitant collateral or meniscal injuries increase the probability of functional instability, thus making a stronger case for surgical intervention, we do not today have unequivocal evidence that these patients are at higher risk for degenerative arthritic changes in life. It is interesting, from our perspective, which includes a significant arthritic population requiring knee replacements, that it is more the rule than the exception that the ACL is present in patients whose severe arthritic changes require a total knee replacement. Thus, while it is theoretically attractive at present to assume that instability enhances the potential for degenerative arthritis, this is not of unequivocal scientific validity.

In general, the younger female patient who is now more aggressive in sports participation has typically more ligament laxity and does not have the muscular "backup" of her male counterpart. With this inherent laxity and lack of muscular potential, it would seem that a more aggressive approach to reconstructing a ligament is warranted in this population. Once again, studies are lacking at the time of this writing, but our impression is that these patients do not do as well nonoperatively.

Societal changes in recreational lifestyles have now even necessitated looking at the much older age population, sometimes with degenerative changes, from a surgical perspective. For the most part, these persons will often change their lifestyles and not require the pivotal demands on their knee and thus obviate the surgical decision or options. For the more demanding older patient, however, there is a place for considering reconstruction of the ACL. When significant arthritic changes and deformity are associated with the instability, however, it remains to be seen whether concomitant osteotomies are indicated in this population. Because repair is not a universal consideration today, there is no urgency to perform an ACL reconstruction and certainly the patient can be observed to see if his or her instability is worsening. In the older population, when one considers ACL reconstruction it is important to assess the patient's complaint, whether it be instability or just discomfort. Although techniques continue to improve, allografts and artificial ligaments (if ever improved significantly) make the procedures easier for older patients to tolerate.

The only absolute contraindication to ACL reconstruction seems to be performing a procedure in the clinical setting of acute sepsis, and in a patient who has a total lack of understanding of the rehabilitation and unreasonable expectations of a successful reconstruction. Potential complications range from 2% to 6%, and failures, which can be as high as 5% or 6%, must be appreciated by the patient prior to any surgical intervention.

While success in the last several decades is truly encouraging, the ideal ACL substitute has yet to be developed. The surgical approaches today require strict adherence to technical details, including preparation, placement, and fixation of the selected substitute.[66] Attention to such details might allow the realization of the goal of any surgical procedure for the deficient ACL, establishing a stable knee with a functional range of motion. Sufficient stability should be sustained for the life of the patient while, theoretically, limiting the potential for degenerative osteoarthritic changes. When the operative approach is considered better for the patient, the surgeon has three options: (1) primary repair, (2) intraarticular reconstruction, and (3) combined intra- and extraarticular reconstruction.

OPERATIVE REPAIR

Results of intrasubstance ACL tears repaired with suture alone are inferior to other operative procedures.[61] Although several earlier studies demonstrated encouraging initial results, recent 5-year follow-up reports showing deterioration of stability have led many to suggest augmentation procedures in addition to primary repair.[18, 67, 69, 77] Several studies have demonstrated good results with augmentation using autogenous grafts[64]; however, a major disadvantage is that insecure fixation of the primary repair with suture requires prolonged postoperative protection. Thus, the potential benefits of saving the ACL to allow for reinnervation and blood supply are outweighed by the morbidity attending lack of early aggressive rehabilitation. The current literature does not support primary repair of intrasubstance ACL tears. Additionally, the earlier contention that repair be performed within 10 days or less has never been supported by clinical studies.[61] In fact, current literature supports allowing 2 to 3 weeks before surgical reconstruction to regain full range of motion and lessen the chances of postoperative arthrofibrosis.[68]

The object of extraarticular reconstructive procedures is to create a check rein to prevent anterior tibial translation. Most procedures described (MacIntoch, Losee, Ellison, Arnold-Coker, James, Andrews) rerouted the iliotibial band (ITB) beneath the fibular collateral ligament to act as a lateral sling.[17, 39, 61, 75] This is done so that the ITB comes to lie just posterior to the transverse center of rotation of the knee. While these procedures constrain the lateral aspect of the knee, the central and medial aspects of the knee are not controlled, and thus this form of ligament substitute is subject to gradual failure as graft tissue is stretched. Currently few surgeons use lateral replacement reconstruction alone. The limited indications include its uses as an adjunct in treating the skeletally immature athlete and in the older, sedentary, less physically demanding patient.[39] Some surgeons continue its use with intraarticular reconstruction in the knee with chronic combined instability.[14]

INTRAARTICULAR RECONSTRUCTION

There are four categories of intraarticular reconstruction: (1) static, (2) static and dynamic autogenous, (3) allografts, and (4) prosthetic. Currently most orthopaedic surgeons use intraarticular static autogenous graft reconstructions in an attempt to duplicate the anatomic ACL.[61] The most popular graft sources are the patellar ligament and the hamstring tendons in various combinations. In choosing an autogenous graft source, one must examine its biomechanical properties: its ability to be placed in a relatively isometric position and to revascularize.

Graft Strength Considerations

The cruciate ligament substitute must be of adequate strength, and several studies have addressed this issue.[41, 49, 50, 78] Noyes et al.[49, 50] reported that a 14-mm-wide bone–patella tendon–bone ligament would withstand a 2,900-N load prior to failure (168% of what it took for the ACL-bone interface to fail). This was the only tissue tested whose maximal load was clearly superior to the ligament being replaced. The semitendinosus tendon measured 1,216 N (70%) and the gracilis, 838 N (49%). The distal iliotibial tract, when taken with 20 mm of adjacent fascia, measured 1,868 N (108%). Woo and colleagues[78] have reported recently that the actual tensile strength of the ACL is closer to 2,500 N which has led many to use a combination of graft sources in an attempt to increase strength. The Kennedy ligament augmentation device (LAD) has a tensile strength of 1,500 N, and its use has been previously described with autografts from patellar tendon, hamstring tendon, and various allograft tissues.[63] There have been reports, however, that persistent effusions may continue in knees augmented with the LAD device.[80] It is interesting to note that no study has specifically addressed the additive nature of combined materials used as ligament substitutes, but it seems reasonable that strength failure would increase. While we often look only at the strength characteristics of a ligament substitute, we must also compare other mechanical properties such as stiffness. While the patella tendon is 300% stiffer in the normal ACL, hamstring tendons and the ITB more nearly replicate the natural stiffness of the cruciate ligament.[50]

Graft Vascularity

During the first several weeks after implantation, intraarticular grafts undergo rapid deterioration of their initial strength.[2] Initially, the patellar tendon autograft was thought to be advantageous when transferred with a vascularized pedicle.[8] Subsequent research by Butler and colleagues[7, 8] showed the mechanical properties of the vascularized ACL graft to be identical to those of the free graft in a monkey model. Arnoszky et al.[2] and others[74, 81] have shown that the healing properties of the free graft take from 2 to 6 months to revascularize, and an additional 2 months to recollagenize. Several studies show that patellar tendon grafts are only at one half their initial strength 1 year postoperatively, and gradually increase to maximal strength at 2 to 3 years.[39, 44, 53] Clancy and colleagues[13-15] and others[60] believe that revascularization may take place more rapidly, but do not take into account the full incorporation of attached bone blocks. Similar studies of the semitendinosus and gracilis tendons by others have shown revascularization complete by 12 to 16 months.[22, 27, 39] However, histologic examination proved that recollagenization was not complete by that time.[39] Zaricznyj et al.[82, 83] have shown that at 7½ years complete transformation to ligament-like tissue has occurred. Vascularity is less of an issue in dynamic tissue transfers.[61] We are not aware of any histologic study confirming transformation of the proximally based ITB into ligament-like material; however, we assume it would within a similar time period. Theoretically, the knee should be protected from maximally deforming forces during this period of revascularization and collagen reorganization.

Isometric Considerations

The anatomy of the ACL has been well documented.[16, 35, 61, 75] The ACL arises from the medial aspect of the intercondylar notch of the posterolateral femoral condyle; it traverses a distance of approximately 38 mm and attaches to a fossa in the anterior tibia just anterior and lateral to the anterior tibial spine. It is approximately 8 to 12 mm wide and is composed of at least two main bundles: the anteromedial and posterolateral. Each bundle is divided into fascicles which are encased in synovium—thus the frequent description of intraarticular but extrasynovial. Neurologic innervation is from a branch of the tibial nerve. Blood supply comes from the medial genicular artery in the form of weblike vessels throughout the course of the ligament. The bone attachments provide little of the blood supply.[61]

Intraarticular reconstruction cannot reproduce the normal anatomy of the ACL. Grafting procedures have attempted to replace the anteromedial band of the ligament which has been shown to be the closest to being isometric.[25, 26, 71] While no fibers of the anatomic ACL are actually isometric, reconstruction techniques attempt to place the graft in a position as close to isometric as possible to result in the least amount of strain ($\Delta l/l$) to the ligament substitute.[28, 59]

Initially, clinical judgment alone was used to determine the isometric "position" within the intercondylar notch, placing the femoral tunnel near the meridian and as posterior as possible. Numerous authors have described the over-the-top position with or without creating a trough in the posterolateral femoral condyle as the "isometric position."[31, 56, 61] Arthroscopic techniques have allowed for better visualization and afford one the ability to place the graft actually "too posterior," creating strain on the ligament as the knee goes into full extension. Isometers have been developed in an attempt to aid in the choice of an appropriate femoral attachment site. A small anchor through which a suture is passed is placed in the intercondylar notch after a trial tibial tunnel has been created. The knee is placed through a range of motion, and the degree of excursion of the suture is measured. If lengthening occurs as the knee is placed into extension, the site chosen is too posterior and should be adjusted. Conversely, tensioning when the knee is placed in flexion would indicate an anteriorly placed femoral site. One must be cautious in interpreting the results of an isometer. The point chosen is just that—a point—and will be overdrilled by 10 mm or so. Additionally, the knee being measured has altered kinematics owing to its inherent cruciate deficiency, and thus measurement once the ligament substitute is placed may be different.[44] In fact, Fleming et al.[21] have shown that isometry correlates poorly with the load measurements made after the new ligament has been fixed in its tunnels.

One must understand the complex three-dimensionality of the ACL attachment sites and use clinical judgment when placing the bone tunnels. Excessive excursion (greater than 2–3 mm) is unacceptable and may lead to early graft failure.[39]

While tibial attachment of the graft is not considered as critical, it should be positioned near anatomic attachments and placed so the graft does not impinge on the roof of the notch with the knee fully extended.

Graft tension is important in restoring normal knee function.[34, 57] Overtensioning will constrain the knee, decrease normal anteroposterior motion, and increase the load within the graft, leading to premature deterioration.[39] Laxity may, on the other hand, allow for excessive translation and lead to instability and possible meniscal tearing.[76] Ideal graft tension is tissue-specific and difficult to determine. Lewis and colleagues[44, 45] measured tensions in cadaver ACLs and compared them to reconstructed ACL grafts. Interestingly, when an anterior load was applied to the tibia, graft tensions were much higher in the reconstructed knees than those of the cadaver knees at all positions tested (0, 30, 60, and 90 degrees).[44, 45] Thus, while we understand graft tension to be important in static reconstruction, specific recommendations cannot be made. The proximally based ITB transfer, on the other hand, functions both as a static and dynamic transfer and tension seems to be less crucial when details of the operative procedure are adhered to.[59–61]

Types of Grafts

Autografts

While several types of autogenous materials have been suggested for use as ACL grafts, including meniscus, free fascia lata, the hamstring tendons, and the proximally based ITB, the central third of the patellar tendon remains the most popular.*

The semitendinosus and gracilis tendons have been used in different ways as intraarticular substitutes, both as free grafts and partially attached (either at proximal or distal ends). More recently, arthroscopic techniques have encouraged their use with tibial and femoral tunnels avoiding the over-the-top position. While clinical success has been reported by several authors, results of hamstring tendon reconstructions are difficult to compare as different series utilize different surgical techniques both in the use of the graft alone and as an augmentation structure.[27, 31, 39] The advantages of using the semitendinosus and gracilis together rather than the patellar tendon include: avoidance of damage to the extensor mechanism (thus less frequent postoperative patellofemoral pain, and quadriceps weakness) and com-

---

*References 32, 33, 36, 40, 53, 61, 73, 83, 84.

plications such as patella fracture or patellar tendon avulsion.[62] In addition, harvesting of the hamstring tendons is technically less demanding than that of the patellar tendon graft.[52] Contraindications include damage to the tendon itself or concurrent medial capsuloligamentous disruptions.[16, 39, 61]

Although several authors prefer the use of the semitendinosus and gracilis tendons, their use is plagued by several inherent disadvantages. Lack of bone-to-bone fixation, increased healing time within the bony tunnels, and the greater likelihood that tendons will stretch by nature of their higher elasticity remain unattractive features.[39, 46, 50, 61] Although it has been suggested that hamstring tendon grafts are associated with less parapatellar pain than patellar tendon grafts, the correlation is not clear. Several factors contribute, including the patient's age, history of previous patellofemoral pain, and type of rehabilitation programs utilized postoperatively.[65, 72, 74] New reports suggest little statistical difference in patellofemoral pain among patients treated conservatively and with the patellar tendon or hamstring reconstruction that have undergone aggressive physical therapy protocols emphasizing early full range of motion and quadriceps strengthening.[39]

The primary advantages of the use of the bone-patellar tendon-bone grafts are their great strength, immediate strong fixation via interference screws, and rapid bone-to-bone healing, thus allowing for an accelerated rehabilitation program.[13, 25, 42, 51, 52, 65, 66] Most surgeons prefer to harvest the central third of the patellar tendon with attached bone blocks from the patella and tibial tubercle. Tibial and femoral tunnels are then created precisely under direct arthroscopic visualization. Endoscopic placement of the graft has done away with the morbidity associated with a second lateral incision. Clancy et al.[13-15] and others[49, 53, 74] have reported clinical success to be consistently 80% to 90% despite frequent technical modifications since its description in 1983.

The intraarticular transfer of the ITB-muscle tendon unit as described by Insall and Scott represents the most commonly used static and dynamic reconstruction for the ACL-deficient knee.[36, 61] This proximally based intraarticular procedure had been independently described by Nicholas and Minkoff,[47] but with distinct technical differences which led to significant patella problems and overall poor results.[61] In the current technique described by Scott and co-workers,[60, 61] the anterior portion of the ITB, in connection with the lateral retinaculum, along with a limited posterior dissection maintaining continuity with a lateral intermuscular septum and fascia overlying the vastus lateralis, is used. This structure is tubed to increase strength and the bony block harvested from Gerdy's tubercle is placed in a central trough created in the interspinous area of the tibial plateau.[60, 61]

The advantages of this technique include primary bone-to-bone fixation which has allowed for immediate passive range-of-motion exercises and early weightbearing without the direct violation of the extensor mechanism. Success has been reported in 85% of patients and in professional basketball players.[60, 61] However, this procedure cannot be performed by a mini-incision with arthroscopic techniques. Parapatellar arthrotomy with dislocation of the patella is required and may lead to increased postoperative morbidity.

Allografts

The use of allograft materials for intraarticular reconstruction has tremendous appeal, but its present status remains investigational.[38, 39] Allografts, like autografts, revascularize, undergo collagen reorganization, and have the potential to respond to injury.[58] The most commonly used allografts are bone-patellar tendon-bone and Achilles tendon with or without attached calcaneus bone block.[70] Techniques of reconstruction are similar to those used for autogenous tissues.

Allografts offer several potential advantages over autografts. There is no donor site morbidity like that associated with autograft harvesting, and the periarticular knee structures are preserved. Second, an autograft is limited in size by the patient's available tissue, whereas an allograft is not and can be made larger and stronger than a graft safely taken from an autogenous source. Third, surgical time may be decreased and cosmesis improved by avoiding incisions needed for autograft harvesting.[38, 85]

While early results are controversial and relate to the method of preservation and preparation, there does appear to be less short-term morbidity. However, results after 1 year or so appear to be no better than those associated with autogenous grafts.[61] Concerns about transmission of viral disease, immunogenicity, and alteration of graft properties with sterilization techniques require further study. It is clear that proper harvesting and banking techniques will be vital to the success and easy availability of allograft tissues.

Prosthetic Ligaments

The use of synthetic material to replace the ACL is not a new concept, and was first described in 1906. Currently there are four general categories of prosthetic ligaments: (1) permanent, (2) stent, (3) augmentation, and (4) scaffold.[61] Gore-Tex (polytetrafluoroethylene) remains the prototypal permanent prosthesis and was first implanted in humans in 1982.[4] The early experience was promising but results deteriorated from the 2- to 5-year follow-up period.[4, 11, 19, 43, 55, 79] The stent type of implant includes the LAD and various Dacron materials. Animal models have proved encapsulation of stents with vascularized fibrous tissue and bony ingrowth within tunnels.[61] Long-term patient series are not available. The LAD is the only approved augmentation type of prosthesis available today. The theoretical advantage of load-sharing during healing stages of autograft or allograft transplant is appealing. However, no long-term investigation has proved its superiority to the use of autogenous tissues alone, and its use has been associated with reports of chronic sterile effusions in up to 7% of patients.[80]

The Leeds-Keio is an example of the scaffold type of prosthesis. Described as a hybrid type of implant, initially it is designed to carry all of the tensile load. As invasion by surrounding tissue matures, it becomes capable of load-sharing and finally is expected to be completely biologic.[61] Its initial strength is greater than that of the ACL at 2,000+ N, and its stiffness and other biomechanical properties are similar.[43] It is now in use in several centers throughout the world after encouraging results in the animal model.[61] Along with arthroscopic techniques of insertion, it may prove to be a viable option in the future. No long-term human studies are yet available.

The use of prosthetic ligaments has been much more extensive in Europe, Japan, and South Africa than in the United States. Clinical performance of these implants is encouraging at best, and these procedures must be considered investigational.[39] No good long-term series are available for comparison with current autogenous techniques. It is hoped that further evaluation and progress will expand current clinical indications, which now include failed intraarticular reconstructions and the symptomatic unstable arthritic knee which requires early full range of motion to prevent further joint deterioration.

SUMMARY

In summary, surgical management of injuries to the ACL remains controversial. While the bone–patellar tendon–bone autogenous graft source combined with arthroscopically assisted techniques remains most popular today, the orthopaedic surgeon treating these injuries must keep abreast of the ever-expanding literature. Undoubtedly, in the coming years, longer-term follow-ups involving other graft sources and new techniques will become available and will influence the trend of surgical management of these injuries.

REFERENCES

1. Andersson C, et al: Surgical or nonsurgical treatment of acute rupture of the anterior cruciate ligament: A randomized study with long-term follow-up, *J Bone Joint Surg [Am]* 71:965–974, 1989.
2. Arnoczky SP, Tarvin GB, Marshall JL: Anterior cruciate ligament replacement using the patella tendon: An evaluation of graft revascularization in the dog, *J Bone Joint Surg [Am]* 64:217, 1982.
3. Arnold JA, et al: Natural history of anterior cruciate ligament tears, *Am J Sports Med* 7:305, 1979.
4. Bruchman WC, Bain JR, Bolton CW: Prosthetic replacement of the cruciate ligaments with expanded polytetrafluoroethylene. In Feagin, JA Jr, editor: *The crucial ligaments: Diagnosis and treatment of ligamentous injuries about the knee*, New York, 1988, Churchill Livingstone, pp 507–515.
5. Buckley SL, Barrack RL, Alexander AH: The natural history of conservatively treated partial anterior cruciate ligament tears, *Am J Sports Med* 17:221–225, 1989.
6. Burnett QM, Fowler PJ: Reconstruction of the anterior cruciate ligament: Historical overview, *Orthop Clin North Am* 16:143–157, 1985.
7. Butler DL: Anterior cruciate ligament: Its normal response and replacement, *J Orthop Res* 7:910–921, 1989.
8. Butler DL, et al: Mechanical properties of primate vascularized vs. non-vascularized patellar tendon grafts; changes over time, *J Orthop Res* 7:68–79, 1989.
9. Butler DL, Noyes FR, Grood ES: Ligamentous restraints to anterior-posterior drawer in the human knee, *J Bone Joint Surg [Am]* 62:259–270, 1980.
10. Campbell WC: Repair of the ligaments of the knee, *Surg Gynecol Obstet* 62:964, 1936.
11. Caulus LE, et al: The Gore-Tex anterior cruciate ligament prosthesis. A long-term follow-up. *Am J Sports Med* 20:246, 1992.
12. Cawley PW, France EP, Paulos LE: The current state of functional knee bracing research. A review of the literature, *Am J Sports Med* 19:226–233, 1992.
13. Clancy WG: Arthroscopic anterior cruciate ligament reconstruction with patella tendon, *Tech Orthop* 2:4, 1988.
14. Clancy WG Jr, et al: Anterior cruciate ligament reconstruction using one-third of the patellar ligament, augmented by extra-articular tendon transfers, *J Bone Joint Surg [Am]* 64:352–359, 1982.
15. Clancy WG Jr, Ray MJ, Zoltan DJ: Acute tears of the anterior cruciate ligament. Surgical vs. conservative

treatment, *J Bone Joint Surg [Am]* 70:1483–1488, 1988.
16. Crenshaw AH: Surgical approaches. In Crenshaw AH, editor: *Campbell's operative orthopaedics,* ed 7, St Louis, 1987, Mosby–Year Book.
17. DeLee JE, Curtis R: Anterior cruciate ligament insufficiency in children, *Clin Orthop* 172:112–118, 1983.
18. Feagin JA, Lambert KL, Cunningham RR: Repair and reconstruction of the anterior cruciate ligament. In Chapman MW, editor: *Operative orthopedics,* Philadelphia, 1988, JB Lippincott.
19. Ferkel RD, et al: Arthroscopic second look at the Gore-Tex ligament, *Am J Sports Med* 17:147–153, 1989.
20. Fetto JF, Marshall JL: The natural history and diagnosis of anterior cruciate ligament insufficiency, *Clin Orthop* 147:29–38, 1980.
21. Fleming B, et al: Isometric vs. tension measurements: A comparison for the reconstruction of the anterior cruciate ligament. Unpublished data.
22. Gartke KA, Portner OT: The semi-tendinosus dynamic transfer for anterior cruciate insufficiency, *J Bone Joint Surg [Br]* 66:305, 1984.
23. Grood ES, Noyes FR, Butler DL: Biomechanics of the knee exercise, *J Bone Joint Surg [Am]* 66:725–734, 1984.
24. Hawkins RJ, Misamore GW, Merritt TR: Followup of the acute nonoperated isolated anterior cruciate ligament tear, *Am J Sports Med* 14:205–210, 1986.
25. Hefzy MS, Grood ES: Sensitivity of insertion locations on length patterns of anterior cruciate ligament fibers, *J Biomed Eng* 108:73–82, 1986.
26. Hefzy MS, Grood ES, Noyes FR: Factors affecting the region of most isometric femoral attachments. Part II: The anterior cruciate ligament, *Am J Sports Med* 17:208–216, 1989.
27. Hendler RC: Intra-articular semitendinosus anterior cruciate ligament reconstruction. In Scott WN, editor: *Ligament and extensor mechanism injuries of the knee: Diagnosis and treatment,* St Louis, 1991, Mosby–Year Book, pp 285–300.
28. Henning CE, Lynch MA, Glick KR, Jr: An in vivo strain gage study of elongation of the anterior cruciate ligament, *Am J Sports Med* 13:22–26, 1985.
29. Hey Groves EW: Operation for the repair of the crucial ligaments, *Lancet* 2:674–675, 1917.
30. Hey Groves EW: The crucial ligaments of the knee joint: Their function, rupture, and the operative treatment of the same, *J Surg Br* 7:505, 1919.
31. Holmes CF, et al: Retrospective direct comparison of three intra-articular anterior cruciate ligament reconstructions, *Am J Sports Med* 19:596, 1991.
32. Hooper GJ, Walton DI: Reconstruction of the anterior cruciate ligament using the bone-block iliotibial-tract transfer, *J Bone Joint Surg [Am]* 69:1150–1154, 1987.
33. Howe JG, et al: Anterior cruciate ligament reconstruction using quadriceps patellar tendon graft. Part I: Long-term followup, *Am J Sports Med* 19:447, 1991.
34. Hunter RE, et al: Graft force-setting technique in reconstruction of the anterior cruciate ligament, *Am J Sports Med* 18:12–19, 1990.
35. Insall JN: Chronic instability of the knee. In Insall JN, editor: *Surgery of the knee,* New York, 1984, Churchill Livingstone.
36. Insall JN, et al: Bone-block iliotibial-band transfer for anterior cruciate insufficiency, *J Bone Joint Surg [Am]* 63:560–569, 1981.
37. Jackson RW: The torn ACL: Natural history of the untreated lesions and rationale for selective treatment. In Feagin JA Jr, editor: *The crucial ligaments: Diagnosis and treatment of ligamentous injuries about the knee,* New York, 1988, Churchill Livingstone, pp 341–348.
38. Jackson DW, Kurzweil PR: Allografts in knee ligament surgery. In Scott WN, editor: *Ligament and extensor mechanism of the knee: Diagnosis and treatment,* St Louis, 1991, Mosby–Year Book, pp 349–360.
39. Johnson RJ, et al: Current concepts review: The treatment of injuries of the anterior cruciate ligament, *J Bone Joint Surg [Am]* 74:140, 1992.
40. Johnson RJ, et al: Five- to ten-year follow-up evaluation after reconstruction of the anterior cruciate ligament, *Clin Orthop* 183:122–140, 1984.
41. Kennedy JC, et al: Tension studies of human knee ligament: Yield point, ultimate failure and disruption of the cruciate and tibial collateral ligaments, *J Bone Joint Surg [Am]* 58:350–355, 1976.
42. Kurosaka M, Yoshiya S, Andrish JT: A biomechanical comparison of different surgical techniques of graft fixation in anterior cruciate ligament reconstruction, *Am J Sports Med* 15:225–229, 1987.
43. Larson RL: Gore-tex anterior cruciate ligament reconstruction. In Scott WN, editor: *Ligament and extensor mechanism injuries of the knee: Diagnosis and treatment,* St Louis, 1991, Mosby–Year Book, pp 319–329.
44. Lewis JL, et al: Factors affecting graft force in surgical reconstruction of the anterior cruciate ligament, *J Orthop Res* 8:514–521, 1990.
45. Lewis JL, et al: Knee joint motion and ligament forces before and after ACL reconstruction, *J Biomech Eng* 111:97–106, 1989.
46. Lipscomb AB, et al: Evaluation of hamstring strength following use of semitendinosus and gracilis tendons to reconstruct the anterior cruciate ligament, *Am J Sports Med* 10:340–342, 1982.
47. Nicholas JA, Minkoff J: Iliofibial band transfer through the infercondylar notch for combined anterior instability (ITPT Procedure, *Am J Sports Med* 6:341-353, 1978.
48. Nichols C, Johnson RJ: Cruciate ligament injuries: Nonoperative treatment. In Scott WN, editor: *Ligament and extensor mechanism injuries of the knee: Diagnosis and treatment,* St Louis, 1991, Mosby–Year Book, pp 227–238.
49. Noyes FR, Barber SD, Mangine RE: Bone–patellar ligament–bone and fascia lata allografts for reconstruction of the anterior cruciate ligament, *J Bone Joint Surg [Am]* 72:1125–1136, 1990.

50. Noyes FA, et al: Biomechanical analysis of human ligament grafts used in knee ligament repairs and reconstructions, *J Bone Joint Surg [Am]* 66:344, 1984.
51. Noyes FR, Mangine RE, Barber S: Early knee motion after open and arthroscopic anterior cruciate ligament reconstruction, *Am J Sports Med* 15:149-160, 1987.
52. Noyes FR, Sonstegard DA: Biomechanical functions of the pes anserinus at the knee and the effect of its transplantation, *J Bone Joint Surg [Am]* 55:1225-1241, 1973.
53. O'Brien SJ, et al: Reconstruction of the chronically insufficient anterior cruciate ligament with the central third of the patellar ligament, *J Bone Joint Surg [Am]* 73:278-286, 1991.
54. O'Donoghue DH: A method of replacement of the anterior cruciate ligament of the knee, *J Bone Joint Surg [Am]* 45:905-924, 1963.
55. Paulos LE, et al: Gore-Tex prosthetic anterior cruciate ligament reconstruction: A long-term follow-up, 57th Annual Meeting of the American Academy of Orthopaedic Surgeons, New Orleans, Feb 8-13, 1990.
56. Reider B: Arthroscopic anterior cruciate ligament reconstruction using patellar tendon. In Scott WN, editor: *Ligament and extensor mechanism injuries of the knee: Diagnosis and treatment,* St Louis, 1991, Mosby-Year Book, pp 239-252.
57. Rosenberg, A, Mikosz RP: Knee biomechanics. In Scott WN, editor: *Ligament and extensor mechanism injuries of the knee: Diagnosis and treatment,* St Louis, 1991, Mosby-Year Book.
58. Sabiston P, et al: Allograft ligament transplantation. A morphological and biochemical evaluation of a medial collateral ligament complex in a rabbit model, *Am J Sports Med* 18:160-168, 1990.
59. Sapega AA, et al: Testing for isometry during reconstruction of the anterior cruciate ligament. Anatomical and biochemical considerations, *J Bone Joint Surg [Am]* 72:259-267, 1990.
60. Scott WN, Ferriter P, Marino M: Intra-articular transfer of the iliotibial tract, *J Bone Joint Surg [Am]* 67:532-538, 1985.
61. Scott WN, Insall J: Injuries of the knee. In Rockwood CA, Green OP, Bucholz RW, editors: *Rockwood and Green's fractures,* ed 3. Philadelphia, 1991, JB Lippincott.
62. Scott WN, Schosheim PM: Intra-articular transfer of the iliotibial band muscle tendon unit, *Clin Orthop* 172:97-101, 1983.
63. Sgaglione WA, et al: Arthroscopic-assisted anterior cruciate ligament reconstruction with the semitendinosus tendon: Comparison of results with and without braided polypropylene augmentation, *J Arthrosc Rel Surg* 8:65-77, 1992.
64. Sgaglione NA, et al: Primary repair with semitendinosus tendon augmentation of acute anterior cruciate ligament injuries, *Am J Sports Med* 18:64-73, 1990.
65. Shelbourne KD, Nitz PA: Accelerated rehabilitation following A.C.L. reconstruction, Annual Meeting of the American Orthopaedic Society for Sports Medicine, Traverse City, Mich, June 18-22, 1989.
66. Shelbourne KD, Nitz P: Accelerated rehabilitation of the anterior cruciate ligament reconstruction, *Am J Sports Med* 18:292-299, 1990.
67. Shelbourne KD, et al: Anterior cruciate ligament injury: Evaluation of intra-articular reconstruction of acute tears without repair. Two- to seven-year follow-up of 155 athletes, *Am J Sports Med* 18:484-489, 1990.
68. Shelbourne KD, et al: Arthrofibrosis in acute anterior cruciate ligament reconstruction. The effect of timing of reconstruction and rehabilitation, *Am J Sports Med* 19:332-336, 1991.
69. Sherman MF, Bonamo JR: Primary repair of the anterior cruciate ligament, *Clin Sports Med* 7:739-750, 1988.
70. Shino K, et al: Reconstruction of the anterior cruciate ligament using allogeneic tendon: Long-term followup, *Am J Sports Med* 18:457-465, 1990.
71. Sidles JA, et al: Ligament length relationships in the moving knee, *J Orthop Res* 6:593-610, 1988.
72. Sweitzer RW, Sweitzer DA, Saraniti AJ: Rehabilitation for ligament and extensor mechanism injuries. In Scott WN, editor: *Ligament and extensor mechanism injuries of the knee: Diagnosis and treatment.* St Louis, 1991, Mosby-Year Book, pp 401-433.
73. Tillberg B: The late repair of torn cruciate ligaments using menisci, *J Bone Joint Surg [Br]* 59:15-19, 1977.
74. Warner JJ, Warren RF, Cooper DE: Management of acute anterior cruciate ligament injury, *Instruct Course Lect* 50:219-232, 1991.
75. Warren RF: Acute ligamentous injuries. In Insall JN, editor: *Surgery of the knee,* New York, 1984, Churchill Livingstone.
76. Warren RF, Levy IM: Meniscal lesions associated with anterior cruciate ligament injury, *Clin Orthop* 172:32-37, 1983.
77. Wickiewicz TL, Kaplan N, Warren RF: Primary surgical treatment of anterior cruciate ligament ruptures: A long-term follow-up study, *Am J Sports Med* 18:354-358, 1990.
78. Woo SL, et al: Tensile properties of the human femur-anterior cruciate ligament-tibia complex. The effects of specimen age and orientation, *Am J Sports Med* 19:217-225, 1991.
79. Woods GA, Indelicato PA, Prevot TJ: The Gore-tex anterior cruciate ligament prosthesis. Two- vs. three-year results, *Am J Sports Med* 19:48-55, 1991.
80. Yamamoto N, et al: Effusion after anterior cruciate ligament reconstruction using ligament augmentation device, *J Arthrosc Rel Surg* 8:303-310, 1992.
81. Yasuda K, et al: Arthroscopic observations of autogeneic quadriceps and patellar tendon grafts after anterior cruciate ligament reconstruction of the knee, *Clin Orthop* 246:217-224, 1989.
82. Zaricznyj B: Reconstruction of the anterior cruciate ligament using free tendon graft, *Am J Sports Med* 11:164, 1983.

83. Zaricznyj B: Reconstruction of the anterior cruciate ligament of the knee using a double tendon graft, *Clin Orthop* 220:167, 1987.
84. Zarins B, Rowe CR: Combined anterior cruciate ligament reconstruction using semitendinosus tendon and iliotibial tract, *J Bone Joint Surg [Am]* 68:160–177, 1986.
85. Zoltan D, Reinecke C, Indelicato P: Synthetic and allograft anterior cruciate ligament reconstructions, *Clin Sports Med* 7:773–784, 1988.

42

Arthroscopic Anterior Cruciate Ligament Reconstruction Utilizing Patellar Tendon

BRUCE REIDER, M.D.

Technique
  General setup
  Portal selection
  Initial diagnostic arthroscopy
  Lateral incision
  Preparation of femoral notch
  Femoral site selection
  Passage of rear-entry drill guide

  Anterior exposure
  Tibial guide placement
  Isometry testing
  Tibial hole preparation
  Harvesting the graft
  Passage of the graft
  Fixation of the graft
  Postoperative care

Reconstruction of the anterior cruciate ligament (ACL) utilizing the central one third of the patellar tendon was first described in the English literature by Kenneth G. Jones of Little Rock, Arkansas, in 1963.[24, 25] Jones recognized the convenience of the patellar tendon autograft and the potential advantage of bone-to-bone healing in the ultimate anchoring of the ligament replacement. However, his procedure differed significantly from its modern descendants in that he did not seek to place the graft exactly at the site of the old ACL. The distal portion of the graft was left attached to its anatomic location on the tibial tubercle and the proximal end, perhaps limited by this anterior placement of the distal end, was "placed in the intercondylar notch just posterior to the margin of the articular cartilage on the low end of the femur . . . While endeavoring to categorize results, it must be appreciated that the procedure under consideration constitutes a substitution for, not a reconstitution of, an anatomical structure which has been irrevocably destroyed. Anatomic normalcy of the structure is, by the nature of the situation, beyond expectation."[25] Most of the subsequent modifications have been aimed at making the procedure as anatomic as possible, although even a champion of the patellar tendon reconstruction technique will admit that a flat tendon will probably never have the anatomic complexity of a normal ACL.

Modifications of Jones's technique utilizing the medial third of the patellar tendon were subsequently described by Bruckner[5] and Eriksson.[13] Although he still left the distal attachment of the patellar tendon in place on the tibial tubercle, Eriksson advocated a more anatomic placement of the reconstruction by creating a tunnel from the anterior tibia to the normal tibial insertion of the ACL and by anchoring the femoral end of the graft in a hole placed at the normal femoral insertion. Marshall and colleagues[31] described reconstruction of the ACL using the middle third of the patellar tendon along with the anterior prepatellar fascia and a portion of the middle third of the quadriceps tendon. Although the authors described the possible use of a femoral drill hole for anchoring the proximal end of the graft, they pointed out the inherent difficulty in placing this hole posteriorly enough on the femoral condyle and suggested the alternative "over-the-top" technique to assure adequate posterior placement of the femoral end of the graft. They did note that grafts placed with the over-the-top technique tended to be tighter in extension than in flexion.[31] MacIntosh[30a] described a similar technique, and Roth[41a] and Fowler[15] have described augmenting such a soft tissue graft with a synthetic ligament augmentation device.

In 1982, Clancy and colleagues[9] published a series of 80 ACL reconstructions utilizing the medial third of the patellar tendon. Clancy led the medial third of the tendon through a tunnel in the anterior tibia and harvested the proximal portion of the graft with a block of patellar bone to permit bony union of the proximal attachment of the ligament reconstruction within a tunnel in the femoral condyle. Clancy subsequently further modified this technique by utilizing the middle third of the patellar tendon and routinely detaching its distal end with a bone block from the tibial tubercle. This established the "bone-tendon-bone" graft which has become standard in patellar tendon reconstruction of the ACL. This procedure has become the basis for most current patellar tendon ACL reconstruction techniques. Clancy reported 94% good or excellent results at 33 months after surgery with all patients relieved of clinical instability over this period of time. Although attempts have been made to establish a vascularized graft, this has not proved to be feasible or necessary.[6,37,38]

Some of the laboratory investigation supporting or refining patellar tendon reconstruction techniques preceded its widespread clinical use, and other laboratory research has followed it. Noyes and colleagues[36] demonstrated that strength to failure of the patellar tendon graft was generally greater than that of other autograft options in clinical use. They found that the strength to failure of a 14- to 15-mm-wide central bone–patellar tendon–bone graft was about 160% of the strength of a normal ACL. It has been assumed, although not proved, that the ultimate strength of the reconstruction may be proportional to the initial strength of the material used. In addition, a strong graft material is believed to be valuable for allowing an aggressive early range-of-motion rehabilitation program.

Important research was done by Clancy and colleagues[10] who published their biologic study of the healing of patellar tendon ACL reconstructions in Rhesus monkeys in 1981. They showed that the transferred tendon was revascularized with time and regained 80% of the tensile strength of the original tendon graft 9 months after the surgery. Amiel and colleagues[1] subsequently promoted the concept of "ligamentization" when they demonstrated that the transplanted patellar tendon subsequently attained the biochemical as well as the structural properties of the ACL.

An anatomic treatise published in 1975 by Girgis and colleagues[17] emphasized that the ACL is a complex structure, with different fiber bundles which tighten in different positions of knee flexion. The intimate relationship between the anatomic attachments of the cruciate ligaments, the complex shape of the femoral condyles, and the normal kinematics of knee motion was described by Kapandji[26] and Goodfellow and O'Connor[18] among others. Mueller[34] emphasized that this relationship dictated that an ACL reconstruction be placed in an anatomic position for optimal function. Because a flat tendon graft can never duplicate the complex anatomy of the normal ACL, which allows different fiber bundles to be tight in different positions, most surgeons have sought to find "isometric" attachment sites which allow the simpler tendon graft to be tight in all positions of the knee. Recent studies by Hefzy et al.,[21] Sidles et al.,[46] and others[33,39] have further delineated the location of such potential isometric attachment sites.

Biomechanical laboratory studies in cadaver knees have shown that patellar tendon reconstruction of the ACL does indeed approximate the function of the normal ligament as intended.[12] Prize-winning research by Arms and colleagues[3] from the University of Vermont in 1984 showed that a properly placed ACL reconstruction exhibited strain behavior similar to the normal anteromedial band of the ACL. More recent force-displacement studies in our own laboratory have shown that patellar tendon reconstruction of the ACL can restore normal anterior stability through a wide arc of motion in the ACL-deficient knee.

Over the last few years, many individuals and groups have perfected methods of performing the intraarticular portion of the operation arthroscopically. When mastered, these techniques have the potential of improving reconstruction placement through enhanced visualization of attachment sites while reducing surgical dissection and subsequent scarring. To achieve optimal results, these surgical methods should be combined with an aggressive rehabilitation program.[43] Our current technique utilizes the ingenious rear-entry drill guide system of Rosenberg et al.[41] and incorporates technical suggestions of Clancy[7] and Graf[19] (Figs 42–1 and 42–2). Rosenberg has also introduced an "endoscopic" drill guide system which eliminates the lateral skin incision by placing the femoral tunnel from the inside outward.

Although only a few cases of patellar fracture or patellar tendon rupture have been reported following ACL reconstruction with patellar tendon autograft,[4,32] some surgeons have begun using cadaver patellar tendon allografts for this procedure. The potential advantages put forward on behalf of allografts are avoidance of whatever morbidity may be associated with autograft harvest and the possibility of using a wider graft. Because clinical follow-up on allograft reconstruction is shorter than that of autograft, and because of the potential for disease transmission with allografts, the use of the autograft remains our standard technique. However, the technique described is equally suitable for allograft use (Fig 42–3).

The timing of the surgery can significantly affect the postoperative course of the patient. Evidence has

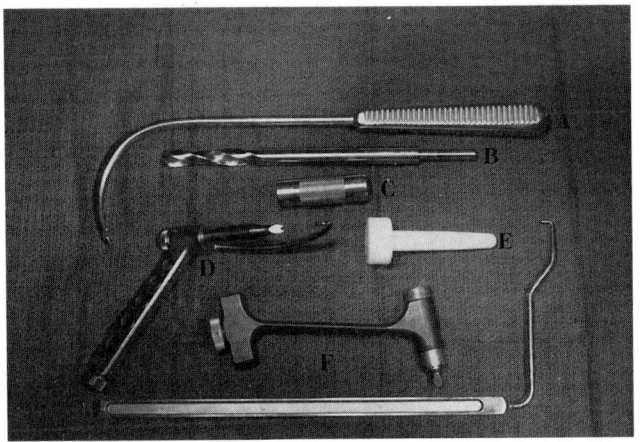

FIG 42–1.
Standard components of the rear-entry drill guide system include (A) the gaff for passing the rear-entry drill guide, (B) 10-mm cannulated reamers, (C) 10-mm bone plug sizer, (D) rear-entry femoral drill guide (assembled with "bullet" aimer inserted), (E) plastic bone plugs, and (F) the two components of the tibial drill guide (aimer).

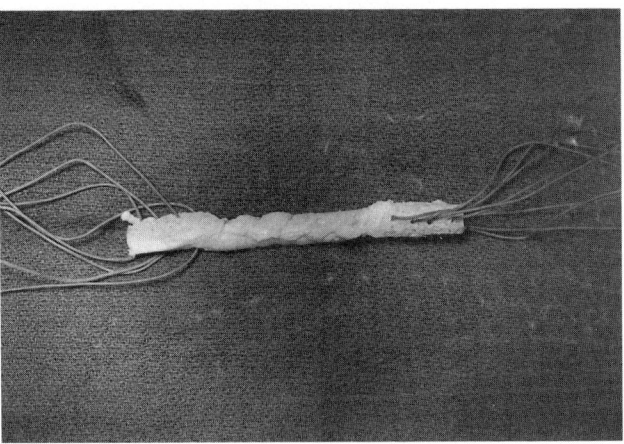

FIG 42–3.
When an allograft is used, the bone blocks are similar in size to those of the autograft, but a 20-mm wide strip of tendon is used and "tubed" with a running suture so that it fits through the 10-mm tunnels.

accumulated that patients who have primary reconstruction of the ACL during the early postinjury period have an increased risk of arthrofibrosis or difficulty regaining full range of motion postoperatively.[4,5] For this reason, we now routinely wait at least 3 or 4 weeks following acute ACL rupture before proceeding with reconstruction. During this period, physical therapy and nonsteroidal anti-inflammatory drugs are used to restore normal range of motion and minimize effusion and inflammation. If significant medial collateral ligament (MCL) laxity is also present, we equip the athlete with a simple lateral hinge brace during this time to support the MCL without restricting the full range of motion necessary to prepare the knee for ACL reconstruction.

TECHNIQUE

General Setup

Any arthroscopy setup that allows full knee motion is suitable for this procedure. The patient may be placed supine on a standard operating table so that the knee projects just distally to the flexion hinge of the "foot" of the table. The requisite flexion in the knee may be obtained solely by dropping the foot of the table, or a Slocum knee block may be placed under the thigh at the beginning of the procedure to increase the amount of knee flexion (Fig 42–4). About 45 degrees of flexion are necessary for surgical exposure. In addition, the surgeon should be able to flex the knee fully to test the isometry of the graft. Draping should be placed proximal enough to allow for adequate exposure of the lateral incision.

Portal Selection

Since both anteromedial and anterolateral portals are used during the procedure, the initial diagnostic arthroscopy may be done through either incision according to the custom of the operating surgeon. The choice of portals for the ligament reconstruction itself is influenced by the need to adequately visualize the posterior portion of the lateral side of the intercon-

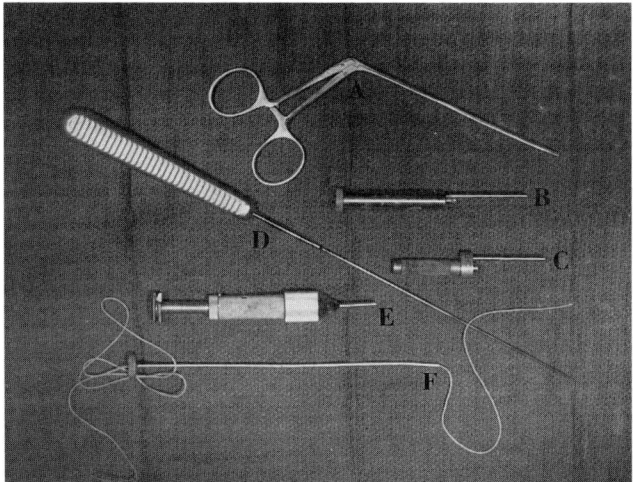

FIG 42–2.
Useful nonstandard accessories include (A) a small arthroscopic grasper, (B) 3-mm and (C) 5-mm parallel drill guides for adjusting guide pin placement, (D) a thin crochet hook for pulling the guide suture through the trial tibial guide pin hole, (E) a Graf isometer, and (F) a single-cannula meniscus suture guide for inserting the guide suture through the femoral tunnel.

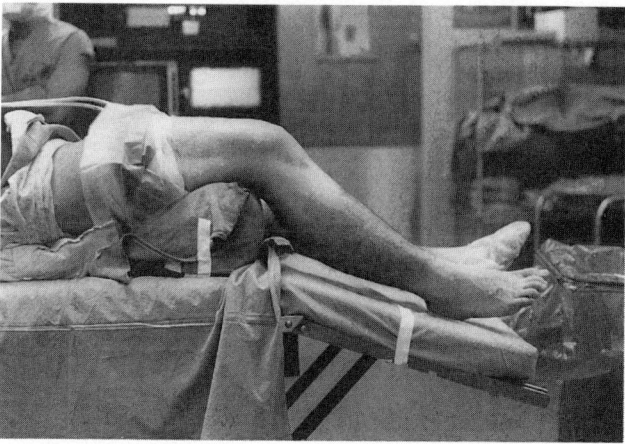

FIG 42-4.
Patient should be positioned so that the knee may be taken through a full range of motion. The setup shown here allows the leg to rest on the table during most of the procedure but leaves the limb free so that the surgeon may test the reconstruction through a full range of motion. The "foot" of the table may be adjusted during the case to change the resting position of the knee.

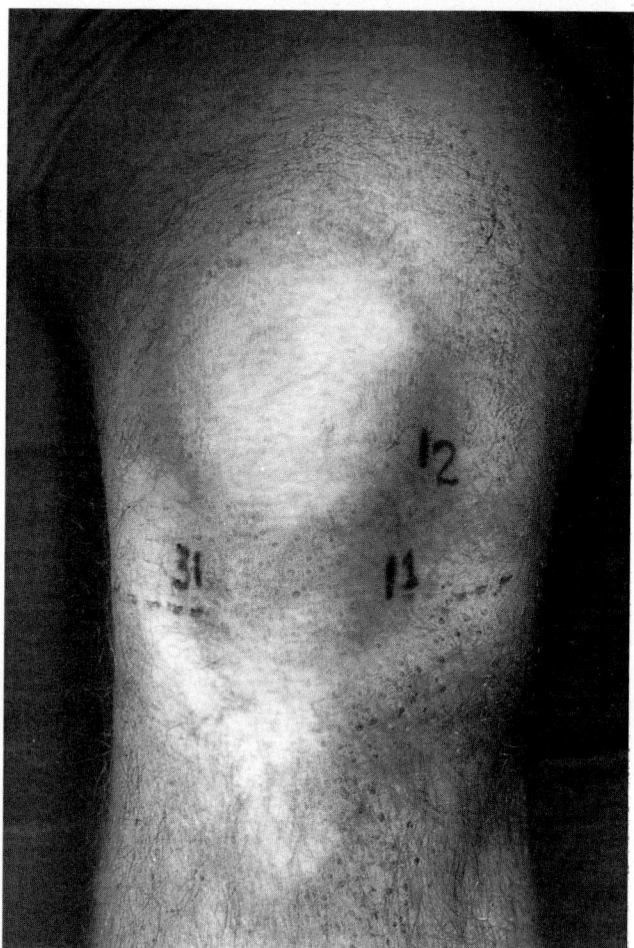

FIG 42-5.
In addition to standard anteromedial *(1)* and anterolateral *(3)* joint line portals, an accessory medial portal *(2)* is excellent for viewing the femoral attachment site of the anterior cruciate ligament while freeing the anteromedial portal *(1)* for the passage of instruments. The surgeon should be careful not to place the accessory medial portal too far medial, or he or she will not be able to visualize the posterior edge of the lateral femoral condyle.

dylar notch and also reach it with operating instruments. The arthroscopic surgeon is faced with a dilemma: the optimal position for both the arthroscope and the instruments needed to establish the femoral tunnel is an anteromedial portal. Some surgeons have solved this dilemma by saving the anteromedial portal for their instruments while placing the arthroscope through the anterolateral portal. Unfortunately, an arthroscope entering anterolaterally glances off the anterior medial edge of the lateral femoral condyle and is directed toward the medial side of the notch. This compromises visualization of the posterolateral notch. The usual solution to this problem is to regain visualization of the posterolateral notch by performing a liberal "notchplasty," resecting portions of the lateral femoral condyle. I prefer to solve this dilemma by operating through two medial portals, creating an accessory medial portal at the junction of the patella and medial femoral condyle for placement of the arthroscope during notch preparation (Fig 42-5). This requires some adjustment on the part of the surgeon because of the proximity of the two portals. However, once the technique is mastered, it provides both optimal visualization and instrument access for the posterior notch.

Initial Diagnostic Arthroscopy

Prior to preparing and draping the patient, we routinely inject 30 mL of 1% lidocaine with 1:100,000 epinephrine into the joint. This provides adequate hemostasis and obviates the need for tourniquet use in most cases. A tourniquet is still routinely applied to the thigh so it is available if hemorrhage obscures visualization more than momentarily.

We routinely perform the diagnostic arthroscopy through the anteromedial portal. Because of the frequent association of meniscus tears with ACL insufficiency, the menisci must be examined carefully. Probably the most common associated meniscus tear is a peripheral longitudinal tear of the posterior horn of the medial meniscus. The surgeon must check for this preoperatively by examining the patient for posteromedial joint line tenderness. Routine utilization of the 70-degree arthroscope to visualize the posteromedial compartment by passing it between the posterior cruciate ligament (PCL) and the medial femoral condyle will help detect most of these tears. If there is any question, a posteromedial portal can be used to provide definitive information. Tears of the posterior horn of the lateral meniscus are also very common, and usually easier to visualize. Our decisions whether to leave meniscus tears alone or treat them with repair or partial meniscectomy are guided by the recommendations of DeHaven.[48] All partial meniscectomies as well as adjunctive procedures such as loose body removal or articular debridement are carried out at the beginning of the procedure. If an arthroscopic meniscus repair is warranted, the appropriate posterior protective incision is made and the sutures are placed prior to reconstruction of the ACL.[8, 23] In order to avoid stressing the repair, the sutures are not tied until the completion of the ligament reconstruction. If a lateral meniscus repair is performed, the posterior protective incision should be placed to allow for anchoring of the femoral attachment of the ACL graft as well. If the surgeon wishes to repair the posterior horn of the medial meniscus through a small posteromedial arthrotomy, as described by DeHaven,[11] we recommend that this procedure be left until the ACL reconstruction is completed.

If a significant ligamentum mucosum is present, it is released from the intercondylar notch to increase exposure of the notch and the tibial attachment of the ACL. Useless tibial stumps of the old ACL, which might cause impingement, may be debrided at this time. However, in the interest of efficiency, the femoral notch is not prepared until the lateral approach to the femur has been performed.

Lateral Incision

The rear-entry drill guide requires a small lateral incision for exposure of the distal lateral femur. This need only be about 3 cm in length (Fig 42–6). This straight incision is positioned at the anterior edge of the iliotibial tract. It should begin about 2 cm proximal to the proximal pole of the patella and proceed proximally. After the subcutaneous tissue is bluntly separated, the fascia lata is divided at the anterior border of the iliotibial tract. This incision should be approximately 7 cm long, extending 2 cm past the skin incision in either direction. The vastus lateralis is separated from the lateral intermuscular septum and retracted anteriorly with a large Slocum or similar retractor placed anterior to the femoral shaft. The lateral femoral cortex is identified. We only coagulate the superior lateral genicular vessels if they are violated during the creation of the femoral tunnel.

Preparation of Femoral Notch

Several clinicians have believed that some patients may be predisposed to ACL tear by a congenitally narrowed intercondylar notch.[2, 16, 22, 35] This hypothesis has not been proved, although recent studies have implicated it as a factor in noncontact ACL tears.[30, 47] On the other hand, the hyaline cartilage of the lateral femoral condyle forms an important articulation with the lateral tibial plateau and the lateral facet of the patella. I therefore do not recommend routine removal of normal portions of the lateral femoral condyle to increase exposure or prevent impingement of the reconstructed ligament.[27] Instead, the surgeon should assess each notch individually to detect an acquired or congenital stenosis. Periarticular osteophytes can sometimes form within 1 year or less of the ACL rupture. These osteophytes form along the edges of the articular surface, and can be visually differentiated by their shape as well as by a subtle difference in color from the adjacent normal hyaline cartilage (Fig 42–7). If such osteophytes are present, they should be removed from the lateral and superior aspects of the notch to return it to its normal size. If the surgeon judges the notch to be congenitally narrow, he should judiciously enlarge its anterior and lateral borders, taking care not to endanger the patellofemoral or tibiofemoral articulations.

The preparation of the notch is done with the knee in about 45 degrees of flexion. The arthroscope is inserted through the accessory medial portal described above. The lateral, superior, and medial borders of the notch and the PCL should be identified to orient the surgeon. A basket forceps is then inserted through the anteromedial incision and used to debride any large remaining fragments of ligament obscuring the lateral wall of the notch. I prefer to do the actual debridement of the notch wall with a large

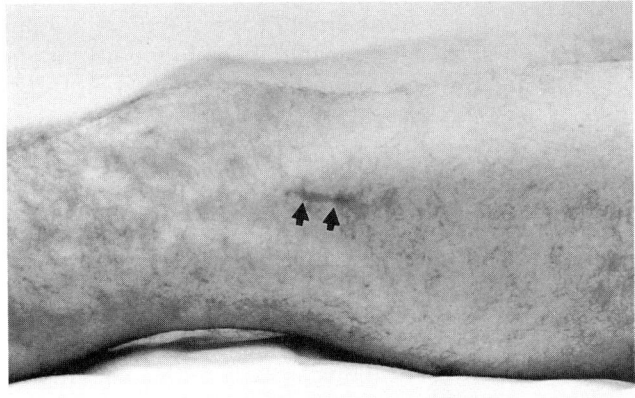

FIG 42–6.
Lateral incision is about 3 cm long and is placed at the anterior edge of the iliotibial tract, beginning about 2 cm proximal to the proximal pole of the patella and proceeding proximally (arrows).

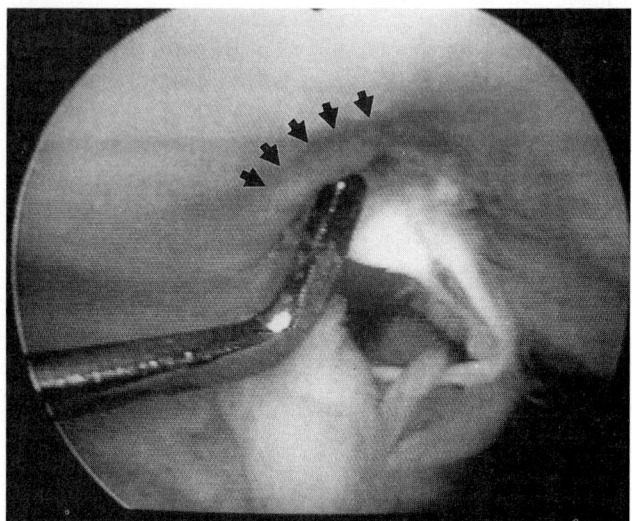

FIG 42–7.
Osteophytes on the lateral and superior aspects of the intercondylar notch should be identified and removed. In this photograph, the probe is palpating a thick rim of osteophytes; the original wall of the notch is indicated by the *arrows*.

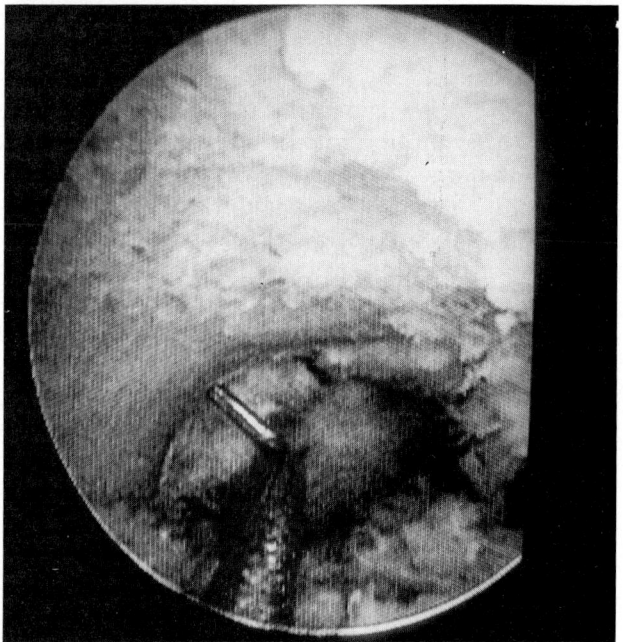

FIG 42–8.
Debridement of the notch exposes the arch joining the lateral "wall" and "roof" of the notch. When a perfect arch-shaped posterior notch is present, the guide pin should emerge slightly above the midpoint between the roof and the lateral wall.

Brun curette. This allows the surgeon to clear the soft tissue from the notch quickly without removing normal bone. If preferred, a motorized synovial resector may also be used for the soft tissue debridement. The curettage should begin at the front of the notch and move from the bottom of the notch to the roof and from the front to the back until the wall and roof of the notch, including the entire femoral cruciate origin, has been cleared. If osteophytes are present, they are removed with the curette at this time. A motorized burr may also be used, but it tends to create more bleeding and does not give the surgeon the same "feel" as a currette. The osteophytes are usually composed of a softer cancellous bone than the normal condyle. The use of the curette will allow the surgeon to feel this distinction between the soft osteophyte and the normal condylar wall when it is reached, allowing him to restore the notch to its normal dimensions without resecting normal bone. Any large pieces of bone loosened during this debridement should be removed from the knee with a pituitary rongeur. A motorized arthrotome is used to remove the loosened synovium and ligament remnants.

The lateral wall of the notch should be debrided until the posterior arch of the notch is clearly visible. The surgeon should be able to see the entire lateral wall and superior roof of the notch in order to select the proper site for the femoral guide pin (Fig 42–8). A ridge of bone is often present on the lateral wall of the notch about 1 cm anterior to the true posterior edge. This has sometimes disparagingly been called the "resident's ridge," implying that the neophyte surgeon will be fooled into thinking that this is the true posterior border of the notch. When the arthroscope is inserted through a medial portal, as described here, the resident's ridge is unlikely to obscure the posterior border of the notch completely. It is usually helpful, however, to curette it away to completely reveal the full arch-shaped posterior margin. Proper identification of the true posterior lip of the notch is extremely important. The most common identifiable error that we encounter in patients with failed ACL grafts done elsewhere is a femoral tunnel that is placed too anterior. Some surgeons will mark the site for the femoral guide pin at this point, but this is actually easier to do once the rear-entry drill guide has been inserted.

Femoral Site Selection

The selection of the site for the femoral guide pin is probably the most crucial step of the operation. Because the femoral drill hole is close to the instant center of the knee, errors of only a few millimeters can make a tremendous difference in the isometry of the resulting reconstruction. The surgeon should remember that it is better to place the pin slightly posterior or superior to the ideal location than too anterior or inferior. Not only is this position better biomechanically, but an error in the superior or posterior direction can always be corrected by enlarging the tunnel anteriorly and inferiorly, since the graft will lie in the anteroinferior portion of the tunnel. When a perfect arch-shaped posterior notch is present, the guide pin should emerge slightly above the midpoint between the roof and lateral wall (see Fig 42–9). It should also be about 5 to 6 mm in front of the posterior cortex. If the intraarticular mouth of tunnel ultimately breaks out of the posterior cortex a bit, this is not a problem since the rest of the tunnel will hold the graft in place. I routinely use a 10-mm reamer for most knees. Since a 10-mm tunnel will be larger in relation to some knees than others, the guide pin should allow for this difference in the size of condyles by being placed a few millimeters higher toward the roof of the notch in a small knee. In the case of a very small-boned patient, such as a female gymnast, or a very large-boned patient, such as a football lineman, smaller or larger reamer sizes can be chosen.

The technique described here uses visual cues to place the femoral tunnel, so thorough familiarity with the correct placement of the femoral guide pin is essential. It is difficult to accurately check the isometry of the femoral hole placement prior to drilling, since the guide pin is actually about 5 mm away from the eventual lip of the femoral tunnel, and 5 mm is a big change in the femoral hole placement. Surgeons who check isometry using the femoral guide pin hole must remember that the actual graft will lie anterior and inferior to this hole.

Passage of Rear-Entry Drill Guide

The gaff for passage of the rear-entry drill guide is then inserted through the anterolateral arthroscopy incision. Its tip should be followed visually into the posterior notch. The instrument is then rotated to allow the tip of the gaff to pass around the femoral condyle and emerge through the lateral intramuscular septum into the lateral incision. The vastus lateralis is then retracted superiorly to allow for visualization of the tip of the gaff. The hook of the appropriate rear-entry drill guide is attached to the gaff. In order to pull the guide into the knee without unseating it from the gaff, the surgeon should place countertension on the guide as he or she rotates the gaff and pulls the guide into the knee. Once the guide has been felt to pop through the posterior capsule, its tip should be visualized so that the gaff can be unhooked and removed from the knee. Failure to do this under direct vision can cause the gaff to break off the tip of the drill guide.

The guide tip is then placed at the site for the femoral guide pin described above. Because the guide pin has a tendency to glance off the tip of the guide and emerge slightly anterior and inferior to the planned entry, the surgeon may wish to place the guide 1 mm posterior and superior to his or her ideal imagined placement. Twisting of the drill guide with resulting inaccuracy of pin placement can be minimized by orientating the handle of the guide within the coronal plane of the thigh (Fig 42–9). The "bullet" portion of the guide is then inserted and pushed down until it meets the lateral femoral cortex. It is then locked in place using the thumbscrew and a 2.4-mm threaded guide pin inserted through the guide into the knee. Error will be minimized if the surgeon does not assume that the guide will automatically place the pin correctly but instead consciously aims down the center of the guide. The drill is then removed from the guide pin and the bullet is detached from the rest of the guide. I recommend that the guide be left in the knee while the surgeon rechecks the position of the guide pin to make sure that it is satisfactory. This avoids the extra step of having to reinsert the drill guide should the first pin placement not be satisfactory. Using adequate retraction, a sharp 10-mm cannulated reamer is then used to create a tunnel over the guide pin. It is relatively easy to bend the pin and break it off during the reaming. Therefore, the surgeon should aim down the shaft of the guide pin with the reamer to avoid cutting into it or bending it. Once the tunnel is placed, it should again be quickly visually checked to verify that it is satisfactory. Any rough edges may be smoothed with a curette and a plug inserted to minimize leakage of fluid through the tunnel.

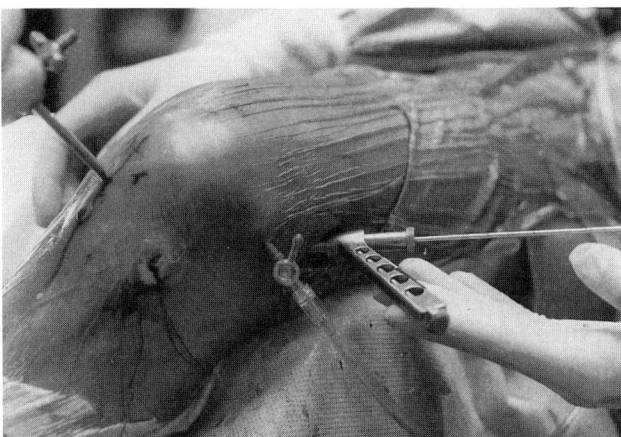

FIG 42–9.
Orienting the rear-entry drill guide as shown will minimize twisting of the guide and result in better accuracy of pin placement.

Anterior Exposure

If an allograft is being used, a 3-cm incision along the medial border of the tibial tubercle just proximal to the superior border of the pes anserinus is sufficient. If an autograft is to be used, this incision is continued to include the anteromedial arthroscopy portal. In a patient with normal looseness of the skin anterior to the knee, this incision can be about 6 to 7 cm. An alternative method is to harvest the graft through two small incisions as described by Purnell,[40] although the technique described here will result in a relatively small and cosmetic incision.

Tibial Guide Placement

Visual cues for correct placement of the tibial guide pin are subtler than those for placement of the femoral guide pin. It is helpful to remember that the ligament normally inserts anterior to the tibial spine at the edge of the articular surface of the medial tibial plateau. Even in chronic cases, the drop-off at the lateral edge of the medial tibial plateau is a reliable landmark for the medial edge of the old ACL insertion. While observing through the same accessory medial portal, the tibial drill guide is inserted through the anteromedial portal. Its tip is inserted in what is judged to be the "footprint" of the old ACL along the lateral margin of the medial tibial plateau. This placement will appear to be too medial when the knee is flexed. However, the normal screw-home mechanism of the knee externally rotates the tibia as the knee is extended, placing the guide in the proper position.

The rest of the drill guide is then assembled and rested against the proximal tibia so that the pin will enter just superior to the pes anserinus and 1 cm medial to the tibial tubercle. This guide is easily twisted out of alignment, so it is important to avoid placing any torque on the guide as the guide pin is drilled into position. When about 10 mm of guide pin is visible in the knee, the tibial drill guide is disassembled and removed. As mentioned, the pin should have emerged in the knee just on the lateral edge of the articular margin of the medial tibial plateau. Placing the guide pin too lateral is a common error.

A visual check at this point is extremely helpful in establishing accurate tibial guide pin placement. With the arthroscope still in the accessory medial portal, the arthroscope is positioned so that it is just lateral to the pin and its 25-degree angle of inclination is looking medially toward the pin. This will allow the surgeon to follow the relationship of the guide pin and the roof of the intercondylar notch as the knee is brought into full extension (Fig 42–10). As the knee is slowly extended, the pin should "tuck inside"

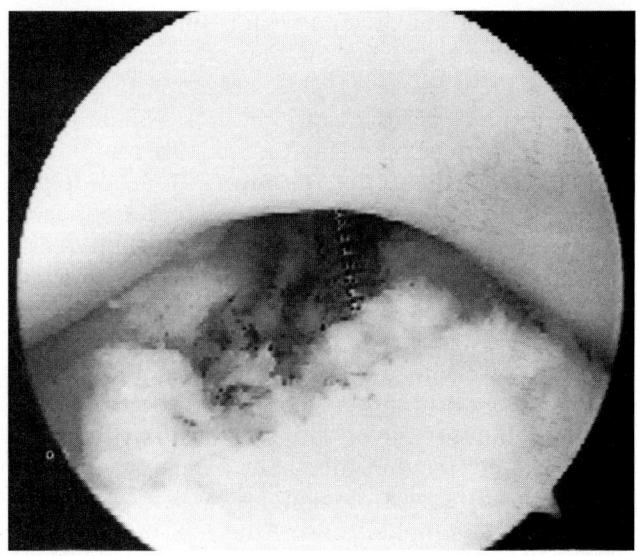

FIG 42–10.
Observing the behavior of the tibial guide pin in relation to the notch as the knee is extended will help the surgeon judge placement and predict impingement.

the roof of the notch, passing posterior to the superior edge of the anterior notch as the knee reaches full extension. If the pin impales the articular cartilage just above the notch as the knee nears extension, the pin placement is either too anterior or the superior notch has been closed down by a rim of osteophytes. If the latter is the case, the osteophytes should be removed with a curette; otherwise, the pin placement should be adjusted. Conversely, if the tip of the guide pin clears the roof of the notch by more than a few millimeters, it has probably been placed too posterior. The pin should appear slightly medial to the center of the notch when the knee is extended. The 3- and 5-mm parallel drill guides are an invaluable way of making controlled minor adjustments in pin placement (see Fig 42–3, B and C). Learning to adjust the tibial placement by visual cues will eliminate time wasted by isometric testing of tibial guide holes, which are far from isometric.

Isometry Testing

Once the clinician feels that satisfactory tibial guide placement has been achieved, the pin is removed from the knee for isometry testing. When the surgeon gains sufficient experience to confidently place the tunnel by visual cues, isometry measurement can be postponed until the actual tibial tunnel has been drilled. If more than one tibial hole has been made, it is important to be able to identify the correct one as it emerges on the anterior tibia. A heavy suture is then passed into the knee through the femoral tunnel. A single-cannula meniscus repair guide makes a handy passer. The suture is simply threaded completely through the guide and inserted into the knee. A small arthroscopic grasper can also be used to pass the suture, which is then visualized entering the knee through the femoral tunnel and grasped with a grasper inserted through the anteromedial portal. A small crochet hook is inserted through the proper tibial guide hole and visualized in the front of the knee. The suture is then hooked and pulled through the tibial guide hole. A large button is tied to the proximal end of the suture. The button is pulled taut against the lateral femoral cortex and the suture is passed through the isometer. After the suture is fixed in the isometer, the knee is taken through a full range of motion several times and the excursion of the isometer is noted. The isometer reading should change by less than 2 mm throughout the range of motion. If the excursion is greater than this, the position of the hole should be reassessed visually to detect the error responsible. Since the suture will represent some fibers of the ultimate graft, the suture itself may be observed for impingement in the roof of the notch near full extension. If the suture impinges, the graft will impinge as well. In addition, the surgeon should observe whether the suture appears to be tented over a hypertrophic tibial spine. In some chronic cases it will be necessary to curette away a portion of a hypertrophied spine to ensure a straight path between the tibial and femoral holes.

If the isometry reading is acceptable, the suture is temporarily withdrawn through the anteromedial arthroscopy portal and a 2.4-mm smooth pin is tapped through the tibial guide hole until it is seen to emerge into the knee. It is important to verify that the guide pin is following the correct path. The guide pin is then overreamed with a 10-mm reamer while the knee is in a flexed position. Again, care must be taken not to bend or break the guide pin while reaming.

Tibial Hole Preparation

A basket forceps is then inserted through the anterolateral incision and used to trim any loose cartilage flaps or fragments of ligament that are still attached to the mouth of the hole. This will help avoid any jamming during passage of the graft. Another technique to predict notch impingement is passing a large curette through the tibial hole into the knee and observing the behavior of the curette as the knee is gradually extended. In this case, the curette acts as a surrogate for the eventual graft. The curette should be able to enter into the notch during extension. The knee should be able to fully extend without impinging on the curette. If impingement exists, it may be necessary to (1) lower a hypertrophied tibial spine, (2) enlarge the tibial hole slightly posteriorly, or (3) enlarge the anterior lip of the notch, depending upon the perceived cause of impingement. The guide suture is then pulled proximally to create slack and again pulled out through the tibial tunnel, this time using either a grasper or crochet hook. If isometry was not assessed earlier, it should be measured now. Interpretation of deviation from ideal isometry should be guided by the figures of Graf and Uhr[20] (Fig 42–11, A and B). Minor deviations from ideal graft isometry can be compensated for by shifting the final graft placement to the appropriate quadrant of the femoral or tibial tunnel, or both, by choice of graft rotation and placement of the interference screw. Larger deviations from ideal isometry can be rescued by expanding the misplaced tunnel in the direction suggested by the tables of Graf and Uhr.[20] In this case, the surgeon may need to harvest a tibial bone block that is thicker than usual to help fill the tunnel and place the tendon in the appropriate quadrant. Extremely large deviations from ideal isometry are corrected by identifying the erroneous tunnel and creating an entirely new one in the proper location.

Harvesting the Graft

To harvest a patellar tendon autograft, the tendon must be clearly exposed and its edges defined. The size of the skin incision necessary to harvest the tendon strip can be minimized by placing the knee in extension during the bone block harvest, thus maximizing the flexibility of the skin. The tibial bone block is harvested first. After the placement of the anchoring sutures in the tibial bone block, the entire graft can be pulled distally to help expose the patella. This technique will usually reduce by several centimeters the proximal extent of the incision necessary to harvest the patellar bone block.

The central 10 mm of the tendon is selected for the graft. Two parallel incisions should be made with a no. 10 scalpel. Each incision should extend about 3 cm past each end of the patellar tendon. Although the ultimate desired length of the bone block is 2.5 cm, it is better to make it a little long initially, thus decreasing the risk of making the bone block too short. Since most patellar tendons have a natural taper, it is important to avoid allowing the graft to taper too much distally or widen too much proximally. If desired, an 11- or 12-mm graft may be harvested in a very large patient and a 9-mm graft in a very small patient. A microsagittal saw (Fig 42–12) is then used to make beveling cuts through the cortical

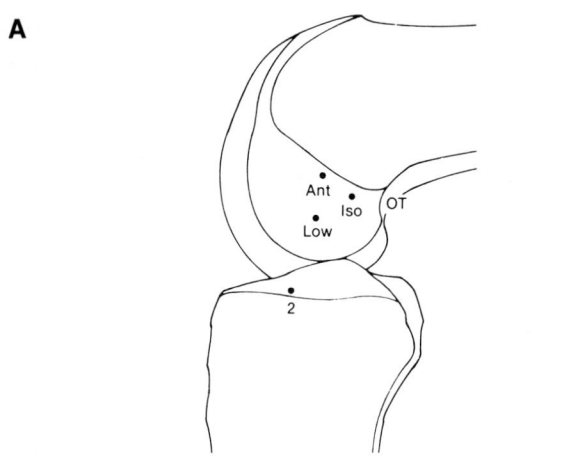

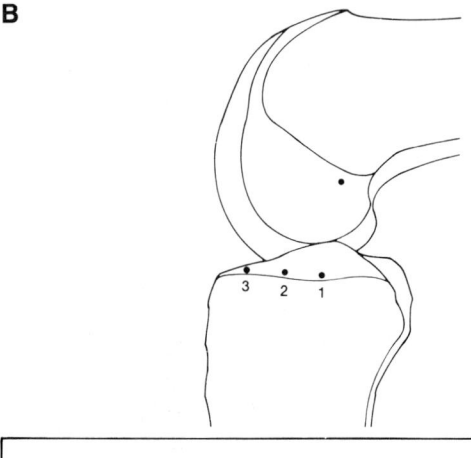

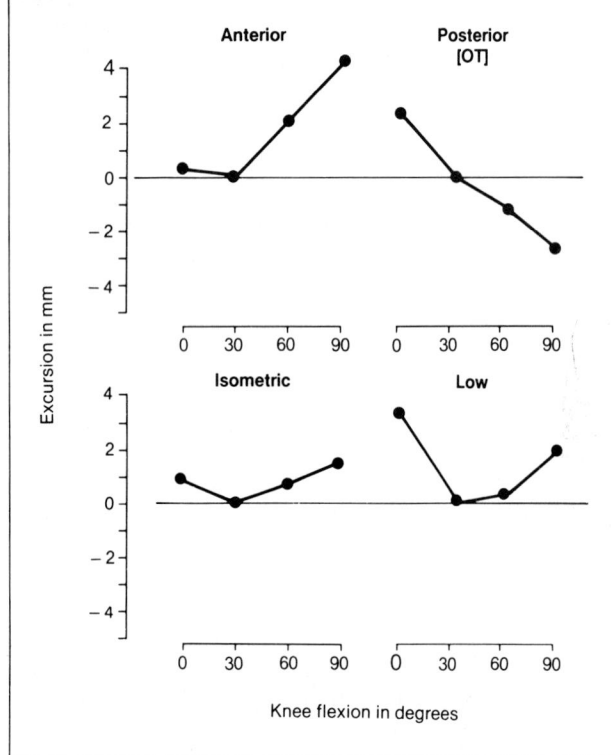

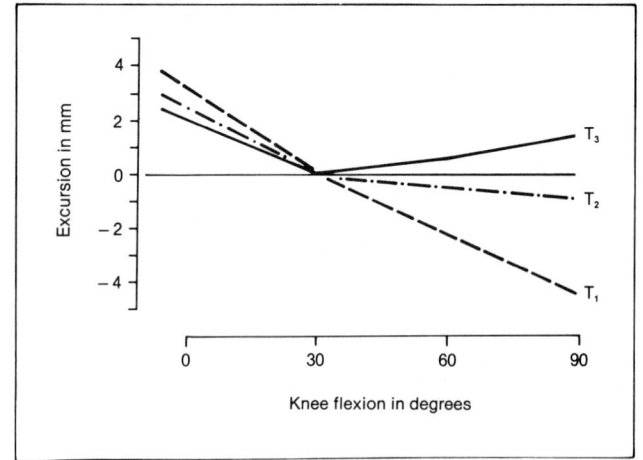

FIG 42–11.
A, comparing the excursion of the isometer to these graphs constructed by Graf and Uhr[20] will allow the surgeon to interpret whether the femoral tunnel is too anterior, too posterior, nearly isometric, or too low. **B,** the location of the tibial tunnel also has an effect on the isometry of the graft, although less than the effect of the femoral tunnel location. Anterior tibial placement makes a given femoral tunnel look more anterior, and posterior tibial placement makes a given femoral tunnel look more posterior. (From Graf B, Uhr F: *Clin Sports Med* 7:840, 1988. Used by permission.)

bone on both sides of each bone block and a vertical cut at the end.

Each bone block is then carefully removed with a curved osteotome. Care must be taken to avoid levering the osteotome while making the cuts, thus fracturing the patella. It is important to remove the entire insertion of the tendon strip at each end of the graft. Each bone block is then trimmed to a length of 2.5 cm using a rongeur. The bone blocks should be sculptured with a rongeur until they have smooth rounded tips and fit easily into a 10-mm guide. Any bits of bone trimmed from the edges should be removed sharply with a scalpel or tissue scissors, since tearing them off with a rongeur may strip significant portions of the tendon graft. If sutures are to be the primary form of fixation, three or four small drill holes are placed at intervals in the bone block and no. 5 Ethibond (nonabsorbable) sutures are passed through each hole. We have found it helpful to tie a single knot in one end of each suture so that the ends can easily be distinguished later. If an interference screw is to be the primary form of fixation, only two drill holes are necessary. Because our laboratory research has shown that grafts fixed with interference screws which are stressed to failure often fail by fracturing through the suture holes, we recommend placing these two holes near the terminal end of each bone block. We also recommend orienting them at 90 degrees to each other to minimize the chance of the interference screw cutting both sutures.

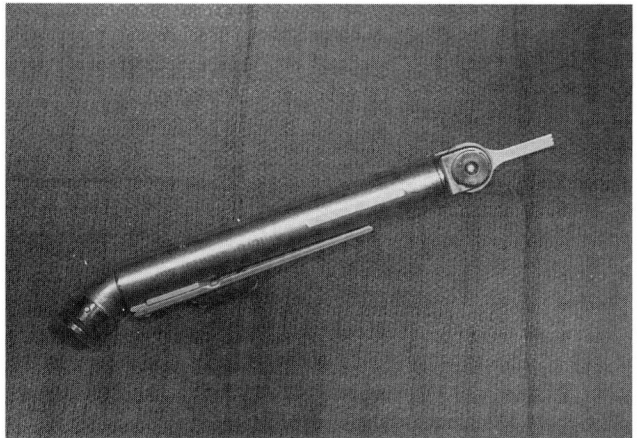

FIG 42-12.
A microsagittal saw is useful for harvesting the patellar tendon autograft.

Whichever bone block passes most easily through the sizer should be chosen as the lead end of the graft during passage. The terminal suture on the lead bone block is tied in a single knot over the end so that it will tend to lead the bone block in the correct path.

Passage of the Graft

The button is then cut off the femoral end of the suture which was used to measure isometry and this suture is tied to the fixation sutures of the lead end of the graft. It is then used to pull the fixation sutures entirely through the knee and out the tibial tunnel. The lead bone block is then fed directly into the lateral opening of the femoral tunnel and the graft is pulled through the knee and into position. If difficulties are experienced in passing the graft, it is usually because the graft is caught as it emerges into the intercondylar notch or as it tries to enter the intraarticular mouth of the tibial tunnel. If the leading bone block is relatively long compared to the width of the femoral notch, the tip of the block will impinge on the PCL before the trailing edge of the block has emerged from the femoral tunnel. Sometimes this can be overcome by visualizing the block and pulling it past the PCL with a probe or other instrument. If this does not work, the impasse can usually be circumvented by withdrawing the graft and shortening the leading bone block by a few millimeters. If the leading bone block is having trouble entering the tibial tunnel, check to see if bits of soft tissue, ligament remnants, or fragments of articular cartilage are causing the graft to jam in the mouth of the tunnel. If this is not the case, the bone block can normally be guided into the tunnel with a probe or other instrument. Often varying the flexion angle of the knee is enough to orient the graft properly and ease its passage into the tibial tunnel.

The isometry of the graft itself may now be evaluated using the "pinch test." To do this, an assistant should stabilize the proximal end of the graft by pinching the sutures between the thumb and index finger where they emerge from the femoral tunnel. The surgeon then brings the knee to full extension and tenses the ligament by pinching the distal sutures tightly between the thumb and index finger where they emerge from the tibial tunnel. The surgeon then takes the knee through a full range of motion, noting whether the sutures pull through his or her fingers into the tibia, indicating tightening of the ligament during flexion, or if the fingers pull away from the tibia, indicating loosening in flexion, or if they maintain a constant relationship to the anterior tibia, indicating isometry. If the ligament varies more than 2 mm from isometry, the surgeon should check for graft impingement or faulty tunnel placement and make the appropriate adjustments. As noted, minor deviations from ideal isometry can be remedied by orienting the graft and placing interference screws appropriately. If the graft is noted to tense near terminal extension, it is important to rule out impingement on the roof of the intercondylar notch. This is done by performing the pinch test while observing the relationship of the graft to the roof of the notch. If the increased tension occurs when the graft appears to touch the notch roof, then impingement is the probable cause and further notchplasty is usually indicated. If this would result in excessive notchplasty, the posterior wall of the tibial tunnel can be curetted to allow the graft to move posteriorly, although this may alter overall isometry. Minor degrees of impingement may respond to pushing the graft to the posterior quadrant of the tibial tunnel by placing an interference screw anteriorly.

Fixation of the Graft

Fixation options include interference screws,[29] fixation sutures through buttons,[9] and fixation sutures tied around posts. All three methods have advantages and disadvantages. The interference screws have been shown in the laboratory to be capable of providing the strongest initial fixation,[28] although it is not known whether bone reabsorption around the screw may weaken this in the weeks following surgery. As noted above, they may also be used to effect minor changes in isometry by adjusting the position of the graft within the bony tunnels. Potential problems with interference screws include inaccurate oblique placement, overtensioning of the graft, and possible difficulty in redoing the fixation should the first placement be deemed unsatisfactory. Some surgeons strive to avoid tensioning problems by using an interference screw at one end of the graft and fixation sutures at the other; however, this would seem to sacrifice the strength advantage of the interference screw, since the strength of the system is only as great as its weakest link.

Fixation sutures can be held in place with buttons or fixation posts. Buttons have the advantage of radiolucency, but cause the fixation sutures to be drawn over the sharp acute edges of the oblique tunnels. Fixation posts allow the sutures to be drawn across the smooth obtuse edges of the tunnels, but do require radiopaque fixation screws. Both these suture techniques depend heavily on the surgeon's ability to set and maintain graft tension while tying the knot. The fixation post screws and knots are more likely to cause subsequent irritation and require later removal than buried interference screws. On the other hand, they are easier to locate and remove should revision be necessary. We are currently using the Kurasaka interference screw technique, although we have used all three techniques successfully. If the fixation post technique is chosen, I recommend 6.5-mm large-fragment AO cancellous screws because their smooth proximal shafts bear no threads which might cut the sutures. It is helpful for a surgeon to be familiar with more than one method should his usual one prove unfeasible in a particular case.

Whichever fixation method is chosen, the femoral end should be fixed first since it is the most difficult to reach. This allows the tension to be adjusted while tightening the more exposed tibial attachment.

If the fixation post method is chosen, a 3.2-mm hole is drilled across both femoral cortices at a point in line with the course of the ligament graft and approximately 2 cm from it. A 6.5-mm AO long-thread cancellous screw of appropriate length and a smooth washer are then inserted. The ends of the fixation sutures are separated into two bundles with one end of each suture contained in each bundle and tied around the post using three or four square throws. Additional knots may be tied among some of the individual sutures to prevent unraveling of these large knots.

If interference screw fixation is chosen, the surgeon has a choice between cannulated or noncannulated types. The length of the screw should be chosen to match the length of each bone block; the diameter may be chosen according to the diameters of the bone tunnels and the bone blocks. The cannulated screw was introduced to reduce the chance of the longitudinal axis of the screw diverging from the axes of the graft and tunnel; such divergence would reduce the strength of fixation by only allowing a few of the screw's threads to engage the graft. We prefer the noncannulated screws, however, since the guide pin used with the cannulated screws can be difficult to remove once the screw is seated. Two technical points can help minimize the chance of screw-graft divergence when using the noncannulated screw. First, the tunnel should be clearly exposed, so the surgeon can visually align the axis of the screw with the axis of the tunnel as the screw is inserted. Second, the surgeon should use minimal pressure and torque when inserting the screw, allowing it to seek the path of least resistance down the tunnel axis. An assistant stabilizes the tibial end of the graft to ensure that it does not shift while the femoral screw is being inserted. The surgeon then places moderate tension on the fixation sutures and inserts the screw as described until its head is flush with the end of the bone block.

Before fixation of the tibial end, the final isometry of the graft itself may be assessed using the pinch test described above. If the graft is truly isometric, the position of the knee at the time of fixation of the tibial end is unimportant. The knee should be cycled through a range of motion several times to remove any slack from the graft. Fixation of the tibial end is then done in the same manner as the femoral end. If the anchoring post technique is used, the bicortical fixation screw is placed just distal to the mouth of the tibial tunnel so that its head will come to rest in the hollow just medial to the tibial tubercle. It is important not to use a screw longer than the depth gauge measurement of the hole to avoid protrusion of the screw tip posteriorly. After the sutures are knotted, the knot may be stuffed into the tibial drill hole to prevent a subcutaneous prominence. If interference screws are used, the tibial screw is inserted in a manner similar to the femoral screw while tension is maintained on the sutures. The optimal amount of tension for graft fixation is not currently known. The sutures are removed after the interference screws are seated. The knee should then be taken through a full range of motion several times and its anterior stability manually assessed at 15-degree intervals. A final visual check is made to verify that the knee can be taken to full extension without graft impingement (Fig 42–13). The knee is then irrigated arthroscopically and the anterior and lateral incisions are irrigated conventionally. Small closed suction drains may be placed in the incisions and exited percutaneously; however, we prefer to use conventional elec-

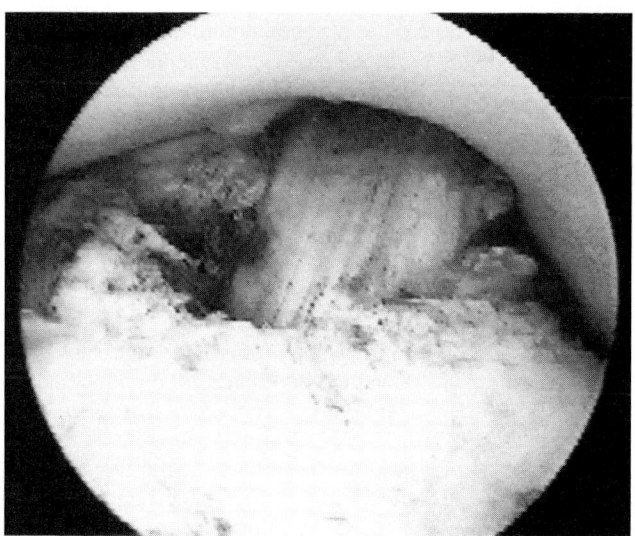

FIG 42-13.
The graft should be observed as the knee is taken to full extension to verify that impingement does not occur.

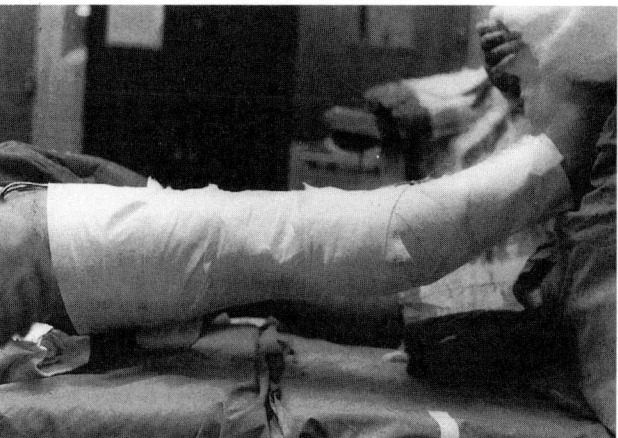

FIG 42-14.
Postoperatively, the knee is placed in full extension to discourage the development of flexion contractures.

trocoagulation for optimal hemostasis and have eliminated the routine use of drains. The incisions are then closed according to the surgeon's preference.

Postoperative Care

The early goals of postoperative rehabilitation include the rapid restoration of full range of motion and the minimization of postoperative muscle atrophy through early weightbearing. The early restoration of motion and weightbearing have not been shown to adversely affect the ultimate stability of the knee.[44] Sachs et al.[42] have shown an association among postoperative flexion contracture, quadriceps weakness, and patellofemoral pain. It is therefore of paramount importance to maintain full extension immediately after surgery, since full extension may be difficult to regain once lost. To minimize the chance of a postoperative flexion contracture, the knee is placed in full extension at the conclusion of surgery in a well-padded Jones dressing or postoperative brace (Fig 42-14). If a Jones dressing is used, it is exchanged the next day for a removable postoperative brace which is locked in full extension. To encourage the maintenance of extension, the patient should elevate the limb with a pillow or two which support the calf but not the knee. The day after surgery, the patient is taught to ambulate with crutches and is allowed full weightbearing as tolerated. He or she is then discharged from the hospital. Patients are taught to remove the brace several times daily and take the knee through a range of motion. This is conveniently done using a continuous passive motion (CPM) machine at home. Alternatively, patients are taught to actively flex their knees up to 90 degrees and to passively extend them. Full weightbearing as tolerated is encouraged; most patients are walking without crutches within 2 or 3 weeks of surgery. The patients continue to wear the brace locked in full extension except when using the CPM machine or performing the range-of-motion exercises. The brace is discontinued 1 month after surgery: patients who are having difficulty achieving flexion or who appear to be at risk for arthrofibrosis are removed from their braces earlier. Once the initial postoperative brace is removed, no further bracing is utilized. Closed-chain kinetic quadriceps exercises which emphasize axial loading, such as partial squats, leg presses, or climbing machines, are started as soon as the patient is able, usually within 3 weeks of surgery. The early weightbearing discourages quadriceps atrophy and improves patient morale; it has not been found to adversely affect the final stability of the knee. Jogging is allowed 3 months after surgery. Because of laboratory studies showing increasing graft strength for the first 9 months following reconstruction, athletes are urged to avoid stressful pivoting and jumping sports for the first 9 months following surgery, although some have violated this guideline without apparent ill effects.

REFERENCES

1. Amiel D, Kleimer JB, Akeson WH: The natural history of the anterior cruciate ligament autograft of patellar tendon origin, *Am J Sports Med* 14:449-462, 1986.
2. Anderson AF, et al: Analysis of the intercondylar notch by computed tomography, *Am J Sports Med* 15:547-552, 1987.
3. Arms SW, et al: The biomechanics of anterior cruci-

ate ligament rehabilitation and reconstruction, *Am J Sports Med* 12:8-18, 1984.
4. Bonamo JJ, Krinick RM, Sporn AA: Rupture of the patellar ligament after use of its central third for anterior-cruciate reconstruction, *J Bone Joint Surg [Am]* 66:1294-1297, 1984.
5. Bruckner H: Eine neue Methode der Kreuzbandplastik [A new method of reconstructing the anterior cruciate ligament]. *Chirurg* 37:413-414, 1966.
6. Clancy WG Jr: Intraarticular reconstruction of the anterior cruciate ligament, *Orthop Clin North Am* 16:181-189, 1985.
7. Clancy WG Jr: Arthroscopic anterior cruciate ligament reconstruction with patellar tendon. In Dorr L, editor: *Techniques in orthopaedics,* Frederick, Md, 1988, Aspen, pp 13-22.
8. Clancy WG Jr, Graf BK: Arthroscopic meniscal repair, *Orthopaedics* 6:1125-1129, 1983.
9. Clancy WG Jr, et al: Anterior cruciate ligament reconstruction using one third of the patellar tendon augmented by extraarticular tendon transfers, *J Bone Joint Surg [Am]* 64:352-359, 1982.
10. Clancy WG, et al: Anterior and posterior cruciate ligament reconstruction in Rhesus monkeys, *J Bone Joint Surg [Am]* 63:1270-1284, 1981.
11. DeHaven KE: Meniscus repair in the athlete, *Clin Orthop* 198:31-35, 1985.
12. Draganich LF, et al: An in vitro study of a combined intra- and extraarticular reconstruction in the anterior cruciate ligament deficient knee, *Am J Sports Med* 18:262-266, 1990.
13. Eriksson E: Reconstruction of the anterior cruciate ligament, *Orthop Clin North Am* 7:167-180, 1976.
14. Reference deleted in galleys.
15. Fowler PJ: Techniques using braided polypropylene as a ligament augmentation device. In Dorr L, editor: *Techniques in orthopaedics,* Frederick, Md, 1988, Aspen, pp 74-80.
16. Gillquist J, Odensten M: Arthroscopic reconstruction of the anterior cruciate ligament, *Arthroscopy* 4:5-9, 1988.
17. Girgis FG, Marshall JL, Al Monajem ARS: The cruciate ligaments of the knee joint: Anatomical function and experimental analysis, *Clin Orthop* 106:216-231, 1975.
18. Goodfellow J, O'Connor J: The mechanics of the knee and prosthesis design, *J Bone Joint Surg [Br]* 60:358-369, 1978.
19. Graf B: Isometric placement of substitutes for the anterior cruciate ligament. In Jackson DW, Drez D, editors: *The anterior cruciate deficient knee,* St Louis, 1987, Mosby-Year Book, pp 55-71.
20. Graf B, Uhr, F: Complications of intra-articular anterior cruciate reconstruction, *Clin Sports Med* 7:835-848, 1988.
21. Hefzy MS, Grood ES, Noyes FR: Factors affecting the region of most isometric femoral attachments. Part II: The anterior cruciate ligament, *Am J Sports Med* 17:208-216, 1989.
22. Houseworth SW, et al: The intercondylar notch in acute tears of the anterior cruciate ligament: A computer graphics study, *Am J Sports Med* 15:221-224, 1987.
23. Jakob RP, et al: The arthroscopic meniscal repair: Techniques and clinical experience, *Am J Sports Med* 16:137-142, 1988.
24. Jones KG: Reconstruction of the anterior cruciate ligament: A technique using the central third of the patellar ligament, *J Bone Joint Surg [Am]* 45:925-932, 1963.
25. Jones KG: Reconstruction of the anterior cruciate ligament using the central one third of the patellar ligament: A follow up report, *J Bone Joint Surg [Am]* 52:1302-1308, 1970.
26. Kapandji IA: *The physiology of the joints. Vol 2. Lower limb,* London, 1970, Churchill Livingstone, p 2.
27. Kieffer DA, et al: Anterior cruciate ligament arthroplasty, *Am J Sports Med* 12:301-312, 1984.
28. Kurosaka M, Yoshiya S, Andrish JT: A biomechanical comparison of different surgical techniques of graft fixation in anterior cruciate ligament reconstruction, *Am J Sports Med* 15:225-229, 1987.
29. Lambert KL: Vascularized patellar tendon graft with rigid internal fixation for anterior cruciate ligament insufficiency, *Clin Orthop* 197:85-89, 1983.
30. LaPrade RF, Burnett QM: Femoral intracondylar notch stenosis and correlation to anterior cruciate ligament injuries: A prospective study. The American Orthopaedic Society for Sports Medicine Specialty Day. Final Program: Book of Abstracts and Outlines, Feb 23, 1992, p 27.
30a. MacIntosh DL: Acute tears of the anterior cruciate ligament over the top repair. Presented at the annual meeting of the American Academy of Orthopaedic Surgeons, Dallas, 1974.
31. Marshall JL, et al: The anterior cruciate ligament: A technique of repair and reconstruction. *Clin Orthop* 143:97-106, 1979.
32. McCarroll JR: Fracture of the patella during a golf swing following reconstruction of the anterior cruciate ligament, *Am J Sports Med* 11:26-27, 1983.
33. Melhorn JM, Henning CE: The relationship of the femoral attachment site to the isometric tracking of the anterior cruciate ligament graft, *Am J Sports Med* 15:539-542, 1987.
34. Mueller W: *The knee. Form, function, and ligament reconstruction,* New York, 1983, Springer-Verlag.
35. Norwood LA, Cross MJ: The intercondylar shelf and the anterior cruciate ligament, *Am J Sports Med* 5:171-176, 1977.
36. Noyes FR, et al: Biomechanical analysis of human ligament grafts used in knee ligament repairs and reconstructions, *J Bone Joint Surg [Am]* 66:344-352, 1984.
37. Noyes FR, et al: Intraarticular cruciate reconstruction. Part I: Perspectives on graft strength, vascularization and immediate motion after replacement, *Clin Orthop* 172:71-77, 1983.

38. Paulos LE, et al: Intraarticular cruciate reconstruction: Replacement with vascularized patellar tendon, *Clin Orthop* 172:78–84, 1983.
39. Penner DA, et al: An in vitro study of anterior cruciate ligament graft placement and isometry, *Am J Sports Med* 16:238–243, 1988.
40. Purnell M: Personal communication, 1989.
41. Rosenberg TD, Paulos LE, Abbott PJ: Arthroscopic cruciate repair and reconstruction: An overview and description of technique. In Feagin JA Jr, editor: *The crucial ligaments,* New York, 1988, Churchill Livingstone, pp 409–423.
41a. Roth JH, et al: Polypropylene braid augmented and non-augmented intra-articulate anterior cruciate ligament reconstruction, *Am J Sports Med* 13:321–336, 1985.
42. Sachs RA, et al: Patellofemoral problems after anterior cruciate ligament reconstruction, *Am J Sports Med* 17:760–765, 1989.
43. Shelbourne D: Anterior cruciate ligament injuries. In Reider B, editor: *Sports medicine: The school age athlete*. Philadelphia, 1991 WB Saunders, pp. 284–316.
44. Shelbourne KD, Nitz PA: Accelerated rehabilitation following anterior cruciate ligament reconstruction, *Am J Sports Med* 18:292–299, 1990.
45. Shelbourne D, et al: Arthrofibrosis in acute anterior cruciate ligament reconstruction, *Am J Sports Med* 19:332–336, 1991.
46. Sidles JA, et al: Ligament length relationships in moving knee, *J Orthop Res* 6:593–610, 1988.
47. Souryal TO, Freeman TR, Evans JP: Intracondylar notch size and ACL injuries in athletes: A prospective study, The American Orthopaedic Society for Sports Medicine Specialty Day. Final Program: Book of Abstracts and Outlines, Feb 23, 1992, p 28.
48. Weiss CB, et al: Non-operative treatment of meniscal tears, *J Bone Joint Surg [Am]* 71:811–822, 1979.

43

Iliotibial Myofascial Transfer

W. NORMAN SCOTT, M.D.
GORDON HUIE, P.A.

History
Anatomy
Theoretical considerations
Contraindications

Surgical technique
Postoperative care
Surgical modification
Results

HISTORY

The iliotibial band has probably accounted for more intraarticular and extraarticular anterior cruciate ligament (ACL) reconstruction than any other supporting structure about the knee.[3, 12, 18] Hey Groves,[2] in 1920, first described the use of the distal portion of the iliotibial band as an intraarticular substitute for the ACL. O'Donoghue[16] later modified the Hey Groves procedure by using the iliotibial band as a distally based transfer. In 1931, Gratz[1] investigated the elasticity and tensile strength of human fascia lata, demonstrating that the structure could withstand significant stresses without becoming elongated or relaxed after the stress ceased. More recently, Jones[5] and MacIntosh[7] reconstructed the ACL using an "over-the-top" repair.

Insall et al.[4] and Nicholas and Minkoff,[12] dissatisfied with existing procedures for treating ACL-deficient knees, independently described an intraarticular transfer of part of Gerdy's tubercle and the iliotibial band. Although the techniques, at first glance, appear similar, they are distinctly different in that a different part of the iliotibial band is used in each procedure.[18] In the Minkoff and Nicholas technique, a central portion of this proximally based transfer was used, with the central defect being closed after the intraarticular transfer. This led to significant patella subluxation problems[9] and a dismal experience for the authors. However, in the Insall technique,[4] the anterior portion of the iliotibial band and its continuous relationship with the vastus lateralis and its interstitial attachment to the lateral intermuscular septum were maintained and "tubed" to increase the cross-sectional area and subsequent strength. Scott et al.[17,20] and Yost et al.[21] described modifications of Insall's technique and published the results of series with long-term follow-up, showing that the intraarticular transfer of the iliotibial band as an isolated procedure is effective for treating ACL insufficiency. The most important modification was the limited posterior dissection of the band and its placement at the interspinous area rather than the anterior margin of the tibial plateau. The advantages of this technique are that it allows immediate range of motion and full weightbearing. The largest published series to date has shown a direct correlation with improved static stability and limited dissection.[20]

Success with the iliotibial band procedure has been reported in almost 85% of patients.[18] This procedure has had unparalleled success in professional basketball players, certainly a true test of the quality of reconstruction.

ANATOMY

Formed from the gluteus maximus and tensor fascia lata muscle, the iliotibial band courses down the lateral side of the leg, sometimes 6 cm wide, with its anterior border coalescing with the lateral retinaculum. Posteriorly, the iliotibial band converges with the lateral intermuscular septum. The vascular supply of the iliotibial band is proximally based. A single dominant vascular pedicle composed of two or three terminal branches enters the deep surface of the tensor fascia lata 8 to 10 cm below the anterior superior iliac spine. This transverse branch is based at the lateral femoral circumflex branch of the profunda femoris artery (Fig 43–1). The iliotibial band also has

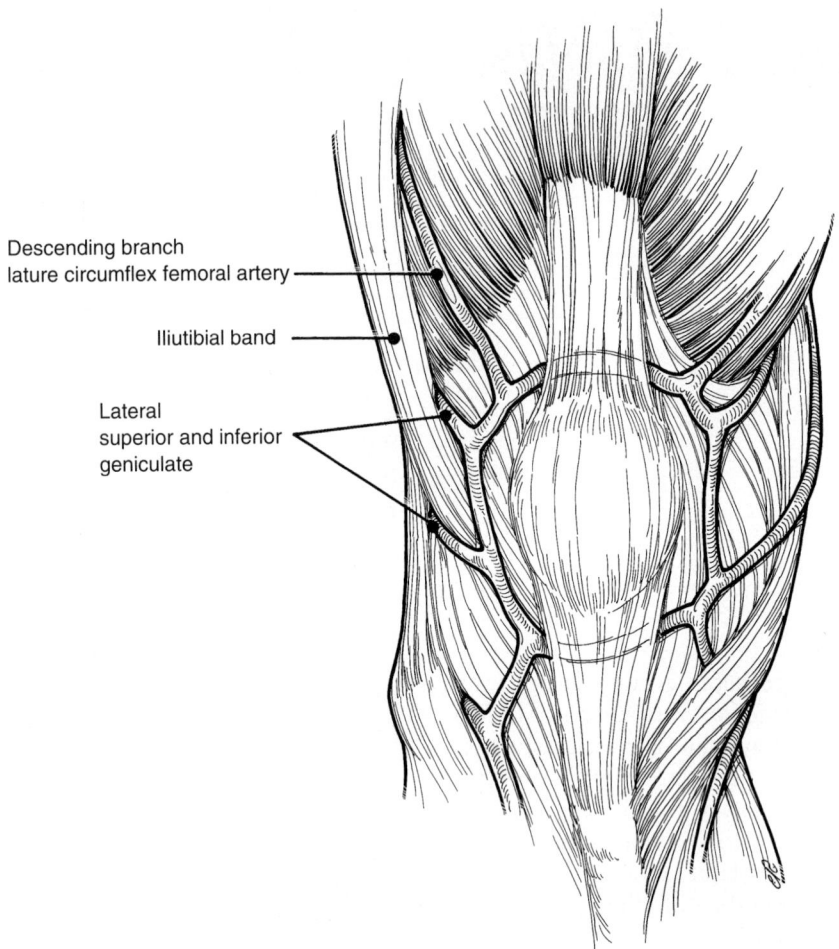

FIG 43–1.
The vascular supply of the iliotibial band.

a prominent supply from the vastis lateralis. Thus, for the proximally based transfer of the iliotibial band, revascularization is unnecessary. Reexamination by arthroscopy or arthrotomy reveals substantial functioning and viable vascular structures in the graft as early as 4 weeks postoperatively, too early for a revascularization process. Distally based or free grafts are not physiologic and would require neovascularization and restructuring of collagen fibrils.

Golgi apparatuses and mechanoreceptors are abundant throughout the length of the iliotibial band, which receives its motor nerve supply from the superior gluteal nerve. The neurovascular supply is undisturbed during the procedure.[8] It has been speculated that this reconstruction might have a dynamic or proprioceptive basis. The gluteus maximus, tensor fascia lata, and vastus lateralis, which normally contract in the stance phase of walking and running, act on the graft, which therefore should function as a dynamic stabilizer of the tibia. On postoperative Cybex testing,[18] the evidence of the iliotibial band as a dynamic stabilizer reinforces our clinical findings in over 800 cases in 15 years of experience.

THEORETICAL CONSIDERATIONS

Biomechanical analysis by Kennedy et al.[6] demonstrated that the iliotibial band is the strongest tissue for a graft about the knee. The iliotibial band has been shown to be stronger than the patellar tendon graft when the latter is tested without bone block fixation. Still, many believe the iliotibial band has insufficient strength to function as a substitute for the ACL.[13–15] Recent testing of part of the iliotibial band yielded only 44% of the maximum load sustained by the ACL. However, the portion of the iliotibial band used in recent studies was different from that used in our surgical procedure because it included neither the proximal muscle attachment nor the distal bone block. Instrom testing of a patellar tendon graft with its proximal and distal bone attachments enhances its strength eightfold. To date, no comparable testing of the iliotibial band has been reported. The anatomic interrelationships of the vastus lateralis, gluteus maximus, and tensor fascia lata provide a formidable and active transfer, which requires in vivo biomechanical analysis.

CONTRAINDICATIONS

Any patient with an ACL-deficient knee without destruction of the lateral quadruple complex is a candidate for iliotibial muscle-tendon unit transfer.[8] An absolute contraindication to use of the iliotibial band for ACL reconstruction is iatrogenic or traumatic destruction of its anatomy.

SURGICAL TECHNIQUE

Strict attention to details cannot be compromised if this procedure is to be a success. There are other procedures utilizing the iliotibial band for ACL-deficient knees, but they differ significantly and should not be confused with this procedure.

After inflating the tourniquet to 300 mm Hg, a straight midline incision is made from the proximal pole of the tibial tubercle to the center of the patella; the length of the incision should not exceed 10 cm (Fig 43-2). The lateral subcutaneous flap is mobilized (Fig 43-3) superficial to the crural fascia, exposing the iliotibial band–myofascial tendon unit (Fig 43-4, A and B).

Using a 1-cm osteotome, a 1- × 1-cm bone block is outlined with a scalpel at the attachment of the iliotibial tract to include Gerdy's tubercle (Fig 43-5, A–C). Once the fibers of the iliotibial band are transected, the corticocancellous bone block is removed

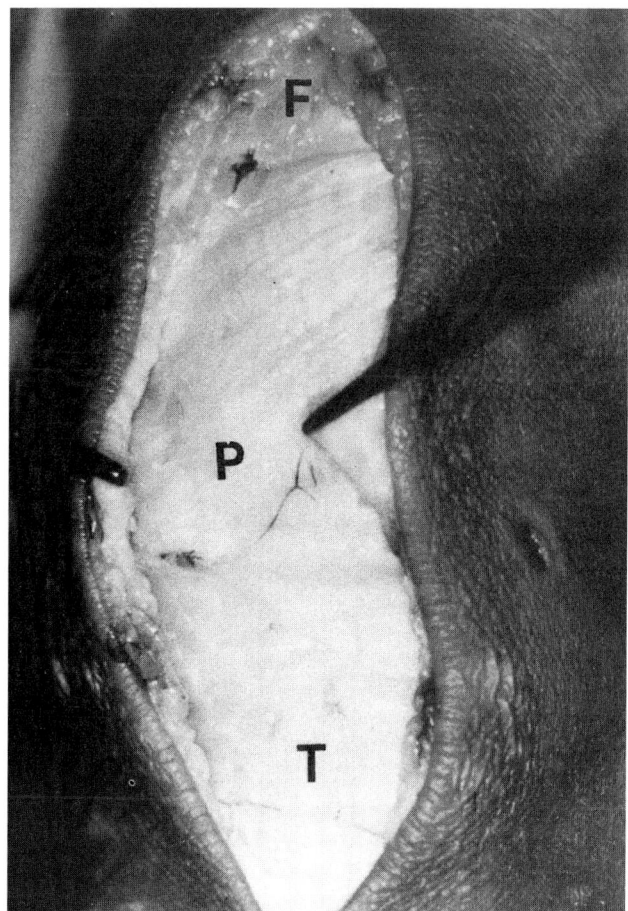

FIG 43-3.
The lateral subcutaneous flap is mobilized. F = femur; P = patella; T = tibia.

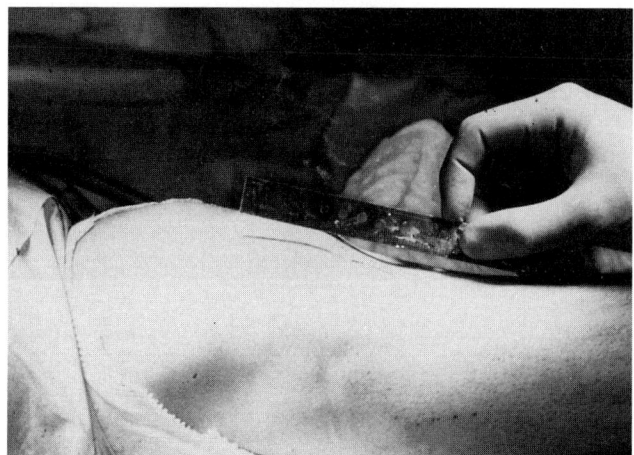

FIG 43-2.
The length of the skin incision is approximately 10 cm.

with a 1-cm osteotome (Fig 43-6). The depth of the bone block should be no less than 1 cm thick (Fig 43-7).

The posterior incision is extended 4 cm proximally (Fig 43-8), terminating at the lateral collateral ligament when the knee is flexed (Fig 43-9, A–C). The posterior half of the iliotibial band is preserved (Fig 43-10). The proximal limit of the posterior dissection is secured with a "rip-stop" stitch of Ethibond (nonabsorbable suture) to prevent propagation along the fibers of the iliotibial band and to create static stability (Fig 43-11, A–C).

The anterior incision extends from Gerdy's tubercle to the lateral border of the patella and extends proximally into the distal fibers of the vastus lateralis.

To facilitate postoperative radiographic analysis, three vascular clips are placed at 1-cm intervals inside the graft prior to the asymmetric "tubing" (Fig 43-12, A and B).

When tubing the graft, the anterior edge is ad-

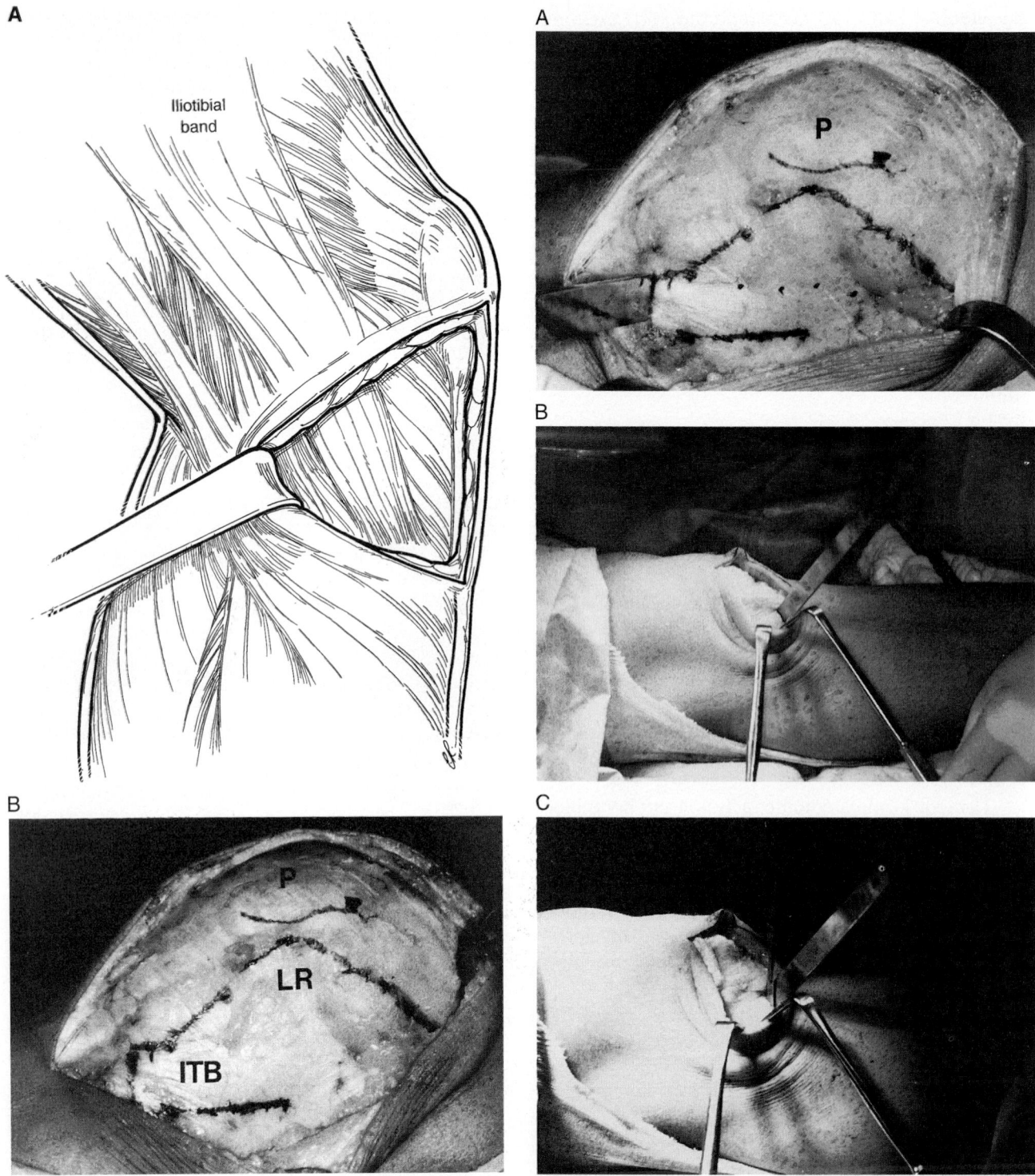

FIG 43-4.
A and **B,** The iliotibial band *(ITB)*–myofascial tendon unit.

FIG 43-5.
A–C, the use of a 1-cm osteotome as a guide for the iliotibial band. *P* = patella.

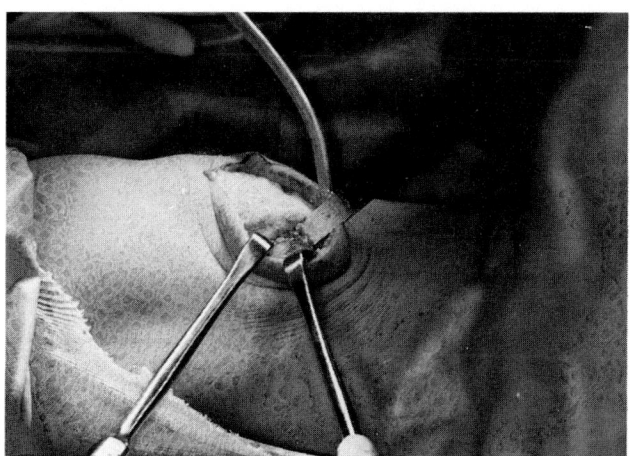

FIG 43–6.
Removal of the corticocancellous bone block.

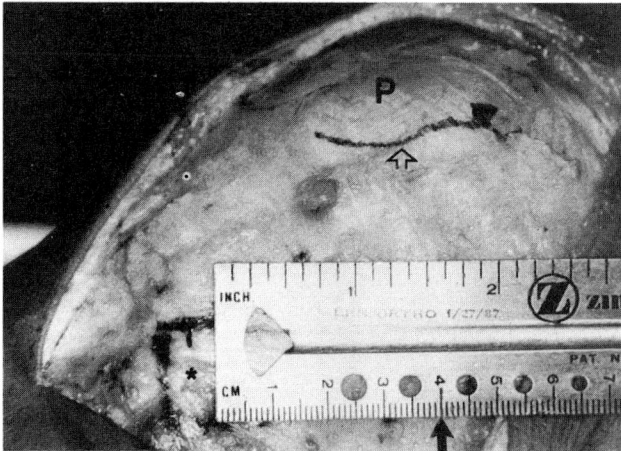

FIG 43–8.
The posterior incision (arrow) is made approximately 4 cm proximally.

vanced distally about 50% on the posterior edge with Ethibond sutures (Fig 43–13, A–D).

The capsule is opened along the lateral edge of the femoral shaft with the electrocautery to access the over-the-top position (Fig 43–14, A–C). This should be just long enough to accommodate the curved periosteal elevator.

Using a curved 1- × 1-cm periosteal elevator, a subperiosteal dissection is performed (Fig 43–15) anterior to the lateral intermuscular septum and posterior to the lateral femoral condyle. To facilitate the over-the-top transfer, the posterolateral capsule and a portion of the lateral head of the gastrocnemius are elevated.

A medial parapatella arthrotomy is performed (Fig 43–16) followed by lateral dislocation of the patella. Note at this point, that until the closure of the arthrotomy it is probably wise to moisten the articular surfaces of the knee with Ringer's lactate every 5

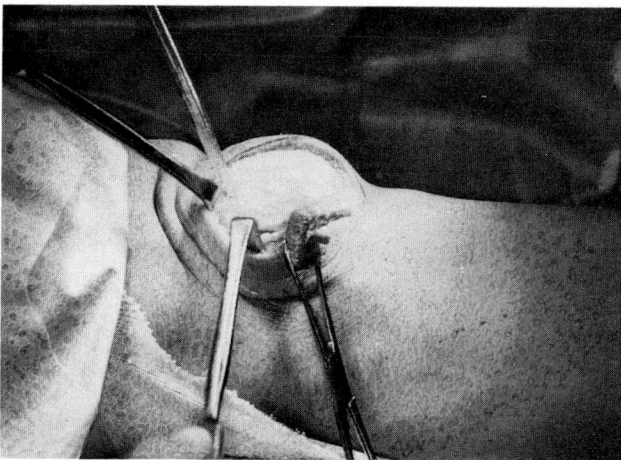

FIG 43–7.
The thickness of the bone block should be no less than 1 cm.

minutes so as not to damage the exposed cartilage through drying and heat.[10]

The ACL remnants are debrided from the medial aspect of the lateral femoral condyle (Fig 43–17, A and B). With careful subperiosteal dissection, the remainder of the posterior capsule is elevated through the intercondylar notch with the knee flexed to 45 degrees. A finger placed posterior to the lateral femoral condyle will help protect against inadvertent vascular injury. On completion of the dissection, a 43-mm uterine dilator should easily pass through the notch.

With the knee flexed to 90 degrees, the infrapatella fat pad is then excised with the knife, and the anterior horns of the menisci are excised with the electrocautery (Fig 43–18, A and B). A trough 1 cm wide by 1 cm deep is made with an osteotome, extending from the interspinous area to the anterior margin of the tibia (Fig 43–19, A–C). The sharp edges of the posterior lip of the trough should be rongeured and curretted. To facilitate later reattachment of the anterior horns of the menisci, two medial and three lateral drill holes (2.0-mm drill bit) are made along the edges of the trough approximately 5 mm apart (Fig 43–20). Nonabsorbable sutures are passed through the holes and menisci (Fig 43–21, A and B).

A 40F chest tube approximately 18 cm in length, with its beveled edge, is passed through the notch, exiting posterior to the lateral femoral condyle (Fig 43–22). A double-0 chromic tag suture is placed through the graft 1 cm proximal to the bone block and then pulled through the chest tube (Fig 43–23). The bone block is then placed into the chest tube (Fig 43–24), which is then pulled through the intercondylar notch, while avoiding twisting of the graft. Distraction of the femur from the tibia at 70 degrees may fa-

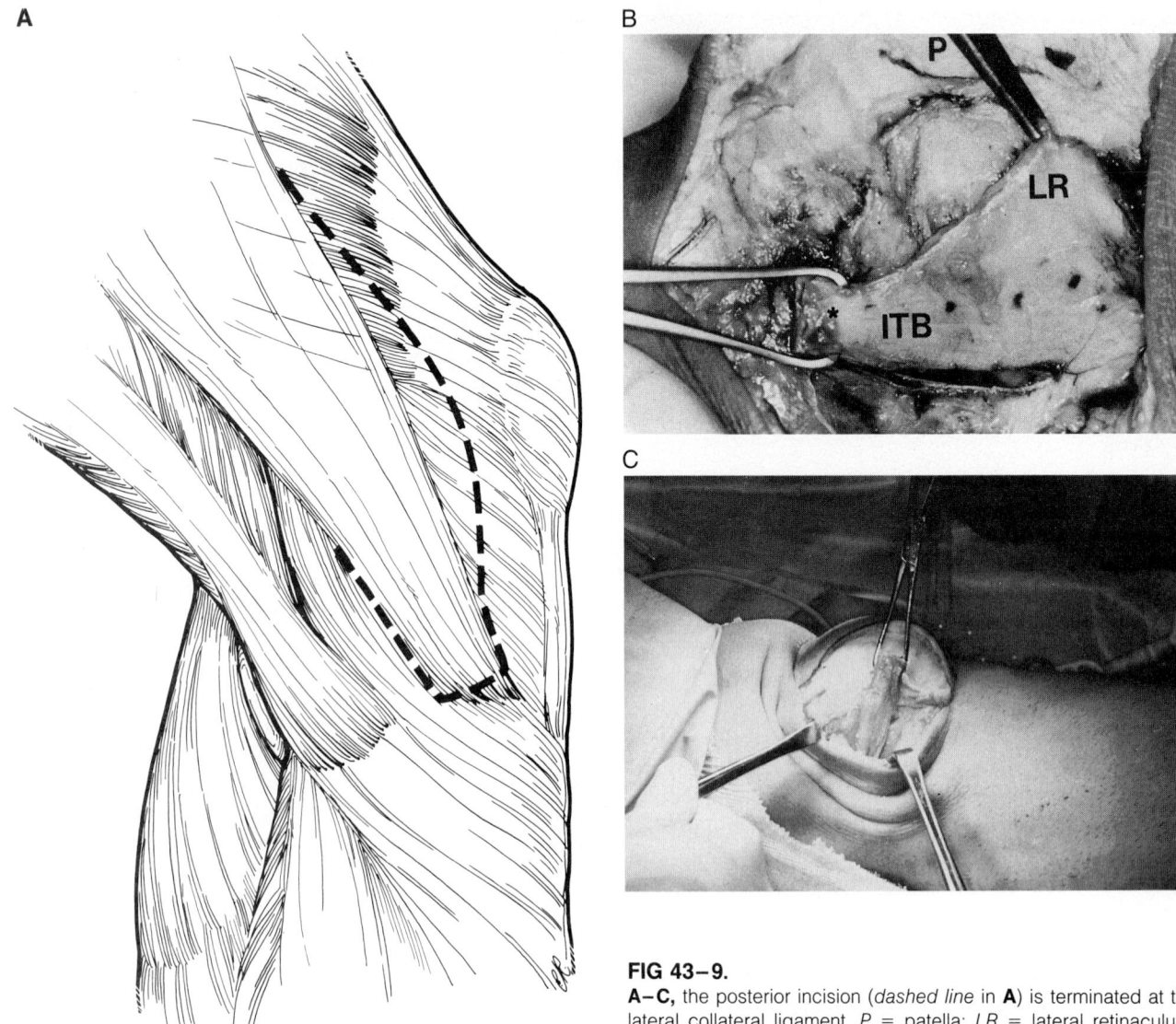

FIG 43-9.
A-C, the posterior incision (*dashed line* in **A**) is terminated at the lateral collateral ligament. *P* = patella; *LR* = lateral retinaculum; *ITB* = iliotibial band.

FIG 43-10.
The posterior half of the iliotibial band *(ITB)* is preserved.

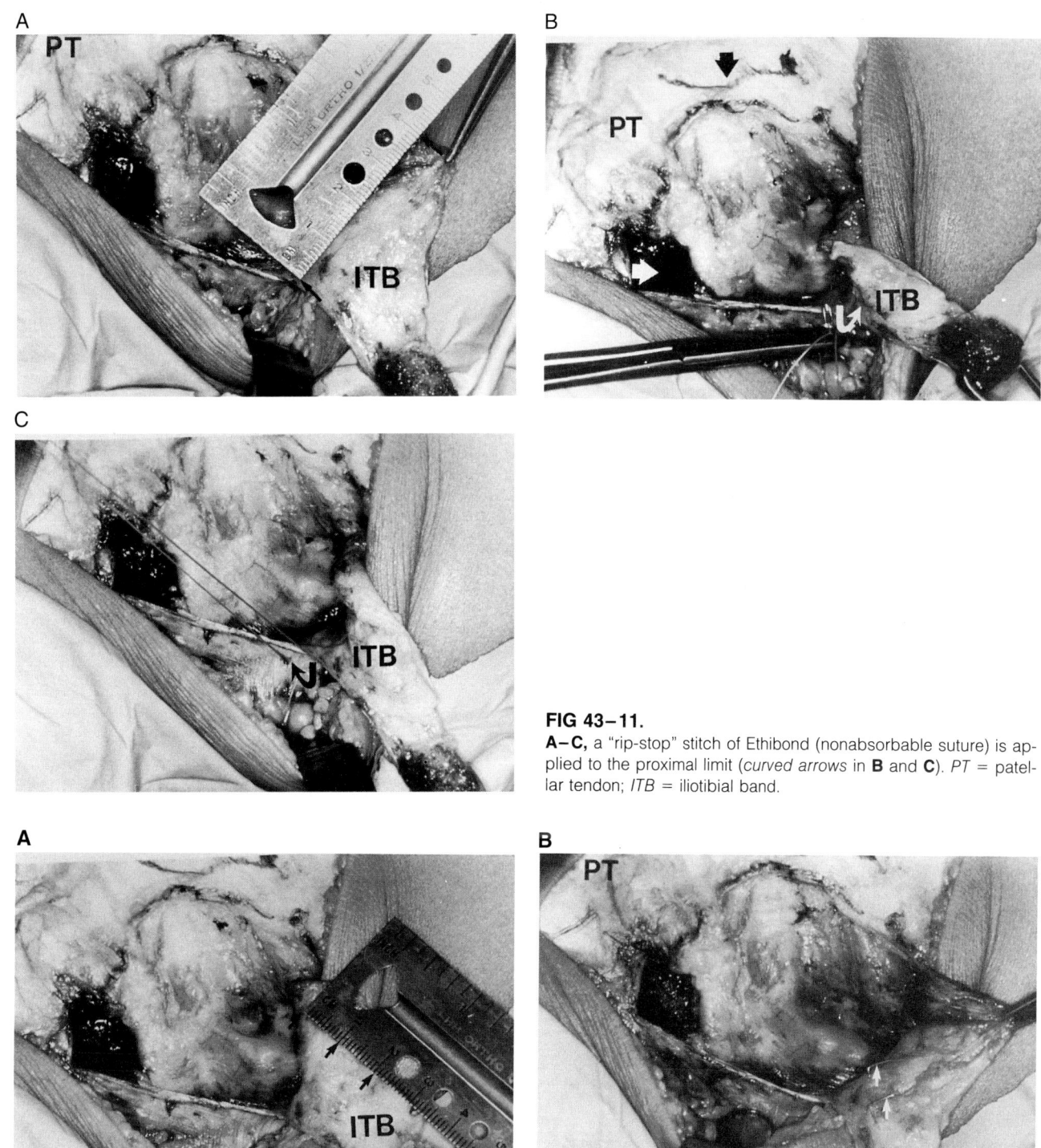

FIG 43-11.
A-C, a "rip-stop" stitch of Ethibond (nonabsorbable suture) is applied to the proximal limit *(curved arrows* in **B** and **C**). *PT* = patellar tendon; *ITB* = iliotibial band.

FIG 43-12.
A and **B,** postoperative radiographic clips are placed at 1-cm intervals *(arrows).*

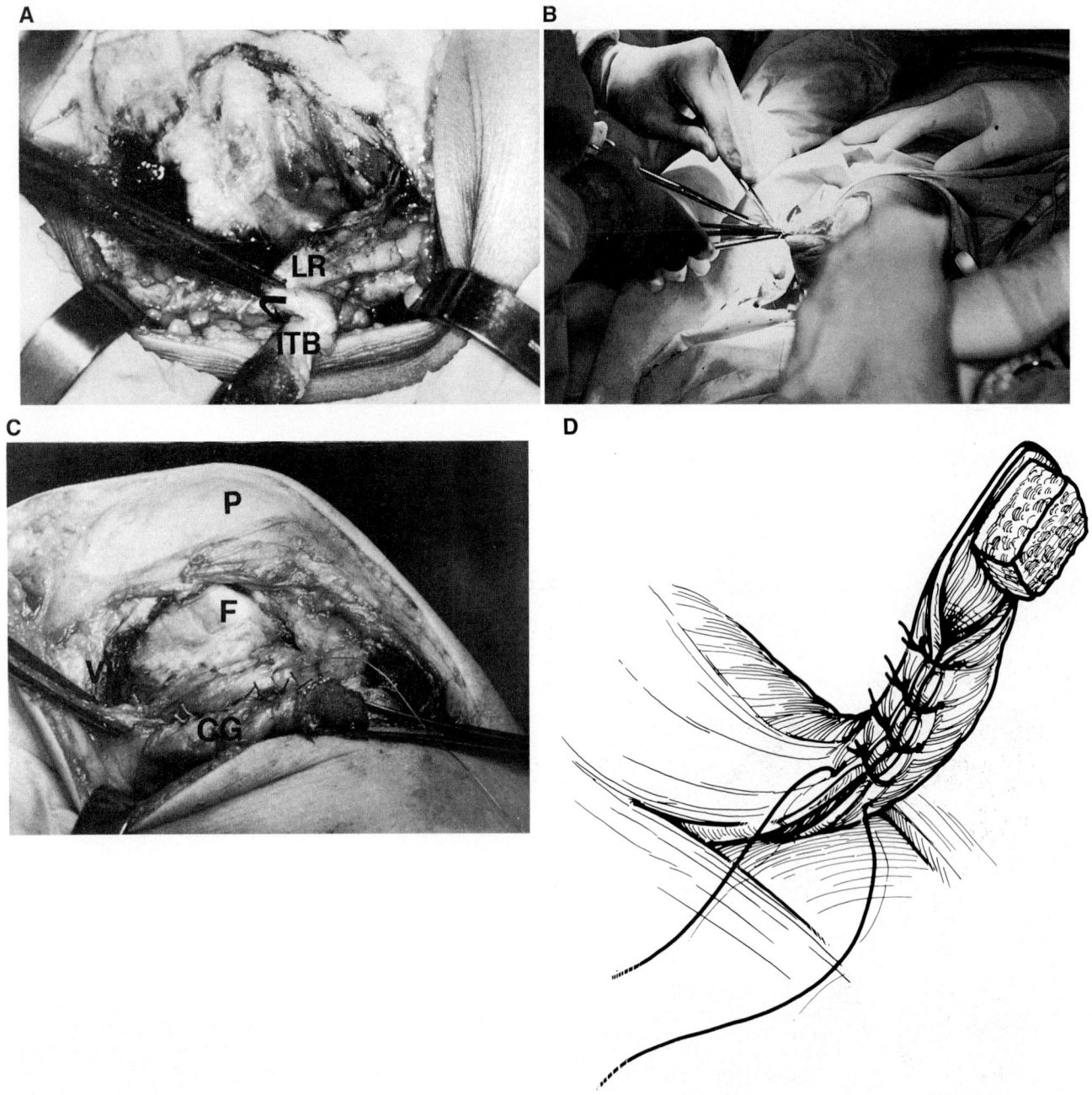

FIG 43–13.
A–D, "tubing" the graft. *LR* = lateral retinaculum; *ITB* = iliotibial band; *P* = patella; *F* = femur; *VL* = vastus lateralis; *CG* = composite graft.

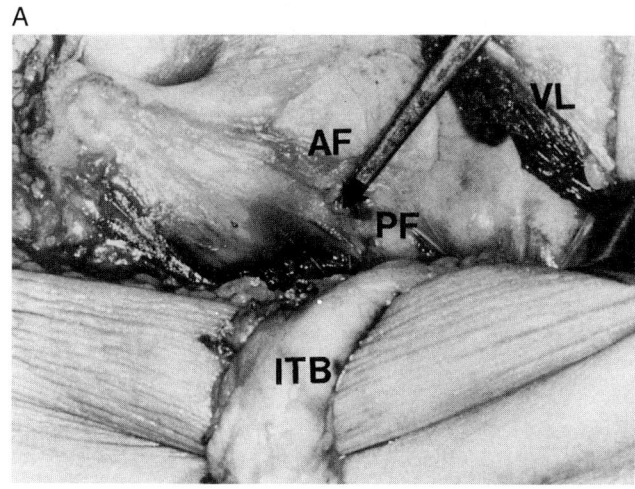

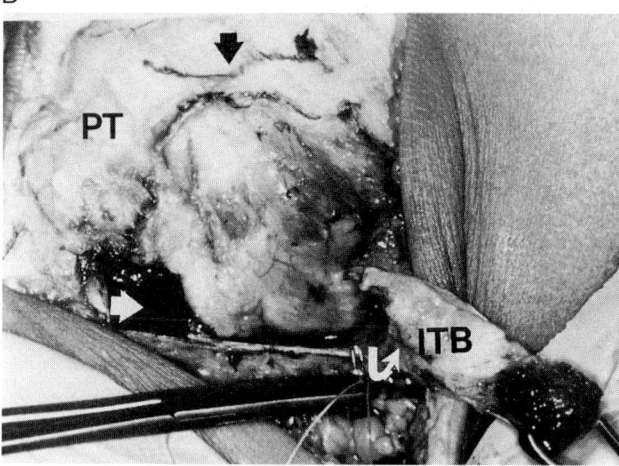

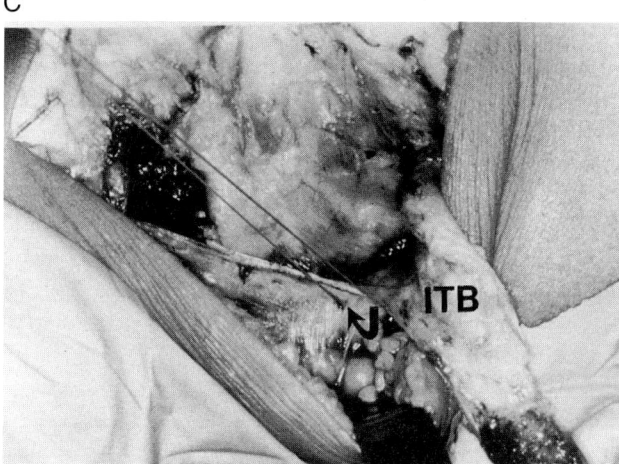

FIG 43–14.
A–C, accessing the over-the-top position. *VL* = vastus lateralis; *AF* = anterior femur; *PF* = posterior femur; *ITB* = iliotibial band.

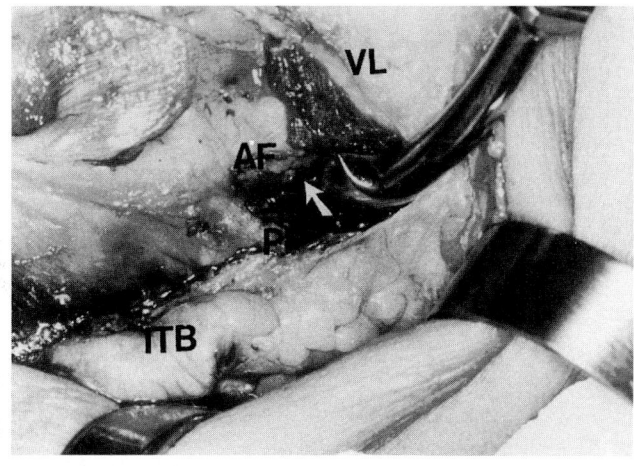

FIG 43–15.
Subperiosteal dissection posterior to the lateral femoral condyle. *VL* = vastus lateralis; *AF* = anterior femur; *PF* = posterior femur; *ITB* = iliotibial band.

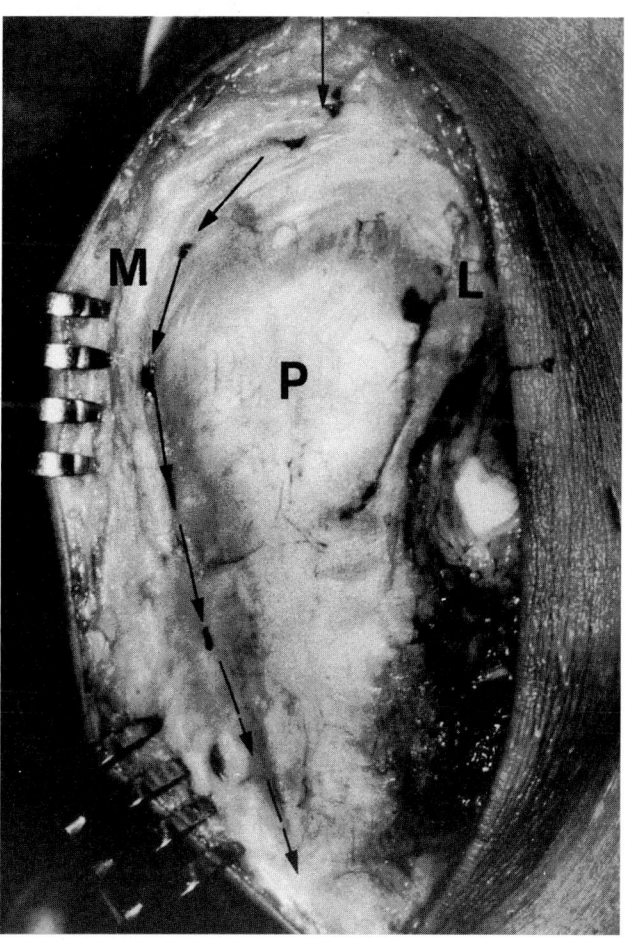

FIG 43–16.
Medial parapatellar arthrotomy. *M* = medial; *L* = lateral; *P* = patella.

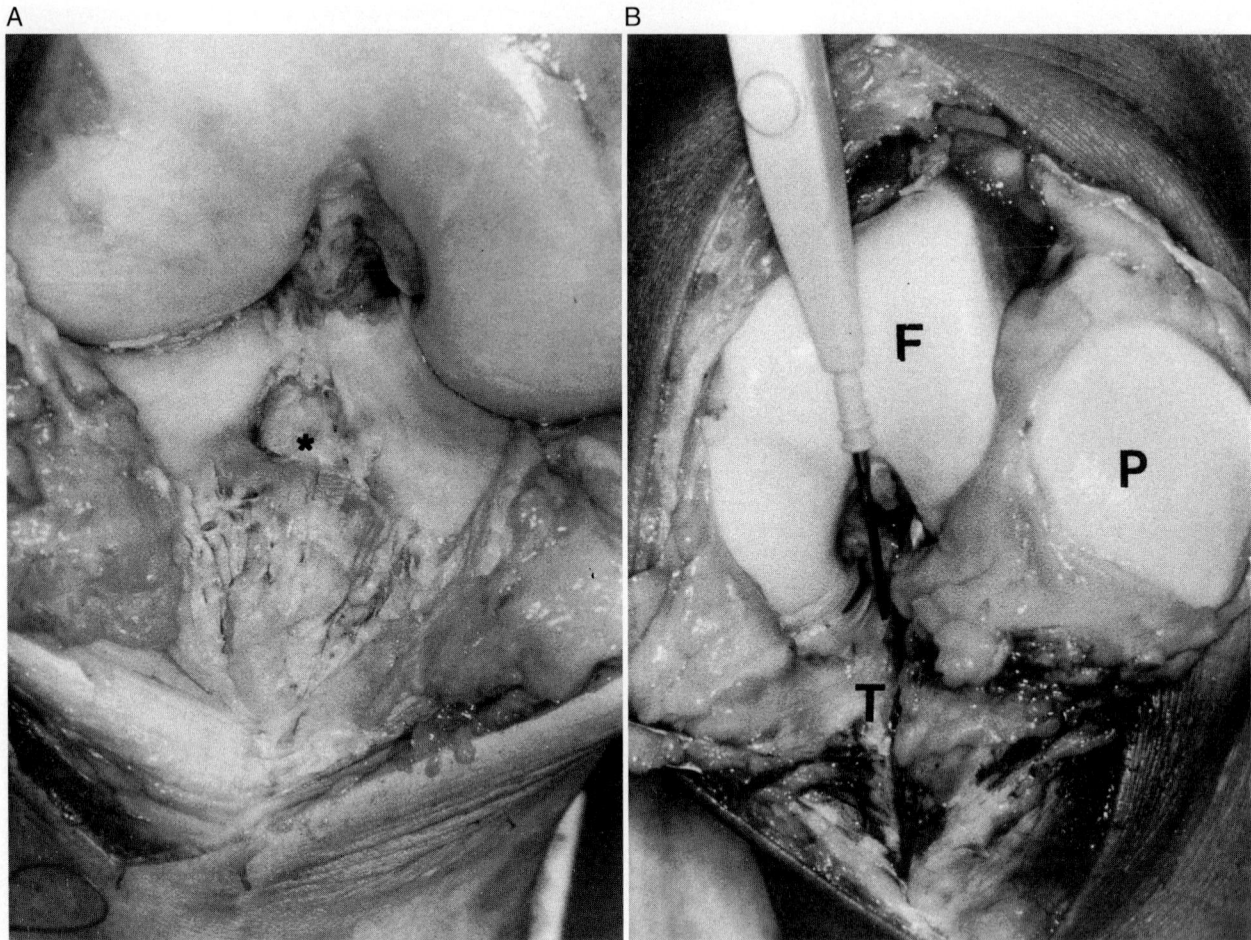

FIG 43–17.
A and **B,** debridement of anterior cruciate ligament remnants. F = femur; P = patella; T = tibia.

cilitate an easier transfer of the graft. The chest tube is removed once the block is visible in the notch.

The block is grabbed by long Allis clamps on its cortical edges and the knee is flexed to 90 degrees (Fig 43–25). Steady traction should be maintained anteriorly to achieve length (Fig 43–26). To achieve additional length of the graft, the tourniquet is then deflated, and traction is maintained until the bone block rests satisfactorily in the trough (Fig 43–27).

With the graft held in the trough, a hole is made (2.0-mm drill bit) in the center of the bone block through the trough until the posterior cortex of the tibia is penetrated. An AO small-fragment (3.5-mm) cancellous screw and washer is used for intraarticular fixation (Fig 43–28, A and B). The preferred position in the interspinous area for screw placement is position 1, as shown in Figure 43–29. The bone block should be secured posteriorly in the tibial trough, thereby ensuring no intraarticular impingement against the femoral notch (Fig 43–30). Laterally, the proximal portion of the composite graft should be visualized going into the over-the-top position accompanied by muscle fibers, thus making it truly both a static and dynamic stabilizer (Fig 43–31).

With the graft securely in place, the anterior horns of the menisci are sutured back to the edges of the trough with the nonabsorbable sutures inserted earlier. Three nonabsorbable sutures are then placed between the composite graft and the anterior edge of the intact iliotibial band and the lateral intermuscular septum (Fig 43–32).

The medial parapatella arthrotomy is repaired using interrupted nonabsorbable sutures. A closed suction drain is placed laterally prior to skin closure. The subcutaneous layer is closed with 2-0 plain catgut and the outer skin closed with an interreticular Prolene (nonabsorbable) suture.

POSTOPERATIVE CARE

Postoperatively in all patients the knee is placed in a Jones dressing for 24 hours, at which time the drains

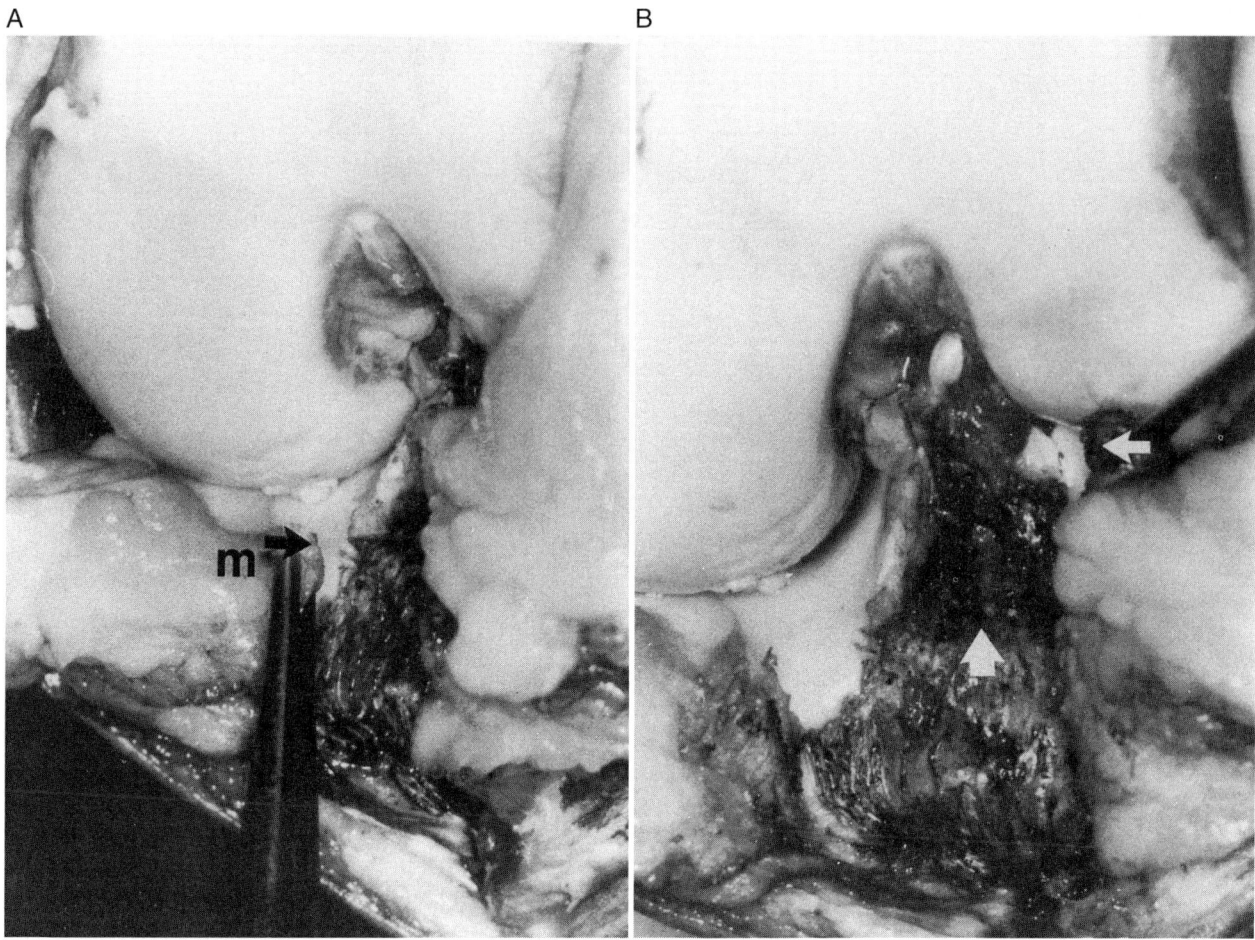

FIG 43–18.
A, excision of the infrapatella fat pad. *m* = meniscus; **B**, elevation of the anterior horns of the menisci with electrocautery.

are routinely removed and the patient is fitted with a Bledsoe type rehabilitation brace (Fig 43–33). The brace is locked with a range of 0 to 60 degrees and continuous passive motion is begun on postoperative day 1 from 0 to 45 degrees and increased 5 to 10 degrees every other day. The goal of the initial range-of-motion program is for the patient to achieve an arc from 0 to 120 degrees of flexion within 3 weeks after surgery. The patient begins weightbearing as tolerated on postoperative day 2. After this, there is no indication for passive mobility because patients will achieve remaining motion on their own through functional activities.

Pain is managed by patient-controlled analgesia for the first 2 days, then analgesia by mouth is begun and continued after discharge home. We have also found that applying cold compressive therapy (Fig 43–34) assists in minimizing the pain and swelling in the immediate postoperative phase.

After 3 weeks, the rehabilitation brace is discontinued and the patient is allowed to wear a sleeve.

At 16 to 20 weeks, the patient is allowed to return to light athletic activities; at 6 to 9 months, the patient is allowed jumping or contact sports. Depending on postoperative stability ratings, certain patients are advised to wear a derotation brace during vigorous activities.

From a rehabilitation perspective, the iliotibial band transfer must be treated differently from other ACL reconstructions. As per the surgical protocol,[8] the lateral retinaculum and distal aspect of the vastus lateralis are incorporated into the graft, diminishing the overall strength of the quadriceps. Physiologically, transferring this anterior structure to a posterior position produces immediate equalization of hamstring strength compared with the contralateral leg. Thus the focus of rehabilitation must be on the quadriceps mechanism, where strength may lag for 6 to 9 months.

Strengthening exercises for the hip flexors, hip abductors, quadriceps, and hamstring muscles are begun within 3 weeks of surgery. The use of exer-

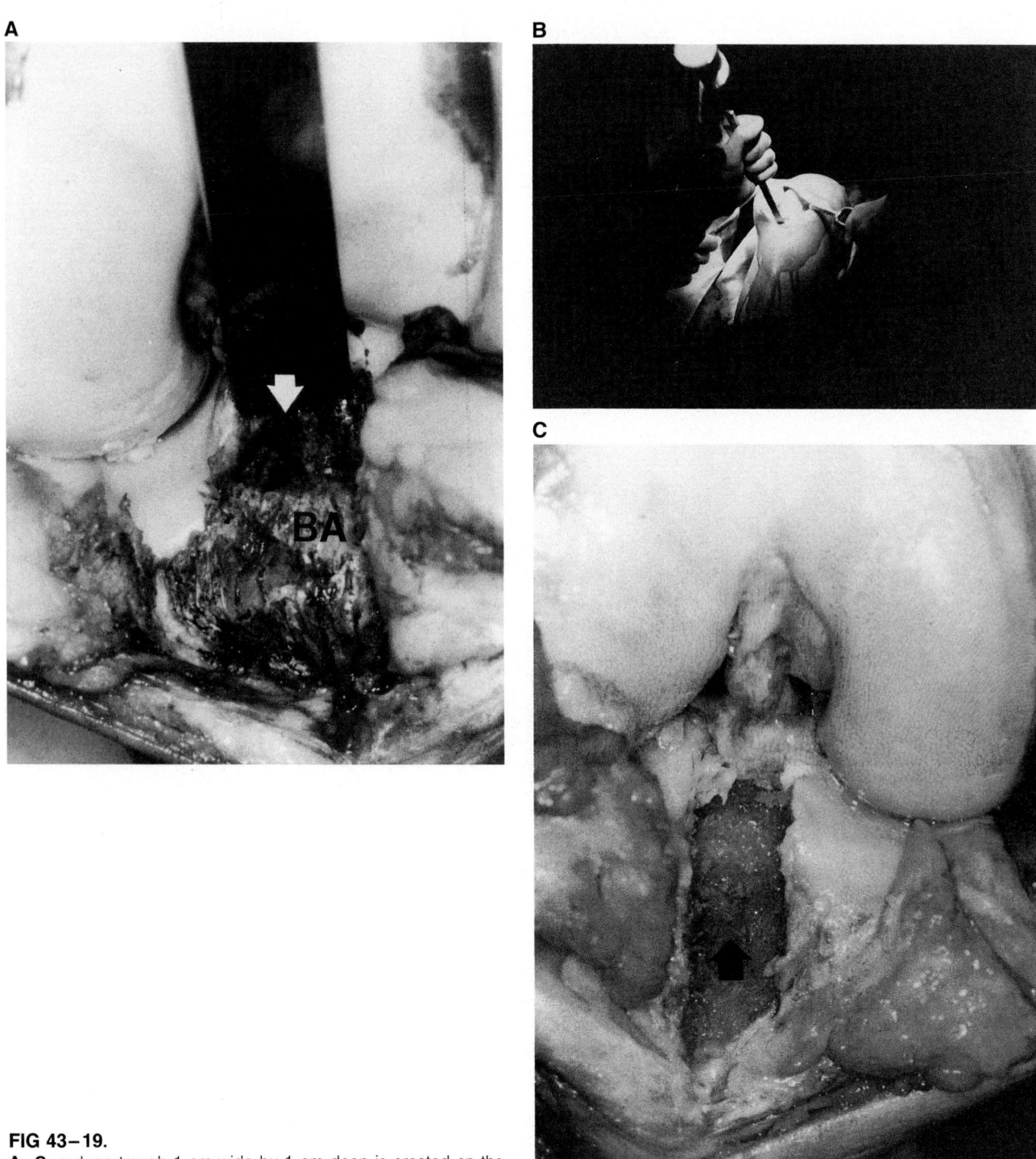

FIG 43-19.
A-C, a deep trough 1 cm wide by 1 cm deep is created on the tibia. *BA* = bare area.

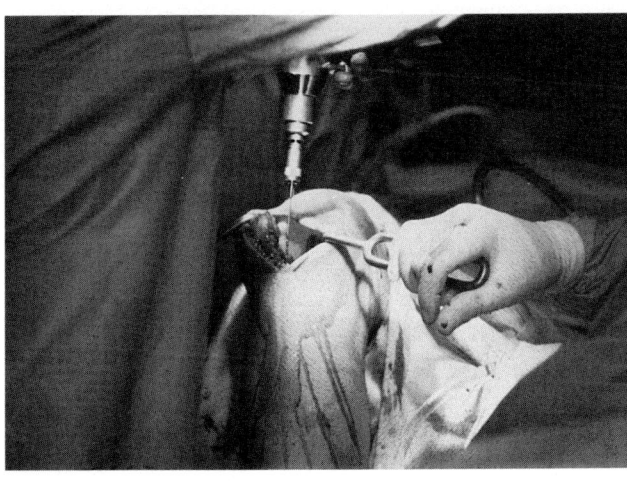

FIG 43–20.
Drill holes (2.0 mm) are made to facilitate menisci reattachment.

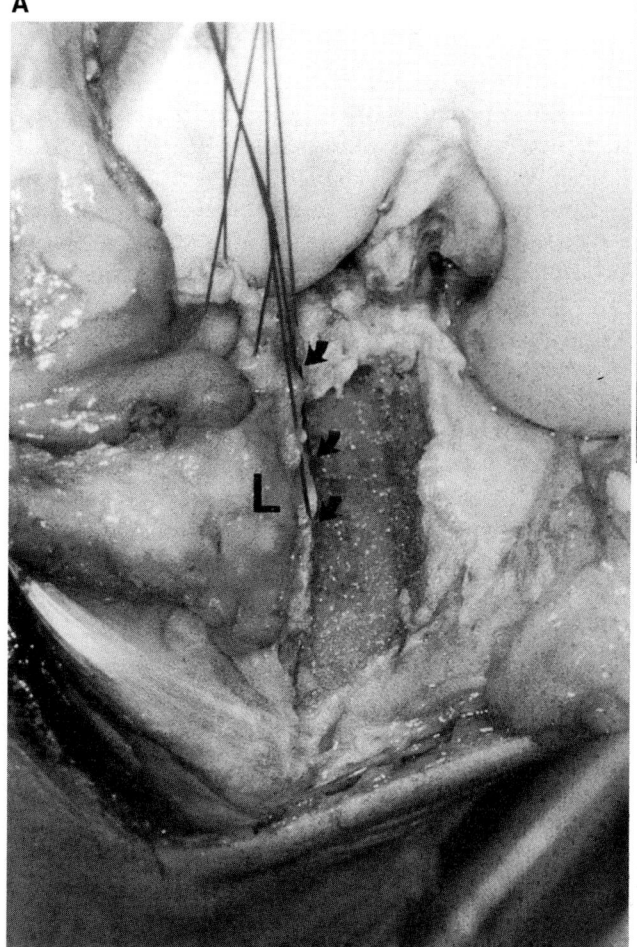

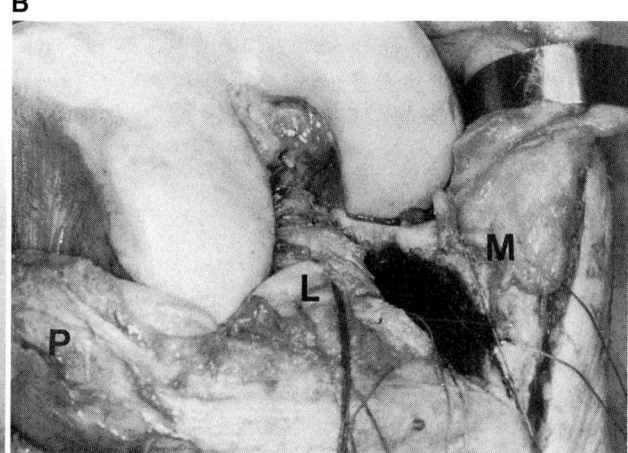

FIG 43–21.
A and **B,** placement of nonabsorbable sutures for menisci reattachment. *L* = lateral; *M* = medial; *P* = patella.

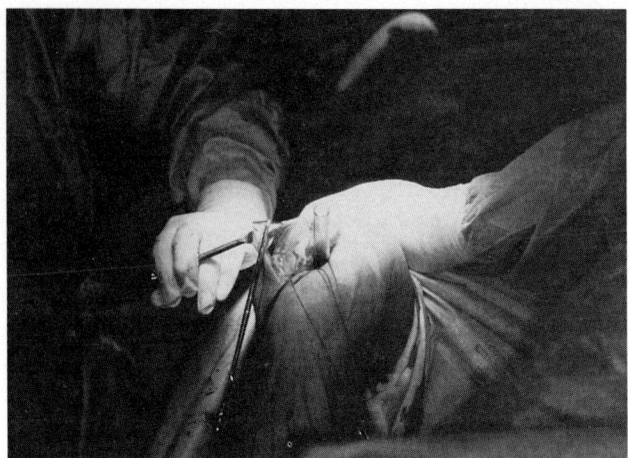

FIG 43–22.
Insertion of 40F chest tube.

cises against resistance is limited until the range of motion of the knee is at least to 90 degrees of flexion and the patient can lift 10 lbs with the knee flexed 5 to 15 degrees.

SURGICAL MODIFICATION

The surgical technique described in this chapter contains important modifications of previously described intraarticular transfers of the iliotibial band.

The AO malleolar screw originally used for intraarticular fixation of the bone block was replaced in favor of a small-fragment AO cancellous screw. The slot in the interspinous area of the tibia, was enlarged into the trough extending from the interspinous area to the anterior margin of the tibia. The trough facilitates optional positioning of the bone block in both the anteroposterior and superoinferior planes.

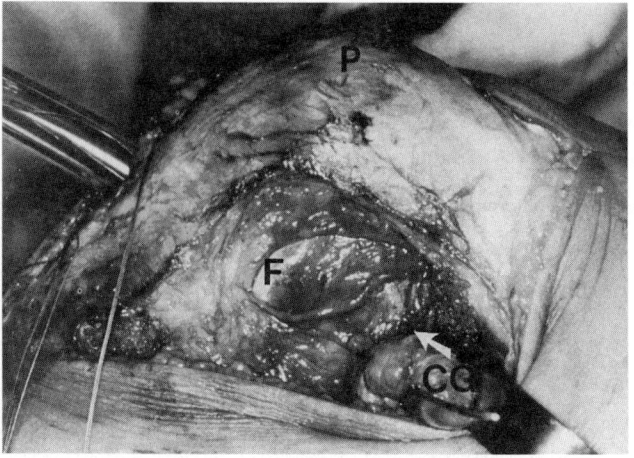

FIG 43–24.
The graft is passed through the chest tube. P = patella; F = femur; CG = composite graft.

The initial operative technique required equal anterior and posterior dissection of the composite graft to 13 cm from Gerdy's tubercle. While the extent of the anterior dissection has not changed, the posterior dissection should only rarely exceed 4 cm, thereby maintaining the graft's strong attachment to the lateral intermuscular septum and restricting its mobility. Subsequently, it is more difficult to reroute the graft than with the original technique; releasing the tourniquet will often decrease the tension in the structure and facilitate intraarticular transfer. A ripstop stitch is placed at the limit of the posterior dissection to prevent proximal propagation along the fibers of the iliotibial tract. Asymmetric advancement of the anterior flap while tubing the graft should bring down the fascia and retinaculum of the vastus lateralis, allowing it to contribute to the dynamic transfer.

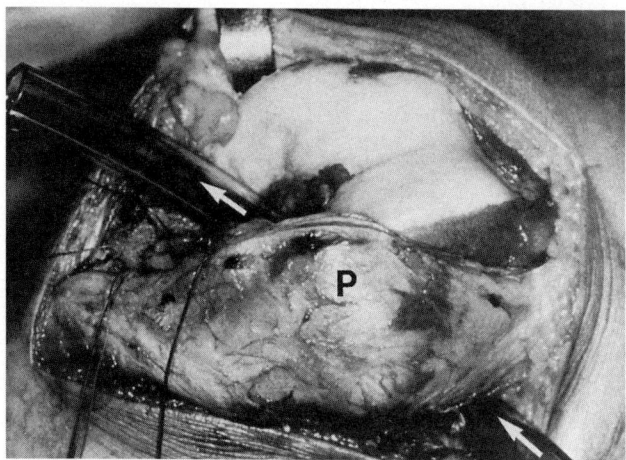

FIG 43–23.
A double-0 chromic tag suture is passed through the chest tube.

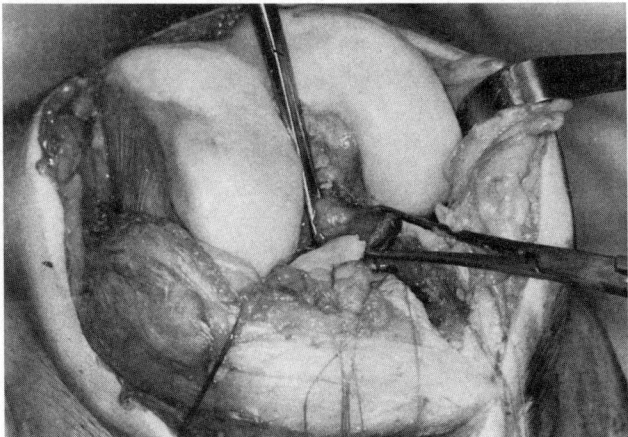

FIG 43–25.
Once the graft is visible at the intercondylar notch, the chest tube is removed and Allis clamps are applied.

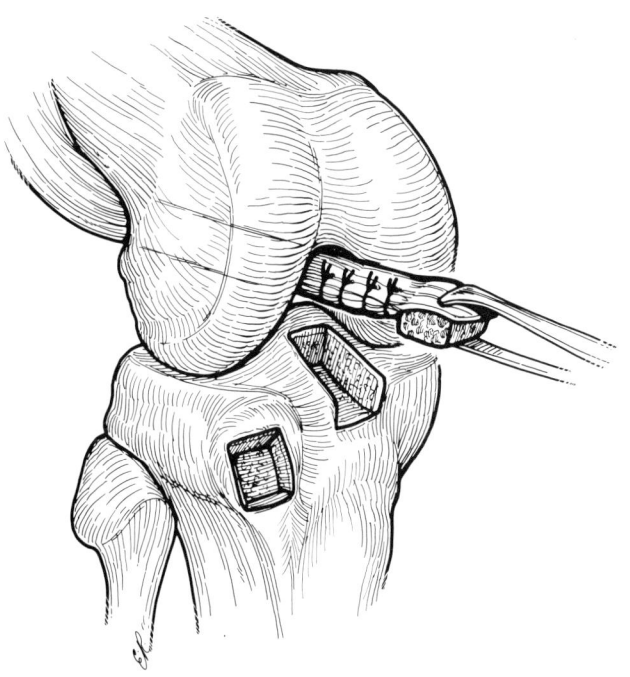

FIG 43-26.
Tension is maintained with long Allis clamps.

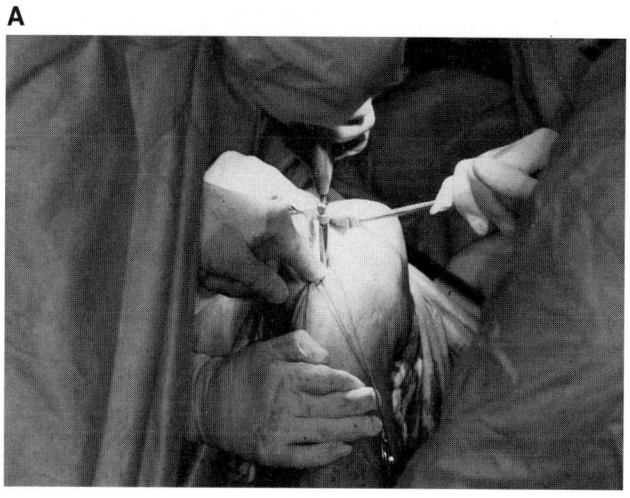

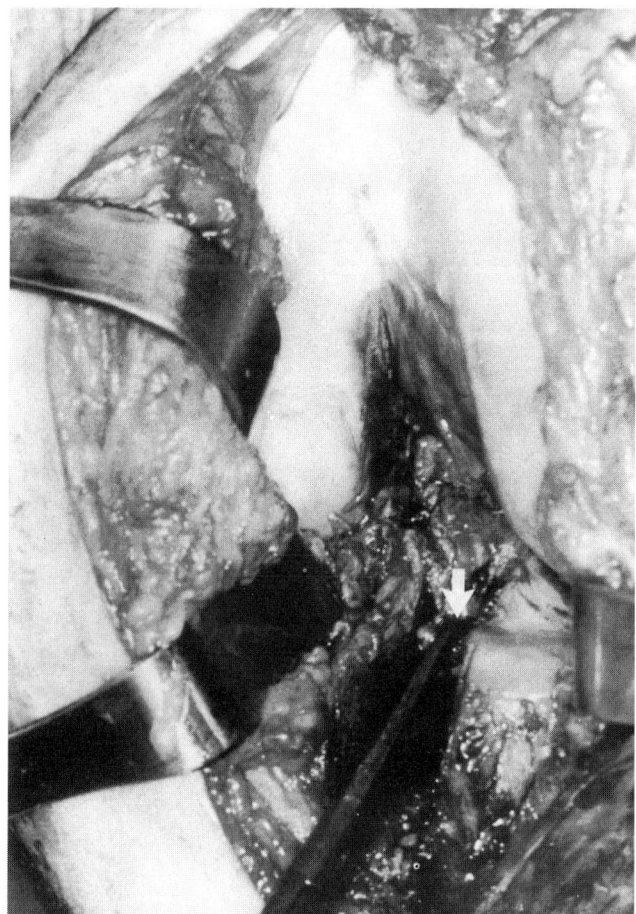

FIG 43-27.
Steady tension is applied as the graft lengthens until it rests in the trough.

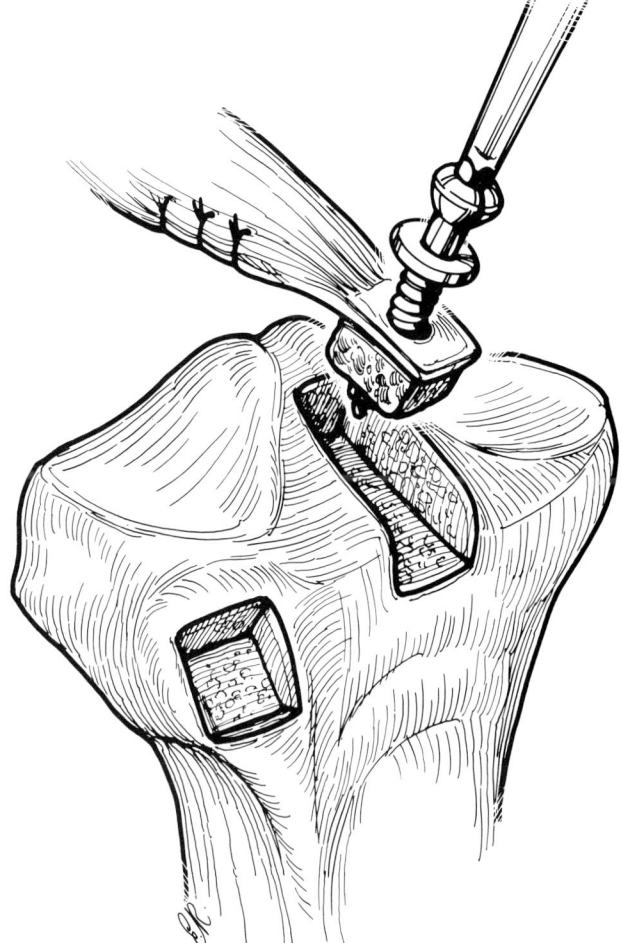

FIG 43-28.
A and **B,** fixation is maintained with an AO small-fragment (3.5 mm) cancellous screw and washer.

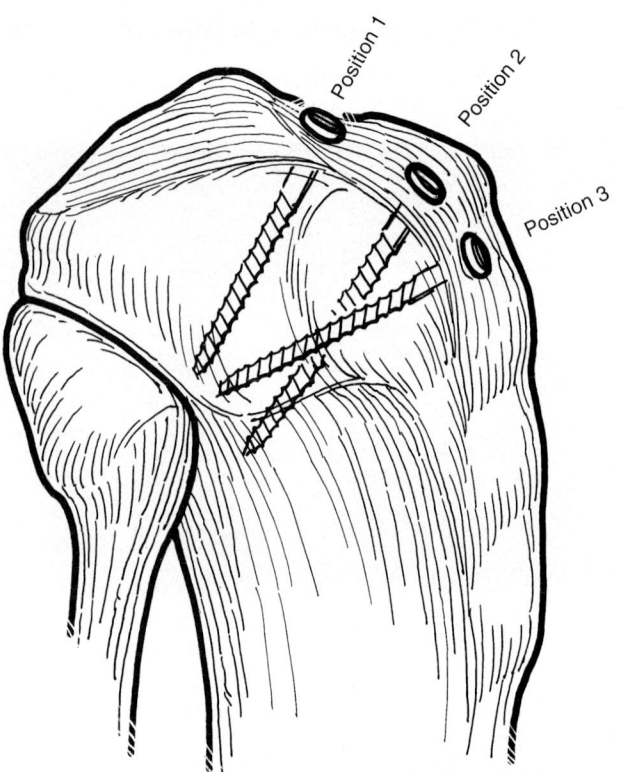

FIG 43–29.
Three positions for screw placement.

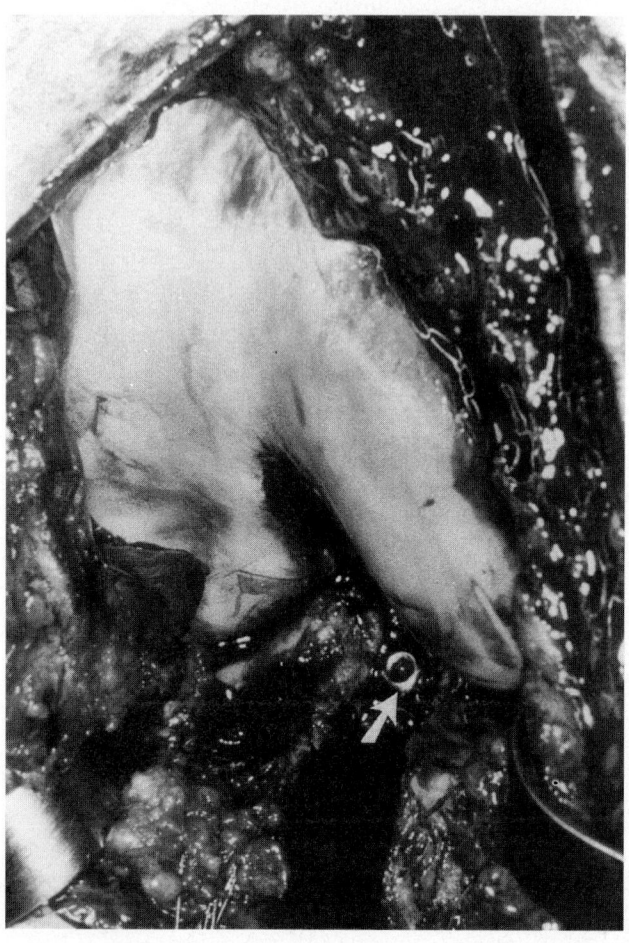

FIG 43–30.
Bone block secured posteriorly *(arrow)*.

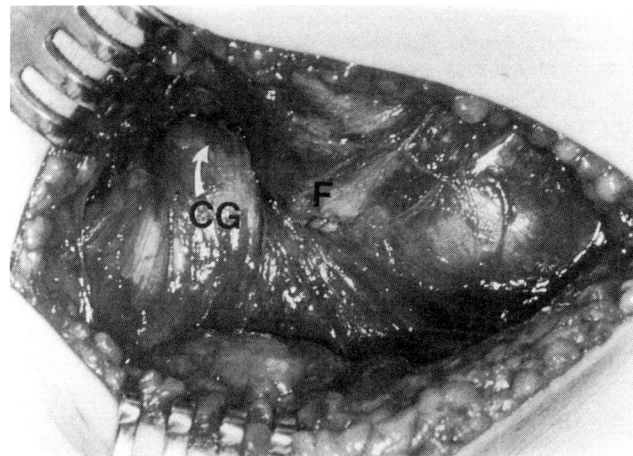

FIG 43–31.
Composite graft (CG)–muscle fibers should be visualized laterally going into the over-the-top position. F = femur.

RESULTS

Several large series published on the use of an intra-articular transfer of the iliotibial band have reported from 85% to 95% good or excellent subjective results.[4, 17, 19] With increasing experience encompassing approximately 750 patients, some with 12 years' evaluation, our subjective combined good and excellent results approaches 90%.

In the series of Insall et al.[4] of 111 knees with a 2- to 7-year follow-up, subjective results were rated using the criteria of Kennedy et al.[6] There were 74% excellent results with no limitation of activities and no discomfort; 21% good results, with postoperative ability to carry out normal activities and return to participation in sports, but with occasional or recurring mild episodes of discomfort or instability; and 5%

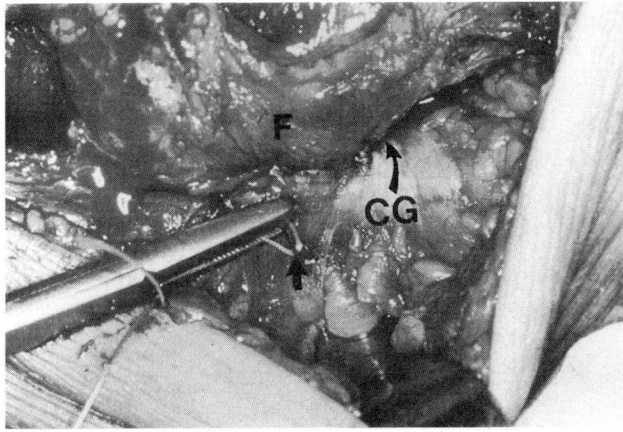

FIG 43–32.
Nonabsorbable sutures are placed between the graft (CG) and anterior edge of the intact iliotibial band to prevent propagation. F = femur.

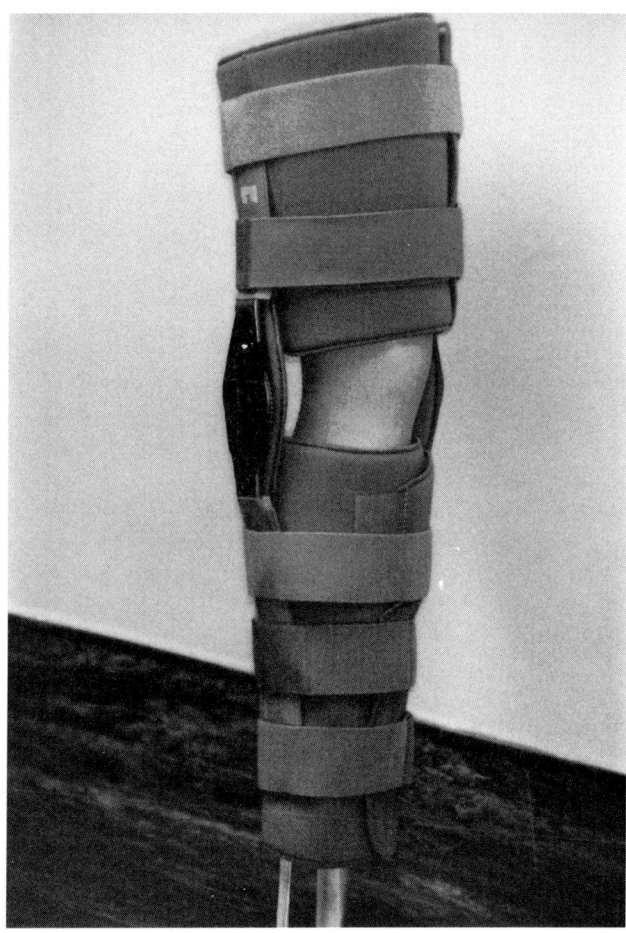

FIG 43–33.
Hinged rehabilitation brace (Bledsoe).

poor results, with persistent discomfort or instability while performing normal activities. An analysis of objective postoperative data revealed that 81% of knees had a negative Lachman test, 84% had an anterior drawer of less than 1+, 94% had a negative pivot shift, 83% had no more than a 1+ valgus stress test, and 93% had no more than a 1+ varus stress test. Approximately 25% of patients had decreased knee extension postoperatively with 20% in the 0- to 5-degree range and 5% in the 6- to 10-degree range. Approximately 40% of patients had some reduction in knee flexion, with only 4% showing more than a 20-degree loss.

The only statistically significant factors that adversely affect outcome are previous operations and a long interval between injury and ACL reconstruction. Virtually all patients operated on within 6 months of injury have good or excellent results. Outcome has not been observed to deteriorate with time; poor results are always apparent within the first year, and are believed to be secondary to problems in surgical technique rather than to rupture of the graft. Intra-

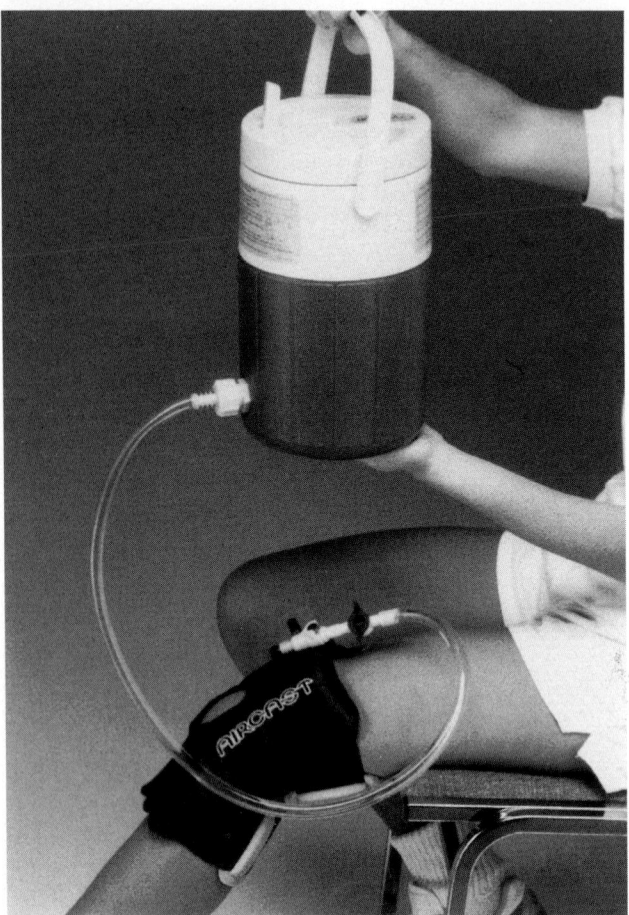

FIG 43-34.
Cold compressive therapy (Aircast).

operatively, the bone block has fragmented in less than 1% of patients, necessitating the use of a Hewson button.

REFERENCES

1. Gratz CM: Tensile strength and elasticity tests on human fascia lata, *J Bone Joint Surg* 13:2, 1931.
2. Hey Groves EW: The crucial ligaments of the knee joint: Their function, rupture and operative treatment of the same, *Br J Surg* 7:505-515, 1920.
3. Insall JN: Chronic instability of the knee. In Insall JN, editor: *Surgery of the knee,* New York, 1984, Churchill Livingstone.
4. Insall JN, et al: Bone-block iliotibial band transfer for anterior cruciate insufficiency, *J Bone Joint Surg [Am]* 63:560-569, 1981.
5. Jones KG: Reconstruction of the anterior cruciate ligament, *J Bone Joint Surg* 45:995, 1963.
6. Kennedy JC, et al: Presidential address. Intraarticular replacement in the anterior cruciate ligament-deficient knee, *Am J Sports Med* 8:1-9, 1980.
7. MacIntosh DL: Acute tears of the anterior cruciate ligament: Over-the-top repair, Annual Meeting of the American Academy of Orthopaedic Surgeons, Dallas, Jan 22, 1974.
8. McMahon M, Scott WN: Intraarticular iliotibial muscle tendon unit transfer for anterior cruciate insufficiency. In Scott WN, editor: *Ligament and extensor mechanism injuries of the knee,* St Louis, 1991, Mosby-Year Book, pp 253-265.
9. Minkoff J, Nicholas JA: Personal communication,
10. Mitchell N, Shepard N: The deleterious effects of drying on articular cartilage, *J Bone Joint Surg [Am]* 71:89-95, 1989.
11. Nahai F: The tensor fascia lata flap, *Clin Plast Surg* 7:51-56, 1980.
12. Nicholas JA, Minkoff J: Iliotibial band transfer through the intercondylar notch for combined anterior instability (ITPT procedure), *Am J Sports Med* 6:341-353, 1978.
13. Noyes FR, et al: Biomechanical analysis of human ligament grafts used in knee ligament repairs and reconstruction, *J Bone Joint Surg [Am]* 66:344-352, 1984.
14. Noyes FR, et al: Intraarticular cruciate reconstruction. I: Perspectives on graft strength, vascularization, and immediate motion after replacement, *Clin Orthop* 172:71-77, 1983.
15. Noyes FR, et al: The symptomatic anterior cruciate-deficient knee. I: The long term functional disability in athletically active individuals, *J Bone Joint Surg [Am]* 65:154-162, 1983.
16. O'Donoghue D: A method for replacement of the anterior cruciate ligament of the knee, *J Bone Joint Surg [Am]* 45:905-924, 1963.
17. Scott WN, Ferriter P, Marino M: Intraarticular transfer of the iliotibial tract, *J Bone Joint Surg [Am]* 66:532-538, 1985.
18. Scott WN, Insall JN: Injuries of the knee. In Rockwood CA Jr, Green DP, Bucholz RW, editors: *Rockwood and Green's Fractures in Adults,* ed 3. Philadelphia, 1991, JB Lippincott, pp 1884-1888.
19. Scott WN, Schosheim PM: Intraarticular transfer of the iliotibial muscle-tendon unit, *Clin Orthop* 172:97-101, 1983.
20. Scott WN, Scuderi G: Intraarticular transfer of the iliotibial muscle-tendon unit for anterior cruciate insufficiency, *Tech Orthop* 2:1-12, 1988.
21. Yost JG, et al: Intraarticular iliotibial band reconstruction for anterior cruciate ligament insufficiency, *Am J Sports Med* 9:220-224, 1981.

44

Intraarticular and Extraarticular Anterior Cruciate Ligament Reconstruction

MEHRDAD M. MALEK, M.D.
GREGORY C. FANELLI, M.D.
JEFFREY V. DELUCA, M.D.

Intraarticular anterior cruciate ligament reconstruction
    Conventional two-incision technique
        Graft harvesting and preparation
        Notchplasty
        Tunnel placement
        Graft fixation
    Single-incision endoscopic reconstruction
        Graft preparation
        Notchplasty
        Tibial tunnel
        Femoral tunnel
        Graft passage
        Graft fixation
        Postoperative care
Extraarticular reconstruction
    MacIntosh procedure
    Losee procedure
    Ellison procedure
    Arnold-Coker procedure
    James procedure
    Andrews procedure
    Pes anserinus transfer
Complications
Summary

The natural history of an untreated anterior cruciate ligament (ACL) tear follows a course of knee deterioration and dysfunction and eventually leads to the classic syndrome of the symptomatic anterior cruciate–deficient knee.[25, 37, 59] The dysfunction and deterioration appear to occur more rapidly in combined injuries involving other intraarticular or extraarticular supporting structures of the knee, particularly when a subtotal or total meniscectomy has been performed or an osteochondral fracture has been present. Nonoperative management of a torn ACL in a young active person has been shown to be inferior to other forms of treatment.[37, 50]

Based on the available embryologic, anatomic, vascular, and biomechanical studies[3, 4, 62] on the ACL, it is our opinion at this time that intraarticular anatomic grafting of the ACL with a strong biologic substitute is necessary to restore the anatomic intraarticular stabilizing structure of the knee.[62, 67] Total stability and function of a normal knee depend also on the contributions of other knee ligaments, the menisci, and on joint geometry.

In recent years, we have also learned lessons in isometry and isometric placement of the ACL substitute, its importance in creating more physiologic load transfer, as well as allowing a full range of motion in the postoperative period.[75]

In spite of all the new information and a better understanding of the anatomy, biomechanics, and function of the ACL and their clinical applications, we should realize that our best intraarticular anatomic grafting of the ACL is only a check rein for excessive joint displacement and not a "fine tuned motion" as described by Noyes et al.[62]

The procedure described by Hey Groves in 1917[31] is the basis of modern intraarticular reconstruction. He used a strip of fascia lata attached distally[30, 31] which was passed through the tibial tunnel and then through the femur. Since the description by Hey Groves, different biologic substitutes used for reconstruction of the ACL have been described.[36, 39, 47–50, 67, 72, 78] New interest was shown after MacIntosh described his extraarticular substitution in 1972.[29, 48] Based on the available biomechanical data[3–5, 10, 58, 59, 62] on mechanical properties of ACL substitutes, we have chosen to use the central third of the patellar tendon with bone attached on either side (bone–patellar tendon–bone unit) as our procedure of choice in reconstruction of the ACL.

Once it was hypothesized that a biologic graft with a vascularized pedicle (vascularized patellar tendon) would undergo less necrosis, thus maintaining greater strength with faster remodeling and maturation.[14, 68] Although the idea was appealing, later studies on ACL blood supply and animal studies have shown that there are no significant differences in any of the measured variables between a vascularized and a nonvascularized graft. These studies suggest that the amount of necrosis, followed by revascularization, remodeling, and finally maturation, is essentially the same in both types of ligaments or tendons.[3, 10] Procedures utilizing the free graft are also easier technically, as described later in this chapter.

We describe two types of arthroscopically assisted ACL reconstruction techniques, and review various extraarticular ACL reconstructions.

INTRAARTICULAR ANTERIOR CRUCIATE LIGAMENT RECONSTRUCTION

Conventional Two-Incision Technique

Intraarticular ACL reconstruction performed as an open or arthroscopically assisted procedure is complex and demands attention to detail. Prior to ACL reconstruction, diagnostic arthroscopy is performed to define additional pathologic changes that are appropriately treated at this time. The remainder of the reconstruction proceeds in sequential order to graft harvesting and preparation, notchplasty, tunnel placement, graft passage, and fixation. We discuss each phase of the intraarticular ACL reconstruction, with emphasis on harvesting and preparation of the central third patellar tendon autograft, preparation of the intercondylar notch, anatomic placement of femoral and tibial tunnels, and secure fixation of a properly positioned graft.

Graft Harvesting and Preparation

The bone–patellar tendon–bone unit is a desirable autogenous tissue for intraarticular reconstruction of the ACL.[62, 63] The graft can be placed isometrically so deformation does not occur. The bone-tendon-bone preparation has the advantage of secure interference fit followed by bone-to-bone healing which provides superior graft fixation[45] and allows early motion and weightbearing.[24]

A midline longitudinal incision is made from 1 cm below the inferior pole of the patella over the patellar tendon to the tibial tubercle. The paratenon is incised and preserved for closure at the end of graft harvesting (Fig 44–1,A). A ruler is used to determine the width of the patellar tendon at the distal tibial end, which is anatomically narrower than the proximal end. The central third of the patellar tendon with patellar and tibial bone blocks attached are harvested as a free graft. The patellar and tibial bone blocks are harvested using an oscillating saw and a sharp osteotome, but the use of the osteotome is minimized on the patella to avoid trauma to the patella articular surface. The bone plugs are 25 to 30 mm long and 9 to 10 mm deep (Fig 44–1,B). The width is determined by the overall width of the patellar tendon.

One third of the patellar tendon rather than a set linear dimension is chosen as the size of the graft. It is also important that the bone plug be no more than one third of the thickness of the patella (see Fig 44–1,B). This will reduce the risk of fracture.[9, 52] The thickness of the patella can be determined on the preoperative axial radiograph taken at 30 degrees of flexion.

The graft is then prepared by suture placement in the bone plugs and tubing of the graft. After harvesting, the graft bone plugs are triangular in shape. A small rongeur is used to round off the cancellous edges of the bone plug to furnish a more rounded and intimate contact with the cancellous bone in the femoral and tibial tunnels (Fig 44–2). A 0.035-in. Kirschner wire is used to make two transverse holes through the cortical and corticocancellous junction. This allows placement of a no. 1 suture through each hole for traction to be applied during graft placement. The transverse suture orientation through the bone plug prevents the suture from being cut during interference fit fixation. The size of the femoral bone plug may be adjusted depending on the fixation technique to be used.

The graft is then tubed into a tight cylindrical shape using 3-0 absorbable suture on a noncutting needle utilizing a running suture pattern (see Fig 44–2). This creates a firm tubular structure of the same diameter or smaller than the bone plugs, facilitating graft passage through the bony tunnel and intercondylar notch. It is important after the graft has been harvested that it is not placed in any solution, but is

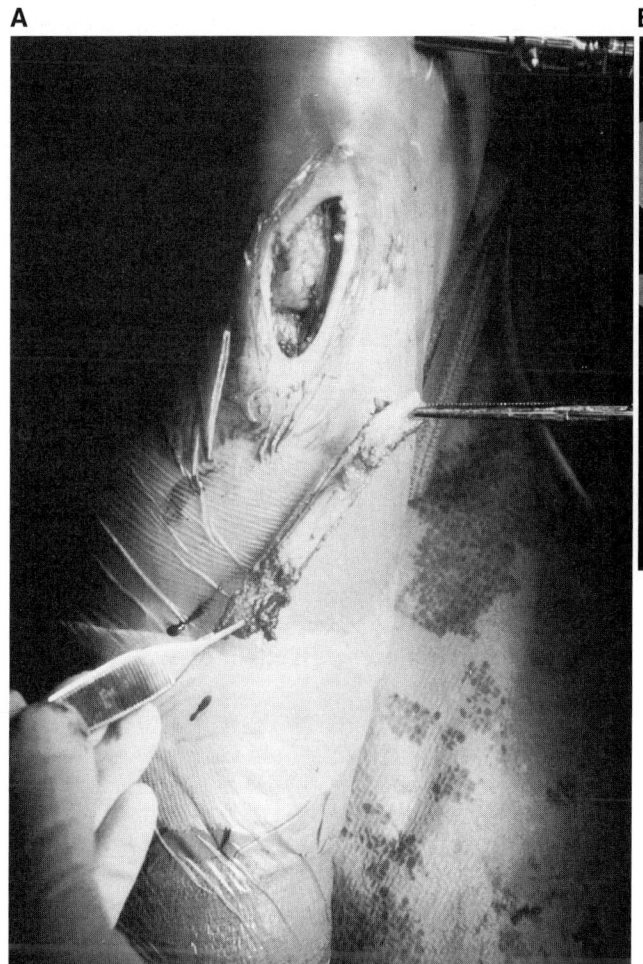
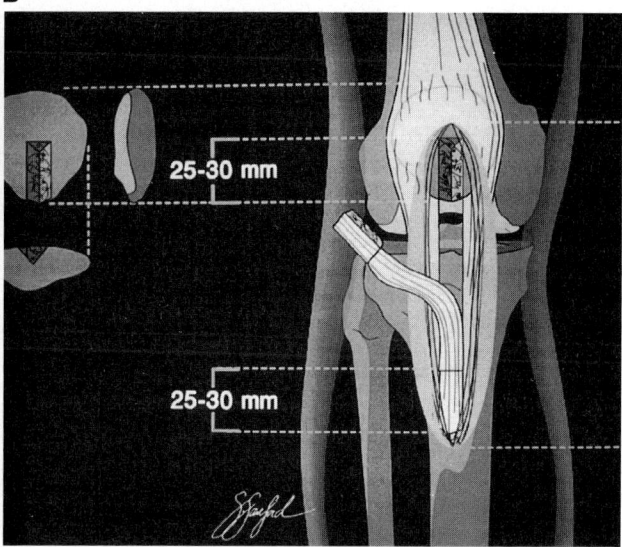

FIG 44–1.
Graft harvesting and preparation. **A,** incision starts at a point 1 cm below the inferior pole of the patella and extends down to the tibial tubercle. The skin and subcutaneous tissues are mobilized for better results and better cosmetics. **B,** location of the incision and harvesting of the substitute are shown schematically. Note the location of the bony plug which is not more than one third of the entire patella thickness.

kept fresh on the back table using a damp sponge. If the graft is soaked in any kind of solution, it will imbibe the fluid, and graft swelling will occur. It will be more edematous, bulky, and much more difficult to pass through the tunnels into the joint. The graft is measured using sizing cylinders provided in most ACL drill guide sets to determine the smallest size of tunnel the graft will pass through (Fig 44–3). It is important to use the smallest tunnel size possible so that maximum interference fit between bone block, femoral or tibial tunnel, and fixation screw is obtained. The placement of the graft in the tunnels is facilitated by using a suture passer from the femoral tunnel, through the joint, and out the tibial tunnel, and then pulling the traction sutures through the tibia, then the joint, into the femoral tunnel, and out the lateral femoral cortical hole. This can also be done the opposite way. The patellar plug is placed in the femur, and the tibial bone plug is placed in the tibia.[24] Technically, however, it is easier to place the tibial bone plug into the femur.

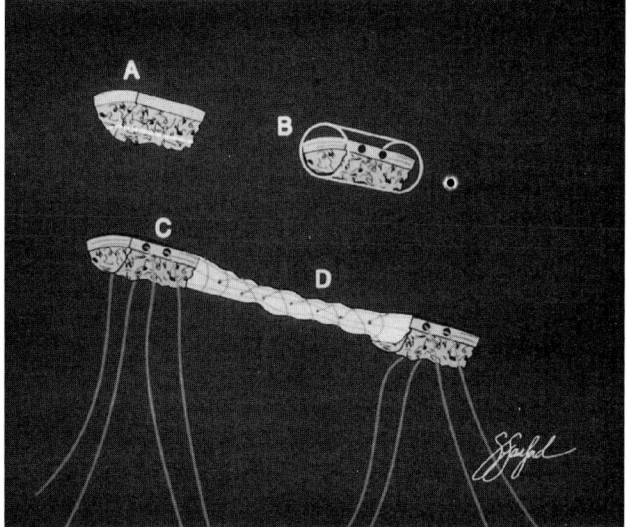

FIG 44–2.
Sculpturing the bone plug for intimate contact with the tunnel. Note the transverse orientation of the bone plug drill holes for fraction sutures.

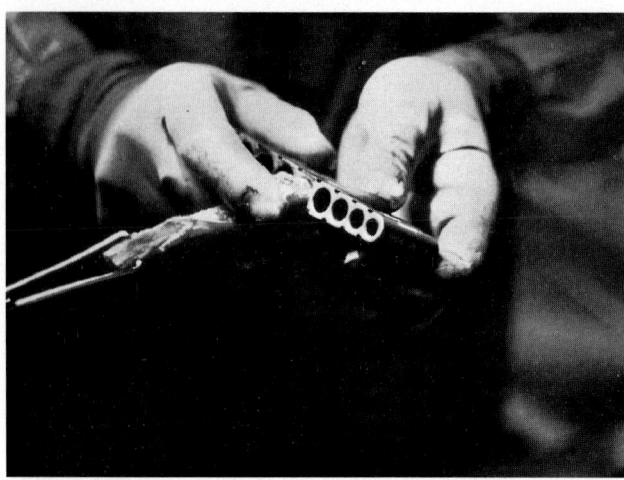

FIG 44–3.
Sizing the graft for the tightest fit possible. In this picture a sizer from the 3M company is being utilized. (Minnesota Mining and Manufacturing Co., St. Paul, Minn.)

Notchplasty

The ACL is in close proximity to the intercondylar notch of the femur when the knee is in full extension. The ACL may contact the femur in the notch with hyperextension and excessive internal rotation causing ACL rupture.[16] In chronic ACL insufficiency, the tibial eminence becomes peaked, and osteophytes narrow the femoral intercondylar notch.[16] This decreases the space available for ACL grafts, and predisposes the graft to rupture by notch impingement.

For these reasons, we recommend notchplasty for all intraarticular reconstructive procedures of the ACL. The methods used to accomplish the notchplasty are varied, but all have the same end point: remove enough bone from the roof and anterolateral edge of the intercondylar notch, and deepen it in a beveled fashion so that there is no graft impingement throughout the range of knee motion. The isometry of the femoral tunnel is preserved by not lateralizing the graft insertion into the femoral tunnel.[16, 30]

When the procedure is performed via arthrotomy, an osteotome and curettes are used to enlarge the notch. At the present time, we perform all of our ACL reconstructions arthroscopically assisted because this gives us superior visualization of the anatomic area, as well as the anatomy of the notch. A motorized burr, synovial shaver, and a small curette are used to perform the notchplasty. Approximately 3 to 5 mm of articular cartilage and bone are removed from the 12-o'clock position around to the posterior medial edge of the lateral femoral condyle. The notch is beveled back to the point of anatomic insertion of the ACL on the femur, on both the medial wall of the lateral femoral condyle and the roof, taking care to protect the posterior cruciate ligament (PCL). This provides sufficient room for graft placement prior to bone plug fixation. Of course, any osteophytes present are shaved or debrided prior to notchplasty.

Tunnel Placement

Anatomic graft positioning demands that the graft points of attachment to the bone remain the same distance from one another during full knee range of motion.[75] Deviations from this positioning will cause the graft to be too tight or too loose, resulting in an inadequate reconstruction.[75] We prefer femoral placement in the posterosuperior portion of the notch, and tibial placement in the center of the anatomic ligament stump[12, 30, 32, 75] (Figs 44–4,A–D)

Drill guides are used to help obtain the anatomic graft placement described above. We believe that an effective drill guide should be easy to position and use, allow exact and reproducible placement of guide pins, and allow for correction of a suboptimally placed guide pin.

The tibial tunnel is made using the tibial drill guide with the goal being to have the ACL graft correspond to the center of the tibial anatomic insertion site of the ACL. The entry point on the tibia is the anteromedial border of the tibia 2.5 cm distal to the joint line, just above the pes anserinus insertion into the tibia. Some of the sartorius fibers may need to be elevated from the tibia subperiosteally during the exposure. Care should be taken to avoid placement too anterior and violating the tibial crest, or placement too medial and interference with the superficial medial collateral ligament. The posterior and lateral edges of the intraarticular portion of the tibial tunnel are chamfered or a radius resector is used to obtain a smooth rounded contour (see Figs 44–4,B–D).

The femoral tunnel is more challenging to place since it requires greater degrees of exposure within the notch to permit adequate visualization. A lateral skin incision is made over the distal lateral femur starting at the lateral epicondyle and proceeding 5 cm proximally. The iliotibial band is split in line with its fibers and the dissection is carried down to the lateral border of the femur posterior to the vastus lateralis and anterior to the lateral intermuscular septum. The over-the-top position is palpated with the gloved finger, and the external portion of the drill guide is positioned so that when drilling is completed a minimum 2-mm rim of sturdy posterior femoral cortex remains for secure fixation of the screw and bone plug (see Fig 44–4,A).

The intraarticular portion of the femoral drill guide is positioned under arthroscopic control with

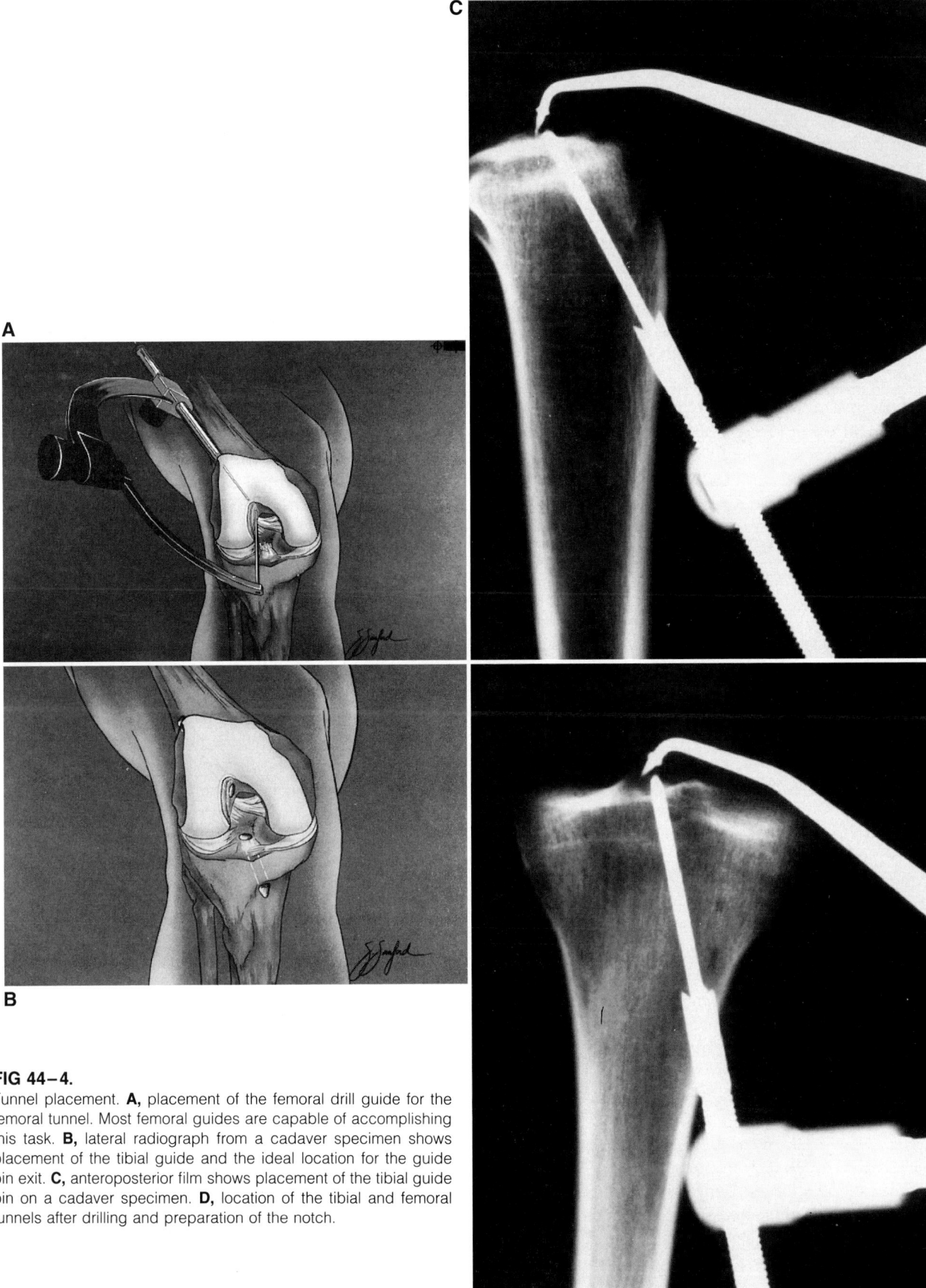

FIG 44–4.
Tunnel placement. **A,** placement of the femoral drill guide for the femoral tunnel. Most femoral guides are capable of accomplishing this task. **B,** lateral radiograph from a cadaver specimen shows placement of the tibial guide and the ideal location for the guide pin exit. **C,** anteroposterior film shows placement of the tibial guide pin on a cadaver specimen. **D,** location of the tibial and femoral tunnels after drilling and preparation of the notch.

several concepts in mind. The notchplasty is performed as described above. Care is taken not to lateralize the medial wall of the lateral femoral condyle,[30] and also to locate and accomodate to the intercondylar shelf.[55] After preparation of the notch, the position of the drill guide tip is located high and posterior in the notch. Clancy[12] advocates positioning the guide pin posterior and superior to the anatomic ACL position. Hewson[30] advocates posterosuperior and medial placement. Sidles et al.[75] recommend high and posterior placement so that the medial edge of the femoral tunnel is at the 12-o'clock position in the notch. We agree with the high and posterior position of the tunnel, because after resecting and chamfering of the edges the tunnel is effectively at the anatomic femoral attachment of the ACL, giving isometric placement. We caution against being too posterior and blowing out the posterior wall of the femoral tunnel since this will compromise interference fixation with screw and bone plug. We prefer to have at least a minimum of 2 mm of posterior femoral cortex to provide firm fixation for our bone plug and screw.

After the tunnels have been made the smoother device from the Gore-Tex ACL kit (W. L. Gore, Inc., Flagstaff, Ariz.) is passed through the femoral tunnel, the notch, and out the tibial tunnel to bevel the tunnel edges and also to check for any notch impingement on the graft. Impingement is checked with direct arthroscopic visualization during knee range of motion, and alterations or modifications of the notchplasty are performed as necessary.

Graft Fixation

Although different techniques have been described in fixation of the ACL substitute, the interference fit fixation described by Lambert[45] appears to be the strongest and most suitable for the bone–patellar tendon–bone unit. This technique is, however, demanding and certain pitfalls should be avoided. The technique allows bone-to-bone healing and solid fixation at both ends, thus allowing early and unrestricted movement of the knee.

The interference fit is obtained first on the femur using the 6.5-mm ASIF cancellous screw (Synthes, Monument, Colo.) or a Kurosaka screw (DePuy, Warsaw, Ind.) in either the 7-mm or 9-mm diameter depending on the size of the bone block, the size of the tunnel, and the discrepancy in size between bone block and tunnel. It is important to have the screw threads in a position perpendicular to the cortical surface of the bone plug, and the shaft of the screw parallel to the bone plug itself. This guarantees that the screw threads engage the cortical bone of the plug, forcing the cancellous bone of the plug to face the cancellous bone of the femoral tunnel. This will theoretically enhance graft incorporation since cancellous bone surfaces are opposed. It is also important to ensure that the screw is positioned parallel to the walls of the tunnel, as well as parallel to the bone plug, and not to choose a divergent pattern. The length of the screw should be at least 5 mm shorter than the plug itself in order not to cause any damage to Sharpey's fibers at the tendon-plug attachment.

At this point, the isometry and pistoning of the graft is tested by placing the knee through a range of motion. We accept 2 mm or less pistoning or excursion of the graft when the knee is placed through a full range of motion. We believe that this amount of excursion is indicative of isometric positioning of the graft. This can be accomplished with or without the use of an isometer. If pistoning or excursion is unacceptable, alterations in the bone plugs or tunnels are made. When graft isometry is obtained, tibial fixation is achieved in the same fashion as for the femoral bone plug. When the graft is truly isometric, the relative position of the knee through flexion and extension would not matter when the graft is tensioned and fixed. We routinely fix our graft under tension at 20 degrees of knee flexion. We do not use a tensiometer for tensioning the graft, but pull on the traction sutures in 20 degrees of knee flexion and have a firm feeling while pulling on the traction sutures. The graft is then secured in place using the interference fit screws on the tibia (Fig 44–5). The sutures are either removed or sewn into the soft tissue for added fixation. Under direct arthroscopic visualization, the knee is placed through a range of motion to make sure there is no impingement of the graft in the intercondylar notch. Final adjustments of the notchplasty are made at this time if necessary.

Single-Incision Endoscopic Reconstruction

Graft Preparation

The first step after examination under anesthesia and diagnostic arthroscopy is graft preparation. Autograft bone–patellar tendon–bone units consist of the central third of the patellar tendon. After harvesting, two no. 5 sutures are placed through the tibial bone plug, and two no. 2 sutures are placed through the patellar bone plug. The no. 5 Ticron sutures are used in the tibial bone plug in case the distal fixation needs to be sutured around a screw and washer. This occurs occasionally when interference fit tibial fixation is not achieved. A no. 2 suture is used in the patellar bone plug since these are the largest sutures that fit through the eye of the Beath pin. The bone plugs are

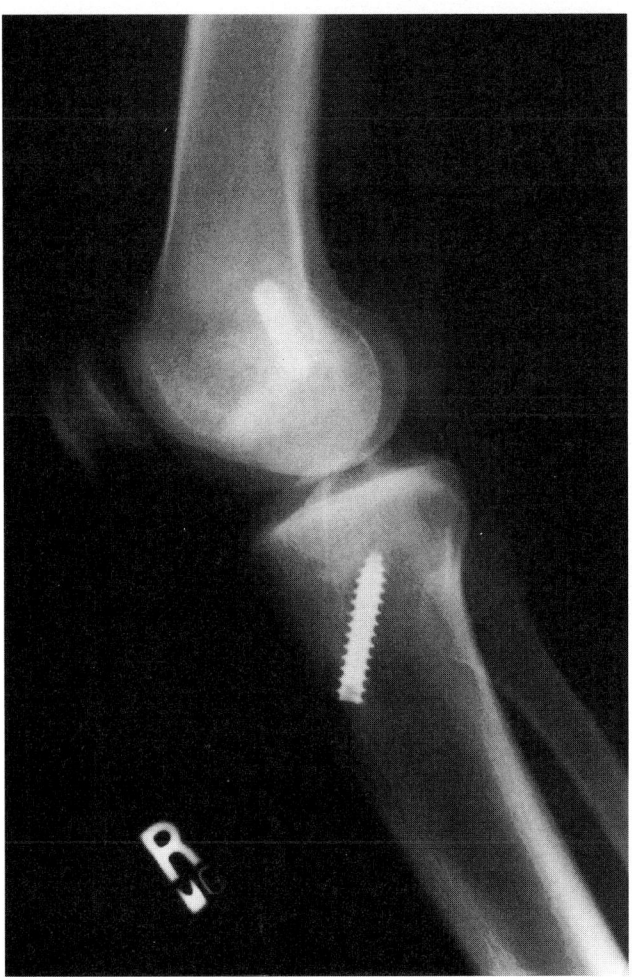

FIG 44–5.
Graft fixation. The two-incision conventional anterior cruciate ligament reconstruction with interference fit fixation screws on the tibial and femoral tunnels.

contoured for intimate fit to the round sizing tubes (see Fig 44–2). The tendon is tubed using 3-0 PDS (polydiaxanone) suture to facilitate synovialization. The completed graft is placed in a damp sponge and saved for later insertion.

Notchplasty

Notchplasty is a critical step in this procedure. A recent study indicated that for ACL substitutes larger than 8 mm in diameter, notchplasty is required to prevent graft impingement.[8] The single-incision technique requires a wide notchplasty to allow adequate visualization of the medial wall of the lateral femoral condyle. Enough bone and articular cartilage must be resected to allow visualization of the anatomic ACL insertion site and the over-the-top position. This wide view facilitates femoral tunnel placement posterior and superior in the intercondylar notch as described by Sidles and Larson.[75] A partial roofplasty is also required to prevent impingement of the intercondylar ridge on the ACL substitute when the knee is in full extension. We routinely use a motorized burr, synovial resector, and hand curettes to perform our notchplasty and remove approximately 3 to 5 mm of bone and articular cartilage from the lateral femoral condyle and roof.

Tibial Tunnel

The tibial tunnel is created using a cannulated reamer of appropriate size over a correctly placed 3/32-in. smooth guide wire. The guide wire is positioned so that the resulting tibial tunnel will be at the center of the tibial stump of the ACL. To ensure proper tibial tunnel length, the guide wire must penetrate the anteromedial aspect of the tibia midway between the anterior tibial crest and the posteromedial border of the tibia at the level of the middle of the tibial tubercle, approximately 4 to 5 cm below the joint line. This positioning allows optimal tunnel length and a sufficiently thick anterior tibial bone bridge (Figs 44–4,C and D, and 44–6). A tibial aimer or guide facilitates guide wire placement; however, the guide wire can be placed freehand by using bony landmarks.

The appropriate size tibial tunnel is made using an endoscopic cannulated and calibrated reamer. The tunnel emerges through the center of the ACL stump (Fig 44–7). The edges of the tunnel are chamfered and rasped to remove sharp bone edges, and a full radius resector is used to remove bone and cartilage, reaming debris from in and around the fat pad. This prevents the free bone and cartilage particles from initiating an inflammatory response in the fat pad with subsequent arthrofibrosis.

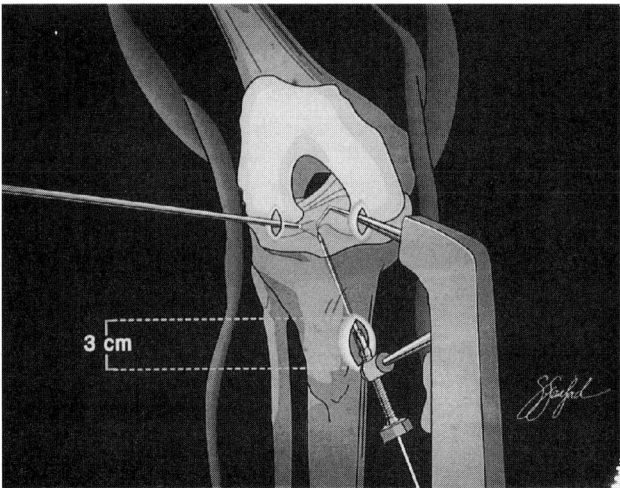

FIG 44–6.
Tibial tunnel. Placement of the tibial guide pin in performing endoscopic anterior cruciate ligament reconstruction. Note the site of pin penetration below the joint line.

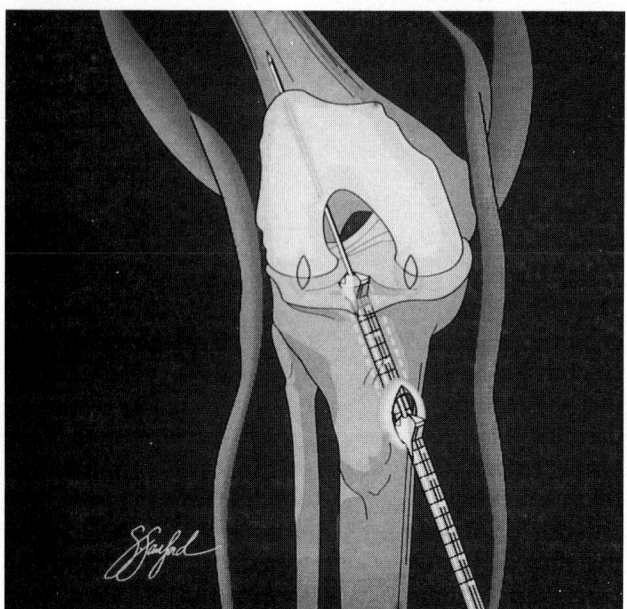

FIG 44–7.
Using cannulated and calibrated reamers, the tibial tunnel is drilled; knee position is at 85 to 90 degrees of flexion.

Femoral Tunnel

The knee is flexed to between 80 and 90 degrees for preparation of the femoral tunnel. A 3/32-in. guide wire is passed through the tibial tunnel to engage the medial wall of the lateral femoral condyle. The guide wire position must respect the following parameters:

First, the over-the-top position must be visualized, which requires a well-performed notchplasty. Second, the guide wire must be positioned far enough distal to the over-the-top position to allow for approximately a 2-mm posterior cortical rim. After the tunnel has been reamed, this provides a firm posterosuperior tunnel wall for interference fit fixation. For example, a 10-mm tunnel has a 5-mm radius. The guide wire will need to engage the medial wall of the lateral femoral condyle 7 mm anterior to the over-the-top position to provide a 2-mm posterior rim after tunnel completion. Third, the guide wire also must be positioned to allow the most medial part of the completed tunnel to lie at the 12-o'clock position in the intercondylar notch. Fourth, the guide wire will be in very close proximity to the PCL fibers (Fig 44–8). We aim to place the guide wire at the 1-o'clock position in the left knee and at the 11-o'clock position in the right knee as the intercondylar notch is viewed with the knee flexed to 90 degrees. The tunnel is drilled to the appropriate length using the cannulated and calibrated reamer (Fig 44–9).

The above femoral tunnel description allows the ACL bone–patellar tendon–bone substitute to assume the most anatomic position and still achieve in-

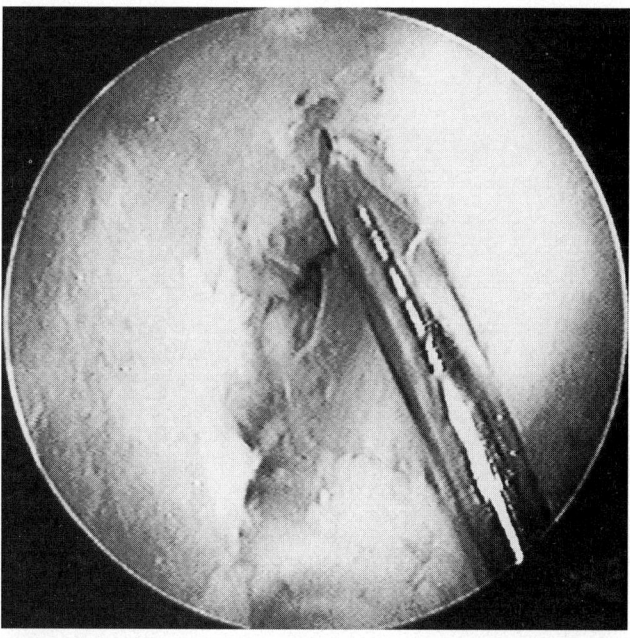

FIG 44–8.
Femoral tunnel. Positioning of the guide wire from the tibial side to engage the superior and posterior position on the femoral condyle. Note the close relationship of this pin to the posterior cruciate ligament (PCL) just behind it (right knee).

terference fit fixation. In our experience, this positioning technique has consistently allowed less than 2 mm of graft excursion with an intraoperative range of motion from 0 to 130 degrees of flexion.

We believe the use of an isometer is not mandatory. The femoral tunnel can only be placed so far posteriorly and superiorly in the intercondylar notch, and still preserve the desired 2- to 3-mm posterior cortical wall of the tunnel. This allows achievement of a secure interference fit fixation. When the femo-

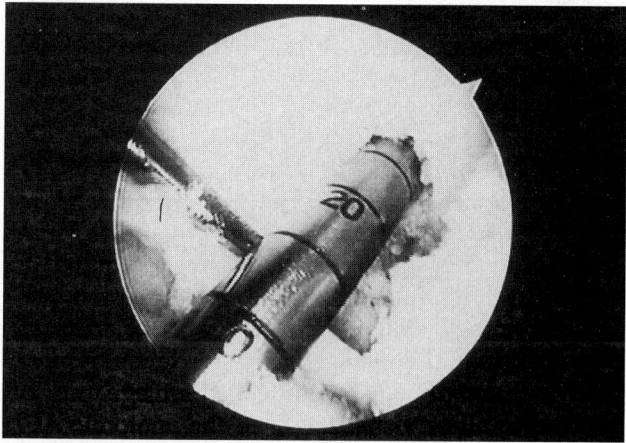

FIG 44–9.
Drilling the femoral tunnel with a cannulated and calibrated reamer to appropriate height. Note placement of the probe behind the reamer to protect the fibers of the PCL.

ral tunnel is positioned using the bony landmarks outlined above, this consistently allows 2 mm or less of graft excursion.

Graft Passage

The bone–patellar tendon–bone unit is pulled through the joint to engage the femoral and tibial tunnels. This is accomplished in three phases. First, the knee is flexed to 80 to 90 degrees. A Beath pin is passed through the tibial tunnel through the joint and into the femoral tunnel. The Beath pin is then driven through the femoral tunnel to emerge through the femoral cortex and skin of the anterolateral thigh. The Beath pin may penetrate the skin of the anterior or anterolateral thigh depending on tunnel direction. Either position is acceptable. Second, the no. 2 sutures attached to the femoral bone plug are passed through the eye of the Beath pin (Fig 44–10). The Beath pin is then pulled out the anterolateral aspect of the thigh, bringing the sutures with it. The sutures should be passed freely before passage of the bone plug into the tunnel to prevent jamming of the sutures in the tunnel. The Beath pin is then disengaged from the sutures (Fig 44–11). Finally, traction is applied to the sutures emerging from the skin in the anterolateral thigh, and the bone–patellar tendon–bone unit is gently pulled into the tibial and femoral tunnels. Contouring the end of the tibial bone plug into a bullet shape will facilitate passage into the

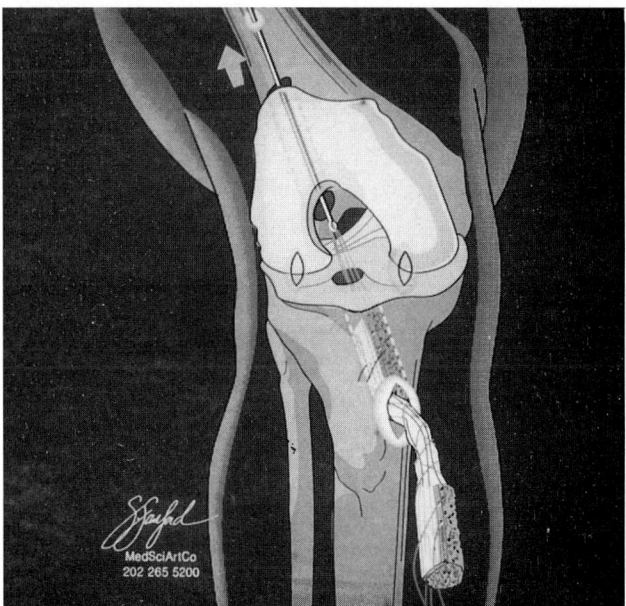

FIG 44–11.
Beath pin is being pulled proximally bringing the prepared graft into the tibial and then the femoral tunnel.

femoral tunnel. The graft is placed so that the tendinous portion is adjacent to the over-the-top position, which means that the cortical surface of the bone plug faces the PCL during graft passage. Traction on the patellar and tibial bone plug sutures allows adjustment and fine-tuning of the graft position. Range of motion and graft excursion can then be tested.

Graft Fixation

Graft fixation is accomplished with an interference fit using cannulated screws (Fig 44–12). In this technique the tibial bone plug is positioned in the femoral tunnel so that the edge of the bone plug is 1 mm medial to the edge of the tunnel. This prevents the tendinous portion of the graft from "hinging" over the tunnel edge or the base of the screw. The bone–patellar tendon–bone unit is positioned so that the tendinous portion is closest to the posterosuperior over-the-top position. The size of the screw used depends on the bone plug–tunnel gap and the bone plug length. When the bone plug–tunnel wall gap is 2 mm or less, a 7-mm-diameter screw is used. Most often a 7-mm × 20-mm interference fit screw is used. It is very important that the screw be positioned to engage the corticocancellous edge of the graft bone plug and not the cortical surface. Engagement of the screw only on the cortical surface of the bone plug would cause laceration of Sharpey's fibers and weakening of the tendon-bone interface.

The flexible guide wire for the cannulated screw is inserted through the inferomedial portal with the

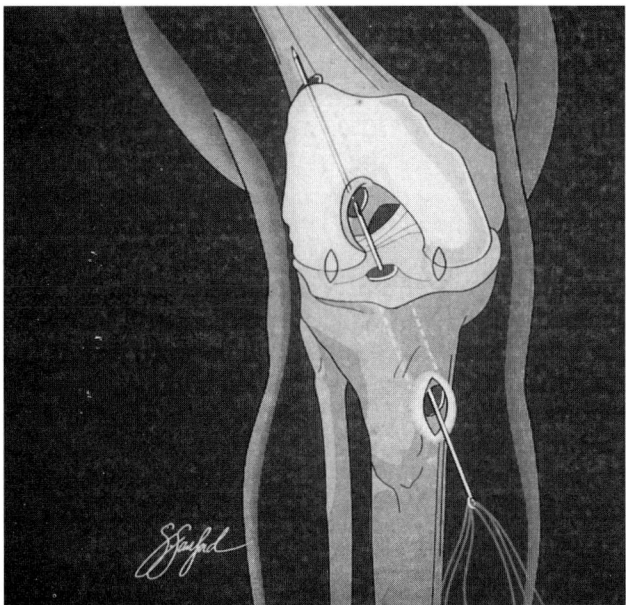

FIG 44–10.
Graft passage. Placement of the Beath pin and passage of the suture through the opening at the end. The other end of the pin has penetrated the lateroanterior cortex of the femur and is through the skin.

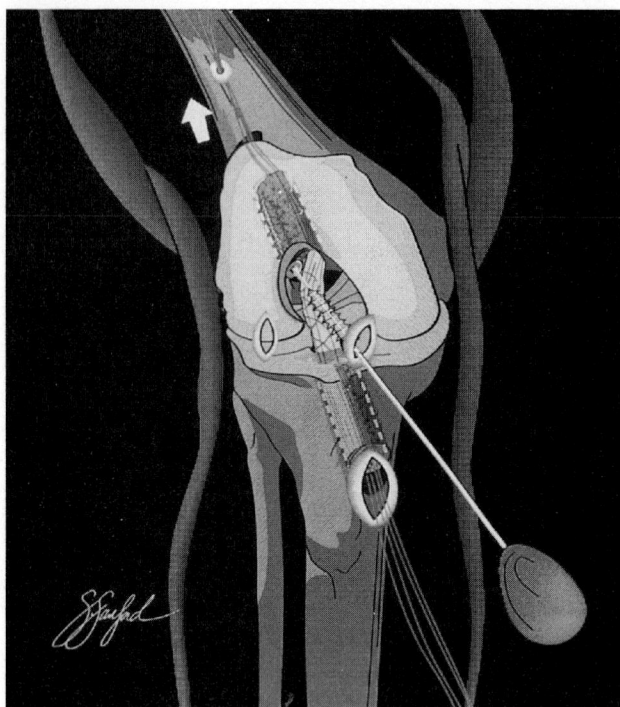

FIG 44–12.
The graft has been pulled into position. This is then fixed with an interference screw from the anteromedial portal for the femoral bone plug. Note the placement of the screw on the lateral side of the bone plug.

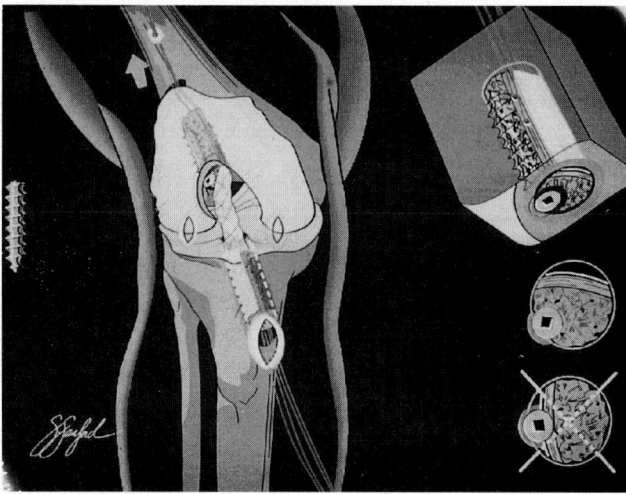

FIG 44–13.
Graft fixation. Tensioning is done and the tibial side is then fixed with an appropriate size of screw. Note the correct placement of the screw.

knee flexed to 110 degrees. The guide wire is placed 5 mm into the plug-tunnel interface at the appropriate position outlined above (Fig 44–12). The cannulated interference screw is then advanced over the guide wire to engage the bone plug–tunnel interface. The base of the screw is positioned flush with the femoral tunnel, but 1 mm lateral to the base of the bone plug so that the graft does not hinge over the screw base.

The knee is placed through a range of motion, and graft excursion and notch impingement are checked for the final time. Tension is applied to the graft with the sutures in the tibial bone plug. The knee is positioned in 20 degrees of flexion and 10 degrees of external rotation of the foot. A strong posterior drawer force is applied, and the tibial bone plug is secured using the appropriately sized cannulated interference fit screw (Fig 44–13). The tibial screw should be slightly shorter than the tibial bone plug. The screw should engage the corticocancellous edge of the bone plug.

The fixation is now complete. Lachman test and pivot shift tests are performed, and if unsatisfactory, the graft is retensioned. When the Lachman test is equal to the normal side, and the pivot shift is eliminated, the sutures are removed and the wound is closed. It is optional whether the patellar bone defect is bone-grafted, and whether the patellar tendon defect is closed.

Postoperative Care

The extremity is placed in a rehabilitation brace locked at 0 degrees of flexion. The patient wears the brace at all times except when on the continuous passive motion (CPM) machine. The knee is also placed in a cryotherapy unit to decrease postoperative swelling. The brace is used to prevent flexion contracture of the knee. The CPM machine begins on the day of surgery at 0 to 30 degrees of flexion and increases by 10 degrees/day to 110 degrees, when it is discontinued. The CPM machine is used to prevent adhesions. The patient is allowed weightbearing as tolerated in the rehabilitation brace. This brace is discontinued at the end of the 6th week. Progressive closed-chain quadriceps and proprioception exercises are initiated immediately. At 6 weeks the patient will be placed in a functional brace which will be worn for up to 6 months after surgery, and is then optional for use in sports participation. Agility and sport-specific drills begin at the 6th postoperative month. Return to sports is at the end of the 9th to 12th postoperative month. This protocol can be adjusted based on individual circumstances and any associated lesions.

EXTRAARTICULAR RECONSTRUCTION

The objective of extraarticular reconstructive procedures for the ACL-deficient knee is to control the anterior subluxation of the lateral tibial plateau by static or dynamic tightening of the lateral support structures of the knee joint during terminal extension.[20] The goal is to maintain the line of pull of the iliotibial band posterior to the sagittal center of rotation, thereby allowing the transferred fascial strip to act as a flexor or restraining band during terminal extension. Owing to the multiple forces across the knee joint, these extraarticular procedures have been used alone and in combination with intraarticular procedures.[6, 11, 15, 21, 38, 47, 48]

Recent biomechanical data on extraarticular reconstructions have been collected by Engebretsen et al.,[23] Draganich et al.,[19] and Sydney et al.[78] Draganich et al.[19] found that iliotibial band tenodesis alone overconstrained internal tibial rotation of the ACL-excised knee between 30 and 90 degrees of flexion. However, it did significantly reduce the anterior laxity between 30 and 90 degrees of flexion, but not to normal. When a combined intraarticular (Clancy[13]) and extraarticular reconstruction was done, there was no significant difference compared with the normal knees in rotatory position or anterior laxity. The authors concluded that because the extraarticular reconstruction shared the load when performed with an intraarticular reconstruction, it would be useful as an adjunct procedure in appropriate clinical situations. They warn, however, that the extraarticular repair should be fixed in place with only enough tension to take up the slack in the tissue without shifting the rotatory position of the tibia in order to both promote load-sharing between the grafts and minimize abnormal rotatory constraints. Sydney et al.,[78] in a cadaver study, showed that iliotibial band tenodesis reduces the occurrence of the pivot shift phenomenon and decreased displacement in the Lachman test by holding the tibia in a position of external rotation during flexion. The tenodesis was nonfunctional at extension, taut between 20 and 60 degrees of flexion, and overly tight at 90 degrees. This biomechanical observation may explain the clinical course seen in some cases in which the tenodesis stretches out and becomes ineffective over time. Engebretsen et al.[23] concluded that the iliotibial band tenodesis reduced the ACL force by an average of 43%. However, they also found that it overconstrained tibial rotation in knee flexion of 90 degrees. The authors were concerned that this may interfere with the screw-home mechanism and lead to abnormal joint loading with possible acceleration of arthrosis.

In the current literature there are a number of studies that review the long-term results of the extraarticular procedures alone, combined intraarticular and extraarticular procedures, and provide a direct comparison between intraarticular procedures with or without extraarticular procedures. Vail et al.[79] reviewed 112 patients in whom a MacIntosh-type procedure was performed with a 7.6-year average follow-up. The authors concluded that although the pivot shift was eliminated in most cases, patients had increased knee swelling and pain over time similar to the symptoms seen in untreated ACL tears. They found that the final clinical rating was not affected by the time lapse between injury and reconstruction because there was no difference between knees reconstructed soon after injury and those reconstructed much later. The authors concluded that there was some doubt whether this procedure truly alters the long-term natural history of the ACL deficiency.

Reid et al.,[71] in an 11-year average follow-up study on isolated Ellison procedures in 36 patients, found 70% of patients had a positive pivot shift and 91% had a positive Lachman test. Odensten et al.[66] reviewed 60 patients using an Ellison modification and found that at 17 months, the Lysholm score was 88 and 80% of knees were stable. However, at 40 months the Lysholm score dropped to 73.1 with increased complaints of instability and pain, and only 42% of knees were stable. After 17 months there were increased meniscal lesions and episodes of subluxation indicating instability. The authors concluded that initially the reconstruction was very good but that the reconstruction stretched out over time with an increase in instability and pain. Frank and Jackson[27] reported a 5-year follow-up of patients reconstructed with a modified MacIntosh procedure and found that 83% continued to have symptoms.

O'Brien et al.[64] had a 4-year average follow-up directly comparing intraarticular reconstruction using the central-third patellar tendon with or without an iliotibial band "lateral sling." By both clinical evaluation and KT-1000 arthrometer measurements, there were no differences between the two groups. In addition, 40% of patients had chronic pain or swelling, or both, related to the lateral sling. Strum et al.[77] reviewed 127 patients with chronic ACL insufficiency and directly compared intraarticular reconstruction alone vs. intraarticular and extraarticular reconstruction using the various techniques of each procedure. The average follow-up time was 45.2 months. There were no significant differences between the two groups in terms of radiographic changes or instrumented laxity testing. They concluded that extraarticular reconstruction is of no benefit provided that the intraarticular substitute is of sufficient strength, and that meticulous attention is given to graft positioning. Roth et al.[72] directly compared intraarticular reconstruction with quadriceps tendon and polypropylene braid augmentation with or without transfer of the biceps femoris tendon. Minimum follow-up was 2 years. There was no significant difference between the groups.

Not all long-term results in the literature on extraarticular reconstructions are negative. Durkan et al.[20] reported on a 51-month follow-up of 104 patients treated with the Ellison procedure. They had 78% good to excellent results and recommend the procedure for the recreational athlete with anterolateral rotatory instability. The authors found a decrease in the pivot shift test, but the majority of their patients (78%) did not develop increased symptoms in the knee over time, as seen in other studies. They did, however, relate their poor results to patients with significant generalized ligament laxity, articular cartilage damage, meniscectomy, and multidirectional instability. Rackemann et al.[70] had a 93% (69/74 patients) satisfactory outcome over an average of 70 months' follow-up in patients treated with middle-third patellar tendon and an extraarticular MacIntosh procedure. Noyes and Barber[57] directly compared bone–patellar tendon–bone allograft with or without an extraarticular modified Losee procedure in 104 patients with chronic ruptures of the ACL, with a 35-month average follow-up. In the patients who had both procedures done there was a significantly better KT-1000 arthrometer test, a higher level of sports activity, and better overall knee scores. The authors concluded that the extraarticular procedure appeared to provide support to the healing intraarticular allograft by reducing deleterious forces and tibial displacement and restoring the secondary restraints provided by the lateral iliotibial band.

Kornblatt et al.[43] found that by adding an extraarticular sling in patients undergoing intraarticular reconstruction using the quadriceps tendon, that the pivot shift was significantly reduced compared to the result after quadriceps tendon reconstruction alone. Their conclusion was that the quadriceps tendon graft is quite weak and needs the extraarticular procedure to improve results. Cross et al.[17] added a modified Ellison procedure to augment acute repair of the ACL in 47 patients. At 21-month average follow-up they had 64% good to excellent results (30/47) and 43 patients (91%) had a negative pivot jerk. The authors considered it necessary to augment all acute ACL repairs extraarticularly so that the healing phase could be protected.

Complications from extraarticular repairs reported in the literature include wound problems, extension loss, "inability to kneel due to tightness in the knee,"[27] tenderness over the lateral sling with pain and swelling,[64] transient peroneal nerve symptoms,[79] hardware pain and loosening,[79] subclinical mild lateral laxity,[17] and early and late herniation of the vastus lateralis through a defect in the iliotibial band (Fig 44–14).

Indications for isolated extraarticular reconstructions to eliminate the pivot shift include a selected group of low-demand patients without previous meniscectomy or generalized ligamentous laxity in whom a more anatomic reconstruction is not possible.[79] Also, patients with open physis or epiphyeal line may benefit from this procedure.[79] Indications for an extraarticular backup procedure with intraarticular reconstruction include severe anterolateral instability,[77] chronic ACL reconstruction with allograft,[57] large patients (>200 lb) who plan early vigorous activity in the postoperative period,[19,23] severely compromised secondary restraints,[19,23] redo reconstructions with no lateral secondary restraints,[23] the use of weak intraarticular grafts,[43,57] and primary repair of an acute ACL tear.[17]

In conclusion, biomechanical studies have shown

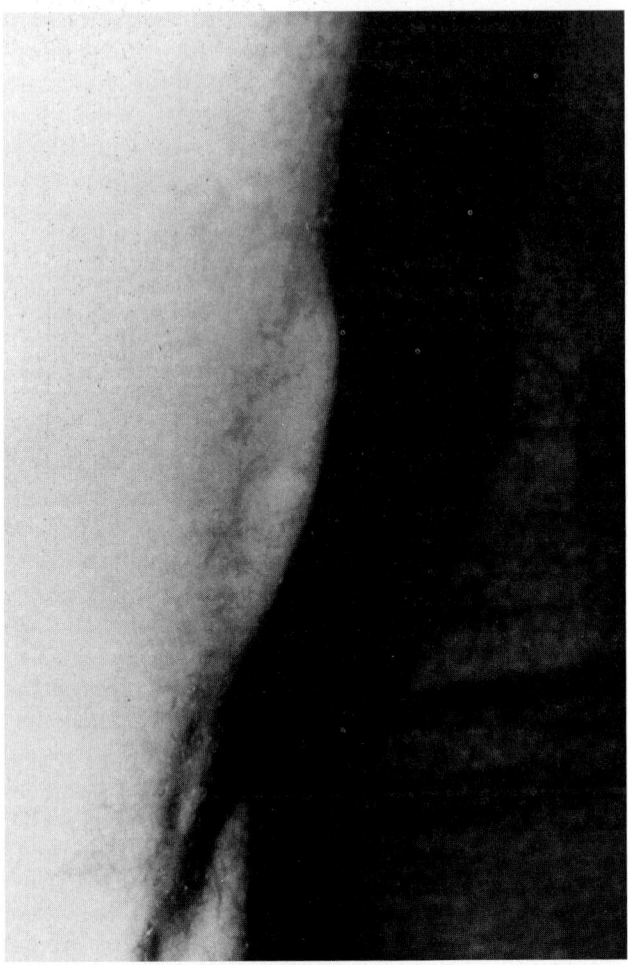

FIG 44–14.
Herniation of the vastus lateralis after harvesting a 2.5-cm iliotibial graft without closure of the defect.

that extraarticular reconstructions alone eliminate somewhat, but not completely, the anterior translation of the tibia in ACL-deficient knees.[19] Most such reconstructions are not isometric and therefore have been shown to be lax in full extension and overly tight in 90 degrees of flexion and thereby may stretch out over time, leading to clinical instability and pain.[27, 65, 71, 78, 79] They also severely constrain internal rotation of the tibia, thereby affecting the normal joint kinematics, which may lead to long-term arthrosis.[23]

The combined intraarticular and extraarticular procedures provide some load-sharing and thereby decrease the stresses to the remodeling intraarticular graft.[19, 23, 57] If the intraarticular graft is of significant strength, then the load-sharing effect of an extraarticular reconstruction has been shown not to be of significant value in the long term.[64, 77] However, if the intraarticular graft is not of significant strength, or there are excessive stresses upon a strong graft due to other factors, then the extraarticular reconstruction has been shown to be of value.[17, 43, 57]

MacIntosh Procedure

In 1972, Galway et al.[29] reported the presence of the lateral pivot shift phenomenon, and its correction, by designing an extraarticular procedure for the ACL-deficient knee utilizing a strip of iliotibial band. In 1976, MacIntosh and Darby[48] reported the results of a lateral substitution for the ACL-deficient knee called the "return lateral loop." A middle strip of iliotibial band measuring approximately 16 cm in length and 1.5 cm in width is dissected and left attached distally to Gerdy's tubercle. This strip is then passed to the posterolateral corner of the knee through a soft tissue tunnel beneath the fibular collateral ligament. It is then brought through an opening which is created at the distal end of the intramuscular septum at the lateral femoral condyle. The strip of iliotibial band is then looped back onto itself again deep to the fibular collateral ligament and then sutured to Gerdy's tubercle with the knee in 90 degrees of flexion and with external rotation of the tibia (Figs 44–15,A–E).

Losee Procedure

In 1978, Losee et al.[47] described a modification of the MacIntosh procedure called the "sling and reef" procedure. The iliotibial band is used to create a sling and the posterior lateral capsule is reefed. As with the MacIntosh procedure a similar strip of iliotibial band is dissected and left with its distal attachment to Gerdy's tubercle. A superficial osseous tunnel is then created beginning at the anterolateral aspect of the femoral condyle at a point anterior to the fibular collateral ligament. The tunnel exits posterolaterally at the insertions of the lateral head of the gastrocnemius tendon and the superior attachment of the posterior capsule. This strip is then pulled tautly through the tunnel from anterior to posterior with the knee flexed to 90 degrees and the tibia externally rotated. The iliotibial band is then woven around the tendon of the lateral head of the gastrocnemius muscle and through the lateral aspect of the arcuate complex and posterolateral corner. The strip is then passed through a soft tissue tunnel deep to the fibular collateral ligament and sutured to Gerdy's tubercle. Tension is maintained on the strip, and reefing sutures are utilized along its course to anchor it to adjacent tissue. As the iliotibial band is woven, it is pulled anteriorly, which further tightens the posterolateral structures. The leg is maintained in a long leg cast with 30 to 45 degrees of flexion and external rotation for approximately 6 weeks. This procedure has been recommended in conjunction with intraarticular ACL reconstructions for severe anterolateral rotary instability with varus laxity[11, 35] (Fig 44–16).

Ellison Procedure

In 1979, Ellison[21] described a distal iliotibial band transfer for anterolateral rotary instability of the knee. A 1.5-cm wide strip of iliotibial band is selected and detached along with a button of bone from Gerdy's tubercle, preserving the proximal blood supply, as well as maintaining the dynamic stabilizing effect of the tensor fascia lata and gluteus maximus musculature contributions. As the iliotibial band is exposed proximally, it is gradually broadened so that the base of the strip is approximately three times as wide as the distal end. A soft tissue tunnel is created beneath the fibular collateral ligament and the lateral capsular ligament is reefed beneath it. The iliotibial band is then passed beneath the fibular collateral ligament and is reattached to a shallow trough which is created in direct line with the pull of the transplanted tissue on the anterolateral tibia. A staple is placed over the strip of iliotibial band just proximal to the button of bone so as to anchor the transplant in its trough. The defect created in the iliotibial tract may be left open or closed. In case the defect is closed, one should be careful not to create an excessive lateral pressure syndrome. In 1980, Ellison[22] reported on supplementing this procedure with a biceps tendon transfer. This was theorized to increase the dynamic stability by providing a powerful posterior restraining force to the proximal tibia. Follow-up evaluations of

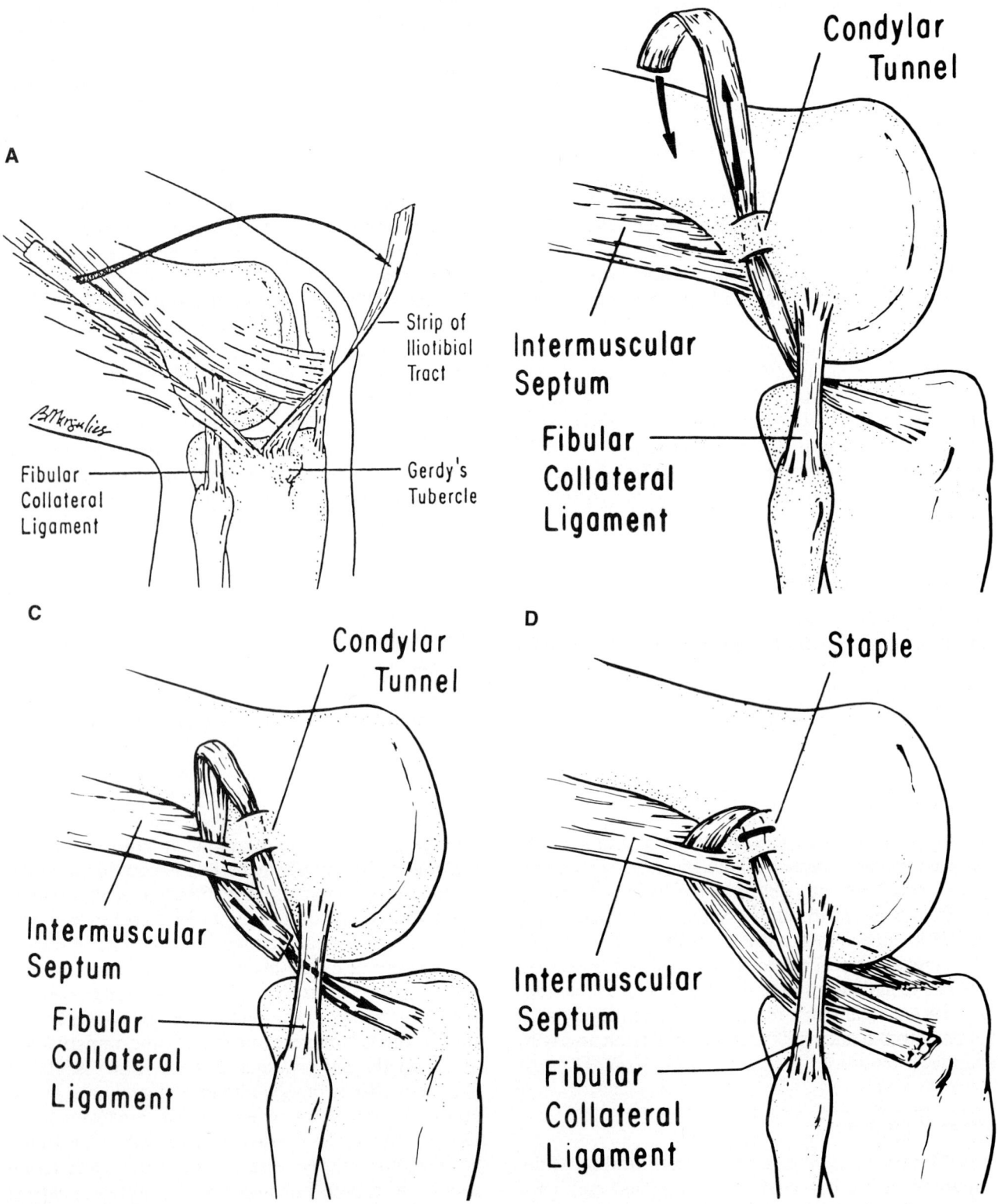

FIG 44–15.
MacIntosh procedure. **A,** a strip of iliotibial tract is separated and based distally. **B,** iliotibial strip is placed under the fibular collateral ligament and through the condylar tunnel. **C,** iliotibial strip is doubled back under the intermuscular septum. **D,** strip is stapled at the condylar tunnel and is returned under the fibular collateral ligament to Gerdy's tubercle. **E,** completed iliotibial tract repair. (From Bassett FH III: *Am J Sports Med* 20:276, 277, 1992. Used by permission.)

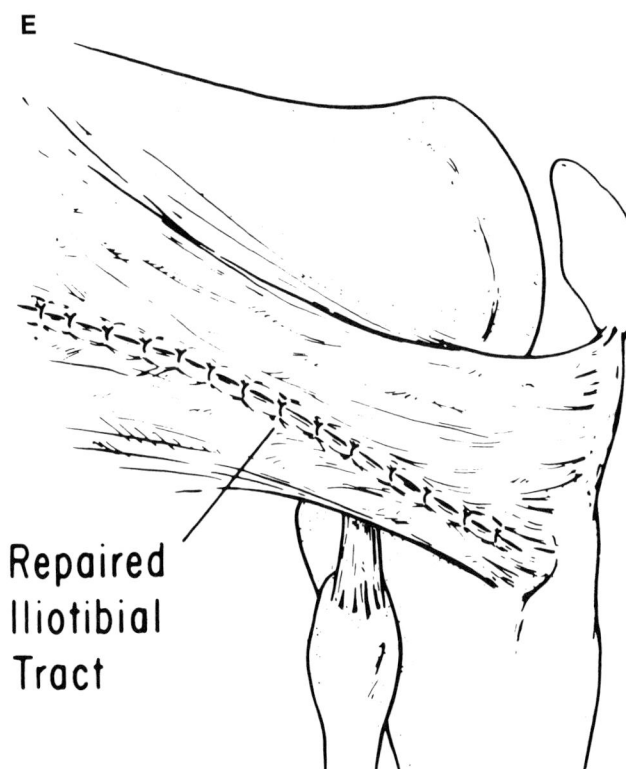

FIG 44–15, cont'd.
For legend see opposite page.

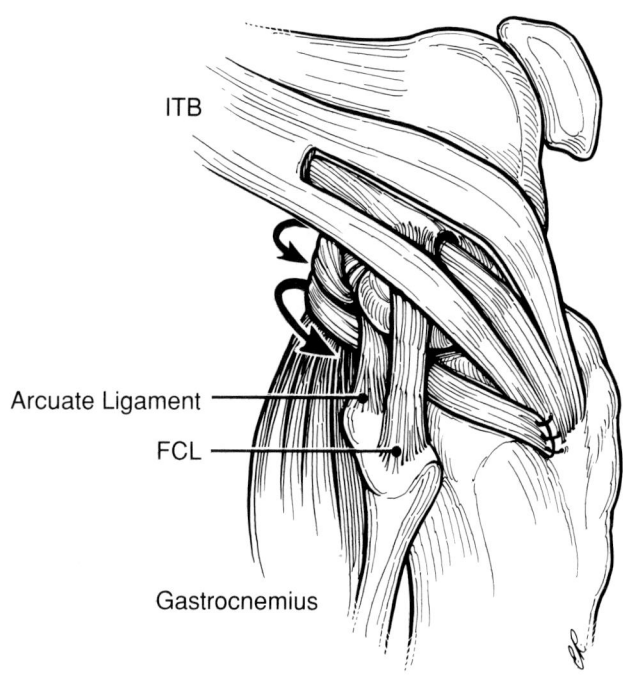

FIG 44–16.
Losee procedure. A proximally detached strip to the iliotibial band (ITB) is passed through an osseous tunnel in the lateral femoral condyle from anterior to posterior. The strip is woven around the tendon of the lateral head of the gastrocnemius and beneath the fibular collateral ligament (FCL), and sutured to Gerdy's tubercle.

the Ellison procedure reveal satisfactory results when the procedure is utilized in combination with an intraarticular reconstruction[16] (Figs 44–17,A–E).

Arnold-Coker Procedure

In 1979, Arnold et al.[6] described a modification of the MacIntosh procedure in which an iliotibial band strip measuring approximately 5 to 10 cm in length and 2 cm in width is created with its distal attachment to Gerdy's tubercle maintained. A soft tissue tunnel is then developed at the posterior edge of the fibular collateral ligament while the knee is maintained in full flexion and external rotation. This tunnel is made approximately 2 cm above the joint line. The iliotibial band is then passed beneath the fibular collateral ligament and stapled just inferior to Gerdy's tubercle. Sutures are utilized to maintain the iliotibial band to its sling around the fibular collateral ligament. Postoperatively, a hinged brace is utilized with an initial range of motion of 55 to 80 degrees. The authors concluded that this procedure had its best results as a delayed repair for anterolateral instabilities[6] (Fig 44–18).

James Procedure

A modification of Losee's procedure was described by James in 1983.[39] Again, the iliotibial tract is maintained distally and the posterolateral corner is tightened by being advanced anteriorly. An iliotibial strip 20 cm long and approximately 2 cm wide is dissected proximally. A soft tissue tunnel is fashioned deep to the fibular collateral ligament and through the gastrocnemius tendon and arcuate complex. The strip is then brought back anteriorly and looped around the same soft tissue tunnel again. This resultant soft tissue loop brings the gastrocnemius tendon and arcuate complex anteriorly toward the fibular collateral ligament, thus producing a tightening effect of the posterolateral corner. The band is then passed from posterior to anterior through an osseous tunnel created in the lateral femoral condyle similar to that described by Losee et al.[47] Finally, the free strip is brought beneath the iliotibial tract, which remains attached to Gerdy's tubercle, and is then sutured under tension to the femoral insertion of the fibular collateral ligament. A long leg cast is fashioned with approximately 30 degrees of knee flexion to be worn for approximately 6 weeks (Fig 44–19,A–C).

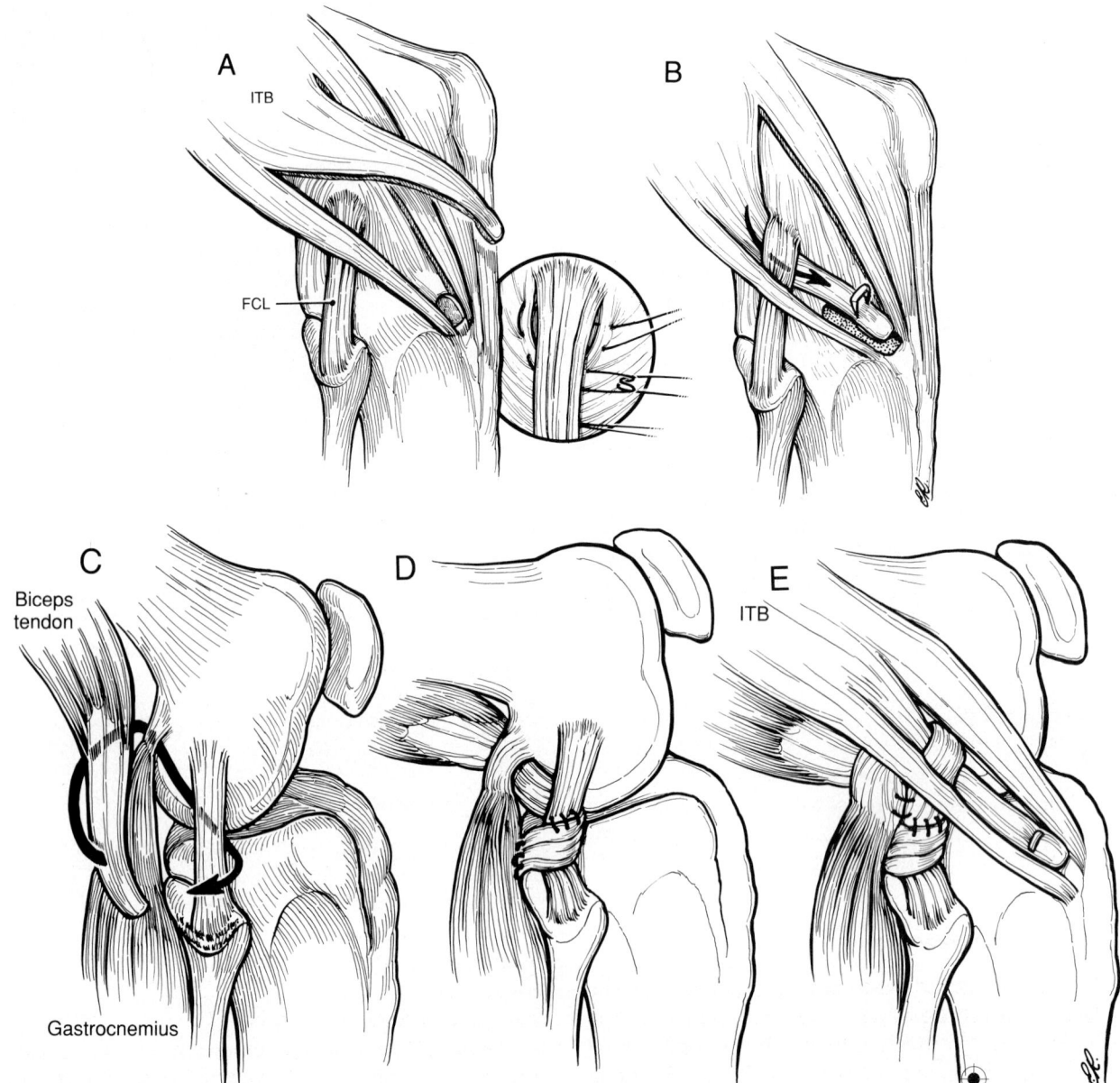

FIG 44–17.
A, Ellison procedure. Strip of the iliotibial band *(ITB)* with a button of bone. *Inset,* the lateral capsule is reefed beneath the fibular collateral ligament *(FCL)*. **B,** iliotibial strip is passed beneath the fibular collateral ligament and reattached. **C,** biceps tendon transfer. The biceps tendon is completely detached from the proximal fibula and passed through the aponeurotic portion of the lateral head of the gastrocnemius and beneath the fibular collateral ligament. **D,** the biceps tendon is then sutured to the capsule of the proximal tibiofibular joint and the insertion of the arcuate complex, and to the fibular collateral ligament. **E,** the Ellison procedure supplemented with biceps tendon transfer. *ITB* = iliotibial band.

Andrews Procedure

In 1983, Andrews and Sanders[1] described a "mini-reconstruction" technique for the treatment of anterolateral rotary instability. In this procedure, tenodesis of the iliotibial tract to the lateral femoral condyle is performed and two isometric bundles are created from the iliotibial tract to duplicate the two bundles of the ACL. The iliotibial tract is divided longitudinally for a length of approximately 10 cm and sutures are placed through its proximal aspect. The lateral femoral cortex is exposed and "fish-scaled" at the distal insertion of the lateral intermuscular septum. Two drill holes are then placed in this area from lateral to medial. The first hole is located at the distal portion of the linea aspera at the junction of the shaft and

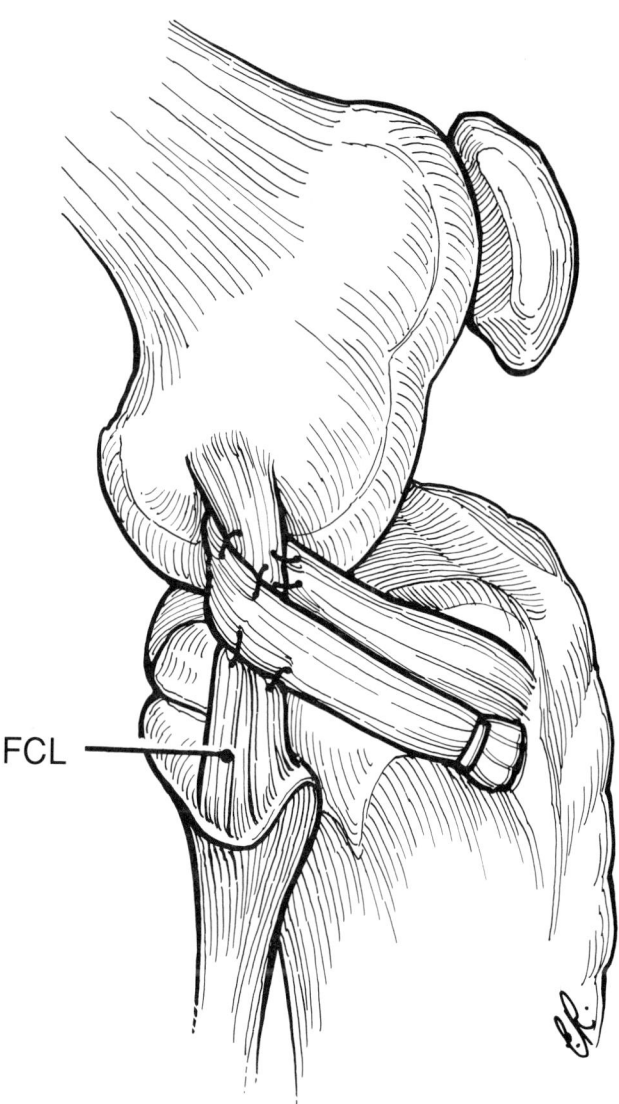

FIG 44–18.
Arnold-Coker procedure. Strip of iliotibial band is freed proximally and passed beneath the fibular collateral ligament *(FCL)* and stapled inferior to Gerdy's tubercle.

the femoral condyle, just anterior to the most posterior border of the cortex. In theory, this drill hole corresponds to the anteromedial bundle of the ACL. The second hole is drilled 1.0 cm anterior and 0.5 cm distal to the first hole corresponding to the posterolateral bundle. The sutures tagging the two ends of the iliotibial tract are then passed through the transverse drill holes from lateral to medial with tension maintained. Stability is tested and if adequate, the sutures are tied down medially over the adductor tubercle. The knee is placed in a cylinder cast with 30 to 40 degrees of flexion for approximately 6 weeks. This procedure is recommended for extraarticular stabilization for moderate to severe acute anterolateral rotary instabilities and mild to moderate chronic anterolateral rotary instabilities.[1, 2, 11] It is advantageous in that the simple longitudinal incision preserves the vascularity of the iliotibial tract. Since the tract maintains its longitudinal arrangement of fibers, there is no loss of strength (Fig 44–20).

Pes Anserinus Transfer

In 1968, Slocum and Larson[76] described a procedure for control of anteromedial knee instability by transferring a portion of the pes anserinus conjoined tendon. Instability is controlled by converting the function of the pes anserinus muscles from flexion to internal rotation of the tibia. This is accomplished by transferring the lower two thirds of the pes anserinus tendon attachment. This portion of the conjoined tendon is elevated and folded over its upper portion to form a double layer of tendon. The elevated portion is then sutured to the periosteum overriding the tibial tubercle and to the medial aspect of the patellar tendon. The knee is then immobilized in 30 degrees of flexion and internal rotation of the tibia for approximately 6 weeks (Fig 44–21, A and B).

This soft tissue procedure for anteromedial instability has been utilized in combination with soft tissue procedures for anterolateral rotary instability, as well as with intraarticular procedures. A follow-up study by Noyes and Sonstegard,[58] which assessed biomechanical function of the pes anserinus and the effect of its transplantation, revealed that internal rotation forces are approximately doubled at 30 to 60 degrees of knee flexion. The authors concluded that the pes anserinus transplant is biomechanically sound and effective for treatment of anteromedial instability.

COMPLICATIONS

The most frequently encountered complication of ACL surgery utilizing the central third of the patellar tendon is failure to regain full range of motion resulting in arthrofibrosis. We recommend gentle manipulation under anesthesia and arthroscopic lysis of adhesions if significant limitation of motion is still present at 12 to 16 weeks postoperatively. Some complications may occur that are not specific for ACL surgery such as postoperative hematoma, infection, deep venous thrombosis, and so forth.

Some complications are basically technique related, and almost always avoidable with systematic approach and meticulous attention to detail. These include patellar fracture,[52] patellar tendon rupture, bone plug loosening or fracture,[8] penetration of the joint with screws, inadequate fixation of bone plugs,

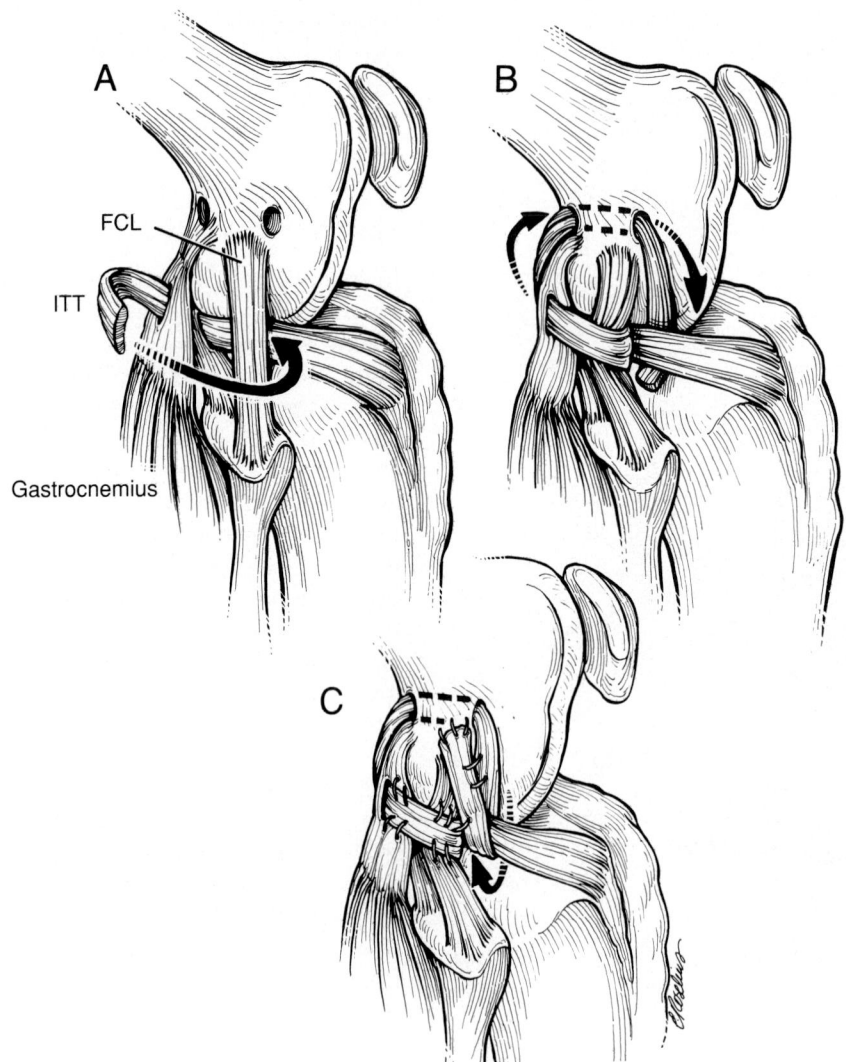

FIG 44–19.
James procedure. A, proximally detached iliotibial strip *(ITT)* is passed through a soft tissue tunnel deep to the fibular collateral ligament *(FCL)* and through the gastrocnemius tendon and arcuate complex. B, the strip is looped around the soft tissue tunnel and passed through the osseous tunnel. C, strip is passed beneath the distally attached iliotibial band and sutured to the femoral insertion of the fibular collateral ligament.

and the use of inappropriate hardware, which may also lead to loosening or joint destruction.

Posttraumatic or postsurgical patellofemoral chondrosis or chondromalacia is now resurfacing on follow-ups of 5 or more years with central-third patellar tendon reconstructions. Infrapatellar contracture syndrome (IPCS) has also been reported[68] to be particularly associated with intraarticular ACL reconstruction. Further studies in this area are needed to identify the exact mechanisms and causes of patellofemoral complications associated with central-third patellar tendon reconstruction.

There is concern about late patellar fracture after harvesting the patella bone block with this procedure. Several cases of intraoperative and late patellar fractures have been reported.[9, 52, 73] Roberts et al.[73] have developed a bone grafting technique for the patella defect. We believe, however, that if the length of the bone plug is no more than 25 to 30 mm, and the thickness is no more than one third the thickness of the patella (as measured on preoperative patellar axial views), even without grafting, remodeling within 4 to 6 months will occur with an extremely rare incidence of fracture.

SUMMARY

We have described our technique of intraarticular ACL reconstruction, as well as several available techniques of extraarticular surgeries. Although in the

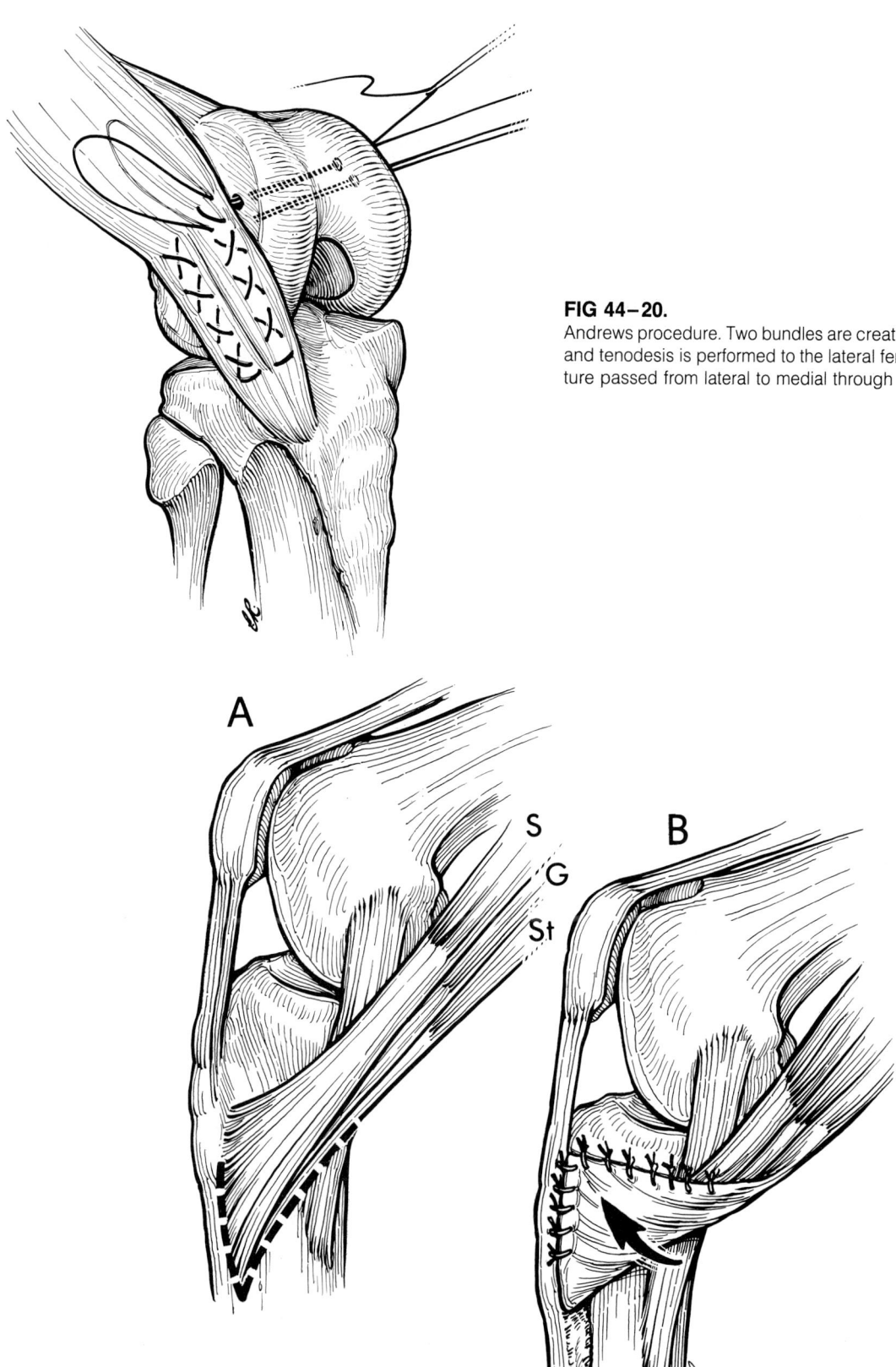

FIG 44–20.
Andrews procedure. Two bundles are created from the iliotibial tract and tenodesis is performed to the lateral femoral condyle with a suture passed from lateral to medial through drill holes.

FIG 44–21.
Pes anserinus transfer. **A,** distal two thirds of the pes anserinus tendon is released. **B,** portion of the conjoined tendon is folded proximally and sutured to the periosteum of the proximal tibia and to the medial aspect of the patellar tendon. S = semimembranosus; G = gracilis; St = semitendinosus.

past, we have combined these two techniques, at the present time, utilizing a strong biologic intraarticular graft, we see no need for additional extraarticular backup surgery. This additional extraarticular substitution may be added only if we are dealing with severe posterolateral instabilities with or without varus deformity. On the other hand, medial extraarticular surgery may also be added in the case of severe medial or posteromedial instabilities. The intraarticular technique described in this chapter has proved to be associated with less morbidity than open conventional reconstructive procedures and has been reproducible in our hands.

Acknowledgement

This work was supported by the National Knee Research and Education Foundation.

We acknowledge the technical assistance of Cindy Smallwood and Karen Knable, A.T.C., in the preparation of this manuscript.

REFERENCES

1. Andrews JR, Sanders R: A mini-reconstruction technique in treating anterolateral rotatory instability (ALRI), Clin Orthop 172:93–96, 1983.
2. Andrews JR, Sanders R, Morin B: Surgical treatment of anterolateral rotatory instability. A follow-up study, Am J Sports Med 13:112–119, 1985.
3. Arnoczky SP: Blood supply to the anterior cruciate ligaments and supporting structures, Orthop Clin North Am, 16:15–28, 1985.
4. Arnoczky SP, Rubin RM, Marshall JL: Microvasculature of the cruciate ligaments and its response to injury, J Bone Joint Surg [Am] 61:1221–1229, 1979.
5. Arnoczky SP, Tarrin GB, Marshall JL: Anterior cruciate ligament replacement using patellar tendon. An evaluation of graft revascularization in the dog, J Bone Joint Surg [Am] 64:217–224, 1982.
6. Arnold JA, et al: Natural history of anterior cruciate tears, Am J Sports Med, 7:305–313, 1979.
7. Bach BR Jr: Arthroscopy-assisted patellar tendon substitution for anterior cruciate ligament insufficiency: Surgical technique, Am J Knee Surg 2:3–20, 1989.
8. Bach BR Jr: Potential pitfalls of Kurosaka screw interference fixation for ACL surgery, Am J Knee Surg 2:76–82, 1989.
9. Bonamo JJ, Krinick RM, Sparn AA: Rupture of the patellar ligament after use of its central third for anterior cruciate reconstruction. A report of two cases, J Bone Joint Surg [Am] 66:1294–1297, 1984.
10. Butler DL, et al: Biomechanical properties of primate vascularized vs. nonvascularized patellar tendon grafts over time, J Orthop Res 7:68–79, 1989.
11. Carson WG: Extra-articular reconstruction of the anterior cruciate ligament: Lateral procedures, Orthop Clin North Am 16:191–211, 1985.
12. Clancy WG Jr et al: Anterior cruciate ligament functional instability: A static intra-articular and dynamic extra-articular procedure, Clin Orthop 172:102–106, 1983.
13. Clancy WG Jr: Intra-articular reconstruction of the anterior cruciate ligament, Orthop Clin North Am 16:181–189, 1985.
14. Clancy WG Jr et al: Anterior and posterior cruciate ligament reconstruction in Rhesus monkeys, J Bone Joint Surg [Am] 63:1270–1284, 1981.
15. Clancy WG Jr et al: Anterior cruciate ligament reconstruction using one-third of the patellar ligament, augmented by extraarticular tendon transfers, J Bone Joint Surg [Am] 64:352–359, 1982.
16. Crenshaw AH, editor: Campbell's operative orthopaedics, ed 7, St Louis, 1987, Mosby–Year Book.
17. Cross MJ, Paterson RS, Capito CP: Acute repair of the anterior cruciate ligament with lateral capsular augmentation, Am Orthop Soc Sports Med 17:63–67, 1989.
18. Daniel DM et al: Instrumented measurement of anterior laxity of the knee, J Bone Joint Surg [Am] 67:720–726, 1985.
19. Draganich LF, et al: An in vitro study of an intraarticular and extraarticular reconstruction in the anterior cruciate ligament deficient knee, Am J Sports Med 18:262–266, 1990.
20. Durkan JA, Wynne GF, Haggerty JF: Extraarticular reconstruction of the anterior cruciate ligament insufficient knee: A long term analysis of the Ellison procedure, Am J Sports Med 17:112–117, 1989.
21. Ellison AE: Distal iliotibial band transfer for anterolateral rotatory instability of the knee, J Bone Joint Surg [Am] 61:330–337, 1979.
22. Ellison AE: The pathogenesis and treatment of anterolateral rotatory instability, Clin Orthop 147:51–55, 1980.
23. Engebretsen L, et al: The effect of an iliotibial tenodesis on intraarticular graft forces and knee joint motion, Am J Sports Med 18:169–176.
24. Feagin JA Jr, editor: Diagnosis and treatment of injuries about the knee, The crucial ligaments: New York, 1988, Churchill Livingstone.
25. Fetto JF, Marshall JL: The natural history and diagnosis of anterior cruciate ligament insufficiency, Clin Orthop 147:29–38, 1980.
26. Fox JM, Orrin HS, Markolf K: Arthroscopic anterior cruciate ligament repair: Preliminary results and instrumental testing for anterior stability, Arthroscopy 1:175–181, 1985.
27. Frank C, Jackson RW: Lateral substitution for chronic isolated anterior cruciate ligament deficiency, J Bone Joint Surg [Br] 407–411, 1988.
28. Galway HR, MacIntosh DL: The lateral pivot shift: A symptom and sign of anterior cruciate ligament insufficiency, Clin Orthop 147:45–50, 1980.

29. Galway RD, Beaupre A, MacIntosh DL: Pivot shift: A clinical sign of symptomatic anterior cruciate insufficiency, *J Bone Joint Surg [Br]* 54:763, 1972.
30. Hewson GF Jr: Drill guides for improving accuracy in anterior cruciate ligament repair and reconstruction, *Clin Orthop* 172:119–124, 1983.
31. Hey Groves EW: Operation for the repair of the crucial ligaments, *Lancet* 2:674, 1917.
32. Hey Groves EW: The crucial ligaments of the knee joint: Their function, rupture, and operative treatment of the same, *Br J Surg* 7:505, 1920.
33. Hughston JC: Complications of anterior cruciate ligament surgery, *Orthop Clin North Am* 16:237–240, 1985.
34. Insall J, et al: Bone block transfer for anterior cruciate deficiency, *J Bone Joint Surg [Am]* 63:560–569, 1981.
35. Jackson D, Drez D, editors: *The anterior cruciate deficient knee: New concepts in ligament repair,* St Louis, 1987, Mosby–Year Book.
36. Jackson DW, Jennings LD: Arthroscopically assisted reconstruction of the anterior cruciate ligament using a patella tendon bone autograft, *Clin Sports Med* 7:785–800, 1988.
37. Jacobsen K: Osteoarthrosis following insufficiency of cruciate ligaments in man, *Acta Orthop Scand* 48:520–526, 1977.
38. James SL: The knee. In D'Ambrosia RD, editor: *Musculoskeletal disorders: Regional examination and differential diagnosis,* Philadelphia, 1977, JB Lippincott, pp 440–486.
39. James SL: Knee ligament reconstruction. In Evarts CM, editor: *Surgery of the musculoskeletal system,* New York, 1983, Churchill Livingstone, pp 31–104.
40. Johnson LL: Lateral capsular ligament complex: Anatomical and surgical considerations, *Am J Sports Med* 7:156, 1979.
41. Jones KG: Reconstruction of the anterior cruciate ligament: A technique using the central one-third of the patellar ligament, *J Bone Joint Surg [Am]* 45:925–932, 1963.
42. Jones KG: Reconstruction of the anterior cruciate ligament using the central one-third of the patellar ligament. A follow-up report, *J Bone Joint Surg [Am]* 52:1302–1308, 1970.
43. Kornblatt IB, Warren RF, Wickiewicz TL: Combined intra-articular quadriceps tendon substitution and extra-articular lateral sling procedure for chronic anterior cruciate ligament insufficiency, *Am J Knee Surg* 4:63–69, 1991.
44. Krackow KA, Brooks RL: Optimization of knee ligament position for lateral extra-articular reconstruction, *Am J Sports Med* 11:293–302, 1983.
45. Lambert KL: Vascularized patellar tendon graft with rigid internal fixation for anterior cruciate ligament insufficiency, *Clin Orthop* 172:85–89, 1983.
46. Larson RV, Sidles JA: Special consideration in graft placement and orientation in ACL reconstruction, Eighth Annual Cherry Blossom Seminar, Washington, DC, 1989.
47. Losee RE, Johnson TR, Southwick WD: Anterior subluxation of the lateral tibial plateau: A diagnostic test and operative repair, *J Bone Joint Surg [Am]* 60:1015–1030, 1978.
48. MacIntosh DL, Darby TA: Lateral substitution reconstruction (abstract), *J Bone Joint Surg [Br]* 58:142, 1976.
49. Malek MM, Fanelli GC, Golden DO: Combined intraarticular and extraarticular anterior cruciate ligament reconstruction. In Scott WN, editor: *Ligament and extensor mechanism injuries of the knee: Diagnosis and treatment,* St Louis, 1991, Mosby–Year Book, pp 267–284.
50. Marshall JL, et al: The anterior cruciate ligament. The diagnosis and treatment of its injuries and their serious prognostic implications, *Orthop Rev* 7:35–46, 1978.
51. Marshall JL et al: The anterior cruciate ligament: A technique of repair and reconstruction, *Clin Orthop* 143:97–106, 1979.
52. McCarroll JR: Fracture of the patella during a golf swing following a reconstruction of the anterior cruciate ligament. A case report, *Am J Sports Med* 11:26–27, 1983.
53. McDaniel WJ, Dameron TB Jr: Untreated ruptures of the anterior cruciate ligament. A follow-up study, *J Bone Joint Surg [Am]* 62:696–705, 1980.
54. Mott HW: Semitendinosus anatomic reconstruction for anterior cruciate ligament insufficiency, *Clin Orthop* 172:90–92, 1983.
55. Mueller W: *The knee: Form, function, and ligament reconstruction,* New York, 1983, Springer-Verlag.
56. Norwood LA, Cross MJ: The intercondylar shelf and the anterior cruciate ligament, *Am J Sports Med* 5:171–176, 1977.
57. Noyes FR, Barber SD: The effect of an extra-articular procedure on allograft reconstructions for chronic ruptures of the anterior cruciate ligament, *J Bone Joint Surg [Am]* 73:882–892, 1991.
58. Noyes FR, Sonstegard DA: Biomechanical function of the pes anserinus at the knee and the effect of its transplantation, *J Bone Joint Surg [Am]* 55:1225, 1973.
59. Noyes FR, et al: Clinical laxity tests and functional stability of the knee, *Clin Orthop* 146:84–89, 1980.
60. Noyes FR, et al: The symptomatic anterior cruciate deficient knee. Part I: The long-term functional disability in athletically active individuals, *J Bone Joint Surg [Am]* 65:154–162, 1983.
61. Noyes FR, et al: The symptomatic anterior cruciate deficient knee. Part II: The results of rehabilitation, activity modification, and counseling of functional disability, *J Bone Joint Surg [Am]* 65:163–174, 1983.
62. Noyes FR, et al: Intra-articular cruciate reconstruction. I: Perspectives on graft strength vascularization, and immediate motion after replacement, *Clin Orthop* 172:71–77, 1983.
63. Noyes FR, et al: Biomechanical analysis of human ligament graft used in knee ligament repairs and reconstruction, *J Bone Joint Surg [Am]* 66:344, 1984.

64. O'Brien SJ et al: The iliotibial band lateral sling procedure and its effect on the results of anterior cruciate ligament reconstruction, *Am J Sports Med* 19:21–25, 1991.
65. Odensten M, Lysholm J, Gillquist J: Long-term follow-up study of a distal iliotibial band transfer (DIT) for anterolateral knee instability, *Clin Orthop* 176:129–135, 1983.
66. O'Donoghue DM: A method for replacement of the anterior cruciate ligament of the knee. Report of twenty cases, *J Bone Joint Surg [Am]* 45:905–924, 1963.
67. Palmer I: On the injuries to the ligaments of the knee joint: A clinical study, *Acta Chir Scand Suppl* 81:53, 1938.
68. Paulos LE, et al: Intra-articular cruciate reconstruction. II: Replacement with vascularized patellar tendon, *Clin Orthop* 172:78–84, 1983.
69. Paulos LE, et al: Infrapatellar contracture syndrome. An unrecognized cause of knee stiffness with patella entrapment and patella infera, *Am J Sports Med* 15:331–341, 1987.
70. Rackemann S, Robinson A, Dandy DJ: Reconstruction of the anterior cruciate ligament with an intra-articular patellar tendon graft and an extra-articular tenodesis, *J Bone Joint Surg [Br]* 73:368–373, 1991.
71. Reid JS, et al: Long-term follow-up of the isolated Ellison procedure for anterior cruciate ligament deficient knees, A.A.D.S. Instructional Course, February 1992, Washington, D.C.
72. Roth JH, et al: Intraarticular reconstruction of the anterior cruciate ligament with and without extra-articular supplementation by transfer of the biceps femoris tendon, *J Bone Joint Surg [Am]* 69A:2, 1987.
73. Roberts TS, Drez DD, Parker W: Prevention of late patellar fracture in ACL deficient knees reconstructed with bone–patellar tendon–bone autografts. A new technique, *Am J Knee Surg* 2:83–86, 1989.
74. Scott WN, Schosheim PM: Intra-articular transfer of the iliotibial muscle-tendon unit, *Clin Orthop* 172:97–101, 1983.
75. Sidles JA, et al: Ligament length relationships in the moving knee, *J Orthop Res* 6:593–610, 1988.
76. Slocum DB, Larson RL: Pes anserinus transplant. A simple surgical procedure for control of rotatory instability of the knee, *J Bone Joint Surg [Am]* 50:226–242, 1968.
77. Strum GM, et al: Intraarticular versus intraarticular and extraarticular reconstruction for chronic anterior cruciate ligament instability, *Clin Orthop* 245:188–198, 1989.
78. Sydney SV, et al: The altered kinematic effect of an iliotibial band tenodesis on the anterior cruciate deficient knee, *Trans Orthop Res Soc* 12:266, 1987.
79. Vail TP, Malone TR, Bassett FH: Long-term functional results in patients with anterolateral rotatory instability treated by iliotibial band transfer, *Am J Sports Med* 20:274–282, 1992.
80. Warren RF: Primary repair of the anterior cruciate ligament, *Clin Orthop* 172:65–70, 1983.
81. Zarins B, Rowe CR: Combined anterior cruciate ligament reconstruction using semitendinosus tendon and iliotibial tract, *J Bone Joint Surg [Am]* 68:160–177, 1986.

45

Intraarticular Semitendinosus Anterior Cruciate Ligament Reconstruction

ROBERT C. HENDLER, M.D.

Semitendinosus as anterior cruciate ligament substitute
Technical considerations
Hendler procedure
Surgical technique
Wound closure and postoperative care
Conclusion

The diagnosis and treatment of the injured anterior cruciate ligament (ACL) has remained a controversial subject among knee surgeons. Many surgical procedures have been designed to correct the problem of the so-called ACL-deficient knee. The complexity of the ACL itself has been a major deterrent to establishment of a standard surgical method of ACL reconstruction. The cruciate ligaments are unique in that they are the only ligaments in the knee that are intraarticular and extrasynovial, without capsular attachments. The ACL is a complex structure with well-defined tibial and femoral attachments that allow at least a portion of the ligament to remain taut and to function with all degrees of knee motion. The intricate anatomy of the ACL has been studied and illustrated in fine detail by Arnoczky[1] and by Girgis et al.[12]

In general, surgical treatment of the ACL can be grouped into three broad categories: extraarticular, intraarticular, and combined procedures. Intraarticular procedures can be further divided into two types: "over-the-top" and transcondylar procedures. In the over-the-top method, the grafted tissue is routed over the lateral femoral condyle, then passed through the posterior joint capsule. In transcondylar procedures the grafted tissue is passed through the lateral femoral condyle via a predrilled bony tunnel. Autogenous tissue, used in intraarticular reconstructions, has included portions of the patellar tendon, fascia lata, iliotibial tract, meniscus, and the medial hamstring tendons. Recently, freeze-dried, or fresh frozen allografts of the patellar tendon, Achilles tendon, foot extensor tendons, and fascia lata have been and are being used as graft substitutes. Experience with bovine xenografts has been disappointing. Prosthetic grafts will probably be used more in the future, but presently only Gore-Tex (polytetrafluoroethylene) and Dacron are commonly used. The ligament augmentation device (LAD) is also being used in the United States as augmentation tissue in ACL substitutions.

Excellent reviews of the medical literature on ACL reconstruction have been contributed by Quinten and Fowler,[42] Rovere and Adair,[46] and Sisk.[49] Intraarticular reconstruction of the ACL utilizing the semitendinosus or gracilis tendon is the subject of this chapter.

SEMITENDINOSUS AS ANTERIOR CRUCIATE LIGAMENT SUBSTITUTE

Before an autogenous tissue can be used as an ACL substitute the graft must fulfill several requirements. At the very least, the size, length, and strength of the graft should be sufficient to be placed in the joint and secured to the tibia and femur. Biologic tissue should be able to revascularize, recollagenize, and attempt to duplicate the function of the ACL. In addition, the tissue must be convenient to harvest, and the resultant absence of the tissue in the donor area must not produce another weakness or deficiency.

Inasmuch as most intraarticular ACL reconstructions usually require a drill hole through the proximal and medial aspects of the tibia, in juxtaposition to the medial hamstring tendons, no extra incisions are needed to harvest the semitendinosus with a tendon stripper. Because no additional incision is needed to harvest the semitendinosus, the patient benefits cosmetically and from less surgical morbidity. The semitendinosus is thus frequently used with the newer arthroscopically assisted procedures.

The anatomic considerations in harvesting the semitendinosus tendon were the subject of a cadaver study by Ferrari and Ferrari.[9] They reported the semitendinosus to have a tendinous portion with an average length of 23 cm. This would thus provide a sufficient graft length for most ACL reconstructions. The anatomy of the distal insertion of the semitendinosus is variable. In a significant percentage of patients, the semitendinosus gave off one or more slips which insert into the gastrocnemius fascia. Thus, when harvesting the semitendinosus with a tendon stripper, the authors recommended that one first cut the slips given off to the fascial attachment of the gastrocnemius prior to stripping. Otherwise the graft diameter could be greatly compromised.

Gomes and Marczyk,[14] however, reported a complication from harvesting the semitendinosus: in four of their first ten patients they noted subcutaneous tissue adherence to the muscle belly of the semitendinosus. In their technique, however, they made a proximal incision, detaching the semitendinosus and suturing it to the semimembranosus during harvesting of the graft. They recommended careful closure over the muscular aponeurosis to prevent this condition.

Loss of the semimembranosus tendon has not led to a decrease, clinically, in overall hamstring strength of the knee.[3] Lipscomb et al.[30] and others, in a retrospective Cybex study of 51 semitendinosus grafts, found that no significant loss of hamstring strength occurred when the semitendinosus and gracilis tendons, alone, or in combination, are used to reconstruct the ACL. The effect of the loss of the semitendinosus and gracilis on medial rotation of the knee has never been assessed.

Cross et al.,[6] with the use of magnetic resonance imaging, electromyographic studies, and strength testing in clinical examination, have demonstrated an apparent regeneration of the tendons of the semitendinosus and gracilis after their use for ACL reconstruction. The results of their study suggest that the tendons of the semitendinosus and gracilis can regrow in a near-anatomic position and are probably functional. Their postulated mechanism for this regeneration is that the regrowth occurs in the distal cut end of the muscle belly following the fascial planes to the popliteal fossa.

The inherent strength and ultimate fate of the semitendinosus tendon apparently make it an adequate intraarticular ACL substitute. Noyes et al.[35, 36] have shown with in vitro laboratory studies that the semitendinosus is approximately 70% as strong as the normal ACL, and the gracilis tendon was found to have 50% of the strength of the ACL. The strength of the semitendinosus (and gracilis) tendon graft can theoretically be doubled by using it in a looped fashion; this conceivably would make the graft stronger than the normal ACL. Kennedy et al.[23] however, demonstrated in an in vivo rabbit semitendinosus tendon study that at 6 months after operation an intraarticular grafted semitendinosus tendon lost 50% of its strength and was still undergoing degeneration.

Lipscomb et al.[28] examined two reconstructed semitendinosus tendons at 11 and 12 months postoperatively at a second operation. They found that the tendon-to-bone healing in both the femur and the tibia was intact. The ruptured tendons had very much the appearance of acute intrasubstance tears of the ACL. Histologic examination of the ruptured tendons showed each to be viable, with normal-appearing collagen and nuclei; few chronic inflammatory cells were present.

Paddu and Ippolito[41] reported a histologic study of an intraarticular portion of a semitendinosus graft at 16 months postoperation. At reinjury the tendon was ruptured 1 cm from its femoral insertion. Microscopic examination of the tendon showed structural changes that rendered the tendon viable as a whole, and it appeared, from a histologic point of view, that the semitendinosus tendon at 16 months was still structurally being converted to a ligament.

Zaricznyj[53] performed a biopsy of a semitendinosus graft specimen 7½ years postoperatively. The histologic study showed well-organized fibrous bundles and cells.

Howell et al.[21] performed serial magnetic resonance imaging of medial hamstring autografts during the first year after implantation. An increased magnetic resonance signal of the ACL graft was observed to be regionalized and confined to the distal two thirds of the intraarticular portion of the graft. They postulated that the increased magnetic resonance signal is related to an increase in the water concentration, representing graft edema. Thus, there may be an inverse relationship with an increase in graft signal indicating a decrease in graft strength over time. However, comparison of the magnetic resonance signal observed in clinically stable and unstable knees failed to show any statistically significant difference. The magnetic resonance signal in the graft could not be used to predict which graft would ultimately fail within the first year of implantation.

From the above it can be shown that the semitendinosus (or gracilis) tendon possesses the basic qualifications to be used as an ACL substitute, and subsequently it has been used in a significant number of surgical techniques. In fact, the semitendinosus and gracilis tendons have probably been used either alone or in combination with other structures more than any other tissue in the intraarticular reconstruction of the ACL.

In the numerous attempts to correct ACL deficiency the semitendinosus tendon has been used in combined intraarticular and extraarticular procedures, either alone or with a gracilis tendon, as a single strand, or in a double loop. It has been used as a free graft or attached either proximally or distally. It has been used in acute repair of the ACL alone or as an augmentation to direct repair of the ACL. In the chronically deficient knee it has been used alone or in combination with extraarticular procedures. Recently, the semitendinosus has been used in arthroscopically aided ACL reconstructions, either in acute or chronic ACL insufficiency.

From the number of operative procedures described using the semitendinosus tendon, it can be seen that in ACL reconstruction in general there is still no single best way to use the semitendinosus tendon to substitute for the damaged ACL. A review of the various semitendinosus tendon techniques that have been used is detailed below.

Attempts have been made to use the semitendinosus (or gracilis) tendon as a dynamic stabilizer of the ACL-deficient knee. Lindemann[27] reported on dynamic intraarticular transfer of the gracilis tendon in ACL reconstruction. DuToit[7] and Thompson et al.[50] used a gracilis tendon in a similar manner. Lange[24] modified Lindemann's operation by using the semitendinosus tendon as a dynamic intraarticular stabilizer in the ACL-deficient knee. Ficat et al.[8] used the semitendinosus and more recently Gartke and Portner[11] reported on the results of their modification of the Heidelberg operation, which transferred the semitendinosus through the knee and into the tibia, where it acted as a dynamic stabilizer. Whether these transfers actually act dynamically to stabilize the ACL-deficient knee remains controversial.

Numerous procedures using the semitendinosus (or gracilis) tendon as a static intraarticular knee stabilizer have been reported in the medical literature. Larsen,[25] Warren,[52] and Sgaglione et al.[47] have described procedures using the semitendinosus tendon to augment repair of the acutely injured ACL. In these techniques the semitendinosus is divided proximally and passed through a drill hole in the proximal tibia, then rerouted over the top of the lateral femoral condyle. Similarly, Horne and Parson,[20] in the chronically ACL-deficient knee, passed a semitendinosus tendon through a tibial drill hole, then over the top of the lateral femoral condyle.

Zarins and co-workers[55, 56] used the semitendinosus tendon and the iliotibial band in a combined intraarticular and extraarticular method of ACL reconstruction in which both the semitendinosus tendon and iliotibial tract are routed from opposite directions over the top of the lateral femoral condyle and through the same oblique drill hole in the proximal part of the tibia (Fig 45–1).

Cho[3] was among the first to use the semitendinosus as a single intraarticular strand to replace a damaged ACL. In his procedure, which was developed to avoid extensive surgical dissection, the semi-

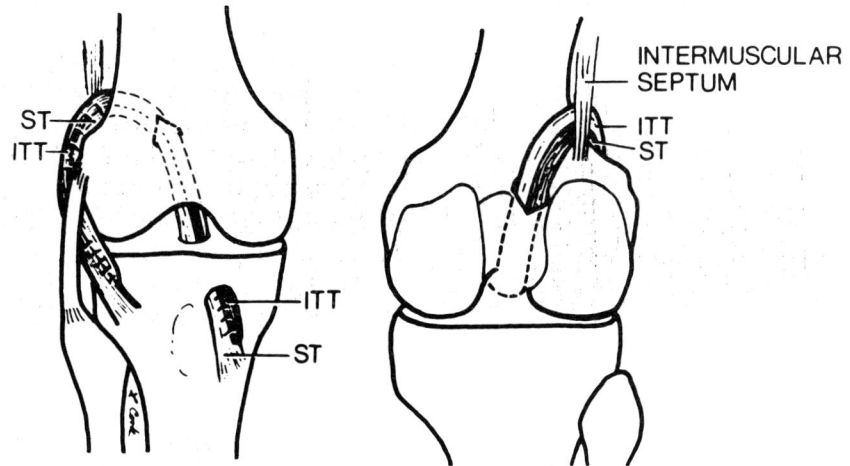

FIG 45–1.
Semitendinosus tendon (ST) and iliotibial band (ITT) are routed from opposite directions over the top of the lateral femoral condyle. (From Zarins B, Rowe C: J Bone Joint Surg [Am] 68:166, 1986. Used by permission.)

tendinosus is divided at its musculotendinous proximal portion and rerouted through the knee through drill holes in the proximal tibia and lateral femoral condyle. The free end of the graft is secured with sutures over the iliotibial band (Fig 45–2).

Lipscomb et al.[29] reported early results using Cho's semitendinosus procedure combined with reefing of the posteromedial capsular ligament. They later modified this technique to use the semitendinosus tendon and gracilis tendon, routing both tendons through drill holes in the tibia and femur. Both tendons were left attached distally on the tibia and secured to the femur with sutures tied subperiosteally on the lateral femoral condyle.

Paddu,[40] in an attempt to retain the flexion and internal rotation functions of the semitendinosus, developed a method of ACL reconstruction in which the distally detached semitendinosus tendon is routed through a proximal medial tibial hole, then enters a tunnel in the lateral femoral condyle. The free end of the graft is sutured to the iliotibial tract (Fig 45–3). All of his cases were associated with extraarticular reconstruction. Sisk[49] modified the Zarins procedure by rerouting the distally detached semitendinosus tendon in a fashion similar to Paddu and combining this with over-the-top placement of the distally based strap of iliotibial band (Fig 45–4).

Gomes and Marczyk[14] used a free graft of a loop of double-thickness semitendinosus tendon to reconstruct the ACL. A single drill hole was made in the tibia and lateral femoral condyle and the graft secured in the drill holes by the trephined plugs of local bone graft. They also combined this procedure with extraarticular repair of the capsular structures.

Zaricznyj[53] reported on 27 patients who underwent intraarticular semitendinosus graft reconstruction of the ACL. He initially routed a free, or distally detached, semitendinosus tendon through a single tibial and femoral drill hole and secured the tendon ends to the tibia and femur with standard bone staples. He later modified this technique[56] and used a loop of semitendinosus tendon through two tibial drill holes and a single femoral drill hole. The graft was secured by tying sutures over the drill hole in the lateral femoral condyle (Fig 45–5).

In an attempt to reconstruct the major anatomic bands of the ACL, Mott[34] developed the semitendinosus anatomic reconstruction (STAR) technique. In this procedure the semitendinosus is routed through two tibial and two femoral drill holes to reproduce the anterior and posterior bundles of the ACL.

Others who have used the semitendinosus or gracilis tendon in ACL reconstructions include Bousquet,[2] Macey,[31] McMaster et al.,[33] and Ramadier and Benoit.[43]

Recently, arthroscopically assisted techniques using the semitendinosus tendon have been used to reconstruct the ACL-deficient knee. Johnson[22] has used a loop of semitendinosus tendon to reconstruct the ACL and to augment the acute repair of the ACL. He arthroscopically routes the semitendinosus into the knee through two tibial drill holes, and then with an arthroscopic staple secures the loop of semitendinosus to the lateral femoral condyle.

Friedman[10] arthroscopically reconstructs the ACL with a double loop of semitendinosus and gracilis tendon passed through a single tibial and femoral drill hole. He attaches the tendinous loops of the graft to the tibial drill hole with a screw and washer, and the more ribbony portion of the composite graft is secured to the lateral femoral condyle with a double-staple technique. In obtaining osseous fixation of the graft in this manner, he is able to use the strongest

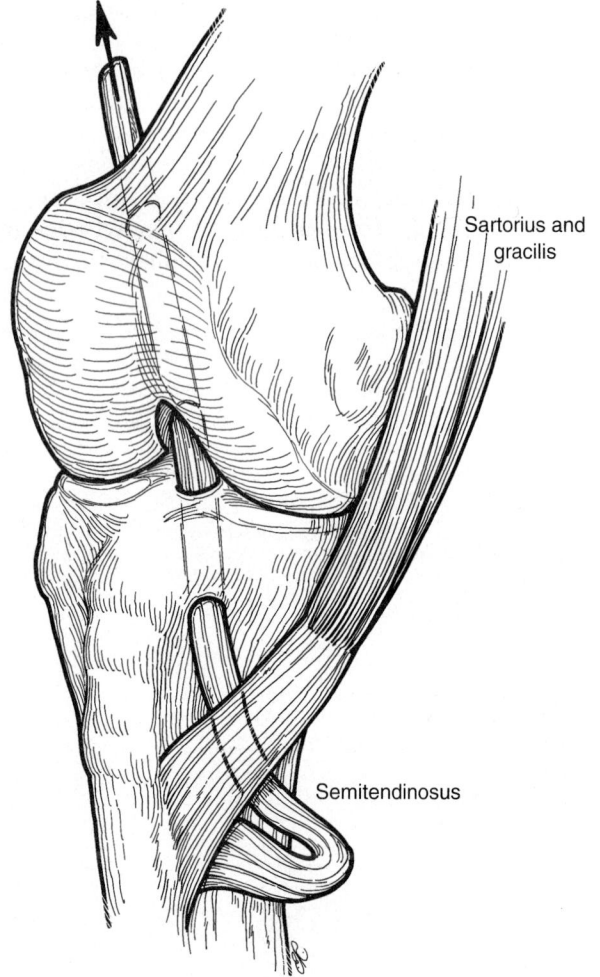

FIG 45–2.
In the technique used by Cho,[3] the semitendinosus is routed through a drill hole in the tibia and femur.

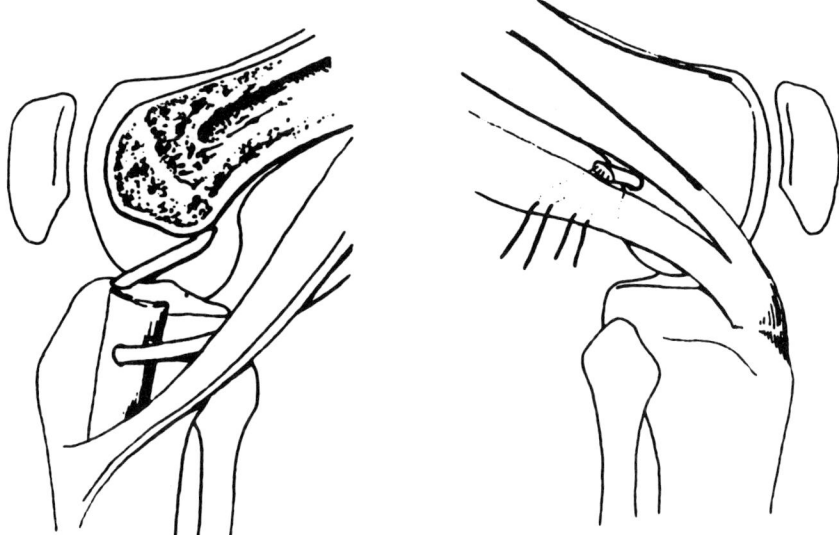

FIG 45-3.
By starting the tibial drill hole more medially, the internal rotation function of the semitendinosus muscle is preserved. (From Paddu G: *Am J Sports Med* 8:15, 1980. Used by permission.)

part of the graft as the intraarticular portion. Sgaglione et al.[48] have reported on the results of a similar procedure, combined with the use of a braided polypropylene augmentation device.

Sisk[49] has developed an arthroscopically aided technique to reconstruct the ACL. In acute cases he uses only the semitendinosus, and in chronic reconstructions the semitendinosus and gracilis tendons are used in combination. In his technique the tendon(s) is left attached distally, then routed through a tibial and femoral drill hole. The free end(s) is secured to the lateral femoral condyle with a screw and washer.

Larsen[26] uses a similar technique of arthroscopically aided reconstruction of the ACL. However, in his technique the semitendinosus is routed over the lateral femoral condyle.

An arthroscopic ACL reconstruction using multiple strands of medial hamstring tendons and a femoral half-tunnel has been reported by Rosenberg[45] (Fig 45-6).

I have developed an arthroscopic semitendinosus ACL reconstruction procedure using a single tibiofemoral tunnel. This procedure is described in detail later in this chapter.

TECHNICAL CONSIDERATIONS

No matter the intraarticular technique used to stabilize the ACL-deficient knee, certain basic principles must be observed. The surgeon must realize that the anatomy and microstructure of the ACL are complex and impossible to recreate. The ultimate goal of surgery is to establish an isometric gross check rein that will function in a similar capacity as the normal ACL. The common goal of the various intraarticular procedures is thus to position the grafted structure isometrically so that its length does not change with range of motion of the knee. To properly position the intraarticular graft, either by arthrotomy or arthroscopically, the surgeon must be familiar with the normal tibial and femoral insertions of the ACL.

Most in vitro and cadaver studies have shown

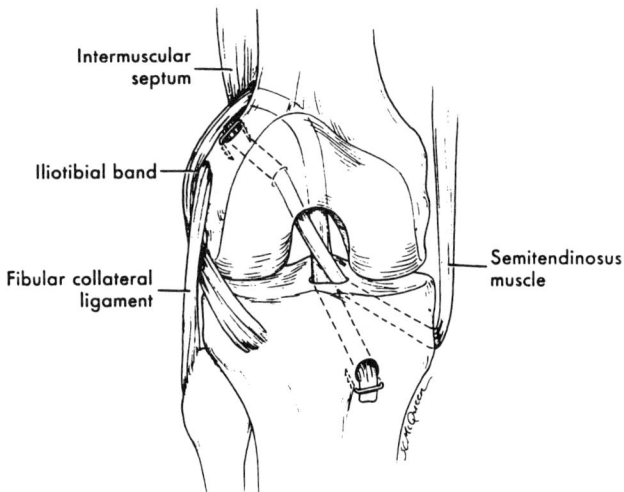

FIG 45-4.
Modified Zarins procedure; see text for discussion. (From Sisk TD: Knee injuries. In Crenshaw AB, editor: *Campbell's operative orthopaedics*, ed 7, vol 3, St Louis, 1987, Mosby-Year Book, p 2283. Used by permission.)

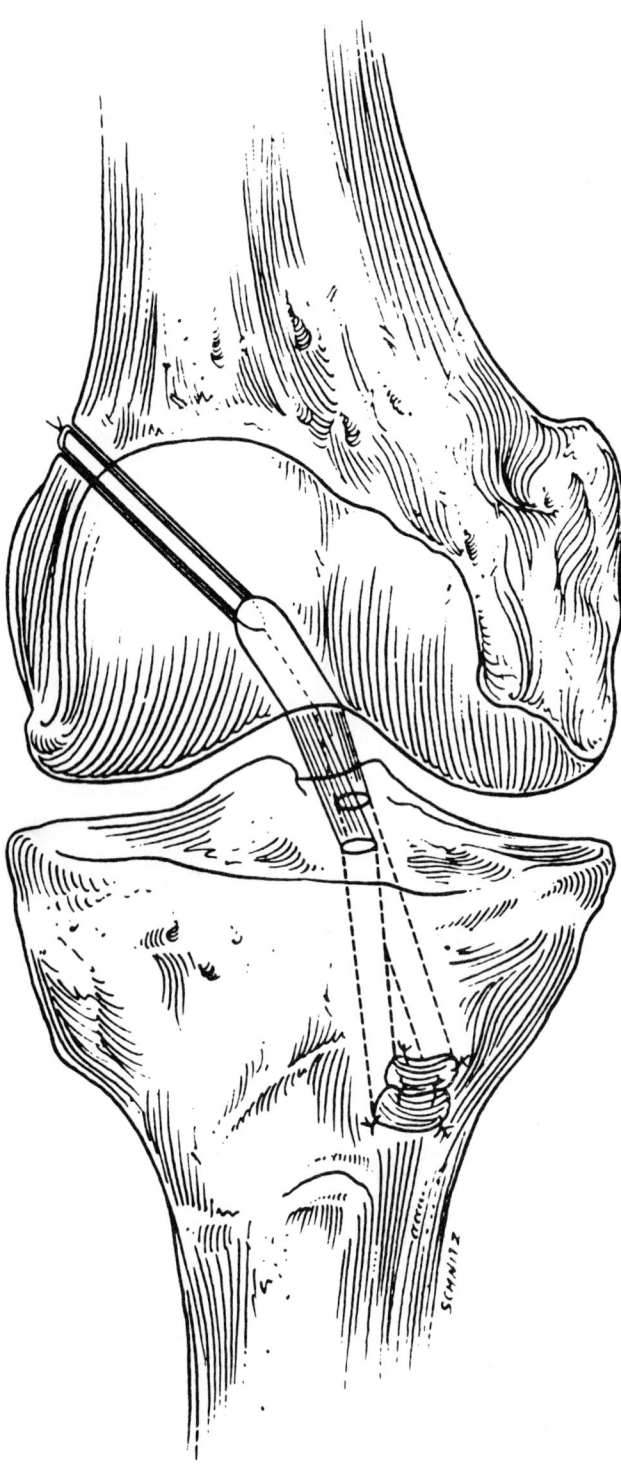

FIG 45-5.
A loop of semitendinosus is passed through the tibia in two different drill holes. (From Zaricznyj B: *Clin Orthop* 220:167, 1987. Used by permission.)

that the optimal isometric position of the intraarticular graft has been with the center of the graft passing through the centers of osseous attachment of the normal ACL.[13, 19, 37] The over-the-top position is considered to be the least favorable with regard to isometry. In actual clinical practice, good results have been reported with over-the-top techniques; however, most of these techniques recommend a grooving or channeling on the superior portion of the lateral femoral condyle in conjunction with passing the graft over the top.

In procedures using drill holes in the tibia and lateral femoral condyle, the surgeon must be able to recognize the "target zones," or tibial and femoral starting points for placement of the guide pin. Normally, the target zones are placed in the centers of attachment of the normal ACL (Figs 45-7 and 45-8). Clancy[4, 5] has demonstrated that as the guide pin is overdrilled the center of the grafted structure shifts posteriorly and laterally in the tibial portion of the tunnel and anteriorly and inferiorly in the femoral bony tunnel. He thus recommends shifting the tibial target zone slightly anterior and medial and the femoral target zone slightly superior and posterior.

The tibial target zone can easily be reached with freehand methods, but drilling a guide pin into the femoral target zone, unless one is passing through the tibia, is difficult, if not impossible, to accomplish from inside the joint. Hoogland and Hillen[19] found this impossible in cadaver knee experiments, but Friedman[10] was able arthroscopically to pass a guide pin into the femoral isometric point. However, to drill over this guide pin it must first be passed retrograde through the lateral femoral condyle; then the cannulated drill is passed over the guide pin from outside the lateral femoral condyle toward the intercondylar notch.

Because the femoral isometric point is difficult to enter from inside the joint, most drill guides, including the new rear-entry models, drill the femoral guide pin from outside the lateral femoral condyle inward. When the femoral tunnel is created from outside to inside (Fig 45-9), the tunnel usually starts too far lateral and approaches the anatomic axis of the normal ACL at an angle. In Figure 45-10 it can be seen that line *B-B'* and line *A-A'* do not coincide with line *AB*, the anatomic center of the normal ACL. The graft will be placed in the joint anatomically; however, the tunnels approaching the graft come in at angles, decreasing the biomechanical advantages of the ACL graft.

Newer methods using a single tunnel, or unitunnel, technique have been developed to drill the femoral tunnel from inside the femoral intercondylar notch outward through the lateral femoral condyle.

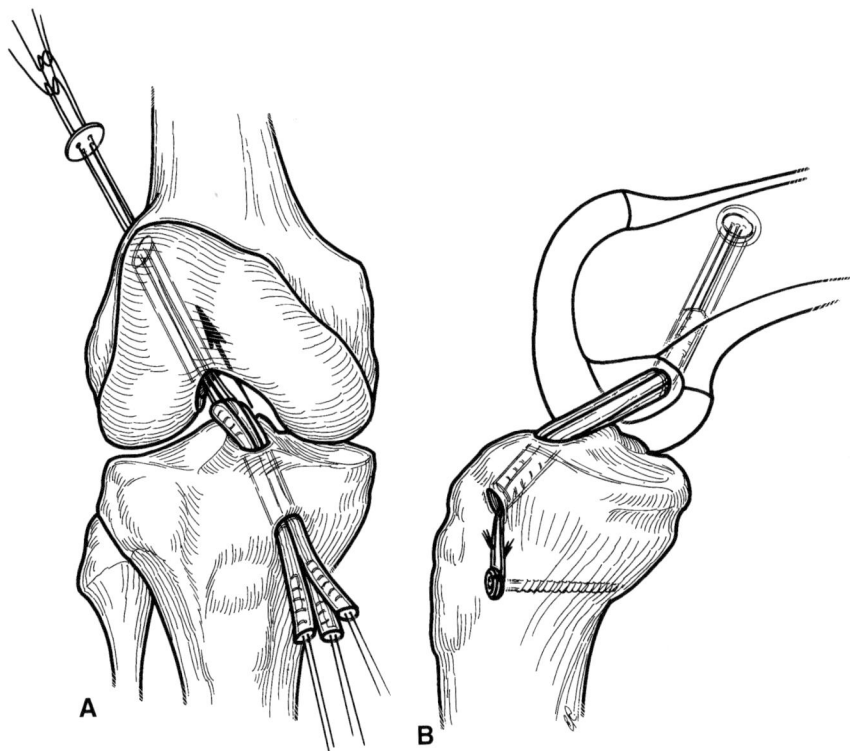

FIG 45-6.
In Rosenberg's endoscopic technique, semitendinosus reconstruction is achieved with triple or quadruple grafts.

With a single-tunnel technique a graft can be placed along the anatomic center of the ACL without creating sharp angles in the graft. Figure 45-11 shows that in addition to the graft being placed anatomically, lines *A-A'* and *B-B'* coincide with the anatomic center of the normal ACL; this optimizes the biomechanical advantages and makes insertion of the graft much easier. A single-tunnel technique may optimize the biomechanical advantages of the graft, and Odensten and Gillquist[38] have postulated that at least the torque forces on the graft in the frontal plane will be reduced. Ease of graft insertion is obvious with the unitunnel technique, because it is a straight pass

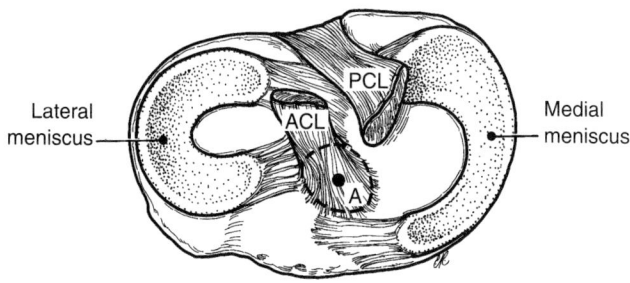

FIG 45-7.
Point *A* represents the anatomic center of attachment of the anterior cruciate ligament *(ACL)* on the tibia. PCL = posterior cruciate ligament.

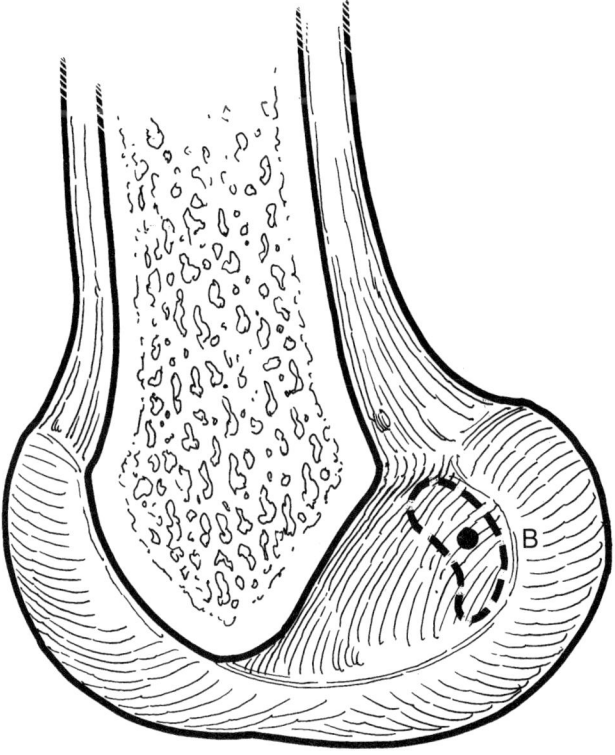

FIG 45-8.
Point *B* represents the anatomic center of attachment of the anterior cruciate ligament on the femur.

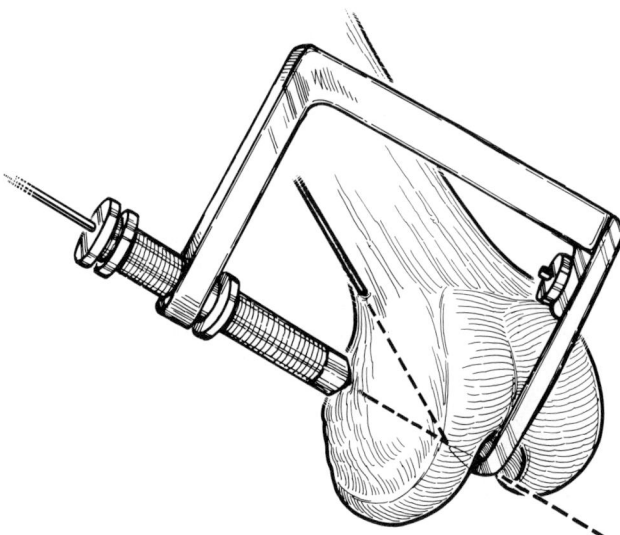

FIG 45-9.
With a standard drill guide, the Kirschner wire is usually started too far laterally.

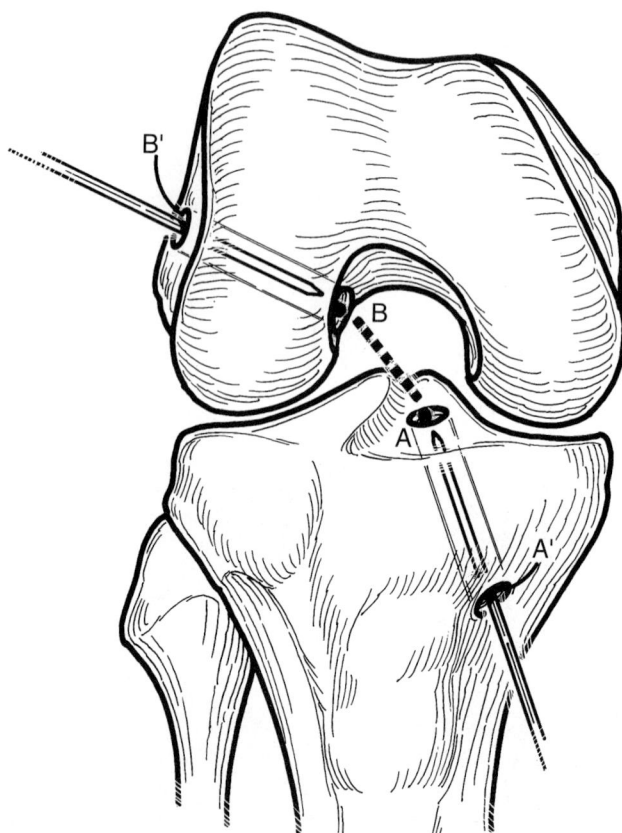

FIG 45-10.
Tunnels approaching the graft come in at angles; see text.

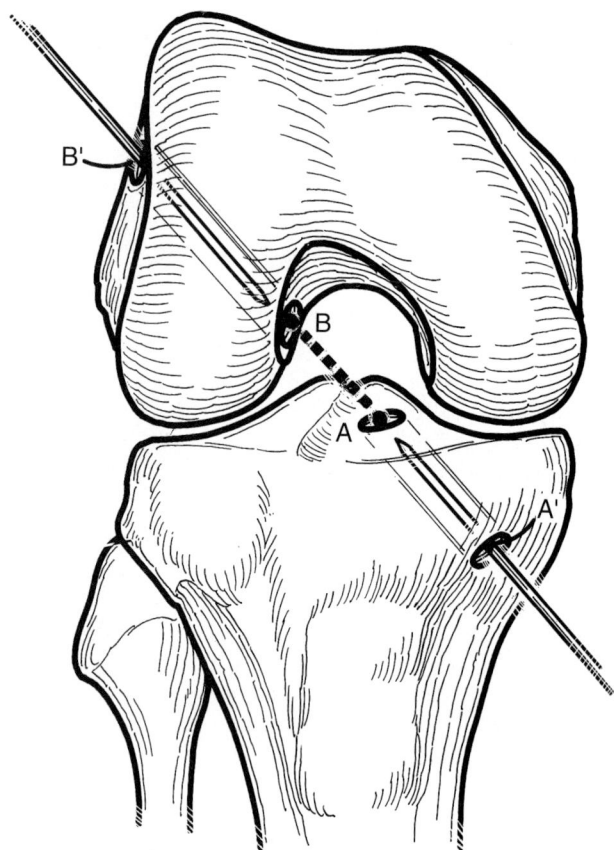

FIG 45-11.
Using a single-tunnel technique, the graft can be placed along the anatomic center of the anterior cruciate ligament; see text.

through both bones and the graft does not have to pass around an angle to enter the femoral bony tunnel.

Several drill guides have been developed for use with a single-tunnel technique. Odensten and Gillquist[38] have developed instrumentation for the unitunnel insertion of an ACL graft; however, their drill guide requires arthrotomy of the knee. Rehm and Schultheis[44] used an arthroscopically assisted method of performing this procedure, but the drill guide used was "extraarticular" and they essentially arthroscopically monitored a "freehand" method of creating a single tibiofemoral tunnel. To eliminate the need for arthrotomy and to facilitate accurate placement of a single tibiofemoral tunnel, I have developed an intraarticular arthroscopic drill guide. The drill guide and my technique are described in detail below.

Goble,[13] Rosenberg,[45] and Wainer et al.[51] have used a technique similar to the unitunnel technique without the use of a drill guide for the femoral portion of the tunnel.

Isometric positioning of the graft, especially the femoral attachment, is probably the single most important technical factor in determining the long-term success of an intraarticular ACL graft. It has been demonstrated that when isometry is tested intraoperatively, the accuracy of graft placement is increased.[17] Recently, tensioning and isometric testing devices have been developed to aid the surgeon in proper positioning of the intraarticular graft.

No matter the intraarticular technique used, certain biomechanical principles must be observed. To eliminate stress points in the graft, an adequate "notchplasty," including the "roof" of the intercondylar notch, must be performed, and it is generally recommended that the intraarticular edges of the bony tunnels be beveled.

Osseous fixation of a semitendinosus graft has been accomplished with a variety of fixation devices, including standard bone staples and orthopaedic screw-and-washer techniques. In several reports,[16, 22, 51] an arthroscopic staple was found to provide adequate fixation of a semitendinosus graft to allow early postoperative motion.

When used as a free graft, the semitendinosus tendon, unlike the patella-tendon graft, has no bone-to-bone healing. Zaricznyj[53, 54] recommends packing bone graft in the tunnels surrounding the semitendinosus graft, and Gomes and Marczyk[14] have used trephined bone plugs to secure the semitendinosus tendon in the bony tibial and femoral tunnels. Perhaps these methods will stimulate more rapid and complete bony ingrowth into the graft, which must ultimately be accomplished to provide the long-term success of a semitendinosus ACL graft. Direct suturing of the free end of the semitendinosus tendon has been used, but usually does not permit early postoperative motion, which is now generally recommended to reduce intraarticular adhesions and to encourage better long-term range of motion of the reconstructed ACL-deficient knee.

HENDLER PROCEDURE

I have developed an arthroscopically assisted unitunnel technique using the semitendinosus tendon to reconstruct the ACL-deficient knee. The essential principle of the unitunnel technique is to create a single tibiofemoral tunnel for placement of a loop of semitendinosus graft so that the central axis of the graft will coincide with the anatomic center of the normal ACL. The procedure requires the use of a specialized drill guide and staple driver for insertion of the semitendinosus graft.

Surgical Technique

After administration of a general anesthetic, the knee is examined for ligamentous laxity and the leg is prepared and draped and the operating room set up as for an arthroscopic procedure. After the landmarks of the knee have been identified, the tibial and femoral incisions are planned. The incision on the tibia should begin 0.75-in. distal to the medial joint line and about 0.75-in. medial to the medial border of the patellar tendon. This cut extends distally, medially, and posteriorly for approximately 2 in., ending at a point over the tract of the semitendinosus tendon. The semitendinosus tendon is then isolated and detached from its tibial insertion. If it appears that the semitendinosus tendon is disproportionately small for the patient's size, then the gracilis tendon is also harvested from the same incision. The cut tendon ends are tagged and passed through the distal end of a tendon stripper. The tendon stripper should be carefully worked proximally into the thigh and the tendon detached at its musculotendinous junction. In a significant number of patients, the distal insertion of the semitendinosus will give off accessory slips attached to the gastrocnemius fascia. These must first be divided with a scissors prior to tendon stripping; otherwise the substance of the tendons could be stripped longitudinally, thus reducing the size of the graft (Fig 45–12).

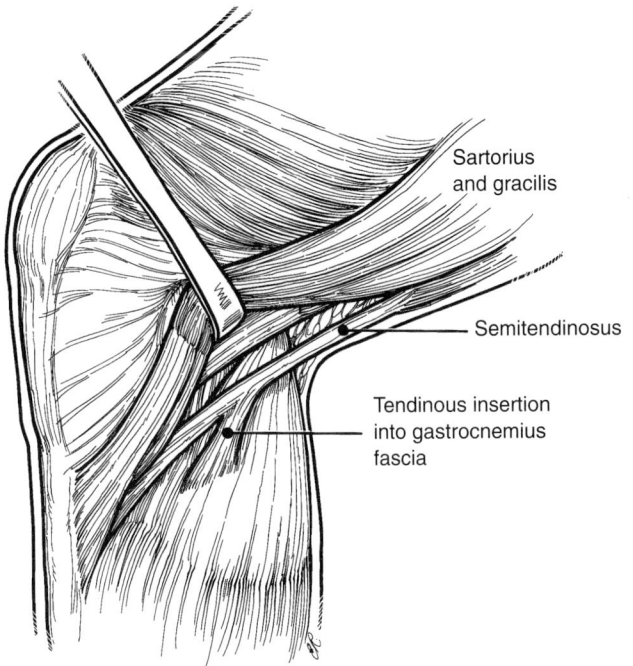

FIG 45–12.
Semitendinosus tendon showing insertion into gastrocnemius fascia which must be divided prior to tendon stripping.

The graft is prepared by removing the muscle fibers from the ribbony portion of the tendons, then "tubing" this area using 4-0 nylon suture. Once prepared, the graft material is stored in a blood-soaked sponge.

A femoral incision is made for later testing the isometry of the graft placement and for using the optional femoral post of the unitunnel drill guide. The lateral femoral condyle is then exposed at the junction of the posterior and lateral borders of the femur, where the metaphysis begins to flare away from the diaphysis of the femur.

After harvesting the semitendinosus graft and making the femoral incision, the arthroscopic portion of the procedure begins. Routine diagnostic arthroscopy and arthroscopic treatment of any associated disorder should be done first, followed by debridement of the soft tissue in the intercondylar notch area. The notch should then be widened with a large motorized abrader and small chisels until there is adequate visualization and no bony areas that could impinge on the graft structure. After the intercondylar notch has been prepared, the intraarticular post of the unitunnel drill guide is introduced into the knee joint. To achieve proper alignment of the guide pin, the semicircular tip of the intraarticular post will rest on the tibial center of the attachment of the ACL or just slightly anteromedial to this point, and the aiming device is then rotated intraarticularly and will touch 2 mm anterior to the femoral center of attachment of the ACL (Fig 45–13). With the knee held in approximately 60 to 90 degrees of flexion, a 3.1-mm guide pin is passed sequentially through the screw mechanism on the tibial guidepost, the proximal portion of the tibia, the semicircular tip of the intraarticular post of the drill guide, and the joint space, and penetrates into the center of the femoral attachment of the ACL and out the lateral surface of the femur. Figure 45–14 demonstrates the proper use of the drill guide on a cadaver knee.

After the guide pin has been passed, the drill guide is disassembled and a channel locator is passed over the guide pin. The guide pin is then removed from the knee joint. A suture is passed along the channel created by the guide pin and attached to an isometer. If the isometry tests normal (i.e., <2 mm excursion of the suture), the suture is removed and the guide pin is reinserted in the same channel. The cannula that introduced the intraarticular portion of the drill guide should remain in the joint to assist in removing the debris generated when the tibial and femoral tunnels are drilled. An 11.1-mm cannulated drill bit should be selected and then passed over the guide pin. For intraarticular fixation with an arthroscopic staple, the single tunnel should extend into the femur to a depth of only 1 cm. The cannulated drill bit is marked at this depth. When the appropriate mark is reached, the drill bit is reversed and forwarded alternately to slightly enlarge the femoral portion of the tunnel. When this has been completed,

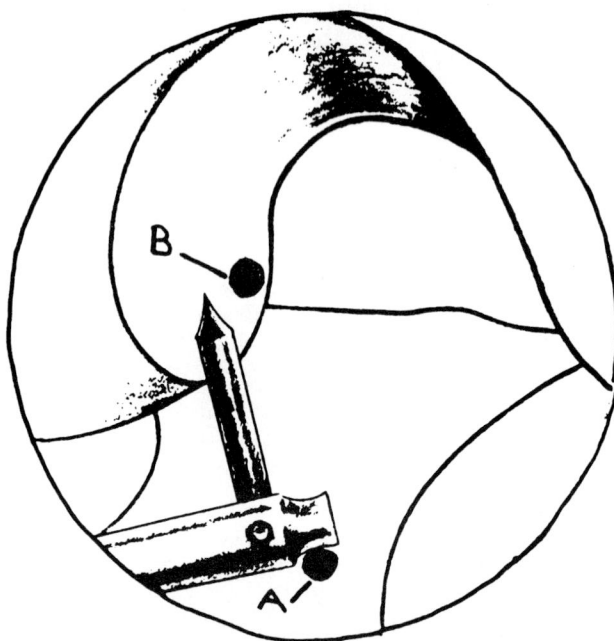

FIG 45–13.
Arthroscopic view of the intraarticular tip of the drill guide. Points A and B represent the tibial and femoral anatomic centers of attachment of the normal anterior cruciate ligament. The tip of the intraarticular post rests on the tibial target zone (point A) and the aiming device is placed slightly forward of the femoral target zone (point B). (From Hendler R: *Tech Orthop* 2:52–59, 1988. Used by permission.)

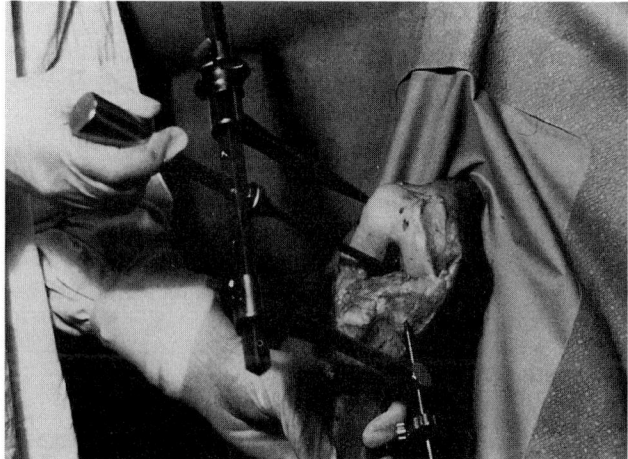

FIG 45–14.
Unitunnel drill guide being used on a cadaver knee. (From Hendler R: *Tech Orthop* 2:52–59, 1988. Used by permission.)

the drill is removed. Once the tunnel is created, the intraarticular space will communicate freely with the external environment. To prevent loss of arthroscopic fluid, a clear plastic cannula and cannulated obturator are passed over the guide pin to plug the tunnel while leaving a working space for passing the graft. The intraarticular openings of the tibial and femoral portions of the tunnel should then be smoothed with an abrader while the obturator is passed only part way through the tibial tunnel. When fixing the graft with an intraarticular staple, the obturator and guide pin should be removed together. This will leave an 11-mm clear plastic cannula in the tunnel for passage of the ACL graft and staple driver. An arthroscopic staple is then placed on a specialized staple driver, and the semitendinosus tendon is looped between the tines of the staple.

When the gracilis tendon is used along with the semitendinosus, both tendons are placed through the tines of the arthroscopic staple and four limbs of tendon graft are created. The limbs are placed 90 degrees circumferentially around the staple driver and sutured to one another with interrupted nylon sutures (Fig 45–15). The "working depth" of the staple with the loop of tendon is approximately 0.625 in. If the staple is driven into the femur past this depth, the graft will be severed; if driven too shallow, the staple will act as a pulley. It is therefore important to control the placement depth of the staple. The staple driver is marked with a series of 0.25-in. reference marks to facilitate this step.

While viewing arthroscopically, the surgeon carefully inserts the loaded staple driver into the cannula until the staple points touch the floor of the femoral portion of the tunnel. At this point the depth guide is locked on the appropriate reference mark. The distance from the end of the cannula to that reference point should be the same as the working length of the staple (Fig 45–16). The driver is then tapped until the depth guide butts against the cannula, indicating that the appropriate depth has been reached. Once secured, the driver is detached from the staple and removed. The graft should be tested for firm placement.

When attachment of the femur is firmly secured, the graft should again be tested for isometry. The surgeon grasps the ends of the semitendinosus tendon graft at the distal opening of the tibial tunnel and, while viewing arthroscopically, places the knee through a range of motion. With the unitunnel technique there should be no tendency for the graft to piston in and out of the tibia.

Once isometric placement is verified, the graft is attached to the tibia under appropriate tension. An

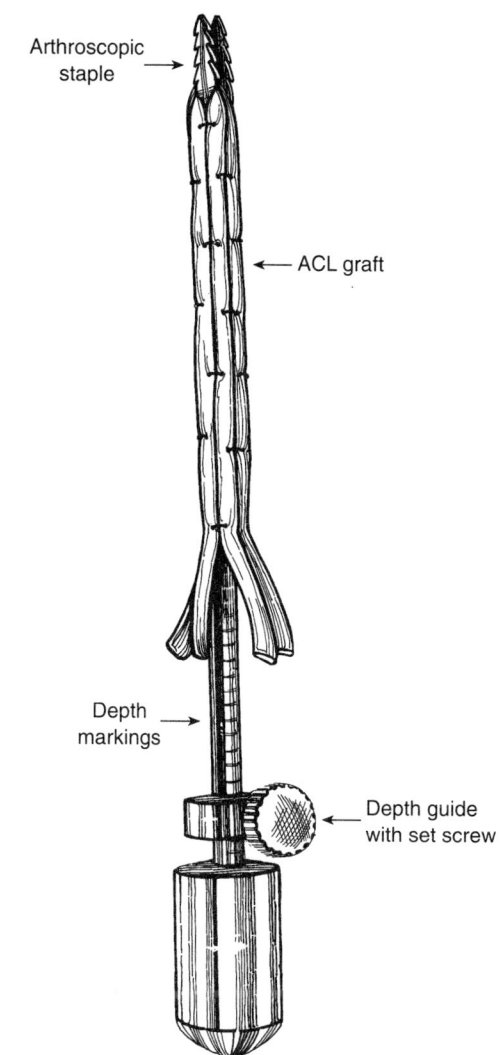

FIG 45–15.
Composite graft of semitendinosus and gracilis tendons affixed to the arthroscopic staple and specialized staple driver with a depth guide to ensure proper penetration of the staple into the lateral femoral condyle; see text. ACL = anterior cruciate ligament.

8-mm bone staple is used, directed so that the tines of the staple are placed within the oval opening of the tibial portion of the tunnel. In this manner, placement is against the posterolateral wall of the tunnel rather than on the flat surface of the proximal medial portion of the tibia. This type of fixation eliminates an additional bend in the graft that could decrease the biomechanical advantages of this technique.

Any excess graft material is excised, and a last arthroscopic look is completed. The final results of this technique are illustrated in Figure 45–17. The correct position of the semitendinosus graft and arthroscopic staple can be seen radiographically in Figure 45–18.

824 SURGICAL MANAGEMENT OF CRUCIATE AND COLLATERAL LIGAMENT INJURIES

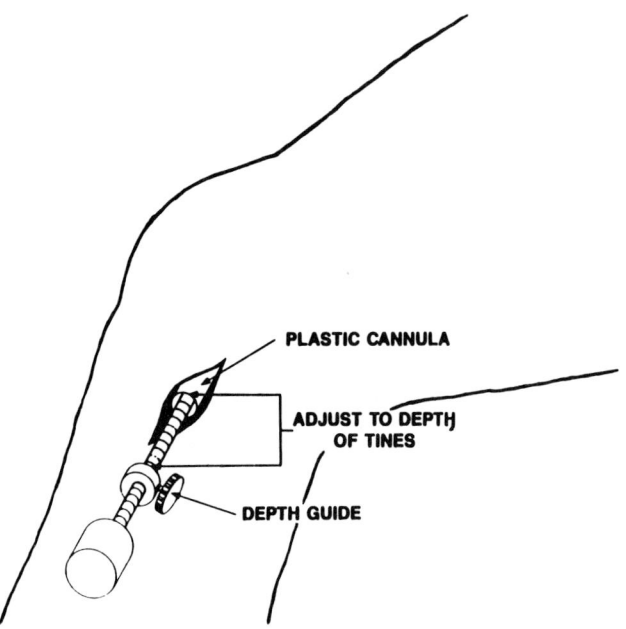

FIG 45–16.
Staple driver in the joint showing its relationship to the clear plastic cannula. The staple driver is driven until the depth guide butts the edge of the plastic cannula, thus assuring proper penetration of the staple tines into the femur. (From Hendler R: *Tech Orthop* 2:52–59, 1988. Used by permission.)

Wound Closure and Postoperative Care

With the graft firmly attached, wound closure can be done in the normal manner. The incisions may be infiltrated with a bupivacaine hydrochloride (Marcaine) and epinephrine solution. The procedure can often be done on an outpatient basis when it has been accomplished with a single tibial incision.

The postoperative immobilization and physical therapy programs are similar to those for routine open ACL reconstructions. It is recommended that a derotation-type brace be worn for activities of daily living for at least 9 months, and indefinitely for strenuous activities such as athletics.

CONCLUSION

In an earlier report, the results of 102 cases using a unitunnel technique for ACL reconstruction, performed at four different centers, was presented.[15] Further personal experience with the above arthroscopic technique of intraarticular semitendinosus grafting has continued to produce encouraging results which greatly reduce surgical morbidity without compromising the surgical result. Longer-term follow-up has shown that the results have not deteriorated with time. It can be seen from the review of the literature that the studies which have used the medial hamstring tendon intraarticularly to reconstruct the ACL have consistently produced, by consensus, good to excellent results. Presently, the so-called gold standard that one uses to compare the results of various intraarticular ACL reconstructive techniques is the middle one third of the patellar tendon. Several studies have compared the use of the semitendinosus and gracilis tendons to the middle third of the patellar tendon. Holmes et al.[18] have done a retrospective direct comparison of the semi-

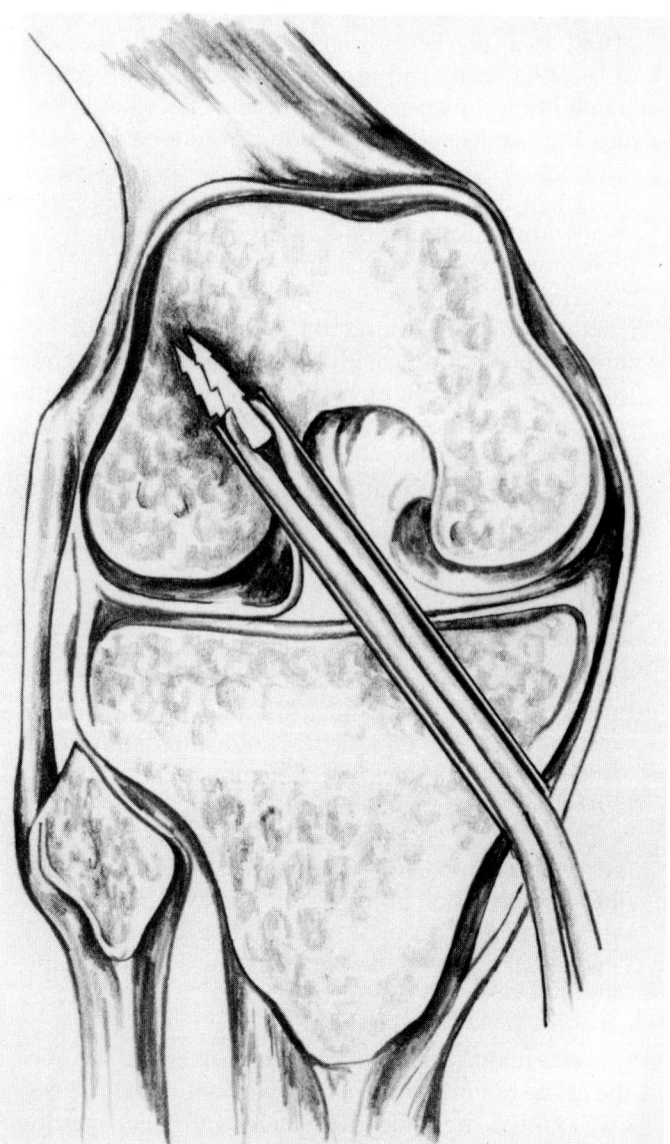

FIG 45–17.
Arthroscopic staple instrument (Instrument Makar, Inc., Okemos, Mich.) affixes a loop of semitendinosus tendon to the floor of the femoral part of the tunnel that has been drilled 1 cm into the lateral femoral condyle. Tibial fixation is obtained with a standard bone staple. (From Hendler R: *Tech Orthop* 2:52–59, 1988. Used by permission.)

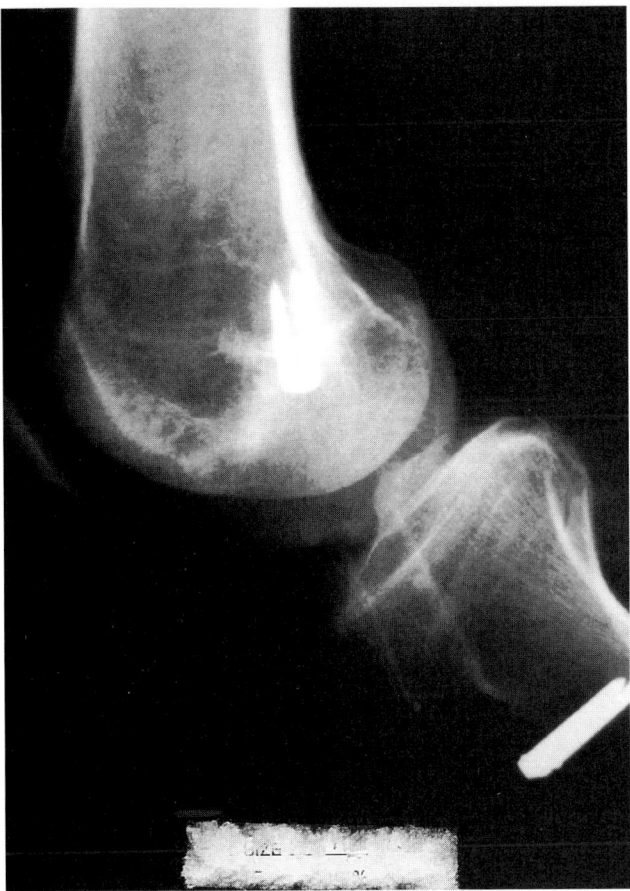

FIG 45-18.
Postoperative lateral radiograph showing the position of the arthroscopic staple. Note the position of the staple just anterior to the posterior cortex of the lateral femoral condyle. (From Hendler R: *Tech Orthop* 2:52-59, 1988. Used by permission.)

tendinosus tendon vs. the middle third of the patellar tendon. They found that the patellar tendon was superior to the semitendinosus tendon in reconstructing chronically unstable knees. However, their technique of intraarticular reconstruction used the over-the-top method, which may have contributed to less-than-optimal results. The semitendinosus, when used in this manner, would not be considered to be isometrically placed and may not have become securely affixed to bone as it would with a transcondylar technique.

Marder et al.[32] reported the results of a prospective evaluation of an arthroscopically assisted ACL reconstruction of the patellar tendon graft vs. the combined semitendinosus and gracilis tendons. In their study, a double-looped semitendinosus and gracilis tendon was passed through the lateral femoral condyle. No significant differences were noted between the groups with respect to subjective complaints, functional level, or objective laxity evaluation. They did, however, find a statistically significant weakness in peak hamstring torque when reconstruction was performed with a double-looped semitendinosus and gracilis tendon.

Otero et al.[39] also presented the results of a comparison study of the semitendinosus vs. patella tendon autograft. The success rate using the double-looped semitendinosus and gracilis graft was 93%, whereas the patellar tendon graft yielded a 96% success rate. In their opinion, the patellar tendon autograft should be considered the gold standard in ACL reconstructions.

At the present time, therefore, the medial hamstring tendons are only one of several options that can be used for an intraarticular ACL reconstruction with autogenous tissue. Although the middle third of the patellar tendon is generally considered the best autogenous tissue, its use as a graft structure is not without complications which have included rupture of the patellar tendon and fracture of the patella; whereas complications from using the medial hamstring tendons as an autogenous tissue graft are rare. Until a biosynthetic material is developed that will produce long-lasting good results, surgeons will still have to make a choice of the appropriate autogenous tissue or allograft tissue to be used for intraarticular ACL reconstruction. The medial hamstring tendons have produced good to excellent results and their use for intraarticular reconstruction of the ACL should remain a part of the surgeon's armamentarium.

REFERENCES

1. Arnoczky SP: The anatomy of the anterior cruciate ligament, *Clin Orthop* 172:19, 1983.
2. Bousquet G: *Chirurgia del ginocchio*, Rome, 1979, Verduci Editore, pp 191-194.
3. Cho KO: Reconstruction of the anterior cruciate ligament by semitendinosus tenodesis, *J Bone Joint Surg [Am]* 57A:608, 1975.
4. Clancy WG: Anterior cruciate ligament functional instability. A static intra-articular and dynamic extra-articular procedure, *Clin Orthop* 172:102, 1983.
5. Clancy WB: Arthroscopic anterior cruciate ligament reconstruction with patella tendon, *Techn Orthop* 2:13, 1988.
6. Cross MJ et al: Regeneration of the semitendinosus and gracilis tendon following their transection for repair of the anterior cruciate ligament, *Am J Sports Med* 20:2, 1992.
7. DuToit GT: Knee joint cruciate ligament substitution. The Lindemann (Heidelberg) operation, *S Afr J Surg* 5:25, 1967.
8. Ficat P, Cuzachq JP, Ricci A: Chirurgie réparatrice des

laxités chroniques des ligaments croisés du genou, *Rev Chir Orthop* 61:89, 1975.
9. Ferrari JD, Ferrari DA: The semitendinosus: Anatomic considerations in tendon harvesting, *Orthop Rev* 20:12, 1991.
10. Friedman MJ: Arthroscopic semitendinosus (gracilis) reconstruction for anterior cruciate ligament deficiency, *Tech Orthop* 2:74, 1988.
11. Gartke KA, Portner OT: The semitendinosus dynamic transfer for anterior cruciate insufficiency, 39th Annual Meeting, Canadian Orthopaedic Association, Quebec City, June 6–9, 1983; abstract *J Bone Joint Surg [Br]* 66:305, 1984.
12. Girgis FG, Marshall JL, Al Monajem ARS: The cruciate ligaments of the knee. Anatomical, functional and experimental analysis, *Clin Orthop* 106:216, 1975.
13. Goble EM: Fluoro-arthroscopic allograft anterior cruciate reconstruction, *Tech Orthop* 2:65, 1988.
14. Gomes JLE, Marczyk RS: Anterior cruciate ligament reconstruction with a loop of double thickness semitendinosus tendon, *Am J Sports Med* 12:199, 1984.
15. Hendler R: A unitunnel technique for arthroscopic anterior cruciate ligament reconstruction. The Triennial Scientific Meeting, International Arthroscopy Association, Sydney, Australia, April 2–4, 1987.
16. Hendler R: A unitunnel technique for arthroscopic anterior cruciate ligament reconstruction, *Tech Orthop* 2:52–59, 1988.
17. Hendler R: Isometric placement of an anterior cruciate ligament graft using a single tunnel technique, Annual Meeting of Arthroscopy Association of North America, Washington, DC, March 24–27, 1988; abstract *Arthroscopy* 4:133, 1988.
18. Holmes PF, et al: Retrospective direct comparison of three intraarticular anterior cruciate ligament reconstructions, *Am J Sports Med* 19:6, 1991.
19. Hoogland T, Hillen B: Intra-articular reconstruction of the anterior cruciate ligament: An experimental study of length changes in different ligament reconstructions, *Clin Orthop* 185:197, 1984.
20. Horne JG, Parson CJ: The anterior cruciate ligament: Its anatomy and a new method of reconstruction, *Can J Surg* 20:214, 1977.
21. Howell SM, Clark JA, Blasier RD: Serial magnetic resonance imaging of hamstring anterior cruciate ligament autografts during the first year of implantation, *Am J Sports Med* 19:1, 1991.
22. Johnson LL: Extrasynovial knee conditions. In Johnson LL, editor: *Arthroscopic surgery: Principles and practice,* ed 3, St Louis, 1986, Mosby–Year Book.
23. Kennedy JC, et al: Presidential address: Intra-articular replacement in the anterior cruciate ligament-deficient knee, *Am J Sports Med* 8:1, 1980.
24. Lange M: Orthopädische-chirurgische Operationslehre, ed 2. Munich, 1962, Bergmann, pp 682–700.
25. Larsen RL: Augmentation of the acute ruptured anterior cruciate ligament, *Orthop Clin North Am* 16:135, 1985.
26. Larsen RL: Technique of arthroscopically aided anterior cruciate ligament reconstruction. In Crenshaw AH, editor: *Campbell's operative orthopaedics,* ed 7, vol 3, St Louis, 1987, Mosby–Year Book, p 2455.
27. Lindemann K: Über den plastischen Ersatz Kreutzbänder durch gestielte Sehnenverpflanzung, *Z Orthop* 79:316, 1950.
28. Lipscomb AB, Johnston RK, Synder RB: The technique of cruciate ligament reconstruction, *Am J Sports Med* 9:77, 1981.
29. Lipscomb AB, et al: Secondary reconstruction of anterior cruciate ligament in athletes by using the semitendinosus tendon: Preliminary report of 78 cases, *Am J Sports Med* 7:81, 1979.
30. Lipscomb AB, et al: Evaluation of hamstring strength following use of semitendinosus and gracilis tendons to reconstruct the anterior cruciate ligament, *Am J Sports Med* 10:340, 1982.
31. Macey HB: A new operative procedure for repair of ruptured cruciate ligaments of the knee joint, *Surg Gynecol Obstet* 69:108, 1939.
32. Marder RA, Raskind JR, Carroll M: Prospective evaluation of arthroscopically assisted anterior cruciate ligament reconstruction, *Am J Sports Med* 19:5, 1991.
33. McMaster JH, Weinert CR, Scranton P: Diagnosis and management of isolated anterior cruciate ligament tears: A preliminary report on reconstruction with the gracilis tendon, *J Trauma* 14:230, 1974.
34. Mott HW: Semitendinosus anatomic reconstruction for cruciate ligament insufficiency, *Clin Orthop* 172:90, 1983.
35. Noyes FR, et al: Intra-articular cruciate reconstruction: I: Perspectives on graft strength, vascularization and immediate motion after replacement, *Clin Orthop* 172:71, 1983.
36. Noyes FR, et al: Biomechanical analysis of human ligament grafts used in knee-ligament repairs and reconstructions, *J Bone Joint Surg [Am]* 66:344, 1984.
37. Odensten M, Gillquist J: Functional anatomy of the anterior cruciate ligament and a rationale for reconstruction, *J Bone Joint Surg [Am]* 67:257, 1985.
38. Odensten M, Gillquist J: A modified technique for anterior cruciate ligament surgery using a new drill guide for isometric positioning of the ACL, *Clin Orthop* 213:154, 1986.
39. Otero AL, Schmidt RH, McDermott KL: Arthroscopic anterior cruciate ligament reconstruction—comparison of results following semitendinosus and gracilis vs patellar tendon autografts, *Arthroscopy* 5:1989.
40. Paddu G: Method for reconstruction of the anterior cruciate ligament using the semitendinosus tendon, *Am J Sports Med* 8:402, 1980.
41. Paddu G, Ippolito E: Reconstruction of the anterior cruciate ligament using the semitendinosus tendon: Histologic study of a case, *Am J Sports Med* 11:14, 1983.
42. Quinten MG, Fowler PJ: Reconstruction of the anterior cruciate ligament: Historical overview, *Orthop Clin North Am* 16:143, 1985.

43. Ramadier JO, Benoit J: Reconstruction des ligaments latéraux et croisés. Syndesmoplasties du genou, *Rev Chir Orthop* 58:78, 1972.
44. Rehm KE, Schultheis KH: Endoscopic replacement of the anterior cruciate ligament, *Orthop Praxis* 2:141, 1986.
45. Rosenberg TD: Multistrand ACL reconstruction with femoral half tunnel, Tenth Annual Meeting of the Arthroscopy Association of North America, San Diego, April 24–27, 1991.
46. Rovere GD, Adair DM: Anterior cruciate–deficient knees: A review of the literature, *Am J Sports Med* 11:412, 1983.
47. Sgaglione NA, et al: Primary repair with semitendinosus tendon augmentation of acute anterior cruciate ligament injuries, *Am J Sports Med* 18:64–73, 1990.
48. Sgaglione NA, et al: Arthroscopic-assisted anterior cruciate ligament reconstruction with the semitendinosus tendon: Comparison of results with and without braided polypropylene augmentation, *Arthroscopy* 8:65–77, 1992.
49. Sisk TD: Knee injuries. In Crenshaw AH, editor: *Campbell's operative orthopaedics,* ed 7, vol 3, St Louis, 1987, Mosby–Year Book, p 2283.
50. Thompson SK, Calver R, Monk CJE: Anterior cruciate ligament repair for rotatory instability: Lindemann dynamic muscle-transfer procedure, *J Bone Joint Surg [Am]* 68:917, 1978.
51. Wainer RA, Clarke PJ, Poehling GG: Arthroscopic reconstruction of the anterior cruciate ligament using tendon allograft, *Arthroscopy* 4:199, 1988.
52. Warren RF: Acute ligamentous injuries. In Insall J, editor: *Surgery of the knee,* New York, 1984, Churchill Livingstone.
53. Zaricznyj B: Reconstruction of the anterior cruciate ligament using free tendon graft, *Am J Sports Med* 11:164, 1983.
54. Zaricznyj B: Reconstruction of the anterior cruciate ligament of the knee using a doubled tendon graft, *Clin Orthop* 220:167, 1987.
55. Zarins B, Barnthouse C: Combined intra-articular and extra-articular anterior cruciate ligament reconstruction, *Tech Orthop* 2:60, 1988.
56. Zarins B, Rowe C: Combined anterior cruciate ligament reconstruction using semitendinosus tendon and iliotibial tract, *J Bone Joint Surg [Am]* 68:160, 1986.

46

Anterior Cruciate Ligament Reconstruction With the Kennedy Ligament Augmentation Device

PETER J. FOWLER, M.D., F.R.C.S.(C.)
SAMUEL W. CAPRA, JR., M.D.

Biomechanics of Kennedy ligament augmentation device
Concept of load-sharing with ligament augmentation device
Infection and synovitis
Clinical results

Augmented anterior cruciate ligament reconstruction using semitendinosus tendon
Procedure

Dr. J. C. Kennedy, in his presidential address[15] to the American Orthopaedic Society for Sports Medicine in 1979, summarized the frustration of the orthopaedic community in dealing with the problem of the anterior cruciate ligament (ACL)–deficient knee. Kennedy noted his concerns over the significant decline in tensile strength and increases in laxity seen with biologic substitutes during the revascularization process. He also noted, from personal experience, that there was not yet a truly satisfactory synthetic ligament to replace the human ACL, because of the difficulties of creep and abrasion failure. Kennedy then reported the initial results of his pioneering research on a composite graft featuring biologic tissue with synthetic augmentation. The ligament augmentation device (LAD; Fig 46–1), as it is now known, is the result of these early studies.

The LAD is manufactured from synthetic material. It is a strap of a braided, biocompatible polypropylene yarn. Its purpose is to provide early tensile strength to the composite graft, protecting the biologic tissue from excessive laxity during revascularization. The LAD is designed as a load-sharing device, taking the major load of the forces seen across the composite graft early in the healing phase. As the autogenous or allograft biologic tissue becomes vascularized and regains tensile strength, the majority of the load passes across this portion of the graft, protecting the synthetic portion from long-term creep failure (Fig 46–2).

The goals of the Kennedy LAD, then, are twofold: the first is to prevent the ligamentous laxity often seen in the first year after ligament reconstruction; the second, serendipitous effect is to allow the surgeon to make use of autogenous donor tissue with less immediate postoperative strength than would be required of a purely biologic donor graft.

The LAD has been previously described with an autograft from patellar tendon with prepatellar periosteum and quadriceps tendon tissue—the Marshall-MacIntosh procedure.[4, 5, 15, 23] The LAD has also been used with the semitendinosus tendon, as well as combinations of semitendinosus and gracilis tendons, and with various allograft tissues.[8, 10, 11, 12]

BIOMECHANICS OF KENNEDY LIGAMENT AUGMENTATION DEVICE

The LAD is a 1.5-mm-thick polypropylene braid of nine tows (strands) of polypropylene yarn, each tow containing 180 polypropylene fibers. These tows are woven together in a flat diamond-weave configuration. The LAD is available in both 6- and 8-mm widths. The ends of the strap of the LAD are heat-sealed to prevent unraveling. Strength studies on this synthetic reveal a tensile strength of 1,500 N.[23] Fatigue testing revealed a decrease in tensile strength of approximately 9% at 500,000 cyclic loads. This is approximately equal to the ultimate failure strength of the human ACL and is twice the normal load range

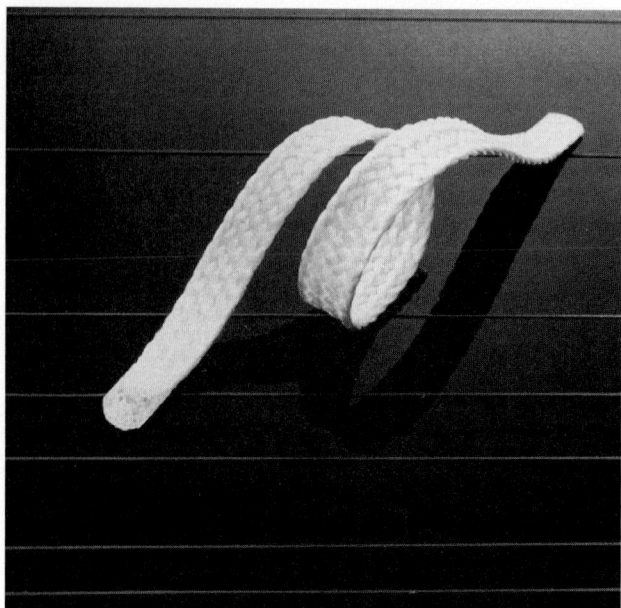

FIG 46–1.
Ligament augmentation device of braided polypropylene.

of the ligament seen in vivo. Cyclic creep test results after 1 million load cycles revealed a mean strain change of 3%.[23]

This suggests that the device should not develop excess laxity in the early postoperative period. The weakest point of the LAD composite construct is found in the suture connection between the synthetic and biologic components. The tensile strength of the suture connection has been shown in animal cadaver studies to be approximately 400 N, more than adequate to allow the load-sharing function of the LAD in the immediate postoperative phase.[20] During the first postoperative year the load-sharing function of the polypropylene is most effective. The biologic graft is still allowed to share some of the load force across the composite, to stimulate collagen organization and maturation of the biologic tissue. As the biologic graft matures and takes more of the load, the LAD is protected from acting as an isolated synthetic ligament replacement. The late problems of pure synthetic grafts, creep laxity and abrasion failure, are thus diminished.

Concept of Load-Sharing with Ligament Augmentation Device

In his initial studies on Marshall-MacIntosh ACL reconstructions in goats, Kennedy tested augmented vs. nonaugmented ACL reconstructions 6 weeks postoperatively.[15] He noted that the augmented reconstruction showed a 74% increase in strength to failure.

Another study using the LAD in combination with a freeze-dried bone-ACL-bone allograft was performed in mature goats.[12] In this model the LAD was released from its tibial fixation at 3 months after operation. Biomechanical, microvascular, and histologic changes were evaluated 1 year after the original procedure. Compared with the same procedure performed without augmentation, the augmented graft was significantly stronger when tested at 1 year. The allograft alone attained approximately 25% of the contralateral normal ACL tensile strength, whereas the augmented allograft was able to obtain 50% of the tensile strength of its contralateral control. At histologic evaluation, cellular repopulation and vascularity of the allograft ACL, with collagen orientation similar to a normal ACL, were noted. Further, there was no evidence of leukocyte infiltration within the allograft and no evidence of synovial inflammation or proliferation in response to the synthetic LAD.

In further support of the load-sharing hypothesis of the LAD is the recent cadaver knee specimen study of Hanley et al.[11] A buckle transducer was used to directly measure the overall force through each portion of two different types of composite grafts. In a

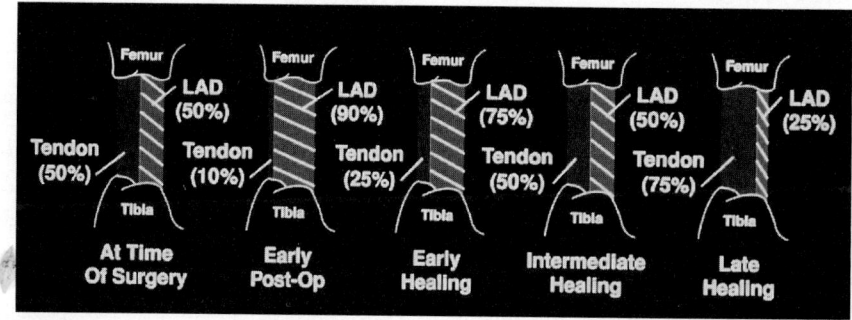

FIG 46–2.
Concept of load-sharing between biologic and synthetic portions of composite graft. Relative widths indicate relative loads. (*Note:* All of total load transfers through tendon attachment to tibia.)

three-segment composite graft of semitendinosus, gracilis, and an LAD, the LAD accepted approximately 45% of the force. In the much stiffer bone–patellar tendon–bone and LAD composite, 28% of the force was transmitted through the LAD.

In a recently completed in vivo study, Fowler and Amendola[8] compared LAD augmented bone-tendon-bone allografts and nonaugmented grafts performed in 50 skeletally mature sheep. Biomechanical testing and quantitative hydroxyproline assays were performed on representative samples of both study groups 4, 16, and 52 weeks postoperatively. The augmented group showed a trend toward increased tensile strength that was statistically significant at both 4 and 16 weeks postoperatively. Anterior laxity showed little difference at the initial postoperative testing, but at 1-year sacrifice the augmented group showed significantly less anterior laxity than the nonaugmented allograft group ($P < 0.02$).

Collagen content as determined by hydroxyproline assay revealed that the presence of an LAD did not affect the collagen content of the biologic graft over time. Histologic evaluation revealed no evidence of any increased inflammatory reaction in the LAD augmentation group as compared with the nonaugmented allograft control group.

INFECTION AND SYNOVITIS

Implantation of any foreign material in the human body is of concern to the orthopaedic surgeon. Does the substance implanted lend itself to an increased incidence of infection? Any intraarticular synthetic ligament must also raise the issue of clinical synovitis related to the implant's immunologic properties. No animal or clinical augmentation series reported to date has revealed an increased infection rate with use of the LAD as compared with a biologic graft alone.[4, 8, 9, 12, 23]

Histologic evaluation in animal studies has occasionally revealed a one- or two-layer macrophage lining surrounding portions of the LAD. Again there has been no correlation with a chronic inflammatory response.[8]

Olsen et al.[21] have shown that all current synthetic ligament materials, including polypropylene, can cause synovial reaction when microfragmented and injected into lapine joints. The reaction caused by polypropylene, measured by host production of collagenases and gelatinases, was similar in magnitude to that produced by the Gore-Tex (polytetrafluoroethylene) and Leeds-Keio synthetic ligaments as well as that from human allograft tissue. The response was markedly less than that brought on by carbon fiber and xenograft (bovine) specimens.

Several authors[4, 9, 23] have noted no clinical evidence of increased incidence of postoperative synovitis with the use of the LAD. This may be due in part to the polypropylene being surrounded by biologic tissue in its intraarticular course, which may lead to a much lower incidence of graft abrasion and particulate release than in a reconstruction with a purely synthetic ligament. Roth et al.[24] reported one case of synovitis secondary to composite graft rupture. At reoperation it appeared that the graft had abraded against the lateral femoral condyle. After removal of the graft tissue the synovitis was noted to resolve, and the patient remains a candidate for a second ACL reconstruction.

CLINICAL RESULTS

The technique of constructing a composite graft of the LAD tubed in a 1-cm strip of quadriceps and patellar tendon, with intervening prepatellar periosteum (Marshall-MacIntosh graft), has been described.[5, 9, 19, 23] The procedure is amenable to either totally open or arthroscopically assisted techniques. The central or medial third of the quadriceps-patellar mechanism can be used.

Between 1979 and his death in 1983, Kennedy performed 143 LAD-augmented ACL reconstructions using the modified Marshall-MacIntosh technique. The initial 43 of these reconstructions were reviewed at a mean follow-up of 4 years.[23] Comparison was made with 45 patients who had undergone the same reconstruction procedure but without augmentation, and with a similar follow-up period. Evaluation included subjective assessment, clinical examination, anterior laxity measurement with the KT-1000 arthrometer, radiographic analysis, Cybex strength analysis, and functional testing by a one-legged hop test. To objective laxity and functional testing the patients with LAD augmentation showed a trend toward better results than those without the LAD. On subjective evaluation, clinical examination, and radiographic analysis, the LAD-augmented group had significantly better results.

A longer follow-up study on the functional stability of 100 of Kennedy's augmented reconstructions was performed by Fowler et al.[9] The results were evaluated at a mean of 7.5 years (range, 5.25–9.0 years) after surgery. Eighty-nine percent of these patients were participating in physical activities at their preinjury stress level, with either no modification or only slight modification of their sports-related activity. Overall evaluation revealed 91% good and excellent functional results. No patient had required a second reconstruction. Ninety-six percent of the patients considered the reconstruction to have been worthwhile.

Results of a multicenter clinical trial of LAD-augmented Marshall-MacIntosh reconstructions performed in the United States were recently released.[4] A long-term prospective clinical trial group of 148 patients with chronic ACL-deficient knees was compared with a group of 31 patients who had undergone nonaugmented Marshall-MacIntosh reconstructions, who served as retrospective controls.

Anterior laxity measurements as tested on the KT-1000 arthrometer, and pivot shift scores were significantly better in the augmented group. Ninety-seven percent of the patients in the LAD-augmented group showed a reduced pivot shift of either grade 0 or grade 1 at an average 3-year follow-up after surgery. Kaplan-Meier statistical failure analysis was performed in the study group, and revealed a 92% probability of successful maintenance of the augmented reconstruction over a 4-year period.

AUGMENTED ANTERIOR CRUCIATE LIGAMENT RECONSTRUCTION USING THE SEMITENDINOSUS TENDON

The semitendinosus tendon is an appealing choice because with its use subtraction from an already abnormal knee may be kept at a minimum. Previous studies have shown no measurable deficit in concentric hamstring strength following semitendinosus harvest.[16] More recently Kramer et al have reported a deficit of 11% in hamstring strength and while this may be significant, normal strength can be restored with rehabilitation.[2]

With semitendinosus tendon substitution, the complex knee extensor mechanism of the knee is not violated. The bone-patellar tendon-bone autograft is of adequate strength, but complications have been reported with its use.[2, 4] Stiffness with infrapatellar contracture and patellofemoral problems are worrisome issues. A canine study by Burks et al which evaluated central third patellar tendon donor sites for morbidity, suggested decreases of up to 30% in patellar tendon tensile strength 6 months after operation.[1] They also reported a 10% average decrease in patellar tendon length. This could lead to potentially disabling alteration in extensor mechanism biomechanics. Aglietti et al have reported a significant increase in patellofemoral crepitus in knees with bone-patellar tendon-bone reconstructions compared to those with hamstring substitution.[1]

Aglietti et al[1] and Marder et al[17] cite that results of hamstring ACL reconstruction are comparable to bone-patellar tendon-bone techniques in subjective and functional levels, and in KT-1000 testing. In addition to synthetic augmentation, the semitendinosus tendon can be used in a single length to augment ACL repair, as a double loop free graft, in triple or quadruple length free grafts, or in combination with the gracilis tendon.

Procedure

The authors' preferred technique is double loop augmented semitendinosus free graft, in which the synthetic device is sandwiched inside the folded tendon and the construct is placed in a groove in the over-the-top position.[6, 7] The composite graft (semitendinosus tendon and LAD) is mechanically fixed to tibia, and the semitendinosus alone is fixed to femur. To prevent abrasion of the synthetic with resulting intra-articular particulate debris, the LAD is completely

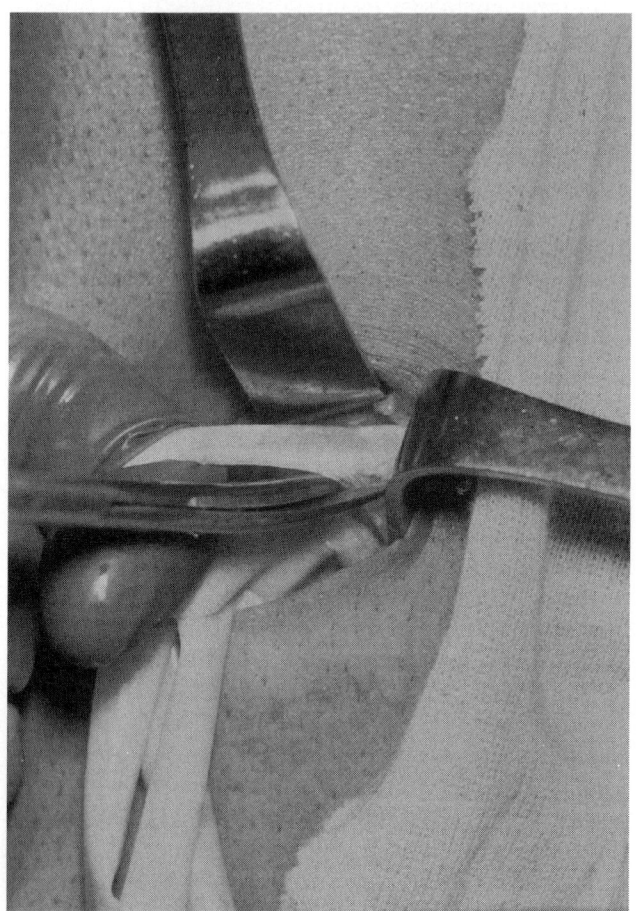

FIG 46–3.
Medial gastrocnemius reflections are resected from the distal, inferior surface of the semitendinosus tendon.

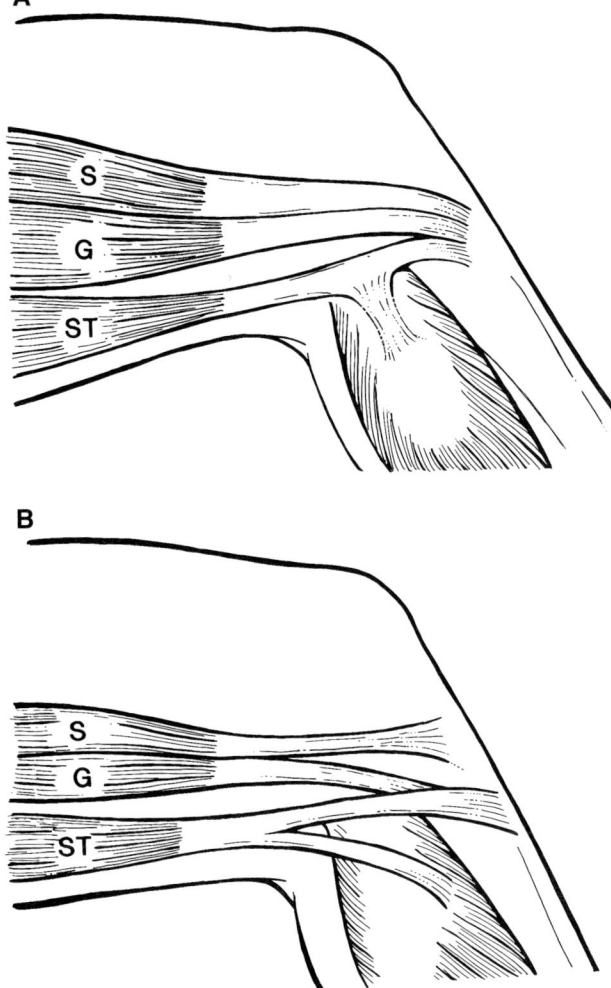

FIG 46–4.
The sartorius (S), gracilis (G), and semitendinosus (St) tendons are represented along with examples of the varying arrangements and size of the fascial connections of the semitendinosus.

surrounded with biological tissue. Proper graft placement will also help avoid abrasion.

Graft harvest is performed through a 3 cm longitudinal incision just a thumb's breadth medial and distal to the tibial tuberosity. The semitendinosus tendon is identified, traction placed on it and all the medial gastrocnemius reflections from its distal, inferior surface are resected (Fig 46–3). This step is emphasized; otherwise the fascial connections which vary in size and arrangement (Fig 46–4) can cause derailing of the tendon stripper with resulting inadequate semitendinosus graft length. An open ended tendon stripper is used to transect the semitendinosus tendon at its proximal musculotendinous junction (see Fig 46–5). It is dissected to its distal insertion and detached from the tibia.

The composite graft is constructed by sandwiching the LAD inside the folded tendon and suturing the two together under tension. To ensure that the femoral fixation will include only biological tissue, the LAD length chosen is about 1 cm less than the length of folded tendon. The suturing technique utilizes a running baseball stitch of a non-absorbable material for approximately 3 cm on the free ends of tendon, with LAD and a second running baseball stitch of absorbable material along the remaining length (Fig 46–6). The composite graft is sized to determine the diameter of the tibial tunnel, and then attached to a tendon leader that will facilitate graft passage.

A longitudinal incision is made over the iliotibial band just proximal to the lateral femoral condyle. The iliotibial band is incised along its fibres, the vastus lateralis is lifted off the intermuscular septum anteriorly, and a 1.5 cm aperture is made posteriorly in the intermuscular septum proximal to Kaplan's fibres. A cancellous screw with low profile washer is inserted anterior to this aperture, and left protruding so that the loop of tendon can be placed over it later (Fig 46–7).

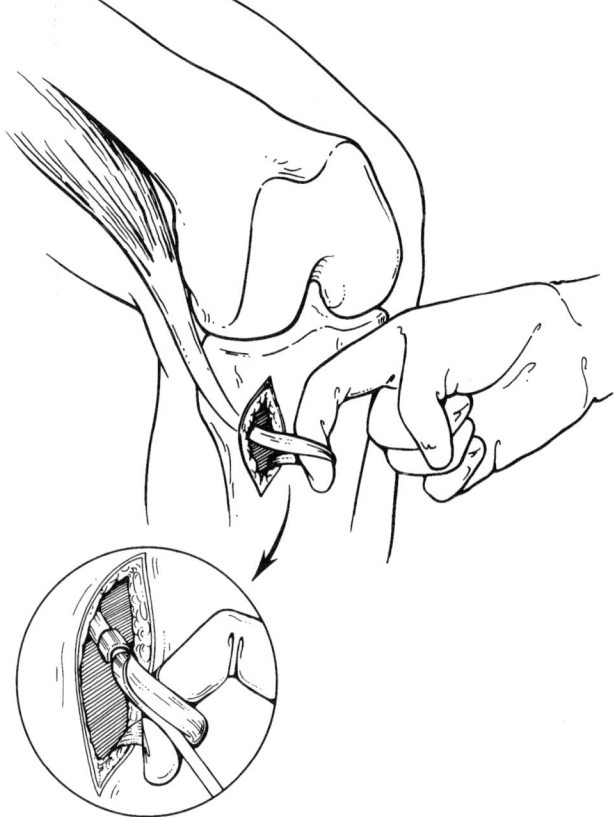

FIG 46–5.
Once the gastrocnemius refections have been resected, tension is applied to tendon and it is completely surrounded with the cutting edge of the open ended tendon stripper.

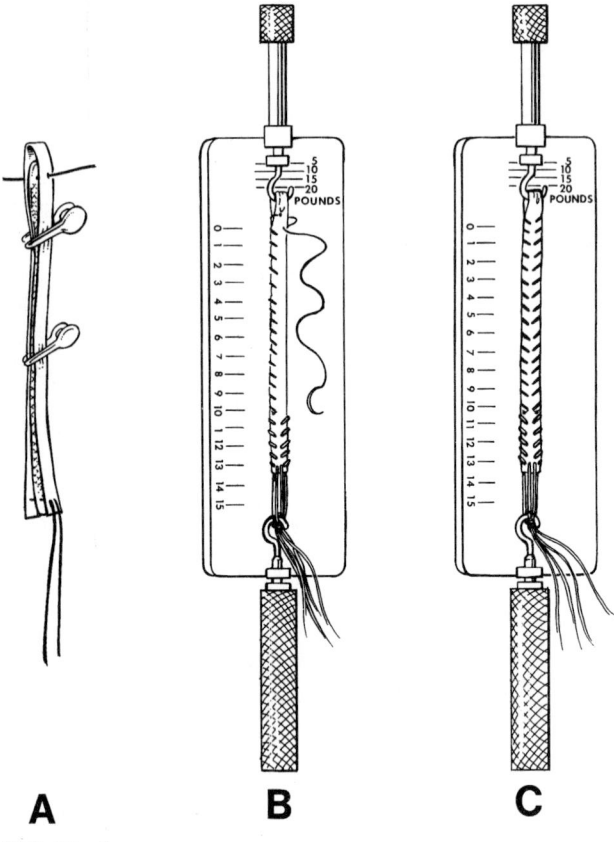

FIG 46-6.
A, the LAD is sandwiched inside the folded tendon and held with bulldog clamps. **B** and **C,** the composite is attached to the tension board and suturing together of the construct is carried out.

A thorough arthroscopic examination of the knee joint is performed and other intraarticular pathology is noted and dealt with appropriately. The over-the-top-position is identified in the notch, a 6 mm groove is developed with a long-handled narrow shaft curette, and chamfered with curved and rounded rasps.

A tibial drill guide is used to position a guide pin in the mid-medial aspect of the ACL insertion through the pretibial incision at angle of 30 degrees to the tibial surface. A tibial tunnel of appropriate diameter is created and chamfered on its posterior and lateral aspects to minimize risk of abrasion (Fig 46-8).

With the 'gaf' hook, a loop of 2-0 stainless is brought from the lateral incision, along the over-the-top position and into the knee (Fig 46-9). It is then brought through the tibial tunnel, and with this as a guide, the composite graft with leader is pulled back through the tibial tunnel, intercondylar notch and into the over-the-top groove, so that the leader and loop of tendon emerge from the lateral incision (Fig 46-10). The loop is placed over the screw and washer and with the composite tensioned distally the screw is tightened, with care taken not to include the LAD in this fixation. The composite graft is held securely at its distal end, and preconditioned by taking the knee through a full range of motion several times. Graft position through a full range of motion is checked arthroscopically (Fig 46-11). The knee is fully extended and composite graft fixation at the

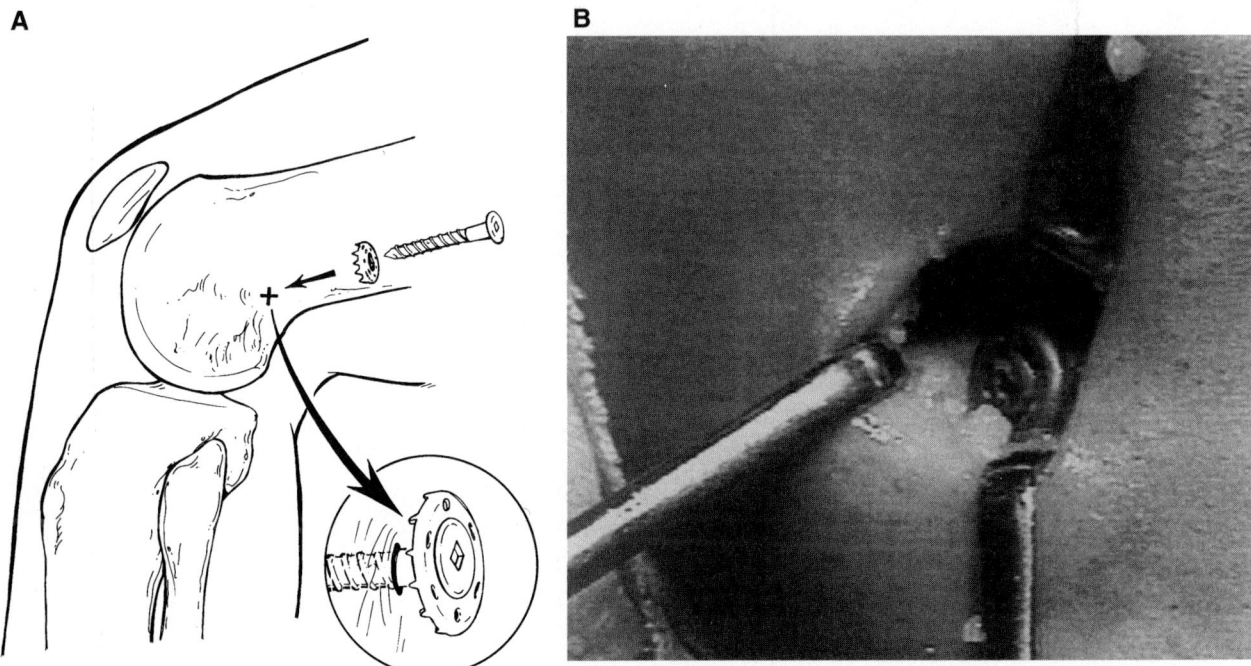

FIG 46-7.
A, a cancellous screw with low profile washer is inserted in the distal femur just anterior to the flare of the notch. **B,** the screw head is left prominent so that the loop of tendon can be placed over it later.

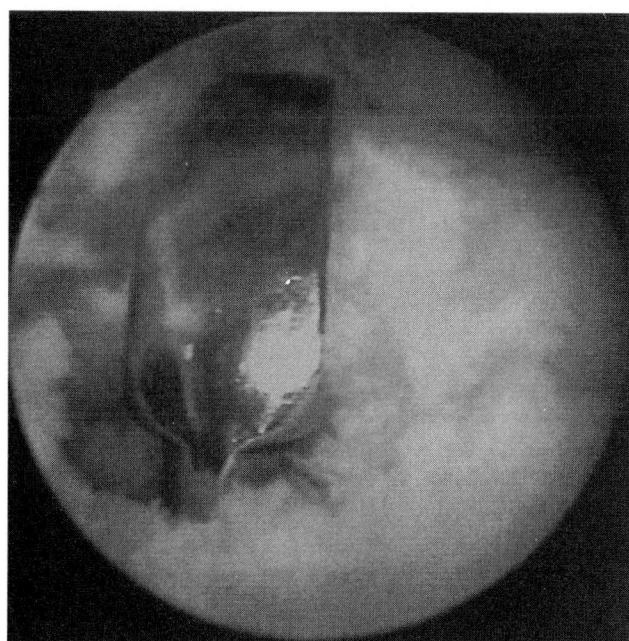

FIG 46-8.
A rasp is used to chamfer posterior and lateral aspects of the tibial tunnel.

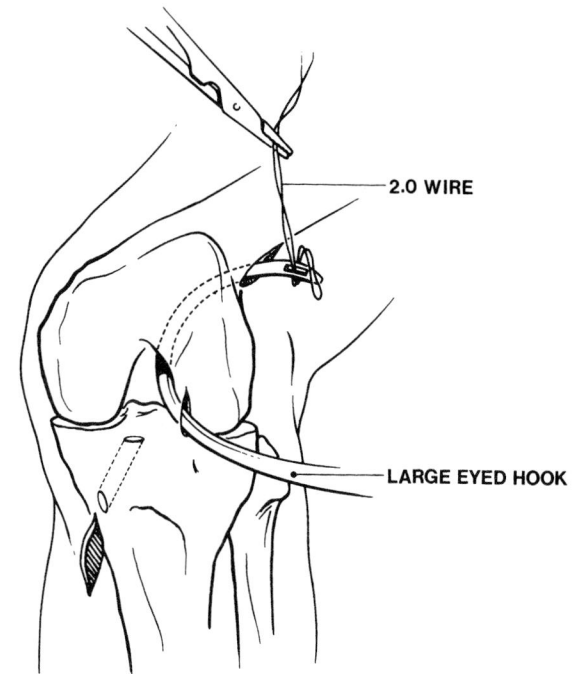

FIG 46-9.
A 'gaf' hook draws a loop of wire into the joint from the lateral incision.

tibia is carried out with multiple low profile staples. To prevent excessive constraint a measured load (average 12 lbs) is applied during fixation (Fig. 46-12). Stability is checked by Lachman and Pivot shift manoeuvres. Instability of an unacceptable degree should be investigated and corrected.

With up-to-date anaesthesia protocols that effectively control post-operative pain and nausea, this procedure can be successfully performed on an outpatient basis.[22] On post-operative day one, the patient returns to clinic for removal of drains and application of a hinged brace.

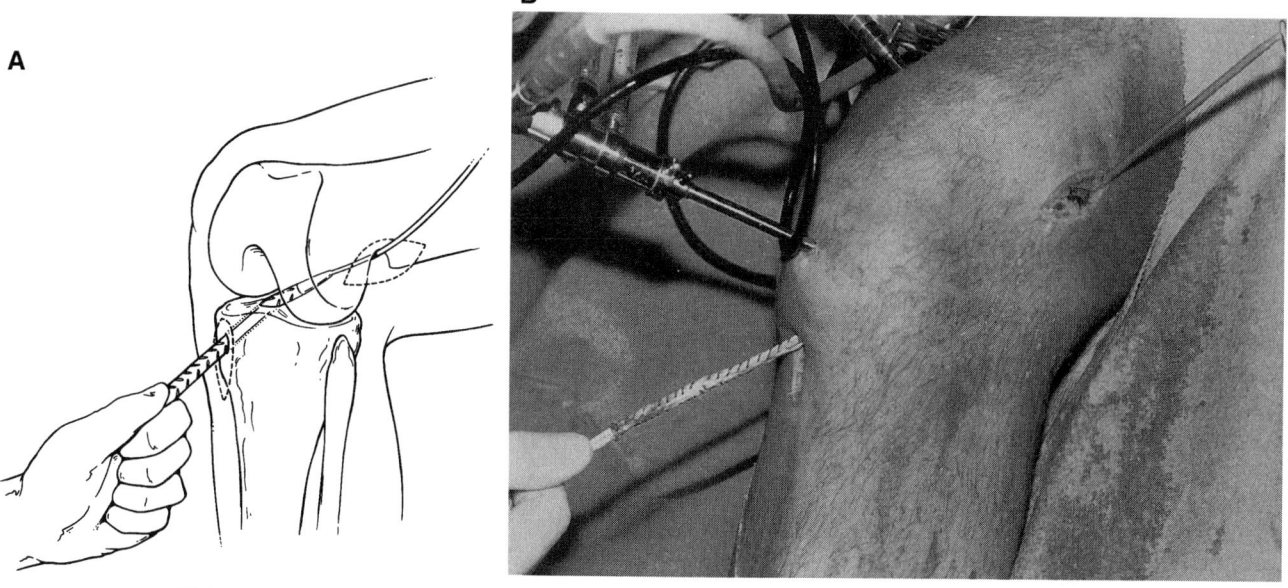

FIG 46-10.
A, drawing and **B,** intraoperative photograph, illustrate the composite graft passing through the tibial tunnel, the intercondylar notch, over-the-top and through the aperture in the intermuscular septum.

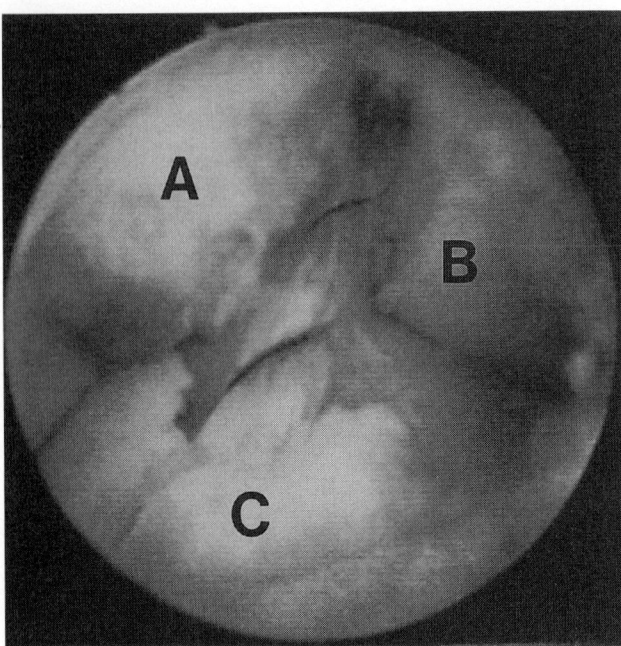

FIG 46–11.
The reconstructed ACL: *(A)* is the posterior cruciate ligament, *(B)* is the lateral femoral condyle, and *(C)* is the ACL footplate.

Rehabilitation is aggressive and includes unlimited motion and protected weightbearing in the immediate post-operative phase. Full rehabilitation should occur by 6 months after surgery and the use of an ACL protective brace is recommended for a minimum of one year after return to any ACL loading activity.

REFERENCES

1. Aglietti P, et al: Patellar tendon vs. semitendinosus and gracilis in ACL reconstruction. Proceedings of the AOSSM, 1992, San Diego, California.
2. Bonamo JJ, et al: Rupture of the patellar ligament after use of its central third for anterior cruciate reconstruction: A report of two cases, *J Bone Joint Surg [Am]* 66:1294–1297, 1984.
3. Burks TR, Haut RC, Lancaster RL: Biomechanical testing of patellar tendon after removal of its central one-third, *Am J Sports Med* 18:148–153, 1990.
4. Daniel DM, et al: The Marshall/MacIntosh anterior cruciate ligament reconstruction with the Kennedy ligament augmentation device: Report of the United States clinical trials. In Friedman MJ, Ferkel RD, editors: *Prosthetic ligament reconstruction of the knee,* Philadelphia, 1988, WB Saunders, pp 71–78.
5. Fowler PJ: Techniques using braided polypropylene as a ligament augmentation device, *Tech Orthop* 2:81–85, 1988.
6. Fowler PJ: Semitendinosus tendon anterior cruciate ligament reconstruction with LAD augmentation, *Orthopaedics* 16(4):449–453, 1993.
7. Fowler PJ: Semitendinosus tendon and the Kennedy ligament augmentation device in anterior cruciate ligament reconstruction, *Operative Techniques in Orthopaedics* 4:117–124, 1992.
8. Fowler PJ, Amendola A: LAD augmented allograft ACL reconstruction in sheep. Residents' presentations: 17th Clinical Seminar in Orthopaedic Surgery, University of Western Ontario, London, Ontario, April 26, 1989 (submitted for publication).
9. Fowler PJ, MacKinlay D, Roth JH: Long term review of intra-articular ACL reconstructions augmented with braided polypropylene. Clinical Residents' Day, University of Western Ontario, April 26, 1989 (submitted for publication).
10. Hales A: Arthroscopically assisted anterior cruciate ligament reconstruction, *AORN J* 49:234–255, 1988.
11. Hanley P, et al: Load sharing and graft forces in anterior cruciate ligament reconstruction with the ligament augmentation device, *Am J Sports Med* 17:414–422, 1989.
12. Jackson DW, et al: Cruciate reconstruction using freeze dried anterior cruciate ligament allograft and a ligament augmentation device (LAD): An experimental study in a goat model, *Am J Sports Med* 15:528–538, 1987.
13. Kramer J, Nusca D, Fowler PJ: Knee flexor and extensor strength during concentric and eccentric muscle actions after anterior cruciate ligament reconstruction using the semitendinosus tendon and the ligament

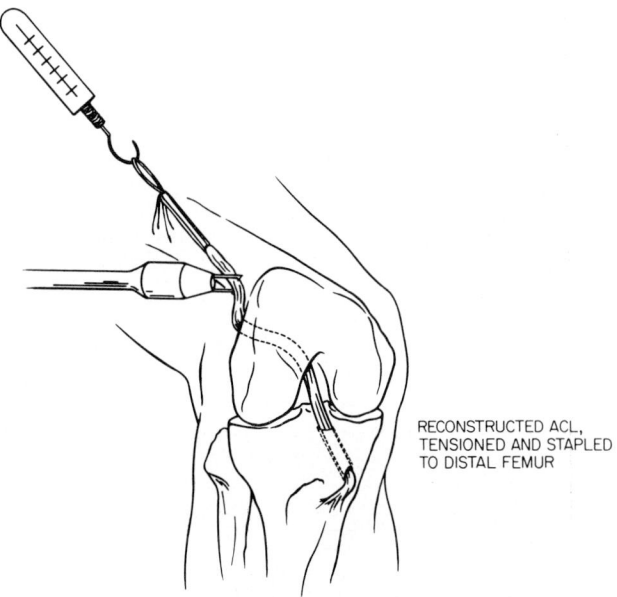

FIG 46–12.
Graft is tensioned to 14 lb of pull, then stapled to lateral femur. Remaining graft is doubled over, and second staple added, in "belt buckle" fashion. *ACL* = anterior cruciate ligament.

augmentation device, *Am J Sports Med* 21(2):285–291, 1993.
14. Kennedy JC, Alexander IJ, Hayes K: Nerve supply of the human knee and its functional importance, *Am J Sports Med* 10:329–335, 1982.
15. Kennedy JC, et al: Presidential address. Intra-articular replacement in the anterior cruciate ligament–deficient knee, *Am J Sports Med* 8:1–8, 1980.
16. Lipscomb B, et al: Evaluation of hamstring strength following use of semitendinosus and gracilis tendons to reconstruct the anterior cruciate ligament, *Am J Sports Med* 10:340–342, 1982.
17. Marder RA, Raskind JR, Carroll PT: Prospective evaluation of arthroscopically assisted anterior cruciate ligament reconstruction. Patellar tendon vs semitendinosus and gracilis tendons, *Am J Sports Med* 19(5):478–484, 1991.
18. MacIntosh D: Acute tears of the anterior cruciate ligament: The over the top repair, Annual Meeting of the American Academy of Orthopaedic Surgeons, Dallas, 1974.
19. Marshall JL, et al: The anterior cruciate ligament: A technique of repair and reconstruction, *Clin Orthop* 143:97, 1979.
20. McPherson GK, et al: Experimental mechanical and histologic evaluation of the Kennedy ligament augmentation device, *Clin Orthop* 196:186–194, 1985.
21. Olsen E, et al: The biochemical and histological effects of artificial ligament wear particles: In vitro and in vivo studies, *Am J Sports Med* 16:558–570, 1988.
22. Rajashingham M, et al: Propofol and keterolac vs inhalational anaesthesia and narcotic analgesia. Outpatient anaesthesia and analgesia for cruciate ligament reconstruction, *Anaesthesiology* 77(3), 1992.
23. Roth JH, et al: Polypropylene braid augmented and nonaugmented intra-articular anterior cruciate ligament reconstruction, *Am J Sports Med* 13:321–336, 1985.
24. Roth JH, Shkrum MJ, Bray RC: Synovial reaction associated with disruption of polypropylene braid–augmented intra-articular anterior cruciate ligament reconstruction, *Am J Sports Med* 16:301–305, 1985.

47
Artificial Cruciate Ligament Reconstruction

BRAD S. TOLIN, M.D.
MARC J. FRIEDMAN, M.D.

Historical perspective
Classification of prosthetic ligaments
FDA approval process
Prosthetic ligaments
  Gore-Tex ligament

Stryker Dacron ligament
Leeds-Keio ligament
Ligastic ligament
Future of prosthetic ligament reconstruction

In the past decade, clinical and biomechanical investigations of prosthetic anterior cruciate ligaments (ACLs) have dramatically increased. The problems inherent with autogenous ACL reconstructions have stimulated the search for alternatives, such as artificial ligaments. Although the results of autogenous reconstructions have been encouraging and are improving, there are several significant disadvantages to the use of autogenous tissues. The use of autogenous bone–patellar tendon–bone grafts may result in complications which include: rupture of the patellar tendon, patellar fracture, infrapatellar contracture syndrome, patellar tendinitis, arthrofibrosis, and alteration of normal patellofemoral biomechanics.* Similarly, use of the semitendinosus and gracilis tendons are not without complications. More important though, is the relative lack of strength of the autogenous ACL grafts when compared with the prosthetic implants. The average strength of the ACL taken from young cadavers was found to be 1,730 (N).[62] Of the autogenous grafts mechanically tested, only the bone–patellar tendon–bone specimens had a strength greater than the in vivo ACL. However, the bone–patellar tendon–bone specimen tested was 14 mm in size, which is significantly larger than the 10-mm graft size usually used in clinical practice. Other studies suggest that the central third of the patellar tendon is stronger than previously reported, with the average strength of a 10-mm graft found to be 2,977 N.[15] Also, rotating the graft 90 degrees was found to significantly increase its strength. When interpreting the biomechanical data, it is important to note that these results reflect graft strength in a static mode with testing and immediately after harvesting. After the graft is implanted, the autogenous tissue undergoes a process of revascularization and remodeling with substitution of new viable collagenous tissue over time.[61] The graft undergoes progressive weakening after implantation and continues to remain significantly weaker than the normal ACL for at least 6 to 12 months postoperatively.[13] As a result, the autogenous reconstructions require protection during this period when the graft is more susceptible to failure.

The use of allograft and prosthetic implants for cruciate ligament reconstruction has developed in an attempt to overcome the problems with autogenous reconstructions. These types of graft replacements allow the ligament reconstruction to be performed without sacrificing the patient's own tissues, avoiding the associated morbidity. Allografts have been used in cruciate ligament reconstruction, but carry the risk of disease transmission and the possibility of subclinical rejection. There is also some evidence that suggests the allograft may require a longer period of time for revascularization than autogenous substitutes, and has a longer period of relative weakness.[4, 39, 56] Conversely, reconstruction using a prosthetic ligament has significant advantages. These include a biomechanically strong graft material which

*References 10, 12, 40, 49, 55, 66, 69, 72.

allows for earlier range of motion of the knee, weight-bearing, and return to full activities. Recent technical improvements in ACL reconstruction (e.g., "notchplasty," isometric placement of the graft, and stronger graft fixation techniques) have reduced the failure rate of autogenous graft reconstruction, but the relative weakness of the graft continues to be the limiting factor for return of the athlete to full competition. Patients with a prior failed autogenous reconstruction present a special problem. These patients will have less autogenous tissue available for a secondary autogenous reconstruction and may have residual strength or range-of-motion deficits as a result of the initial reconstruction. In these patients, prosthetic ligament reconstruction may be beneficial as the high-strength graft will allow a faster return to activities. Despite these theoretical advantages, the prosthetic ligaments continue to have inherent problems. Currently, the use of prosthetic ligaments for ACL reconstruction has been limited to those patients with prior failed autogenous reconstructions, but further research is necessary to further define the role of these implants.

HISTORICAL PERSPECTIVE

One of the earliest descriptions of prosthetic reconstruction of the ACL was that of Corner[16] in 1914. He used a loop of silver wire to replace a torn ACL, but no long-term follow-up was reported. In 1918, Smith[76] used multiple sutures through channels in the tibia and femur to reconstruct the torn ACL. The sutures were removed at 11 weeks post reconstruction because of severe inflammatory reaction. Von Mironova[82] used a ligament composed of Lavsan, a type of polyester, to reconstruct the ACL. He claimed 91% satisfactory results in 262 patients over 15 years of study.

The Proplast ligament substitute (Vitek Inc., Houston) was originally intended to be used as a stent, or temporary internal splint, to provide instability while an associated extraarticular reconstruction was healing. This prosthesis was approved by the Food and Drug Administration (FDA) for implantation in 1973. James and associates[41] reported results in 15 patients in whom the ligament was implanted as a salvage procedure for chronic anterior laxity. Only 7 (47%) of the patients had satisfactory results and ligament breakage occurred in 8 of the 15 patients. Most of the failures occurred during the first postoperative year. The ligament is no longer available for implantation in the United States.

In 1976, the Richards Polyflex system (Richards Manufacturing Co. Memphis) was the only prosthetic ligament marketed in the United States. The prosthesis was constructed of ultrahigh-molecular-weight polyethylene and stainless steel tubes that were fixed with a threaded nut augmented with polymethyl methacrylate cement. Initial biomechanical studies performed with the Polyflex ligament raised concern over the ability of the implant to resist in vivo forces in the young active patient without sustaining any permanent deformation.[36] Biomechanical[14] and clinical[20, 23] studies confirmed these suspicions. The failure rate was over 50% within the first year of implantation.[20] In November 1977, Richards ceased commercial production and distribution of the device. The experience with this ligament resulted in the FDA forming an advisory panel to study the prosthetic ligament and ultimately led to the development of the guidelines used in the approval process today.[22]

Jenkins,[42] in 1978, began to use flexible carbon fibers to reconstruct the ACL. The carbon was thought to act as a temporary scaffold which encouraged the ingrowth of fibroblastic tissue and subsequently produced new collagen. The clinical results reported by Rushton and colleagues[71] demonstrated a high percentage of patients had persistent pain and effusions which necessitated removal of the carbon fiber implant. Also, no ingrowth of organized fibroblastic tissue was observed and free carbon fibers were found within the joint. Bercovy and associates[6] also highlighted the problems with these uncoated carbon ligaments. Of concern was the migration of the carbon fibers from the ligament to regional lymph nodes. In an attempt to reduce the shedding of the carbon particles and improve its handling characteristics, the carbon fiber implants were coated with a polylactate acid polymer. This ligament was known as the Integraft stent (Osteonics Biomaterials, Livermore, Calif.). The composite allows for reabsorption of the copolymer shortly after implantation. The carbon fibers then undergo a more prolonged mechanical degradation while simultaneously gradually transferring the forces to the newly formed collagen tissue. This graft was used to augment standard autogenous ACL reconstruction and was designed to be completely covered by the autogenous grafted tissue when implanted. Initially, the Integraft ligament (Fig 47–1) was woven through a strip of iliotibial band which had been detached distally and passed through the posterior capsule of the knee and then through a tibial tunnel. The graft was fixed to the tibia with a carbon–polylactate acid fastener. Further studies showed that the carbon fiber was found in the lymph nodes after implantation of the uncoated carbon material, but coating the carbon decreased the fragmen-

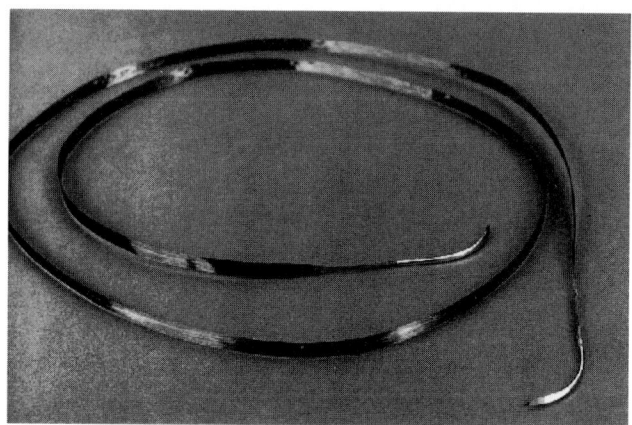

FIG 47–1.
The Integraft stent. (From Rusch RM: Integraft anterior cruciate ligament reconstruction. In Friedman MJ, Ferkel RD, editors: *Prosthetic ligament reconstruction of the knee.* Philadelphia, 1988, WB Saunders. Used by permission.)

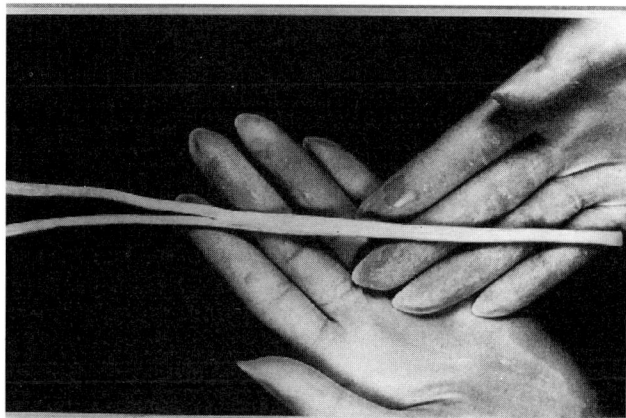

FIG 47–2.
Xenotech anterior cruciate ligament prosthesis.

tation and particle migration.[6] Preliminary clinical studies demonstrated satisfactory results in patients that underwent reconstruction with this ligament as a salvage procedure.[83] Another study showed no apparent difference at 1 year postoperatively between patients undergoing ACL reconstruction with the central one third of the patellar tendon, or the semitendinosus tendon augmented with the Integraft prosthesis, and those patients that had a nonaugmented autogenous reconstruction.[77] The ligament was never given market approval by the FDA and remains unavailable for use.

In July 1981, clinical trials began using the Pro-Col xenograft bioprosthesis (Xenotech Laboratories, Irvine, Calif.) which was composed of bovine extensor tendons treated with glutaraldehyde (Fig 47–2). The glutaraldehyde treatment protects the collagen bundles from proteolytic enzyme degradation by cross-linking adjacent molecules. This process produces an implant that has a greater modulus of elasticity and does not undergo remodeling; thus the ligament is considered to be a permanent prosthesis. Results of implantation with the xenograft have generally been disappointing.[1, 18, 34] In the patients in whom the ligament was implanted arthroscopically, the reconstruction failed in 31% and 29% developed a sterile synovitis.[84] Failure of the graft usually occurred during the first postoperative year. Tietge and Rojas[80] examined 18 patients after implantation over an 18-month period. Ten of the patients had recurrent effusions and only one patient was stable by KT-1000 arthrometer testing. Nine grafts had been removed at the time of the report and the majority had demonstrated a chronic inflammatory response with foreign body giant cell granulomatous reactions. In the same group of patients, with a longer follow-up averaging 44 months, 78% of the grafts (14/18) had already been removed.[79] Van Steensel and associates[81] retrospectively reviewed 40 knees in which a tendon xenograft was implanted to replace the torn ACL. Five of the first 30 patients (17%) developed a severe synovitis within 8 months of implantation, which necessitated graft removal. The rinsing procedure for xenograft preparation was modified in the last 10 patients, with only one case of synovitis developing in this group. The single case of synovitis occurred in a patient in whom the original rinsing procedure was done inadvertently. There was no synovitis present in any knee in which the graft ruptured. The authors concluded that the glutaraldehyde was possibly the causative factor responsible for the severe synovitis, rather than particulate debris from the ruptured xenograft. Others have implicated graft particulate matter or mechanical overload of the graft as the cause of the adverse reactions.[7, 63] As a result, the FDA in May 1987 reported that the ProCol bioprosthesis was "not approved" for release, citing concern over the high incidence of complications. This prosthesis is currently not available in the United States.

CLASSIFICATION OF PROSTHETIC LIGAMENTS

Prosthetic ligaments are generally classified into three types: permanent ligaments, stents, or scaffold. Permanent ligaments include the Gore-Tex and Stryker Dacron ligaments and are designed with high strength and increased resistance to fatigue failure. These ligaments rely on their inherent mechanical properties to withstand forces over a prolonged period of time without any contribution from autogenous tissues or tissue ingrowth into the ligament.

The second type of prosthetic ligament, the stent, functions to augment the strength of an intraarticular autogenous reconstruction. These devices, such as the Kennedy LAD (ligament augmentation device), increase the security of fixation of the autogenous tissue and increase the immediate strength of the complete reconstruction. These ligaments are usually fixated at only one end of the graft to allow the transfer of stress to the underlying autogenous tissue reconstruction. Theoretically, as the autogenous tissue strength increases, the role of the LAD becomes less important.

The third type of prosthetic ligament, the scaffold device, allows ingrowth of tissue. This ligament depends on autogenous tissue ingrowth which is derived from the fibroblasts within the postsurgical knee. The collagen tissue may either grow into the existing graft, as in the Leeds-Keio ligament, or may actually replace the graft tissue as it is slowly degraded, as with the carbon ligaments. In these cases, the new collagen tissue matures into a replacement ligament which can theoretically last indefinitely without fatigue. Table 47-1 lists the various prosthetic ligaments in this classification scheme.

Each type of prosthetic ligament has inherent advantages and disadvantages. The ideal prosthetic ligament would have high tensile strength, would be inserted arthroscopically with minimal tissue dissection, and allow early range of motion and immediate weightbearing without immobilization. In addition, the graft would eventually be replaced by autogenous tissue with strength characteristics similar to the normal ACL. None of the currently available types of prosthetic ligaments are able to meet all of these basic criteria.

FDA APPROVAL PROCESS

Currently, there are only three prosthetic ligament devices approved by the FDA for use in ACL reconstruction. The FDA follows a systematic process before approving prosthetic devices for implantation[22] (Fig 47-3). Manufacturers are required to notify the FDA before marketing a new device. These premarket notification submissions are referred to as 510 K(S). During this 90-day period, the FDA determines whether the device is similar to a previously approved device. If the device is not substantially equivalent, it is required to undergo the approval process prior to marketing.

These devices must then be tested in laboratory and animal studies and found to be reasonably safe and effective. This first phase includes biomechanical studies performed in animal models. The prosthetic ligaments are implanted and the animals are routinely examined for evidence of adverse reactions. The prosthetic ligament also undergoes biomechanical testing to determine its inherent properties. In contrast to autogenous reconstruction in which continuous remodeling of the collagen occurs, prosthetic

TABLE 47-1.
Classification of Prosthetic Ligaments

Permanent prosthesis	Gore-Tex ligament
	Stryker Dacron ligament
	Richards Polyflex ligament*
	ProCol xenograft bioprosthesis*
	Ligastic ligament (E series)*
Stent	Kennedy ligament augmentation device
	Integraft stent*
Scaffold	Leeds-Keio ligament
	Ligastic ligament (NE series)*

*Not currently available in the United States.

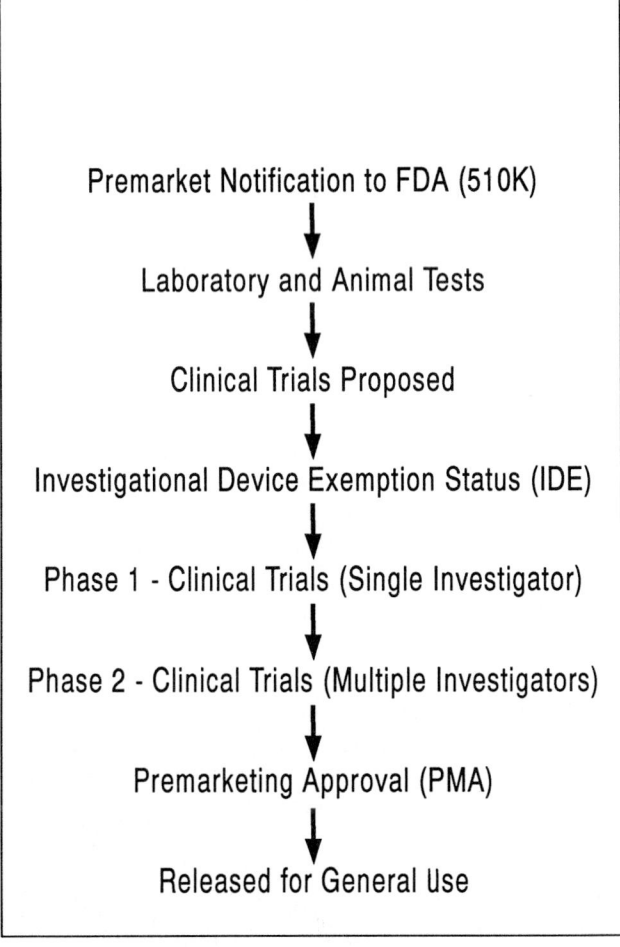

FIG 47-3.
Steps in FDA approval of a ligament prosthesis. See text for discussion.

ligaments have no method to remodel once implanted. An important characteristic of these ligaments, therefore, is the measurement of fatigue failure which is usually measured as million of cycles to failure (average cycles per year, 1.4 million). From these data an estimate of the life expectancy of the ligament in humans may be calculated. The measurement of ligament strength and stiffness is also an important variable. The ultimate tensile strength measures the force required to cause complete rupture of the ligament. The measurement of stiffness reflects the compliance of the prosthetic ligament or its ability to temporarily elongate without rupture. Table 47–2 demonstrates the comparative biomechanical testing results for the normal ACL and four different prosthetic ligaments.

Although the biomechanical and animal testing data are helpful, interligament comparison is difficult. There can be marked variability in the animal models used in evaluation, in addition to differences in the duration of ligament implantation and the postoperative rehabilitation. Nor do the biomechanical tests accurately detect the true in vivo situation that the ligament experiences. The predicted fatigue life of the ligament does not take into account the effects of extrinsic factors that can influence the success or failure of the reconstruction. For example, abrasion of the ligament on the edges of the bony tunnels may drastically decrease the life span of the implant. Also, the strength of the graft will be less important if the fixation of the implant to host tissues is the weakest link of the reconstruction. Thus, the differences in the experimental protocols and the method by which each ligament is implanted compound the difficulty in accurately comparing the individual ligaments.

The next step for FDA approval involves submitting a proposed clinical trial with sufficient numbers and adequate follow-up to allow statistical determination of safety and efficacy. At this point, the device may be granted an "investigation device exemption" (IDE) status. Phase I clinical trials are then begun which are confined to a single clinical investigator. In phase II, multicenter trials are conducted using a common protocol. During phase I and II trials the device is not available for general use. After the data from the clinical trials have been evaluated, the FDA may grant premarketing approval (PMA) status. A PMA status means that a decision from the FDA is expected within 6 months. Only after analysis of the clinical trials has been completed and a panel of experts have approved the ligament, is it released for general use. At this point, the ligament is available to all orthopaedic surgeons, but it may be marketed only for the indications specifically approved by the FDA. For example, the Gore-Tex and Stryker ligaments are approved only for use in patients with a previously failed intraarticular reconstruction. The LAD, as of September 1991, has been approved for use with an iliotibial, semitendinosus, and patellar tendon ACL reconstruction as a result of a multicenter phase II US study. The individual surgeon may still use an approved ligament outside of the FDA guidelines but needs to thoroughly discuss with the patient and document the reasons for the choice of a prosthetic ligament as opposed to an autogenous reconstruction. Also, the medicolegal implications of using a device for a non-FDA approved use needs to be considered.

PROSTHETIC LIGAMENTS

Gore-Tex Ligament

Concept

The Gore-Tex prosthesis (Fig 47–4) is intended to serve as a permanent replacement for the ACL. The ligament is composed of expanded polytetrafluoroethylene (PTFE). The prosthesis is composed of a single strand of the material which is wound into multiple loops. The strands are then woven into a three-bundle multifilament with fixation eyelets incorporated at each end of the ligament. The eyelets

TABLE 47–2.

Biomechanical Testing Results for Normal Anterior Cruciate Ligament and Five Prosthetic Ligaments

	Normal ACL	Prosthetic Ligament			
		Gore-Tex	Stryker Dacron	Leeds-Keio	Ligastic
Type of prosthesis		Permanent	Stent	Ingrowth	Permanent (E series) Ingrowth (NE series)
Material		Polytetrafluoroethylene	Dacron fabric	Dacron mesh	Polyethylene knitted
Ultimate tensile strength (N)	1,730	>4,448	3,110–3,631	2,000	1,800–4,200
Stiffness (N/mm)	182	322	39	>182	180–420 (daN)
Ultimate strain (%)	60	9	18	35	15–30

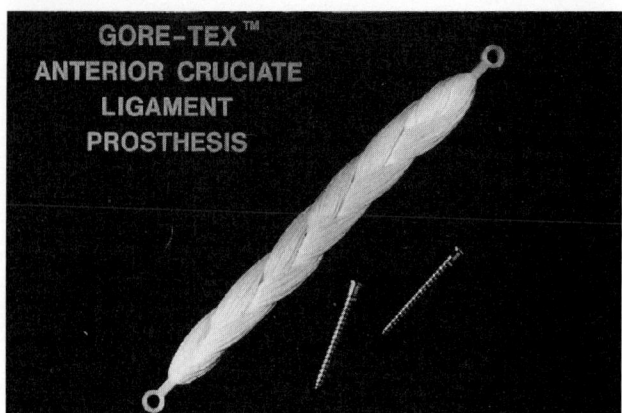

FIG 47-4.
The Gore-Tex ligament prosthesis.

allow fixation at each end of the prosthesis with cortical screws into the host bone. The screw fixation is intended to supply the initial fixation of the ligament, while permanent fixation is provided by tissue ingrowth into the strands of ligament contained in the bony tunnels. This ingrowth is estimated to take at least 6 months to occur. Bolton and Bruchman[9] performed static and cyclic creep tests measuring the in vivo loading stresses in the normal ACL. They found that ligament strength of approximately 4,400 N was necessary to prevent clinically significant elongation in vivo. The Gore-Tex prosthetic ligament is able to withstand a greater maximum load with approximately 8% to 10% elongation at failure.[50] The fatigue life of any prosthetic ligament is a concern prior to implantation. To address this issue, biomechanical tests were performed using a load equivalent to approximately 20 years of in vivo use and demonstrated that the ligament was resistent to fatigue failure. All testing performed in a sheep animal model showed the maintenance of joint stability and excellent bony ingrowth within the tunnels for ligament fixation. Also, no significant effects on the synovial tissues within the joint were noted. Based on the encouraging preliminary biologic studies, clinical trials of the device were initiated in the United States in October 1982 under an IDE. As part of the study, 1,021 patients had a Gore-Tex ligament implanted for ACL insufficiency by 20 groups of investigators. The prospective study was performed with patients being evaluated at 3-month intervals for the first year and at 6-month intervals until 5 years' postoperative follow-up were obtained. The preliminary results of this study were satisfactory and formal FDA approval was obtained in October 1986.

Technique

Routine knee arthroscopy is performed to evaluate the menisci and articular surfaces of the joint.[9, 24] The intercondylar notch is then evaluated and a notchplasty is performed using a curved gouge, mechanical abraders, and shavers. Attention is directed to the superior aspect of the notch which can impinge on the Gore-Tex ligament when the knee is completely extended. A 3-cm vertical incision is made 1 cm medial to the tibial tubercle and 2 to 3 cm distal to the joint line. An arthroscopic ACL guide is used to drill a guide wire through the tibia onto a point on the tibial plateau that is slightly anterior and medial to the insertion of the normal ACL. After the position of the guide wire is judged to be satisfactory, the tibial tunnel is drilled using an 8-mm reamer (Fig 47-5). After the tibial tunnel has been made, a chamfering device is used to round off the posterior edges of the tibial tunnel. This is an important technical point because the edges of the bony tunnels may cause abrasion and subsequent failure of the graft. A 5-cm incision is made on the lateral aspect of the distal femur, proximal to the lateral femoral epicondyle. The iliotibial band is split longitudinally in line with the incision and the vastus lateralis is elevated anteriorly from the intermuscular septum. A 3.2-mm drill bit is used to perforate the femoral cortex in the superolateral aspect of the wound. A guide wire is then drilled

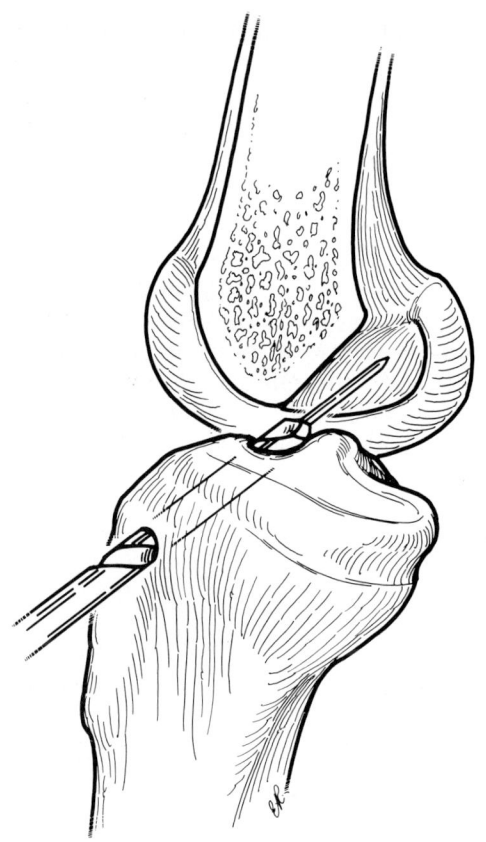

FIG 47-5.
Proper placement of the tibial guide wire followed by reaming.

through this hole in an oblique direction aiming along the posterolateral aspect of the femur, 1 cm medial to the insertion of the lateral head of the gastrocnemius muscle (Fig 47–6). This hole is drilled under direct vision with the knee flexed to prevent neurovascular injury. A flat periosteal elevator is used at all times during any drilling or reaming to prevent neurovascular drainage. After the guide wire has been satisfactorily positioned, an 8-mm reamer is again used to enlarge the tunnel. Internal and external chamfering of the extraarticular lateral femoral tunnel is performed as described for the tibial tunnel.

The arthroscope is then reinserted and a curved passer is placed through the anteromedial portal along the posterolateral aspect of the notch to perforate the posterior capsule (Fig 47–7). The capsular hole is progressively enlarged with dilators of increasing size to a 9-mm diameter. A Gore-Tex smoother is then passed through the tibial tunnel and into the notch and out through the perforation of the posterior capsule along the lateral femoral incision. The wire-braided portion of the Gore-Tex smoother is pulled proximally and distally to rasp the bony tunnels as the knees move through 0 to 60 degrees of flexion. The smoother serves to remove any residual soft tissue in the posterior capsular hole and along the intercondylar notch superiorly. A Red Robinson catheter is passed through the lateral femoral tunnel and an umbilical tape is passed through the catheter and pulled back through the tunnel. The Gore-Tex smoother is tied to the tape which is then used to pull the smoother out through the lateral femoral extraarticular tunnel. Further smoothing of the femoral and tibial tunnels and the posterior capsule hole can be performed if necessary. The smoother is marked to determine the proper Gore-Tex graft length. The prosthesis is tied to the tibial end of the Gore-Tex smoother which is pulled through the tibial tunnel across the joint and out through the posterolateral capsule along the extraarticular femoral tunnel. The femoral end of the prosthesis is fixated by drilling through both lateral and medial femoral cortices. A depth gauge is used to determine screw length. The holes are tapped and the cortical screw is then passed through the femoral end of the graft, securing one end of the prosthesis.

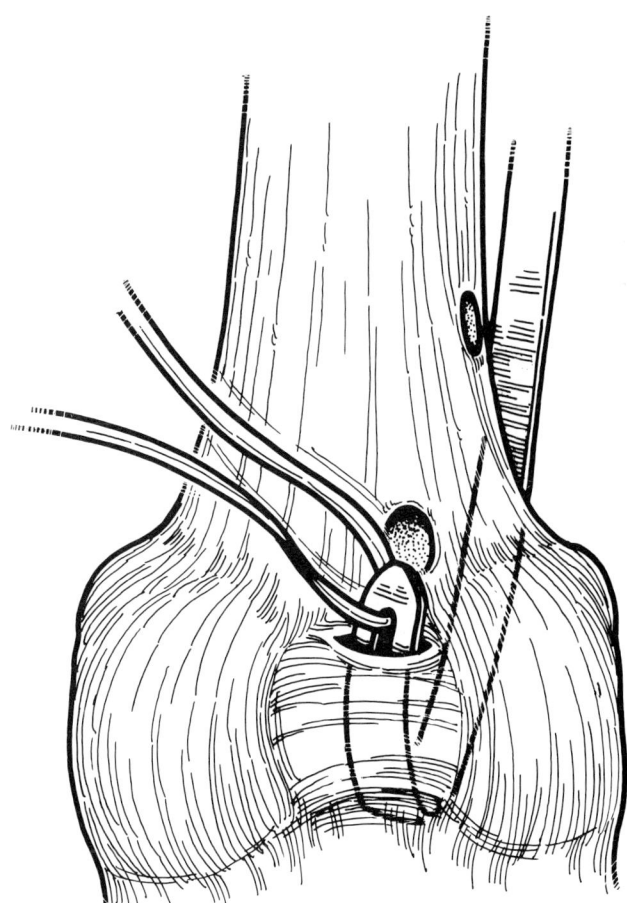

FIG 47–7.
Perforation of the posterior capsule with a curved passer.

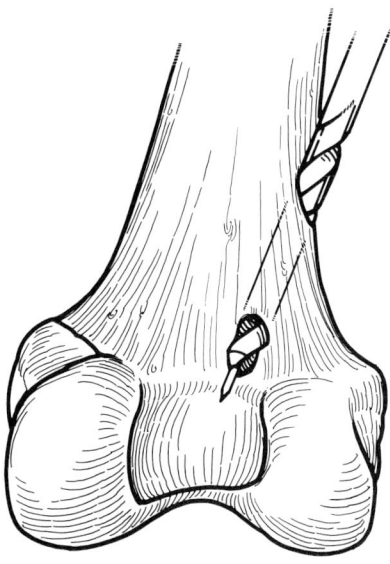

FIG 47–6.
Placement of the femoral drill hole.

After the femoral end of the graft has been fixated, the Gore tensiometer is applied to the tibial eyelet and 40 lbs of tension is applied while the knee is taken through 20 cycles of full flexion and extension. This maneuver eliminates any inherent laxity within the graft and is called "preconditioning." With the knee in full extension and maintaining 40 lbs of tension applied to the prosthesis, a bone punch is used to mark the site for the tibial hole. As with the femoral drill hole, both cortices are drilled with a 3.2-mm drill and a depth gauge is used to determine the length of the screw. After both ends of the Gore-Tex ligament have been fixed, the arthroscope is reinserted and a careful evaluation of the ligament is performed as the knee is flexed and extended. Particular attention is paid to the notch area to ensure that there is no graft impingement present. It is also important to evaluate the posterior portion of the intraarticular tibial tunnel and the superior roof of the intercondylar notch, as these areas may cause abrasion of the ligament. Motion of the knee is checked to assure that full extension can be obtained. If complete extension cannot be obtained, this indicates that the Gore-Tex ligament has been implanted incorrectly and it will be impossible to obtain complete extension in the postoperative period. In this situation, repositioning of the fixation screws is necessary. A careful ligamentous examination of the knee should be performed after implantation.

Postoperatively, the patient can bear weight as tolerated. Range of motion of the knee is not restricted. The patient is not allowed to return to sports activities for at least 6 months which allows for additional fixation of the ligament within the intraosseous tunnels. After the 6-month period, the patient can return to athletic activities when the strength of the operative leg is at least 85% of that of the noninjured knee.

The Gore-Tex ligament can be readily inserted with arthroscopic-assisted techniques, but careful attention to technical details is required for optimal results. Specifically, these include chamfering the edges of the bony tunnels, a notchplasty to minimize abrasion and impingement of the ligament, preconditioning of the graft to remove the inherent laxity in the multifilament ligament, and tensioning to improve the efficacy in stabilizing the knee. Also, it is important to visualize the ligament arthroscopically after the reconstruction is completed to ensure that these objectives have been met.

Results

The Gore-Tex ligament has been implanted in over 18,000 patients worldwide. The W.L. Gore company has reported the results of Gore-Tex ligament reconstruction in 186 patients included in the original study with at least 5 years of follow-up.[35] The average age of the patients was 27.5 years. Seventy-six of these patients had prior surgical procedures on the involved knee. Objective examination preoperatively demonstrated that 84% of the patients had a Lachman grade of 2+ or greater and 83% of the patients had a positive pivot shift. After insertion of the Gore-Tex ligament, 30% of the patients had a Lachman grade of 2+ or greater and only 24% had a residual positive pivot shift. The incidence of giving-way symptoms decreased from 89% before reconstruction to only 11% postoperatively. Complications occurred in 14.3% of patients. Thirty-eight patients had the graft removed (3.8%), with 18 patients having actual failure of the graft (1.8%). An infection developed in 13 patients (1%) which required removal of the prosthesis in 10 patients. Recurrent instability developed in 8 patients (0.8%) without evidence of graft failure, with 5 of these 8 patients subsequently reconstructed successfully.

Recently, the original Gore-Tex investigators have individually published the results of reconstruction in their patients. Ahfeld and associates[2] reported on 30 patients with an average follow-up of 2 years. They noted improvement of instability in 26 (87%) patients and satisfactory results in 25 (83%). Glousman and colleagues[33] evaluated 82 patients who underwent Gore-Tex ligament reconstruction with a mean follow-up of 18 months. The objective analysis, which included Lachman, anterior drawer, and pivot shift testing, demonstrated improvement at final follow-up in comparison with the patients' preoperative status. Complications noted in their study included four ligament ruptures, four chronic sterile effusions, two patients with partial attenuation of the ligament, one infection, and one loose body. Fourteen patients subsequently required additional surgery. The authors considered the results satisfactory but cautioned that longer-term follow-up was necessary. Of concern was a deterioration of the objective data when evaluated at 6-month intervals. The investigators speculated that the trend of graft loosening may be the result of some resorption of the bone tunnels adjacent to the graft due to interposed soft tissue, ligament creep, or possibly actual loosening of the graft. It is interesting that the subjective scores have not significantly changed in these patients. Johnson[43] reported on 59 patients that underwent a Gore-Tex ACL reconstruction with a minimum of 2 years follow-up. Fifty-five patients (93%) were satisfied with the procedure. There were 12 objective failures with all these patients asymptomatic. Only 3 (5%) patients were considered subjective failures. KT-1000 arthrometer testing demonstrated a side-to-side difference of 2.0 mm at 2-year follow-up and 1.5 mm at a 3-year follow-up. The authors suggest that this is evidence that the results did not deteriorate over time, but there were only 13 patients included in the 36-month follow-up group. Complications included 11% who had effusions and 5% who required secondary reconstruction after failure of the graft.

Indelicato et al.[38] reported on 39 patients who underwent a Gore-Tex ligament reconstruction with a minimum of 2 years' follow-up. Thirty-four patients (87%) had a satisfactory result which allowed a return to activities without symptoms of pain or instability in the reconstructed knee. Four patients subsequently had a rupture of the Gore-Tex prosthesis and nine patients developed postoperative complications which included at least a single episode of a sterile effusion. Six of the patients had recurrent effusions and five underwent rearthroscopy for evaluation. The arthroscopy demonstrated partial tears of the Gore-Tex graft in all cases. Synovial biopsies obtained showed PTFE particulate debris within the synovium. The authors believe that strict adherence to technical factors such as adequate notchplasty and graft tensioning may reduce the incidence of complications in future reconstructions. In a subsequent paper[87] involving the original group of patients, the authors compared 2- and 3-year results of the Gore-Tex ACL reconstruction. Thirty-three patients were evaluated with a 36-month follow-up. Of those 33, 5 patients had an acute injury while 28 patients had a chronically ACL-deficient knee. At a 48-month follow-up, there were an additional 7 patients that had a graft failure. When combined with the 4 patients that had failure at the 24-month follow-up, the overall failure rate was 33%. All of the graft failures were in the reconstructions performed on the chronically ACL-deficient knee. The average time to failure after implantation of the graft was approximately 32 months. Only three of the failures could be associated with a traumatic event. Twenty-eight percent of the patients had at least one episode of a sterile effusion. A survival analysis of the graft was performed and demonstrated an 82% probability of graft survival at 48-month follow-up and only 44% survival at a 62-month follow-up after implantation. The role of notchplasty was evaluated to determine if this played a part in graft failure. Fourteen of the 39 patients had a notchplasty performed. A graft failure rate of 14% was seen in the notchplasty group (2/14) compared to 36% (9/25) in those patients that did not have a notchplasty, though this was not statistically significant. Subjectively, 93% of the patients felt that the knee was normal or improved. The authors suggest that the results did not support the concept of a slow deterioration in the results, as the successful patients at 2- and 3-year follow-ups did not differ in either subjective or objective evaluations.

Ferkel and associates[21] reported the results of an arthroscopic second look in 21 knees that had arthroscopic-assisted implantation of the Gore-Tex prosthesis. Eight of the arthroscopies were performed for complaints of knee pain post reconstruction, while two were for giving-way symptoms, three for recurrent effusions, and eight were done at the time of screw removal. The time interval from implantation to rearthroscopy was, on average, 11 months. The ligament was found to be intact in 11 knees, partially ruptured in six and completely ruptured in four patients. The majority of the patients had synovitis present at the time of the second-look arthroscopy, but this was similar in intensity to the synovitis present at the time of the original surgery and not thought to be due to a reaction to the graft. No PTFE particles were appreciated on histologic evaluation of the synovium when the Gore-Tex ligament was intact. Particulate debris was found only when ruptured strands of the graft were present. However, there appeared to be no relation between the integrity of the graft and the presence of a synovial reaction. The authors believe that the Gore-Tex ligament was inert and did not cause any significant synovial reaction or effusion when either intact or ruptured.

Despite the encouraging preliminary results of Gore-Tex ligament reconstruction, the results of 4- to 5-year follow-up of many studies have demonstrated an apparent deterioration in both subjective and objective results. Karzel et al.[44] reported on 61 patients with a 4-year follow-up. A progressive increase in side-to-side differences on KT-1000 testing was noted with longer follow-up, though 48 (79%) patients had good or excellent subjective results. There was a relatively high complication rate, involving 30 (49%) patients, although most were minor. Seventeen percent of the patients subsequently required that the Gore-Tex ligament graft be removed. Of interest was that approximately one third of the patients that subjectively were scored as good to excellent had side-to-side differences of greater than 5 mm. The authors noted that the subjective results did not always correlate well with the objective evaluation.

Rosenberg[70] reported an overall failure rate of 17.5% of patients within a group of 234 patients that underwent Gore-Tex prosthesis reconstruction. Of those failures, there was an acute rupture in 22 patients, residual symptomatic instability in 7 patients, a recurrent effusion requiring removal of the prosthesis in 7 patients, and infection in 5 patients. Eleven percent of the patients demonstrated objective failures on KT-1000 testing, but were asymptomatic. Of the ruptured ligaments that underwent rearthroscopy, the ligament rupture was found in the intraarticular portion of the ligament or at the inlet to the femoral tunnel. Paulos and associates[67] had a 76% complication rate with the Gore-Tex reconstruction in patients with a previous intraarticular reconstruction and a 42% failure rate. The patients that had excellent results tended to be female, older, and less active.

Sledge and colleagues[75] prospectively evaluated 81 patients of whom 54 were available for a 5-year follow-up. The mean age at the time of the Gore-Tex ligament implantation was 27.6 years and the time interval from injury to reconstruction was 43.6 months. Objective examination demonstrated improvement postoperatively with the Lachman test improving from a grade of 2.5 to 1.2 and the pivot shift from 2.0 to 0.7. KT-1000 testing at 89 N showed a side-to-side difference of 2.3 mm. Objectively, 54 (93%) of the patients were satisfied at a 5-year follow-up, although 12 (22%) had major complications. Analysis of the eight graft failures found all occurred within the fourth and fifth postoperative year. Nordt and Terry[60] had 21 graft failures (23%) in 90 Gore-Tex reconstructions. Willis and Collins[86] reviewed 99 reconstructions 2 to 6 years postoperatively. In 38% of the patients, the knee became increasingly lax with longer follow-up. KT-1000 testing at maximum manual load showed a side-to-side difference of 5.1 mm. Removal or replacement of the prosthesis occurred in only 6% of the patients, despite a 32% reoperation rate for other reasons.

Moseley and associates[59] evaluated 57 patients that underwent reconstruction after a 4-year follow-up. Seventy-eight percent of the patients had satisfactory subjective results, but objective examination showed that all of the results deteriorated with time. KT-1000 testing at 4-year follow-up showed a side-to-side difference of 4.3 mm, which was close to the average preoperative value of 4.8 mm. The overall failure rate in this series was 18%, and again satisfactory subjective results did not necessarily correlate with the objective results.

The primary concern with the use of the Gore-Tex ligament is the progressive increase in laxity of the ligament with longer periods of follow-up and the relatively high incidence of sterile effusions found in the postreconstruction knee. In the results of the clinical trials of the Gore-Tex ligament, approximately one third of the patients had increasing laxity on Lachman testing from 3 months after ligament implantation to approximately 12 to 18 months after surgery. This increased laxity was equivalent to a shift in 1 grade on the Lachman test. Glousman and colleagues[33] found that 98% of the knees 3 months postoperatively often had a Lachman grade of 0 or 1+, whereas at 18 months, 88% met this criterion. Likewise, Strum and associates[78] evaluated anteroposterior stability in 11 patients after Gore-Tex reconstruction. Six patients (55%) had residual anterior laxity greater than 8 mm with a side-to-side difference between injured and noninjured greater than 2 mm at 1-year follow-up. The Lachman test had relatively firm end points, but there was more anterior tibial translation than expected.

Since biomechanical testing predicted minimal elongation of the device over time, the reason for this increased laxity was not apparent. Moore and Markolf[58] subsequently tested Gore-Tex ligaments implanted in fresh cadaver knees. They subjected the ligament to repeated 200-N anteroposterior load cycles that produced an increase of 5 to 7 mm in laxity of the ligament. The laxity could be eliminated if the knee were flexed and extended 30 times between 0 and 90 degrees with a constant 200-N force applied to the tibial eyelet after fixation of the femoral side of the graft. After the tibial eyelet was secured, the testing demonstrated no increase in laxity of the ligament. This process, called preconditioning, led to a recommendation that the maneuver be performed at the time of implantation. A subsequent study by Markolf and associates[54] evaluated 20 patients who had undergone previous Gore-Tex ACL reconstruction. They found that the difference in anterior laxity between the injured and normal knee was unchanged 2 months postoperatively when compared with the amount of laxity in the injured knee before operation. All patients had an anterior laxity on the reconstructed knee of greater than 8 mm and 90% had a side-to-side difference of greater than 2 mm at 2-year follow-up. Clinically, all of these patients demonstrated improvement in both subjective and objective ratings. There was found to be no significant correlation between the clinical parameters evaluated and instrumented test measurements. A comparison study of those patients who had undergone a preconditioning of the Gore-Tex ligament at the time of implantation has not yet been performed. The current recommendation for prestressing the ligament is to maintain approximately 40 lbs of tension on the ligament while moving the knee through 20 cycles of flexion and extension prior to fixing the ligament on the tibia.

Another area of concern is the relatively high rate of recurrent sterile effusions in the postreconstruction knee.[70] These effusions generally present as an acutely inflamed knee. Synovial fluid analysis demonstrates an elevated white blood cell count, consisting primarily of polymorphonuclear leukocytes. Cultures of the fluid are invariably negative. These patients will often respond to initial conservative treatment which includes rest, ice, and anti-inflammatory medications. In arthroscopic evaluation of these cases, the ligament may be partially ruptured. Analysis of the synovial fluid by the ligament manufacturer has not demonstrated a direct relationship between the number of PTFE particles in the synovium and the degree of the effusion. In recalcitrant cases the prosthesis may have to be removed to alleviate the chronic and recurrent effusions. Attention to the technical factors previously alluded to may help reduce the ligament abrasion and subsequent release of PTFE particles. The synovial reaction to particulate debris may not be a problem limited solely to the Gore-Tex prosthesis. Olson and associates[63] demonstrated that injection of wear particles from the Gore-Tex, Stryker-Dacron, Carbone Versigraft, Kennedy LAD, ProCol xenograft, Leeds-Keio, and human patellar tendon allografts into animal synovial cell tissue cultures all produced a similar reaction. These synoviocytes were found to produce destructive enzymes which may contribute to the development of degenerative changes in the joint. Fu[26] has proposed a protocol for synovial fluid analysis and failed ligament retrieval for use by orthopaedic surgeons in the general community. The protocol consists of:

1. Documentation of the events, signs, and symptoms leading to explant (e.g., reinjury or chronic synovitis with effusions).
2. Radiographic evaluation.
3. Synovial fluid analysis prior to ligament removal, with attention to fluid appearance, volume, presence of wear particles, and cytologic features.
4. Synovial fluid cultures and sensitivities.
5. Photographic documentation of the failed ligament in situ, with attention to where the ligament failed (e.g., drill hole edge or narrow intercondylar notch).
6. Photograph of the failed ligament specimen.
7. The retrieved ligament specimen should be placed in 10% neutral buffered formalin, together with any attached tissue.
8. Several synovial biopsies of the knee, not limited to regions of apparent inflammation. Juxtaarticular synovial folds should be biopsied because wear particles tend to accumulate in these regions. The region biopsied should be noted for each specimen (e.g., retrofemoral synovial fold).
9. Histologic examination of the ligament explant to characterize the cell population around the ligament's fibers (e.g., fibroblasts, monocytes, macrophages, multinucleated giant cells, lymphocytes, polymorphonoculear cells, vascularity).
10. Histologic examination of the synovial biopsies and tissue surrounding the intraarticular portion of the ligament for the location of particulate matter and characterization of the cell population around it.
11. Use of polarized light microscopy to aid in the identification of particulate matter.
12. Evaluation of the size of the particulate matter present.
13. No meaningful biomechanical tests can be performed on the failed ligament.

Another concern is the formation of a tibial bone cyst adjacent to the Gore-Tex prosthesis in the tibial tunnel.[25] These cysts appear to represent a foreign body reaction, but they can be confused with a neoplasm. In most cases, once a tibial cyst is present, it will be necessary to remove the Gore-Tex prosthesis, after which the cyst will subsequently resolve.

Summary

With doubts regarding the ultimate longevity of the Gore-Tex ligament, the apparent failure of the ligament after implantation with longer follow-up, and the recurrent and chronic effusions, a judicious approach to Gore-Tex prosthetic ligament implantation would appear to be justified. Currently, the ligament is approved by the FDA only for use in the previously failed autogenous reconstruction. In a young active patient with ACL deficiency, an autogenous ligament reconstruction should be the initial choice, rather than a Gore-Tex prosthetic replacement. In the chronically ACL-deficient knee, there is some evidence that reconstruction with the Gore-Tex ligament may result in a higher incidence of failure than reconstruction after an acute ACL injury. The Gore-Tex ligament should be reserved for patients that have had previous failed autogenous reconstructions or those not athletically active. A possible indication for Gore-Tex reconstruction may be an older patient with ACL deficiency who has disabling functional instability associated with degenerative changes within the knee. In this particular instance, a more rapid rehabilitation can be permitted, possibly decreasing the chance of postoperative knee stiffness. Another indication may be in an older, less active, sedentary patient with disabling functional instabilities with activities of daily living who wishes to avoid the morbidity of autogenous reconstruction and the potential of disease transmission with an allograft. Also included in this group would be those patients that are not able to commit to an extensive prolonged rehabilitation program which is necessary when using an autogenous ACL reconstruction. With the success of autogenous and allograft reconstructions, the use of the Gore-Tex prosthesis has become less appealing and

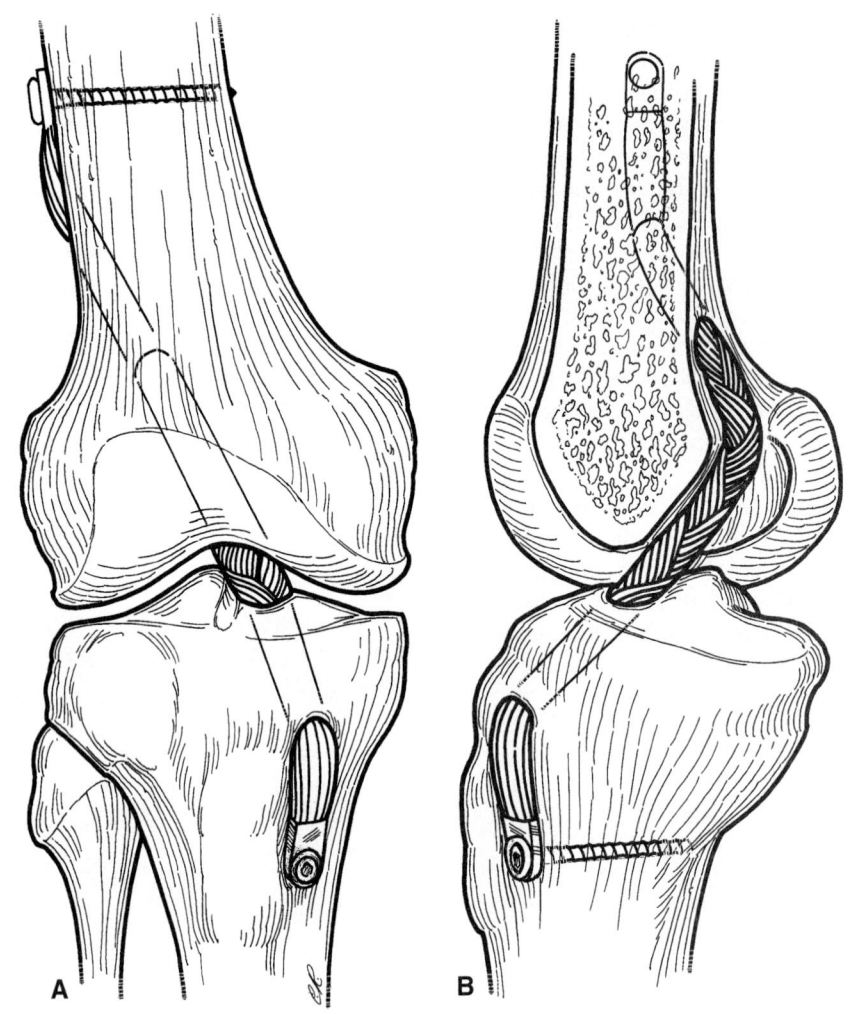

FIG 47–8.
Frontal **(A)** and cross-sectional **(B)** view of the implanted Gore-Tex ligament demonstrating proper placement of the graft.

more strictly defined in its indications for use. When using the Gore-Tex ligament, careful attention to the technical factors previously alluded to is necessary to optimize the results of reconstruction.

New developments in the Gore-Tex ligament with the advent of the Gore-Tex II prosthesis may improve the results of prosthetic reconstruction. The Gore-Tex II ligament (Fig 47–9) addresses some of the biomechanical problems inherent in the original prosthesis. This prosthesis has been changed by compacting the diameter of the ligament with a tighter weave configuration, compared to the Gore-Tex I ligament, which may help prevent abrasion of the ligament on the bony edges in the intercondylar notch. This, theoretically, may increase the longevity of the implant and reduce PTFE shedding. Further, in vitro testing has demonstrated that the prototype Gore-Tex II prosthesis has approximately twice the wear resistance and residual strength of the old Gore-Tex ligament. This ligament is currently being tested in Canada and is not commercially available in the United States.

Stryker Dacron Ligament

Concept

The Stryker Dacron ligament prosthesis is a composite of four Dacron tapes surrounded by a woven Dacron velour sleeve (Fig 47–10). The components are combined to form a single prosthesis. The ends of the device are covered with plastic tips that facilitate passage of the graft within the knee. The development of the Stryker Dacron ligament for use in orthopaedic surgery was preceded by the safe use of Dacron in vascular surgery. The implant was initially designed to be used as an augmentation device with the

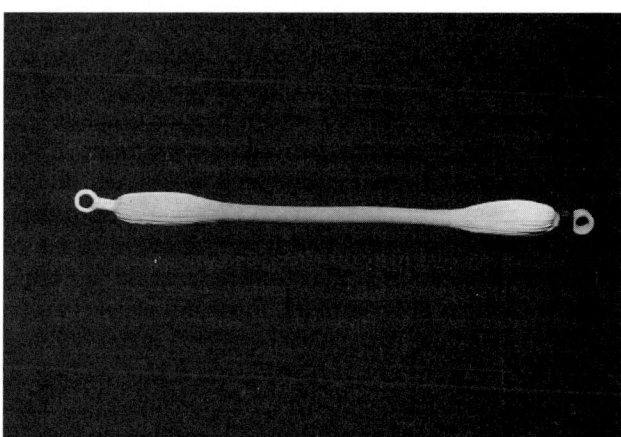

FIG 47–9.
The compact diameter Gore-Tex ligament (Gore-Tex II).

iliotibial band in ACL reconstructions, but the high strength of the ligament has led to its use as a permanent prosthesis. Animal studies in dogs had demonstrated significant bone and fibrous tissue ingrowth when used as an augmentation device.[64, 65] When used as a permanent type of prosthesis, no synovial tissue ingrowth is noted intraarticularly.[73] Mechanical testing has demonstrated the ultimate tensile strength of the ligament to be 3,631 N.[65] Fatigue testing showed the ability to withstand 134,000 fatigue cycles at 1,730-N force.[8] This amount of force would presumably disrupt a normal ACL after a single cycle. The estimated in vivo life expectancy from the fatigue testing data is 8.5 years. The ligament can be used for combined intraarticular and extraarticular reconstruction and is manufactured in an 8-mm diameter with an overall length of 70 cm.

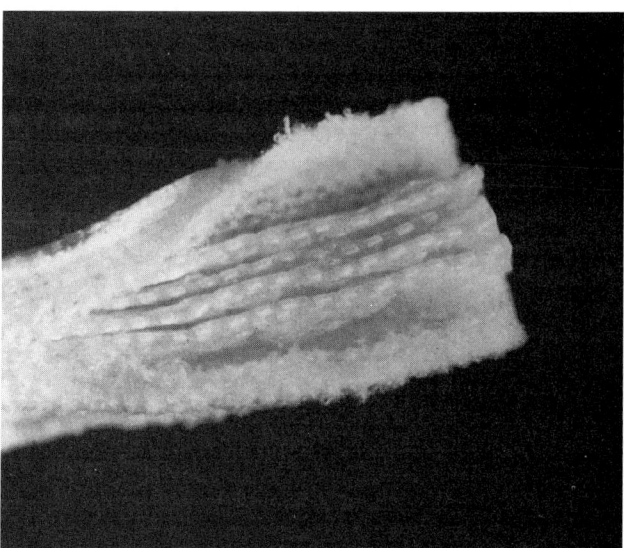

FIG 47–10.
Close-up of the Stryker Dacron ligament.

Technique

The reconstruction is performed with the knee at approximately 90 degrees of flexion.[17] An anterior medial incision, 3 to 5 cm in length, is made medial to the patella. This allows visualization for a notchplasty to be performed and insertion of the drill guide. Special retractors are placed in the incision to retract the patella laterally. This allows visualization of the intercondylar notch and the tibial plateau. The manufacturer has developed a notch-measuring device which is used to determine the amount of notchplasty for implantation of the prosthesis. This device creates a width of 21 mm between the medial and femoral condyles. An osteotome or gouge can be used to remove the appropriate amount of bone. Care is taken not to remove excessive bone at the ACL insertion site on the lateral femoral condyle, as this would tend to lateralize the insertion point of the graft. After completion of the notchplasty, the isometric drill guide frame is positioned. Two small pins on the lower portion of the distal end of the guide handle are positioned within the remnants of the original ACL attachment site on the tibial plateau. If the guide is positioned correctly, the transverse line on the superior surface of the isometric guide should lie directly above the junction of the anterior horn of the medial meniscus. The patellar retractor is removed during this step to prevent rotation of the tibia during guide alignment. The guide handle is rotated until the intraarticular portion of the guide handle comes into contact with the medial wall of the lateral femoral condyle. Care is taken to maintain the guide handle in a horizontal position parallel to the long axis of the femur. When the guide has been positioned correctly, the guide tube is advanced through its holder on the inferior surface of the guide handle. When the guide tube has been advanced to the anterior medial surface of the tibia, it is lightly tapped into the surface of the tibia with a mallet to secure the guide handle position. The locking screw on the guide tube is then tightened firmly. At this point, proper positioning of the guide handle can be confirmed with an image intensifier. The guide has been designed so that the intraarticular portion of the guide handle replicates the original 28-degree angulation of the ACL with respect to the tibia and its mean length of 31 mm. When the guide is properly positioned on the tibia, the distal end of the guide handle will be within the last 20 degrees of Blumensaat's line on the lateral radiograph.

A guide pin is positioned within the guide tube and advanced to the tibia. The knee is held at 90 degrees of flexion and the tibia in neutral position while the pin is advanced. The guide pin directs the pin automatically toward the intraarticular portion of the guide handle. The pin then passes through the guide handle and into the opposing lateral femoral cortex. As the pin begins to pass through the outer lateral femoral cortex, a second incision is made to expose the guide pin and protect the soft tissues.

The guide pin used in the reconstruction is specially designed and has a flat portion in the midsection. It is important to put the flat portion of the guide pin in a vertical orientation. The next step is confirming the isometric placement of the guide pin. The guide pin is removed and an ejector rod is inserted through the tibial hole and through the lateral femur. With the knee maintained at 90 degrees of flexion, the ejector rod should follow the same course as the guide pin. The distal end of the ejector has a hole through which a no. 1 steel suture can be positioned. The objector is then pulled back through the tunnels bringing the suture with it. The suture is clamped firmly on the posterolateral aspect of the femur. A strain gauge and tensioning device is used to confirm proper guide placement. The strain gauge is secured to the cortex on the periosteum on the anterior medial tibia by rotating the collar on the proximal end until adequate contact is achieved. The suture is held within the strain gauge and clamped firmly at the proximal end. The wide locking collar is then turned to create tension of 15 to 20 N in the steel suture. The knee is passed through a full range of motion and the excursion of the strain gauge is noted. A total excursion of less than 3 mm indicates that the guide pin has been properly positioned. If more than 3 mm of excursion is obtained, the guide handle and pin must be repositioned in order to determine the isometric point. After the guide pin channel has been confirmed to be in its isometric position, the suture is removed and the pin is reinserted. The guide pin is then overdrilled using the 5-mm cannulated reamer. Low-speed reamers are used to prevent bone necrosis. After the tunnels have been made, the holes are chamfered.

The implant is then inserted through the tibial drill hole opening on the medial side and passed intraarticularly into the femoral tunnel. A minimum of 10 mm of the prosthesis should be left leading from the tibial tunnel to facilitate later attachment of the strain gauge tensioning device. A staple is used to fix the implant securely to the lateral aspect of the femur and the strain gauge and tension device is then attached to the portion of the implant protruding from the tibial tunnel. The locking collar aligns the strain gauge and tensioning device in the same plane as the bony tunnel. Three newtons of tension is applied to the implant and a Lachman test is performed with the strain gauge and tension device locked in place. Tension can be adjusted as necessary in an attempt to restore stability to the knee. With the ligament implant maintained under proper tension, the locking collar is loosened to allow alignment of the strain gauge and tension device cylinder within the tibia. This allows sufficient clearance to permit placement of a fixation staple while the implant is maintained under tension. After the strain gauge and tensioning devices are removed, a second staple can be placed to further fixate the ligament. After wound closure, the extremity is placed into a hinged brace.

This procedure can also be performed arthroscopically.[64] The isometric drill guide system is placed through the anteromedial portal which may need to be slightly enlarged. The remainder of the steps are similar to those described for the miniarthrotomy technique. Postoperatively, the patient starts range-of-motion exercises of the knee during the first 3 postoperative days. A continuous passive motion (CPM) machine can also be used. The patient is kept nonweightbearing for 4 weeks to allow for bony ingrowth into the prosthesis and assure additional fixation into the interosseous tunnels. Return to sports activities is not permitted until full muscle strength is regained, which usually is within 3 to 6 months post implantation.

Results

Lukianov and colleagues[52] reported results of ACL reconstructions for chronic instability using the Stryker Dacron ligament in 513 patients from 19 investigational centers. Three hundred thirty patients were available for at least 2 years of postoperative follow-up. Ninety-seven percent of these patients had a negative pivot shift at follow-up compared to 11% preoperatively. Complications included ligament rupture, which occurred in 3.8% of the cases; infection in 2.3%; and synovitis in 1.5%. Lysholm scores improved from an average of 59 preoperatively to 93 at 2 years' final follow-up.

Bartolozzi and associates[5] followed 53 patients with chronic ACL deficiency that underwent Stryker Dacron ligament reconstruction with a mean follow-up of 29 months. Subjectively, 44 (83%) patients had excellent or good results, 4 (7.5%) fair, and 5 (9.5%) poor. The percentage of poor subjective results tended to increase with longer follow-up. Objectively, only 35% of the patients had Lachman grades of 1+ or less. The jerk test was 1+ or less in 61.5%, and 70.5% of patients had a residual positive jerk test. These particular parameters were found not to deteriorate significantly with time. The KT-1000 testing data showed a side-to-side difference of 3 mm or greater in approximately two thirds of the cases. Complications were present in 13% of the patients. There were no cases of persistent synovitis but on radiographic evaluation after at least 1 year of ligament reconstruction, 85% of the patients demonstrated periligamentous femoral osteolysis which was primarily located at the intraarticular portion of the distal femoral tunnel. In this series, patients over the age of 25 years tended to have worse overall results than younger patients.

Anderson and co-workers[3] prospectively evaluated 57 patients with chronic laxity that underwent Dacron ligament reconstruction. The mean follow-up in this series was 34 months. There were 71% excellent or good results. Twenty-two percent of the patients had a negative Lachman test and 42% had a negative anterior drawer postoperatively. There were ten ruptured grafts, six of which occurred within the first 12 months and four within the next 12 months. Six of the ruptures were in the proximal portion of the graft, while four were midsubstance disruptions. Additional complications included cases of postoperative infection, chronic synovitis, and one case of reflex sympathetic dystrophy. Only 15 patients were able to regain their preinjury activity level. Guarda and colleagues[37] evaluated 34 patients after an average follow-up of 3 years. The graft was inserted in the over-the-top position by an arthrotomy. Overall functional results demonstrated 82.4% (28/34 patients) excellent or good results, 5.7% fair (2), and 11.8% (4) poor. Sixty-five percent of the patients had 0 to 1+ Lachman grades. Five cases of breakage of the radial marker occurred, but only three had objective signs of recurrent instability. Only half of the patients were able to resume sports activities at their prior level.

Longer-term follow-up studies have recently appeared in the literature and demonstrate further deterioration of results. Lopez-Vazquez and co-workers[51] viewed 54 patients that underwent Dacron prosthetic ligament implantation. Nineteen of these patients had acute ACL injuries while 36 had chronic tears. Follow-up ranged from 2 to 5 years. Twenty-six patients (48%) had either detachment or elongation of the prosthesis. The majority of the failures occurred between the second and fourth postoperative years with no predilection for acute or chronic reconstructions. The Lysholm and Gillquist scores demonstrated deterioration with time. The authors concluded that the prosthesis was not a durable substitute for ACL replacement or supplementation.

Richmond and associates[68] reported their results of reconstruction in 35 patients with a mean follow-up of 50 months. They divided their patients into two groups: patients with isolated ACL instability only, and patients with a previously failed ACL reconstruction or other rotational laxity. In the first group, the pivot shift test was negative, and the anterior drawer and Lachman tests were 1+ or less at 2 years. At the final follow-up, 96% of the patients had Lachman tests of less than 1+. KT-1000 testing at 89 N showed a mean 1.2-mm side-to-side difference. Nineteen percent of the patients had a difference greater than 3 mm. There was a 27% failure rate in this group, all occurring after the 2-year follow-up. In the second group, there was a positive pivot shift in one third of the patients at final follow-up. The anterior drawer and Lachman tests were 2+ or greater in 11% of patients at 2 years and in 33% at final follow-up. KT-1000 testing revealed a mean side-to-side difference of 4.2 mm and two thirds of the patients had a side-to-side difference greater than 3 mm. There was a 78% failure rate in the group at 2-year follow-up. There was functional improvement based upon the Lysholm and Tegner scores but deterioration in the overall performance of the patient occurred in the reconstructions at longer follow-up. As part of a larger prospective multicenter study, Wilk and Richmond[85] reported on 84 patients who underwent reconstruction with the Dacron ligament in the chronic ACL-deficient knee. These patients were followed for at least 5 years and were placed into two groups as in the previous study. The overall failure rate in this study was 35.7% (30/84 patients), compared with the 2.5% failure rate at 2 years. Again, this showed a significant deterioration of the results during the follow-up intervals.

Gillquist and associates[32] have performed reconstruction with the Dacron prosthesis in 150 patients, of whom 70 had at least a 5-year follow-up. The difference in laxity between the reconstructed and normal knee at 5-year follow-up was 2 mm or less in two thirds of the patients with an intact ligament. The remaining 34% of the patients were considered to have a nonfunctioning ligament. The reconstructed knees also demonstrated a slow progressive increase in laxity up to 3 years postoperatively which then appeared to stabilize. Lysholm scores increased from 50 preoperatively to 90 postoperatively, which was maintained at final follow-up. The mean Tegner activity rating also increased but did not usually reach preinjury levels. Sixteen patients (23%) had ruptures of their ligaments and 14 of these had prosthetic ligaments reinserted. The authors emphasize careful attention to the technical factors of implant insertion to minimize rupture rates.

Tissue ingrowth into the ligament was evaluated in two cases in which the Dacron ligament, used as a prosthesis, ruptured.[73] The histologic and electron microscopic evaluation demonstrated fibroblasts and elastic fibers in a lax connective tissue stroma immediately adjacent to the Dacron threads. Fibroblasts and collagen fibrils were located further from the Dacron threads. The periprosthetic tissue did not demonstrate the biomechanical properties or morphologic characteristics necessary to resist tension stresses. Also noted was the infrequent occurrence of inflammatory cells in the synovial membrane, which indicated the relative inertness of the Dacron material.

Summary

The Stryker Dacron ligament was approved for general use in failed intraarticular ACL reconstructions by the FDA in January 1989. Recent studies demonstrate a significant failure rate at 5 years. Initially, the ligament was designed to act as a scaffold to allow soft tissue ingrowth which would then ultimately provide its own tensile strength while simultaneously decreasing the role of the graft material. Subsequent investigations have demonstrated no significant differences of function and stability in the knees that underwent reconstruction with or without augmentation.[64] This suggests that the Dacron ligament functions as a true prosthesis rather than a scaffold type of implant. Since the graft material is biologically inert, there has been a lower incidence of synovitis than has been reported with the Gore-Tex ligament reconstructions. The results of the Stryker Dacron ligament reconstruction appear to be similar to those of the Gore-Tex, with continued deterioration and failure over time.

Leeds-Keio Ligament

Concept

The Leeds-Keio ligament is not a prosthesis, although the implant is permanent and initially carries all of the load of the device. The device is meant to act as a scaffold to allow ingrowth of collagenous tissue. As the collagen matures, aligns, and becomes capable of bearing the load of the implant, the importance of the prosthetic ligament is decreased. The implant is not designed to biodegrade and will retain a considerable portion of its initial strength over time. The ligament is composed of polyester fibers that are woven to form a mesh structure consisting of two main sections: one tubular and one flat (Fig 47–11). At the end of the tubular portion of the ligament, a cord is attached to facilitate passage through the bone tunnels. One of the ends of the implant has a pouch where the bone plug is inserted to anchor to the substitute into the bone tunnel. The other end is split open. The

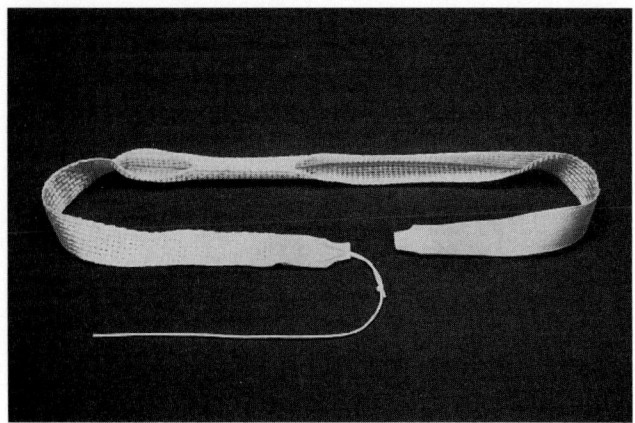

FIG 47–11.
The Leeds-Keio Ligament. (Courtesy of Dr. Bahaa B. Seedhom, University of Leeds, England.)

diameter of the tubular portion of the ligament is 11 mm. The graft is available in two separate lengths: one is suitable for intraarticular reconstruction alone; the other, longer implant allows a combined intraarticular and extraarticular reconstruction to be performed. The implant was designed through collaboration between groups at Leeds University in England and Keio University in Japan. Biomechanical testing has demonstrated that the ligament has a strength in excess of 2,000 N.[74] Studies have also shown a strain rate at low-loading levels similar to that of the normal ACL. Fatigue testing has demonstrated that the implant is able to withstand 94 million cycles between 50 and 700 N, with a residual strength of 1,380 N.[27]

A unique aspect of the Leeds-Keio ligament is the method of anchoring the ligament to bone (Fig 47–12).[29] The ligament is designed to be implanted between two bony surfaces. Theoretically, as the bony surfaces heal, they unite through the holes in the implant and securely lock the ligament into place. The anchoring is achieved by securing the implant between the bone tunnel and the bone plug with the difference in diameter between the plug and the hole being large enough to accommodate the size of the implant. The bone plug is obtained with a special instrument that cuts the bone plug sharply and removes it from the tunnel. The bone plug is approximately 9.5 mm in diameter and 20 to 25 mm in length. The harvested bone plug is then placed into the pouch at the end of the Leeds-Keio ligament and pushed back into the tunnel to secure the graft. Recently, staples have also been used in addition to the bone plug fixation, to transfix the ligament at the tibial and femoral tunnels. The staples provide initial mechanical support of the graft, so that a more aggressive postoperative rehabilitation program can be

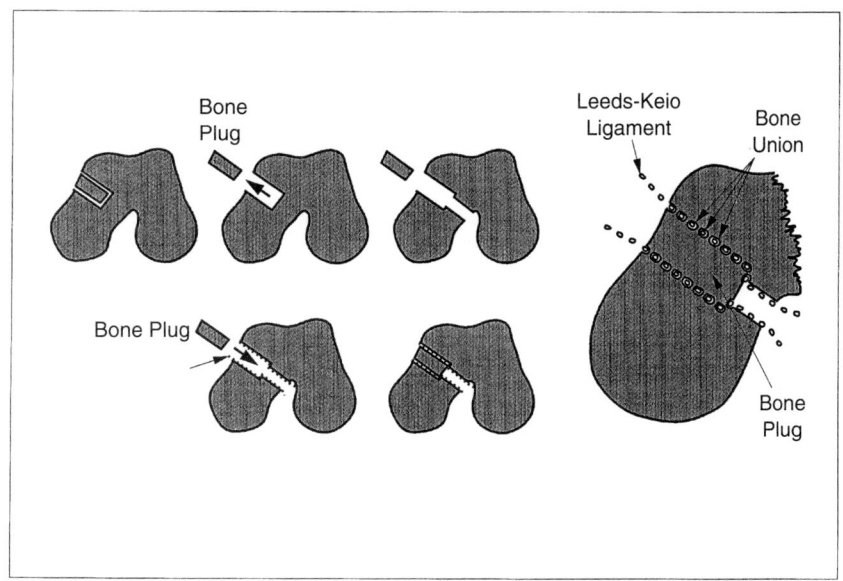

FIG 47–12.
Anchoring system of the Leeds-Keio ligament. (Courtesy of Dr. Bahaa B. Seedhom, University of Leeds, England.)

undertaken. Since the implant is a loosely woven polyester, it is highly susceptible to damage and snagging against the bones as it is pulled through the bony tunnels. For this reason, the implant is placed within a polyethylene tubular sheath during passage through the tunnels. After placement of the graft, the sheath is removed.

The Leeds-Keio ligament has been implanted in over 14,000 patients worldwide but the ligament has not yet been approved for use in the United States.

Technique

The Leeds-Keio ligament is designed so that it can be implanted intraarticularly or in combination with an extraarticular reconstruction. The procedure is performed with specially designed instruments including reamers, ligament guides, bone plug extractors, and introducers (Fig 47–13). The technique described here is that of one of the designers of the ligament, Dr. Kyosuke Fujikawa.[27, 31]

Initially, two incisions are made for access to the knee. The first incision is made along the lateral aspect of the distal femur and is extended through the subcutaneous tissue and the iliotibial band. The vastus lateralis is reflected anteriorly and the lateral femoral metaphysis is exposed. The second incision is then made along the anteromedial aspect of the proximal tibia with an arthrotomy to visualize the anterior articular placement of the guides. The patella is not everted during the procedure. A ligament guide is used and first placed on the lateral femoral condyle. A guide pin is then placed in an isometric position located posteriorly and superiorly in the intercondylar notch. A reamer is used to make a bony tunnel 11 mm wide and 20 to 25 mm long. The special extractor allows for removal of the bone plug of this length from within the tunnel. An 11-mm drill sleeve is placed in the tunnel and a second, smaller 6-mm hole is drilled through the remaining bone into the isometric point. A similar procedure is then undertaken for placement of the tibial tunnel. A hole is drilled medially into the tibial insertion of the ACL. Again, a bone plug is removed after reaming the tunnel using the bone plug extractor. A smaller tunnel

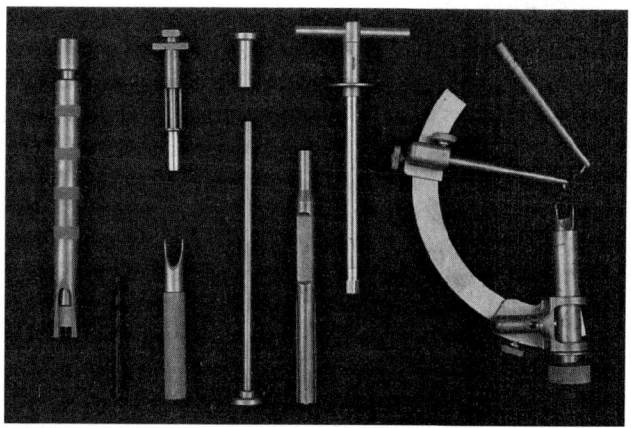

FIG 47–13.
Instrumentation for anterior cruciate ligament reconstruction *(right to left):* universal clamp, reamer, bone plug extractor, drill bit guide and push rod, bone plug introducer and bone pindenter, 0.25-in. drill bit, staple introducer. (Courtesy of Bahaa B. Seedhom, B.Sc, Ph.D, University of Leeds, England.)

is drilled to 6.5 mm in diameter. The manufacturer does not recommend performing a notchplasty. A notchplasty is thought to be unnecessary given the small diameter of the ligament used and because the sharp edges created from the notchplasty expose cancellous bone that may abrade the implant. In an intraarticular reconstruction, the ligament is passed antegrade through the femoral tunnel and out the tibial tunnel. The passage of the implant through the bony tunnels is facilitated by a plastic covering over the ligament and a loop of polyester at the end of the ligament. The ligament is pulled through the bone until the closed pouch at the femoral end is adjacent to the tunnel, at which point the previously obtained bone plug is placed into the pouch of the ligament. The ligament is then pulled distally, locking the bone plug securely through the femoral tunnel (Fig 47–14, A and B). After passage of the ligament through the tibial tunnel, tension is maintained and the second bone plug is impacted firmly within the tibial tunnel securing the ligament (Fig 47–15). A staple and buckle plate are used to fixate the ligament at both ends of the implant.

In those cases in which an extraarticular procedure is added to the intraarticular reconstruction, the longer Leeds-Keio ligament is used. The procedure is as previously described with the exception that the ligament is passed intraarticularly in a retrograde manner, i.e., from the tibial tunnel, then out through the femoral tunnel. The bone plug is then placed in the closed end of the ligament, which is the tibial side of the implant. The femoral portion of the graft is fixated with a bone plug while the knee is at 30 degrees of flexion. The Leeds-Keio ligament is then passed subcutaneously along the lateral side of the joint under the iliotibial tract and lateral collateral ligament. A third bony tunnel, approximately 5 mm in diameter, is drilled from the anterosuperior aspect of

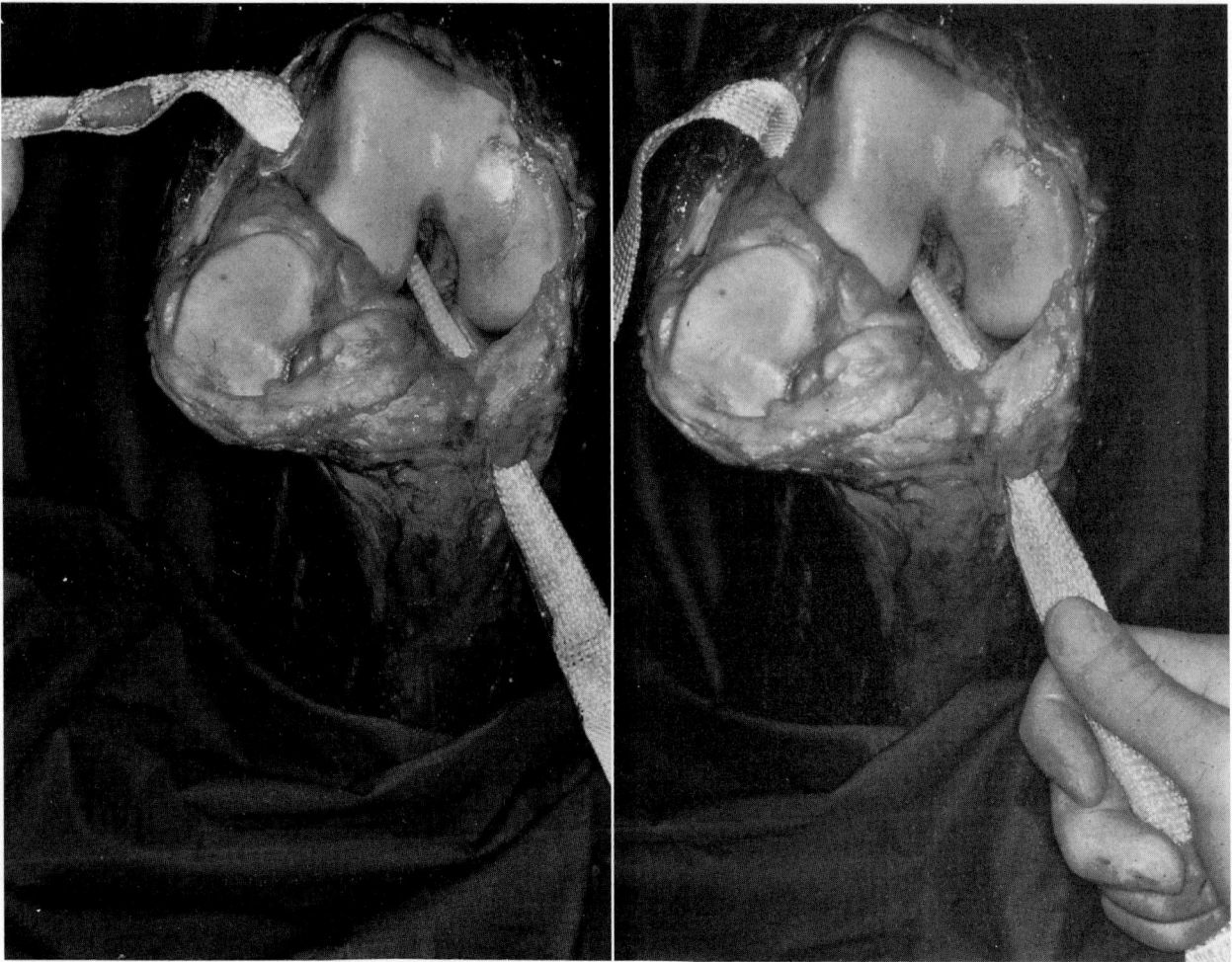

FIG 47–14.
A and **B,** anchoring the ligament at the distal femoral tunnel with a bone plug as the ligament and sheath are pulled distally.

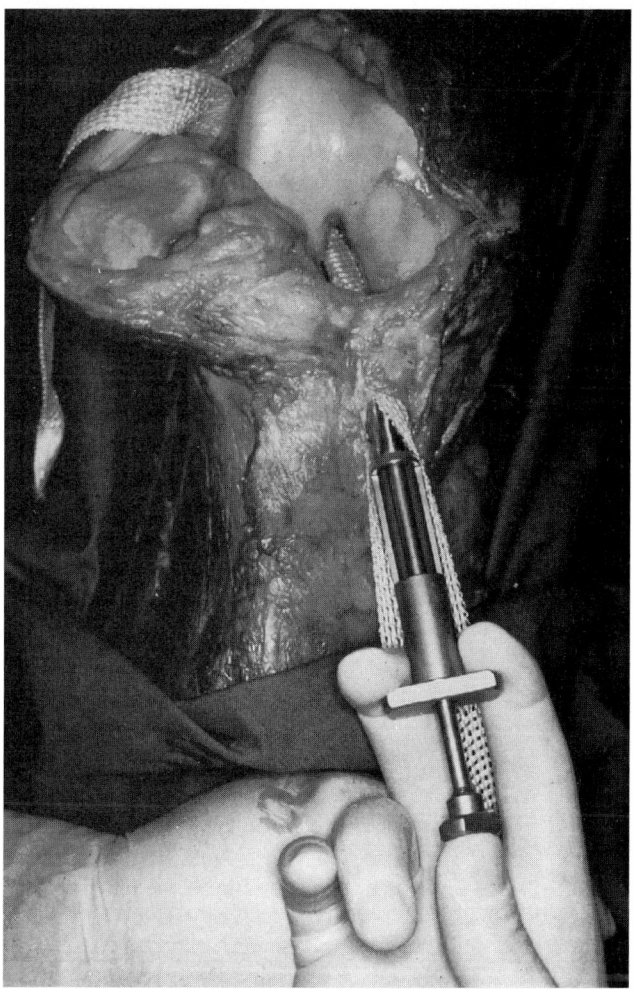

FIG 47–15.
The tibial bone plug is introduced within the ligament and pushed into the tunnel. (Courtesy of Dr. Bahaa B. Seedhom, University of Leeds, England.)

Gerdy's tubercle to the medial side of the tibia. The implant is passed through the tunnel and then stapled in place, while the tibia is externally rotated. Recently, arthroscopic-assisted techniques with modified instrumentation have been developed.

Postoperatively, the knee is placed on a CPM machine immediately after surgery, allowing a range of motion of approximately 20 to 60 degrees. The range of motion is increased up to 90 degrees of flexion after 1 week. Partial weightbearing is allowed at 3 to 4 weeks post implantation and at 6 to 10 weeks flexion and extension in the brace are no longer restricted. Jogging is begun in the brace at 12 weeks, and sports activities are progressively incorporated in the postoperative rehabilitation program at 3 to 5 months. Despite the relative strength of the ligament found on biomechanical testing, it is believed that 3 to 4 weeks of protective activity is essential to allow healing of tissue around the bony tunnels and to prevent abrasion or damage to the implanted ligament. During this time, some bony fixation will occur to the ligament and bone plug, providing additional fixation prior to initiating vigorous activity. Denti and associates[19] evaluated the ligament and bone plugs after implantation of the Leeds-Keio ligament with magnetic resonance imaging (MRI) scans. They recommended that the implant not be fully loaded for at least 45 days after surgery to permit bony anchorage and stabilization of the prosthesis.

Results

The Leeds-Keio study group has implanted more than 450 artificial ligaments since February 1982. Fujikawa[28] reported the results of 152 cases that had 4 years of postoperative follow-up. Preoperatively, all of the patients had evidence of gross instability and giving way. Objective evaluation with the Lachman test, anterior drawer test, and pivot shift tests in all patients were between 1 and 2+, which improved postoperatively. The Lachman and anterior drawer tests were negative or less than 1+ in 90.1% and 82.2% of patients, respectively. The pivot shift test was negative in 80.3% and trace-positive in 3.9% of the patients. There was a normal or nearly normal knee range of motion in 71.7% of patients and only 4.6% of patients demonstrated a loss of more than 21 degrees of forward motion. No patient had evidence of chronic joint effusion, synovitis, or infection. There were five incidences (3.3%) of ligament rupture requiring revision.

Denti and associates[19] viewed 26 patients that underwent implantation of the Leeds-Keio ligament with a 2- to 4-year follow-up. Twenty-four patients were high-level athletes. The time from initial injury to reconstruction averaged 26.6 months. Postoperatively, the pivot shift test was negative in 23 of the 26 patients. KT-1000 testing at 20 lb demonstrated a 2.1 mm side-to-side difference. The Lysholm scores improved 51%. Overall, 14 patients were rated excellent, 10 good, 1 fair, and 1 poor. There were no significant complications except for two ligament ruptures which occurred after 12 to 20 months of implantation. One of the ruptures was due to a technical error in placement of the implant. There were no cases of synovitis noted.

Evaluation of the tissue ingrowth and the fate of the ligaments post implantation can be assessed with arthroscopy. Fujikawa and colleagues[30] performed postimplantation arthroscopy in 42 cases. Nineteen ligaments had a biopsy taken from the tissue implant from 3 to 24 months post reconstruction. The majority of cases had shown satisfactory tissue ingrowth around the artificial ligament at 3 to 4 months post surgery, and the implant was noted to be covered with immature fibrous tissue and an extensive vascular network. After 6 to 7 months, the tissue was firmly fixed to the implant with the vascular supply visible on the surface of the ligament (Fig 47–16). By 12 to 14 months, the new ligament looked like the natural ACL in overall shape and thickness. However, the vascular network was less prominent. Histologic evaluation demonstrated collagenous fibers running parallel and longitudinal to the axis of the ligament with the surrounding tissue slightly hypercellullar in comparison to that seen in normal ligamentous tissue. By 18 to 24 months, the implanted ligament arthroscopically resembled a normal ACL. Mollica and colleagues[57] reexamined six patients after implantation with the Leeds-Keio ligament. They noted that there was a greater vascularity in the proximal and distal areas of the ligament with a relative absence in the intermediate portion of the graft, which indicated that the vascular proliferation initiated at the bony tunnels and extended centripetally along the ligament. Marcaci and co-workers[53] performed histologic and ultrastructural studies of tissue ingrowth into the Leeds-Keio ligament in a patient that had a ruptured graft at 18 months following implantation. The collagen fibers along the periphery of the ligament tended to be parallel along the axis of the implant. There was no specific orientation of the fibers in the central portion of the graft. The new collagen was found to be primarily type I. The authors concluded that growth of host tissue occurred in and around the Leeds-Keio ligament in response to tensile stresses.

Summary

The Leeds-Keio ligament has several potential advantages over other prostheses. The ligament is strong and relatively compact allowing an arthroscopic-assisted technique for insertion, without the need for a notchplasty. Most important, the ligament has the potential for soft tissue ingrowth which would allow for long-term survival of the implant. The ligament also allows the option of combining an intraarticular and extraarticular procedure at the time of reconstruction. The method of fixation of the implant within the bony tunnels is innovative and appears to allow incorporation of the ligament into the bony tunnels for secure fixation. Backup staple fixation allows a more rapid rehabilitation by providing rigid fixation of the implant while the bone plug–ligament complex heals. The designers of the ligament emphasize the importance of placing the implant under tension so that the induced tissue can organize along the lines of stress and serve a load-bearing function. Also, current recommendations include attaching a piece of synovium to the ligament at the time of implantation to expedite tissue ingrowth.

Although the short-term results are encouraging, longer-term studies are necessary to determine the ultimate fate of soft tissue ingrowth. Of concern is the quality of the soft tissue ingrowth into the ligament. If ingrowth actually does occur, as recent studies suggest, and occurs reproducibly with a strong collagen tissue, this obviously would be an advantage over previous prosthetic ligament reconstructions. The evidence of tissue ingrowth is primarily based on animal studies with only a few recent reports in the literature of results after ligament implantation in humans. Unfortunately, these cases represent only a small number of the ligaments implanted. Further long-term follow-up studies from groups other than the original investigators are necessary to determine the actual efficacy of the Leeds-Keio ligament. Likewise, further investigation as to whether ingrowth does occur reproducibly and whether the collagen tissue obtained provides a structural support to the graft are needed. The Leeds-Keio ligament has gained widespread acceptance in Europe and Asia.

Ligastic Ligament

Concept

The Ligastic ligament, made of polyethylene terephtalate, is unique in its knitted structure (Figs 47–17 and 47–18). The fibers of the ligament are oriented

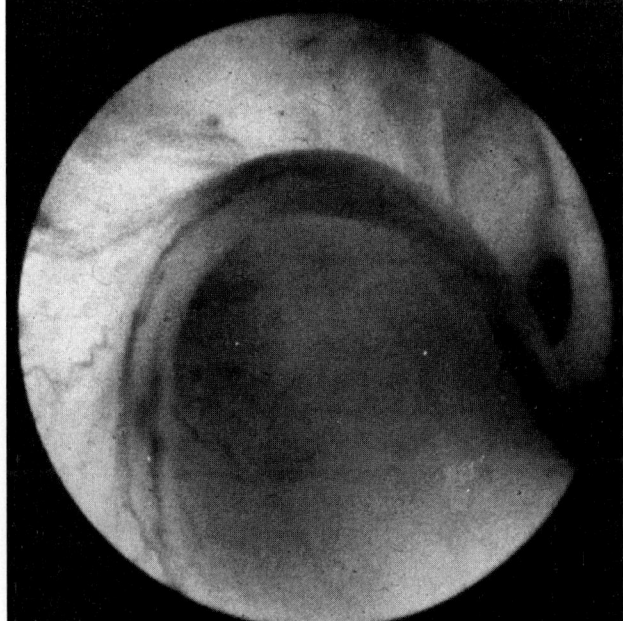

FIG 47–16.
Arthroscopic appearance of the ligament 7 months postoperatively. (Courtesy of Dr. Bahaa B. Seedhom, University of Leeds, England.)

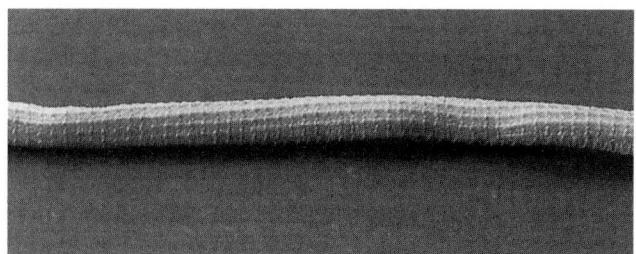

FIG 47–17.
The Ligastic ligament. (Courtesy of Gerard Dericks, Jr., M.D., Honolulu.)

longitudinally to maintain maximal fiber length and eliminate plastic lengthening which can occur with woven or braided prosthetic ligaments. As a result of the design, the ligament has a porosity of 400 μm, which can allow tissue ingrowth to occur when performed with suturing of the residual cruciate ligament suture to the prosthesis. There are three types of ligaments available: the noncoated ligament (NE series), the coated ligament (E series), and the Ligastic HX series (noncoated two-bundle ligament). The noncoated ligament is used in acute ligament ruptures or in situations in which host-tissue ingrowth is warranted. The coated ligament, now rarely used, is considered a true prosthesis. Its mechanical properties tend to duplicate those of the in situ human ACL. No fibroblastic tissue ingrowth occurs in this ligament owing to the intraarticular portion of the ligament being coated with a polyurethane resin. Biomechanical testing[45] (see Table 47–2) of the ligaments demonstrated maximum strength values ranging from 1,800 to 4,200 N depending on the diameter of the ligament used. Fatigue testing with 300-N sinusoidal free application extended up to 11 million cycles had only a 0.6% permanent deformation of the ligament. The ligament also has demonstrated suitable elasticity characteristics under physiologic and traumatic stress conditions.

Technique

The surgical technique for ACL reconstruction is performed through a medial parapatellar arthrotomy after evaluation of the joint by arthroscopy.[46] Using a tibial tunnel guide, a point just posterior and medial to the ACL insertion is identified. A 5-mm drill is then used to create the tibial tunnel. The site for the femoral tunnel is chosen using an isometric guide. The guide is introduced into the intercondylar notch and placed along the posterior border of the lateral femoral condyle. An additional incision is made along the distal lateral femoral condyle and the femoral drill guide is then slid down the lateral femoral condyle. The direction of passage of the ligament is dependent upon the level of the ACL rupture. The ligament is passed retrograde if the tear is near the femoral insertion and antegrade if the rupture is adjacent to the tibial insertion. The cords, which are located at the ends of the plastic portion of the Ligastic ligament, are pulled through the tunnel using a metal wire as a passer. The stump of the ACL is then sutured using absorbable material. This is done in an attempt to preserve any proprioceptive function of the torn ligament in addition to expediting tissue in-

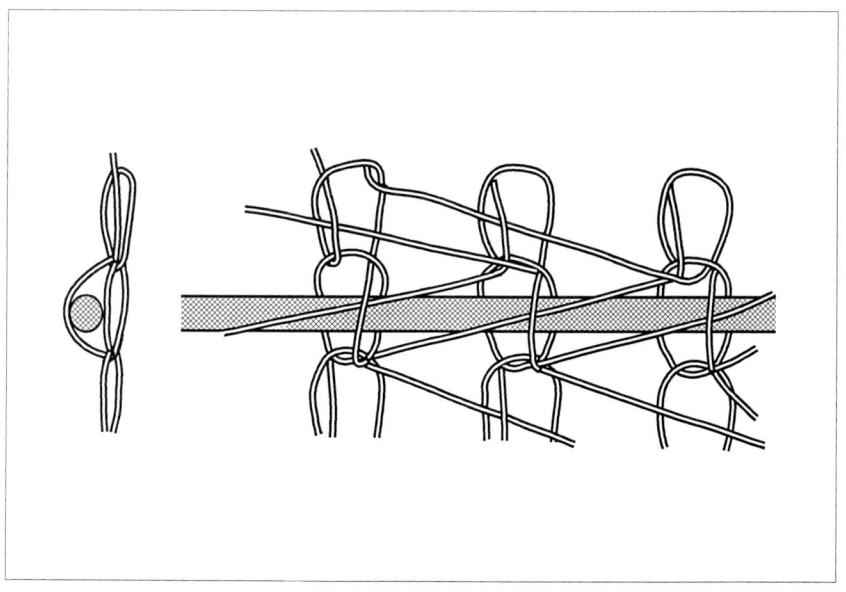

FIG 47–18.
Ligastic knitting structure. (Courtesy of Gerard Dericks, Jr., M.D., Honolulu.)

growth. Also, the residual ACL stump helps to protect the prosthesis. The designers of the Ligastic ligament do not recommend excessive tensioning of the ligament prior to fixation. Manual traction is applied to the ligament when passage of the ligament through the intraosseous tunnels is performed such that the ligament is taut. No additional tension is recommended. The ligament is anchored either by using a double-staple fixation technique at each end or with bone plugs. Postoperatively, gradual mobilization of the knee is performed with ambulation, and an extension block brace is encouraged after 2 days. Quadriceps exercises are initiated, but dynamic resistance exercises are avoided. The brace is discontinued when full active extension of the knee is obtained. Strengthening exercises are continued during the first 2 months with jogging, bicycling, and swimming started after this time. Return to full activities is allowed after 3 months.

Posterior cruciate ligament (PCL) reconstruction using the Ligastic ligament is performed with a non-coated double-bundled ligament.[47] After arthroscopic evaluation, an anteromedial arthrotomy is made extending approximately to the quadriceps tendon and distally to the pes anserinus. The vastus medialis is retracted to expose the distal medial femoral condyle. The intercondylar notch is debrided to the posterior edge of the tibial plateau and the lateral aspect of the medial femoral condyle is visualized. Two diverging femoral tunnels are made using a 5-mm drill inside-out. The tunnels should diverge by approximately 3 cm to form a bony bridge between their points of emergence. The tibial tunnel is made using a tibial guide with the knee at 90 degrees of flexion. The tip of the guide should slide over the posterior tibial plateau. Two tunnels are created by drilling obliquely, posteriorly, and proximally. Prior to drilling, Kirschner wires are inserted through the guide to confirm the correct position. After drilling the tunnels, a looped metal wire is then placed through the tunnels to assist in passage of the prosthesis. The two ends of the prosthetic ligament are pulled through the two femoral tunnels from outside-in forming a U over the bony bridge of the medial femoral condyle, thus requiring no formal femoral fixation. The two free ends of the ligament are pulled through the intercondylar notch and out the individual tibial tunnels by the two metal loops. Tension in the ligament is adjusted manually until the ACL is observed to be under tension, which indicates that the posterior displacement of the tibia has been corrected. The knee is then taken through a range of motion and the ligament is fixed to the tibia with a 6-mm staple on each bundle. A third staple is used to fix the two bundles together.

The remnants of the PCL can then be attached to the artificial ligament with an absorbable suture. Postoperatively, weightbearing is allowed with the knee splinted in extension. Range-of-motion exercises are avoided until after 4 days. Again, early active traction of the quadriceps is initiated and resistive exercises are avoided. The splint is removed when knee extension is obtained. Physical therapy is continued for 2 months and return to sports can be started after 3 months.

Results

Laboureau and colleagues[46] have reported on 225 patients that have undergone Ligastic ligament reconstruction for an acute ACL deficiency. Three separate groups were evaluated based upon the length of follow-up. In group I (>3 years of follow-up) the drawer was less than 5 mm in 85% of the patients, the jerk test was negative in 92%, and the Lachman test was less than 5 mm in only 37%. In groups II (>2 years follow-up) and III (<2 years follow-up) the anterior drawer was less than 5 mm in 88% of group II and 87% of group III patients. A negative jerk test was found in 95% of patients in both group II and III. Only the Lachman test was less than 5 mm in 70% of cases in group II and 79% in group III. The poor results noted with the Lachman test with longer follow-up (group I) was believed to be due to an imprecise, nonisometric method of femoral implantation of the ligament. Functionally, the results were rated as 88% good, 9% satisfactory, and 3% poor. Subjectively, 94% of the patients were satisfied with the procedure. Complications in this series included six cases of thrombophlebitis, nine cases of arthrofibrosis, and two cases of reflex sympathetic dystrophy. There were no cases of acute synovitis noted although three patients developed a chronic synovitis as a result of an abrasion of the prosthesis on the intercondylar notch. Seventeen patients were reevaluated post implantation by arthroscopy or arthrotomy. At 1 year, the prosthetic ligament was found to be completely covered by fibrous tissue. Biopsies of the ligament demonstrated encapsulation with dense connective tissue 1 to 2 mm thick. The fibrous tissue was found among the fascicles of the ligament. The three documented cases of traumatic ligament rupture occurred in the midportion of the ligament, without disruption along the intraosseous tunnels.

Over a 2-year period from 1989 to 1991, Laboureau and Dericks[48] performed 105 Ligastic ligament reconstructions using an arthroscopic technique. Approximately half of these were performed within 6 months from time of injury. Two thirds of the patients had a previous surgery on the involved knee, with 20% having a failed ACL reconstructive procedure. Preoperatively, all patients had a Lachman grade of greater than 1+, 74% had a positive anterior drawer, and 72% had a positive pivot shift. Postoperative evaluation with an average follow-up of 12 months demonstrated an absent Lachman, anterior drawer, and pivot shift test in greater than 90% of patients. The patients that had a positive Lachman, drawer, or pivot shift test postoperatively had chronic ACL insufficiency. Complications included one infection, two hematomas, three postoperative effusions, and one ligament rupture at 20 months postoperatively.

The results of PCL reconstruction using the two-bundle Ligastic ligament have been reported.[47] Sixty-six patients were reviewed with a 1- to 9-year follow-up (average, 3.75 years). Included in this series were 44 patients with chronic deficiency (group I) and 22 patients with acute PCL ruptures (group II). In both the acute and chronic groups, the posterior drawer was greater than 5 mm in all cases. Postoperatively, 86% of the acutely reconstructed group had a posterior drawer of less than 5 mm compared to 70% of the chronic group. Subjectively, the chronic group was rated as 53% excellent, 32% good or fair, and 15% poor. The acutely reconstructed group had 82% excellent results, 14% good or fair, and 4% poor. Complications included two cases of thrombophlebitis, three cases of arthrofibrosis that required manipulation, and one case of reflex sympathetic dystrophy, which resolved. There were no infections present in this series, although there were complications as a result of technical errors which included a partial tibial nerve lesion. A single graft rupture occurred as a result of a traumatic event. Approximately 10% of the patients were examined arthroscopically between 6 months and 3 years postoperatively. The ligament was found to be completely covered by vascularized fibrous tissue that was approximately 2 mm thick. Collagen deposition was noted throughout the entire anterior ligament with longitudinal orientation of the fibers. Infrequent macrophages were noted, which was thought to demonstrate the knee's tolerance to the polyester.

Summary

The Ligastic ligament with its unique design combines desirable biomechanical properties with porosity, promoting collagen tissue ingrowth and intraosseous anchorage. A significant biomechanical characteristic of this ligament is the absence of significant elongation during fatigue testing. Early results of implantation of the ligament for PCL deficiency by the original investigators are encouraging, with better results in the acutely reconstructed group. In ACL reconstructions using the Ligastic ligament, the Lachman test was positive with longer follow-up. The authors believed that this was a technical error in placement of the femoral portion of the graft in a nonisometric position since further analysis of the group followed for longer than 3 years did not demonstrate deterioration of the anterior drawer, Lachman, or pivot shift tests when reevaluated at 6- to 12-month intervals. Thus the objective results appeared to remain stable over this time.

As with the Leeds-Keio ligament, soft tissue ingrowth is another area where further study is necessary. Specifically, the quality of fibrous ingrowth and its ultimate mechanical function are areas that need further investigation. Longer-term follow-up is necessary to determine the ultimate efficacy of the use of this ligament. At this time, experience with implantation using the Ligastic system is limited, with only the designers of the ligament reporting their results of reconstruction. The ligament is currently being used in centers in Europe and Canada.

FUTURE OF PROSTHETIC LIGAMENT RECONSTRUCTION

The prosthetic cruciate ligaments that are currently available all have significant potential drawbacks. The ideal artificial ligament substitute has not yet been developed. The desire to shorten the recovery period allowing rapid return to athletic activity, in addition to arthroscopic insertion, which would avoid the morbidity of soft tissue dissection and graft harvesting, is an attractive alternative to autogenous reconstructions. The variety of prosthetic ligament substitutes currently available and the differences in design and implantation techniques suggest that the optimal synthetic material and implant design have not been found. However, the role of prosthetic replacements in cruciate ligament reconstruction will continue to evolve. The ideal cruciate ligament prosthesis should provide[11] (1) simple insertion with minimal resultant surgical morbidity, (2) reproduction of the "normal" biomechanics and kinematics of the knee, (3) immediate mobility to avoid the detrimental effects of immobilization, (4) success rates equal to or greater than other types of reconstructions, and (5) long-term biologic compatibility of the prosthesis within the intraarticular and intraosseous environments. While all artificial substitutes may ultimately be expected to fail, it is important to continue development of prosthetic ligaments, especially those that would allow for the gradual transfer of stresses to new collagenous ingrowth material which could then mature into ligamentous tissue and be able, theoretically, to resist tensile loading indefinitely. Many critical questions remain unanswered regarding the use of prosthetic ligaments and the safety and long-term effects of the various synthetic materials on the joint. The theoretical advantages of using a synthetic material for cruciate ligament reconstruction are apparent, but until future investigations provide further understanding of the behavior of synthetic ligaments, the search for the "ideal" cruciate replacement will continue.

REFERENCES

1. Allen PR, et al: Evaluation of preserved bovine tendon xenografts: A histological, biomechanical and clinical study, *Biomaterials* 8:146–152, 1987.
2. Ahfeld SA, Larson RL, Collins HR: Anterior cruciate reconstruction in the chronically unstable knee using an expanded polytetrafluoroethylene (PTFE) prosthetic ligament, *Am J Sports Med* 15:326–330, 1987.
3. Anderson HN, Brunn C, Sondergard-Petersen PE: Reconstruction of chronic insufficient anterior cruciate ligament in the knee using a synthetic Dacron Prosthesis: A prospective study of 57 cases, *Am J Sports Med* 20:20–23, 1992.
4. Arnoczky SP, Warren RF, Ashlock MA: Replacement of the anterior cruciate ligament using a patella tendon allograft. An experimental study, *J Bone Joint Surg [Am]* 68:376–385, 1986.
5. Bartolozzi P, Salvi M, Velluti C: Longterm follow-up of 53 cases of chronic lesions of the anterior cruciate ligament treated with an artificial Dacron Stryker ligament, *Ital J Orthop Traumatol* 16:467–80, 1990.
6. Bercovy M, et al: Carbon-PGLA prosthesis for ligament reconstruction, *Clin Orthop* 196:159–168, 1985.
7. Berg WS, et al: Mechanical properties of bovine xenograft, *Orthop Trans* 7:279, 1983.
8. Bhate AP, et al: Durability characterization of Stryker Dacron prosthetic ligaments, Sixth International Symposium on Advances in Cruciate Ligament Reconstruction of the Knee, Los Angeles, March 3–5, 1985.
9. Bolton CW, Bruchman WC: The Gore-Tex expanded polytetrafluoroethylene prosthetic ligament, *Clin Orthop* 186:202–213, 1985.
10. Bonamo JL, Krinick RM, Sporn AA: Rupture of the patellar ligament after use of its central third for anterior cruciate reconstruction. A report of 2 cases, *J Bone Joint Surg [Am]* 66:1294–1297, 1984.
11. Bruchman WC, Bolton CW, Bain JR: Design considerations for cruciate ligament prosthesis. In Jackson DW, Drez D, editors: *The anterior cruciate deficient knee: New concepts in ligament repair,* St Louis, 1987, Mosby–Year Book, pp 254–272.
12. Burks RT, Haut RC, Lancaster RL: Biomechanical and histological observations on the dog patellar tendon after removal of its central one-third, *Am J Sports Med* 18:146–153, 1990.
13. Butler DL, et al: Mechanical properties of primate vascularized vs. nonvascularized patellar tendon grafts: Changes over time. *J Orthop Res* 7:68–79, 1989.
14. Chen EH, Black J: Materials design analysis of the prosthetic anterior cruciate ligament, *J Biomed Mater Res* 14:567–586, 1980.
15. Cooper DE, et al: Strength of the Central Third Patellar Tendon Graft: A Biomechanical Study, Annual Meeting of the American Academy of Orthopaedic Surgeons, Washington, DC, Feb 21, 1992.
16. Corner EM: Notes of a case illustration of an artificial anterior cruciate ligament, demonstrating the action of that ligament, *Proc R Soc Med* 7:120–121, 1914.
17. *Dacron ligament prosthesis surgical technique.* Sunnyvale, Calif, 1989, Stryker Endoscopy Co.
18. Dahlstedt LJ, Netz P, Dalen N: Poor results of bovine xenograft for cruciate ligament repair, *Acta Orthop Scand* 60:3–7, 1989.
19. Denti M, et al: Preliminary assessment of anterior cruciate reconstruction with the Leeds-Keio artificial ligament, *Am J Knee Surg* 3:181–186, 1990.
20. FDA Orthopaedic Device Classification Panel. Initial survey of Richards Polyflex cruciate ligament prosthesis, Washington, DC, November, 1978.
21. Ferkel RD, et al: Arthroscopic "second look" at the Gore-Tex ligament, *Am J Sports Med* 17:147–153, 1989.
22. Ferl JG, Goldenthal KJ, Mishra NK: FDA Regulation of prosthetic ligament devices. In Friedman MJ, Ferkel RD, editors: *Prosthetic ligament reconstruction of the knee,* Philadelphia, 1988, WB Saunders, pp 202–208.
23. Fox J: Report on the clinical results of Polyflex ligament replacement, presented to FDA Orthopedic Panel, April 15, 1977.
24. Friedman MJ: Gore-Tex anterior cruciate ligament reconstruction, *Tech Orthop* 2:36–43, 1988.
25. Friedman MJ: Prosthetic anterior cruciate ligament, *Clin Sports Med* 10:499–513, 1991.
26. Fu FH: Evaluation of prosthetic debris, Seventh International Symposium on Advances in Cruciate Ligament Reconstruction of the Knee: Autogenous vs. Prosthetic. Palm Desert, Calif, March 1990.
27. Fujikawa K: Clinical study of anterior cruciate ligament reconstruction with the Leeds-Keio artificial ligament, In Friedman MJ, Ferkel RD, editors: *Prosthetic ligament reconstruction of the knee,* Philadelphia, 1988, WB Saunders, pp 132–139.
28. Fujikawa K: Clinical study on ACL reconstruction with the Leeds-Keio artificial ligament, Sixth International Symposium on Advances in Cruciate Ligament Reconstruction, Los Angeles, March 3–5, 1989.
29. Fujikawa K, Iselie F, Seedhom BB: Leeds-Keio artificial ligament. The anchoring system to the bone, *Knee* 8:240–246, 1983.
30. Fujikawa K, Iselie F, Seedhom BB: Arthroscopy after anterior cruciate reconstruction with the Leeds-Keio ligament, *J Bone Joint Surg [Br]* 71:566–570, 1989.
31. Fujikawa K, Iselie F, Seedhom BB: Anterior Cruciate Reconstruction with the Leeds-Keio Artificial Ligament. In Scott WN, editor: *Ligament and extensor mecha-*

nism injuries of the knee, St Louis, 1991, Mosby–Year Book, pp 311–318.
32. Gillquist J, Odensten M: Reconstruction of the anterior cruciate ligament with a Dacron prosthesis: A prospective analysis of complications and stability in a minimum five year followup, Annual Meeting, American Academy of Orthopaedic Surgeons, Anaheim, Calif, March 8, 1991.
33. Glousman R, et al: Gore-Tex prosthetic ligament in anterior cruciate deficient knees, Am J Sports Med 16:321–326, 1988.
34. Good L, et al: Failure of a bovine xenograft for reconstruction of the anterior cruciate ligament, Acta Orthop Scand 60:8–12, 1989.
35. Gore-Tex cruciate ligament prosthesis: 5-year clinical results, Flagstaff, Ariz, 1989, WL Gore & Associates.
36. Grood ES, Noyes FR: Cruciate ligament prosthesis: Strength, creep and fatigue properties, J Bone Joint Surg [Am] 58:1083–1088, 1976.
37. Guarda E, De Laurentiis L, Andreani A: The use of artificial ligaments in anterior cruciate ligament reconstruction, Ital J Orthop Traumatol 16:323–330, 1990.
38. Indelicato PA, Pascale MS, Huegel MO: Early experience with the Gore-Tex polytetrafluoroethylene anterior cruciate ligament prosthesis, Am J Sports Med 17:55–62, 1989.
39. Jackson DW, et al: Freeze dried anterior cruciate ligament allograft, Am J Sports Med 15:295–302, 1987.
40. Jackson DW, Schaefer RK: Cyclops syndrome: Loss of extensor following intraarticular anterior cruciate ligament reconstruction, Arthroscopy 6:171, 1990.
41. James SL, et al: Cruciate ligament stents in reconstruction of the unstable knee, Clin Orthop 143:90–96, 1979.
42. Jenkins DM: The repair of cruciate ligaments with flexible carbon-fibre, J Bone Joint Surg [Br] 60:520–522, 1978.
43. Johnson DH: Arthroscopic reconstruction of the anterior cruciate ligament with Gore-Tex graft, Am J Sports Med 19:540, 1991.
44. Karzel RP, et al: Four year experience with the Gore-Tex prosthetic ligament in anterior cruciate deficient knees, Annual Meeting of the American Academy of Orthopaedic Surgery, New Orleans, February 1990.
45. Laboureau JP, Cazenave A: The Ligastic ligament, Seventh International Symposium on Advances in Cruciate Ligament Reconstruction of the Knee: Autogenous vs. Prosthetic, Indian Wells, Calif, March 1990.
46. Laboureau JP, Cazenave A, Dericks GH: Acute ruptures of the anterior cruciate ligament: Reconstruction by suture and a synthetic reinforcement. Results after a five year experience, Unpublished data.
47. Laboureau JP, Cazenave A, Dericks GH: Two bundles prosthetic plasty for reconstruction of the posterior cruciate ligament: 9 year followup, Unpublished data.
48. Laboureau JP, Dericks GH: 105 anterior cruciate ligament reconstruction cases using the Ligastic reconstruction system—by arthroscopic technique. Update 1992: New Perspectives in Arthroscopy and Sports Medicine, Palm Springs, Calif, March 1992.
49. Langan P, Fontanetta AP: Rupture of the patellar tendon after use of its central third, Orthop Rev 16:61, 1987.
50. Larson RL: Prosthetic replacement of knee ligaments: Overview. In Feagin JA Jr, editor: The crucial ligaments: Diagnosis and treatment of ligamentous injuries about the knee, New York, 1988, Churchill Livingstone, pp 495–506.
51. Lopez-Vazquez E, et al: Reconstruction of the anterior cruciate ligament with a Dacron prosthesis, J Bone Joint Surg [Am] 73:1294–1300, 1991.
52. Lukianov AV, et al: A multicenter study on the results of anterior cruciate ligament reconstruction using a Dacron ligament prosthesis in "salvage" cases, Am J Sports Med 17:380–386, 1989.
53. Marcacci M, et al: Histologic and ultra structural findings of tissue ingrowth: The Leeds-Keio prosthetic anterior cruciate ligament, Clin Orthop 267:115–121, 1991.
54. Markolf KL, et al: Instrumented measurements of laxity in patients who have a Gore-Tex anterior cruciate ligament substitute, J Bone Joint Surg [Am] 71:887–893, 1989.
55. McCarroll JR: Fracture of the patella during a golf swing following reconstruction of the anterior cruciate ligament, Am J Sports Med 11:26–27, 1983.
56. Mirolan PK, Seaver AV, Guttan RR: Anterior cruciate ligament allograft transplantation: Long-term function, histology, revascularization, and operative technique, Am J Sports Med 14:348–360, 1986.
57. Mollica O, et al: The biological evolution of the Leeds-Keio ligament in the human race, Ital J Orthop Traumatol 14:501–512, 1988.
58. Moore RC, Markolf RL: Measurement of stability of the knee and ligament force after implantation of a synthetic anterior cruciate ligament, In vitro measurement, J Bone Joint Surg [Am] 70:1020–1031, 1988.
59. Mosely JB, Shields CL, Glousman RE: Four year follow-up on the Gore-Tex ACL reconstruction, Annual Meeting of the American Academy of Orthopaedic Surgery, New Orleans, February, 1990.
60. Nordt WE, Terry GC: Gore-Tex prosthetic ligament replacement. A report on 112 patients, Orthop Trans 14:241, 1990.
61. Noyes FR, et al: Intra-articular cruciate reconstructions: Perspectives on graft strength vascularization and immediate motion after replacement, Clin Orthop 172:171–177, 1983.
62. Noyes FR, et al: Biomechanical analysis of human ligament grafts used in knee ligament repairs and reconstruction, J Bone Joint Surg [Am] 62:687–695, 1980.
63. Olson EJ, et al: The biomechanical and histological effects of artificial ligament wear particles: In vitro and in vivo studies, Am J Sports Med 16:558–570, 1988.
64. Parke JP: Dacron ligament prosthesis for anterior cruciate ligament reconstruction. In Scott WN, editor: Ligament and extensor mechanism injuries of the knee, St Louis, 1991, Mosby–Year Book, pp 331–339.

65. Parke JP, Grana WA, Chitwood JS: A high-strength Dacron augmentation for cruciate ligament reconstruction. A two-year canine study, *Clin Orthop* 196:175–185, 1985.
66. Paulos LE, et al: Intrapatellar contracture syndrome, *Am J Sports Med* 15:331–341, 1987.
67. Paulos LE, et al: The Gore-Tex cruciate ligament prosthesis: A longterm followup, *Orthop Trans* 14:617, 1990.
68. Richmond JC, et al: Anterior cruciate reconstruction using a Dacron ligament prosthesis: A longterm study, *Am J Sports Med* 20:24–28, 1992.
69. Roberts TS, Drez D, Banta CJ: Complications of anterior cruciate ligament reconstruction. In Brigg NF, editor: *Complications in arthroscopy*, New York, 1989, Raven Press, pp 169–177.
70. Rosenberg T: Data presented at Sixth International Symposium on Advances in Cruciate Ligament Reconstruction of the Knee, Los Angeles, March 3–5, 1989.
71. Rushton N, Dandy DJ, Naylor CPE: The clinical arthroscope and histological findings after replacement of the anterior cruciate ligament with carbon-fibre, *J Bone Joint Surg [Br]* 65:308–309, 1983.
72. Sachs RA, Daniel DM, Stone ML, et al: Patellofemoral problems after anterior cruciate ligament reconstruction, *Am J Sports Med* 17:760–765, 1989.
73. Salvi M, et al: Ultra structure of periprosthetic Dacron knee ligament tissue, *Acta Orthop Scand* 62:174–197, 1991.
74. Seedhom BB: The Leeds-Keio Ligament: Biomechanics. In Friedman MJ, Ferkel RD, editors: *Prosthetic ligament reconstruction of the knee,* Philadelphia, 1988, WB Saunders, pp 118–131.
75. Sledge SC, et al: Five-year followup with the Gore-Tex polytetrafluorethylene anterior cruciate ligament prosthesis, *Am J Sports Med* 19:539, 1991.
76. Smith A: The diagnosis and treatment of injuries of the cruciate ligaments, *Br J Surg* 6:176–189, 1918.
77. Strum GM, Larson RL: Clinical experience and early results or carbon fiber augmentation of anterior cruciate ligament reconstruction of the knee, *Clin Orthop* 196:77–85, 1985.
78. Strum GM, et al: In vitro AP stability measurements of patients with synthetic anterior cruciate ligaments, *Orthop Trans* 10:253, 1986.
79. Tietge RA: Experience with bovine xenobioprosthesis. In Scott WN, editor: *Ligament and extensor mechanism injuries of the knee,* St Louis, 1991, Mosby–Year Book, pp 339–347.
80. Tietge RA, Rojas F: Anterior cruciate ligament reconstruction using a bovine xenograft prosthesis, American Orthopaedic Society of Sports Medicine, Atlanta, Feb 8, 1984.
81. Van Steensel CJ, et al: Failure of anterior cruciate ligament reconstruction using tendon xenograft, *J Bone Joint Surg [Am]* 69:860–864, 1987.
82. Von Mironova SS: Spätresultate der Rekonstruktion des Bandapparates des Kniegelenks mit Lawson. *Zentralbl Chir* 103:432, 1978.
83. Weiss AB, et al: Ligament replacement with an absolute copolymer carbon fiber scaffold—early clinical experience, *Clin Orthop* 196:77–85, 1985.
84. Whipple TL: Arthroscopic anterior cruciate ligament reconstruction with ProCol xenograft bioprosthesis. In Friedman MJ, Ferkel RD, editors: *Prosthetic ligament reconstruction of the knee,* Philadelphia, 1988, WB Saunders, pp 112–117.
85. Wilk RM, Richmond JC: Dacron reconstruction in chronic anterior cruciate ligament insufficiency: Five year followup, American Academy of Orthopaedic Surgeons, Washington, DC, Feb 21, 1992.
86. Willis RP, Collins HR: Two to six year followup of Gore-Tex prosthetic anterior cruciate ligament reconstruction, *Orthop Trans* 14:241, 1990.
87. Woods GA, Indelicato PA, Prevot TJ: The Gore-Tex anterior cruciate ligament prosthesis: Two versus three year results, *Am J Sports Med* 19:48–55, 1991.

48
Allografts in Knee Ligament Surgery

DANA G. SELTZER, M.D.
STEPHEN J. LOMBARDO, M.D.

Donor screening and prevention of disease transmission
Graft procurement and storage
Secondary sterilization
Allograft immunogenicity
Allograft histology
Allograft biomechanics
Indications for allograft use in ligament reconstruction
Allograft anterior cruciate ligament technique

Two-incision rear-entry guide technique
Postoperative management
Allograft posterior cruciate ligament technique
Postoperative management
Human allograft reconstruction results
Other frontiers
Summary

The number of anterior cruciate ligament (ACL) reconstructions performed in the United States has skyrocketed over the past 10 years for several reasons. The fitness boom and increased opportunities for adults to participate in organized, competitive sports have generated an epidemic of serious knee ligament injuries in patients who desperately want to maintain their health by remaining active. The elucidation of the natural history of the ACL-deficient knee, with its propensity for meniscal injury and early degenerative arthritis, has swayed many orthopaedic surgeons from conservative treatment toward early surgical intervention in the athletically active young adult with an unstable, ACL-deficient knee. Long-term studies showing superior results with reconstructions, as opposed to primary repairs, have led to the acceptance of ligament substitution as the standard of operative care. Improved techniques and tools for ACL reconstruction have allowed us to advance from open reconstructions to arthroscopically-assisted procedures. Newer endoscopic techniques allow for ACL reconstruction utilizing a single incision at the site chosen for harvesting the autograft tissue to be used as a ligament replacement. A clearer understanding of the biology and biomechanics of both the intact ACL and the various graft substitutes has led to drastic improvements in the technical aspects of our operative procedures, as well as in the postoperative rehabilitation of our patients. This, in turn, allows us to offer patients predictably good results, less agonizing rehabilitation, and an earlier return to competitive athletics. With more postoperative patients returning to the arena of competition, the number of repeat knee injuries has increased, giving surgeons the unique opportunity to "salvage" deranged knees that have been operated on before. This perpetual cycle seems to assure that the trend toward increased surgery to enhance quality of life is likely to persist, and there is reason to believe that the number of posterior cruciate ligament (PCL) reconstructions that will be performed during the next decade will rise in a similar fashion.

Though autograft tissues are considered by most experts to be the optimal substitute for either ACL or PCL reconstructions, alternatives do exist and rightfully hold a place in the armamentarium of the sports medicine surgeon. Though many authors still consider allografts and synthetics experimental, both groups currently have a well-defined role in knee ligament surgery that is likely to expand in the future. The role of artificial ligament substitutes was explored in Chapter 47. The purpose of this chapter is to define the role of allografts, characterize their benefits and weaknesses, provide the basic knowledge necessary for their judicious use, and supply the reader with ACL and PCL reconstruction techniques that take advantage of the strengths of allografts.

DONOR SCREENING AND PREVENTION OF DISEASE TRANSMISSION

Tissue banks were established in the 1940s for collecting and processing human tissue for the purpose of transplantation, and bone banks have arisen out of necessity, along with the popularity of massive allografts and limb salvage surgery for total joint reconstructions and tumor surgery. Encouraging early reports on soft tissue allograft reconstructions[10] sparked an interest in allograft ACL reconstructions in the 1980s. The major deterrent to widespread use of allografts for ACL reconstructions has been a concern, on the part of both patients and surgeons, over disease transmission, particularly human immunodeficiency virus (HIV) disease and acquired immunodeficiency syndrome (AIDS). With many authors reporting promising results for allograft ACL and PCL reconstructions, it is reasonable to believe that elimination of disease transmission as a possible complication would greatly enhance the acceptance of this technique.

Centers for Disease Control (CDC) estimates place the number of HIV-infected persons in the United States at approximately 1.5 million.[6, 89] As of December 31, 1991, the CDC had collected 202,921 reported AIDS cases in the United States.[45] Earlier CDC estimates placed the number of AIDS cases at 365,000 by December 31, 1992.[44] The actual number of reported cases, however, will likely be in the neighborhood of 250,000 at that time. Of these, over 60% have already died.[45] Using the method described by Buck et al.[13] for estimating the risk of a patient receiving an allograft from an unrecognized HIV-seropositive donor, a wide range of figures are possible based upon varying screening procedures. Lack of screening places the risk in the neighborhood of 1:161, while use of all screening tools available lowers the estimated risk to 1:1,667,600. Each screening test that is omitted drops the risk closer to the lower estimate. For example, reliance on HIV-antibody (HIV-Ab) testing, initial donor screening, and limited proxy tests (i.e., HBsAg) places the risk at 1:12,392,[13] significantly higher than the risk from a single-unit blood transfusion.[20]

The ideal donor of allograft tissues for ligament reconstruction is a young adult, 15 to 30 years of age, who is likely to be a victim of vehicular trauma or penetrating trauma in the urban setting. This population overlaps considerably with the 25- to 44-year-old age group that has the highest HIV seroprevalence rate in the country.[19] If CDC estimates of HIV prevalence in the United States are correct,[89] then 1 of every 96 persons across the country in the age range of 15 to 50 years is HIV seropositive.[13] Prevalence rates vary greatly by region, as evidenced by numerous accounts in the literature, but are generally higher in urban and metropolitan areas. A recent sentinel hospital study surveying seroprevalence rates around the country reported unrecognized HIV infection rates between 0.1% and 7.8%.[94] The Johns Hopkins University Hospital emergency room studies have reported unrecognized HIV infection rates of approximately 4%.[3, 56, 57] HIV seroprevalence rates among trauma victims have been reported to be 1.67% at the Maryland Shock Trauma Center[101] and 5.1% at the University of Miami/Jackson Memorial Medical Center.[40] The orthopaedic seroprevalence studies performed at the University of Miami/Jackson Memorial Medical Center revealed HIV infection rates of approximately 9% for victims of major orthopaedic trauma.[95]

Though it has long been suspected that bone and soft tissue allografts were capable of HIV transmission,[14] only recently was this suspicion clinically confirmed. The first incident involved a young woman who received a bone graft for a spinal fusion in 1984 from a fresh frozen femoral head allograft removed from a 52-year-old man during routine primary hip arthroplasty. She developed *Pneumocystis carinii* pneumonia and AIDS 4 years later. HIV testing was not available at the time of this operative inoculation, but retrospective investigation revealed that the donor had a history of intravenous drug use. A simple risk factor history would have excluded this patient from the donor pool.[108] The second case, the so-called LifeNet incident, recently came to light. In this case, 58 bone and soft tissue allografts were obtained from a single donor in 1985. This donor was HIV-Ab negative at the time of graft procurement, but was apparently in the "window period," generally thought to be the 6-week period after infection with HIV and prior to the detectable production of antibodies to HIV. A retrospective evaluation with the polymerase chain reaction (PCR) test, which detects genetic fragments of HIV and effectively cuts the window period down to approximately 2 to 4 days, performed on his marrow was positive. Fifty-two allograft recipients were identified, and 35 submitted to HIV testing. Two patients that received fresh frozen femoral head allografts seroconverted, and a third patient who received a bone–patellar tendon–bone (BTB) allograft in 1985, seroconverted in 1987. None of the patients tested after receiving freeze-dried, ethanol-treated freeze-dried, or irradiated freeze-dried bone or soft tissue allografts seroconverted. Food and Drug Administration (FDA) approval of the PCR test and its routine use by tissue banks could have averted this tragic incident.[9, 65]

Evidence to support the potential for disease

transmission via bone and soft tissue allograft transplantation, though not abundant, is readily available. Buck et al.[14] were able to culture virus from three of five fresh bone specimens of AIDS victims. HIV could also be recovered from bone after deep freezing or freeze-drying. HIV cultures were positive for only two of five tendon specimens, and virus could not be recovered from any tendons after freezing. This study documents the presence of HIV in musculoskeletal tissues and suggests that freezing may help to decrease the risk of viral transmission, though it does not sterilize the grafts. The authors suggest that the estimated risk of HIV transmission can be dropped even further, perhaps as low as 1 in 8 million, if grafts are frozen.[14] More than 200,000 fresh frozen and freeze-dried allografts have been implanted since 1982, many of which were obtained from donors prior to the availability of HIV testing and without current multifaceted screening protocols, yet only two donors have been reported to have transmitted HIV disease to recipients. It seems likely that several other donors must have been HIV carriers, so Malinin and Buck[65] postulate that freezing may partially inactivate the virus and help to diminish the risk of HIV transmission from allograft reconstructions.

Though each tissue bank has an ethical and moral responsibility to provide allografts that are safe and useful, there is no uniform set of standards required of tissue banks for the procurement and preparation of their grafts. The American Association of Tissue Banks provides guidelines for its constituents and has published standards for donor selection, as well as tissue procurement, processing, sterilization, preservation, storage, labeling, and distribution.[103, 106] The Southeastern Organ Procurement Foundation has also published guidelines for bone banking,[38] and the American Academy of Orthopaedic Surgeons has addressed the issue of prevention of HIV transmission from allograft transplantation.[105] The risk of HIV transmission is directly related to the methods of donor selection and exclusion followed at each individual tissue bank. Therefore, it is extremely important that every surgeon be familiar with the methods utilized by his allograft supplier in order to determine whether he is placing his or her patients at unacceptable risk for disease transmission when performing an allograft ligament reconstruction. The knowledgeable surgeon can minimize risks and maximize the probability of a satisfactory end result by evaluating several different banks and deciding exactly what type and form of graft he or she wishes to implant.

The process of donor selection is the critical issue in the safety of allograft surgery. The screening process must begin with a detailed medical and social history. Potential candidates at high risk for AIDS should automatically be excluded from the donor pool. High-risk categories include intravenous drug abusers, homosexual and bisexual males, prostitutes, persons with hemophilia, persons receiving multiple transfusions or any transfusions before 1985, and sexual partners of anyone in these risk groups.[95] A thorough review of the medical history and circumstances surrounding death is necessary to identify potential donors with significant diseases or conditions that might adversely affect the recipients of their tissues. For instance, any medical evidence of systemic infection is cause for rejection as a tissue donor.

Laboratory tests that should be performed routinely include aerobic and anaerobic cultures of blood and all harvested tissues, serologic tests for syphilis and all three forms of detectable viral hepatitis, and screening tests for HIV (both antibody and antigen) and human T-cell lymphotrophic virus type 1 (HTLV-1). These tests serve as either direct identifiers or proxies for identifying HIV-Ab-negative carriers, aside from identifying patients with significant transmissible diseases. In addition, postmortem examinations should be performed in an attempt to identify significant diseases that were not suspected clinically, paying particular attention to lymph nodes. Node histologic findings consistent with HIV disease should be a criterion for rejection of a potential donor.[65]

The University of Miami undertook an unpublished study of their first 1,000 consecutive accepted bone donors. Of this group, 1 patient was excluded for a positive HIV antibody test sequence and HIV antigen test. Seven patients were excluded because of the presence of HBsAg, and 48 others were rejected owing to the presence of HBcAg. Eight patients had positive syphilis serology as the reason for their exclusion. Screening for hepatitis C only recently became available and was not a cause for exclusion of any patients during this study period. In addition, 14 potential donors were turned away because of autopsy findings, including two patients with lymph node findings consistent with early HIV disease.[65]

GRAFT PROCUREMENT AND STORAGE

Soft tissue allografts can be harvested under clean, nonsterile conditions or under aseptic conditions in an operating suite. Nonsterile tissue procurement decreases the initial costs but necessitates secondary sterilization, whereas aseptically harvested grafts can be transplanted without secondary treatment. Regardless of the method utilized, the objective remains to provide a graft that is free of transmissible disease without compromising the structural or biomechanical integrity of the tissues.

The preferred procurement method is the use of standard operating room techniques. The safety of tissue harvested in this manner is directly dependent upon strict donor selection and exclusion criteria. Buck et al.[13, 14] have described the risks of HIV transmission from grafts procured in this fashion to range from 1:161 if only HIV antibody testing is performed to 1 in 8 million if all available screening methods are utilized along with freezing of the specimen. Buck and colleagues believe that "bone allografts prepared from carefully selected and closely monitored donors do not, at this time, carry a significant risk of HIV transmission."[65]

The shelf life of allograft bone and soft tissues is greatly prolonged by preserving the graft using either a fresh frozen or freeze-dry process. Grafts to be fresh frozen are wrapped immediately after harvest and deep-frozen at −70° to −80° C, and can be stored for up to 6 months prior to clinical use.[33, 50] Storage at higher temperatures decreases the useful storage time. The alternative is to lyophilize the frozen tissue to a residual moisture of 3% to 5% with subsequent packaging in a vacuum-sealed container. Tissues stored in this manner have greatly extended shelf lives of 2 years or more.[31, 33, 50]

Another alternative for storage whose value is promising, but as yet unproven, is cryopreservation. In this procedure, the graft is frozen at a controlled rate in the presence of specific cryoprotective agents, subsequently stored in vapor or liquid-phase nitrogen, and then thawed for clinical use. This method of preservation has been useful for maintenance of viable cells in both articular[31] and meniscal cartilage,[29, 66] and several reports of 45% to 80% cell viability in ACL allografts performed in animals have been presented recently.[59, 68, 73]

SECONDARY STERILIZATION

The tremendous pressure to produce allograft tissues free from the risk of transmission of HIV has led to the controversy surrounding the question of secondary sterilization. Though it is mandatory only for grafts harvested in a clean, nonsterile fashion, many tissue banks have initiated secondary sterilization of their aseptically harvested grafts at the requests of the surgeons they supply, in order to allay concerns about HIV transmission to patients undergoing elective procedures, such as ACL or PCL reconstructions, aimed solely at improving the quality of life. Numerous techniques of secondary sterilization have been proposed, including boiling, autoclaving, irradiation, antibiotic soaking, and chemical sterilization with products such as ethylene oxide. Even tissue banking specialists are not in agreement as to whether secondary sterilization is necessary, and it has become readily apparent that certain techniques of secondary sterilization adversely affect the outcome of allograft ACL reconstruction[49, 50, 90] or the biomechanical and biologic properties of the grafts.[11, 16, 34, 42, 50, 60, 84] Others, such as antibiotic soaking, have simply proved to be ineffective.[22] At the present time, ethylene oxide and gamma irradiation are the two most popular secondary sterilization methods in evaluation or use.

HIV is a heat-labile virus that is sensitive to irradiation,[102] but is more resistant to inactivation in the dried state.[104] Currently, irradiation appears to be the most promising method of secondary sterilization. Preliminary reports had also favorably commented on the effects of ethylene oxide on HIV eradication, but early clinical uses resulted in many complications and side effects, including the loss of osteoinductive potential in allograft bone,[43] persistent intraarticular effusions believed to be secondary to either an immunogenic rejection phenomenon or a reaction to the toxic byproducts ethylene chlorhydrin and ethylene glycol,[49, 50] extensive bone resorption in the tunnels with cyst formation,[50, 90] and the "applesauce reaction" with characteristic delayed dissolution of the graft over time.[25, 49, 50, 83, 84] For these reasons, the use of ethylene oxide for secondary sterilization of allograft tissues is not recommended at this time.

The effective dose of gamma irradiation for tissue sterilization and the eradication of HIV remains a matter of debate. The International Atomic Energy Association has proposed 2.5 Mrads as the appropriate dose for sterilization of medical products, though others have demonstrated that less than 2.0 Mrads is adequate for medical product sterilization.[33] The American Association of Tissue Banks holds 1.5 to 2.5 Mrads as its standard for allograft sterilization.[106] Contrary to these findings, Conway et al.[21] showed that 0.4 Mrad delayed HIV infectivity without eliminating it, and they postulated that 3.6 Mrads would be necessary to inactivate free HIV virus, with larger doses being necessary to eradicate intracellular virus. In addition, Winthrow and colleagues[116] demonstrated that a related retrovirus, the feline leukemia virus (FeLV), was not routinely eliminated by 2.9 Mrads or any of several other secondary sterilization techniques.

There is a consensus among researchers that the deleterious effect of gamma irradiation on allograft tissue properties is dose-dependent. Studies done on frozen, allograft bone have uniformly shown that doses below 3 Mrads do not significantly alter the compression, torsional, or bending strength.[10, 86, 109] Other studies of BTB allografts have shown significant reductions in stress and strain above 3 Mrads, though less than 2 Mrads did little to alter the material properties. Some authors also commented that irradiation of freeze-dried allografts caused significantly greater decline in properties.[42, 84] Thus, it appears that the optimal dose of gamma irradiation is something less than 3 Mrads, and it is wise to freeze the allograft tissue after irradiation.

ALLOGRAFT IMMUNOGENICITY

Early concerns about rejection of allograft ligament substitutes were assuaged by experimental and clinical studies showing few instances of rejection. However, further study recently has pointed out that subtle immune responses to allograft tissues may be occurring either systemically or compartmentally. Furthermore, these reactions may affect the ultimate rate of graft transformation into a functional ACL. Fortunately, there appear to be a number of methods to control, if not eliminate, an immunogenetic response by the host to the allograft tissue.

The primary source of immunogenetic potential in the allograft appears to be the major histocompatibility complex (MHC), which is present as surface antigens on the cellular components of allograft tissues. Certain matrix components, such as proteoglycans, may also be sources of an immune response, though collagen demonstrates only weakly immunogenetic potential. Fresh allografts have been shown by several investigators to provoke graft rejection via an immune response,[2, 26, 30] but other investigators have demonstrated significantly diminished immune response to allografts prepared using current preservation techniques, including deep-freezing,[26, 30, 36, 74] freeze-drying,[26, 30] and gamma irradiation.[27, 30] The mechanism by which these methods decrease immunogenetic potential is not entirely understood, but may be related to the elimination of viable cells and the denaturation of the MHC surface antigens. Even clinical trials have not related failures of allograft ACL reconstructions to immune rejection responses,[33, 50] but occasionally to inflammatory responses related to the methods of tissue preservation and sterilization.[25, 49, 50] There are also sparse reports of immunomodulated rejection of ACL allografts in humans.[87, 88] Recent studies have also made it apparent that host response is a graded response, not an all-or-none phenomenon of acceptance vs. rejection. Vasseur et al.[111] demonstrated with frozen bone-ligament-bone allografts in dogs that the knee joint, as a separate compartment, can contain detectable levels of antidonor leukocyte antibodies in the synovial fluid that are not detectable in the serum. Another study revealed a sensitization reaction to a lymphocyte blast transformation test in four of eight patients receiving freeze-dried allograft BTB ACL reconstructions.[87] This study is unfortunately flawed by the use of ethylene oxide for secondary sterilization of the grafts, as the effect of ethylene oxide on the immunogenetic potential of the graft must be questioned.[50]

All portions of the allograft tissue are not equally immunogenetic. Bone carries more antigens than tendon or ligament, and therefore has a higher potential for causing an inflammatory response.[50] Histocompatibility plays a major role in bone graft incorporation, and enhanced incorporation of bone grafts with histocompatibility matching has been demonstrated,[7, 8] presumably by diminishing host sensitization. Numerous studies have documented greatly reduced immunogenetic potential of allograft bone after deep-freezing,[26, 30, 36, 74] with near complete elimination of immunogenicity after freeze-drying.[26, 30] Gamma irradiation also weakens the immune response of the host.[27, 30] The immunogenicity of the allograft is also dose dependent, with larger bone plugs causing a proportionately greater immune response.[50] More prolonged clinical follow-up is necessary to determine the effect of these subtle immune responses on the ultimate fate of transplanted allograft tissues.

ALLOGRAFT HISTOLOGY

There is very little histologic difference between the patterns of healing seen in allograft ligament reconstructions vs. autograft reconstructions. The phases of healing occur in the same sequence and the final result is the same, but it is apparent that allograft healing lags slightly behind autograft healing in terms of timing.[1, 2, 25, 100] The sequence has been well documented in various animal models and begins with initial graft necrosis, proceeding to revascularization, fibroblast replacement and ingrowth, new collagen synthesis, and finally collagen maturation with realignment of collagen fibers along the lines of stress.[2, 25, 33, 50, 96, 114] Initially, the graft swells as it imbibes fluid and undergoes avascular necrosis, with death of all native fibroblasts. At 4 weeks there is evidence of vascular invasion at either end of the graft,[33] with vascularization appearing on the surface of the graft by 6 to 8 weeks.[2, 25, 33, 50, 78, 97, 99] Revascularization of the central core of the graft lags behind the changes seen in the periphery, but takes place by 12 to 16 weeks.[33, 50-52]

The blood supply appears to initiate from the infrapatellar fat pad and the synovium that envelops the graft.[33] A hypervascular state develops within the graft substance that abates over the ensuing months in favor of a fibroplasia with new collagen synthesis that begins to align fibers along the longitudinal axis of stress.[33] By 12 to 18 months the graft vascularity has returned to normal, resembling that of the natural ACL. The graft histologically resembles a mature ligament at this time.[33, 50, 78, 96, 97, 99] Though the sequence is thought to be similar in humans, the progression undoubtedly occurs over a more extended period of time. Levitt et al.[63] performed 53 biopsies in humans at postoperative intervals of 8 weeks to 5 years, and they demonstrated consistent completion of the transformation between 18 and 24 months. The graft increases in cross-sectional area as it matures and revascularizes.[50, 53] However, unlike the natural ACL, the graft matures with small-diameter collagen fibers rather than the more desired large-diameter fibers,[50] possibly accounting for the necessity of increasing the cross-sectional diameter of the allograft. The healed autograft has a similar configuration.[50]

The bone plugs of the grafts that contain bone-tendon interfaces also heal at a slower rate than their autogenous counterparts.[50, 111] Early new bone formation is followed by a period of necrosis, which is then gradually replaced by osteogenesis that results in graft incorporation. The bone graft supplies a scaffold for creeping substitution that eventually replaces the necrotic bony trabeculae of the graft with viable bone that supports the re-creation of a normal interface between the newly formed ACL and its bony origin and insertion. There is evidence that immunologic response of any sort may lead to delayed incorporation of the donor bone, and limiting the possibility of an immune response to the major histocompatibility complex may prove to be important for obtaining early graft healing and incorporation.[50] Fahey and Indelicato[28] recently reported bone tunnel enlargement in femoral and tibial bone tunnels after fresh frozen allograft ACL reconstructions which is unrelated to clinical outcome. These allografts were not secondarily sterilized with ethylene oxide, and the authors postulated that this phenomenon might be a resorptive immune response.[28] They are currently investigating this curiosity further.

ALLOGRAFT BIOMECHANICS

For allografts to be considered a rational alternative to autografts for ligamentous reconstruction of the knee, their biomechanical properties must be similar to autograft tissues. Ideally, the graft tissue utilized should have stiffness similar to and strength greater than or equal to the natural ACL. The classic description of graft strength vs. normal ACL strength was published by Noyes and colleagues.[81] Using the in vitro strength of the normal ACL as 100%, they compared various allograft tissues commonly used for reconstructions, and noted that a 13.8-mm-wide central-third BTB graft could withstand a force of 2,734 N in vitro and exhibited strength equal to 158% of the normal ACL at the time of implantation. All other tissues tested had strengths less than the normal ACL at the time of implantation.[81] It is extremely important to perform allograft reconstructions with tissues that will withstand the forces placed on the ACL during normal activities,[32, 37, 50, 75, 76] and the mechanical properties of the allograft tissues are maximal at the time of implantation.[50] The forces generated during normal daily activities range to nearly 500 N for the ACL and 1,200 N for the PCL, while forces generated during jogging are in the neighborhood of 630 N for the ACL. Therefore, we must assume that the forces generated while playing basketball or football are significantly closer to the figure reported by Noyes et al. of 1,725 N for stress at failure.[81] A more recent study suggested that patellar tendon grafts are stronger than reported by Noyes et al. Cooper and associates[23] reported average tensile strengths of 15-mm, 10-mm, and 7-mm grafts to be 4,389 N, 2,977 N, and 2,238 N, respectively. Both of these studies report in vitro measurements exacted from mechanical devices that do not represent the normal mode of failure, however, and may not necessarily have direct correlations to clinical results.

Data concerning the change in strength of implanted autografts and allografts with time are conflicting. There is a consensus, however, that any graft, regardless of its source or derivation, is strongest at the time it is implanted. It then decreases in strength, only to regain some, but not all, of its strength at maturation. Allografts and autografts follow similar patterns, both being weakest at the 6- to 12-week period.[50] Autograft animal studies show maximal force to failure of 15% to 28% at 6 months after implantation, advancing to only 30% to 52% of contralateral ACL controls at 1 year.[15, 17, 18, 92] Fresh frozen allografts utilized by Shino et al.[96] showed mean maximal tensile strength of only 30% of controls at 30 weeks after implantation, while Vasseur et al.[111] found loads to failure of only 15% compared with controls at 9 months after implantation. Several other investigators have corroborated these results.[25, 52, 114] Another group, however, measured the mechanical strength of fresh frozen ACL allografts in dogs at 8, 16, 24, 36, and 78 weeks after implantation and reported minimum strength of 50% of controls at 8 weeks with return to 90% of controls at 36 weeks. There was no statistical difference between autograft and allograft ACL reconstructions at any time period.[78] Several investigators have stated that the method of preservation does not significantly alter the mechanical properties of the graft, but rather that the weakening occurs during the remodeling of the graft.[4, 78, 114, 115] The important message is to implant a tissue for reconstruction that is stronger than the natural ACL, in order to achieve a final product that closely matches the biomechanical properties of the native ligament.

INDICATIONS FOR ALLOGRAFT USE IN LIGAMENT RECONSTRUCTION

Though the threat of disease transmission, particularly HIV disease and AIDS, has recently curtailed the widespread use of soft tissue allografts for ligamentous knee reconstructions, many indications and relative indications exist for the use of these tissues in knee surgery. Undoubtedly, as screening procedures, harvesting and storage techniques, and sterilization methods improve, allograft ligament reconstructions will regain their popularity. In addition, a vaccine against HIV would likely alleviate the fears of patients and physicians who are now reluctant to accept allograft tissues for reconstruction when safer autograft tissues can be utilized.

At the present time, situations that merit consideration of allograft reconstruction include the following:

1. Patients with failed autograft reconstructions (i.e., salvage cases), to avoid harvesting tissues from the contralateral limb or utilizing less optimal tissues from the injured extremity.
2. Patients over 40 years of age with gross instability that diminishes their quality of life and does not respond to conservative treatment.
3. Patients with small patellar tendons (less than 25 mm in width), moderate to severe patellofemoral chondrosis, patellofemoral malalignment syndrome, patella baja, or hyperelastic tissues, in an attempt to diminish the risks of postoperative patellofemoral complaints and recurrent instability.
4. Patients with knee dislocations and multidirectional instability that require multiple grafts for reconstruction or extensive surgery, in whom autograft harvests will increase operative and tourniquet time and perhaps boost the potential for postoperative stiffness or arthrofibrosis. Patients presenting with concurrent ACL rupture and either partial or complete hamstring or patellar tendon rupture are candidates for allograft reconstruction.
5. Patients with PCL injuries requiring reconstruction, because the long, broad Achilles tendon allograft provides a larger, stronger graft substitute.
6. Patients who request allograft reconstructions whether on cosmetic or medical grounds, as there is a growing body of literature supporting these techniques as viable alternatives to autograft reconstructions.

Other indications for allograft use will certainly emerge in the near future, such as the possibility of controlling posterolateral rotatory instability by reconstructing the fibular collateral ligament from the fibular head to an isometric point on the lateral femoral condyle employing a BTB allograft. At this time, however, it is important to emphasize that autograft reconstructions remain the gold standard of care, and long-term studies from academic centers on allograft reconstructions should be reviewed critically as they appear in the literature over the next several years. The most valuable studies will obviously be randomized, prospective comparisons of allograft vs. autograft reconstructions using similar techniques.

In the meantime, orthopaedic surgeons should make judicious use of allografts for knee ligament reconstructions. A sound understanding of the physiology of allografts, and the inherent differences between these tissues and their autogenous counterparts, is of utmost importance in this regard. For instance, the use of allografts for routine, primary reconstructions in athletes in order to reduce rehabilitation time is not supported by current literature on either theoretical or clinical grounds. Allograft reconstructions should be performed when their unique properties increase the potential for a successful final outcome. Our current allograft techniques and rehabilitation protocols are described below.

ALLOGRAFT ANTERIOR CRUCIATE LIGAMENT TECHNIQUE

After the decision has been made to utilize an allograft for ACL reconstruction, a determination must be made concerning the type of graft to be utilized. The surgeon should have a strong understanding of the differences between fresh frozen and freeze-dried soft tissue grafts, as well as being familiar with the methods of harvest and graft sterilization employed by the tissue bank(s) supplying the grafts. Next, the question of the graft source must be resolved. We prefer BTB, but we have also utilized Achilles tendon–bone with good success. Other, less routinely harvested potential sources include bone-ACL-bone, bone-PCL-bone, quadriceps tendon–bone, fascia lata or iliotibial band, medial hamstring tendons, and extensor tendons of the foot or hand. This by no means exhausts the list of potential sources. In fact, Shino et al.[97] mentioned that one cadaver donor could conceivably yield 22 separate grafts for use in ligament reconstructions.

The surgeon should be assured at least 24 hours in advance that an adequate specimen of the requested allograft tissue is available in the operating room and ready for implantation. On occasion, the choice of graft source may be limited owing to the law of supply and demand in the community. In such cases, a surgeon must decide whether to postpone the operation until the preferred graft is available, or to compromise his initial choice. The surgeon has many more options if this discovery is made the day prior to the scheduled procedure.

Once the surgeon is satisfied that everything is in order for the allograft ACL reconstruction, a technique that takes advantage of the benefits of the allograft over autograft tissues should be utilized for the procedure. Our endoscopic technique described below makes use of minimal incisions, thereby minimizing the iatrogenic trauma to soft tissues and bone, resulting in decreased postoperative pain. Operative time, and therefore anesthetic time, is decreased since no surgical time is spent harvesting or preparing the graft. In addition, the size and shape of the graft is not limited by the size of the patient's patellar tendon, and can be manipulated to meet the demands of the surgeon. For example, reconstruction of the stronger, more stout PCL can be completed using a 13- to 15-mm graft that more closely resembles the normal ligament diameter, if desired.

Allograft reconstructions preserve host tissues and negate the possibility of intraoperative or postoperative complications, which can be associated with harvesting autogenous tissues. For instance, complications such as patellar tendon rupture,[5] patella fracture,[35, 67, 110, 113] extensor mechanism dysfunction (e.g., patella baja),[85] patellar tendinitis,[12, 35, 46, 93] patellofemoral pain,[39, 54, 58, 91] and iatrogenic disruption of the infrapatellar branch of the saphenous nerve[12] that have been reported after autograft BTB ACL reconstructions can be avoided. However, it must be recognized that this list of complications is simply exchanged for another list of potential problems that includes graft resorption, bone cyst formation,[49] sterile effusions,[49] the applesauce reaction,[25, 49, 83, 84] graft rejection, bone tunnel enlargement,[28] and disease transmission.[9, 65] Lastly, cosmetically, this procedure causes scarring similar to that of routine arthroscopy, with three arthroscopic portals and a 1.5- to 2.0-cm transverse incision in Langer's lines over the proximal medial tibia (Fig 48–1) for reaming the tibial and femoral tunnels, plus insertion and fixation of the graft. Other advantages include the option of performing ACL reconstructions on an outpatient basis because of the reduced

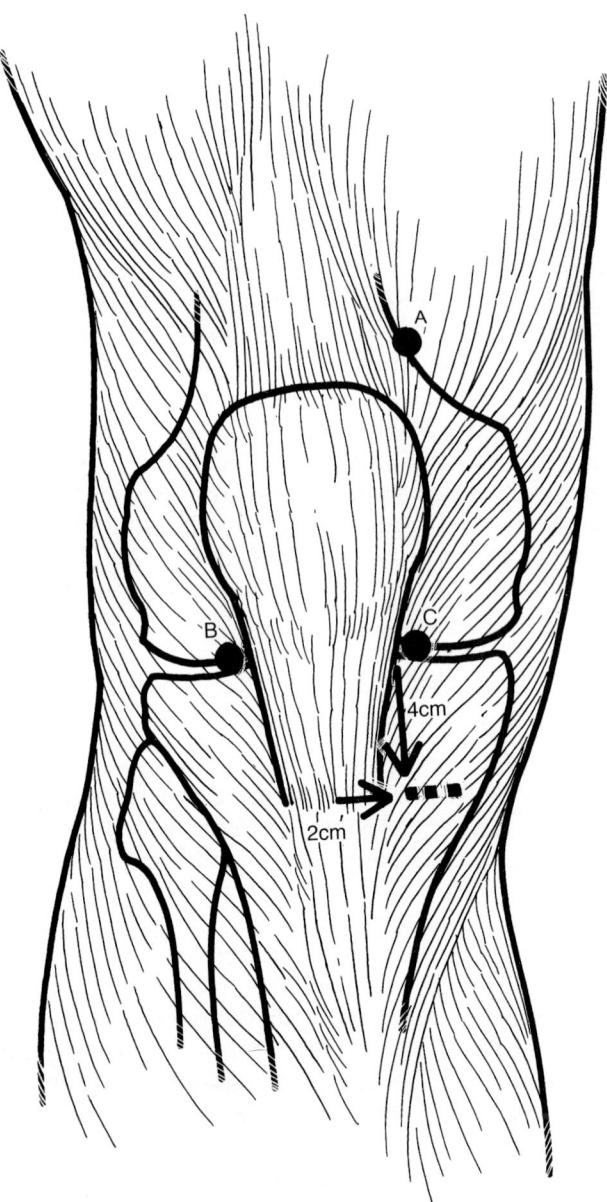

FIG 48–1.
Incisions utilized for endoscopic allograft anterior cruciate ligament reconstruction include three standard arthroscopy portals (A, B, and C) and a 2-cm transverse incision over the proximal medial tibia, just proximal to the pes anserinus insertion, which is necessary for reaming the tibial tunnel and insertion of the graft.

pain, and the increased tolerance of patients to immediate postoperative motion in their rehabilitation program because of decreased surgical morbidity. A current description of our endoscopic technique is detailed stepwise below:

1. The graft should be prepared prior to placing the patient under anesthesia to minimize anesthetic time, provided there is little question about the diagnosis of an ACL-deficient knee. The bone plugs of the thawed BTB allograft are shaped into triangular wedges that measure 10 to 11 mm in their largest diameter. If the bone plugs are of disparate size, the smaller plug will be placed into the femoral tunnel. The bone plugs should be a minimum of 20 mm and a maximum of 30 mm in length. We strive to make both approximately 25 mm long. A single small drill hole is placed transversely in the femoral bone plug, and two similar drill holes are placed in the tibial plug. A no. 5 Ticron suture is placed through each of the drill holes, and each is then tagged with hemostats. A surgical marker is used to mark the bone-tendon interfaces of both bone plugs, and is especially important for the femoral plug, for identification during the arthroscopic insertion of the graft. The diameter of the bone plugs is then checked using the appropriate cylindrical sizer with either a 10- or 11-mm inner diameter, assuring that the graft fit is tight, while still passing with minimal effort (Fig 48–2). The graft should then be wrapped in a moist Ray-tec and left in a kidney basin on the back table while the initial stages of the surgery are being per-

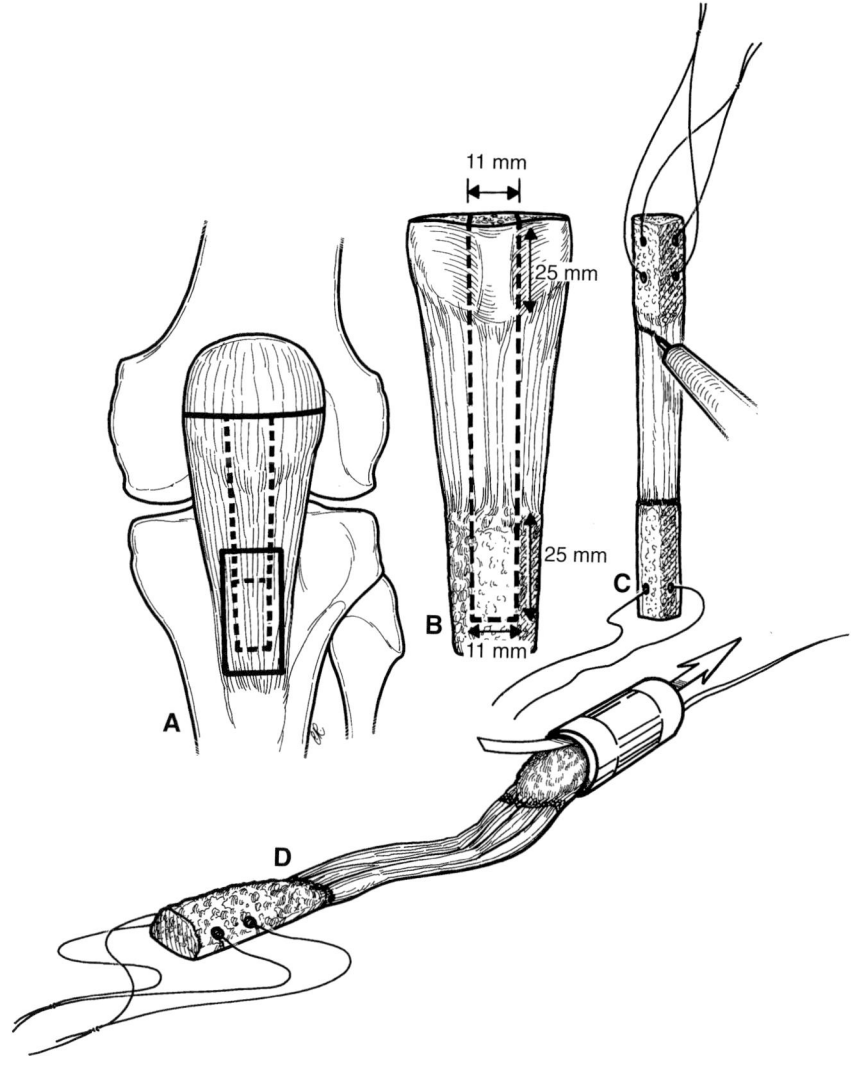

FIG 48–2.
Bone–patellar tendon–bone allografts can either be harvested in their entirety (outlined in *A* and *B*) or in a more finished fashion with bone plugs of standard length and width (*dashed lines* in *A* and *B*). The graft is then pared to the desired dimensions, and the bone-tendon interfaces are highlighted with a surgical marker *(C)*. The graft is then pulled through a cylindrical sizer to assure smooth graft passage *(D)*.

formed. If desired, the graft can be preloaded at 10 to 15 lb on a tension board while the diagnostic arthroscopy is performed. We do not currently follow this routine.

2. The patient can then be anesthetized and an examination under anesthesia performed to confirm the original diagnosis and compare the injured with the contralateral extremity.

3. A standard diagnostic arthroscopy should be performed in every case, looking for coexisting abnormalities. Videographic or photographic documentation of intraarticular pathologic changes, including the ACL rupture, is judicious. Any indicated arthroscopic procedures, such as loose body removal, partial meniscectomy or meniscal repair, or chondroplasty, should be performed at this time.

4. We perform a notchplasty in every case after debriding the ACL stump. Enough of the lateral wall must be removed to prevent abrasion of the graft during range of motion, and enough of the roof must be removed to allow for full extension of the knee without anterior impingement of the graft. The amount of notchplasty necessary varies with the size and shape of the notch in the given patient. All remaining soft tissue should be removed from the lateral wall so that identification of the over-the-top position and placement of the femoral guide pin is facilitated.

5. A 1.5- to 2.0-cm transverse incision along Langer's lines is made approximately 2 cm medial to the midtibial tubercle, and carried sharply down to bone. This corresponds roughly to 4.0 to 5.0 cm distal to the medial joint line (see Fig 48–1). A small elevator is used to raise periosteal flaps and enhance visualization of the tibial bone tunnel.

6. Using the Acufex Pro-Trak guide set at a 45-degree inclination and inserted through the medial portal, the intraarticular portal of entry for the tibial tunnel at the site of the tibial attachment of the ACL is marked. A smooth guide pin is then drilled into the joint under arthroscopic visualization, until the tip is just protruding into the joint (Fig 48–3).

7. With a curette placed over the tip of the guide pin to protect the PCL, the cannulated reamer corresponding to the size of the tibial bone plug is employed to create the tibial tunnel (Fig 48–4). It is desirable for the anterior wall of the tibial tunnel to be at least the length of the tibial bone plug, and it is preferable to have a 4- to 5-cm tunnel.

8. All bone and soft tissue debris created by the reaming must then be removed from the proximal end of the tunnel, and the posterior margin of the tunnel is then chamfered with a motorized backcutting reamer or hand-held rasp to prevent mechanical abrasion of the graft (Fig 48–5).

9. The over-the-top position is then palpated with a probe, and at the 1-o'clock position in a left knee, or the 11-o'clock position in a right knee, the femoral insertion site for the graft is marked with a burr.

10. A smooth beeth pin with an eyelet serves as the femoral guide pin and is directed up the tibial tunnel with the knee flexed to approximately 60 degrees. This pin should enter the femur 5 to 6 mm anterior to the over-the-top position at either the

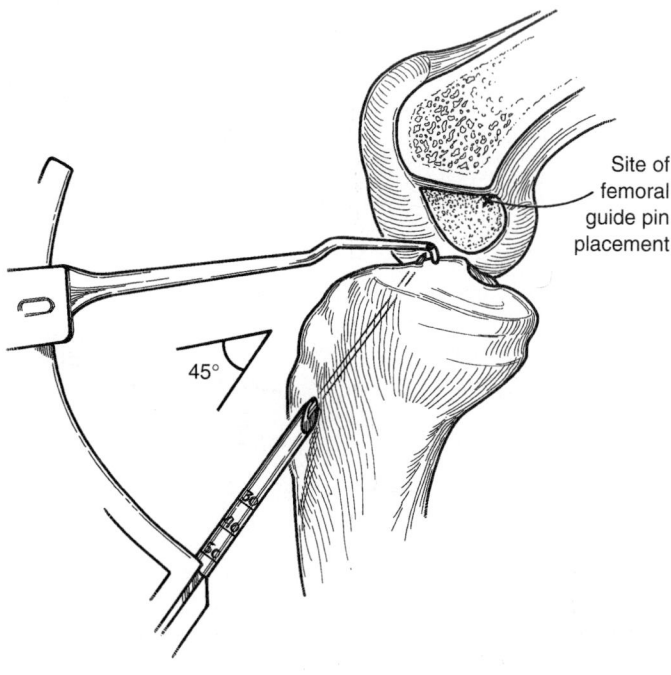

FIG 48–3.
The tibial guide directs the guide pin to a point just posterior to the anterior horn of the medial meniscus and just medial to the midpoint between the tibial spines. Care is taken to provide an adequate anterior wall to the tibial tunnel.

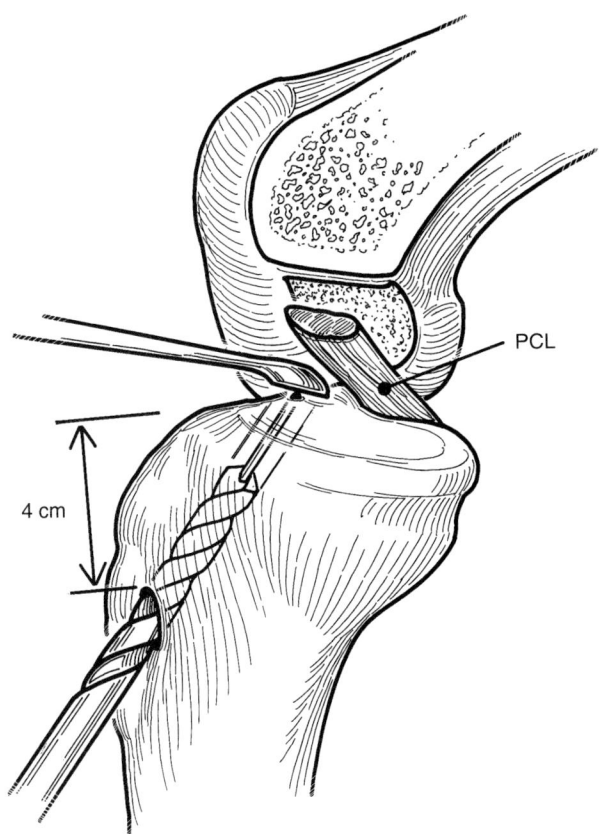

FIG 48-4.
With a curette over the tip of the guide pin to protect the posterior cruciate ligament (PCL), a cannulated reamer prepares the tibial tunnel.

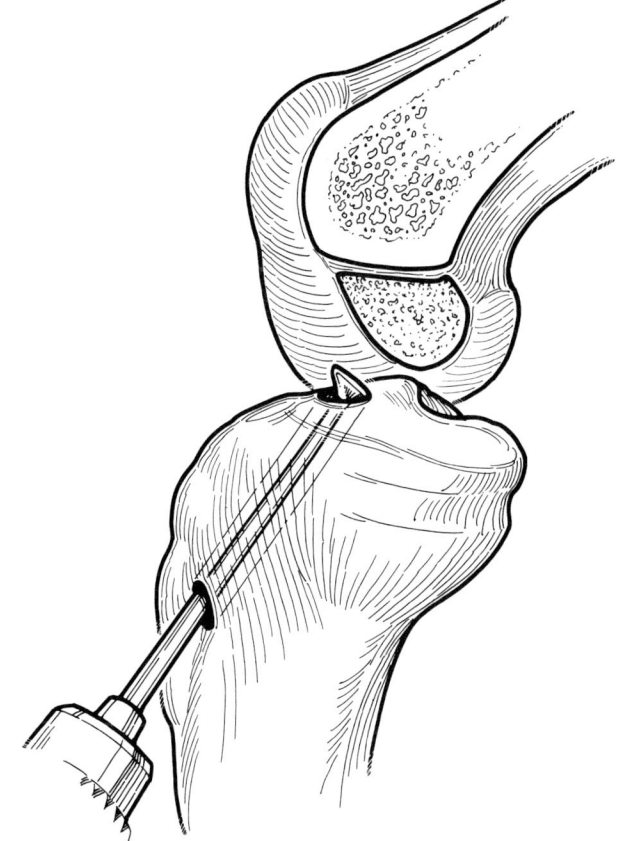

FIG 48-5.
A motorized backcutting reamer, or hand rasp, chamfers the posterior wall of the tibial tunnel, removing all sharp edges that can cause graft abrasion and early failure.

1-o'clock or 11-o'clock position. This is the most critical and difficult portion of the procedure, and the guide pin should not be advanced until the placement is correct. The guide pin is then drilled through the lateral cortex of the femur to exit the distal lateral thigh (Figs 48-6 and 48-7).

11. The cannulated reamer corresponding to the diameter of the femoral bone plug is then placed over the guide pin and turned manually until it advances to the level of the lateral femoral condyle. This calibrated reamer is then drilled to a depth of 30 mm (or 5 mm longer than the bone plug) and removed (see Fig 48-7). Bony debris can be removed by suctioning the femoral tunnel, and the tunnel should be inspected to assure that there is bone on all sides. This can best be performed by inserting the arthroscope through the tibial tunnel. The posterior wall should be a thin 1 to 2 mm if the position is chosen correctly.

12. The graft is then passed through the tibial tunnel by placing the solitary suture through the eyelet of the guide pin, which is then removed, leaving the sutures protruding through the distal lateral thigh. A hemostat inserted through the medial portal can help guide the bone plug into the femoral tunnel, and the plug should be advanced until the surgical pen mark at the bone-tendon interface is barely visible at the entrance of the tunnel (Figs 48-8 and 48-9).

13. The screwdriver is then inserted through the medial portal, and a mallet is used to gently notch the anterosuperior edge of the tunnel for initiation of screw insertion.

14. A 7- × 20-mm interference screw is then inserted with a tonsil clamp through the medial portal and held on the superior surface of the graft. Meanwhile, under arthroscopic visualization, the screwdriver is inserted into the joint through the tibial tunnel along the anterior surface of the graft, and the screw is engaged. The tonsil is then placed between the graft and the screw to protect the graft as it is inserted anterior to the graft at the site of the notch (Fig 48-10). This pushes the graft into the more anatomic posterior position. An appropriate amount of tension must be maintained on both ends of the graft during

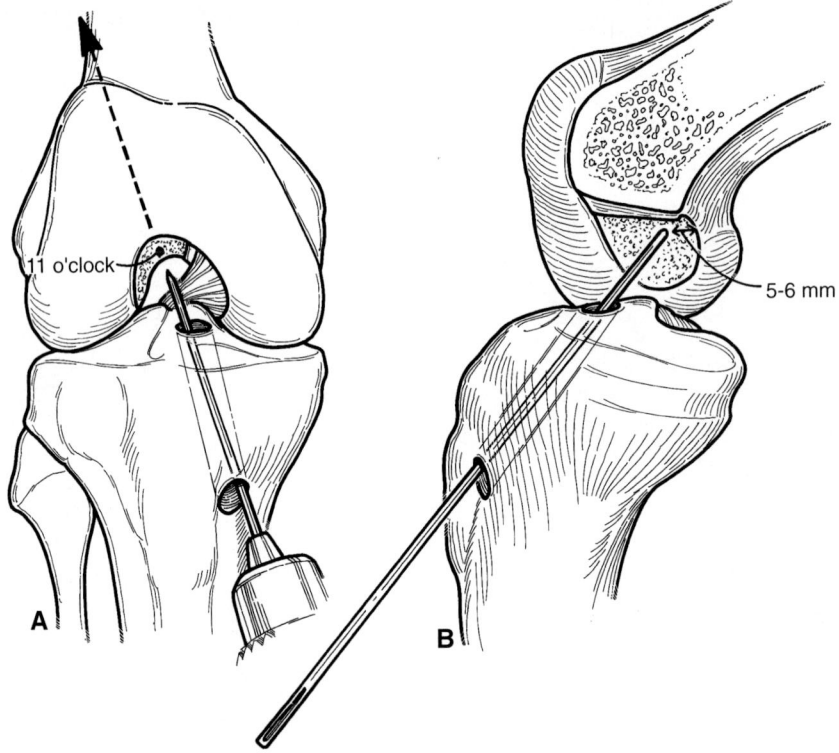

FIG 48–6.
With the knee flexed to 60 to 90 degrees, a smooth Beath pin with an eyelet is directed to a spot 5 to 6 mm anterior to the over-the-top position, at the 11-o'clock position in this right knee, and advanced until its tip exits the distal lateral thigh. This serves as the femoral guide pin.

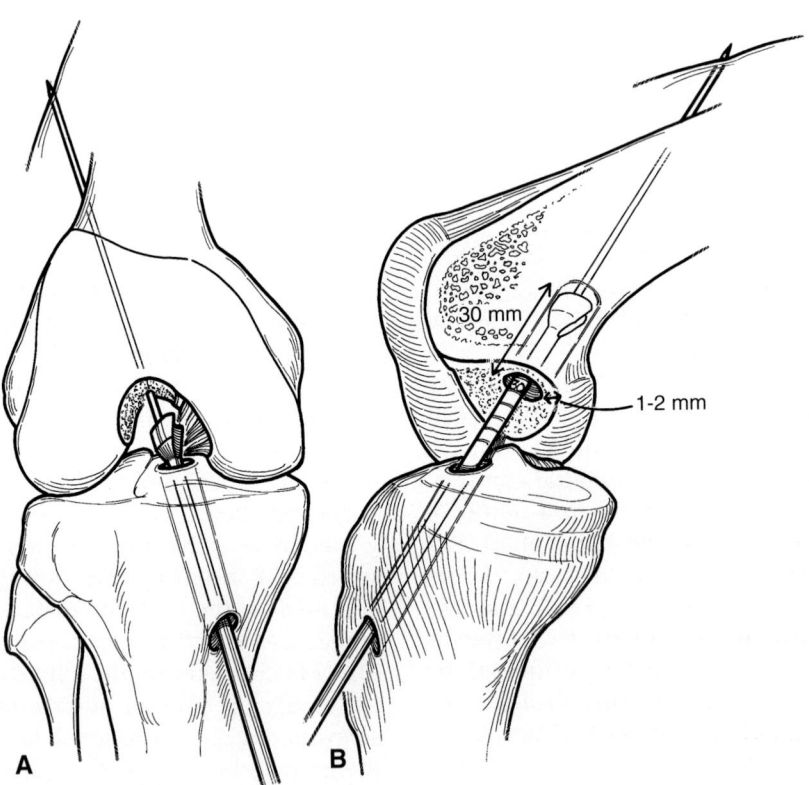

FIG 48–7.
A calibrated, cannulated femoral reamer then prepares a femoral tunnel that is approximately 5 mm longer than the femoral bone plug (generally 30 mm deep). The tunnel created should have a complete, but thin, posterior wall if the placement is correct.

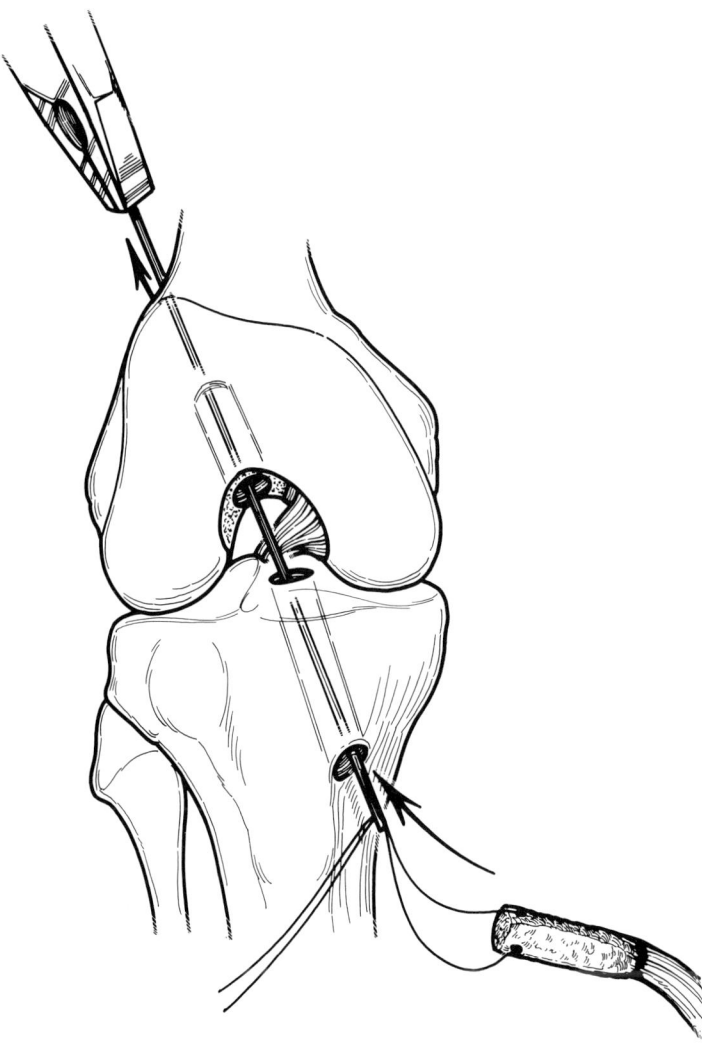

FIG 48–8.
With the suture of the femoral bone plug threaded through the eye of the *beeth* needle, the femoral guide pin is removed from the distal lateral thigh, leaving the sutures protruding from the location where the pin was removed.

screw insertion to avoid having the bone plug advance into the femoral tunnel with the screw.

15. The knee is then taken through a range of motion several times with tension on the femorally fixed graft to preload the allograft, as well as to check isometry. Ideally, the tibial bone plug should not move during the range of motion, though it may be pulled into the joint 1 to 2 mm as the knee is brought into full extension. Arthroscopic visualization of the graft throughout the range of motion and with the knee in full extension should reveal a graft free of impingement laterally and in the superior notch. If any impingement is noted, the notchplasty should be augmented prior to tibial fixation of the graft.

16. While a posterior drawer is placed on the knee and tension is maintained on the sutures attached to the tibial bone plug, a 9- × 20-mm interference screw is placed on the posterolateral aspect of the bone plug for fixation. This prevents the graft from abutting the lateral wall, tightens the graft, and decreases the potential for mechanical abrasion on the posterior lip of the tibial tunnel (Fig 48–11,A). A 90- to 180-degree twist can be placed in the graft[23, 77] if the surgeon believes this adds to the strength of the graft. We are not presently twisting our grafts. Occasionally, the graft is too long, and interference fixation is not possible in the tibia. We then create a triangular trough in the proximal tibia with a rongeur, and dual staple fixation is then utilized. This fixation can also be reinforced by tying the sutures over a post (Fig 48–11,B).

17. The knee is then taken through a range of motion to assure that full extension and at least 90 degrees of flexion can be achieved. A gentle Lachman test is performed to test stability, and tension of the graft is checked under arthroscopic visualization. Any questions about the adequacy of fixation should be addressed at this time. Intraoperative anteroposterior (AP) and lateral radiographs can be helpful but are not routinely necessary.

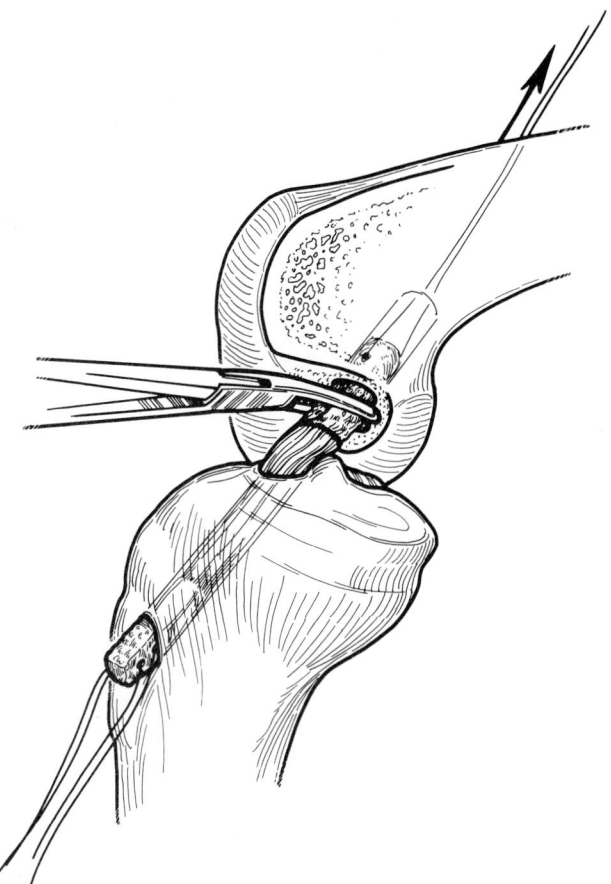

FIG 48-9.
Traction on the femoral suture advances the bone plug into the femoral tunnel. A hemostat is used to position the cortical bone of the plug posteriorly and direct the plug into the tunnel.

18. The periosteum is closed over the tibial tunnel, and an interrupted subcutaneous polyglactin 910 (Vicryl) closure with Steri-Strips (3M Company, St. Paul, Minneapolis) leaves a good cosmetic appearance. Nylon sutures or a subcuticular nonabsorbable suture (Prolene) can also be used.

Two-Incision Rear-Entry Guide Technique

Though the endoscopic technique provides optimal cosmesis for allograft surgery, the two incision rear-entry guide technique remains a viable option. The procedure is similar to that described above, except that a 4- to 5-cm incision over the iliotibial band is required for placement of the rear-entry guide, as well as reaming the femoral tunnel and fixation of the femoral bone plug with an interference screw (Fig 48-12). This technique allows placement of the tibial guide pin just posterior to the anterior horn of the medial meniscus (see Fig 48-12). The endoscopic technique forces us to place the guide pin slightly

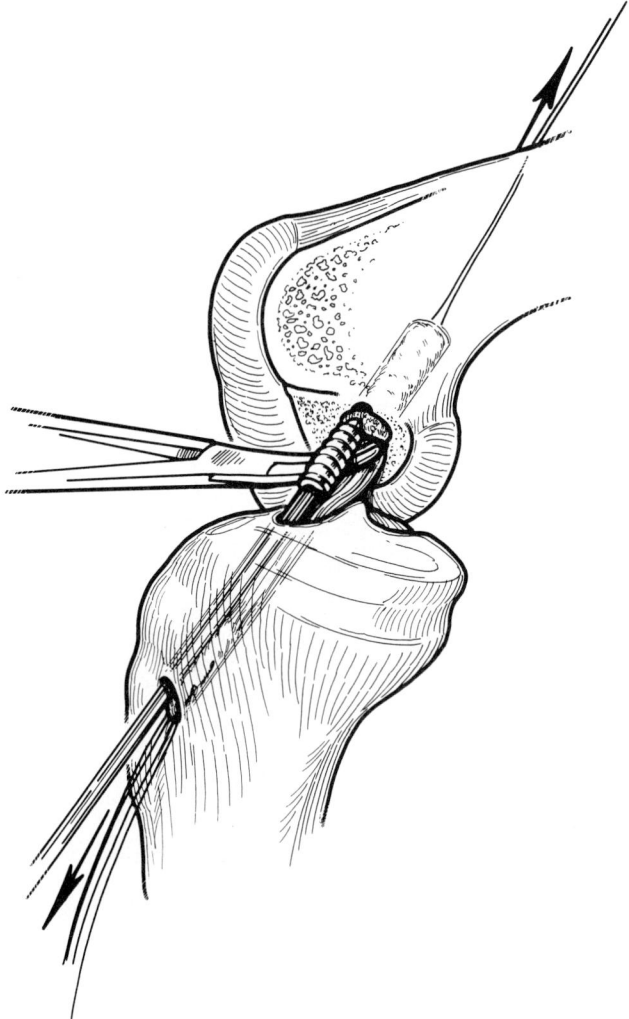

FIG 48-10.
A 7- × 20-mm interference screw is placed on the superior surface of the graft using a tonsil clamp, and skewered with the corresponding screwdriver, which is inserted through the tibial tunnel anterior to the graft. This parallel position of the screwdriver allows for nondivergent screw insertion and optimal graft fixation. The notch placed in the anterosuperior edge of the tunnel permits easy insertion of the screw tip between the bone plug and the tunnel when initiating screw implantation.

more posterior on the tibia, in order to place the femoral guide pin through the tibial tunnel. Studies are underway to ascertain whether this significantly affects isometricity. If proper placement of the femoral guide pin cannot be achieved through the tibial tunnel, then the rear-entry guide should be utilized for production of the femoral tunnel (see Fig 48-12). One advantage of the rear-entry technique is the ability to use a 9-mm interference screw for femoral fixation. Both techniques can be used to perform reliable ACL reconstructions with either autograft or allograft tissues.

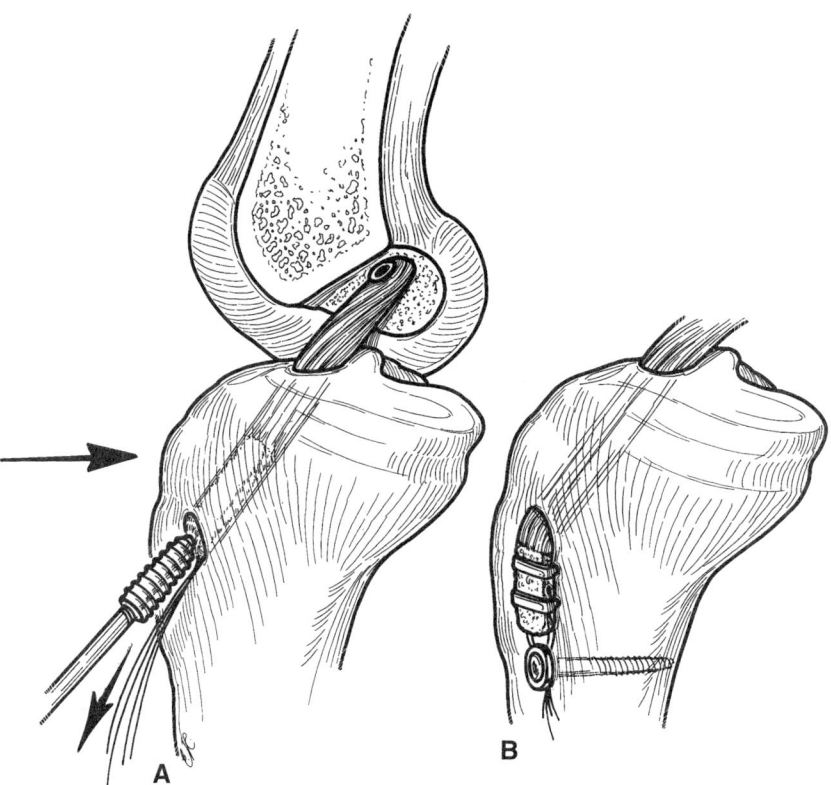

FIG 48–11.
Tibial interference fixation is generally feasible and can be performed with the larger 9- × 20-mm screw **(A)**. If the graft is too long, and the bone plug protrudes from the tunnel so that interference fixation is impossible, a triangular trough is created with a rongeur or burr and dual staple fixation is employed. Supplemental fixation with sutures tied around a post can reinforce fixation if desired **(B)**.

Postoperative Management

Patients are placed in a knee immobilizer in the operating room, which is removed when they are placed on a continuous passive motion (CPM) machine in the recovery room. Patients are instructed by the physical therapist in gait training, weightbearing as tolerated, with the knee in the immobilizer, and are discharged home within 24 hours. They are given home CPM for 1 to 3 weeks and instructed to place the heel on a rolled towel several times per day to maintain full passive knee extension. Patients begin formal physical therapy after 5 to 7 days when their sutures are removed. Crutches are discontinued after 6 to 8 weeks, and patients are placed in range-of-motion braces locked at 0 to 90 degrees for ambulation until their strength is 80% of the normal knee. Early emphasis is on regaining extension, and range of motion in general, and strengthening is added to the program gradually as range of motion approaches normal. Straight-ahead activities, such as jogging, are allowed at 3 to 4 months, and patients are allowed to return to competitive sports at 7 to 8 months provided they have full range of motion and at least 90% of the strength of the contralateral limb.

When we have performed allograft ACL reconstructions in an outpatient setting, we have discharged our patients in knee immobilizers without CPM machines. Patients are telephoned the day following surgery for a postoperative check, and they return to the office 3 to 4 days after surgery for suture removal, if necessary. Physical therapy and home CPM are started at that time. Otherwise the treatment is unchanged.

ALLOGRAFT POSTERIOR CRUCIATE LIGAMENT TECHNIQUE

Posterior cruciate ligament reconstructions are performed far less commonly than ACL reconstructions, generally being executed primarily when combined injuries are noted on examination, and rarely for isolated PCL injuries. Though autografts remain the gold standard replacement, the need for a larger, stronger graft than is necessary for ACL reconstructions to replace the more stout PCL makes allograft reconstruction of the PCL enticing. We have utilized BTB autografts for PCL reconstructions in the past, but our current protocol is to replace the PCL with

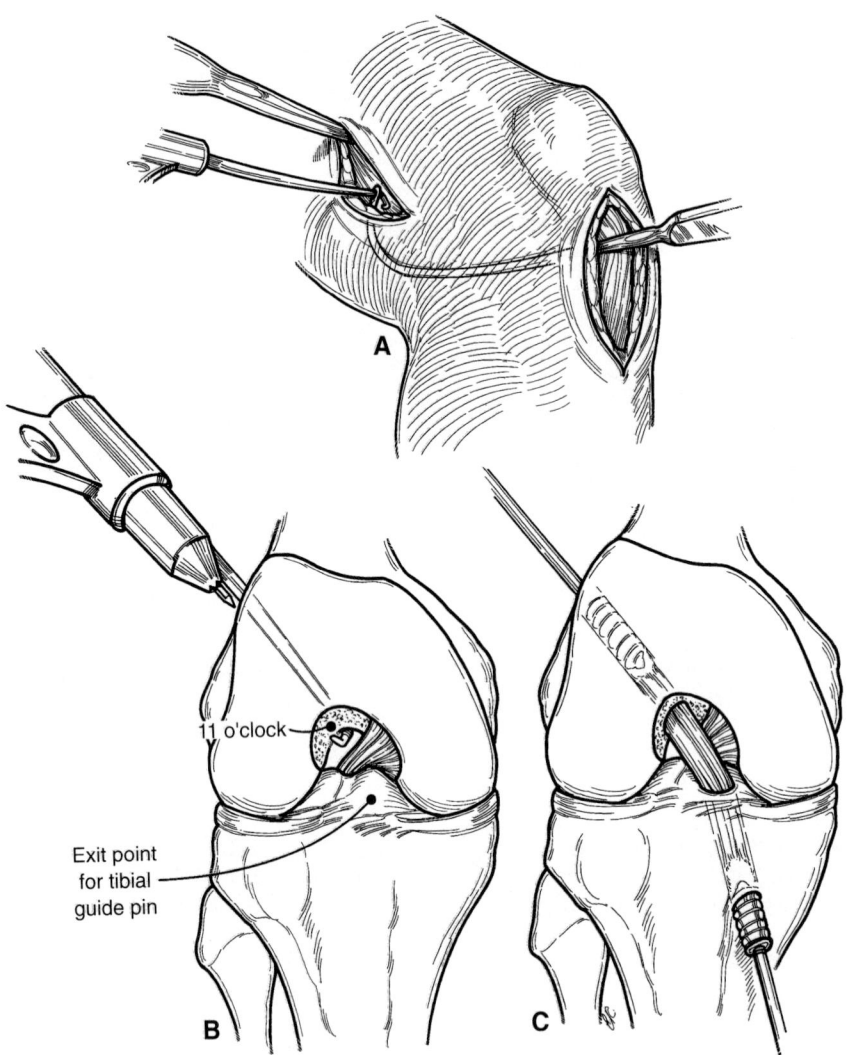

FIG 48–12.
The rear-entry technique utilizes a 4- to 5-cm lateral incision over the iliotibial band and a two-part guide system. The guide passer is inserted through the lateral portal and hooked around the over-the-top position to exit the lateral incision, where the guide is hooked into the eye of the passer **(A)**. The passer then pulls the guide into the joint, and after disengaging the guide from the passer, the tip of the guide is placed 5 to 6 mm anterior to the over-the-top position at 11 o'clock in this right knee **(B)**. The femoral guide pin is then advanced, and the femoral tunnel is reamed with a cannulated reamer. The graft can then be fixed with two 9- × 20-mm interference screws, both inserted externally under direct visualization **(C)**.

the stronger and stiffer fresh frozen Achilles tendon allograft using an arthroscopically-assisted technique as described below.

1. The graft should be prepared prior to beginning the operative procedure to minimize anesthetic time to the patient. The bone plug of the thawed Achilles tendon graft is shaped into a triangular wedge approximately 30 mm in length with a maximum diameter of 11 to 13 mm. The bone plug diameter should roughly correspond to the largest diameter of the rolled Achilles tendon graft. The Achilles tendon is rolled into a tube and secured with a single no. 2 nonabsorbable suture using a baseball-type stitch throughout its length. The suture ends are tagged for later use in passing the graft. A single transverse drill hole is placed in the bone plug and a no. 5 Ticron suture is placed through the hole and tagged (Fig 48–13). The graft is then wrapped in a moist Ray-tec and placed on the back table in a kidney basin until needed. We have not routinely preloaded our grafts, though this can be performed on a tension board at this time if desired.

2. The patient is then anesthetized and an examination under anesthesia is performed to confirm the PCL rupture, document any concurrent ligamentous abnormalities, and compare the injured with the contralateral extremity.

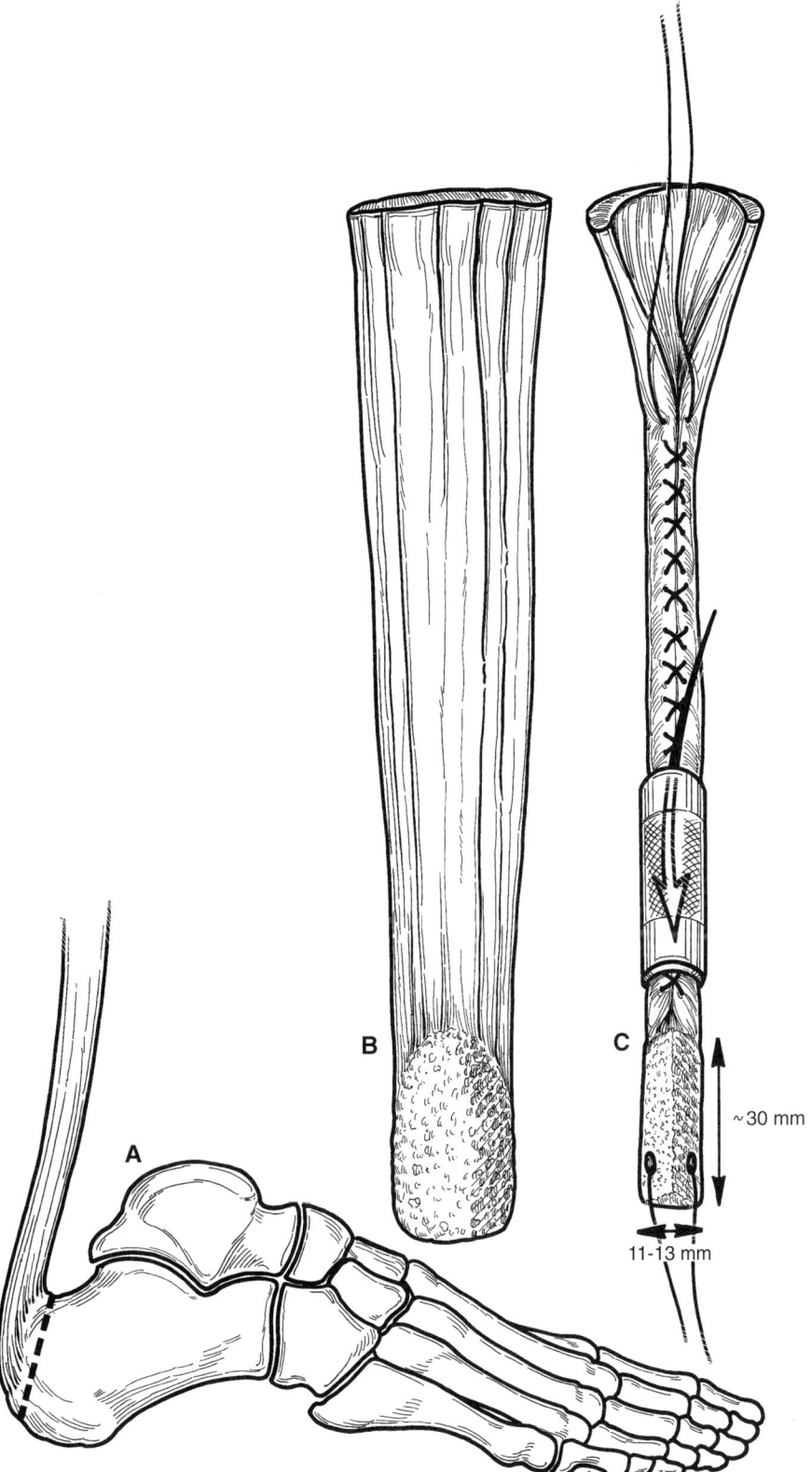

FIG 48-13.
The Achilles tendon allograft is generally procured with a large, irregular bone block and a wide tendon graft **(A** and **B)**. The bone block requires shaping, and the tendon requires tubulation. A cylindrical sizer measures the diameter of the graft and bone plug and assures smooth passage of the graft **(C)**.

3. A routine diagnostic arthroscopy is then performed to document and treat any coexisting lesion, as mentioned in step 3 of the ACL reconstruction technique.

4. A notchplasty is not as important in PCL reconstructions, but good visualization cannot be obtained unless the ligamentum mucosum, the PCL stump, and all remaining soft tissues are completely debrided from the medial wall and the posterior notch of the tibia. Tight intercondylar notches may require medial and posterior notchplasty with a motorized burr to prevent abrasion of the large graft. A posteromedial instrument portal and a 70-degree arthroscope may be necessary to completely debride the tibial insertion of the PCL.

5. A 3- to 5-cm vertical incision is made just medial to the inferior aspect of the tibial tubercle approximately 8 to 10 cm distal to the joint line (Fig 48–14). Periosteal flaps are elevated and retracted for visualization of the tunnel and tibial fixation of the graft. The incision can also be placed just lateral to the tibial tubercle if preferred, and this site is preferable if an ACL reconstruction is needed as well.

6. The Acufex posterior cruciate tibial guide is inserted through the medial portal, and correct placement of the guide in the posterior compartment is confirmed using a 70-degree arthroscope from the lateral portal or a 30-degree arthroscope from a posteromedial portal. With the knee flexed to 90 degrees and the guide pin directed at a 45-degree angle, the guide pin is drilled under lateral fluoroscopic visualization until the tip has barely protruded through the posterior cortex (Fig 48–15). Care must be taken to avoid premature penetration of the posterior cortex. For less experienced arthroscopists or surgeons who prefer not to use fluoroscopy, a 6- to 8-cm posteromedial incision can allow for dissection down to the posterior capsule, digital palpation of the guide, and protection of neurovascular structures with a malleable retractor.

7. Under arthroscopic visualization or fluoroscopic control, or both, the cannulated tibial reamer matching the size of the rolled Achilles tendon graft is used to prepare the tibial tunnel. Care must be taken to avoid plunging through the posterior cortex and injuring posterior structures. A curved curette placed over the end of the guide pin can be helpful (Fig 48–16).

8. All bone and soft tissue debris are then removed from the tibial tunnel and its entrance into the joint using motorized equipment. A plug is then placed in the tunnel to prevent extravasation of irrigation fluid during the remainder of the arthroscopy.

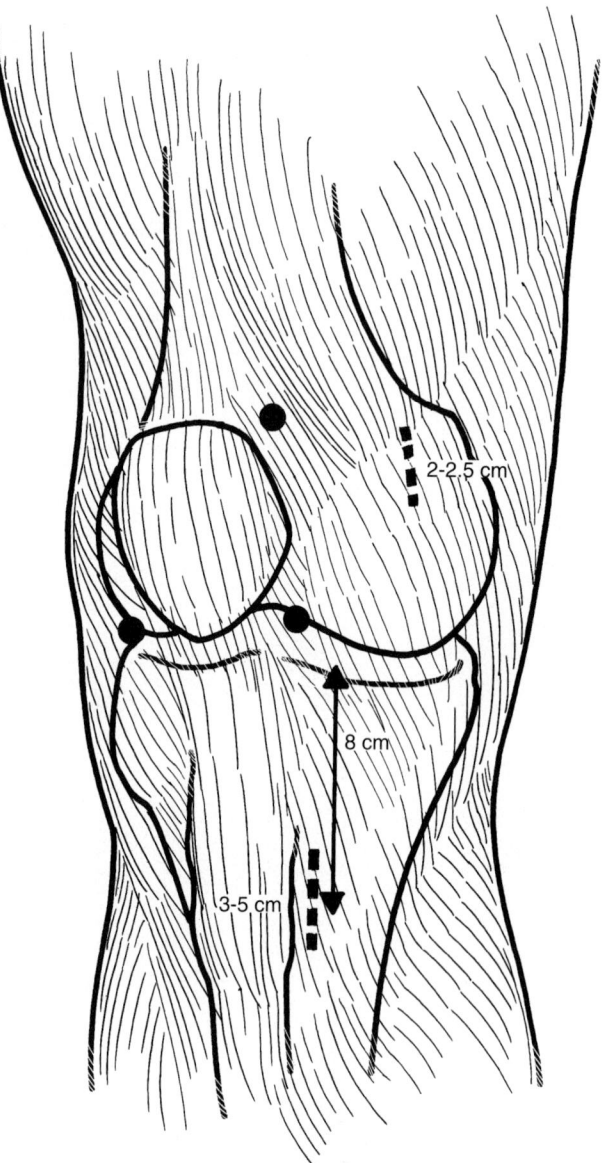

FIG 48–14.
Incisions for allograft posterior cruciate ligament reconstruction consist of the three standard arthroscopy portals, plus an additional 3- to 5-cm vertical incision over the proximal medial or lateral tibia and a 2.5-cm longitudinal incision over the medial femoral condyle for preparation of the tibial and femoral tunnels, respectively.

9. A 2.0- to 2.5-cm incision over the medial femoral condyle is carried down to bone without penetrating the joint capsule (see Fig 48–14). Periosteal flaps are raised with an elevator for adequate visualization of the tunnel.

10. The femoral guide is inserted through the medial portal and placed in the anatomic femoral origin site of the PCL, approximately 6 to 7 mm posterior to the articular surface of the medial femoral condyle in the 1-o'clock position in the right knee or the 11-o'clock position in the left knee. Once the guide

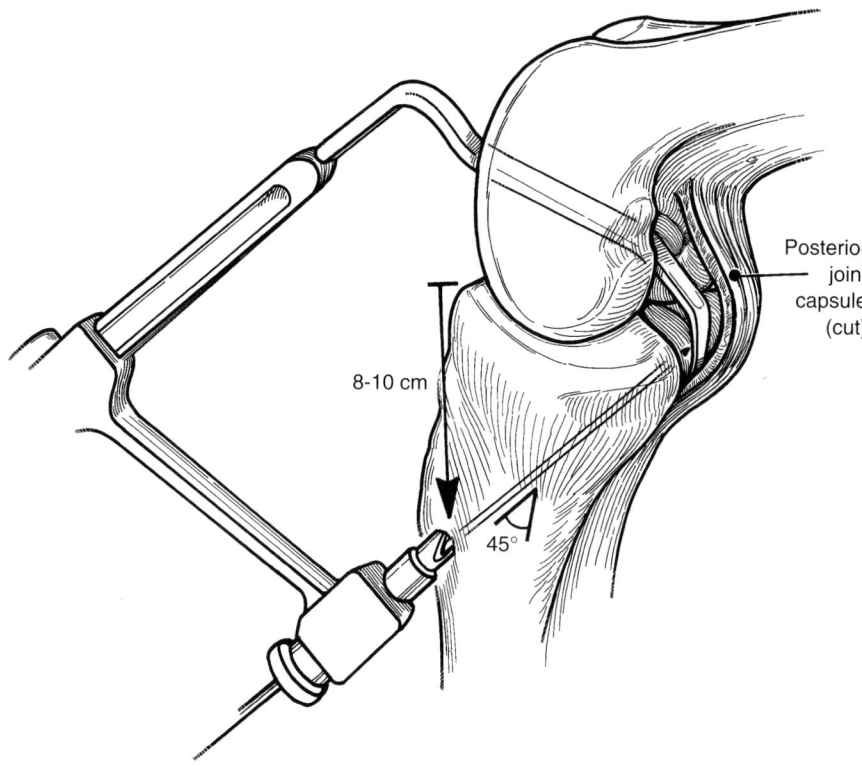

FIG 48-15.
Under fluoroscopic control, the tibial guide pin is inserted, making sure not to penetrate the posterior tibial cortex prematurely. Correct placement of the tibial guide can be accomplished using a 70-degree arthroscope through the lateral portal or a 30-degree arthroscope through a posteromedial portal.

is engaged, the guide pin is inserted under arthroscopic visualization (Fig 48-17).

11. With a curette placed over the tip of the guide pin to protect the ACL, the cannulated reamer matching the diameter of the femoral bone block is used to create the femoral tunnel (Fig 48-18). Once again, all bone and soft tissue debris must be removed from the tunnel and its exit site in the notch.

12. The Gore smoother is then passed from the tibial tunnel into the joint, grasped with a tonsil clamp, and passed to a second tonsil clamp inserted through the femoral tunnel. This device is then used in a gentle, sawing fashion to smooth and chamfer the posterior wall of the femoral tunnel and the anterior wall of the tibial tunnel to minimize the risk of graft abrasion.

13. The graft is then secured to the Gore smoother using the suture in the bone plug and pulled through the tibial tunnel and the joint into place with the aid of a hemostat for guidance of the bone plug into the femoral tunnel (Fig 48-19). Generally, a significant tendinous portion of the graft will remain exposed when the bone plug of the graft is flush with the extraarticular edge of the femoral tunnel (Fig 48-20).

14. The femoral bone plug is secured in place with a 9- × 25-mm interference screw placed posterior to the bone plug while maintaining tension on both ends of the graft. This maintains the graft in the more anatomic anterior position in the tunnel. Ideally, the bone-tendon interface of the graft should be at the level of the entry of the femoral tunnel to the notch to minimize abrasion of the graft on the posterior aspect of the femoral tunnel, as it takes a sharp turn toward the tibial tunnel (see Fig 48-20).

15. On the tibial side, fixation can be either with a 6.5-mm AO cancellous screw and soft tissue washer or a staple technique. We prefer a pants-over-vest dual Richards soft tissue staple technique. The tubed Achilles tendon is opened as it exits the tibial tunnel, and the flat graft is placed against the anteromedial cortex of the tibia. An anterior drawer is placed on the tibia, and the knee is placed through a range of motion six to ten times to check isometry of the graft and to preload the graft prior to final fixation. With the knee flexed to 20 to 30 degrees and an anterior drawer applied, the first staple is placed through the graft perpendicular to the tibial cortex, making sure both tines are engaged in bone. The graft is then folded over itself, and the second staple

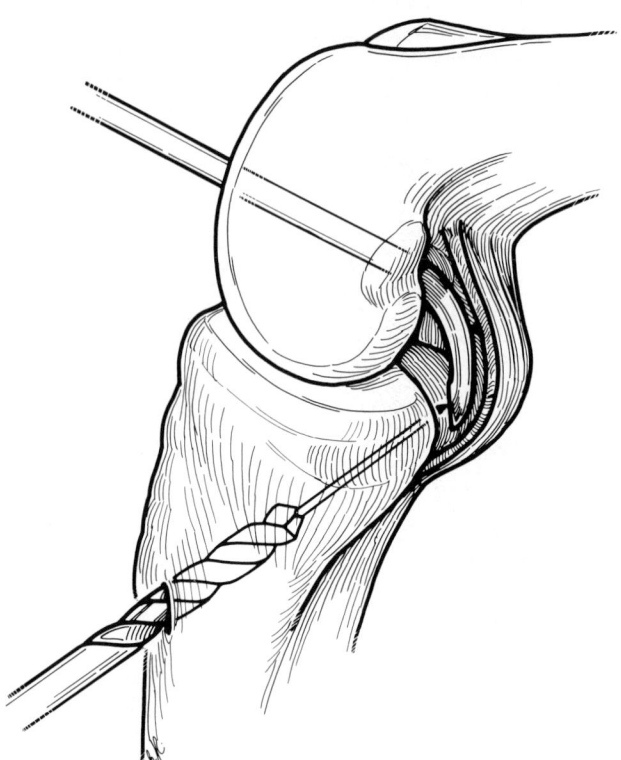

FIG 48–16.
Protecting against pin penetration with a curved curette and observing closely with the arthroscope or fluoroscopy, a cannulated reamer prepares the appropriately sized tibial tunnel.

is placed proximal to the first staple in the same manner. If desired, the sutures can also be tied over a post for additional fixation (Fig 48–21).

16. The knee is then gently taken through a range of motion, assuring that full extension and at least 90 degrees of flexion can be obtained. A gentle posterior drawer is performed to assess the amount of laxity present in the reconstruction. Tension of the graft is checked under arthroscopic visualization while performing the drawer maneuver.

17. Excess graft tissue can be trimmed after fixation, and the incisions can be closed in a standard fashion. The staples on the tibia can be prominent and bothersome in some patients, and there is no detrimental effect to their removal at 12 to 18 months postoperatively.

Postoperative Management

Patients are placed in a knee immobilizer in the operating room. The immobilizer is removed when the patient is placed in a CPM machine in the recovery room. Patients are instructed by the physical therapist in gait training, weightbearing as tolerated on the extremity that was operated on, with crutches and

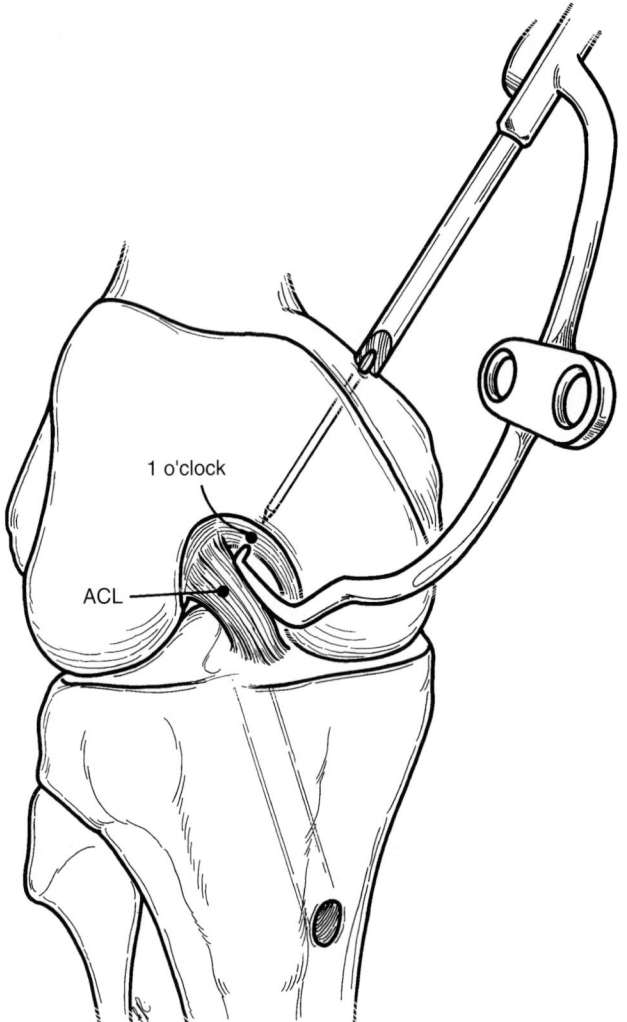

FIG 48–17.
The femoral guide is inserted through the medial portal and placed 6 to 7 mm posterior to the articular edge of the medial femoral condyle in the 1-o'clock position in this right knee. The femoral guide pin is then inserted. ACL = anterior cruciate ligament.

the knee in the immobilizer. They are discharged home on postoperative day 2, and a CPM machine is ordered for home use, 6 to 8 hr/day. Patients work on passive and active extension, as well as gentle passive flexion for the first 3 to 6 weeks, after which active assisted flexion is instituted. As with ACL rehabilitation, early emphasis is on regaining extension, and the patient's heels are placed on rolled towels for 1 hour three times daily initially. Crutches are discontinued at approximately 8 weeks, and a range-of-motion brace locked at 0 to 90 degrees is utilized for ambulation until limb strength is 80% of the contralateral limb. Quadriceps strengthening is added when range of motion reaches 90 degrees, and hamstring strengthening is begun at 4 to 6 months after full range of motion is achieved and quadriceps strength

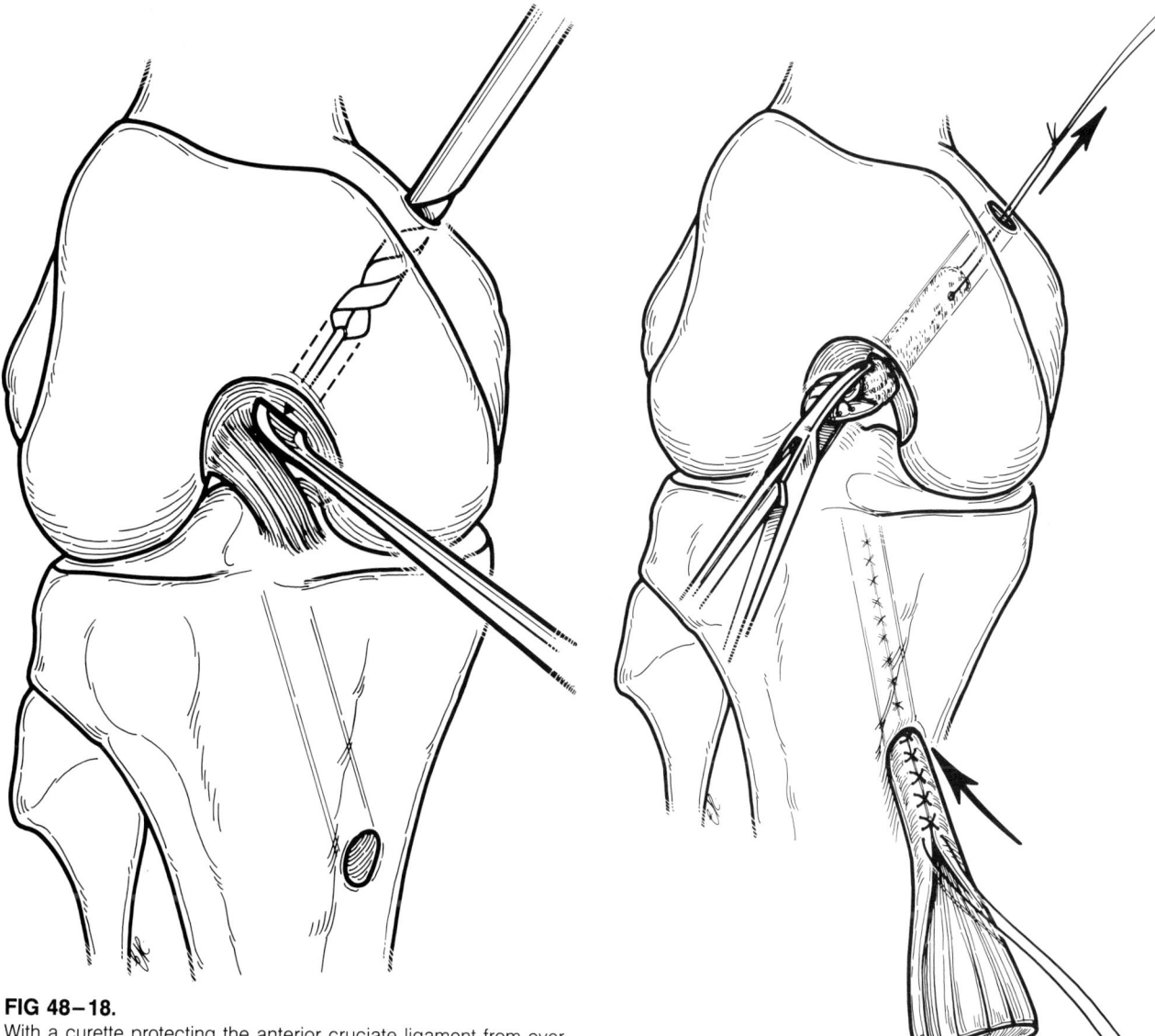

FIG 48–18.
With a curette protecting the anterior cruciate ligament from over-penetration, a cannulated reamer prepares the appropriately sized femoral tunnel.

FIG 48–19.
Use of a hemostat is essential to maneuvering the bone plug through the tortuous course of the posterior cruciate ligament.

approaches normal. Patients are allowed to resume straight-ahead activities, such as jogging, at 4 to 6 months, and may return to competition at 8 to 9 months provided they have full range of motion and at least 90% of the strength of the contralateral limb.

HUMAN ALLOGRAFT RECONSTRUCTION RESULTS

It is only recently that long-term follow-up reports on allograft ligamentous reconstructions of the knee have been presented at regional and national meetings, and few have appeared in the literature. However, the next several years will provide us with a plethora of data on the complications and results of reconstructions utilizing different allograft techniques, and, it is hoped, supply us with some prospective studies comparing allograft and autograft reconstructions in matched populations. For now, the data available are limited, but encouraging.

Levitt and Malinin[62] reported their experience using fresh frozen and freeze-dried Achilles tendon and BTB allografts in a consecutive series of 300 patients undergoing arthroscopically assisted ACL reconstruction over a 6-year period. Chronic instability was the indication for surgery in the vast majority of their patients, and 53 patients required follow-up arthroscopy for arthrofibrosis (18), secondary joint lesions including meniscal tears (15), painful hardware (13),

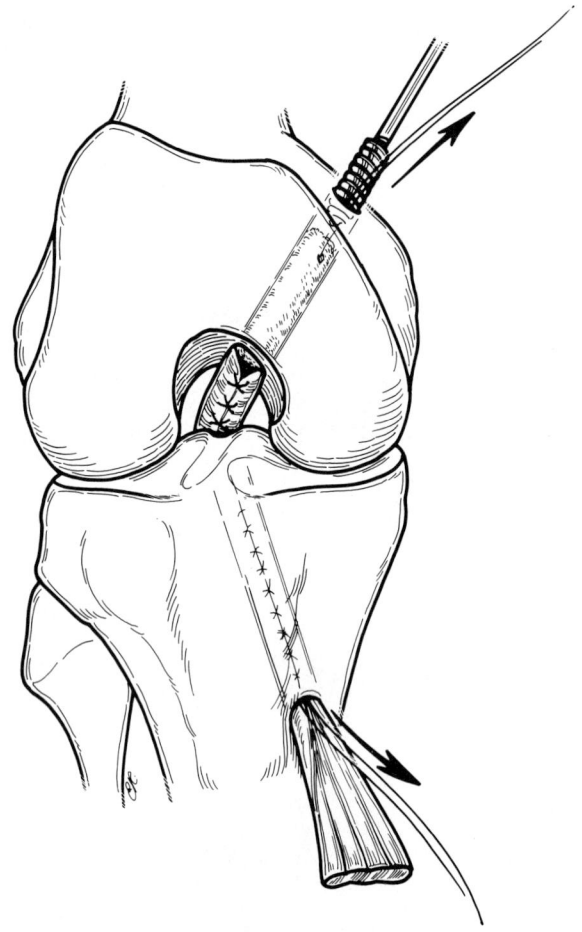

FIG 48–20.
Femoral fixation is provided with a 9- × 25-mm interference screw. A significant tendinous portion of the graft is exposed on the tibial side after femoral fixation is achieved.

synovitis associated with anterior impingement and graft fraying (4), and allograft ruptures (3). Biopsies of the grafts taken at the time of second-look arthroscopy from 8 weeks to 5 years after the reconstruction revealed that revascularization and mature cellular ingrowth with linear orientation of collagen bundles was completed by 18 to 24 months. They noted improvement in their results as measured by a modified Feagin scoring system, from 69% satisfactory in 1984 to 89% satisfactory in 1990 as their techniques and rehabilitation protocols improved, and 87% of their patients were noted to have 20-lb KT-1000 arthrometer scores with less than 5-mm side-to-side difference at 1-year follow-up. Furthermore, the authors reported that results stabilized at 1 year follow-up, with no deterioration on longer follow-up as measured by the KT-1000 arthrometer. They reported slightly better results in reconstruction of acute injuries as opposed to chronic instability and with fresh frozen grafts vs. freeze-dried grafts, though these differences were not statistically significant. Results using Achilles tendon and BTB allografts were virtually identical. All allografts for this study were harvested under sterile conditions, and no secondary sterilization was performed. There were no instances of disease transmission noted.[62] Long-term follow-up averaging 45 months confirmed these original findings.[63]

Meyers et al.[69, 71, 72] began performing allograft ACL reconstructions as early as 1983, and they reported their results using primarily 10- to 12-mm-diameter freeze-dried double fascia lata allografts. Their study included 54 patients with minimum 2-year follow-up evaluated with a Lysholm scale and KT-1000 arthrometer. They obtained 78% satisfactory results, and 87% of their patients were satisfied with the outcome of their surgery. Only 2 of the 54 patients had side-to-side differences of greater than 4 mm on testing with 20 lb of force using the KT-1000 arthrometer. Twenty-eight of the patients underwent second-look arthroscopy for assessment of articular cartilage changes, as well as evaluation of the allograft ligament. The graft failed in 2 patients, showed fraying as evidence of lateral wall impingement in 2, was lax despite clinical stability in 2, revealed dense fibrous scarring in the retropatellar and intercondylar regions in 6, and was entirely normal in appearance in the remaining 18 patients. Nine patients exhibited worsening of articular cartilage during their postoperative course, 6 of whom had deterioration of their medial compartment after partial medial meniscectomy performed in conjunction with the ACL reconstruction. No patients showed evidence of intraarticular reaction to the allograft tissue.[69, 71, 72] The authors believed that allograft ACL reconstruction compared favorably with their prior report on the outcome and effect of open autograft ACL reconstructions, though they admitted that the two procedures were not directly comparable.[70]

Indelicato and colleagues[48] performed a prospective study comparing the results of freeze-dried BTB allografts performed in 14 patients to fresh frozen BTB allografts in 27 patients using identical arthroscopically assisted techniques and rehabilitation protocols. There was no clinical evidence of graft rejection in any of the patients, and there were two clinical failures at minimum 2-year follow-up. Four patients had second-look arthroscopies and biopsies, including 1 for a ruptured graft. Interestingly, 3 patients with biopsies at 8, 9, and 20 months showed vascularization and collagenization in the peripheral biopsy specimens, while the ruptured graft biopsied 48 hours after rupture and 26 months after implantation exhibited poor vascularity and reorganization.

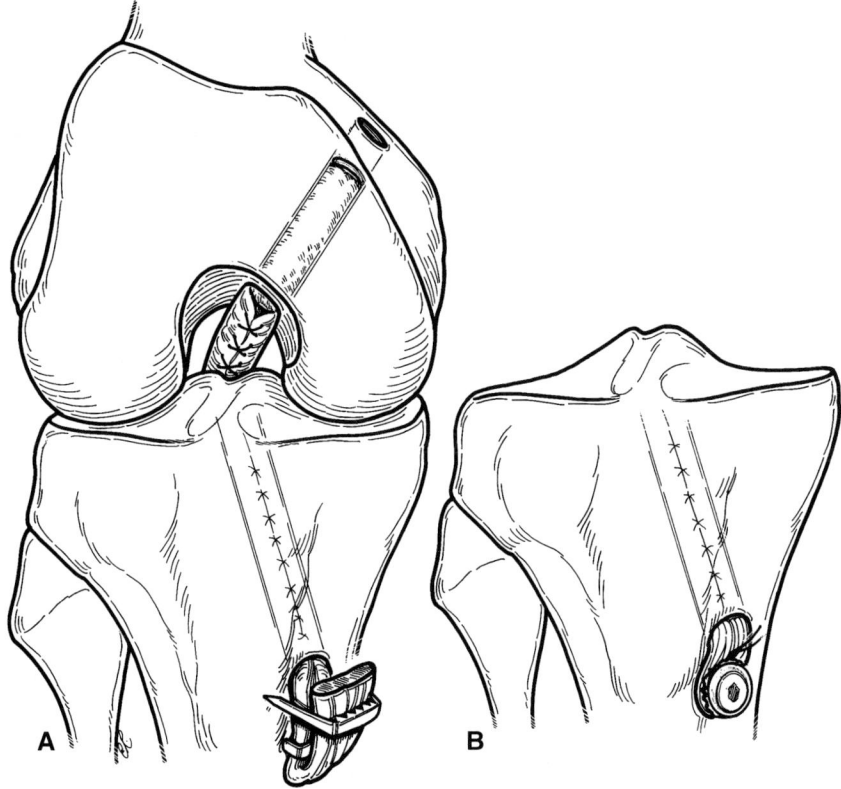

FIG 48-21.
A pants-over-vest staple fixation technique provides secure tibial fixation while an anterior drawer is applied to the knee and tension is maintained on the graft **(A)**. Alternatively, screw and washer fixation can be utilized **(B)**. Excess tendon tissue is removed after fixation is accomplished.

Owing to the small patient populations, only three parameters were noted to be statistically different between the two groups: patients with fresh frozen allografts described less instability and less giving way, and clinically were less likely to have a pivot shift. It should be emphasized, however, that 20-lb KT-1000 testing showed no statistical difference between the two groups, and no patient had greater than a 4-mm side-to-side difference. Overall, 64% of the patients who received freeze-dried allografts had satisfactory results, compared with 81% of those with fresh frozen allografts.[48]

Indelicato et al.[47] also reported their results for fresh frozen BTB allografts used in knee reconstructions of patients with chronic, isolated ACL deficiency. Follow-up was obtained on 41 of 73 patients in this prospective, consecutive series. Nearly half of these patients had undergone arthroscopic meniscectomies earlier, and 3 patients had undergone extraarticular reconstructions. The grafts were all harvested under sterile conditions, the tendinous portion of the graft measuring 14 to 20 mm in diameter, and all were implanted using an arthroscopically assisted "mini-arthrotomy" technique. Approximately half of the patients had meniscal lesions treated at the time of ACL reconstruction. Two patients had traumatic graft failures and a third patient had an atraumatic graft failure, but no patients developed any symptoms consistent with graft rejection. Although 93% of the patients claimed that their knee was either normal or improved from their preoperative status at the time of follow-up, only 49% of the patients were able to return to their preinjury level of athletic competition. Objectively, 92% of the patients had a side-to-side difference of 5 mm or less on testing with the KT-1000 arthrometer using 20 lb of force. Overall, 30 (73%) patients achieved satisfactory results, and the authors believed that their results were comparable to those achieved with autogenous BTB grafts.[47]

Harner et al.[41] recently presented their experience using allografts for cruciate ligament reconstructions at the University of Pittsburgh. They performed 506 allograft ACL reconstructions between 1985 and 1991, but only presented retrospective follow-up on 28 patients with fresh frozen allograft reconstructions. These patients ranged in age from 16 to 51 years, with minimum follow-up of 30 months and average follow-up of 44 months. Five patients had bilateral reconstructions; therefore 33 knees were rated, but only 23 patients had KT-1000 testing. Four patients had anterior translation greater than 5 mm on 20-lb testing and 11 patients had grade 2 or greater pivot shifts, but only 3 patients reported gross knee instability. Despite the fact that at least one third of the study patients reported difficulty with certain athletic tasks and one third showed greater than 10% deficits on objective testing, 73% of the study patients reported being able to return to their preoperative activities at a similar level. Two patients had flexion contractures greater than 10 degrees, and 27% of the patients had trace to moderate effusions. They concluded that sterilely harvested, deep-frozen allografts do not exhibit complications reported for ethylene oxide–sterilized or freeze-dried grafts, and they believe that their allograft results provide evidence that an acceptable functional level was maintained, despite acknowledging that their allograft reconstructions deteriorated with time.[41, 82]

In a separate study by the same group, quadriceps testing using a Cybex isokinetic testing device, functional performance tests, and measurements of thigh circumference were obtained in patients at least 1 year post allograft or autograft ACL reconstruction to assess the effect of graft harvest on outcome. There was no significant difference in mean thigh circumference, performance testing, or any strength or power parameters measured between the two groups.[61] We must conclude that there may not be any functional compromise to the quadriceps mechanism secondary to graft harvest, as was originally thought.

Shino et al. have reported on several occasions their results for ACL reconstructions using various sources of fresh frozen tendon allografts.[97, 98, 100] None of their 84 patients showed signs of graft rejection, and 79 (94%) patients achieved satisfactory results at minimum 3-year followup. Only 12% of patients showed clinical signs of instability on physical examination. Three patients ruptured their reconstructions. Some of the patients had undergone concomitant extraarticular reconstruction consisting of pes anserinus transfer medially and iliotibial band tenodesis laterally, but this reinforcement appeared to have no effect on the final results.[100] Second-look arthroscopy performed on 51 patients revealed two failed grafts and four reconstructions that could not be visualized owing to retropatellar scarring. Patellofemoral chondromalacia was found in 90% of patients, despite a lack of anterior knee pain. Tibiofemoral disease was noted primarily in patients who had undergone partial meniscectomies at the time of their reconstruction. With follow-up as long as 6 years, the authors did not note increasing laxity of the reconstructed ligaments with time.[98]

Noyes et al.[80] published a prospective study of their fresh frozen BTB and fascia lata allografts with minimum 2-year follow-up. Only 5% of their patients had side-to-side differences greater than 5 mm on 20-lb testing with the KT-1000 arthrometer, and they reported 89% satisfactory results. They also had no patients demonstrating evidence of graft rejection, and they stated that their BTB allograft reconstructions showed significantly less AP translation than their fascia lata allografts. One of the 47 patients developed frank giving way after experiencing failure of his fascia lata allograft, but all patients were able to obtain range of motion from 0 to 135 degrees postoperatively.[80] A second study by this group[79] explored the effect of extraarticular reconstruction using an iliotibial band tenodesis on the outcome of allograft BTB reconstructions for chronic ACL instability. They showed significant improvement for the combined procedure in overall knee scores, return to preinjury level of athletics, and on KT-1000 arthrometer testing. Their overall rate of failure was 11%, but the addition of the extraarticular reconstruction significantly decreased the failure rate from 16% to 3%.[79]

Gibbons and Bartolozzi[33] mentioned in their review article that 6- to 40-month follow-up in their 52 patients undergoing ACL reconstructions with fresh frozen, irradiated BTB allografts revealed only 4% of patients with AP displacement greater than 5 mm on 20-lb KT-1000 testing. Subjectively, satisfactory results were achieved in 90% of patients.[33]

Jackson et al.[50] reported on their results with over 200 allograft ACL and 50 allograft PCL reconstructions between 1985 and 1989. The authors stated a preference for utilizing BTB grafts for ACL reconstructions and Achilles tendon–bone grafts for PCL reconstructions. An earlier report on their initial allograft reconstructions with ethylene oxide–sterilized BTB allografts in 109 patients revealed numerous complications, including cyst formation in the bone tunnels and persistent synovial effusions in seven patients that resolved with removal of the grafts. For this reason, they recommended against using ethylene oxide–sterilized tissues for reconstructions.[49] They describe no intraarticular reactions or cyst formation with fresh frozen allografts. Their PCL reconstructions have reported improvement of posterior instability in 80% of patients, though many patients have close to 5 mm of side-to-side AP translation differences and 20-degree loss of flexion. In addition, another 5% had graft failure due to trauma.

The fresh frozen ACL allografts, on the other hand, are more predictable, with approximately 80% showing side-to-side differences of less than 3 mm on 20-lb testing with the KT-1000 arthrometer.[50]

A single other report documents the poor results and numerous complications seen with ethylene oxide–sterilized allograft ACL reconstructions. Roberts et al.[90] described eight failures in this group of 36 patients, all of whom showed complete dissolution of their graft on repeat arthroscopy and demonstrated large femoral cysts on radiographs. Only 17 patients were considered to be clinical successes based on their return to their desired activity levels, but even these patients had an average side-to-side difference of 5.9 mm on testing with the KT-1000 arthrometer at 30 lbs of force. The authors also recommended against the use of ethylene oxide–sterilized grafts for ligament reconstructions.[90]

Cox[24] recently presented his personal experience with over 400 freeze-dried fascia lata allograft ACL reconstructions performed since April 1981. He claimed better results than with autograft reconstructions and denied any graft failures, rejection, or cystic bone tunnel changes.[24] This, however, was strictly an anecdotal report and not a formal study of his results.

Several other small studies have appeared in the literature. Wainer et al.[112] reported on 23 patients undergoing freeze-dried allograft ACL reconstructions, and stated that all patients had improved knee ratings postoperatively. All of their patients followed for a minimum of 20 months had returned to their pre-injury activity levels.[112] Malek and Fields[64] reported their preliminary results on 27 consecutive arthroscopically assisted freeze-dried Achilles tendon allograft ACL reconstructions with 9- to 21-month follow-up. They reported minimal morbidity and complications without elucidating them, and claimed 75% satisfactory results.[64]

OTHER FRONTIERS

The most important area of research on allografts must be the arena of graft sterilization. The widespread use of allografts for knee reconstructions will not take place until surgeons and patients can be assured that the risk of disease transmission, particularly HIV disease, is negligible. For this to occur, a technique for sterilization must be found that routinely eradicates the free and intracellular virus without significantly altering the mechanical properties of the graft. This single advance will allow for a blossoming of clinical research that may lead to other improvements in allograft reconstruction techniques.

Improvement in techniques of implantation and better understanding of the immune response to soft tissue transplantation for ligamentous reconstruction of the knee will allow for advancement of biomedical engineering and tissue engineering. This, in turn, may allow us in the near future to direct specific cell lines for remodeling of implanted allografts that more closely resemble native ligamentous tissue.

Transplantation of viable tissue, be it autograft or allograft, always holds a theoretical advantage, so cryopreservation of allograft tissues to be used for ACL reconstructions will no doubt get a serious look during the upcoming decade. Bypassing the phases of necrosis, revascularization, and cellular replacement could theoretically mean stronger ACL grafts in the early postoperative period, theoretically allowing for safer early return to competitive sports.

A technique devised by Tibone and El Attrache at the Kerlan-Jobe Orthopaedic Clinic in Inglewood, Calif., for the BTB allograft reconstruction of the lateral ligamentous complex in combined instabilities has shown promise clinically.[107] Kan and colleagues are presently working to experimentally define a reproducible isometric point for this lateral reconstruction.[55]

SUMMARY

The key to providing safe allograft surgery is to secure a tissue bank for supplying grafts that maintains high-quality control standards and utilizes all of the means available for identifying and excluding potential HIV carriers and patients with other transmissible diseases from the donor pool. Surgeons using allografts for knee ligament reconstructions should obtain fresh frozen or freeze-dried grafts from these reliable banks and forego the use of secondarily sterilized grafts until researchers determine the dose of gamma irradiation that consistently eradicates HIV from the graft without dramatically altering its properties or until another safe and effective method of secondary sterilization is found. Grafts sterilized secondarily with ethylene oxide should not be used for reconstructions at this time.

Surgeons utilizing allografts for ligamentous reconstructions of the knee should have a sound understanding of the biology and biomechanics of allograft healing and choose allografts that are initially stronger than the native ACL, as weakening of the graft does occur with maturation. The technique used for ACL or PCL allograft reconstruction should take advantage of the benefits of allograft tissue over autografts, and indications for allograft use in reconstruction should be followed. Patients should receive informed consent prior to receiving allograft tissue for reconstruction, and the advantages and disadvantages of allograft vs. autograft should be discussed thoroughly with the patient.

There is a definite role for the use of allograft tissue in ligamentous reconstruction of the knee, and the indications for its use will undoubtedly increase over the next decade. However, despite the encouraging results presented here, autograft reconstructions should still be considered the gold standard for knee reconstructions, and anyone implanting allografts must consider the potential disadvantages, particularly the risk of disease transmission, when implanting these tissues in elective procedures.

REFERENCES

1. Andreefe I: A comparative experimental study on transplantation of autogenous and homogenous tendon tissue, *Acta Orthop Scand* 38:35–44, 1967.
2. Arnoczky SP, Warren RF, Ashlock MA: Replacement of the anterior cruciate ligament using a patellar tendon allograft. An experimental study, *J Bone Joint Surg [Am]* 68A:376–385, 1986.
3. Baker JL, et al: Unsuspected human immunodeficiency virus infection in critically ill emergency patients, *JAMA* 257:2609, 1987.
4. Barnd S, Cuband HE, Rodrigo JJ: The effect of storage at −80C as compared to −4C on the strength of rhesus monkey anterior cruciate ligament, *Trans Orthop Res Soc* 7:378, 1982.
5. Bonamo JJ, Krinick RM, Sporn AA: Rupture of the patellar ligament after use of its central third for anterior cruciate reconstruction. A report of two cases, *J Bone Joint Surg [Am]* 66A:1294–7, 1984.
6. Booth W: CDC paints a picture of HIV infection in the U.S., *Science* 239:253, 1988.
7. Bos GD, et al: The effect of histocompatibility matching on canine frozen bone allografts, *J Bone Joint Surg [Am]* 65A:89, 1983.
8. Bos GD, et al: Immune responses to frozen bone allografts, *J Bone Joint Surg [Am]* 65A:239, 1983.
9. Bottenfield S: HIV transmission incidence described by Lifenet's Bottenfield, *Am Assoc Tissue Banks Newslett* 14:1–2, 1991.
10. Bright RW, Green WT: Freeze-dried fascia lata allografts. A review of 47 cases, *J Pediatr Orthop* 1:13–22, 1981.
11. Bright RW, Smarsh JD, Gambill VM: Sterilization of human bone by irradiation. In Friedlander GE, Mankin HJ, Sell KW, editors: *Osteochondral allografts: Biology, banking, and clinical applications,* Boston, 1981, Little & Brown, pp 223–232.
12. Brown HR, Indelicato PA: Complications of anterior cruciate ligament reconstruction, *Operative Tech Orthop Surg* 2:125–135, 1992.
13. Buck BE, Malinin TI, Brown MD: Bone transplantation and human immunodeficiency virus: An estimate of risk of acquired immunodeficiency syndrome (AIDS), *Clin Orthop* 240:129–136, 1989.
14. Buck BE, et al: Human immunodeficiency virus cultured from bone, *Clin Orthop* 251:249–253, 1990.
15. Butler DL, et al: Biomechanics of cranial cruciate ligament reconstruction in the dog. II. Mechanical properties, *Vet Surg* 12:113–118, 1983.
16. Butler DL, et al: Biomechanics of human knee ligament allograft treatment, *Trans Orthop Res Soc* 12:128, 1987.
17. Butler DL, et al: Mechanical properties of primate vascularized versus nonvascularized patellar tendon grafts: Changes over time, *J Orthop Res* 7:68–79, 1989.
18. Clancy WG, et al: Anterior and posterior cruciate ligament reconstruction in rhesus monkeys: A histological, microangiographic, and biomechanical analysis, *J Bone Joint Surg [Am]* 63A:1270–1284, 1981.
19. *Clinical manual on HIV and AIDS,* Jacksonville, 1989, Florida Medical Association.
20. *Consumers development conference statement,* Bethesda, Md, 1988, National Institutes of Health.
21. Conway B, et al: Effects of gamma irradiation on HIV-1 in a bone allograft model, *Trans Orthop Res Soc* 15:225, 1990.
22. Cooper DE, Arnoczky SP, Warren RW: Contaminated patellar tendon grafts: Incidence of positive cultures and efficacy of an antibiotic solution soak—an in vitro study, *Arthroscopy* 7:272–274, 1991.
23. Cooper DE, et al: Strength of the central third patellar tendon graft: A biomechanical study. American Academy of Orthopaedic Surgeons Annual Meeting, Washington, DC, 1992.
24. Cox JS: Graft selection, isometry, and fixation of grafts, American Academy of Orthopaedic Surgeons Course, Arthroscopically-Assisted ACL Reconstructions, San Antonio, 1992.
25. Curtis RJ, DeLee JC, Drez DJ: Reconstruction of the anterior cruciate ligament with freeze-dried fascia lata allografts in dogs, *Am J Sports Med* 13:408–414, 1985.
26. Czitrom AA, et al: Bone and cartilage allotransplantation. A review of 14 years of research and clinical studies, *Clin Orthop* 208:141–145, 1986.
27. Esses S, et al: The effect of the immune response on the healing of bone allografts, *Orthop Trans* 5:246, 1981.
28. Fahey M, Indelicato PA: Bone tunnel enlargement in allograft anterior cruciate ligament reconstruction, American Orthopaedic Society for Sports Medicine Annual Meeting, San Diego, 1992.
29. Flandry F, et al: Viability and function of meniscal allografts harvested by cryopreservation in a canine model. American Orthopaedic Society for Sports Medicine Specialty Day Meeting, New Orleans, 1990.

30. Friedlander GE: Immune responses to osteochondral allografts. Current knowledge and future directions, *Clin Orthop* 174:58–68, 1983.
31. Friedlander GE, Tomford WW: Approaches to the retrieval and banking of osteochondral allografts. In *Bone and cartilage allografts,* Park Ridge, Ill, 1991, American Academy of Orthopaedic Surgeons, pp 185–192.
32. Fu FH, et al: The science of anterior cruciate ligament implants—1989, American Academy of Othopaedic Surgeons Annual Meeting, Las Vegas, 1989.
33. Gibbons MJ, Bartolozzi AR: Anterior cruciate ligament reconstruction using allografts: A review of the important issues. *Operative Tech Orthop* 2:76–85, 1992.
34. Gibbons MJ, et al: Effects of gamma irradiation on the initial mechanical and material properties of goat bone–patellar tendon–bone allografts, *J Orthop Res* 9:209–218, 1991.
35. Graf B, Uhr F: Complications of intra-articular anterior cruciate reconstruction, *Clin Sports Med* 7:835–848, 1988.
36. Graham WC, et al: The use of frozen stored tendons for grafting, *J Bone Joint Surg [Am]* 37:624, 1955.
37. Grood ES, Noyes FR: Cruciate ligament prosthesis: strength, creep, and fatigue properties, *J Bone Joint Surg [Am]* 58A:1083, 1976.
38. *Guidelines and standards for excision, preparation, storage and distribution of human tissue allografts for transplantation,* Richmond, Va, 1987, Southeastern Organ Procurement Foundation.
39. Halperin N, et al: Anterior cruciate ligament insufficiency syndrome, *Clin Orthop* 179:179–184, 1983.
40. Hammond JS, et al: HIV, trauma, and infection control: Universal precautions are universally ignored, *J Trauma* 30:555, 1990.
41. Harner CD, et al: The use of fresh frozen allograft tissue in knee ligament reconstruction: Indications, results, and controversies, American Academy of Orthopaedic Surgeons Annual Meeting, Washington, DC, January, 1992.
42. Haut RC, Powlison AC: Order of irradiation and lyophilization on the strength of patellar tendon allografts, *Trans Orthop Res Soc* 14:154, 1989.
43. Herron LD, Newman MH: The failure of ethylene oxide gas–sterilized freeze-dried bone graft for thoracic and lumbar spinal fusion, *Spine* 14:496–500, 1989.
44. Heyward WL, Curran JW: The epidemiology of AIDS in the United States, *Sci Am* 259:72, 1988.
45. *HIV/AIDS surveillance,* Atlanta, January 1992, Centers for Disease Control.
46. Huegel M, Indelicato PA: Trends in rehabilitation following anterior cruciate ligament reconstruction, *Clin Sports Med* 7:801–811, 1988.
47. Indelicato PA, Linton RC, Huegel M: The results of fresh-frozen patellar tendon allografts for chronic anterior cruciate ligament (ACL) deficiency of the knee, Submitted for publication.
48. Indelicato PA, et al: Clinical comparison of freeze-dried and fresh frozen patellar tendon allografts for anterior cruciate ligament reconstruction of the knee, *Am J Sports Med* 18:335–342, 1990.
49. Jackson DW, Windler GE, Simon TM: Intraarticular reaction associated with the use of freeze-dried ethylene oxide–sterilized bone–patella tendon–bone allografts in the reconstruction of the anterior cruciate ligament, *Am J Sports Med* 18:1–10, 1990.
50. Jackson DW, Rosen M, Simon TM: Soft tissue allograft reconstruction: The knee. In Czitrom AA, Gross AE, editors: *Allografts in orthopaedic practice,* Baltimore, 1992, Williams & Wilkins, pp 197–216.
51. Jackson DW, et al: Freeze dried anterior cruciate ligament allografts, *Am J Sports Med* 15:295, 1987.
52. Jackson DW, et al: Cruciate reconstruction using freeze dried anterior cruciate ligament allograft and a ligament augmentation device (LAD), *Am J Sports Med* 15:528, 1987.
53. Jackson DW, et al: The effects of in situ freezing on the anterior cruciate ligament. An experimental study in goats, *J Bone Joint Surg [Am]* 73A:201, 1991.
54. Johnson RJ, et al: Five to ten year follow-up evaluation after reconstruction of the anterior cruciate ligament, *Clin Orthop* 183:122–140, 1984.
55. Kan D: personal communication, January 1992.
56. Kelen GD, et al: Unrecognized human immunodeficiency virus infection in emergency department patients, *N Engl J Med* 318:1645, 1988.
57. Kelen GD, et al: Human immunodeficiency virus infection in emergency department patients, *JAMA* 262:516, 1989.
58. Kieffer DA, et al: Anterior cruciate ligament arthroplasty, *Am J Sports Med* 12:301–312, 1984.
59. Kirkpatrick JS, et al: Biomechanical, histological, and microvascular properties of cryopreserved ACL allografts 3 and 6 months post-transplantation. Orthopaedic Research Society Annual Meeting, New Orleans, 1990.
60. Lane JM, et al: The effect of storage and radiosterilization on the osteoinductive properties of demineralized bone matrix (DBM), *Orthop Trans* 8:227–228, 1984.
61. Lephart SM, et al: Effects of two selected anterior cruciate ligament reconstructions on the quadriceps mechanism functional status of athletes, Arthroscopy Association of North America Annual Meeting, Boston, 1992.
62. Levitt RL, Malinin T: Allograft reconstruction of the anterior cruciate ligament: A six-year experience with 300 allografts (abstract), *Arthroscopy* 7:318–319, 1991.
63. Levitt RL, Posada A, Malinin T: Allograft reconstruction of the anterior cruciate ligament: Six year experience with 181 cases, Submitted for publication, 1992.
64. Malek MM, Fields RH: Arthroscopic reconstruction of anterior cruciate deficient knee using achilles tendon allograft—preliminary results, *Am J Sports Med* 15:398–399, 1987.
65. Malinin TI, Buck BE: Allograft safety: Problems with HIV infections. *Instruct Course Lect* 128:1992.

66. McCaa C, et al: Transplantation of viable cryopreserved menisci. Society for Biomaterials Annual Meeting, Charleston, SC, 1990.
67. McCarroll JR: Fracture of the patella during a golf swing following a reconstruction of the anterior cruciate ligament. A case report, *Am J Sports Med* 11:26, 1983.
68. McCarthy JA, et al: Cryopreserved allogenic ACL reconstruction, biomechanics and histology. Orthopaedic Research Society Annual Meeting, Anaheim, Calif, 1991.
69. Meyers JF: Allograft reconstruction of the anterior cruciate ligament, *Clin Sports Med* 10:487–498, 1991.
70. Meyers JF, et al: Arthroscopic evaluation of anterior cruciate ligament reconstructions, *Arthroscopy* 2:155–161, 1986.
71. Meyers JF, et al: Arthroscopic evaluation of allograft anterior cruciate ligament reconstructions (abstract), *Arthroscopy* 6:148–149, 1990.
72. Meyers JF, et al: Arthroscopic evaluation of allograft anterior cruciate ligament reconstruction. Submitted for publication, 1992.
73. Milton JL, et al: Cryopreserved, anterior cruciate ligament transplantation. American Association of Tissue Banks Annual Meeting, Baltimore, 1989.
74. Minami A, et al: Effect of the immunological antigenicity of the allogeneic tendons on tendon grafting, *Hand* 14:111–119, 1982.
75. Morrison JB: Bioengineering analysis of force actions transmitted by the knee joint, *Biomed Eng* 3:164, 1968.
76. Morrison JB: The mechanics of the knee joint in relation to normal walking, *J Biomech* 3:51, 1971.
77. Munns SW, Jayaraman G, Luallin S: Effects of pretwist on biomechanical properties of canine patellar tendons. Arthroscopy Association of North America Annual Meeting, Boston, 1992.
78. Nikolaou PK, et al: Anterior cruciate ligament allograft transplantation. Long term function, histology, revascularization, and operative technique, *Am J Sports Med* 14:348–360, 1986.
79. Noyes FR, Barber SD: The effect of an extra-articular procedure on allograft reconstructions for chronic ruptures of the anterior cruciate ligament, *J Bone Joint Surg [Am]* 73:882–892, 1991.
80. Noyes FR, Barber SD, Mangine RE: Bone-patellar ligament-bone and fascia lata allografts for reconstruction of the anterior cruciate ligament, *J Bone Joint Surg [Am]* 72:1125–1136, 1990.
81. Noyes FR, et al: Biomechanical analysis of human ligament grafts used in knee ligament repairs and reconstructions, *J Bone Joint Surg [Am]* 66:344–352, 1984.
82. Olson EJ, et al: Anterior cruciate ligament reconstruction with sterilely harvested, fresh frozen allograft: Four year results, Arthroscopy Association of North America Annual Meeting, Boston, 1992.
83. Paulos LE, Rosenberg TD, Gurley WD: Prosthetic ligament reconstruction of the knee. In *Anterior cruciate ligament allografts,* Philadelphia, 1988, WB Saunders, pp 25–26.
84. Paulos LE, et al: Comparative material properties of allograft tissues for ligament replacement. Effect of type, age, sterilization, and preservation, *Trans Orthop Res Soc* 12:129, 1987.
85. Paulos LE, et al: Infrapatellar contraction syndrome, an unrecognized cause of knee stiffness with patella entrapment and patella infera, *Am J Sports Med* 15:331–341, 1987.
86. Pelker RP, Friedlander GE, Markham TC: Biomechanical properties of bone allografts, *Clin Orthop* 174:54–57, 1983.
87. Pinkowski JL, Reiman PR, Suio-Ling C: Human lymphocyte reaction to freeze-dried allograft and xenograft ligamentous tissue, *Am J Sports Med* 17:595, 1989.
88. Prolo DJ, Pedroytti PW, White DH: Ethylene oxide sterilization of bone–dura mater and fascia lata for human transportation, *Neurosurgery* 6:529–539, 1980.
89. Quarterly report to the Domestic Policy Council on the prevalence and rate of spread of HIV and AIDS—United States, *MMWR* 37:377, 1988.
90. Roberts TS, et al: Anterior cruciate ligament reconstruction using freeze-dried, ethylene oxide–sterilized, bone–patellar tendon–bone allografts. Two year results in thirty-six patients, *Am J Sports Med* 19:35–41, 1991.
91. Roth JH, et al: Intra-articular reconstruction of the anterior cruciate ligament with and without extra-articular supplementation by transfer of the biceps femoris tendon, *J Bone Joint Surg [Am]* 69:275–278, 1987.
92. Ryan JR, Droupp BW: Evaluation of tensile strength of reconstructions of the anterior cruciate ligament using the patellar tendon in dogs, *South Med J* 59:129–134, 1966.
93. Sachs RA, et al: Patellofemoral problems after anterior cruciate ligament reconstruction, *Am J Sports Med* 17:760–765, 1989.
94. St Louis ME, et al: Seroprevalence rates of human immunodeficiency virus infection at sentinel hospitals in the United States, *N Engl J Med* 323:213, 1990.
95. Seltzer DG, Campbell DR, Zych GA: Human immunodeficiency virus infection in orthopaedic emergency room patients at a level-one trauma center, American Academy of Orthopaedic Surgeons Annual Meeting, Anaheim, Calif, 1991.
96. Shino K, et al: Replacement of the anterior cruciate ligament by an allogeneic tendon graft. An experimental study in the dog, *J Bone Joint Surg [Br]* 66:B672–681, 1984.
97. Shino K, et al: Reconstruction of the anterior cruciate ligament by allogenic tendon graft: An operation for chronic ligamentous insufficiency, *J Bone Joint Surg [Br]* 68:739–746, 1986.
98. Shino K, et al: Arthroscopic follow-up of anterior cru-

ciate ligament reconstruction using allogeneic tendon, *Arthroscopy* 5:165–171, 1989.
99. Shino K, et al: Anterior cruciate ligament reconstruction using allogeneic tendon. A long term followup, *Am J Sports Med* 17:714, 1989.
100. Shino K, et al: Reconstruction of the anterior cruciate ligament using allogeneic tendon, *Am J Sports Med* 18:457–465, 1990.
101. Soderstrom CA, et al: HIV infection rates in a trauma center treating predominantly rural blunt trauma victims, *J Trauma* 29:1526, 1989.
102. Spire B, et al: Inactivation of lymphadenopathy associated virus by heat, gamma rays, and ultraviolet light, *Lancet* 1:188–189, 1985.
103. *Standards for tissue banking,* McLean, Va, 1989, American Association of Tissue Banks.
104. Strong DM, Sayers MH, Conrad EU: Screening tissue donors for infectious markers. In *Bone and cartilage allografts,* Park Ridge, Ill, 1991, American Academy of Orthopaedic Surgeons, pp 193–209.
105. Task Force on AIDS and Orthopaedic Surgery: *Recommendations for the prevention of human immunodeficiency virus transmission in orthopaedic surgery practice,* Park Ridge, Ill, 1989, American Academy of Orthopaedic Surgeons.
106. *Technical manual for surgical bone banking,* McLean, Va, 1987, American Association of Tissue Banks.
107. Tibone JE: Personal communication.
108. Transmission of HIV through bone transplantation, *MMWR* 37:597–599, 1988.
109. Triantafyllou N, Sotiropoulos E, Triantafyllou J: The mechanical properties of the lyophilized and irradiated bone grafts, *Acta Orthop Belg* 41:35–44, 1975.
110. Uribe JW: Personal communication.
111. Vasseur PB, et al: Replacement of the anterior cruciate ligament with a bone-ligament-bone anterior cruciate ligament allograft in dogs, *Clin Orthop* 219:268, 1987.
112. Wainer RA, Clarke TJ, Poehling GG: Arthroscopic reconstruction of the anterior cruciate ligament using allograft tendon, *Arthroscopy* 4:199, 205, 1988.
113. Wang JB, Hewson GF: Anterior cruciate ligament reconstruction using the lateral one third of the patella tendon, *Tech Orthop* 2:23–27, 1988.
114. Webster DA, Werner FW: Freeze-dried flexor tendons in anterior cruciate ligament reconstruction, *Clin Orthop* 181:238–243, 1983.
115. Webster DA, Werner FW: Mechanical and functional properties of implanted freeze-dried flexor tendons, *Clin Orthop* 180:301, 1983.
116. Withrow SJ, et al: Evaluation of the antiviral effect of various methods of sterilizing/preserving corticocancellous bone, *Trans Orthop Res Soc* 15:226, 1990.

49

Posterior Cruciate Reconstruction With Bone–Patellar Tendon–Bone Autografts

JAMES R. ANDREWS, M.D.
STEPHEN R. SOFFER, M.D.

Evolution of patellar tendon autograft
Indications for posterior cruciate ligament reconstruction
Surgical technique
    Examination under anesthesia
    Graft harvest
    Graft preparation

Tunnel placement
Passage and fixation
Postoperative rehabilitation
Clinical experience
Appendix

EVOLUTION OF PATELLAR TENDON AUTOGRAFT

The first reported reconstruction of the posterior cruciate ligament (PCL) was by Hey Groves in 1917 using the semitendinosus tendon through femoral and tibial drill holes.[23] He later modified the procedure, using the gracilis and semitendinosus tendons.[24] A similar type of procedure was described by Gallie and LeMesurier in 1927,[21] by Lindemann in 1950,[35] and by Kennedy and Grainger in 1967.[32] In 1980 Trickey described a technique using semitendinosus and gracilis tendons as free grafts passed through drill holes in the femur and tibia; however, no results were reported.[54] The following year, the use of proximally detached gracilis and semitendinosus tendons for PCL reconstruction was reported by Lipscomb in 15 patients with 87% good results (13/15).[37] However, the postoperative data regarding posterior laxity were absent, and 12 of these 15 patients had concomitant anterior cruciate ligament (ACL) reconstructions which influenced the data. More recently, Wirth and Jager[60] in 1984 reconstructed 12 PCLs using distally detached gracilis and semitendinosus tendons through femoral and tibial drill holes. They considered this a "dynamic" replacement of the PCL, given that the hamstring tendons were left proximally attached to their muscular origins. All patients returned to some athletic activity; however, all had a posterior drawer sign. In summary, in evaluating all of these reports on semitendinosus and gracilis reconstructions, one realizes that there is either a lack of postoperative data or disappointing postoperative objective results.

The use of other hamstring tendons for PCL reconstruction is quite limited. Southmayd and Rubin[50] reported a case using a proximally detached semimembranosus tendon through a femoral drill hole. The patient returned to athletics; however, he continued to have positive (1+) posterior drawer test results.

Prior to the 1980s, various other structures about the knee were implemented for PCL replacement. In 1939, Cubbins et al.[15] used a slip of iliotibial band with limited success. Barfod in 1971[2] and McCormick et al.[40] in 1976 used a proximally detached popliteus placed through a femoral drill hole. This resulted in subjectively stable knees. However, postoperative objective determination of laxity was lacking. In 1969, Lindstrom[36] reported two cases using the lateral meniscus as a PCL substitute. In the next decade Collins et al.[13] Tillberg,[52] and Hughston et al.[28] also used either the lateral or medial meniscus. No objective results were reported by Collins et al. or Tillberg in their respective series. In the study of Hughston et al., primary repair was performed in 11 patients and primary repair and meniscal augmentation in 9 patients. The authors found that 13 of 20 patients had a negative posterior drawer sign, and 16 had good functional results. However, the results specifically of the 9 patients with meniscal augmentation were not described. Also, most of these patients had concomitant ACL or other ligamentous disruptions that were repaired, thus influencing the results.

Since the early 1980s, several series describing primary repair for PCL injuries have been published.[4, 28, 38, 41, 45, 51, 57] Moore and Larsen[41] found 83% residual instability in 20 patients. Bianchi[4] reported only 48% good objective results in 27 cases (13/27). Pournaras and Symeonides[45] described posterior instability in all 20 patients after primary PCL repair. They concluded that direct suture repair of the PCL will not restore PCL function. This conclusion is well supported by the aforementioned literature and is now widely accepted.

Multiple series concerning the use of the proximally detached medial head of the gastrocnemius as a dynamic transfer for PCL reconstruction were also reported in the 1980s. Hughston[26] first described this technique in 1969, then reported the results in 29 patients in 1982.[27] However, 40% of patients had a 2+ posterior drawer after surgery. Results of the procedure by Clendenin et al.,[12] Kennedy and Galpin,[31] and Insall and Hood[29] corroborated these less than satisfactory results. Finally, in 1988, Roth et al.[47] reported poor results in 31 patients after medial gastrocnemius transfer and concluded that this procedure was not recommended for primary PCL reconstruction.

Use of the patellar tendon then became popular in the late 1980s and early 1990s. Augustine[1] described a technique of PCL reconstruction using a distally detached portion of the patellar tendon placed through a tibial bone tunnel intraarticularly. Clancy et al.,[9] in an elegant basic science study, first reported the use of a free bone–patellar tendon–bone autograft for ACL and PCL reconstruction in Rhesus monkeys in 1981. Encouraged by successful basic science results, bone–patellar tendon–bone autografts were utilized in humans for ACL reconstruction with excellent results.[10] In 1983, the first series of bone–patellar tendon–bone autografts for PCL reconstruction in humans was reported by Clancy et al.[11] Twenty-one of 23 patients in this study had good to excellent objective results after PCL reconstruction with bone–patellar tendon–bone free graft. With these impressive results, the patellar tendon graft became widely used for PCL reconstruction.

Other types of grafts have since been reported without much success. Eriksson et al.[19] in 1986 used a proximally detached, long flap of quadriceps and patellar tendon through femoral and tibial drill holes. Their results were poor, probably owing to failure of the quadriceps tendon flap at the junction of the quadriceps tendon and the patella. Prosthetic ligaments have been employed in PCL reconstructive surgery[3, 34, 56, 61]; however, results were also less than optimal. (Prosthetic cruciate ligament reconstruction is thoroughly discussed in Chapter 47.) Thus, the bone–patellar tendon–bone autograph has continued to be a likely graft source for PCL reconstruction through the 1980s and into the early 1990s.

INDICATIONS FOR POSTERIOR CRUCIATE LIGAMENT RECONSTRUCTION

The indications for PCL reconstruction are quite controversial.[3, 5, 14, 16, 20, 44, 53, 55] This is in part due to the lack of knowledge as to the true natural history of the PCL-deficient knee. Proponents of a nonoperative approach claim that functional instability tends not to be a symptom in these patients and that many may lead active lives with minimal untoward consequences. An inability for many surgeons to consistently reproduce satisfactory results in PCL reconstruction also sways many toward a conservative treatment plan in these patients. Interestingly, some well-respected sports medicine specialists have become such strong advocates of conservative treatment of PCL-injured knees that they emphatically deny the importance of the PCL. Many patients without functioning PCLs complain of pain and sometimes instability. Degenerative arthritis of the patella and medial femoral condyle has been reported as a late sequela of PCL tears.[6, 11, 14, 44] This tends to sway one toward an operative approach in these patients, especially if one believes that stabilizing the knee may prevent or least retard the arthritic process.

We believe the PCL is important to knee biomechanics and that the PCL-injured knee is *not* a normal knee. It seems obvious that a ligament that is in the center of the knee joint, 13 mm wide, and biomechanically stronger than the ACL must be an important structure. The question is not whether the PCL is important, but rather whether we are able to make the PCL-deficient knee significantly better through surgery. The other important question is upon which patients with PCL insufficiency should we operate.

To answer the first question, in our hands we are able to improve the PCL-deficient knee by at least one grade with surgery. (Our results are discussed in detail at the end of this chapter.) To determine the patients best served by surgery, we classify PCL-injured patients by tibial translation posteriorly on the femur at 90 degrees of knee flexion[7] (Figs 49–1 and 49–2). This flexion angle is chosen because posterior translation is maximum at 70 to 90 degrees of flexion in

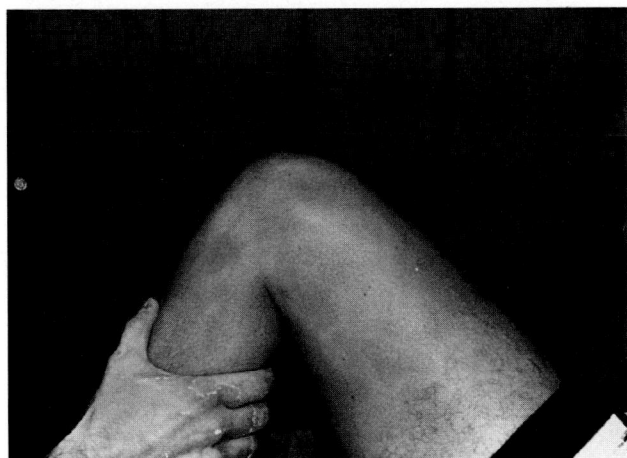

FIG 49–1.
Normal tibial step-off. Tibial plateau is anterior to femoral condyles.

TABLE 49–1.
Posterior Cruciate Ligament (PCL) Deficiency Grading System*

Grade		Examination (at 90 Degrees of Knee Flexion With Tibia in Neutral Rotation)
I	Partial PCL disruption	Palpable but diminished tibial step-off (tibial plateau anterior to femoral condyles)
II	Complete PCL disruption (or significant interstitial PCL stretch)	No palpable tibial step-off (tibial plateau flush with femoral condyles)
III	Combined injury: complete PCL disruption + other major ligament injury	No palpable step-off and tibial plateau posterior to femoral condyles

*Classification based on data from Clancy WG-Personal Communication, 1992.

the PCL-deficient knee.[53] Also, the posterior capsule is lax at 90 degrees, and posterior translation better reflects the status of the PCL than at 30 degrees where the capsule is tauter. The grading system that we use is described in Table 49–1.

In general, we tend to take a conservative approach with grade I injuries and an operative approach with grade III injuries. The disability from grade I injuries is not extensive, and the results from conservative treatment are excellent in our experience. Also, we are unable to improve these patients significantly with surgical intervention. Thus, we take a nonoperative approach in this situation.

Management of grade III injuries, however, is quite different. These are combined ligamentous injuries. The PCL is insufficient along with another important ligamentous structure.[49] These patients usually become functionally unstable after injury and ultimately require surgical intervention. Furthermore, surgical reconstruction will improve a grade III to a grade II or even a grade I translation. Thus, this type of patient will benefit from operative stabilization.

In terms of grade II injuries, this is a "gray zone," and we tend to individualize treatment for these patients. We consider age, activity, associated injury, symptoms, objective laxity, and injury acuteness. For example, a concomitant significant medial meniscus injury will sway us toward a more aggressive approach because this patient is at high risk for developing medial compartment arthritis. Also, an acute or subacute (less than 6 weeks) PCL tear will incline us toward surgical treatment. These patients tend to have more predictable results after surgery than more chronic PCL-injured patients. In older, less active patients with mild laxity, we recommend a conservative approach. A physical therapy protocol emphasizing rehabilitation of the quadriceps, the dynamic stabilizer of the PCL-deficient knee, is utilized. The patient may be followed with serial bone scans which indicate early patellofemoral or medial compartment degenerative changes.

We presently use an arthroscopically assisted bone–patellar tendon–bone autograft technique for our PCL reconstruction. This has produced the most reliable and predictable results in our hands. The technique is described below.

SURGICAL TECHNIQUE

Examination Under Anesthesia

After the patient is placed under general anesthesia, a complete knee examination is performed to deter-

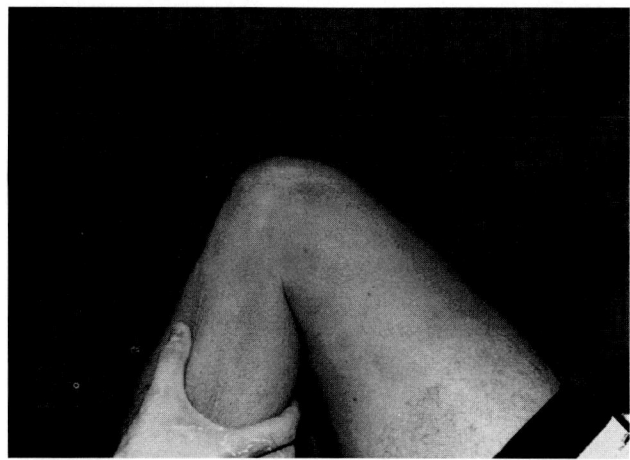

FIG 49–2.
Loss of tibial step-off. Tibial plateau is flush with femoral condyles.

mine other ligamentous injuries. One must check the medial and lateral tibial step-off at 90 degrees of flexion, and the posterior drawer at 90 degrees with the tibia at neutral. One must also evaluate for concomitant ACL injury with a Lachman and pivot shift test. Posterolateral instability, frequently associated with PCL injury, must be determined. Associated instabilities are often best addressed at the time of PCL reconstruction.

Graft Harvest

A sandbag is taped onto the operating room table so that when the knee is flexed approximately 70 degrees, the foot sits on the sandbag to support it. The patient is prepared and draped in the usual sterile fashion. The tourniquet is elevated to 300 mm Hg. The knee is flexed to approximately 70 degrees. A midline incision is made from the tip of the patella to a point 3 cm distal to the tibial tubercle (Fig 49–3, A and B). Dissection through the subcutaneous tissue to the patellar tendon sheath is performed sharply. The plane between the subcutaneous fat and the sheath is developed medially and laterally. The patellar tendon sheath is incised in the midline and separated from the tendon sharply. The sheath is preserved so that it may be repaired at the conclusion of the operation.

The width of the patellar tendon is measured. If we use an autogenous graft alone, we take a 12-mm graft at this point. If we use a patellar tendon graft in conjunction with a ligament augmentation device (LAD) (such as the Kennedy LAD), we take a 10-mm graft at this point.

Using a double-barreled scalpel of the appropriate width (DePuy, Warsaw, Ind.), the middle one third of the patella, patellar tendon, and tibial tubercle is incised longitudinally. A hemostat is placed at the junction of the incised tendon and the tip of the patella. The hemostat indicates the distal end of the patellar bone plug. A distance of 2 cm is measured proximal to this point and marked transversely on the patella with a scalpel. Thus, a 2-cm-long patellar bone plug is outlined. Similarly, on the tibial side of the patellar tendon, a point 3 cm distal to the tibial tendon insertion is marked transversely with a scalpel on the tibia. Thus, a 3-cm-long bone plug is outlined on the tibial side. A powered saw is used to cut the bone plugs along the outlined scalpel markings. The saw is tilted 10 degrees from perpendicu-

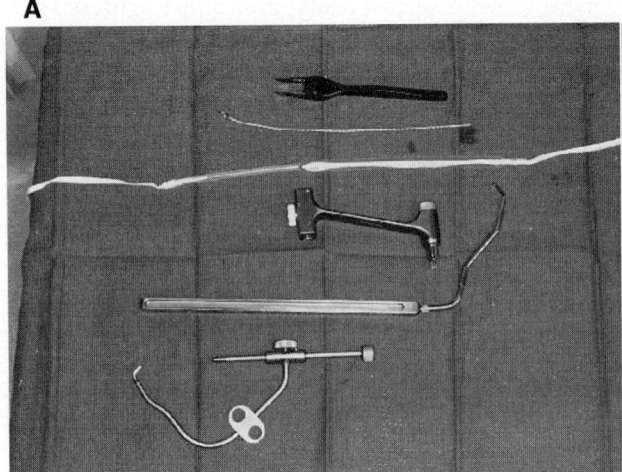
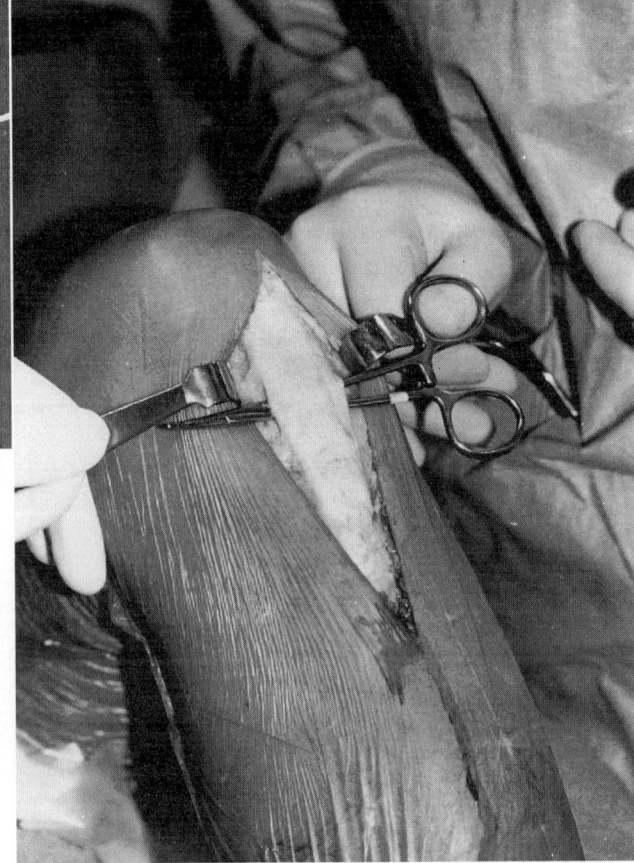

FIG 49–3.
A, equipment for posterior cruciate ligament (PCL) reconstruction. *Top to bottom:* double-barreled scalpel for graft harvest, wire loop, DePuy graft passer, drilling outrigger, tibial drill guide, femoral drill guide with drill sleeve. **B,** skin incision for PCL reconstruction. Hemostat is under patellar tendon.

lar when making the longitudinal cuts so that trapezoidal bone plugs are formed. A 0.25-in. curved osteotome is used to complete the bone cuts and remove the bone plugs. The bone–patellar tendon–bone graft is carefully passed to the back table where it is prepared. Cancellous bone is removed from the tibial bone plug donor site (proximal tibial metaphysis) using a specifically designed dowel (Instrument Makar, Okemos, Mich.) or a curette. The bone is placed in the patellar bone plug donor site. The patellar tendon and sheath are closed with absorbable sutures.

Graft Preparation

The 12-mm-wide bone plugs are trimmed with a rongeur so that they smoothly pass through a sleeve of 12-mm caliber. The length of each bone plug is measured. The bone plugs should measure 2 and 3 cm long and are trimmed appropriately.

Using a small drill bit, three holes are drilled through each bone plug (Fig 49–4). A no. 5 braided, nonabsorbable suture is placed through each hole. The graft with sutures attached should slip easily through a 12-mm-caliber sleeve. A methylene blue pen is used to mark the tendon-bone interface of both ends of the graft (Fig 49–5). After this is performed, a hemostat is placed over the sutures at each end of the bone plugs. A moist sponge is placed over the graft, and the graft is placed in a tray safely on the back table.

Tunnel Placement

A thorough diagnostic arthroscopy is now performed with a 30-degree angled arthroscope. Beneath the midline incision, anteromedial and anterolateral portals are established in the standard fashion. Articular lesions and meniscal injuries are recorded and treated appropriately.

The PCL is evaluated. One may note that at times the PCL may appear macroscopically intact while the preoperative examination indicates complete disruption. This is due to microscopic collagen fibril failure prior to macroscopic tearing.[33] Probing of the PCL often reveals a lax ligament in this situation.

The PCL remnant is excised. The PCL femoral insertion and femoral condyle are debrided with a shaver or cutting cautery (Fig 49–6). One must be careful not to injure the intact ACL.

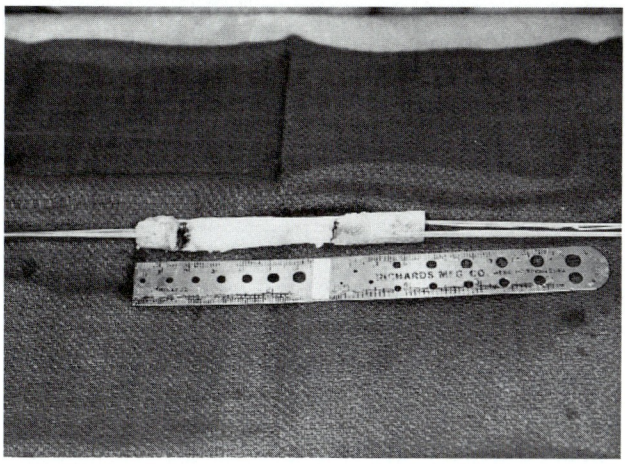

FIG 49–5.
Prepared bone–patellar tendon–bone graft. Tibial bone plug is on *right*; patellar bone plug is on *left*.

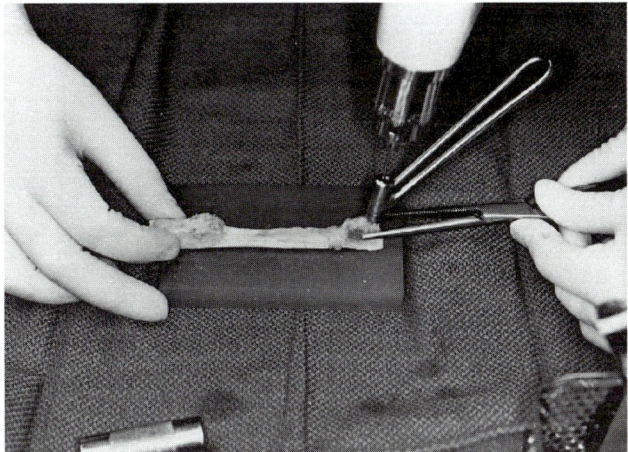

FIG 49–4.
Bone–patellar tendon–bone autograft. Three drill holes are made into each bone plug.

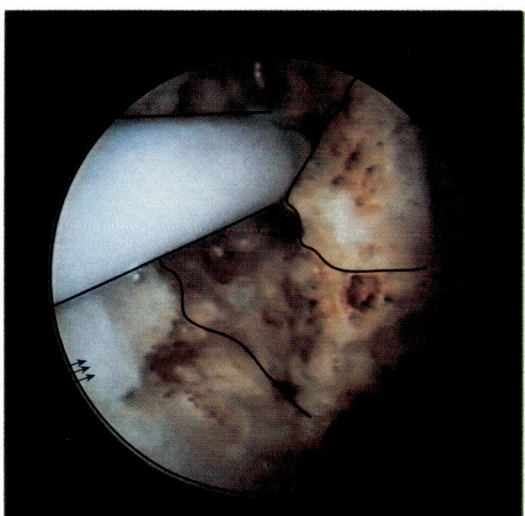

FIG 49–6.
Debridement of posterior cruciate ligament (PCL) (arthroscopic view). *Single arrow,* cautery; *double arrow,* PCL remnant; *triple arrow,* medial femoral condyle.

At this point, we prefer to drill the tibial tunnel prior to the femoral tunnel. The tibial tunnel is the more difficult of the two tunnels to establish. Distention and visualization of the posterior aspect of the joint is critical. However, once the first tunnel is drilled, water may extravasate from the hole. Distention is lost, and visualization is impaired. Thus, drilling the tibial tunnel first affords the best visualization for the more difficult of the two tunnels to establish.

The arthroscope is placed into the posteromedial corner of the knee with the knee in 70 to 90 degrees of flexion. A posteromedial portal is established in the following fashion. The posteromedial joint line is palpated while visualizing this area arthroscopically. A spinal needle is placed in this area (Fig 49-7,B). The location of the spinal needle is evaluated to be certain that it is proximal and posterior enough so that when a shaver is placed through this portal, it can easily reach the posterolateral side of the tibia. A common error is to place the portal too distal or too anterior so that one is unable to reach the PCL tibial insertion. After ideal placement of the spinal needle, the skin is cut with a no. 11 scalpel and a blunt trocar and sheath are placed posteromedially (Fig 49-8,B). A shaver is exchanged for the trocar, and debridement of the remains of the PCL tibial insertion is begun from the central tibia (Fig 49-9,B). The soft tissue should be removed about 2 cm distal to the lateral tibial plateau. This is where the PCL fibers attach to the posterior central sulcus or fovea of the tibia (Fig 49-9,C). Also removed is the soft tissue slightly posterolateral to the central sulcus.

The Acufex tibial drill guide is placed through the anteromedial portal onto the appropriate point on the posterior tibial cortex (Fig 49-10,A and B). This point is approximately 2 cm distal to the lateral plateau and about 0.5 cm lateral to central on the tibia. In other words, this area is where the most inferior and lateral fibers of the PCL insert (the inferolateral aspect of the posterior central sulcus). After the tibial guide tip is placed at this point, the drilling outrigger is passed onto the guide and secured with the set knob. The calibration on the tibial guide is noted. This represents the distance between the drilling outrigger lying on the anterior tibial cortex and the tip of the tibial drill guide lying on the posterior cortex. The guide pin is marked with methylene blue at this specific distance from its point (e.g., if the calibration on the tibial guide measures 100 mm, one marks the pin with methylene blue 100 mm from its tip). The pin is placed through the drilling outrigger and onto the anterior tibia so that it passes through the tibial bone plug donor site. (We choose this point anteriorly because it is easier to drill through this defect than through the thick, anterior tibial cortex elsewhere. Also, if the guide pin is placed through the anterior tibial cortex, as one drills through the hard bone the drill may deviate and shear off or break the pin.) The pin is drilled approximately to the methylene blue mark. The pin will penetrate the posterior tibial cortex at this point. This should be visualized through

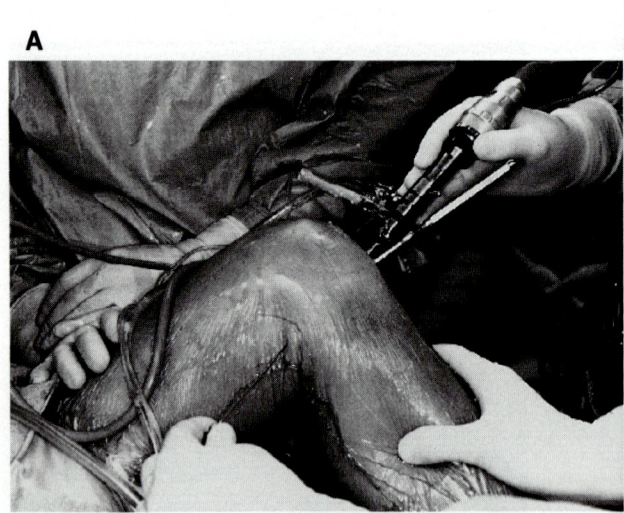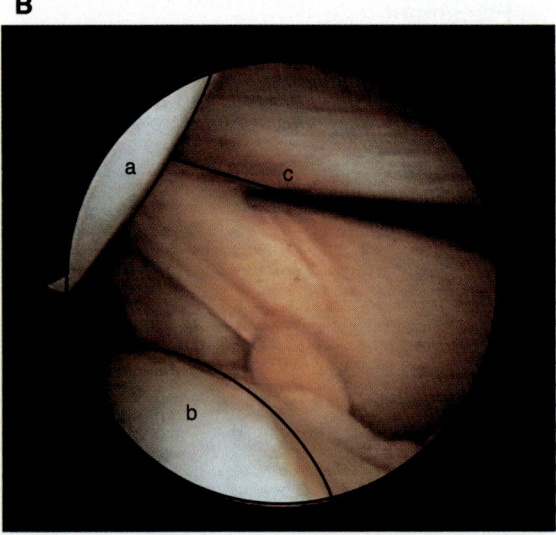

FIG 49-7.
A, spinal needle is placed at the posteromedial joint line to establish the posteromedial portal. **B,** intraarticular location of spinal needle (arthroscopic view): *(a)* medial condyle of femur, posterior aspect; *(b)* tibial plateau, posterior aspect; *(c)* spinal needle through posterior capsule.

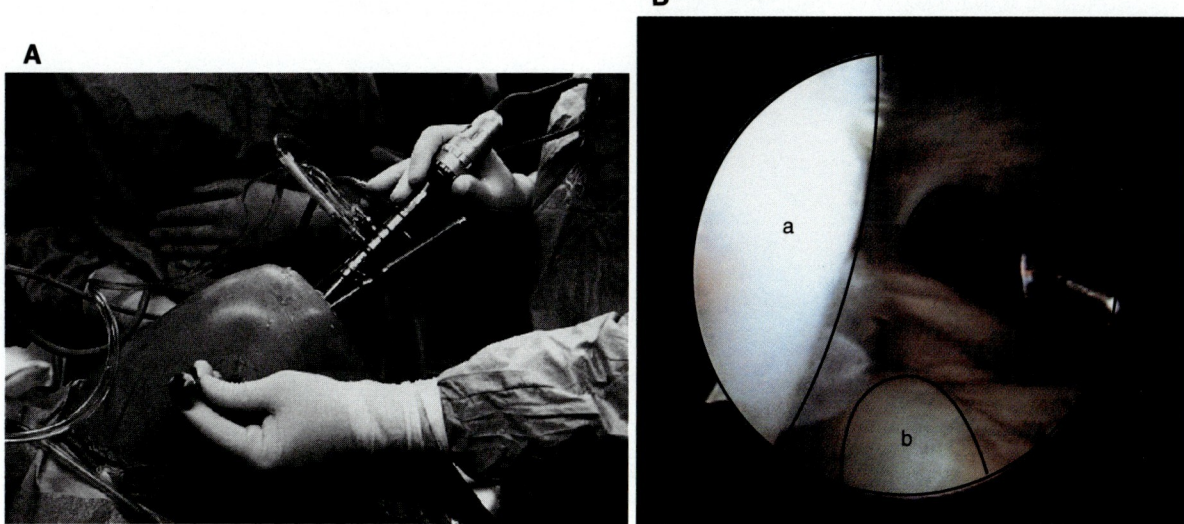

FIG 49–8.
A, a blunt trocar in the posteromedial portal. **B,** arthroscopic view: *(a)* medial condyle of femur, posterior aspect; *(b)* tibial plateau, posterior aspect; *(c)* trocar through posteromedial portal.

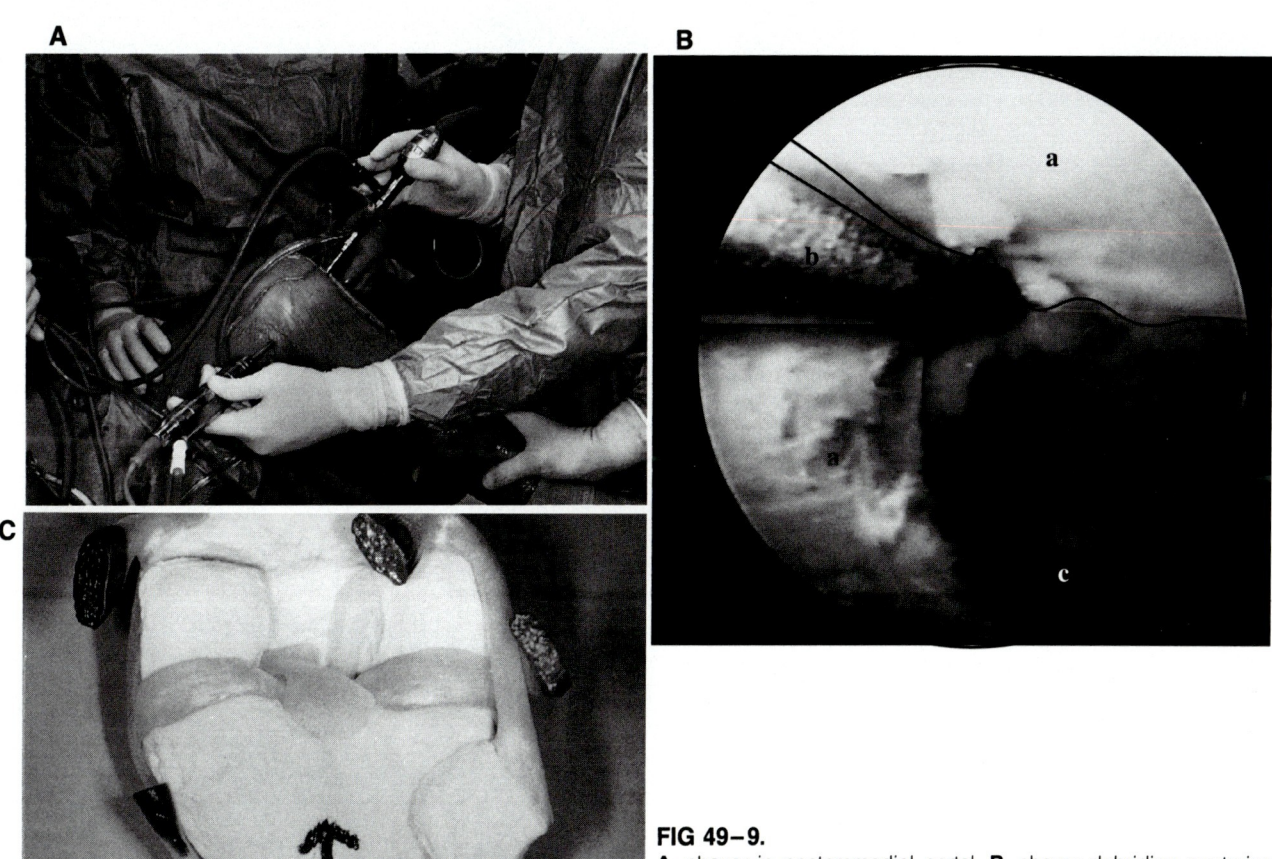

FIG 49–9.
A, shaver in posteromedial portal. **B,** shaver debriding posterior cruciate ligament tibial stump (arthroscopic view): *(a)* posterior capsule; *(b)* shaver; *(c)* posterior cortex of tibia. **C,** posterior central sulcus of tibia.

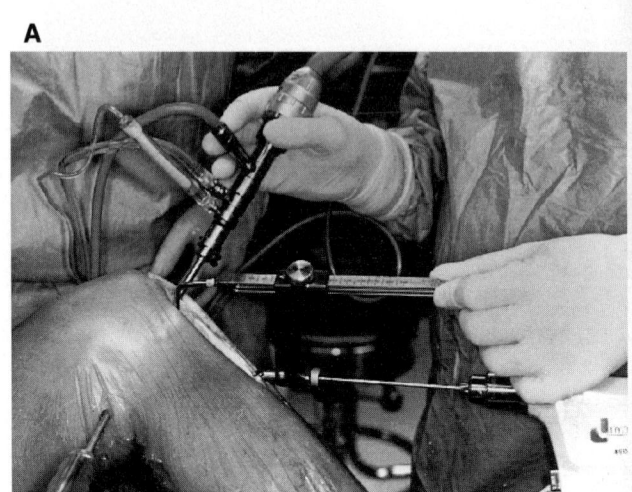

FIG 49–10.
A, tibial drill guide in anteromedial portal. Pin is about to be drilled through guide. **B,** tibial drill guide on posterior tibial cortex (arthroscopic view): *(a)* posterior capsule; *(b)* posterior tibial cortex; *(c)* tibial drill guide.

the arthroscope. Thus, marking the pin prevents one from drilling through the posterior cortex and into the popliteal fossa.

One may better visualize pin penetration of the posterior tibial cortex utilizing the following technique. The 70-degree–angled arthroscope may be placed through the anterolateral portal, through the intercondylar notch, and into the posterior aspect of the knee. To aid visualization of the posterior central sulcus, the shaver is placed through the posteromedial portal and retracts the posterior capsule posteriorly. This maneuver allows excellent visualization of the pin penetrating the posterior tibial cortex. Alternatively, the 70-degree–angled arthroscope may be placed through the posteromedial portal to visualize pin penetration.

The tibial guide system is removed. Pin placement is checked with the arthroscope in the anterolateral portal and then in the posteromedial portal to confirm proper placement. If the pin placement is correct, the pin is overreamed with a cannulated 6-mm reamer, and then with a 12-mm reamer (Fig 49–11). The shaver tip is placed through the posteromedial portal and over the end of the pin to prevent further advancement of the pin posteriorly while reaming. This prevents injury to the popliteal fossa neurovascular structures. We use the 6-mm reamer prior to the 12-mm reamer because the tibial bone is often very thick and difficult to ream initially with a 12-mm reamer. The other advantage of reaming first with the 6-mm reamer is that it allows one to make minor adjustments of the tibial exit posteriorly with the 12-mm reamer. After the 12-mm tunnel is made, the superior edge of the tunnel is rasped (so that the graft will not lie on a sharp edge). A rubber plug is placed in the tibial tunnel anteriorly.

The femoral tunnel is then established A vertical 3-cm incision centering over the adductor tubercle and parallel to the anterior midline incision (in line

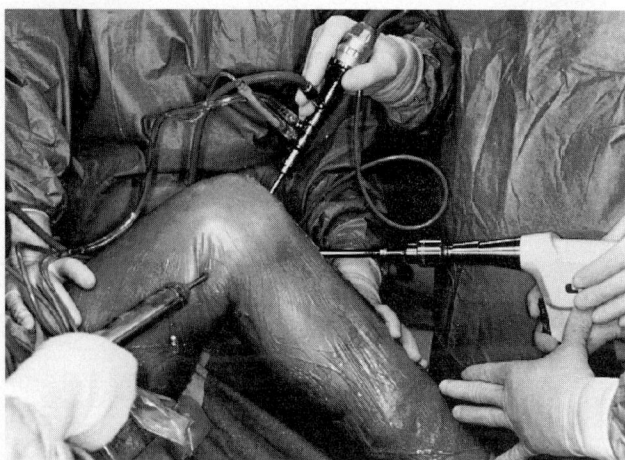

FIG 49–11.
A 6-mm cannulated reamer is being drilled over the pin. The shaver end is placed over the pin to protect the popliteal fossa.

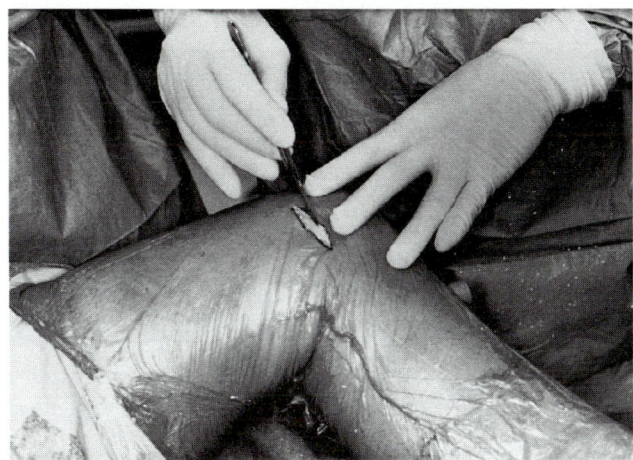

FIG 49–12.
Medial incision for femoral tunnel.

with the tibia) is made (Fig 49–12). The vastus medialis is dissected from the medial intermuscular septum for a distance of 2 to 3 cm. This is the point at which the femoral tunnel will exit. The Acufex PCL femoral guide is placed through the anteromedial portal and onto the appropriate point on the medial femoral condyle (PCL femoral insertion) (Fig 49–13,B). The ideal position for the femoral guide pin in our experience is at the roof of the intercondylar notch, approximately 9 to 12 mm from the articular edge of the medial femoral condyle. This is at the 11-o'clock position in the left knee. One places the pin through the drill sleeve of the femoral guide and through the medial incision (Fig 49–14,B). The vastus medialis is retracted so that the guide pin is flush on bone. Guide placement is checked; one must be posterior enough on the condyle so as not to break out anteriorly through the medial femoral condyle. (One should err inferiorly on pin placement so as to reduce the angle the graft will take as it exits the femur and enters the tibial tunnel.) The guide pin is then drilled. The guide system is removed, and the pin position is evaluated. If the pin placement is correct, a cannulated 6-mm reamer and then a 12-mm reamer are placed over the femoral pin. A rasp is used on the inferior and posterior edges of the tunnel to remove the rough edge where the graft is likely to lie. Sometimes the bone is very hard, and a burr is needed to smooth over these edges.

Femoral tunnel placement for PCL reconstruction is still controversial. Ogata and McCarthy[43] recently reported the isometric area of the PCL to be 10 mm proximal (i.e., "posterior" in the flexed femur) to the edge of the articular cartilage at the 10-o'clock position (for the left knee). We agree and thus place the femoral tunnel 9 to 12 mm from the articular edge of the medial femoral condyle. Clancy and colleagues[8, 11] agree with this location for the isometric area; however, they believe the femoral tunnel should be placed eccentrically so that the inferoposterior circumference of the tunnel coincides with the anatomic center of the PCL. In other words, they place the guide pin 5 mm posteriorly from the anterior edge of the articular surface of the medial femoral condyle at the 10:30-o'clock position (left knee).[8] The patellar tendon graft will then exit the femoral tunnel and tend to lie posteroinferiorly and thus approximate the isometric area of the PCL.[11, 22]

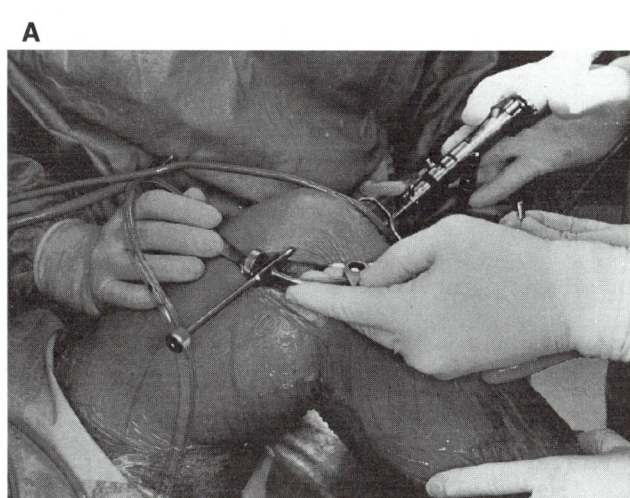

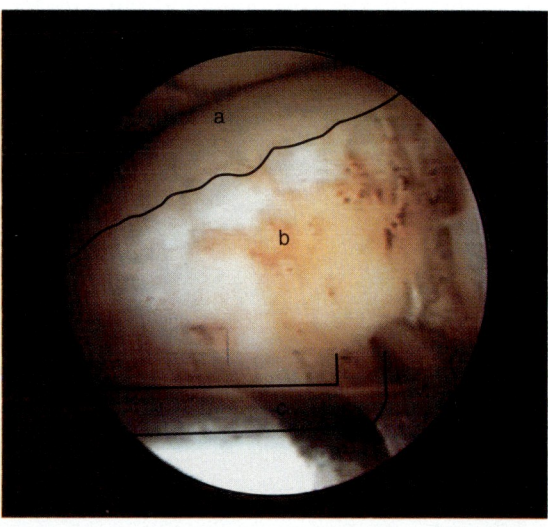

FIG 49–13.
A, femoral drill guide being placed into the anteromedial portal. **B,** position on medial femoral condyle for femoral tunnel placement (arthroscopic view): *(a)* medial femoral condyle; *(b)* posterior cruciate ligament insertion, debrided; *(c)* femoral drill guide.

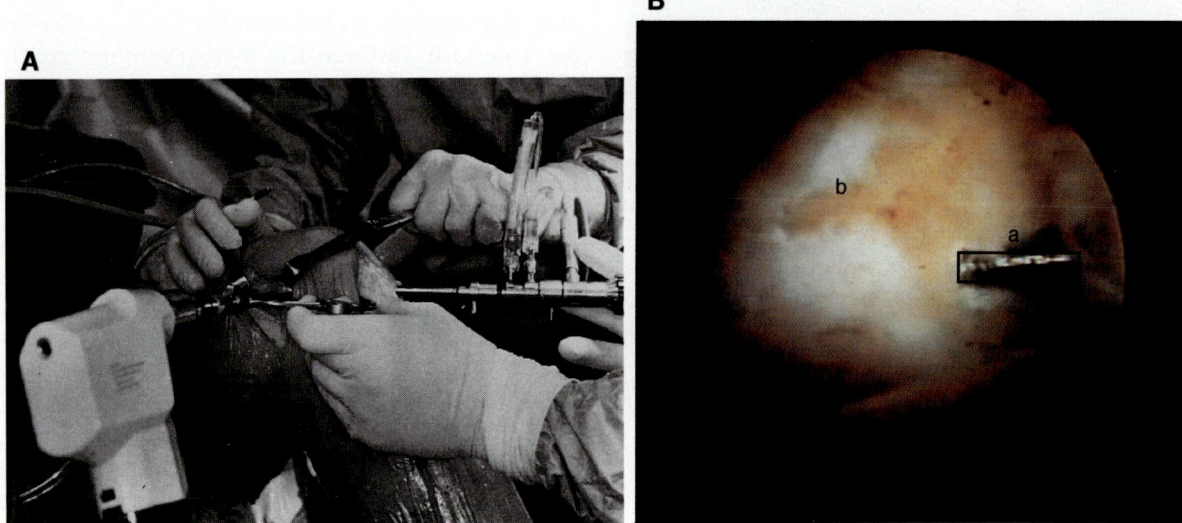

FIG 49-14.
A, pin being placed through the femoral guide. **B,** intraarticular view of pin in medial femoral condyle (arthroscopic view): *(a)* pin; *(b)* medial femoral condyle.

Graft Passage and Fixation

The DePuy graft passer is cut to an appropriate length so that it accepts the patellar bone plug. The shorter bone plug and its sutures are fed through the graft passer (Fig 49-15). An 18-gauge wire twisted into a loop at its end is passed through the tibial tunnel from anterior to posterior. A 70-degree-angled arthroscope is placed through the anterolateral portal, and a grasper is placed through the anteromedial portal to the posterior aspect of the knee. The loop is grasped and pulled anteriorly into the intercondylar notch. Another grasper is then placed through the femoral tunnel into the knee joint and the wire loop is pulled out through the femoral tunnel to the outside of the knee. The sutures attached to the patellar bone plug are placed through the wire loop (Fig 49-16). (We pass the shorter bone plug, the 2-cm patellar bone plug, through the femur initially for two reasons. Firstly, because it is shorter than the 3-cm tibial bone plug, it will pass through the intercondylar notch back to the posterior aspect of the knee easier. Secondly, it will pass into the tibial tunnel posteriorly much easier than the 3-cm bone plug for the same reason.) The wire is pulled from the tibial tunnel anteriorly, and the sutures are passed through the knee joint and out through the tibial tunnel. The 30-degree-angled arthroscope visualizes this process to be certain the sutures do not tangle in soft tissues or become caught at the tunnel edges. Then the sutures

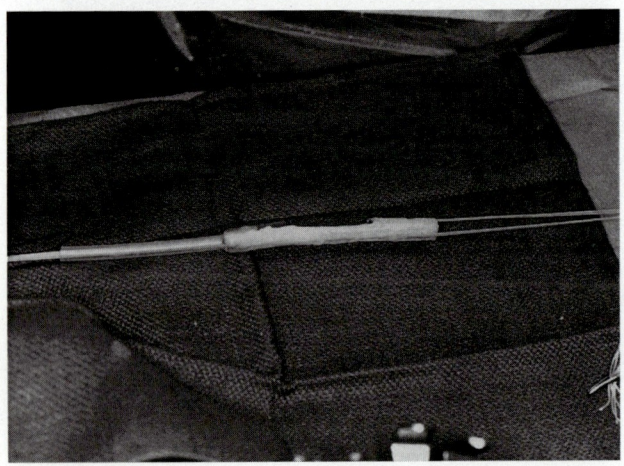

FIG 49-15.
Bone-patellar tendon-bone graft within graft passer.

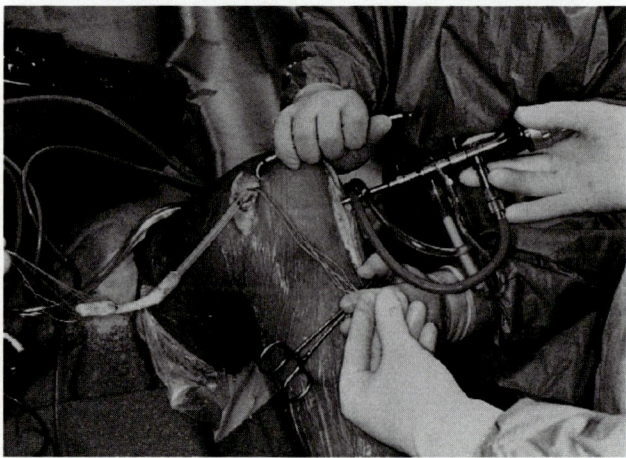

FIG 49-16.
Sutures attached to patellar bone plug passed through wire loop.

emerging from the tibial tunnel are grasped and pulled anteriorly. The bone plugs are rotated so that the tendon lies anteriorly in the femoral tunnel. In this way the tendon will not contact and be injured by the posterior edge of the tunnel because it is protected by the cancellous portion of the bone plug. The rest of the graft is pulled through the knee joint. Again, the patellar bone plug is visualized with the arthroscope as it enters the tibial tunnel posteriorly, making certain it does not get entangled or caught on the edge of the tibial tunnel. The DePuy graft passer is seen emerging from the tibial tunnel anteriorly (Fig 49–17,A). It is removed from the graft with a Kocher clamp.

At this point, the femoral bone plug may be secured. The location of the methylene blue mark on the femoral bone plug is checked. This mark should be at the edge of the femoral tunnel exit into the knee joint. The femoral bone plug is secured using a 9-mm cannulated interference screw (see Fig 49–17,B). Alternatively, the femoral bone plug sutures may be tied over a post, i.e., a 6.5-mm cancellous bone screw

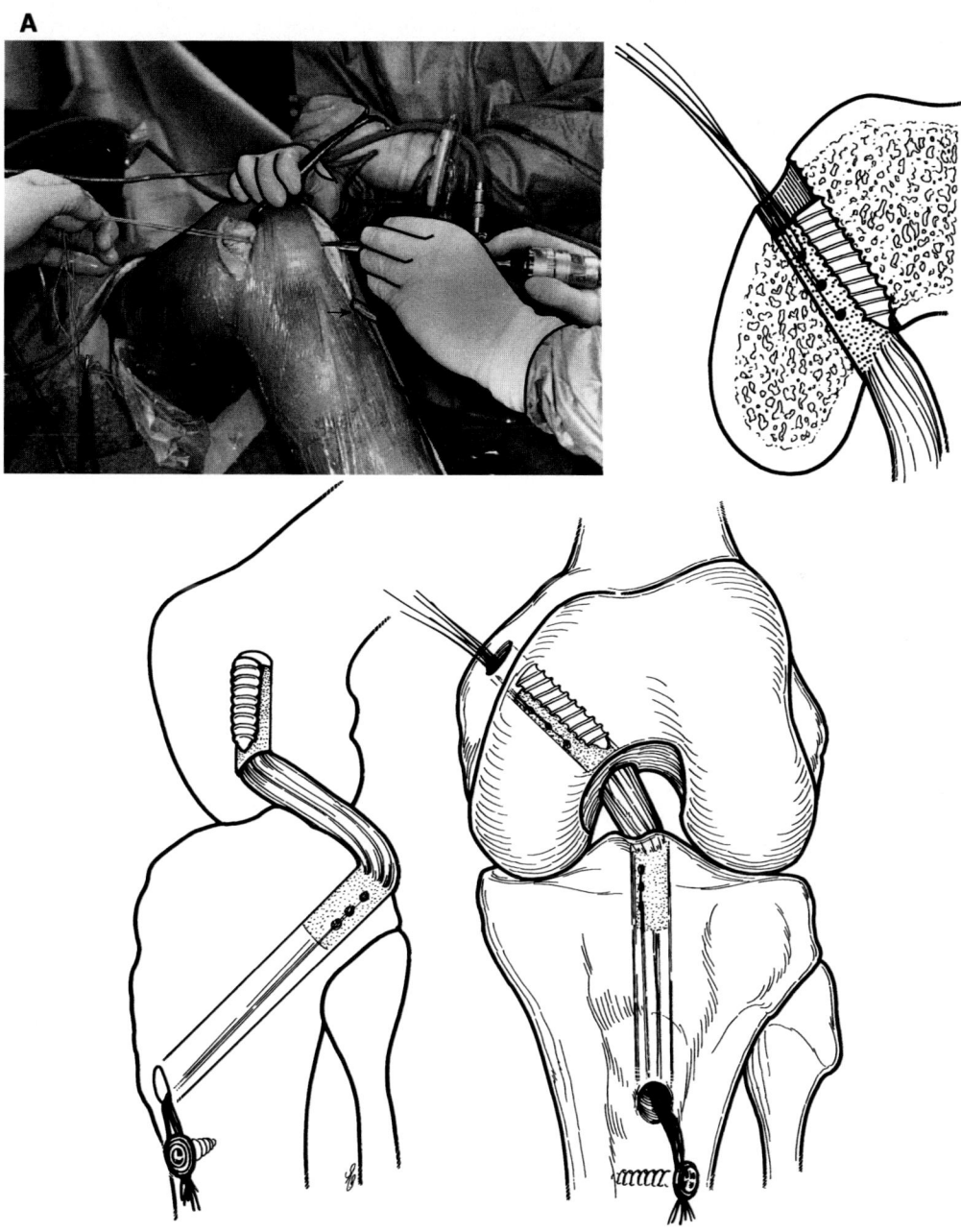

FIG 49–17.
A, graft passer *(arrow)* emerging from tibial tunnel. B_1–B_3, illustrations of bone plugs within bone tunnels after graft fixation.

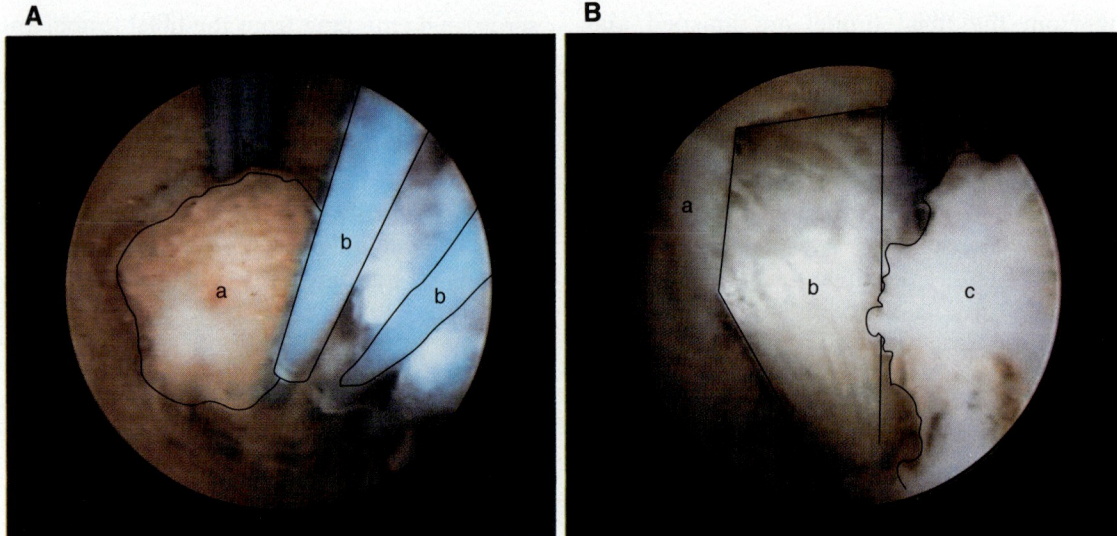

FIG 49-18.
A, arthroscopic view of bone plug within tibial tunnel: *(a)* bone plug; *(b)* sutures. **B,** arthroscopic view of medial femoral condyle showing patellar tendon graft in place: *(a)* medial femoral condyle; *(b)* graft; *(c)* anterior cruciate ligament.

and washer placed proximal to the femoral bone tunnel.

The arthroscope is then placed into the tibial tunnel from anterior to posterior in order to visualize the bone plug (Fig 49–18, A and B) and ensure that the bone plug lies within the tunnel. If the bone plug is not in the tunnel, then it is caught on the outer edge of the tunnel posteriorly. When the bone plug is confirmed to lie within the tunnel, the sutures may be secured to a post in the tibia. A 3.2-mm bicortical drill hole is made 1 cm distal to the tibial bone plug donor site from lateral to medial. The hole is depth-gauged. A screw is selected 3 to 4 mm longer than this length. With the knee flexed to 90 degrees, the sutures are tied over this screw and washer while an anterior drawer is placed on the tibia. After the first few knots are tied and the screw secured, the knee is extended to be certain the knee can achieve full extension with the graft in place. The arthroscope is placed back into the flexed knee and the patellar tendon graft is probed and evaluated for laxity (Fig 49–18, B). The ACL should also be taut if the knee is properly reduced. At this point, the remaining knots of the tibial sutures may be tied. A drain is placed intraarticularly and in the anterior wound. Standard closure is performed. Appropriate dressings are applied over the wounds. The knee is placed in a hinged, postoperative brace locked at 0 degrees of extension while the patient is still under anesthesia.

Postoperative Rehabilitation

The rehabilitation process following reconstructive surgery of the PCL plays a significant role in the patient's ultimate functional outcome. Improving the dynamic stabilizing power of the quadriceps femoris muscle is critical.

Our program consists of a five-phase progression to full, unrestricted activities between 6 to 8 months following surgery. The detailed program can be found in Appendix 49–1. The ultimate goal of the rehabilitation program is a gradual return to functional activities while maintaining joint stability and preventing further joint surface degeneration. During the rehabilitation process the clinician must continuously reevaluate the patient to monitor the rehabilitation program so that the patient does not overdo his or her program.

Immediately post surgery, the patient is placed in a knee brace locked at 0 degrees of extension. This brace is worn for ambulation only, and range of motion is encouraged from 0 to 60 degrees. Continuous passive motion (CPM) is begun on postoperative day 1 from 0 to 70 degrees. The CPM is used 30 to 45 minutes, five to six times per day. The CPM device is used to nourish the articular cartilage, neuromodulate joint pain, and to improve patient compliance with the rehabilitation program.[42, 48] In addition, active knee extensions and full passive terminal knee extension exercises are employed. Immediate weight-bearing as tolerated is allowed with two crutches. Usually patients discontinue crutch use by 2 weeks; however, the 0-degree locked brace is used for ambulation for 6 weeks.

Early quadriceps strengthening exercises are initiated the day after surgery to prevent quadriceps atrophy and provide dynamic stability to the knee. Quadriceps sets, straight leg flexion raises, multiangle isometric knee extensions (60, 40, and 20 degrees), and active resisted knee extension (60 degrees to 0 degrees) are employed. The use of electrical muscle stimulation assists in the reeducation and hypertrophy of the quadriceps muscle during active exercise.[18] Patellar mobilization is performed four to five times per day to improve patellar mobility which will prevent patella infera and facilitate passive knee extension. Superior patellar mobility is critical in obtaining full passive knee extension and in preventing loss of motion.[57-59]

Quadriceps muscle strengthening plays a significant role in the rehabilitation process following PCL surgery and has been emphasized in many PCL rehabilitation programs.[6, 14, 16, 39, 58, 59] Active knee extensions from 60 to 0 degrees will create an anterior shear force at the tibiofemoral joint, and thus are safe for the healing PCL. Conversely, active knee extension from a knee flexion angle of greater than 75 degrees produces a posteriorly directed shear force which may overstress the healing PCL graft.[17, 25, 30, 46] Therefore, the safe range in which to perform active resisted knee extension exercises or isometrics is from 60 to 0 degrees.

Resisted hamstring curls are not permitted until 6 to 8 weeks post surgery. During resisted knee flexion from 70 degrees and greater, the tibia is pulled posteriorly and creates a shear force on the PCL graft. In addition, during closed-chain exercises, such as minisquats, leg press, step-ups, and Stairmaster exercises, the knee flexor muscle group contracts to control the hip flexion angle. This knee flexor muscle contraction provides a posterior drawer to the tibia on the femur. Thus, closed-chain exercises should be delayed until the physician thinks adequate stability has been obtained. Often in our program, these closed-chain exercises are delayed until 4 to 6 weeks or until significant quadriceps muscle control or force has been reestablished. Thus, with the PCL-reconstructed knee we emphasize open-chain exercises immediately, then progress to closed-chain exercises. This represents a contrast to our ACL program in which closed-chain exercises are begun on postoperative day 1.[57]

During the first 2 months, bimonthly assessments of knee stability are performed using a computerized knee arthrometer (KT-2000, Medmetric, San Diego) to document objectively anteroposterior tibia translation. These tests are performed at 70 to 20 degrees of knee flexion. Testing posterior tibial translation at 20 degrees may reflect posterior capsule tightness and not necessarily PCL stability; thus testing at 70 to 90 degrees of knee flexion may prove to be a more accurate assessment of PCL stability.

Running is usually initiated at 4 to 5 months after surgery, and noncontact sports are allowed at 6 months. For a return to high-demand sports, (e.g., football, skiing, soccer), functional return occurs in 6 to 8 months. The PCL-reconstructed patient is encouraged to continue a strengthening program for 1 to 2 years after surgery. This program is usually performed three to four times per week and includes an aggressive quadriceps-strengthening program and vigorous endurance routine. The emphasis of this maintenance program is closed-chain exercise while carefully monitoring patellofemoral and medial tibiofemoral degenerative changes.

CLINICAL EXPERIENCE

In our extensive review of the literature, we found only one article on the results of bone-patellar tendon-bone autografts for PCL reconstruction. This well-documented article by Clancy et al. describes results in 23 patients with a minimum 2-year-follow-up after an open bone-patellar tendon-bone autograft procedure.[11] Twenty-one of 23 patients had good or excellent results based on functional as well as static or objective criteria. All 10 patients with acute PCL tears had good to excellent results and returned to their preinjury level of athletic activity without symptoms of instability, pain, or effusions. Of the 13 patients with chronic PCL insufficiency, 11 had good to excellent results with 6 returning to sports activities with minimal symptoms. One must consider that probably several of these patients with chronic PCL-deficient knees had not been participating actively in sports for many months after their initial injuries. Thus, return of these 6 patients and of all 10 of the acutely injured patients are truly remarkable results.

In the 1983 series of Clancy et al.,[11] good to excellent results were achieved in over 90% of patients. The results of our experience with bone-patellar tendon-bone PCL reconstruction have not been as outstanding. We have found functional and subjective improvement in the majority of our patients. They have no complaints of instability, pain, or loss of motion. Objectively, we are able to improve static stability by one grade. In other words, a patient with grade II tibial translation and a nonpalpable tibial step-off will be improved to a grade I tibial translation with a palpable though diminished tibial step-off. Better results are obtained in acute rather than chronic PCL-injured patients. Results are also more reliable if there is no concomitant posterolateral laxity. Many of our athletic patients are able to return to competitive sports. To our knowledge we have not worsened the condition of the knee in any of our patients, though this is certainly a possible outcome of this type of surgery.

In conclusion, orthopaedists have progressed significantly since Hey Groves's initial description of PCL reconstruction. Much has been learned concerning the anatomy and biomechanics of the PCL. Natural history studies of patients with PCL-deficient knees are beginning to emerge in the literature. Operative procedures with arthroscopic assistance and aggressive rehabilitative methods have been developed that yield better results than earlier studies. In time, we believe that as the techniques for PCL reconstruction continue to improve and we become more able to consistently normalize the PCL-deficient knee, a more aggressive surgical approach will be utilized. With basic science and clinical research efforts, there will be better understanding of the PCL-deficient knee, optimizing the treatment program for these patients.

REFERENCES

1. Augustine RW: The unstable knee, Am J Surg 92:380, 1956.
2. Barfod B: Posterior cruciate ligament reconstruction by transposition of the popliteal tendon (abstract), Acta Orthop Scand 42:438, 1971.
3. Barrett GR, Savoie FH: Operative management of acute PCL injuries with associated pathology: Long-term results, Orthopedics 14:687, 1991.
4. Bianchi M: Acute tears of the posterior cruciate ligament: Clinical study and results of operative treatment in 27 cases, Am J Sports Med 11:308, 1983.
5. Cain TE, Schwab GH: Performance of an athlete with straight posterior knee instability, Am J Sports Med 9:203, 1981.
6. Clancy WG: Repair and reconstruction of the posterior cruciate ligament. In Chapman MW, editor: Operative orthopaedics, vol 3, Philadelphia, 1988, JB Lippincott, pp 1651–1666.
7. Clancy WG: Personal communication, February 1992.
8. Clancy WG, Smith L: Arthroscopic anterior and posterior cruciate ligament reconstruction technique, Ann Chir Gynaecol 80:141, 1991.
9. Clancy WG, et al: Anterior and posterior cruciate ligament reconstruction in Rhesus monkeys. A histological microangiographic and biochemical analysis, J Bone Joint Surg [Am] 63:1270, 1981.
10. Clancy WG, et al: Anterior cruciate ligament reconstruction using one third of the patellar ligament augmented by extra-articular tendon transfers, J Bone Joint Surg [Am] 64:352, 1982.
11. Clancy WG, et al: Treatment of knee joint instability secondary to rupture of the posterior cruciate ligament. Report of a new procedure, J Bone Joint Surg [Am] 65:310, 1983.
12. Clendenin MB, DeLee JC, Heckman JD: Interstitial tears of the posterior cruciate ligament of the knee, Orthopedics 3:764, 1980.
13. Collins RH, et al: The meniscus as a cruciate ligament substitute, Am J Sports Med 2:11, 1974.
14. Cross MJ, Powell JF: Long-term follow-up of a posterior cruciate ligament rupture: A study of 116 cases, Am J Sports Med 12:292, 1984.
15. Cubbins WR, Callahan JJ, Scuderi CS: Cruciate ligaments. A resume of operative attacks and results obtained, Am J Surg 43:481, 1939.
16. Dandy DJ, Pusey RJ: The long-term results of unrepaired tears of the posterior cruciate ligament, J Bone Joint Surg [Br] 64:92, 1982.
17. Daniel DM, et al: Use of quadriceps active test to diagnose posterior cruciate ligament disruptions and measure posterior laxity of the knee, J Bone Joint Surg [Am] 70:386–390, 1988.
18. Eriksson E, Haggmark T: Comparison of isometric muscle training and electrical stimulation supplementing isometric muscle training in the recovery after major knee ligament surgery, Am J Sports Med 7:169–171, 1979.
19. Eriksson E, Haggmark T, Johnson RJ: Reconstruction of the posterior cruciate ligament, Orthopedics 9:217, 1986.
20. Fowler PJ, Messieh SS: Isolated posterior cruciate ligament injuries in athletes, Am J Sports Med 15:553, 1987.
21. Gallie WE, LeMesurier AB: The repair of injuries to the posterior cruciate ligament of the knee joint, Ann Surg 85:592, 1927.
22. Grood ES, Hefzy MS, Lindenfield TN: Factors affecting the region of most isometric femoral attachments. Part 1: The posterior cruciate ligament. Am J Sports Med 17:197, 1989.
23. Hey Groves EW: Operation for the repair of the crucial ligaments, Lancet 2:674, 1917.
24. Hey Groves EW: The crucial ligaments of the knee-joint. Their function, rupture, and the operative treatment of the same, Br J Surg 7:505, 1919.
25. Hirokawa S, et al: Anterior-posterior and rotational displacement of the tibia elicited by quadriceps contraction, Am J Sports Med 20:299–306, 1992.
26. Hughston JC: The posterior cruciate ligament in knee joint stability, J Bone Joint Surg [Am] 51:1045, 1969.
27. Hughston JC, Degenhardt TC: Reconstruction of the posterior cruciate ligament, Clin Orthop 164:59, 1982.
28. Hughston JC, et al: Acute tears of the posterior cruciate ligament. Results of operative treatment, J Bone Joint Surg [Am] 62:438, 1980.
29. Insall JN, Hood RW: Bone-block transfer of the medial head of the gastrocnemius for posterior cruciate insufficiency, J Bone Joint Surg [Am] 64:691, 1982.
30. Jurist KA, Otis JC: Anteroposterior tibiofemoral displacements during isometric extension efforts, Am J Sports Med 13:254–258, 1985.
31. Kennedy JC, Galpin RD: The use of the medial head of the gastrocnemius muscle in the posterior cruciate-deficient knee, Am J Sports Med 10:63, 1982.
32. Kennedy JC, Grainger RW: The posterior cruciate ligament, J Trauma 7:367, 1967.

33. Kennedy JC, et al: Tension studies of human knee ligaments. Yield point, ultimate failure, and disruption of the cruciate and tibial collateral ligaments, *J Bone Joint Surg [Am]* 58:350, 1976.
34. Kennedy JC, et al: Posterior cruciate ligaments, *Orthop Digest* 7:19, 1979.
35. Lindemann K: Über den plastischen Ersatz der Kreuzbänder durch gestielte Sehnenverpflanzungen, *Z Orthop* 79:316, 1950.
36. Lindstrom N: Cruciate ligament plastics with meniscus, *Acta Orthop Scand* 29:150, 1959.
37. Lipscomb AB, Johnston RK, Snyder RB: The technique of cruciate ligament reconstruction, *Am J Sports Med* 9:27, 1981.
38. Loos WC, et al: Acute posterior cruciate ligament injuries, *Am J Sports Med* 9:86, 1981.
39. Mangine RE, Eifert-Mangine MA: Postoperative posterior cruciate ligament reconstruction rehabilitation. In Engle RP, editor: *Knee ligament rehabilitation*, New York, 1991, Churchill Livingstone, pp 165–176.
40. McCormick WC, et al: Reconstruction of the posterior cruciate ligament. Preliminary report of a new procedure, *Clin Orthop* 118:30, 1976.
41. Moore HA, Larsen RL: Posterior cruciate ligament injuries. Results of early surgical repair, *Am J Sports Med* 8:68, 1980.
42. Noyes FR, Mangine RE, Barber S: Early knee motion after open and arthroscopic ACL reconstruction. *Am J Sports Med* 15:149–160, 1981.
43. Ogata K, McCarthy JA: Measurements of length and tension patterns during reconstruction of the posterior cruciate ligament, *Am J Sports Med* 20:351, 1992.
44. Parolie JM, Bergfeld JA: Long-term results of nonoperative treatment of isolated posterior cruciate ligament injuries in the athlete, *Am J Sports Med* 14:35, 1986.
45. Pournaras J, Symeonides PP: The results of surgical repair of acute tears of the posterior cruciate ligament, *Clin Orthop* 267:103, 1991.
46. Renstrom P, Arms SW, Stanwyck TS: Strain within the anterior cruciate ligament during hamstring and quadriceps activity, *Am J Sports Med* 14:83–87, 1986.
47. Roth JH, et al: Posterior cruciate ligament reconstruction by transfer of the medial gastrocnemius tendon, *Am J Sports Med* 16:21, 1988.
48. Salter RB, Simmonds DF, Malcolm BW: The biological effects of continuous passive motion on the healing of full thickness defects of articular cartilage. *J Bone Joint Surg [Am]* 62:1231–1251, 1980.
49. Seebacker JR, et al: The structure of the posterolateral aspect of the knee, *J Bone Joint Surg [Am]* 64:536, 1982.
50. Southmayd WW, Rubin BD: Reconstruction of the posterior cruciate ligament using the semimembranosus tendon, *Clin Orthop* 150:196, 1980.
51. Strand T, et al: Primary repair in posterior cruciate ligament injuries, *Acta Orthop Scand* 55:545, 1984.
52. Tillberg B: The late repair of torn cruciate ligaments using menisci, *J Bone Joint Surg [Br]* 59:15, 1977.
53. Torg JS, et al: Natural history of the posterior cruciate ligament-deficient knee, *Clin Orthop* 246:208, 1989.
54. Trickey EL: Injuries to the posterior cruciate ligament. Diagnosis and treatment of early injuries and reconstruction of late instability, *Clin Orthop* 147:76, 1980.
55. Warren RF: The posterior cruciate ligament, American Academy of Orthopaedic Surgeons 58th Annual Meeting, Anaheim, Calif, March 12, 1991.
56. Weiss AB, et al: Ligament replacement with an absorbable copolymer carbon fiber scaffold—early clinical experience, *Clin Orthop* 196:77, 1985.
57. Wilk KE, Andrews JR: Current concepts in the treatment of anterior cruciate ligament disruptions. *J Orthop Sports Phys Ther* 15:279–293, 1992.
58. Wilk KE, Clancy WG, Andrews JR: *The posterior cruciate ligament,* La Crosse, Wisc, 1992, Orthopaedic Section of American Physical Therapy Association.
59. Wilk KE, Price S: *The posterior cruciate ligament, injury and treatment,* Shirley, NY, 1988, Biodex Clinical Advantage Series.
60. Wirth CJ, Jager M: Dynamic double tendon replacement of the posterior cruciate ligament, *Am J Sports Med* 12:39, 1984.
61. Woods DW, et al: Proplast leader for use in cruciate ligament reconstruction, *Am J Sports Med* 7:79, 1979.

APPENDIX

Posterior Cruciate Ligament (PCL)–Patellar Tendon Graft Reconstruction Rehabilitation Protocol

KEVIN WILK, P.T.

I. **Immediate Postoperative Phase**
   A. **Postoperative day 1:**
      1. *Brace:* locked in 0 degrees of extension.
      2. *Weightbearing:* Two crutches as tolerated (less than 50%).
      3. *Exercises:*
         a. Ankle pumps.
         b. Quadriceps sets.
         c. Straight leg raises.
      4. *Muscle stimulation:* Muscle stimulation to quadriceps (4 hr/a day) during quadriceps sets.
      5. *Continuous passive motion (CPM):* 0–60 degrees.
      6. *Ice and elevation:* Continue with ice and elevation 20 minutes out of every hour and elevate with knee in extension.
   B. **Postoperative day 2–5:**
      1. *Brace:* brace locked at 0 degrees.
      2. *Weightbearing:* Two crutches as tolerated (50%).
      3. *Range of motion (ROM):* Intermittent ROM out of brace 4–5 times daily (0–60 degrees).
      4. *Exercises:*
         a. Multiangle isometrics at 60, 40, 20 degrees (Quadriceps only).
         b. Intermittent ROM (4–5 times daily).
         c. Patellar mobilization.
         d. Ankle pumps.
         e. Straight leg raises.
         f. Hip abduction, adduction.
         g. Continue quadriceps sets.
         h. Toe raises with knee in extension.
      5. *Muscle stimulation:* Electrical muscle stimulation to quadriceps (6 hr/day) during quadriceps sets, multiangle isometrics, and straight leg raises.
      6. *CPM:* 0–60 degrees.
      7. *Ice and elevation:* Continue with ice and elevation 20 minutes of every hour and elevate with knee in extension.

II. **Maximum protection phase (week 2–6):**
   Goals:
   - Absolute control of external forces to protect graft.
   - Nourish articular cartilage.
   - Decrease swelling.
   - Decrease fibrosis.
   - Prevent quadriceps atrophy.
   A. **Week 2:**
      1. *Brace:* locked at 0 degrees. Continue to perform intermittent ROM exercises.
      2. *Weightbearing:* As tolerated (≥50%).
      3. *KT-1000 test:* Performed at 15-lb maximal force.
      4. *Exercises:*
         a. Multiangle isometrics (60, 40, 20 degrees).
         b. Quadriceps sets.
         c. Knee extension (60–0 degrees).
         d. Intermittent ROM (0–60 degrees (4–5 times daily).
         e. Patellar mobilization.
         f. Well leg bicycle.
         g. Proprioception training.
         h. Continue electrical stimulation to quadriceps.
         i. Continue ice and elevation.
   B. **Week 4:**
      1. *Brace:* locked at 0 degrees.
      2. *Full weightbearing:* No crutches, or one crutch if necessary.
      3. *KT-1000* arthrometer testing performed.
      4. *Exercises:*
         a. Weight shifts.

b. Minisquats (0–40 degrees).
c. Intermittent ROM (0–90 degrees).
d. Knee extension (90–40 degrees).
e. Pool walking.
f. Initiate bicycling.
5. *Fit* for functional PCL brace.

III. **Controlled ambulation phase (week 7–12):**
Goals:
- Control forces during ambulation.
- Increase quadriceps strength

A. **Week 7:**
1. *Discontinue* locked brace, brace opened 0–125 degrees.
2. *Criteria for full weightbearing* with knee motion:
   a. Active assertive ROM 0–115 degrees.
   b. Quadriceps strength 70% of contralateral side (isometric test).
   c. No change in KT-1000 test.
   d. Decreased joint effusion.
3. *Ambulation* with functional knee brace.
4. *Exercises:*
   a. Continue all exercises listed above.
   b. Initiate hamstring curls (low weight).
   c. Initiate swimming.
   d. Initiate vigorous stretching program.
   e. Increase closed-chain rehabilitation.

B. **Week 8:**
1. *KT-1000* testing.
2. *Continue* all exercises.

C. **Week 12:**
1. *Discontinue* ambulation with brace.
2. *Brace* used for strenuous activities.
3. KT-1000 testing.
4. *Exercises:*
   a. Begin isokinetics (100–40 degrees ROM).
   b. Continue minisquats.
   c. Initiate lateral step-ups.
   d. Initiate pool running (forward only).
   e. Bicycle for endurance (30 minutes).
   f. Begin walking program.

IV. **Light activity phase (3–4 months):**
Goals:
- Development of strength, power, endurance
- Begin to prepare for return to functional activities

1. *Exercises:*
   a. Begin light running program.
   b. Continue isokinetics (light speed, full ROM).
   c. Continue eccentrics.
   d. Continue minisquats/lateral step-ups.
   e. Continue closed-chain rehabilitation.
   f. Continue endurance exercises.
2. *Tests:*
   a. Isokinetic test (week 15).
   b. KT-1000 test (prior to running program).
   c. Functional test (prior to running program).
3. *Criteria for running:*
   a. Isokinetic test interpretation satisfactory.
   b. KT-1000 test unchanged.
   c. Functional test 70% of contralateral leg.

V. **Return to activity (5–6 months):**
Advance rehabilitation to competitive sports.
Goals:
- Achieve maximal strength.
- Further enhance neuromuscular coordination and endurance.

1. *Exercises:*
   a. Closed-chain rehabilitation.
   b. High-speed isokinetics.
   c. Running program.
   d. Agility drills.
   e. Balance drills.
   f. Polymetrics initiated.

VI. **Follow-up:**
A. **6-month follow-up:**
1. *Tests:*
   a. KT-1000 test.
   b. Isokinetic test.
   c. Functional test.

B. **12-month follow-up:**
1. *Tests:*
   a. KT-1000 test.
   b. Isokinetic test.
   c. Functional test.

50

Posterior Cruciate Ligament Reconstruction With Semitendinosus and Gracilis Tendons

A. BRANT LIPSCOMB, JR., M.D.
ALLEN F. ANDERSON, M.D.

Technique
Clinical results

Discussion

The posterior cruciate ligament (PCL) functions to resist posterior translation of the tibia on the femur as well as assist in posterolateral stability.[1,6] In addition, the integration of the PCL with the anterior cruciate ligament (ACL) in the four-bar cruciate linkage system ensures the physiologic rolling and gliding mechanism in flexion and extension of the knee.[8]

Despite the tensile strength of the PCL and its restraint to posterior translation of the tibia, controversy exists over treatment of an "isolated" PCL injury. Some reports[3,5,13] suggest that with quadriceps strengthening, functional instability can be minimized despite significant objective residual posterior instability. Others[2] report severe articular damage involving the medial compartment in knees that undergo PCL reconstruction. The premise is that loss of the normal gliding and rollback mechanism with loss of the PCL causes significant shearing, resulting in articular damage, particularly to the medial femoral condyle.

Our experience and success using the semitendinosus and gracilis tendons as a reconstructive substitute for a torn ACL[9] kindled our enthusiasm for their utilization as a secondary reconstruction for a torn PCL. Their length, excellent bony attachment distally, technical ease of harvesting, as well as sparing of the quadriceps mechanism, make them attractive as a substitute for the PCL.

The purpose of this chapter is to describe our technique of PCL reconstruction using the semitendinosus and gracilis tendons as an intraarticular substitution as well as describe an extraarticular procedure that was developed to assist the intraarticular reconstruction. In addition, our clinical experience with this reconstruction for acute and chronic isolated PCL tears is discussed.

TECHNIQUE

After adequate relaxation by anesthesia, a complete examination of the affected knee is performed to confirm the preoperative diagnosis.

A long, medial parapatellar incision is made. The quadriceps tendon is split, and the patella is subluxated laterally. With the knee flexed to 90 degrees, the synovial sleeve of the PCL is incised longitudinally and carefully preserved for suture around the newly reconstructed ligament. The semitendinosus and gracilis tendons are dissected free in the distal thigh, divided at the musculotendinous junction, and sutured together using a Bunnell stitch of no. 1 nonabsorbable material. The muscle bellies are allowed to retract.

A long, curved lateral incision is made ending over Gerdy's tubercle. A vertical 2.5-cm incision is then made through the posterolateral capsule entering the joint. The point of the Lipscomb-Anderson drill guide (Richards Medical Co., Memphis, Tenn.) is inserted through this incision. It is pushed inferiorly and secured in bone in the center of the posterior intercondylar fossa about 1.9 cm below the level of the tibial plateau at the anatomic origin of the PCL. The position of the drill guide is confirmed by placing a right-angled clamp through the intercondylar

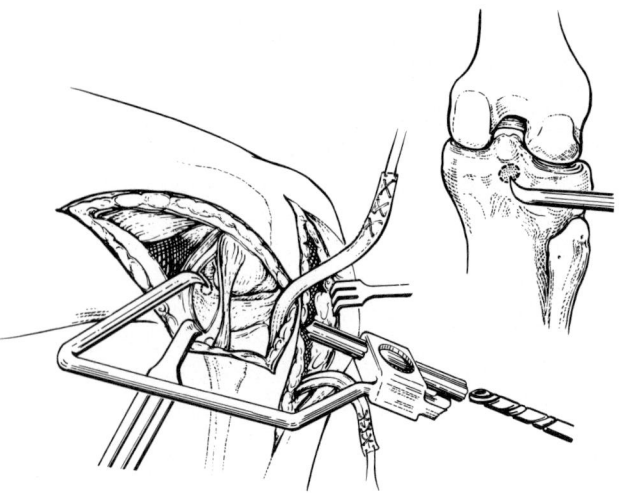

FIG 50–1.
Vertical 2.5-cm incision is made through the posterolateral capsule. The point of the Lipscomb-Anderson drill guide is inserted through this incision, secured in bone at the anatomic origin of the posterior cruciate ligament, and a 0.79-cm drill hole is made front to back through the anteromedial tibia.

PCL on the femur (Fig 50–2), a position most consistently isometric, as has been shown by Sidles et al.[14]

The semitendinosus and gracilis tendons are then passed from front to back through the tibial drill hole, up through the notch, and out the drill hole in the medial femoral condyle. They are fixed to the medial femoral condyle with a small barbed staple under moderate tension (approximately 20 lb) with the knee at 45 degrees of flexion and the tibia resting anteriorly on the femur (Fig 50–3). If a substantial portion of the torn PCL is present, a gathering suture is placed in its end, drawn through the drill hole, and sutured to the periosteum. However, no attempt is made to do a primary repair of mop-end intrasubstance tears. These fibers are sutured over the newly reconstructed PCL along with the synovium.

The medial parapatellar incision is then closed to maintain normal patellofemoral alignment. The vertical incision in the posterolateral capsule is closed by advancing the arcuate complex superiorly and dis-

notch and palpating the point of the drill guide. A 0.79-cm drill hole is made front to back through the anteromedial tibia exiting at the tibial attachment origin of the PCL (Fig 50–1). Using the drill guide, a 0.79-cm drill hole is made through the medial femoral condyle, entering the joint high in the intercondylar notch slightly posterior to the insertion of the

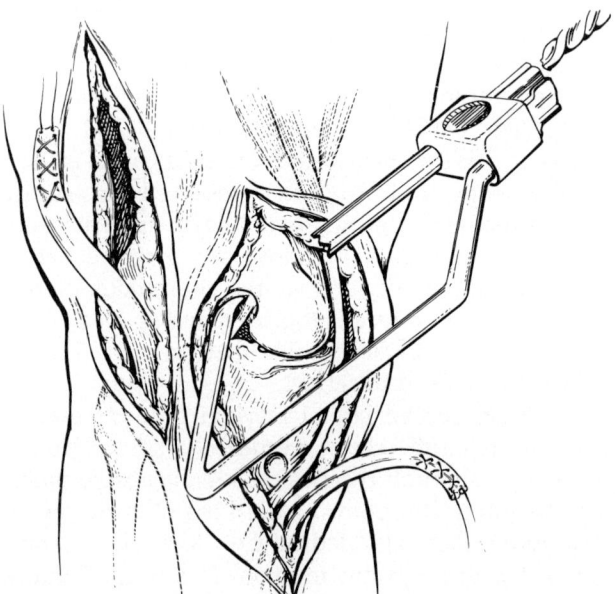

FIG 50–2.
Drill guide is used to make a 0.79-cm hole through the medial femoral condyle, entering the joint slightly posterior to the anatomic insertion of the posterior cruciate ligament.

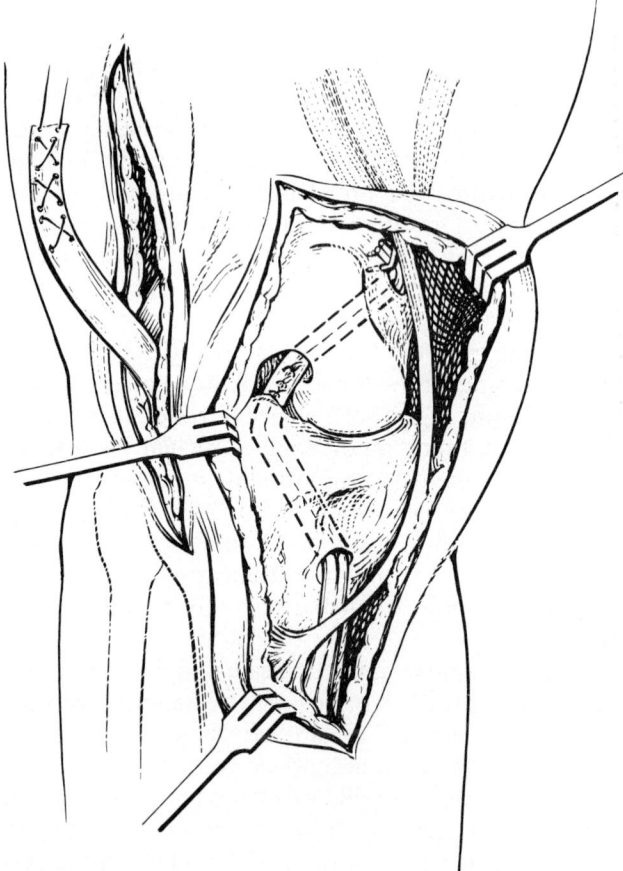

FIG 50–3.
Semitendinosus and gracilis tendons are passed from front to back through the tibial drill hole, up through the notch, and out the hole in the medial femoral condyle. They are secured to the medial femoral condyle with a small barbed staple.

tally. The previously described intraarticular technique can be performed arthroscopically; however, it is of paramount importance that there be adequate visualization of the posterior intercondylar fossa in order to prevent injury to the popliteal neurovascular structures.

Initially, the Losee lateral compartment reconstruction[10] was added to the intraarticular procedure to reduce posterior instability and tighten the arcuate complex. When it became appreciated that this procedure was more effective in reducing anterior tibial displacement as opposed to posterior displacement, a modification of Muller's lateral reconstructive extraarticular procedure[12] was devised to reduce posterior displacement.

A strip of iliotibial tract measuring approximately 30 cm in length and 3.8 cm in width is mobilized from proximal to distal leaving it attached at Gerdy's tubercle. The proximal attachment of this strip at Gerdy's tubercle is released.

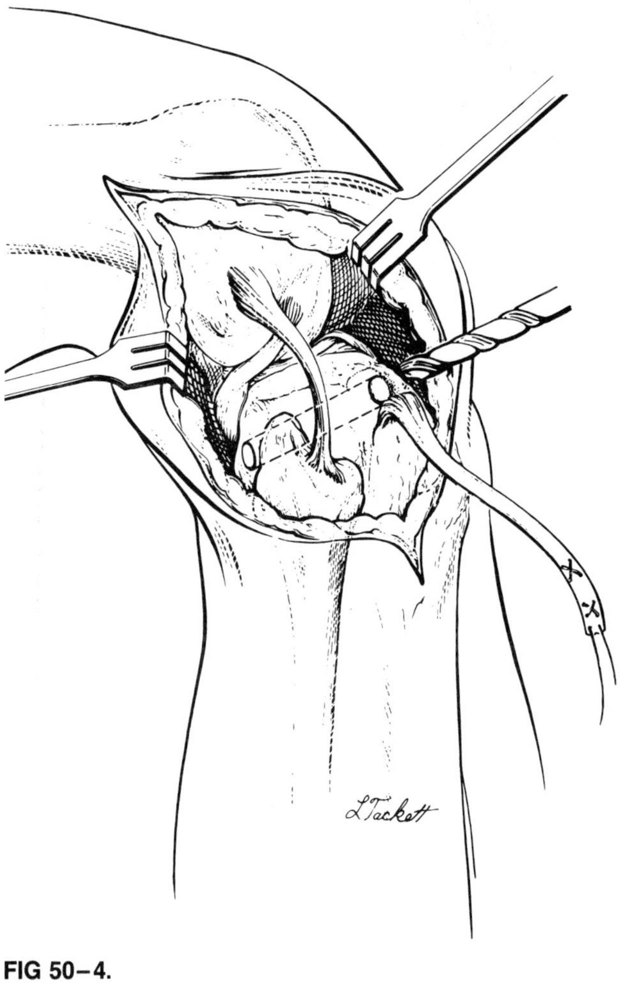

A 0.79-cm drill hole is then made through Gerdy's tubercle from anterior to posterior, exiting inferiorly to the articular surface, just medial to the fibula (Fig 50–4). The strip of iliotibial tract is passed from front to back through the tibia (Fig 50–5), placed under tension, and stapled to a groove in the lateral femoral condyle (Fig 50–6). The groove is angled at 45 degrees to the long axis of the femur and located just superior to the origin of the fibular collateral ligament. The remainder of the strip is then brought back on itself, passed through the tibial drill hole from posterior to anterior, and stapled to Gerdy's tubercle (Fig 50–7). Care is taken not to entrap the peroneal nerve.

Postoperatively, the knee is immobilized in 20 degrees of flexion. Active range-of-motion exercise is begun at 3 weeks from 30 to 60 degrees and advanced to full range of motion at 8 weeks.

Weightbearing is begun at 4 weeks, followed by swimming and bicycling at 4 months. Full activity is limited generally until 9 to 12 months postoperatively.

FIG 50–4.
A 0.79-cm drill hole is made through Gerdy's tubercle from anterior to posterior exiting inferior to the articular surface, just medial to the fibula.

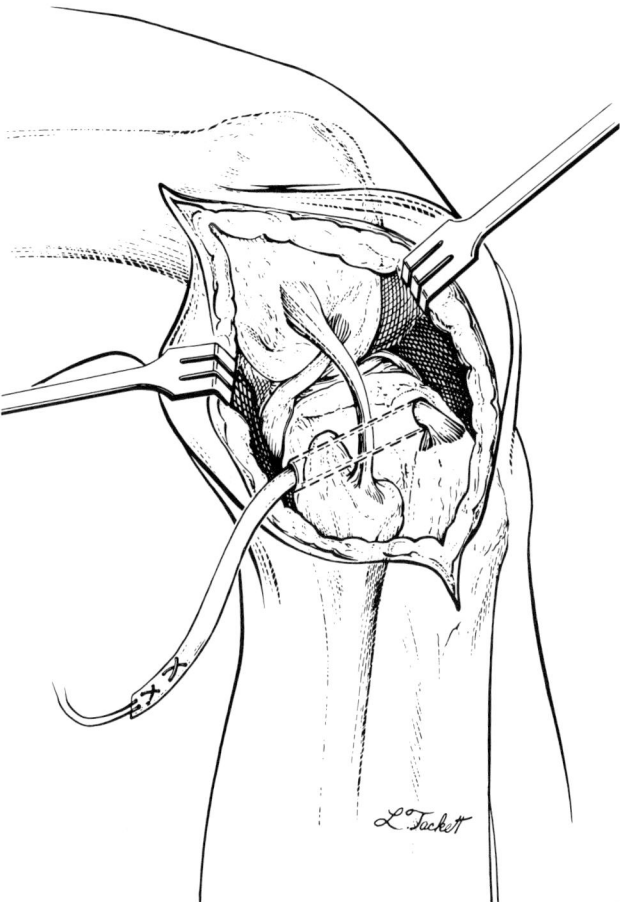

FIG 50–5.
Strip of iliotibial tract is passed from front to back through the tibia.

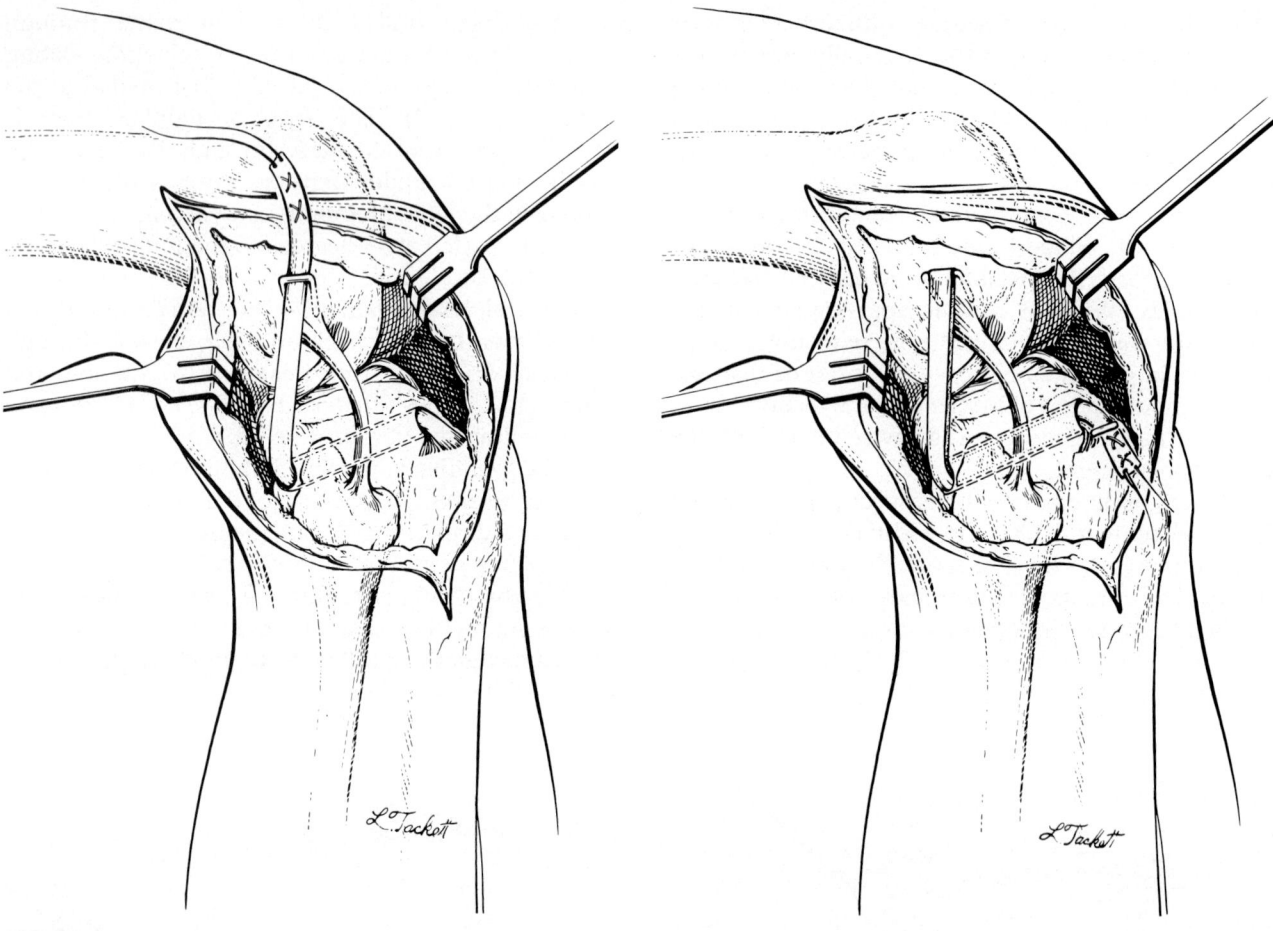

FIG 50–6.
Strip is placed under tension, and stapled to a groove in the lateral femoral condyle. The groove is angled at 45 degrees to the long axis of the femur and located just superior to the origin of the fibular collateral ligament.

FIG 50–7.
Remainder of the iliotibial tract is brought back on itself, passed through the tibial drill hole from posterior to anterior, and stapled to Gerdy's tubercle.

CLINICAL RESULTS

From the years 1973 to 1987, 28 patients underwent secondary reconstruction for isolated PCL tears utilizing both the described intra- and extraarticular procedures. Twenty-five of these patients were available for follow-up at a mean of 7 years. Fourteen patients sustained acute tears while 11 patients sustained chronic tears.

Of the 14 patients with acute tears, 2 subsequently underwent repeat reconstruction with allografts for continued instability. Follow-up examination in the 12 remaining patients revealed posterior drawer examinations in 90 degrees of flexion and neutral rotation averaging 2+, a finding not appreciably different from the average preoperative examination. KT-1000 (Medmetric, San Diego) arthrometric measurements were performed at 89 N, with the knee in the quadriceps neutral position.[4] The average corrected posterior drawer was 6.32 mm greater than the uninvolved limb, indicating minimal improvement in posterior restraint.

Similar evaluations in the 11 patients who underwent reconstructions for chronic PCL tears revealed little improvement in stability on posterior drawer examination. In addition, KT-1000 measurements at 89 N, with the knee in the quadriceps neutral position, averaged greater than 7 mm, a measurement comparable to an unreconstructed chronic PCL tear.

More important, radiographic evaluation revealed degenerative changes in the medial compartment in greater than half of these 25 patients, confirming that significant articular damage occurs with residual posterior instability.

DISCUSSION

Due to its location, function, and strength, the PCL has been emphasized to be the primary posterior stabilizer of the knee. Logically, it would appear that secondary reconstruction of this ligament would be indicated to help maintain the normal biomechanical linkage of the knee.

Unfortunately, operative series[7, 11] regarding particular reconstructive methods for midsubstance isolated PCL tears have been small, and the overall results, with the exception of the report of Clancy et al.,[2] have been only fair.

In addition, Parolie and Bergfeld[13] and Dandy and Pusey,[3] as well as Fowler and Messieh,[5] have advocated conservative treatment of isolated PCL midsubstance tears. Subjectively, their patients seem to do well, yet objectively there remains significant residual posterior instability. In addition, Parolie and Bergfeld's[13] study describes mild to moderate degenerative radiographic changes involving primarily the medial femoral condylar region, a finding corroborated in the study of Clancy et al.[2]

Our retrospective study adds to the list of secondary reconstructive procedures which do not effectively limit posterior translation of the tibia following isolated midsubstance PCL tears. Inadequate graft strength of the semitendinosus and gracilis in comparison to the PCL appears to be the main factor in the failure of this procedure. In addition, despite the optimistic subjective reporting of our patients, significant posterior instability remains, as confirmed by both manual and KT-1000 testing. More important, at 7 years' follow-up, significant degenerative radiographic changes were present in the majority of these knees, which had intact menisci.

It appears that residual posterior instability is not totally benign. Despite adequate quadriceps rehabilitation, the abnormal surface velocities leading to inefficient sliding of the knee following PCL disruption would predispose the knee to abnormal articular forces resulting in degenerative changes. Whether these degenerative changes continue to progress is unclear at this time.

Acknowledgment

We thank H. David Hovis, M.D., David L. Brown, M.D., and Emily D. Norwig, R.P.T., for their assistance, as well as Marilyn Holt and Lana Tackett in the preparation of this manuscript and the illustrations.

REFERENCES

1. Butler DL, Noyes FR, Grood ES: Ligamentous restraints to anterior-posterior drawer in the human knee. A biomechanical study, *J Bone Joint Surg, [Am]* 62:259–270, 1980.
2. Clancy WG, et al: Treatment of knee joint instability secondary to rupture of the posterior cruciate ligament. Report of a new procedure, *J Bone Joint Surg [Am]* 65:310–322, 1983.
3. Dandy DJ, Pusey RJ: The long-term results of unrepaired tears of the posterior cruciate ligament, *J Bone Joint Surg [Br]* 64:92–94, 1982.
4. Daniel DM, et al: Use of the quadriceps active test to diagnose posterior cruciate ligament disruption and measure posterior laxity of the knee, *J Bone Joint Surg [Am]* 70:386–391, 1988.
5. Fowler PJ, Messieh SS: Isolated posterior cruciate ligament injuries in athletes, *Am J Sports Med* 15:553–557, 1982.
6. Grood ES, Stowers SF, Noyes FR: Limits of movement in the human knee. Effect of sectioning the posterior cruciate ligament and posterolateral structures, *J Bone Joint Surg [Am]* 70:88–97, 1988.
7. Hughston JC, Degenhardt TC: Reconstruction of the posterior cruciate ligament, *Clin Orthop* 164:59–77, 1982.
8. Kapandji IA: *The physiology of the joints. Annotated diagrams of the mechanics of the human joints. Lower limb,* ed 2, vol 2, London, 1970, Livingstone.
9. Lipscomb AB, Anderson AF: Anterior cruciate ligament tears in the skeletally immature knee, *J Bone Joint Surg [Am]* 68:19–29, 1986.
10. Losee RE; Johnson TR, Southwick WO: Anterior subluxation of the lateral tibial plateau. A diagnostic test and operative repair, *J Bone Joint Surg [Am]* 60A:1015–1030, 1978.
11. McMaster WC: Isolated posterior cruciate ligament injury: Literature review and case reports, *J Trauma* 15:1025–1029, 1975.
12. Muller W: *The knee. Form, function and ligament reconstruction,* New York, 1983, Springer-Verlag, pp 246–248.
13. Parolie JM, Bergfeld JA: Long-term results of nonoperative treatment of isolated posterior cruciate ligament injuries in the athlete, *Am J Sports Med* 14:35–38, 1986.
14. Sidles JA, et al: Ligament length relationships in the moving knee, *J Orthop Res* 6:593–610, 1988.

PART XII

Rehabilitation, Bracing, and Nursing Care for Cartilage and Ligamentous Injuries

51

Rehabilitation of Cartilage Lesions

RONALD W. SWEITZER, P.T.
DANIA A. SWEITZER, P.T.
ANTHONY J. SARANITI, P.T.

Prehabilitation evaluation
   Subjective information
   Objective information
      Biomechanical analysis of functional activities
   Assessment
Rehabilitation and biomechanical rationale for treatment of chondromalacia patellae and patellofemoral pain syndrome
   Inflammation
      Muscular inhibition secondary to edema
   Flexibility
   Strengthening
      Isometric quadriceps sets
      Vastus medialis obliquus exercise
      Terminal knee extension
      Neuromuscular electrical stimulation
      Manual resistance exercise
   Taping
   Stationary bicycle
   Proprioceptive training
   Isokinetic exercise
   Open-chain and closed-chain activities
      Functional closed-chain vastus medialis obliquus training
   Electromyographic biofeedback
      Sitting
      Partial squats
      Lunge
   Resistive closed-chain exercise
   Stair climber vs. stairs
   Patient education
Physical therapy after arthroscopic procedures
Physical therapy after patellar realignment
Osteochondritis dissecans
   Typical treatment
      Non-weight-bearing
      Partial weight-bearing
      Full weight-bearing
Meniscal repairs

The patellofemoral and tibiofemoral joints are subjected to repetitive loads of varying intensities which are dependent on activity. In the healthy joint, there is good mechanical alignment of segments, intact ligaments and menisci, and normal synovial membrane. When these components are damaged, the joint is no longer able to safely tolerate the loads that would be expected of a healthy joint. The rehabilitation of injured articular cartilage must be based on biomechanical principles that reduce joint stresses to allow healing and prevent continued or repeated articular deterioration. This is accomplished by improving the musculoskeletal biomechanics through proper exercise and functional retraining, and by activity modification through patient education.

PREREHABILITATION EVALUATION

A thorough patient evaluation is the first step in providing the most appropriate rehabilitation program. The examination should include segments adjacent to the knee to find deficient components of the musculoskeletal link segment that will affect the knee. A comprehensive evaluation should include but not be limited to the following.

Subjective Information

A description of the patient's complaints must be obtained for consideration in the establishment of the rehabilitation goals and program.

- What is the chief complaint? Pain, swelling, giving way, locking?
- What makes it worse or better?

This information is useful for determining the initial stage of rehabilitation and the types of activities for the patient to avoid.

- What is the patient's occupation? What recreational activities does the patient participate in?

This information is necessary for later determining realistic goals for the patient.

- What is the patient's general health? Is he or she on any medications? What laboratory tests have been done?

These data are necessary to customize the rehabilitation so that other medical conditions are not aggravated.

Objective Information

Static observation of the knee for contour is used to screen for effusion, atrophy, and discoloration. Static structural alignment in the fixed standing position allows evaluation of static alignment while in a bilateral weightbearing position. Ease and symmetry of stance, including weight-shift patterns, are observed. The tibiofemoral relationship is examined for rotational (joint) or torsional (within the bone) variations. If a foot malalignment is found, a temporary correction should be made with a subsequent reexamination of static and dynamic alignment.

Static patellar orientation is determined with respect to glide, tilt, rotation, anteroposterior (AP) position, proximal-distal position (alta or baja), and Q (quadriceps) angle.

Dynamic patellar orientation must be assessed and related to the static alignment. Dynamic alignment is the more significant factor in the formulation of the rehabilitation program. It is the bony articulations during movement that determine the articular points of contact and subsequent pain patterns. The patient should be instructed to report any increase in symptoms during the activities being performed and to specify at what point in the activity symptoms occur. This is considered a positive sign and is used for reassessment.

The patient should be observed during walking at different speeds, stepping up and down steps of various heights (Fig 51–1), standing on a single leg, and squatting. Other functional movements may be added at the examiner's discretion. The patient's balance, willingness to move, and general motor control must be analyzed in conjunction with the observed joint alignment and muscular asymmetries caused by atrophy, hypertrophy, or inhibition patterns.

Biomechanical Analysis of Functional Activities

Walking. Patients with patellofemoral problems have less pain when walking slowly as compared to walking fast. During slow walking, the ten-

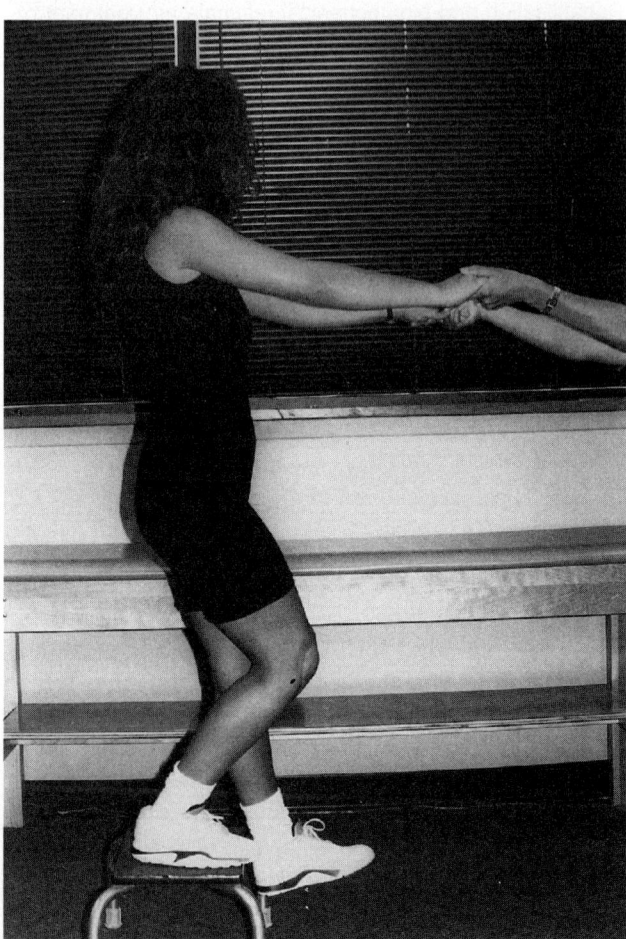

FIG 51–1.
Assisted step-up and step-down for evaluation and exercise.

dency to flex the knee after heel strike is minimal; consequently there is little patellofemoral joint reactive force (PFJRF). As the walking speed increases to 90 to 100 steps per minute, the knee flexes to as much as 15 degrees. The resultant PFJRF increases to 0.3 to 0.5 times body weight. Another possible reason for an increase in patellofemoral pain with fast walking is the increased quadriceps activity following toe-off to enhance knee extension during the following swing phase.[39, 85] During level walking, joint reactive forces (JRF) through the tibial condyles vary from two times body weight at the beginning of stance phase to almost four times body weight just before push-off.

Stair Climbing. Stair climbing probably is the first activity that patients with patellofemoral dysfunction report as being painful. It is also the first activity they are told to avoid. Because of the increase in flexion required during stair climbing, PFJRF reaches 3.3 to 3.5 times body weight or 7 to 10 times the force produced during slow walking. While ascending stairs, tibiofemoral JRF may reach 4.25 times body weight. As in the patellofemoral joint, the JRF of the tibiofemoral joint increases when resistance is applied in the flexed position.[63] When questioned carefully, patients usually report that descending stairs is more painful than ascending stairs. At least two factors contribute to this finding. The knee joint flexes between 50 and 60 degrees during the weight-bearing phase of ascending stairs that are 7 to 7½ in. high. Descending stairs requires approximately 80 degrees of flexion during the full weightbearing phase, which produces a greater PFJRF.[39] When ascending stairs, the subject tends to lean forward, which shifts the center of gravity anteriorly. The anterior shift reduces the flexion movement at the knee and therefore requires less quadriceps contraction to elevate the body. When descending stairs, the subject tends to lean backward, thereby increasing the flexion movement and consequently requiring more quadriceps contraction to control the descent.[1]

Squats. The patient with patellofemoral dysfunction is unable to squat comfortably. The extreme squat, or deep knee bend, has been shown to increase PFJRF to as high as 7.6 times body weight.

Running. Running is another activity which is stressful to the patellofemoral joint for several reasons. During running overall knee joint motion is greater than during walking. Running produces greater knee flexion at the moment of foot contact. Increased flexion at the knee and hip with increased ankle dorsiflexion help somewhat to absorb the added impact produced during running, but the ground reaction force upon unilateral foot impact during running has been shown to be about 2.5 times body weight compared to 0.8 during walking. Much of this added load will result in greater PFJRF at greater angles of flexion. Running also produces repetitive stress problems. If a 150-lb man walked 1 mile with average step lengths, he would have taken about 2,110 steps and absorbed about 63.5 tons on one foot. If the same man ran, he would have had to take only 1,175 steps, but would have absorbed 110 tons.[47] This information may be helpful in convincing patients with biomechanical and degenerative problems of the risks associated with running.

Flexibility must be assessed carefully. Proper positioning and stabilization of proximal segments while applying a constant tension to the tested muscle is critical to finding subtle length differences and obtaining reliable results. Shortened musculature may impair normal joint function by (1) producing a variation in the proprioceptor firing pattern, thereby altering motor unit activation patterns; and (2) producing increased tautness in connective tissue structures around the joint. For example, a shortened tensor fascia lata (TFL) increases tension in the ilio-tibial band and lateral retinaculum. This factor may increase lateral tibiofemoral compressive forces and cause the patella to track more laterally.

Muscular strength assessment may be performed in a variety of ways. Standard gross manual muscle testing should be performed initially. For more precise evaluation of muscle strength differences, a hand-held myometer or computerized dynamometer should be used. Muscular assessment should not stop here. Although dynamometer assessment for strength may be relatively symmetric for peak torque, torque graphs throughout the range and fatigue tests may show asymmetries. Abnormal torque curves may accompany a painful arc where sensitive tissue is only irritated through a limited arc of motion such as a local condylar or patellar facet lesion.

Muscular firing patterns may be altered because of neurophysiologic inhibition secondary to edema and chronic dysfunction. Muscular inhibition may be assessed by palpation and electromyography (EMG). When used appropriately, a multichannel EMG biofeedback system can provide valuable information about motor unit activation patterns among muscle groups. This information can then be used to enhance the rehabilitation functional training sessions.

Active movement testing includes flexion and extension and internal and external rotation. Testing provides the link between muscle activation and strength as related to the available range of motion

(ROM). For example, if active terminal knee extension is less than passive extension, an extension lag exists. The examiner must then look for the cause, such as muscular inhibition, weakness, or patella restriction. Smidt[74] observed that in the arthritic patient the functional ROM is often less than the active ROM. If this is the case, the rehabilitation program should address this discrepancy.

Passive physiologic movement testing of the above-mentioned motions should be performed. Note the presence of a capsular, bony, or springy end feel. Passive mobility testing should be performed at the patellofemoral joint to evaluate the amount of patellar glide, tilt, and rotation. This information is critical for the treatment of patients with patellofemoral disorders and should be considered in the prevention of patellofemoral irritation in other knee rehabilitation patients.

Palpation is used in the examination to further identify tight, painful, and swollen tissues.

Standard ligament and meniscus tests are performed to assess joint stability.

Proximal and distal segment assessment must be performed. The foot greatly influences the knee by its ability to absorb shock by pronating; produce functional shortening by pronating; produce increased tibial medial rotation by pronating; and produce greater valgus forces by pronating. Be aware that the converse may apply. Knee malalignment may produce a compensatory foot alignment. This finding may be determined from a thorough lower extremity biomechanical evaluation including temporary orthotic correction with subsequent static and dynamic reevaluation.

Assessment

The assessment includes a review of all positive findings and a patient interview to determine the goals for this individual. Short-term goals are established primarily from the clinical and test findings. The long-term goals need to be carefully established based on the patient's lifestyle demands tempered by the limitations produced by the physical condition. The physician and physical therapist must listen to the patient. If this is a person who only wants to be able to walk around a shopping mall or climb a flight of stairs occasionally, we set our rehabilitation toward that goal. If the patient is a competitive athlete who wants to run a marathon, but has significant knee joint degeneration, we have to caution him or her as to the deleterious effects that type of activity would have on the knee. The clinician must help the patient find other physically challenging and rewarding activities that are not detrimental.

REHABILITATION AND BIOMECHANICAL RATIONALE FOR TREATMENT OF CHONDROMALACIA PATELLAE AND PATELLOFEMORAL PAIN SYNDROME

Rehabilitation of the patellofemoral joint is based on the biomechanical factors that change the stresses on the involved joint structures. Patients with chondromalacia patellae or patellofemoral pain syndrome (PFPS) have areas of degenerative and irritated articular cartilage. From the initial examination, it has been determined what activities cause pain, what part of the ROM is painful, and how much muscular force can be exerted throughout the range without producing pain. Although hyaline cartilage is aneural, as it degenerates pain from synovial irritation may occur. Also, as the articular cartilage softens and erodes, the pressure distribution to the innervated subchondral bone intensifies and produces pain.[25] The rehabilitation process should progress without causing pain.[58, 73]

The therapeutic plan is to (1) decrease areas of excessive pressure, (2) reduce inflammation of irritated tissue, (3) improve joint biomechanics by stretching tight structures that disturb normal tracking, (4) increase strength and endurance of the lower extremity musculature, and (5) improve motor control of the lower extremities, particularly of the vastus medialis obliquus (VMO), through functional retraining. This plan removes the irritating forces and applies normalized, progressive stresses to stimulate healing and restore function. The description of exercises and activities proceeds from the least to the most stressful. A successful treatment progression must be based on a thorough initial clinical assessment and constant monitoring and reevaluation of clinical signs and functional performance.

Inflammation

The acutely involved patient will present with pain, edema, a real or perceived loss of motion, and decreased functional strength. Reduction of inflammation is the highest priority. Decreasing stressful activities; cold applications; transcutaneous electrical nerve stimulation in various forms, including neuromuscular electrical stimulation (NMES);[71] low intensity ultrasound; massage; and elevation of the extremity may all be helpful in reducing pain and edema. The reader is referred to the references for techniques that have been shown to be effective.[40, 46, 51, 54, 77]

Muscular Inhibition Secondary to Edema

Edema reduction is very important to allow for efficient motor control and strengthening of the quadriceps. DeAndrade et al.[15] showed that there is decreased quadriceps motor unit activity from reflex inhibition in human knees distended with nonirritating plasma. Others have reported similar findings, including Spencer et al.[78] who discovered that the VMO is more easily inhibited than the vastus lateralis or rectus femoris. Two to three times more saline had to be injected into the knee joint to inhibit the vastus lateralis and rectus femoris. EMG biofeedback training and NMES are valuable techniques used to overcome this inhibition.

Flexibility

The lengthening of shortened contractile and noncontractile tissues must begin at the onset of the rehabilitation program.[27, 38] Connective tissue shortening leads to increased joint compressive forces, bony malalignment, and restriction of motion. The structures on the lateral side of the leg, such as the iliotibial band and lateral retinaculum, are commonly hypomobile. Iliotibial band shortening may contribute to a variety of lower extremity problems other than patellofemoral dysfunctions.[30] The iliotibial band can be stretched by placing the leg in a position of neutral rotation and adduction. Myofascial release in this position is also effective, especially at the distal insertion to Gerdy's tubercle. The lateral retinaculum can be more directly stretched by patellar mobilization including a medial glide and medial tilt (Figs 51–2 and 51–3) of the patella. This may be combined with deep friction massage to increase tissue extensibility.[12]

As the iliotibial band and the lateral retinaculum are stretched, the lateral static forces on the patella are reduced and the patella is positioned more centrally. Doucette and Goble[20] found that iliotibial band stretching in combination with joint mobility exercises and VMO strengthening improved patellar tracking as evaluated by Merchant's congruence angle.[50] As the patella moves medially, there is also a reduction in the chronic stress on the medial retinaculum. This is helpful in preventing medial retinaculitis. The more central position of the patella places the VMO at a better mechanical advantage, and in a position more receptive to neuromuscular reeducation.

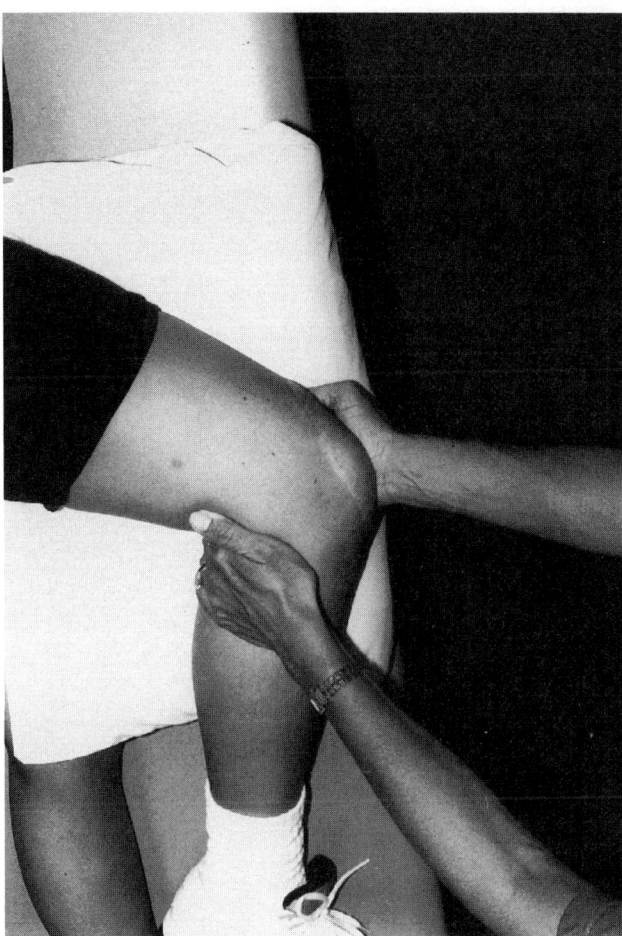

FIG 51–2.
Medial tilt to stretch deep lateral retinaculum.

Stretching of the hamstrings (Fig 51–4) and the quadriceps is also important in the treatment of patellofemoral disorders. Tight hamstrings may cause the quadriceps to work harder during knee extension, particularly in a flexed hip posture. This subjects the patellofemoral joint to excessive compressive forces. Tightness of the rectus femoris reduces inferior patellar movement during knee flexion, further increasing the compression of the patella against the femur.

Gastrocnemius and soleus flexibility is important because of the interrelationship of the foot, ankle, and knee. A tight gastrocnemius-soleus complex causes increased pronation, which causes increased internal tibial rotation, which increases the dynamic Q angle, which ultimately causes the patella to track more laterally.[13]

Strengthening

A total lower extremity strengthening and functional activity program is an integral part of the treatment

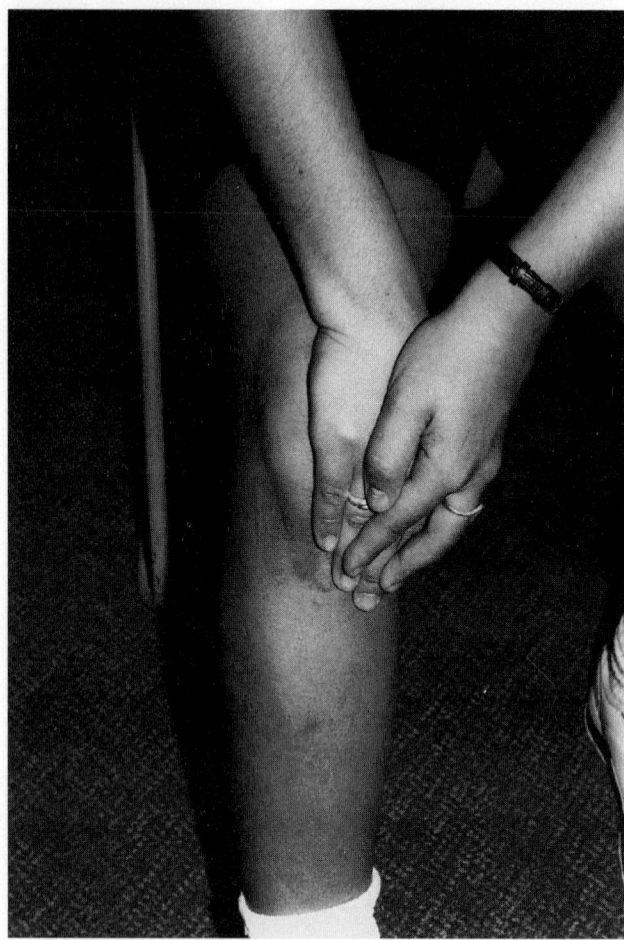

FIG 51–3.
Self-stretch of deep lateral retinaculum.

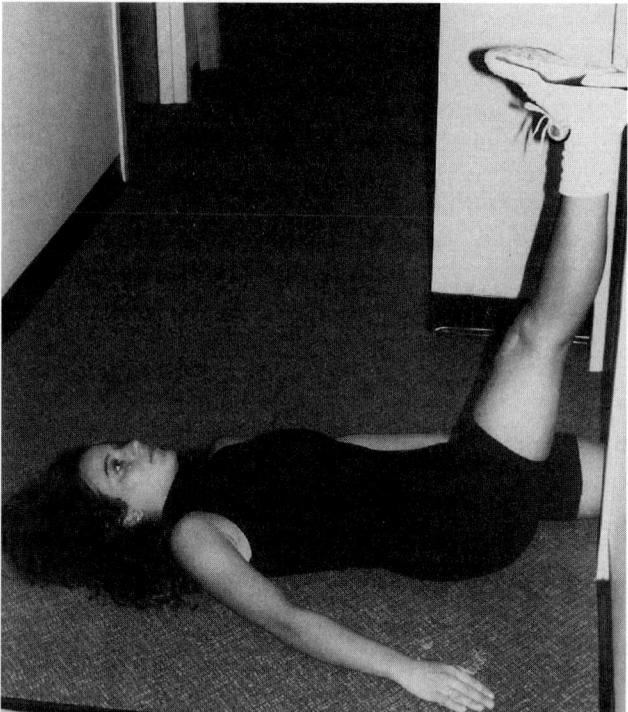

FIG 51–4.
Hamstring stretch.

plan. The joints of the lower extremity do not function independently. A dysfunction at one joint can effect the joints distal and proximal to it.

There are two schools of thought regarding the nonoperative management of patellofemoral disorders. One method is to strengthen all muscle groups around the pathologic joint, including the quadriceps, through active knee extension exercises. The rationale to include active knee extension exercise is that knee extension is the most efficient exercise for strengthening the quadriceps and training the VMO. The other school believes in strengthening all muscle groups around the pathologic joint without having the patient perform active knee extension.[36] This is based on the concept that performing knee extension against a resistive load places excessive stress on the patellofemoral joint. Patients experiencing patellofemoral pain and dysfunction commonly have poor patellar alignment. If this type of patient repeatedly extends the knee joint, there may be increases in compressive and shearing pressures, and exacerbation of the patient's signs and symptoms. Although this nonextension approach is logical and useful in the acute stage, it does not prepare the knee for the functional demands that arise on a daily basis.

It is advisable to begin a complete lower extremity–strengthening program without performing knee extension and flexion in the acute phase. While the knee is painful, the patient's exercise regimen should be limited, to prevent further irritation and pain. The physical therapist must control and vary the level of muscular contraction, ROM, and training velocity. A proximal muscle group–strengthening program, which includes supine straight leg raises, prone straight leg raises, side-lying hip abduction and side-lying hip adduction, and sitting hip flexion, may be initiated immediately. It should be noted that these exercises contribute to the strengthening of the quadriceps by requiring co-contraction to stabilize the knee. These exercises cause the cartilaginous surfaces of the patella and femur to come into contact with each other intermittently, providing a pumping action for synovial fluid to enter and nourish the articular cartilage and perhaps provide a stimulus for regeneration and repair.

Each exercise requires activation of two joint muscles that cross and influence the function of both the hip and knee. These exercises produce only mild patellofemoral compressive forces and minimal meniscal shear forces. Although greater tibiofemoral compressive forces are produced, they are less irritating than those occurring during walking. By increasing strength and endurance these exercises allow for more effective functional and closed-chain activities in the next stage of rehabilitation.

Supine straight leg raises with the knee extended recruit the quadriceps and hip flexors while producing minimal PFJRF. The patella makes no significant contact with the femoral condyles until 10 to 20 degrees of flexion. When the knee begins to flex, the initial patellar contact occurs on the inferior pole, on a relatively small surface. As flexion continues, contact on the patella moves superiorly and onto a greater surface area up to 90 degrees. The medial patellar facet does not come into contact with the femur until 135 degrees of flexion. It then shares the load with the lateral facet while the midpatella has no contact with the femur.[26, 29, 65]

Initially, the patient is directed to perform each exercise for five sets of ten repetitions with the maximum amount of weight he or she can comfortably lift. Cuff weights of increasing resistance are applied to the ankle,[18] with the goal for each patient being the ability to lift 10% to 15% of the body weight for each exercise. If there is knee pain the weight is reduced or moved proximal to the knee joint to decrease the stresses on the knee ligaments. When the patient is able to perform five sets of ten repetitions with 5 lbs comfortably, the patient can be progressed to performing the same exercises on an isokinetic system, such as the Orthotron II.[43] The proximal muscle groups may also be strengthened in the upright position by using a variable resistive weight machine such as the Cybex Multi-Hip or by using the resistance of a pulley system.[21]

Isometric Quadriceps Sets

Quadriceps setting exercises are also beneficial in the early stage of knee rehabilitation. Although straight leg raising is a good initial quadriceps exercise, it is not the most efficient way to recruit maximum vastus medialis, lateralis, and intermedius contraction. When subjected to equal workloads or maximal effort trials, the vastus muscles are twice as active as the rectus femoris during quadriceps setting, whereas the rectus femoris is significantly more active than the vastus muscles during straight leg raising.[31, 75]

Vastus Medialis Obliquus Exercise

Exercises specifically intended to facilitate the VMO are also paramount in the rehabilitation program. The function of the VMO is to realign the patella medially during extension of the knee.[4, 20, 44, 83] It is also the only medial dynamic stabilizer of the patella. Any insufficiency of the VMO will allow increased lateral patellar translation. By having the patient perform a straight leg raise with the lower extremity in slight external rotation at the hip, a greater demand is placed on the medial musculature.[4] The adductor magnus is the origin for the majority of the VMO fibers; therefore, strengthening the adductor muscles will help to provide a dynamic medial glide of the patella and prevent lateral tracking. Working the adductors also lessens the pull of the tensor fascia lata through its attachment into the iliotibial band by preventing femoral internal rotation and abduction. One exercise incorporating this concept is performed in the hook-lying position. The patient is asked to squeeze a small pillow or ball between the knees, isometrically contracting the adductors and quadriceps. This exercise can be performed at various angles of knee flexion. Hanten and Schulthies[35] demonstrated an increase in VMO rather than vastus lateralis activity during resisted hip adduction exercise, while they found no increase in the VMO during resisted medial tibial rotation exercise.

Quadriceps setting exercises should include VMO training. The patient may begin isometric quadriceps exercises at various pain-free points in the range. In the neutral position, the least amount of patellofemoral compression occurs. Angles of 30, 50, 70, and 90 degrees should also be performed if pain-free. Lieb and Perry[44] found that VMO recruitment occurred at higher levels during multiangle isometrics between 0 and 90 degrees of flexion. The isometric mode of a dynamometer may be used to give the patient and clinician objective data about the ability of the quadriceps to generate torque at various points in the range. We also recommend closed-chain isometric quadriceps and gluteal contractions from the sitting position with the foot on the floor (Fig 51–5). In this position, the patient can focus on VMO recruitment while preparing the lower extremity for better control of the sit-to-stand maneuver.

Terminal Knee Extension

Most patients can perform terminal knee extension (TKE) from 20 degrees of flexion to neutral painlessly because of the small PFJRF in this range. The exercise can be performed in an open-chain fashion supine with a quadboard or a towel roll under the knee. If this exercise is painful, it usually indicates extreme inflammation, a lesion on the inferior patellar facet, or patella alta. Terminal knee extension can also be performed in a closed-chain fashion while standing. The patient allows the knee to flex 15 to 20 degrees

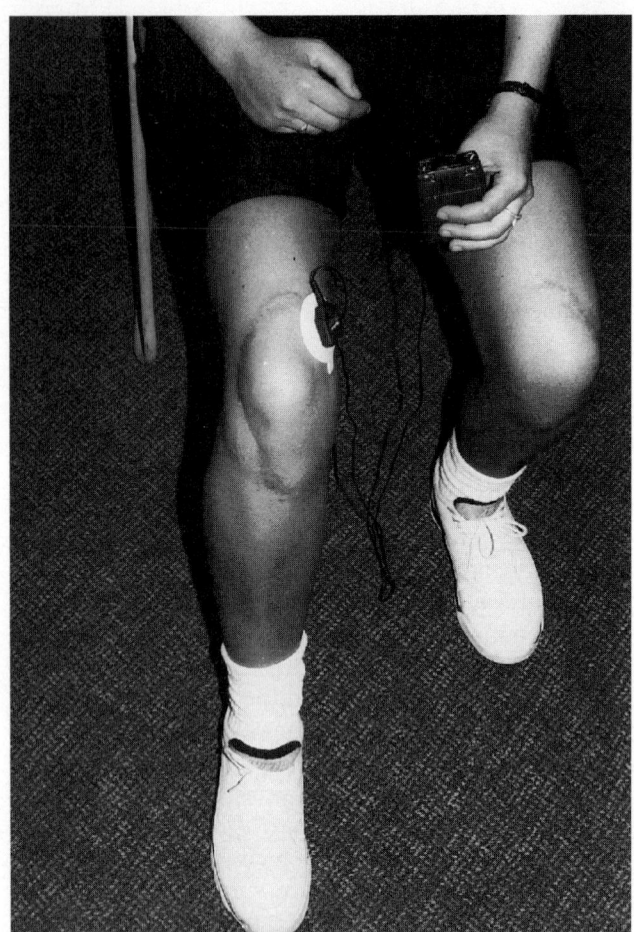

FIG 51–5.
Vastus medialis obliquus training in sitting with biofeedback.

and then extends the knee fully, but not into hyperextension. Resistance may be applied to the posterior thigh with an elastic band (Theraband) or pulleys to create a flexion moment at the knee joint (Fig 51–6). The Cybex Multi-Hip machine can also be set for weight-bearing resistive terminal knee extension.

When analysis of vectors is performed throughout the knee joint ROM, the patellar compression component or PFJRF is significantly lower in the extended, not hyperextended, position. The changing angular relationship of the quadriceps tendon to the patellar tendon produces increasing PFJRF as the knee flexes. Nordin and Frankel[56] used a theoretical example to calculate PFJRF at various degrees of flexion for a subject maintaining a constant quadriceps muscle force. The authors determined that if the quadriceps force was constant at 1,000 N with the knee in 5 degrees of flexion, the PFJRF would be about 600 N, at 45 degrees about 1,000 N, and at 90 degrees about 1,275 N.

TKE exercises recruit the VMO more easily than straight leg lifts.[31, 75] Approximately 60% more quad-

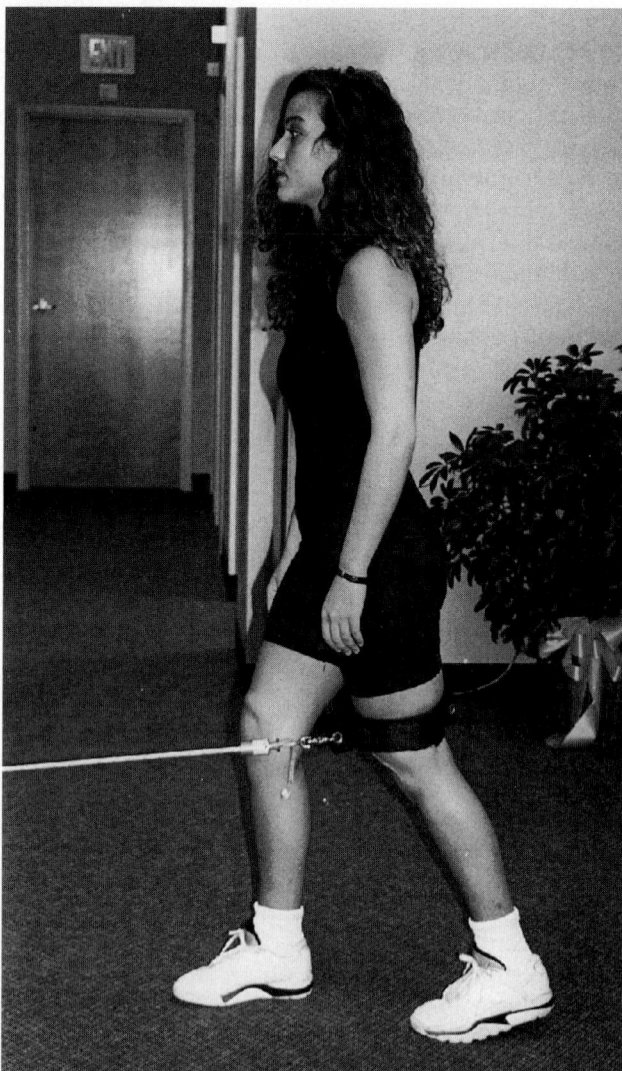

FIG 51–6.
Resistive closed-chain knee extension to regain full-extension range of motion.

riceps muscle force is required for the last 15 degrees of knee extension. Therefore, more quadriceps motor units are recruited in a range that has very low PFJRF.[44]

Neuromuscular Electrical Stimulation

Neuromuscular electrical stimulation (NMES) is used to facilitate muscular contraction in a muscle group in which the patient is having difficulty producing a voluntary contraction.[3, 5, 23, 86] Precise electrode placement is essential to maximize the efficiency of the contraction.[3] A proper training technique that incorporates the patient's concentration is critical to producing carryover into functional use. The patient must be instructed to contract the muscle as soon as he or she feels the stimulus. Since this is not a passive activity, the patient must focus on gaining voluntary control of the muscle.

A variety of neuromuscular stimulators are now available to assist with retraining proper timing of the VMO and to facilitate proper balance within the quadriceps. By electrically stimulating the VMO first, and then the lateral quadriceps, a preset protocol enables the patient to contract the quadriceps more efficiently.

Manual Resistance Exercise

Manual resistance exercises have the advantage of providing the therapist with more control over the patient's movement pattern and the degree of resistance throughout the ROM. Resistance can be applied at an isolated joint, as in knee extension, or in a pattern, such as hip extension, knee extension, and ankle plantar flexion. Motion can be in a cardinal plane or in a functional diagonal plane as prescribed in proprioceptive neuromuscular facilitation techniques.[82] Manually resisted diagonal patterns are useful for providing controlled rotational and varus and valgus forces on the knee to condition the appropriate neuromuscular responses in preparation for more advanced functional rehabilitation activities.

Taping

In the biomechanically normal knee, as flexion occurs from the neutral position, both the PFJRF and patellofemoral contact area increase. Therefore, surface pressure does not necessarily increase as the PFJRF does. Hyaline cartilage is damaged by excessive local pressure or mechanical overload.[59] If the mechanical load is distributed over a larger area, there should be no deleterious effect on the joint surfaces. This rationale supports the use of resistive activities through the flexed position. If the criteria of normal biomechanics are not met, the articular surfaces are at risk. Dynamic malalignment of the patellofemoral joint does not allow for normal weightbearing and resistive knee extension activities. To rehabilitate the knee, the alignment must be restored to the greatest degree as soon as possible.

Patellar taping, as developed by McConnell,[48, 49] has proved to be a very effective supplemental procedure that allows patients to increase activity without aggravating their symptoms. The taping procedure is specific and must be learned from a competent instructor. The patient is taped to correct the tilt (Fig 51–7), glide (Fig 51–8), rotational (Fig 51–9), or AP malalignment that was found in the examination. The step-up and step-down, which

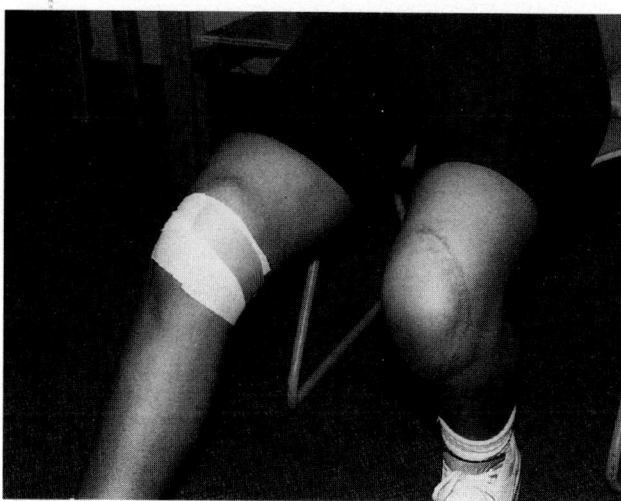

FIG 51–7.
McConnell taping to correct lateral tilt.

yielded a positive sign, are used to evaluate the initial effectiveness of the taping (Fig 51–10). An immediate increase in the ability to perform the motion without pain, both concentrically and eccentrically, should occur.

The patient should report a decrease in pain and a more stable feeling. If this does not occur, the tape needs to be readjusted until the motion can be performed appropriately. Patients must be able to apply and adjust the tape themselves to allow for daily use for several weeks or when activities warrant it. Taping does work. There are at least two mechanisms that may explain its effectiveness. First, the tape produces mechanical changes on the patella which improve tracking and pressure distribution. These changes would certainly be difficult to maintain with the amount of soft tissue mobility between the tape and the bone. The second mechanism may be a neurophysiologic one in which stimulation to skin afferent fibers and deeper proprioceptive fibers allows the patient to retrain the musculature in a manner that produces better tracking.

Stationary Bicycle

The stationary bicycle offers the patient a safe, comfortable means of exercise with rhythmic, bilateral, and reciprocal muscle activation through a safe ROM. The seat is generally kept high to reduce excessive flexion and the tension is kept low to reduce PFJRF. The first session should be only 5 minutes so that the response may be evaluated. Moran et al.[53] and Wozniak Timmer[87] give comprehensive reviews of cycling related to rehabilitation and the mechanics associated with road cycling.

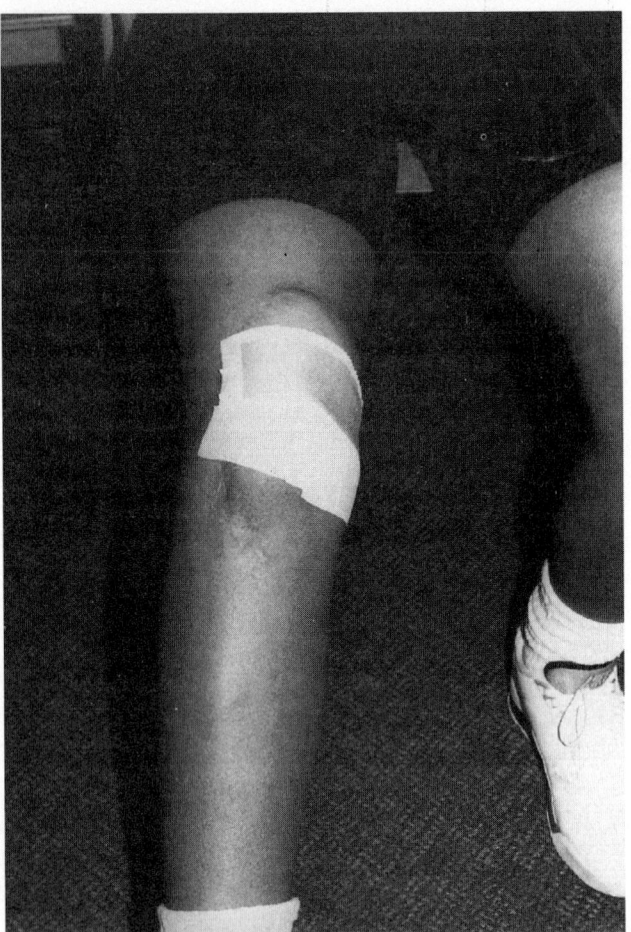

FIG 51–8.
McConnell taping to correct lateral glide.

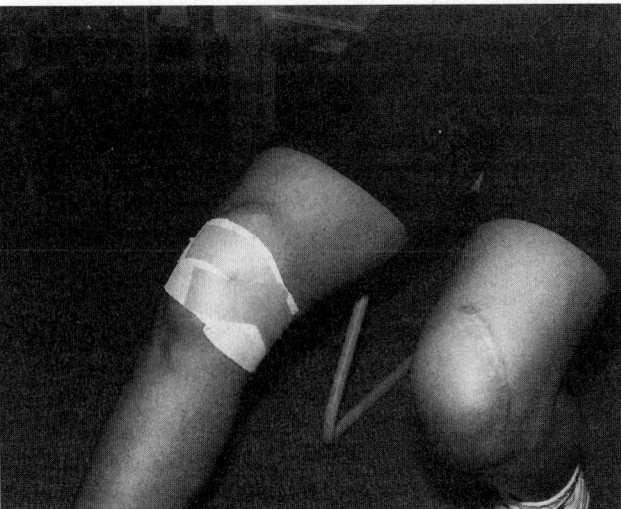

FIG 51–9.
McConnell taping to correct patellar glide and rotation.

Proprioceptive Training

Proprioceptor-stimulating exercises are performed to activate joint and muscle mechanoreceptors that have been traumatized or inhibited secondary to inactivity. The work of Wyke[88] emphasizes the importance of activation of mechanoreceptors by providing stimulatory stresses. Proprioceptor exercises are designed to produce controlled stress at different rates on all aspects of the joint capsule and ligament and on all the muscles that cross and protect the knee. Devices such as the Biomechanical Ankle Platform System (BAPS) (Camp International Inc., Jackson Miss.) (Fig 51–11), kinesthetic ability training (KAT) (Breg Vista, Calif.), and the Fitter (Fitter International Inc., Calgary, Alta., Canada) (Fig 51–12) can be used to provide a changing ground surface, which will be translated through the foot, ankle, and knee to trigger reflex muscular contraction to control movement in that direction. Proprioceptive exercises must begin gradually, with controlled ROM and at low velocity in single planes. When this stage has been mastered, the patient may progress through a greater ROM at higher velocities and into multiplanar patterns. Progression may begin in the seated position and end with standing on one limb.

Isokinetic Exercise

Isokinetic knee extension and flexion exercises may be used in the rehabilitation of patellofemoral dysfunction if the following concepts are considered:

1. High rather than low velocity should be used. High-velocity knee extension produces lower PFJRF. When angular velocity increases, the muscle tension generation ability decreases.[22, 28]

2. The arc of motion that is chosen should be specific to the patient's condition. As emphasized previously, the arc of motion should not cause further aggravation of symptoms. Traditionally, short-arc TKE exercise has been advocated while resisted motion in greater degrees of flexion have been avoided because of the increased PFJRF.[16, 45, 61, 83] High-velocity isokinetic exercise often allows the patient to exercise through a full arc of motion which under low-velocity conditions would cause pain. Sczepanski et al.[70] and Brownstein et al.[8] have demonstrated, respectively, that the VMO is more selectively recruited in the range of 60 to 85 degrees and 60 to 90 degrees.

3. Taping or other realignment devices should be considered to allow for pain-free isokinetic exercise with increased torque development. McConnell[48] has demonstrated increased performance of isokinetic exercise with taping. Conway et al.[11] compared the McConnell taping protocol to the use of the Palumbo

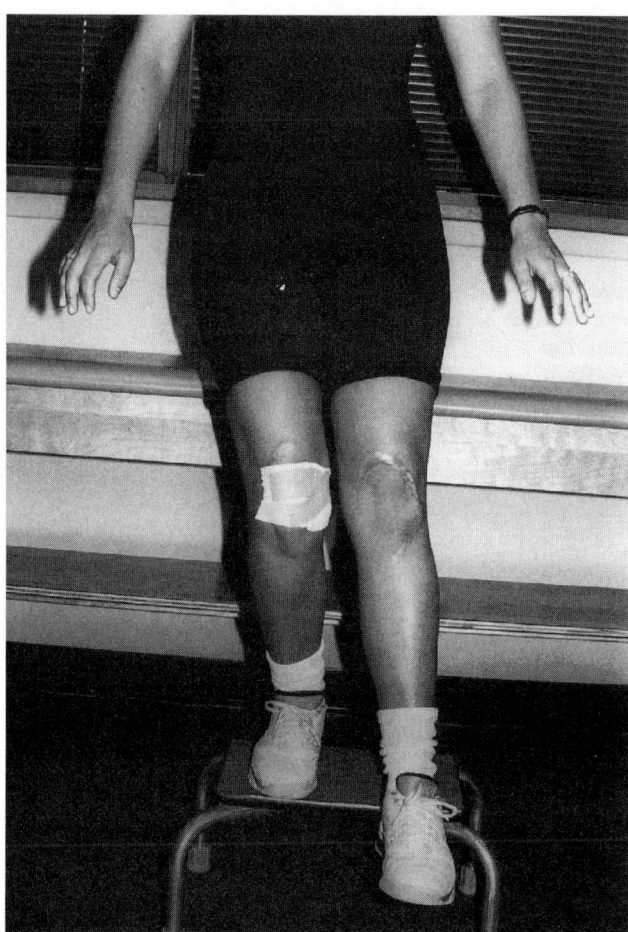

FIG 51-10.
Step-up exercise with McConnell taping.

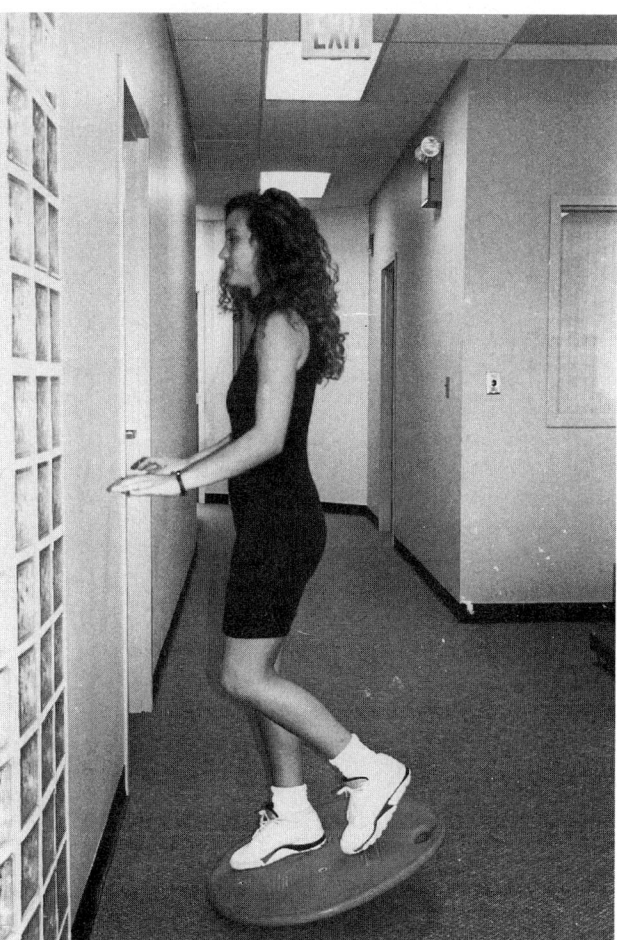

FIG 51-11.
Proprioceptive training using the BAPS board.

brace and found that both increased the subject's ability to generate isokinetic torque at 60 degrees per second eccentrically, but only taping allowed improved torque concentrically at the same speed.

4. The velocity and type of contraction (concentric vs. eccentric) may be significant in VMO recruitment. A recent study found that concentric isokinetic knee extension at 120 degrees per second produced a greater VMO–vastus lateralis EMG ratio than eccentric contractions at the same velocity or than concentric contractions at 60 degrees per second. At 60 degrees per second, neither type of contraction was more significant than the other in improving the VMO–vastus lateralis ratio.[70] Although 120 degrees per second is faster than 60 degrees per second, it is still in the low- to mid-velocity range. This initial study on normal subjects adds another dimension of support for the use of high-velocity isokinetic exercise for the patient with patellofemoral dysfunction.

Eccentric isokinetic training has been shown to increase both eccentric and concentric strength at speeds other than the training speed for the hamstrings.[6, 66] Eccentric isokinetic training produced no significant gains in concentric isokinetic strength for the quadriceps.[6, 80] These studies compared velocities between 60 degrees per second and 180 degrees per second. The VMO was found to be almost twice as active as either the rectus femoris or vastus lateralis during eccentric activation at 30 degrees per second.

Open-Chain and Closed-Chain Activities

The exercises previously described are considered open-chain exercises because the distal portion of the extremity is free to move and has no weightbearing load through it. These exercises, in which the foot is free to move, such as leg lifts, and isometric, isokinetic, and isotonic knee extension and flexion exercises, continue to have their place in the rehabilitation of the knee. They may be used to enhance strength and endurance, particularly while the patient is in a nonweightbearing status. The compre-

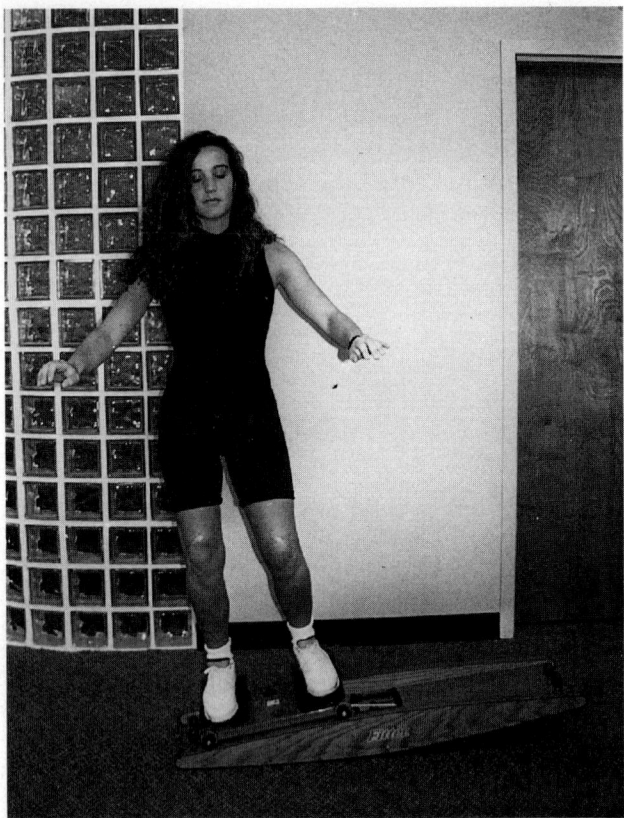

FIG 51–12.
Proprioceptive training using the Fitter.

hensive rehabilitation program will use a combination of exercises based on the requirements, both physical and emotional, of the individual patient.

Closed-chain activities are widely used at this time for rehabilitation of many types of knee problems.[5] Closed-chain activities require that the end segment, in this case the foot, be fixed. Activities such as step-ups, partial squats, leg presses, and exercise on an independent-action stair climber all meet this criterion. The obvious benefits of this type of exercise include: (1) it is functional; (2) it allows for varying velocities depending on the activity requirement; (3) it occurs in all three planes; (4) it encourages synergistic muscle contractions; (5) it facilitates normal proprioceptive feedback mechanisms[33, 34]; and (6) it produces less anterior tibial translation during extension.[87]

Functional Closed-Chain Vastus Medialis Obliquus Training

Vastus medialis obliquus strengthening and training must continue in a closed-chain weightbearing manner to provide functional dynamic medial stability to the patella. NMES, biofeedback, self-palpation, and training in front of a mirror are all techniques that should be incorporated into the rehabilitation and home training sessions to get the patient to recruit and maintain contraction of the VMO during functional exercises and activities. The following maneuvers are designed to train the patient to gain VMO and quadriceps control of the knee by applying gradually increasing stresses. Functional closed-chain activities have the advantage of requiring both concentric and eccentric contractions. Eccentric contractions are important in maximizing the functional control of the knee required for activities of daily living (ADLs) and sports.[25]

Electromyographic Biofeedback

Electromyographic biofeedback may be used to enhance the contraction or relaxation of any muscle accessible to surface electrode placement. This discussion focuses on the use of biofeedback to enhance the recruitment pattern of the VMO as it relates to the vastus lateralis. McConnell[48, 49] discusses the use of simultaneous VMO and vastus lateralis EMG monitoring. She finds that patients with PFPS frequently have less than a 1:1 VMO–vastus lateralis ratio and often the VMO is recruited after the vastus lateralis. EMG biofeedback training should include not only high-intensity VMO recruitment but also early VMO recruitment. The use of biofeedback allows the patient to acquire a motor skill in combination with strengthening the muscle.

VMO biofeedback monitoring can be done during any of the exercises the patient is to perform. The use of biofeedback during functional activities, such as step-up and step-down (Fig 51–13), sit-to-stand, and walking, will be the most beneficial. The patient's loss of ability to reach the EMG threshold is a sign of fatigue and is the patient's cue to stop the activity until recovery occurs. This approach keeps the patient focused on the target muscle and does not allow him or her to develop a muscle substitution pattern.

Sitting

The patient sits with the knee comfortably flexed with the foot on the floor. He or she palpates the VMO and contracts the quadriceps. This should be performed in varying degrees of flexion and with adduction to facilitate the VMO.

Partial Squats

The patient begins with quarter-squats while maintaining good lower extremity and upper body alignment (Figs 51–14 and 51–15). The lower extremity must be controlled to prevent excessive pronation, tibial rotation, and varus or valgus deviation at the knee. The depth of the squat is increased as the pa-

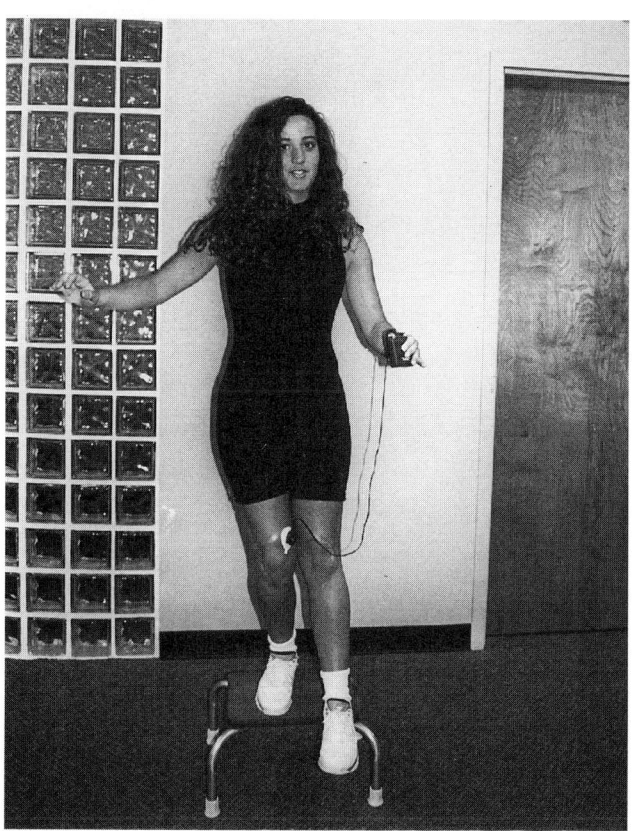

FIG 51-13.
Closed-chain step-up with biofeedback for the Vastus medialis obliquus.

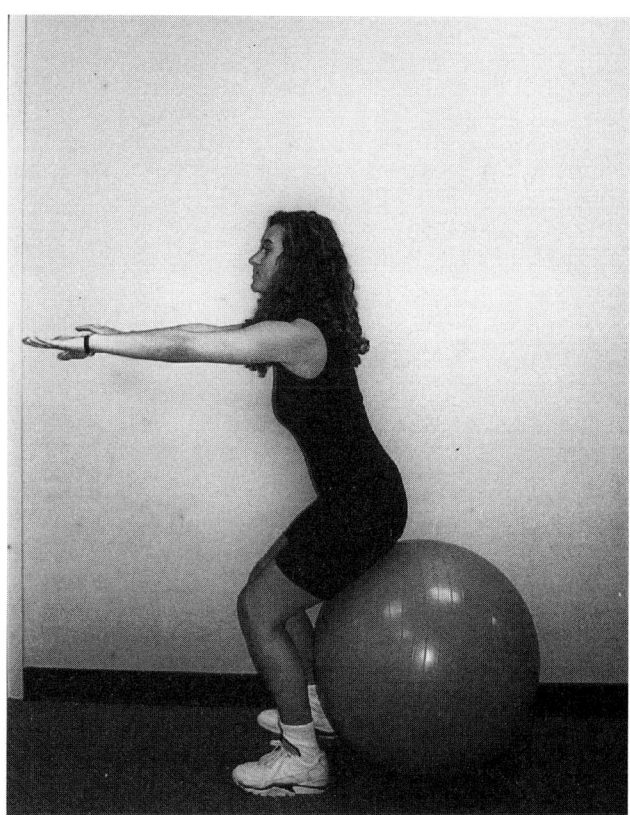

FIG 51-14.
Closed-chain partial squat.

tient becomes able to perform it without pain. The quality rather than the quantity of exercise must be encouraged. If form is deteriorating and the VMO is fatiguing, as demonstrated by EMG monitoring, the exercise should be stopped. Another set should be attempted after a rest. It is best to begin by performing multiple sets of low-stress repetitions to build control and endurance. Resistance is added as the biomechanics improve and there is no pain (Fig 51-16).

Lunge

Single leg lunges in the forward plane may begin if the patient has successfully completed partial squats. The lunge should occur with the knee moving forward in the midsagittal plane of the foot. The degree of flexion begins at 20 to 30 degrees, with progression to greater degrees as appropriate for the individual's condition and goals.

Resistive Closed-Chain Exercise

The partial squats and lunges initially use body weight for resistance. Elastic tubing or a pulley system may be used to increase the resistance for the more advanced patient (Figs 51-17 and 51-18). The same principles of retraining and biomechanical alignment apply to the use of those systems. Pulleys provide a preset constant tension throughout the exercise for easier monitoring, whereas tubing provides increasing resistance as it stretches. Tubing therefore provides a maximum resistance at the terminal portion of the movement pattern. The use of tubing may be advantageous in an exercise such as the squat where less resistance in the more flexed range and greater resistance in the terminal upright portion of the activity may be wanted. The use of a pulley system may be preferable for performing resisted gait through several cycles of the gait pattern in which a constant resistance throughout all cycles is required.

Stair Climbers vs. Stairs

A variety of stair-climbing machines are available for professional and home use. Mechanical stair-climbing exercise can be a valuable tool when used in moderation and with proper supervision. The patient must learn to limit and vary the ROM appropriately, step symmetrically, and use the proximal and distal musculature in a balanced manner (Fig 51-19). Taping and biofeedback may be helpful initially to aid in proper motor control (Fig 51-20).

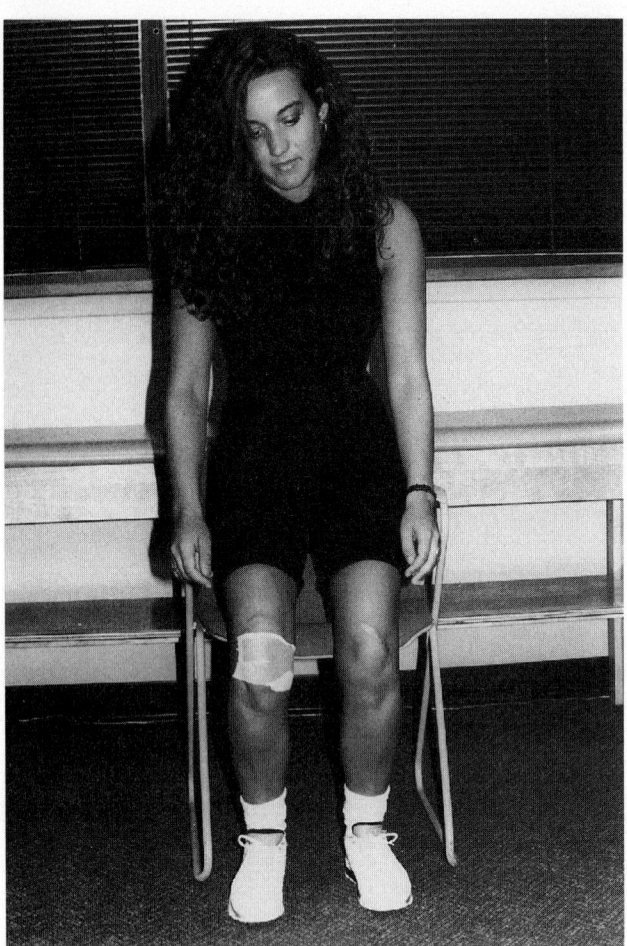

FIG 51–15.
Modified squat exercise with McConnell taping.

A thorough analysis of mechanical stair climbers as related to ROM and joint compression forces is not available at this time. In its absence, some assumptions must be made. (1) The knee extension forces and consequent PFJRF and tibiofemoral compression forces required to take a step on a stair climber are less than those required to lift a person's body weight up a step of equal height. On a stair climber, the body is not lifted, and the foot pedal is pushed away with forces that may be a fraction of the body weight. (2) The muscular forces may be reduced on the stair climber by increasing the speed of the pedals. The degree of knee flexion required is related not only to the height of the step but also to the foot position and ankle plantar flexion pattern. The greater the degree of ankle plantar flexion, the less ROM required at the knee. Therefore, patients should be instructed on symmetric movement patterns throughout all joints bilaterally. DeCarlo et al.[14] examined EMG and joint movements during use of the StairMaster and found significant concentric co-contraction of the quadri-

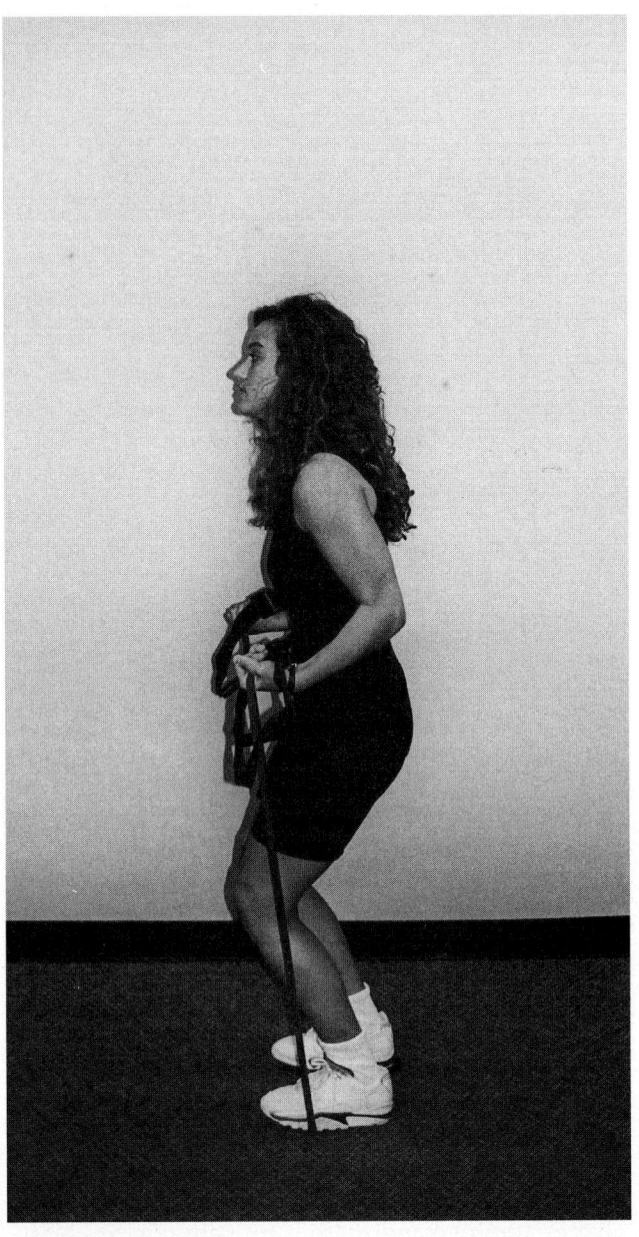

FIG 51–16.
Closed-chain resistive partial squat with elastic cord.

ceps and hamstrings during the climbing cycle. Co-contraction results in decreased anterior shear forces at the tibiofemoral joint, reducing stresses on the meniscus and anterior cruciate ligament.

Patient Education

We believe our role as patient educators is a vital one. Patients who are taught the mechanism of their injury or the biomechanics of their condition will have a greater understanding of how to avoid further pain and progression of their dysfunction. Patients are taught which portions of their ROM to avoid and

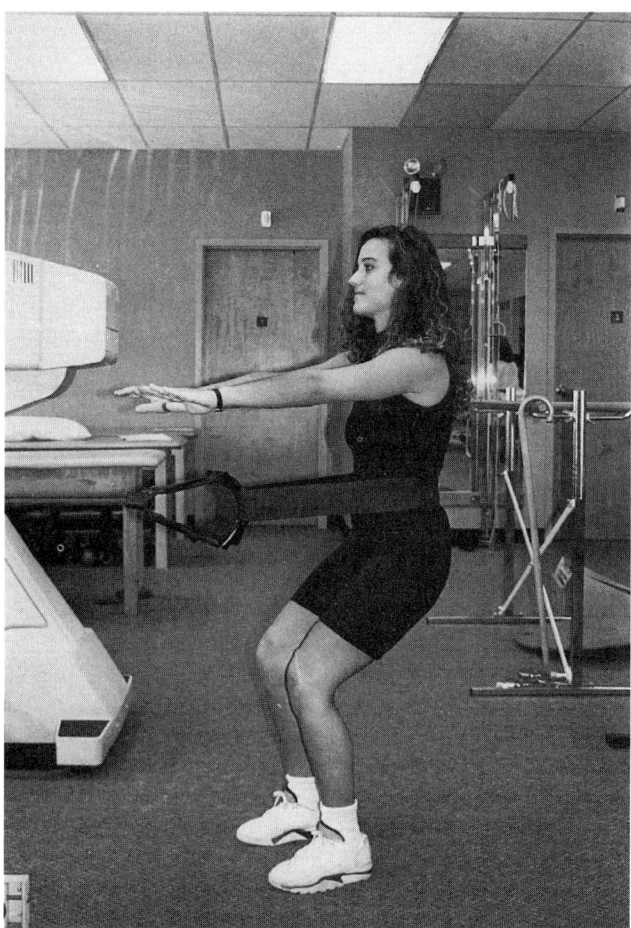

FIG 51–17.
Resistive closed-chain quadriceps exercise.

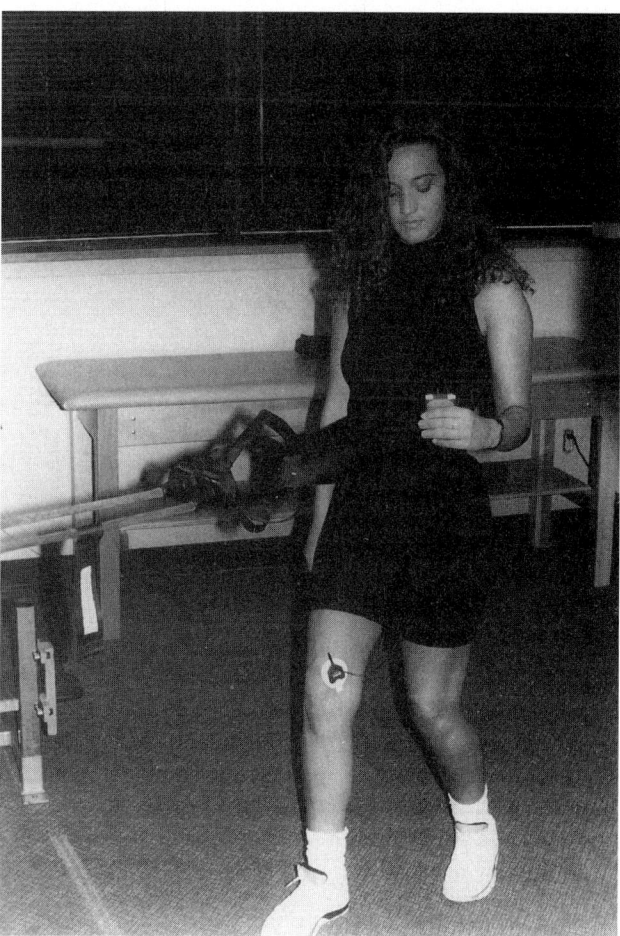

FIG 51–18.
Resistive closed-chain quadriceps exercise with biofeedback.

which activities are stressful to the knee. Patients should be advised of the importance of weight control to reduce the excessive forces carried by the knees of an overweight person. An evaluation of patients' activities at their workplace, home, and recreational site should be performed. Patients are advised as to which routine activities put them at risk for further injury and pain. If possible, they are helped to find a way to continue performing those activities in a nonstressful manner. If a patient is told to avoid an activity like running, he or she is guided toward a different activity, such as biking or swimming, which will provide the same physical benefits and eventually the same emotional ones.

Patients should be instructed in how to perform a self-examination of their knees to look for signs of inflammation and effusion. This practice will be especially important as activities are altered. Patients are also instructed in the need for continuing strength, endurance, and flexibility programs to maintain proper motor control of the knee and to maintain good weight control. The more information patients have about their condition, the more active roles they are prepared to play in their rehabilitation.[52]

PHYSICAL THERAPY AFTER ARTHROSCOPIC PROCEDURES

Patients who undergo an arthroscopic procedure can usually begin the rehabilitation program at home with isometric quadriceps setting exercises the same day. The next day the patient can begin to strengthen all muscle groups in the lower extremity with a straight leg raise exercise program. When the patient can actively flex the knee to approximately 70 degrees, hip flexion in the sitting position can be added.

In the initial visit to the physical therapist's office, common findings include a knee that is warm to the touch, joint effusion, muscle atrophy, and a decrease in muscle tone and strength (especially in the quadriceps and in the VMO in particular). Nodules or a build-up of adhesions or scar tissue over the arthroscopic incisions, a loss of ROM, and tenderness

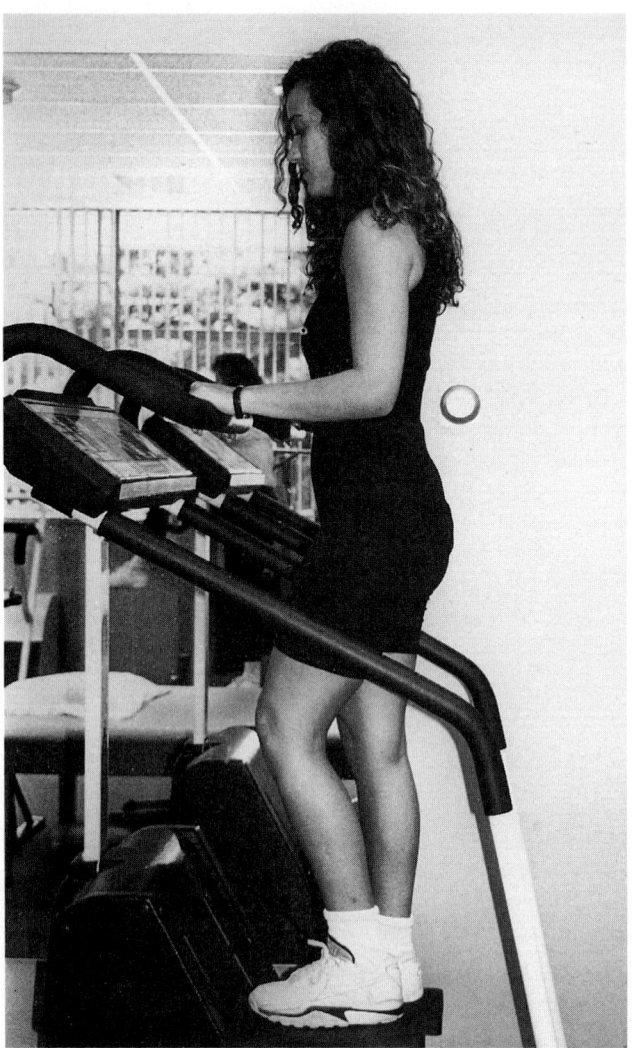

FIG 51–19.
Stair climbing closed-chain exercise.

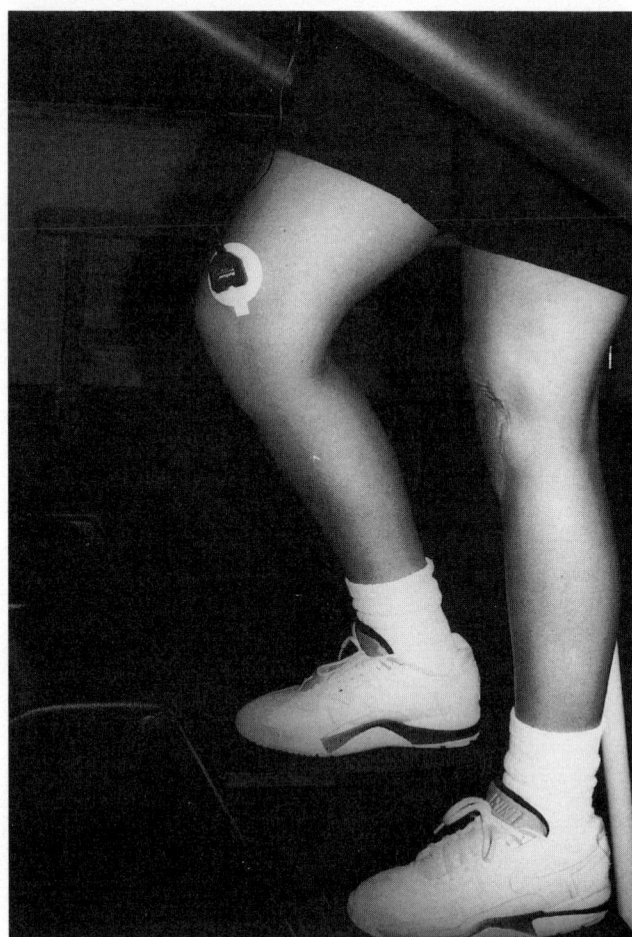

FIG 51–20.
Stair-climbing exercise with biofeedback training for the vastus medialis obliquus.

in the medial and lateral compartments of the knee (especially over the medial and lateral arthroscopic incisions) are also common. In rare cases, the patient will be unable to perform a straight leg raise or will have an extensor lag.[62]

In terms of the stretching and strengthening exercise program, the treatment is similar to that discussed above. However, the treatment program will vary in relation to the surgery itself. Upon completion of the active exercises, if there is no active swelling, heat is applied to the knee for approximately 10 to 15 minutes to promote relaxation of the musculature and tight soft tissues.[42] Patellar mobilization and knee ROM exercises follow.[12, 41] Usually, the patient will require (1) inferior glides of the patella for increased knee flexion, (2) superior glides for extension, and finally (3) medial glides to stretch the lateral patellar static and dynamic stabilizers. If there is an extensor lag, more effort should be directed to superior glides to stretch any tight peripatellar tissues that can bind the patella. After patella mobilization is performed, active and passive ROM exercises such as wall slides and prone flexion with a tire tube or extension over the end of a treatment plinth are introduced to increase knee flexion or extension.

If the patient has painful adhesions or scar tissue under the arthroscopic incision, 3-MHz ultrasound and transverse friction massage are used to reduce the size and tenderness of the adhesions.[12, 51, 86] If there is moderate to severe effusion in the knee, electrical stimulation combined with ice, compression, and elevation is helpful. The Cryocuff Aircast C is an excellent modality for simultaneously applying cold and compression. Medial or lateral compartment pain can be managed by various forms of electrical stimulation.[40, 54, 76]

As the patient progresses, he or she is taken off therapeutic modalities. The rehabilitation program focuses on strength, closed-chain, and endurance exercises. The patient may use patellar taping, a patellar restraining brace, or a horseshoe-shaped felt pad placed around the patella and secured with a woven elastic (Ace) bandage to provide better tracking and pain relief during physical activity.

Giving the athlete the go ahead to return to sports participation can be a difficult decision. Objective parameters of fitness or performance should be used to give the athlete permission to return to sports. Our criteria for permitting a patient to return to sports include: (1) the quadriceps and hamstrings on the injured leg at least 90% as strong as on the noninjured side at both low (60 degrees per second) and midspeed (180 degrees per second) testing as measured by an isokinetic dynamometer; (2) the performance of agility drills without pain or effusion; and (3) the completion of training sessions on various types of closed-chain equipment without pain or effusion. If the patient has met these criteria, he or she is permitted to return to sports-specific drills on a daily basis which are gradually increased in intensity and duration. Over a few weeks the athlete may return to sports participation without restriction.

PHYSICAL THERAPY AFTER PATELLAR REALIGNMENT

Patients that have undergone a proximal or distal patellar realignment are usually referred to physical therapy approximately 1 to 3 weeks postoperatively. The patient is placed in an ROM-limiting brace that provides support and stability to the knee.[69] A continuous passive motion (CPM) unit is commonly prescribed immediately after surgery. This machine enables the knee and patellofemoral joint to begin moving much earlier, helping to prevent arthrofibrosis.[40, 57, 67] Patients using the CPM obtain increased ROM of the knee and increased patellar mobility without as much scarring and adhesion formation in the suprapatellar pouch and medial and lateral compartments of the knee.[9] Common findings in these patients include a loss of muscle tone, moderate atrophy with a concomitant loss of muscle strength, loss of motion, and an extensor lag.

After this more invasive procedure, the physical therapy program is similar to that following other arthroscopic surgery. However, the initial emphasis is on restoring ROM and eliminating any extension lag, rather than on obtaining muscle strength.

How quickly ROM is obtained postoperatively varies from person to person. It is clearly advantageous to restore ROM as soon as it is safely possible. The early establishment of normal patellar mobility and knee ROM reduces the incidence of complications such as pain, atrophy, extension lag, and arthrofibrosis. If the knee is stiff, the goal is to gain at least 5 degrees of flexion every 2 days.

Immediately after surgery, the patient is encouraged to perform isometric quadriceps exercises. By the second postoperative day, the patient can add straight leg raises to the program. If the patient is unable to perform a straight leg raise, the physical therapist may try eccentric or descending straight leg raises. If the patient is unable to perform a descending straight leg raise, electrical stimulation or biofeedback may be helpful to reeducate and facilitate the quadriceps. When the patient is discharged from the hospital the goal for the patient is to achieve approximately 45 degrees of flexion and have the ability to perform straight leg raises and hip abduction and adduction. The patient is also instructed to continue the rehabilitation program at home until he or she starts on an outpatient physical therapy program.

Physical therapy usually begins about 1 to 3 weeks postoperatively. The treatment program is centered around increasing patellar mobility, ROM of the knee, and muscle strength of the entire leg. By 6 weeks postoperatively, the patient should have at least 0 degrees of extension to over 90 degrees of flexion. At 9 to 12 weeks, the ROM should be within normal limits, the strength training program should be progressing well, and the patient should be performing closed-chain work without complications (i.e., pain, effusion). Walking on a treadmill, the Nordic-Track ski machine, and agility drills are incorporated into the treatment program as tolerated by the patient.

The progression of the treatment program and the criteria for returning to sports participation is as outlined in the discussion of physical therapy after arthroscopy, above.

OSTEOCHONDRITIS DISSECANS

Osteochondritis dissecans and chondral fractures present with similar clinical signs and symptoms. The degree of severity may vary from that of the developing lesion of osteochondritis dissecans to complete separation of the osteochondral body. The chondral fracture may be detectable only upon probing in the incomplete stage or may have progressed to a large flap or crater of exposed subchondral bone.[7, 37, 79] The rehabilitation of these cartilage lesions must progress gradually to prevent further disruption and to promote healing.

The goal of nonsurgical treatment is to create a healing environment with minimal stress that promotes restoration of congruent joint surfaces. If the lesion is stable, eliminating all stressful activities, such as running, jumping, excessive walking, and full stair climbing, may be adequate to allow healing. If after 4 to 6 weeks symptoms persist, a weightbearing brace or nonweightbearing ambulation with a knee immobilizer may be prescribed for the next 6 weeks.[32] The knee immobilizer may be removed several times a day for gentle ROM exercises.

Typical Treatment

Nonweightbearing

Inflammation: Treat inflammation with anti-inflammatory drugs, compression, elevation, cold.

Range of motion: Begin gentle ROM exercises as indicated.

Patellar mobilization: To prevent shortening of peripatellar tissue.

Lying proximal muscle group program: Straight leg lifts in all four planes; add a 1-lb weight if the patient is able to do five sets of 10 repetitions or three sets of 20 repetitions.

Standing proximal muscle group program: Standing on the noninvolved leg to exercise the involved extremity on the Cybex Multi-Hip or with a wall pulley system.

Isometrics: Multiangled isometric exercises may be performed in the range that does not permit compression of the articular defect until it is stable. VMO training should be included.

Terminal knee extension: TKE exercises incorporating VMO training should be implemented to prevent an extensor lag.

Stationary bike: Low resistance with the seat high for 5 to 10 minutes; patients may choose a comfortable cycling speed.

Pool exercise: Active knee extension and flexion, proximal muscle group exercises in water; gentle flutter kicks.

Flexibility: Hamstring, quadriceps, iliotibial band, gastrocnemius, soleus, lateral patellar retinaculum, and other structures as indicated.

Lower leg strengthening: All ankle motions may be exercised with elastic bands or manual resistance.

Partial Weightbearing

Stationary bike: Resistance may be increased to a moderate level as tolerated.

Pool program: Walking forward, backward, and from side to side in water may begin if the patient is allowed 50% weightbearing.

Proprioceptive training: The patient may begin using the BAPS, KAT, or other proprioceptive training system in the sitting position or standing bilaterally with hand supports.

Manual resistance: Manual resistance of hip and knee extension and flexion patterns, including proprioceptive neuromuscular facilitation (PNF) diagonals and rhythmic stabilizers, are used to activate synergistic muscle groups in functional movement patterns.

Partial weightbearing minisquats: Bilateral quarter-squats with handrail support are begun to prepare the musculature and joint for the full weightbearing stresses soon to follow.

Isokinetic exercise: High-speed isokinetic exercise produces less JRF than low-speed sessions. Nissell et al.[55] found that tibiofemoral compression forces produced during isokinetic knee extension at 30 degrees per second could be nine times body weight. When the speed of the exercise was increased to 180 degrees per second, JRF decreased to five times body weight.

Full Weightbearing

Wall sit: The patient may perform an isometric wall-sitting exercise at various angles. The patient keeps the lower legs perpendicular to the floor, leans back against a wall, partially squats, and holds until the quadriceps fatigue.

Partial squats: The patient may progress to bilateral half-squats without hands.

Lunge: A program of quarter-squat lunges are begun when the patient is able to successfully complete three sets of 20 bilateral squats.

Sit-to-stand: The patient should progress from a high seat to a low seat during the sit-to-stand exercise.[60]

Step-ups: Low-height step-ups should begin with emphasis on smooth weight transfer and lift. When the patient is able to perform four sets of 10 repetitions, he or she progresses to the next height.

Proprioceptive exercises: Full weightbearing, simple BAPS exercises with the knee straight and in 15 to 20 degrees of flexion may begin. Fitter and side-slide activities may also be initiated.

Resistive cord: Lunges, partial squats, and controlled gait activities may begin with resistive cord.

Ski machine: The ski machine may be used as an aerobic exercise device to replace running.

MENISCAL REPAIRS

This description of rehabilitation is for the patient who has just undergone meniscus repair without having serious ligament damage or repair. If ligaments have been injured, this factor must be taken into account when implementing a rehabilitation program. Because of the advantages of maintaining the menisci rather than removing them, a repair is performed when possible.[2, 19, 68, 84] The harmful effects of high JRF are more likely if there is an abnormal pressure distribution in the knee. Normally, the tibiofemoral weightbearing surface is larger in extension than in flexion and greater on the medial tibial plateau. The menisci play a major role in pressure distribution by enlarging the intact area by two to three times. Therefore, if the menisci are removed, the pressure at the point of tibiofemoral contact may be two to three times greater than with the menisci intact.[74] Rehabilitation following meniscus repair must focus on reducing the strong shear and compressive forces associated with ROM and weightbearing. Therefore, early management of the postoperative patient must limit both of these components. The following guidelines are suggested.

During the first 2 to 3 weeks, the knee is braced at between 30 and 45 degrees of flexion while the patient ambulates with a nonweightbearing gait. The patient should begin submaximal co-contraction isometric exercises of the quadriceps and hamstrings while in the brace. The proximal muscle group–strengthening program of straight leg lifts should also begin.

During postoperative weeks 3 through 6, gentle ROM exercises in the midrange should begin. Partial weightbearing ambulation should progress as strength improves.[10, 17]

During weeks 6 through 8, ROM should increase from 0 to 120 degrees, and weightbearing should progress to full weightbearing. Weights are added to the proximal muscle group program. Midrange isotonic knee extension and flexion should be tolerated without pain. If these exercises are performed without pain or swelling, mild bicycling and swimming exercises should commence around the eighth week.

Over the next 2 to 6 months, the patient can progress through the previously described exercise continuum. Low-level closed-chain activities begin with partial weight shifting to minisquats. Submaximal isokinetic knee extension and flexion should begin with a range-limiting device to protect the terminal extension range and progress through the range of tolerance.

By the fifth month the patient may begin straight jogging at half-speed if the quadriceps strength is 85% to 90% of that of the nonoperative extremity. The patient now progresses through advanced-level activities in preparation for return to sports. If the patient successfully completes the advanced-level rehabilitation program and sports-specific drills, he or she is ready to return to unrestricted sports between the sixth and ninth postoperative month.

REFERENCES

1. Andriacchi TP, et al: A study of lower-limb mechanics during stair climbing, *J Bone Joint Surg [Am]* 42:749–757, 1980.
2. Baratz ME, Rehak DC, Rudert MJ: Peripheral tears of the meniscus: The effect of open versus arthroscopic repair on intra-articular contact stresses in the human knee, *Am J Sports Med* 16:1–6, 1988.
3. Barnett S, Cooney K, Johnston R: Electrically elicited quadriceps femoris muscle torque as a function of various electrode placements, *J Clin Electrophysiol* 3:5–8, 1991.
4. Basmajian JV, DeLuca CJ: *Muscles alive: Their functions revealed electromyographically,* ed 5, Baltimore, 1985, Williams & Wilkens.
5. Binder-Macleod SA, Guerin T: Preservation of force output through progressive reduction of stimulation frequency in human quadriceps femoris muscle, *Phys Ther* 70:32–38, 1990.
6. Bishop KN et al: The effect of eccentric strength training at various speeds on concentric strength of the quadriceps and hamstring muscles, *Orthop Sports Phys Ther* 13:226–230, 1991.
7. Bradley J, Dandy DJ: Osteochondritis dissecans and other lesions of the femoral condyles, *J Bone Joint Surg [Br]* 71:518–522, 1989.
8. Brownstein BA, Lamb RL, Mangine RE: Quadriceps torque and integrated electromyography, *J Orthop Sports Phys Ther* 6:309–314, 1985.
9. Brunet M, Stewart G: Patellofemoral rehabilitation, *Clin Sports Med* 8:319–329, 1989.
10. Cannon WD Jr, Vittori JM: The incidence of healing in arthroscopic meniscal repairs in anterior cruciate ligament–reconstructed knees versus stable knees, *Am J Sports Med* 20:176–181, 1992.
11. Conway A, Malone T, Conway P: Patellar alignment/tracking alteration: Effect on force output and perceived pain, *Isokinetics Exerc Sci* 2:9–17, 1992.
12. Cyriax J, Russell G: Textbook of *orthopaedic medicine,* ed 11, vol 2, Tindall, 1984, London.
13. D'Amico JC, Rubin M: The influence of foot orthosis on the quadriceps angle, *J Am Podiatr Med Assoc* 76:337–340, 1986.
14. DeCarlo M, et al: Electromyographic and cinemato-

graphic analysis of the lower extremity during closed and open kinetic chain exercise, *Isokinetics Exerc Sci* 2:24–29, 1992.
15. DeAndrade JR, Grant C, Dixon A: Joint distension and reflex muscle inhibition in the knee, *J Bone Joint Surg [Am]* 47:313–332, 1965.
16. DeHaven KE, Dolan WA, Mayer PJ: Chondromalacia patellae in athletes, *Am J Sports Med* 7:5–14, 1979.
17. DeHaven KE, Sebastian WJ: Meniscal Tears. In Rider R, editor: *Sports medicine—The school-age athlete,* Philadelphia, 1991, WB Saunders.
18. DeLorme TL, Watkins AL: Techniques of progressive resistance exercises, *Arch Phys Med* 29:263–273, 1948.
19. Deutsch AL, et al: Peripheral meniscal tears; MR findings after conservative treatment or arthroscopic repair, *Radiology* 176:485–488, 1990.
20. Doucette SA, Goble EM: The effect of exercise on patellar tracking in lateral patellar compression syndrome, *Am J Sports Med* 20:434–440, 1985.
21. Engle R: Knee ligament rehabilitation, *Clin Manage,* 10:36–39, 1990.
22. Enoka RM: *Neuromechanical basis of kinesiology,* Champaign, Ill. 1988, Human Kinetic Books.
23. Ercole MA, et al: Knee extensor dynamic torque production during neuromuscular electrical stimulation, *J Clin Electrophysiol* 3:17–20, 1991.
24. Ficat RP, Hungerford DS: *Disorders of the patellofemoral joint,* Baltimore, 1977, Williams, & Wilkens.
25. Fiebert I, Hardy CJ, Werner KL: Electromyographic analysis of the quadriceps femoris during isokinetic eccentric activation. *Isokinetics Exerc Sci* 2:18–23, 1992.
26. Fujikawa K, Seedhem BB, Wright V: Biomechanics of the patello-femoral joint. I: A study of the contact and the congruity of the patello-femoral compartment and movement of the patella, *Eng Med* 12:3–11, 1983.
27. Gajdosik RL: Effects of static stretching on the maximal length and resistance to passive stretch of short hamstring muscles, *J Orthop Sports Phys Ther* 14:250–255, 1991.
28. Ghena DR, et al: Torque characteristics of the quadriceps and hamstring muscles during concentric and eccentric loading, *J Orthop Sports Phys Ther* 14:149–154, 1991.
29. Goodfellow J, Hungerford DS, Zindel M: Patellofemoral joint mechanics and pathology, *J Bone Joint Surg [Br]* 58:287–290, 1976.
30. Gose IC, Schweizer P: Iliotibial band tightness, *J Orthop Sports Phys Ther* 10:399, 1989.
31. Gough JV, Ladley G: An investigation into the effectiveness of various forms of quadriceps exercises, *Physiotherapy* 5:356, 1971.
32. Graf BK, Large RH: Osteochondritis dissecans. In Rider R, editor: *Sports medicine—The school-age athlete,* Philadelphia, 1991, WB Saunders.
33. Gray G: *Chain reaction,* Kirkland, Wash, 1989, Wynn Marketing.
34. Gray G, et al: Plane sense, *Fitness Manage* 30–33, April, 1992.
35. Hanten W, Schulthies S: Exercise effect on electromyographic activity of the vastus medialis oblique and vastus lateralis muscles, *Phys Ther* 70:561, 1990.
36. Henry J: Conservative treatment of patellofemoral subluxation, *Clin Sports Med* 8:261–278, 1989.
37. Hopkinson WJ, Mitchell WA, Curl WW: Chondral fractures of the knee: Cause for confusion, *Am J Sports Med* 13:309–312, 1985.
38. Humphrey D: Flexibility for the knees. *Physician Sportsmed* 18:137–138, 1990.
39. Inman V, Ralston H, Todd F: *Human walking,* Williams & Wilkens. 1981, Baltimore.
40. Kahn J: *Principles and practice of electrotherapy,* New York, 1991, Churchill Livingstone.
41. Kaltenborn F: *Manual therapy of the extremity joints,* Oslo, 1976, Olaf Norlis Bokhandel.
42. Lentell G, Eagan J, Hetherington T: The use of thermal agents to influence the effectiveness of a low load prolonged stretch, *J Orthop Sports Phys Ther,* 15:48, 1992.
43. Lesmes GR et al: Muscle strength and power changes during maximal isokinetic training, *Med Sci Sports* 10:266, 1978.
44. Lieb F, Perry J: Quadriceps function: An anatomical and mechanical study using amputated limbs, *J Bone Joint Surg* 50:1535–1548, 1968.
45. Malek MM, Mangine RE: Patellofemoral pain syndromes. A comprehensive and conservative approach, *J Orthop Sports Phys Ther* 2:108–116, 1981.
46. Manheimer JS, Lampe GN: *Clinical transcutaneous electrical nerve stimulation,* Philadelphia, 1984, FA Davis.
47. Mann R: Biomechanics of running. In D'Ambrosia R, Drez D Jr, editors: *Prevention and treatment of running injuries,* Thorofare, NJ, 1982, Charles B Slack.
48. McConnell J: The management of chondromalacia patellae: A long term solution, *Aust J Physiother* 32:215-223, 1986.
49. McConnell J: *McConnell patellofemoral treatment plan course notes.* Santa Ana, Calif, 1991, McConnell Seminars.
50. Merchant AC, et al: Roentgenographic analysis of patellofemoral congruence angles, *J Bone Joint Surg [Am]* 56:1391–1396, 1974.
51. Michlovitz SL: *Thermal agents in rehabilitation,* Philadelphia, 1986, FA Davis.
52. Milgrom C, et al: Patellofemoral pain caused by overactivity, *J Bone Joint Surg [Am]* 73:1041–1043, 1991.
53. Moran GT, Hall JM, Robertson RN: The use of stationary cycling with biomechanically adjustable pedals in the rehabilitation of ankle and knee injuries, *J Orthop Sports Phys Ther;* 15:46, 1992.
54. Nelson RM, Currier DP: *Clinical electrotherapy,* East Norwalk, Conn, 1987, Appleton-Century-Crofts.
55. Nisell R, et al: Tibiofemoral joint forces during isokinetic knee extension, *Am J Sports Med* 17:49–54, 1989.
56. Nordin M, Frankel V: *Basic biomechanics of the musculoskeletal system,* Philadelphia, 1989, Lea & Febiger.

57. Noyes FR, et al: Intra-articular cruciate ligament. I: Perspectives on graft strength, vascularization and immediate motion after replacement, *Clin Orthop* 173:71, 1983.
58. O'Neill DB, Micheli LJ, Warner JP: Patellofemoral stress: A prospective analysis of exercise treatment in adolescents and adults, *Am J Sports Med* 20:151–156, 1992.
59. Ohno O, et al: An electron microscopic study of early pathology in chondromalacia of the patella, *J Bone Joint Surg* 70:883–899, 1988.
60. Pai Y, Rogers MW: Segmental contributions to total body momentum in sit-to-stand, *J Orthop Sports Phys Ther* 14:128, 1991.
61. Paulos L, et al: Patellar malalignment: A treatment rationale, *Phys Ther* 60:1624–1632, 1980.
62. Paulos LE, et al: Infrapatellar contracture syndrome, an unrecognized cause of knee stiffness with patella entrapment and patella infra, *Am J Sports Med* 15:331–341, 1987.
63. Perry J, Antonelli D, Ford W: Analysis of knee-joint forces during flexed-knee stance, *J Bone Joint Surg [Am]* 57:961–967, 1975.
64. Rhodes VJ: Physical therapy management of patients with juvenile rheumatoid arthritis, *Phys Ther* 71:42, 1991.
65. Rosenberg A, Mikosz RP: Knee biomechanics. In Scott WN, editor: *Ligament and extensor mechanism injuries of the knee—Diagnosis and treatment,* St Louis, 1991, Mosby–Year Book.
66. Ryan LM, Magidow PS, Duncan PW: Velocity-specific mode-specific effects of eccentric isokinetic training of the hamstrings, *J Orthop Sports Phys Ther* 13:33–39, 1991.
67. Salter RB: The biologic concept of continuous passive motion of synovial joints, *Clin Orthop* 242:12–25, 1989.
68. Scott GA, Jolly BL, Henning CE: Combined posterior incision and arthroscopic intra-articular repair of the meniscus, *J Bone Joint Surg [Am]* 68:847–850, 1986.
69. Scuderi G, Cuomo F, Scott WN: Lateral release and proximal realignment for patellar subluxation and dislocation, *J Bone Joint Surg [Am]* 70:856–861, 1988.
70. Sczepanski TL, et al: Effect of contraction type, angular velocity, and arc of motion on VMO: VL EMG ratio, *J Orthop Sports Phys Ther* 14:256–262, 1991.
71. Section on Clinical Electrophysiology, American Physical Therapy Association: *Electrotherapeutic terminology in physical therapy,* Alexandria, V, 1990, American Physical Therapy Association.
72. Shelbourne KD, Nitz P: Accelerated rehabilitation after anterior cruciate ligament reconstruction, *J Orthop Sports Phys Ther* 15:265–269, 1992.
73. Shelton GL, Thigpen LK: Rehabilitation of patellofemoral dysfunction: A review of literature, *J Orthop Sports Phys Ther* 14:243–249, 1991.
74. Smidt GE: Gait in Musculoskeletal Abnormalities. In *Gait in rehabilitation,* New York, 1990, Churchill Livingston.
75. Soderberg GL, Cook TM: An electromyographic analysis of quadriceps femoris muscle setting and straight leg raising, *Phys Ther* 63:1434, 1983.
76. Snyder-Mackler L, Robinson AJ: *Clinical electrophysiology, electrotherapy and electrophysiologic testing,* Baltimore, 1989, Williams & Wilkins.
77. Snyder-Mackler L, et al: Electrical stimulation of the thigh muscles after reconstruction of the anterior cruciate ligament, *J Bone Joint Surg,* 73:1025–1036, 1991.
78. Spencer JD, Hayes KC, Alexander IJ: Knee joint effusion and quadriceps reflex inhibition in man, *Arch Phys Med Rehabil* 65:171–177, 1984.
79. Terry GC, et al: Isolated chondral fractures of the knee. *Clin Orthop* 234:170–177, 1988.
80. Tomberlin JP, et al: Comparative study of isokinetic eccentric and concentric quadriceps training, *J Orthop Sports Phys Ther* 14:31–36, 1991.
81. Voight M, Bell S, Rhoades D: Instrumental testing of tibial translation during a passive Lachman test and selected closed chain activities in the anterior cruciate deficient knee, *J Orthop Sports Phys Ther* 15:49, 1992.
82. Voss DE, Ionta MK, Myers BJ: *Proprioceptive neuromuscular facilitation,* ed 3, New York, 1985, Harper & Row.
83. Wallace L: Rehabilitation following patellofemoral surgery. In Davies GJ, editor: *Rehabilitation of the surgical knee,* Ronkonkoma, NY, 1984, Cypress.
84. Weiss CB, et al: Non-operative treatment of meniscal tears, *J Bone Joint Surg* 17:811–821.
85. Williams M, Lissner H: *Biomechanics of human motion,* Philadelphia, 1962, WB Saunders.
86. Wood EC: *Beards massage. Principles and techniques,* Philadelphia, 1974, WB Saunders.
87. Wozniak Timmer CA: Cycling biomechanics: A literature review, *J Orthop Sports Phys Ther* 14:106–113, 1991.
88. Wyke B: Articular neurology: A review, *Physiotherapy* 58:94, 1972.

52
Knee Rehabilitation After Knee Ligament Injury or Surgery

LONNIE E. PAULOS, M.D.

Patient differentiation
Procedure selection
Surgical techniques
Rehabilitation
Effects of disuse and immobilization on musculoskeletal tissue
Characteristic changes in musculoskeletal tissue
Healing of musculoskeletal tissue
General protocol for rehabilitation
    Immobilization and bracing
    Range-of-motion phase
    Progressive weight-bearing
    Isometric exercises
    Isotonic or progressive resistive exercises

Return to activities and sports
Functional exercises
Isokinetic exercises
Specific procedure protocols
    Anterior cruciate ligament reconstruction
    Posterior cruciate ligament reconstruction
Failure to progress
Summary
Appendix
    ACL protocol
    Semitendinosus protocol
    ACL patellar tendon autograft
    PCL protocol
    PCL and PLRI protocol

The ultimate goal after knee ligament injury or surgery is to restore the knee to full function without loss of motion or long-term impairment. Meeting this goal requires effective communication between members of the health care team—the physician, physical therapist, athletic trainer, *and* the patient. It is the physician who initiates the type and course of treatment, a course designed by him upon evaluation of the injured patient. This course, or "treatment chain," begins with patient differentiation, then moves to a selection of specific procedures or surgical techniques, proceeds to a rehabilitation protocol, and ends with a return to normal function (Fig 52–1).

At all stages of the treatment course the nature of the musculoskeletal tissues and their manner of healing is fundamental to the means of correction, rehabilitation, and ultimate function of the knee after an injury. Thus, the biologic foundation is an integral part of our study on knee injuries.

PATIENT DIFFERENTIATION

Individual characteristics will determine the procedure selected and surgical techniques chosen by the surgeon for an individual patient. Age is a major determinant. For example, prepubescent patients who have potential growth in their knees will require a different type of surgical procedure for anterior cruciate ligament (ACL) reconstruction than that designed for more mature patients. In fact, older patients may require no surgery at all, in light of the functional demands on their knees following rehabilitation.

Patients' morphologic characteristics are another major factor in determining which type of procedures to use. Patients who are loose-jointed tend to heal more slowly and ultimately exhibit greater laxity after ligament reconstruction. These patients require more extensive surgery (particularly in regard to the secondary ligamentous restraints), a prolonged period of time on crutches, and increased work throughout the rehabilitation phases. By contrast,

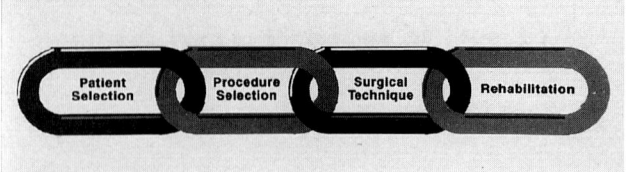

FIG 52–1.
Chain of treatment decisions.

some patients who present after injury or surgery with very stiff swollen knees will require vigorous and less protected therapy to regain normal range of motion. Because of these differences, it is paramount that the physician "read" the soft tissues after major knee injury and prior to undertaking surgery. These differences will affect the timing of surgery as well, for there is now strong evidence that ligamentous surgery within the first 3 to 4 weeks after injury will lead to a more prolonged recovery and loss of motion.[27, 50, 54, 59] Thus, surgery should be delayed for patients with swollen, painful knees, but can be performed immediately in others.

Finally, the patient's athletic prowess and his or her emotional makeup will influence the choice of surgical procedure. Patients who have injured their knees in nonathletic accidents and who tend to be less active should be selected for less invasive procedures, requiring less rehabilitative effort. By contrast, high-intensity athletes desirous of returning to full sports participation will probably require more extensive surgery to better stabilize the knee and, because of their ambition, may better assume the mental and physical demands of a detailed, vigorous, and time-consuming rehabilitation protocol.

Both the poorly motivated and the ambitious patient can compromise the best-laid surgical and rehabilitation plans, since a fine-tuned combination of movement and relaxation are needed for healing musculoskeletal tissue. Many studies have shown that the healing tissues must undergo stress to promote the healing process, yet at the same time overload must be avoided. The overly ambitious patient flirts with disaster secondary to overload, whereas the overly cautious patient may suffer the effects of disuse and immobility. A moderate course between stress and immobility is the ideal route.

PROCEDURE SELECTION

When the physician selects surgery as the better treatment, the procedure chosen should be tailored to the patient's age, the time from presentation to surgery, the patient's physical habitus, and his or her ultimate goal. For example, repair of a torn ACL using a central-third patellar tendon graft is far riskier than using a semitendinosus tendon or allograft. The strong, more inelastic patellar tendon must be accurately placed and demands that patients attain immediate, full range of motion so as to avoid loss of extension, subsequent quadriceps weakness, and patellar entrapment. Patients unlikely to comply with a vigorous rehabilitation program are poor candidates for this type of graft. Timid patients are better candidates for a semitendinosus graft, which is more compliant, requires less accurate anatomic placement, and tolerates a less demanding rehabilitation program.

The decision to perform extraarticular procedures in combination with an intraarticular cruciate reconstruction should be made as a function of the patient's determination and willingness to cooperate in rehabilitative phases designed to diminish loss of motion. Less extensive extraarticular surgery is more appropriate for patients who are less motivated or have less time to spend in the physical therapy unit.

Posterior cruciate ligament (PCL) injuries may be treated conservatively, i.e., without surgery, and with rehabilitative exercises only. These procedures are selected for patients who are less demanding or who cannot devote an extended time on crutches and in physical therapy. Extraarticular surgery is required for the majority of PCL injuries. For this reason, the demands are far greater than for other types of ligament surgery.

SURGICAL TECHNIQUES

Regardless of the patient or procedure selected for surgery, isometric placement of a strong ligament, well fixed to allow early range of motion, should always be the objective. Surgical techniques that result in weaker fixation, such as sutures tied to buttons, should not be used for patients who will undertake physical therapy more aggressively in anticipation of an early return to sports activity. Bone-tendon-bone grafts with interference screw fixation are appropriate for these patients, as this technique is the strongest and can withstand a more rapid rehabilitation program. In cases where meniscal repair is also required, and the goal of the patient is to return to sports quickly, a combined arthroscopic and open meniscal procedure may be preferable; arthroscopic meniscal repair alone requires more protection than open meniscal repair.

Because arthroscopic ligament surgery is less invasive than arthrotomy, the surgeon may consider extending the indications for ligament surgery to patients who would otherwise be poor candidates for an open procedure. Many times, the surgeon can offer the marginal patient an arthroscopic or endoscopic cruciate ligament reconstruction, thereby shortening the rehabilitation time, while providing the patient with a more functional knee and less risk.

REHABILITATION

Early and complete range of motion should be the ultimate goal of a rehabilitation program after a knee ligament injury or surgery. Although there are instances when this goal is unreachable because of multiple ligamentous injuries, the surgeon and physical therapist should make every effort to initiate immediate passive range-of-motion exercises that extend through flexion and extension of the knee. Exceptions to this include collateral ligament repairs, as they are more likely to be nonisometric and require early motion protection during the initial fixation phases of healing. Also, rehabilitation following repair of an unstable meniscus must be modified. Flexion should be delayed for the initial few weeks of meniscal healing because the knee is more unstable in flexion.

As noted above, a more aggressive range-of-motion program is required after grafting with the central-third patellar tendon. Fortunately, this type of program is safe because the bone-tendon-bone graft can be fixed rigidly to the bone tunnels.

One frequent mistake of physicians, physical therapists, and patients is to confuse rehabilitation modalities with those designed for training and return to activities. The knee must *not* be overloaded; cartilaginous surfaces, which have been exposed first to injury and then to surgical trauma, must be allowed to heal. Irrespective of the patient's final goal, rehabilitation phases are the same for all. These phases are designed to reduce swelling from the joint as soon as possible, to return complete passive range of motion to the joint with equal efficiency, and to relieve pain, thereby restoring muscular control. It is not safe to employ overload-type training techniques such as isokinetic, open-chain, and neuromuscular-facilitating exercises before the knee has entered its anabolic state.

The time patients must remain in rehabilitative phases varies in accordance with the procedure selected and the surgical techniques employed. In general, 4 to 6 weeks suffice, after which training modalities can be slowly initiated. At this time, certain patients may elect a less vigorous physical therapy program undertaken at home, in large part, with intermittent supervision by the physical therapist. Patients who are very athletic and wish to return to sports as soon as possible may prefer a more formal training program in a physical therapy setting where isotonic, isokinetic, and other types of rehabilitation devices are available. Since this option is obviously more time-consuming and expensive, it should be undertaken with the full knowledge and cooperation of the patient.

The rehabilitation programs we prescribe are phased in accordance with the procedures and surgery employed, the processes and progress of healing, and the individual patient's goals. If the physician and therapist have laid the proper foundation and framework for the rehabilitation protocol, a successful outcome can be anticipated.

Because our protocol and the approach we take towards rehabilitation are grounded upon the nature of musculoskeletal tissue and the basic principles that govern its healing, a discussion of the biologic foundation for this protocol will precede a detailed exposition of rehabilitation and its phases.

EFFECTS OF DISUSE AND IMMOBILIZATION ON MUSCULOSKELETAL TISSUE

No musculoskeletal tissue can escape the atrophic effects of disuse, whether atrophy be secondary to immobilization in a cast or failure to voluntarily use a limb. Since irreversible changes in these tissues may occur within a short time,[1, 3, 24, 25, 34, 66] every effort must be made to minimize the deleterious effects of immobility. As early as 5 weeks after surgery, effects such as quadriceps atrophy up to a 40% decrease in muscle mass have been observed.[22, 32] Another study[21] has shown that immobilization of a muscle in a shortened position appears to accelerate atrophic change,[32] affecting, in particular, fast-twitch oxidative and slow-twitch endurance fibers. Joint effusion can lead to inhibition of the neuromuscular apparatus and further contribute to atrophy.[20, 62]

There appears to be a point at which the effects of muscle atrophy become irreversible. Where there is significant atrophy, we have observed prolonged deficits in strength despite isokinetic observations showing that strength has returned to normal levels.[49]

It was hoped that neuromuscular stimulators would reduce the effects of disuse and counteract muscle atrophy early in the postoperative course during which isotonic, isokinetic, and functional exercises are contraindicated. Many studies have shown mixed results.[33, 44, 54, 61] Our own controlled study examining the effect of neuromuscular stimulators (NMS) on strength, atrophy, and mobility after ACL reconstruction shows that NMS promotes motion, especially in relation to patellar mobility.[54] Consequently, NMS may be useful in preventing postoperative arthrofibrosis. It does not however, prevent muscle atrophy, but merely retards its development. We found no enhancement of strength after the use of NMS.

CHARACTERISTIC CHANGES IN MUSCULOSKELETAL TISSUE

Motion and weightbearing are fundamental needs of healthy articular (hyaline) cartilage and subchondral bone. Loss of these stresses is rapidly followed by alterations in cartilage fluid dynamics, as demonstrated by rabbit studies that recorded histologic changes as early as 6 days after immobilization. The changes that were recorded included decreased metachromasia (proportional to the loss in chondroitin sulfate), decreased water content, and increased metabolic activity.[63] This study showed that these changes can be permanent after 8 weeks of immobility. Early motion, however, may effectively reverse these changes.[23, 24, 57] Long-term immobility produces chondrocyte clumping and atrophy of the chondral-subchondral unit, after which ulceration at the bone-cartilage interface can occur.[23, 25] After prolonged immobility, we have also observed additional ulcerations secondary to adhesions that are mobilized through manipulation. It appears that the damaging effect of these lesions depends on the length of immobilization.

The ligament-bone junction is also sensitive to disuse and immobilization. In particular, the insertion site is prone to stress deprivation as well as to the effects of resorption after immobilization.[42, 65] With the loss of physiologic stress, collagen that is deposited along lines of stress is randomly deposited and remodeled, resulting in decreases in compliance and tensile strength.[4] Noyes et al.,[46] whose work has shed much light on the effects of immobilized ligaments, have shown that after 8 weeks of immobility, a loss of strength of 40% and loss of stiffness of 30% may occur. More unfortunate is evidence that reversal of these deficiencies may not be complete at 1 year after reinstitution of biologic stress.[46] A process similar to the randomization of collagen deposition in remodeling ligamentous structures can also occur in the periarticular tissues. If it occurs at the immobilized joint, permanent shortening can ensue. Joint stiffness may occur where randomization of collagen is coupled with articular surface adhesions.[1-3, 6, 23, 34, 55] Extreme effort must be used at this juncture since a significant increase in torque is required to move a stiff joint through its range of motion. Increases of up to 12 times normal have been seen by 12 weeks after surgery.[23]

While the necessity of initiating early motion to reduce these adverse effects is obvious, the mode of early motion is less obvious. Although continuous passive motion (CPM) has been advocated as one mode of early motion,[13, 45, 47] we have found that CPM does not encourage patient involvement in rehabilitation. It is not only expensive but requires meticulous attention to range-of-motion settings which can be disturbed by the patient's movements. Inaccurate settings pose a risk to graft integrity in the immediate postoperative period. Hence, early active or passive motion, or both, with *patient involvement* in the range-of-motion program are recommended.

In summary, an early active and passive range-of-motion program is indicated and must be tailored to operative considerations, such as the type of tissue selected for a cruciate ligament graft. The goal is to deliver a safe level of stress to the knee joint and its healing tissues, thereby avoiding the multiple deleterious effects of disuse and immobility.

HEALING OF MUSCULOSKELETAL TISSUES

Injury to hyaline cartilage can occur via the loss of matrix molecules (e.g., proteoglycans) in response to factors such as trauma or surgical arthrotomy, immobilization, infection, and loss of synovial fluids which may occur during joint irrigation with arthroscopy. Mechanical injuries can also occur secondary to blunt or penetrating trauma. Reversal of this type of injury depends primarily on chondrocyte viability and a reestablishment of the vasculature.

Repair of defects of the hyaline cartilage superficial to subchondral bone is limited to chondrocyte proliferation and localized matrix repair. The defect, however, usually remains and may even expand. Unfortunately, the surgeon's ability to modify the healing capabilities of superficial hyaline lesions is limited.[18, 43, 58] On the other hand, should an injury penetrate the subchondral bone, the classic healing response of the subchondral bone produced elsewhere in the body is seen within the cartilage defect. It is nevertheless an imperfect response owing to the long-term inferiority of the regenerated cartilage.[28] Thus, it is important to stimulate healing of these defects through drilling or abrasion chondroplasty. Early motion after this procedure encourages healing of the defect. As illustrated by the classic studies on rabbits by Salter et al.,[57] small defects heal with the benefit of CPM. In our experience, however, large defects in high-stress weightbearing zones affected by chronic knee laxity or instability, such as the patellofemoral joint, do not heal well.

Research on meniscus healing has demonstrated that regeneration occurs in the peripheral vascular zone of the meniscus.[8, 10, 15, 35, 64] This form of healing is extrinsic in nature and depends upon the migration of reparative cells from the vascular bed. The cells are transformed into fibroblasts which in turn produce collagen and heal the defect via a fibrocartilaginous scar. This transformation will occur if the environment is protected from shear stress secondary to extensive motion or weightbearing.

The intrinsic sources of meniscal healing are now the focus of some interest. The term *intrinsic sources* refers to the inherent capability of meniscal cells, nourished by synovial fluid diffusion, to initiate a healing response in the "white zone," or the area independent of an extrinsic vascular supply.[12, 64] A fibrin clot is used to augment this particular healing response, whose mechanism seems to act by virtue of a platelet-derived growth factor.[11, 64]

Ligament healing is dependent on a number of variables. The first consideration is the strength of the initial fixation of a ligament graft. An inverse relationship exists between the strength of this fixation and the healing of the graft at the fixation site. Factors contributing to the initial loss of fixation strength are cyclic loading, tissue creep, suture migration, and tissue necrosis at the fixation site. The superiority of interference bone screws for bone plug-to-bone tunnel fixation over staples or sutures has been documented by several studies.[19, 40, 41] The healing response of bone-to-bone healing has been shown to be superior to the response of soft tissue-to-bone healing.[9, 17, 41] Such superior fixation techniques have allowed earlier motion and weightbearing with decreased residual morbidity and reduced arthrofibrosis,[16] and have accounted for the near-universal acceptance of the patellar tendon autograft as the standard for ACL reconstructions at the present time.

The choice of semitendinosus or gracilis graft, or both, for reconstruction is controversial with concerns centering principally on their method of healing within bony tunnels. Several reports have noted that the histologic healing patterns of soft tissue to bone resemble fracture healing, i.e., enchondral ossification.[60, 61] Initial fixation of these tendon grafts is dependent upon non-interference screw techniques such as suture or screw and washer fixation, both of which have the potential to create local soft tissue necrosis and stress riser effects at tunnel margins. To counter these adverse effects, alterations in screw and washer configurations have been tested.[38, 49, 56] However, much more experimentation on ligament fixation and graft-to-bone healing remains to be done.

Consideration must be given to the course of ligament tissue healing (Fig 52–2). The healing response of soft tissues can be divided into three phases.[14] The first phase is the acute inflammatory phase lasting only 72 hours. The second phase, repair and regeneration, occurs between 48 hours and 6 weeks and is characterized by fibroblastic proliferation and migration. It is coupled to new collagen meshwork production, i.e., type III collagen. The third phase is characterized by remodeling and maturation and can begin as early as 3 weeks and proceed for many months. This phase is highlighted by replacement of type III collagen by type I mature collagen and the remodeling of collagen patterns along lines of stress.

The strength of tendon and ligament substitutes at 3 to 12 months after implantation has been tested in numerous animal studies. Results at 1 year show maximal strength to be approximately 50% of the original strength measurement.[5, 14, 17, 29, 38, 39, 48] Allograft tissues apparently undergo a healing process similar to that of autografts, as noted above.[9, 60] However, the healing time may actually be prolonged with the use of larger allografts, such as the entire patellar tendon or Achilles tendon grafts, owing to the larger cross-sectional area.

Our observations show further that the ligamentous healing response is patient dependent. We have observed a spectrum of healing capabilities, ranging from patients with lax ligament to scar formers. The former present signs of diffuse joint laxity with hyperextension of knees, elbows, and other joints, and may require more careful protection than the scar-former, who seems to be at greater risk for arthrofibrosis and generalized stiffness due to an aggressive healing response. Scar-formers may require a more aggressive rehabilitative protocol, as primary patellar

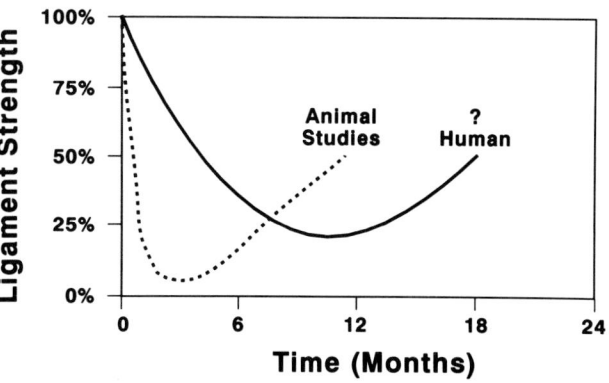

FIG 52–2.
Time course of ligament healing after reconstruction.

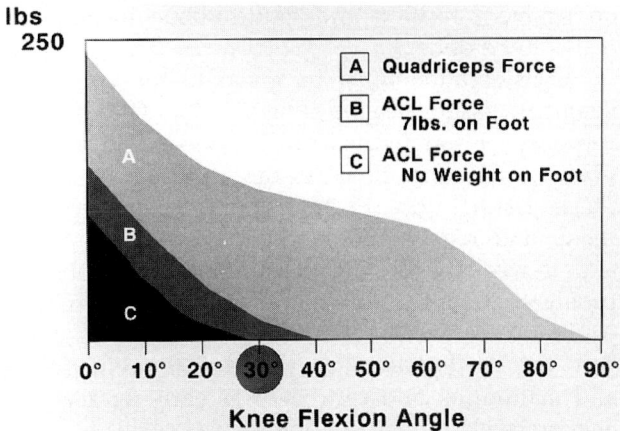

FIG 52–3.
Force on the anterior cruciate ligament (ACL) reconstruction is minimized by avoiding active knee extension past 30 degrees.

entrapment syndrome may develop in patients in this category.[53]

Biomechanical considerations are another factor in ligamentous healing. Several modes of mechanical failure which must be prevented include excessive acute overload due to reinjury, cyclic stress creating fatigue cycles at stress points (e.g., the margins of bony tunnels), and stretching beyond the elastic limit.[52] Several studies have shown that graft tension increases with knee extension exercises, particularly in the range of 0 to 30 degrees of extension (Fig 52–3), due to the anterior tibial drawer produced by the action of the quadriceps and patellar tendon.[7, 31, 51] The forces on the ligaments that occur during functional activities must also be considered.

Harmful effects of these biomechanical stresses on ACL reconstructions can be avoided by careful, isometric positioning of the graft and avoidance of active knee extension (particularly from 30 degrees to full extension).

The latest attempts to protect reconstructed ligaments involve graft tensioning at the time of implantation. Although the proper tension of a ligament reconstruction is unknown, it will most likely be a function of the type of tissue and the specific implant location. The relatively stiff patellar tendon graft[26, 48] probably requires less tensioning than more compliant tissues such as the semitendinosus, gracilis, and Achilles tendon. In my judgment, these latter tissues require higher pre-tension at insertion.

GENERAL PROTOCOL FOR REHABILITATION

In selecting the rehabilitative protocol it is vital that the healing factors discussed above be clearly kept in mind. The various forms we use when planning a patient's knee rehabilitation are illustrated in the appendix to this chapter. Our approach starts with an initial protective period, which is omitted in simple arthroscopic procedures, such as meniscectomy or debridement, and prolonged in the most extensive procedures, such as PCL reconstruction. The forms provide a guideline and format for the patient and therapist alike. The specific protocols on each form are derived from the surgeon's knowledge of the healing factors involved in the particular operative procedure and the goals of the surgery, and are designed to meet the individual patient's needs and concerns.

The forms serve as the initial rehabilitation prescription. As the patient proceeds through the recovery phase, it is important that the physician assess soft-tissue healing responses and adjust the prescription accordingly.

Immobilization and Bracing

The initial protective phase should be as short as possible. In general, immobilization should last no longer than 3 to 4 weeks, and at most, 6 weeks. In most cases, complete immobilization rarely exceeds 10 days. Exceptions include PCL and posterolateral reconstructions which may be protected for a 3 to 4 week period.

The angle at which knee flexion in immobilization is allowed depends upon the procedure employed. For example, an angle of 15 degrees is appropriate after PCL reconstruction and an angle of 30 degrees is appropriate after ACL reconstruction. A rehabilitative-type knee brace that is easy to apply, permits wound inspection, facilitates patellar mobilization, and has a hinge mechanism that may be easily adjusted for change in range of motion should be used in this initial phase (Fig 52–4).

Range-of-Motion Phase

Passive range of motion exercises should be initiated as early as possible postoperatively. Flexion should be limited to 0 to 90 degrees immediately after ACL reconstruction and from 0 to 40 degrees after PCL reconstruction.

Early active motion must be limited, especially active extension following ACL reconstruction and active flexion after PCL reconstruction. For meniscal repairs, range-of-motion exercises should be modified 4 to 5 weeks postoperatively, depending on the location of the tear.

In reference to CPM, patient-initiated passive and active range-of-motion exercises stimulate pa-

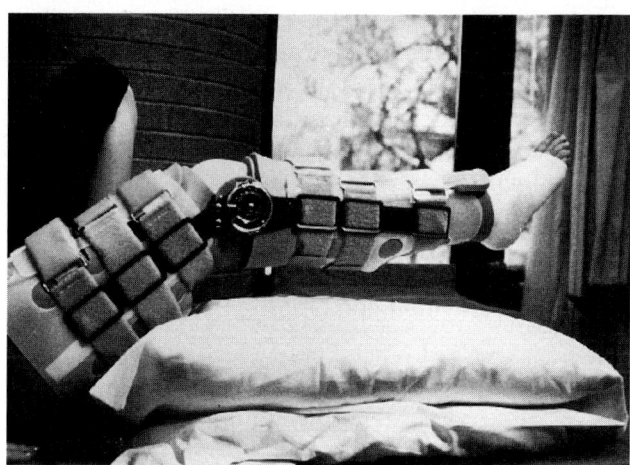

FIG 52–4.
Rehabilitative knee brace allows early, safe, active flexion exercises for anterior cruciate ligament reconstruction under a controlled range of motion.

tient involvement and reduce the risk of graft failure during the initial rehabilitation phases in comparison to CPM. Exercises such as wall slides and contralateral, leg-assisted, extension maneuvers allow patient feedback and produce an enhanced sense of well-being for the patient actively engaged in his or her rehabilitation program.

Progressive Weight-bearing

The initiation of weightbearing into the postoperative rehabilitation protocol requires a specific strategy that is dependent on the patient's condition. Prohibitive or partial weightbearing practices are important for protecting early healing of grafts within tunnels, whether bone-tendon-bone or tendon-bone grafts. Level walking alone may generate up to 40 lb of force on the ACL.[52]

With exceptions made for specific cases, full weightbearing is usually permissible when nearly full extension has been achieved (−5 degrees), swelling has been minimized, no quadriceps lag is present, and there is sufficient quadriceps strength to maintain a normal gait. Full weightbearing after abrasion and drilling chondroplasty should be delayed for a minimum of 6 weeks. This allows for clot adherence and fibrocartilage metaplasia and protects fibrocartilage loss due to the axial loading and shear stresses of weightbearing.

Isometric Exercises

Isometric exercises are the earliest strengthening techniques that may be introduced and undertaken immediately after any surgical procedure on the knee. We favor the use of spectrum isometrics and co-contractions to protect ACL and PCL reconstructions. To minimize antagonistic shear forces, early isometric exercises should be undertaken with the brace locked at 30 to 40 degrees of extension (Fig 52–4) for ACL and 10 degrees for PCL reconstructions. Although electrical muscle stimulation may help in regaining early motion after knee surgery, it does not enhance strength. It does, however, retard atrophy, aids in maintaining patellar mobility, and reduces the incidence of arthrofibrosis.[54]

The "cross-over effect," intended to strengthen the operative limb through isometric exercise of the well leg, has been demonstrated to be successful.[36, 37] Thus, attention to the opposite limb is important, especially during the early phases of rehabilitation.

Isotonic or Progressive Resistive Exercises

The timing and control of isotonic strengthening is important. In our opinion, full motion, antagonist muscle progressive resistive exercises (PREs) must be delayed for as long as 3 months after ACL and PCL reconstruction. We also recommend supervision during the rehabilitation phases to avoid reversing the early healing response. The range of motion and forces utilized must be carefully controlled during PREs as well.

Leg presses should be used to permit a more physiologic co-contraction of antagonist groups. Leg presses can be introduced earlier than leg extension exercises owing to the potential overload on the patellofemoral joint from leg extension exercises.

The necessity of controlling motion and force mandates the use of rehabilitative braces with isotonic exercise. A good starting point for isotonic exercises is 10% of body weight for hamstring and quadriceps exercises with slow progression. In the presence of arthrosis, caution should be used when prescribing isotonic exercises to avoid increasing joint reactive forces.

Functional Exercises

Closed-chain functional exercises are usually introduced at the same time as early weightbearing. Among the advantages of functional exercises are their physiologic nature, the benefits to coordination and proprioception, and the positive feedback to the patient. Braces to control knee motion should be worn while performing these functional exercises. At a minimum of 3 weeks after ACL surgery, sports cords (Fig 52–5) and minisquats are allowed. Station-

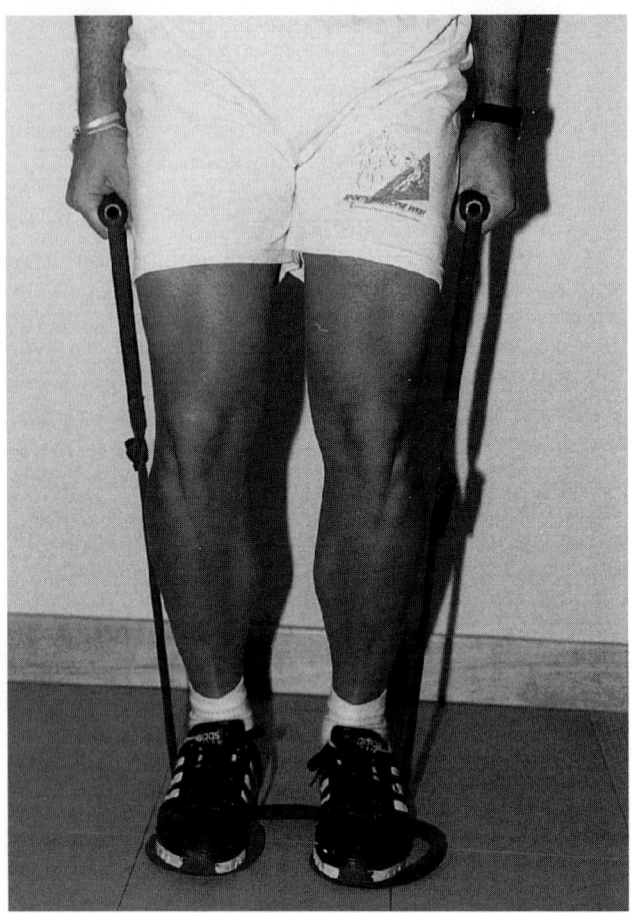

FIG 52–5.
Early introduction of sports cord functional exercises allows hamstrings strengthening after anterior cruciate ligament reconstruction. A brace is preferred.

ary cycling and swimming can begin earlier. Although the pogo ball, balance board, and trampoline have been shown to be beneficial, these activities should be delayed 3 months and then performed with a knee brace for protection.

Isokinetic Exercises

Isokinetic exercises are introduced last in the sequence of strengthening phases; they are usually deferred for at least 20 to 24 weeks after reconstructive procedures. A good time to begin is generally after isotonic exercises are performed pain-free with 10% to 20% of body weight resistance.

High-speed settings should be used to improve strength and coordination after the patient has progressed through the previous phases. Low-speed settings should be deferred until very late in the rehabilitative protocol because of significant force generated at the joint and potential exacerbation of chondrosis. Placement of the pad on the tibia is another important criterion to take into account when prescribing isokinetic exercises. Generally, the pad should be placed on the upper tibia after ACL surgery and on the distal tibia after PCL surgery (Fig 52–6). Isokinetic exercise is more risky in patients with symptomatic patellofemoral joints.

Return to Activities and Sports

The final phase of rehabilitation, which includes a return to activities and sports, must also be governed by specific procedures or conditions. For example, running in place against the resistance of a sports cord can be started as early as 4 weeks after ACL surgery or 24 weeks after PCL surgery, if other factors, such as strength, motion, and stability, are satisfactory. Typically, jogging is begun 16 weeks after ACL reconstruction, sprints as early as 20 weeks afterward, and figure-eight drills deferred until 24 weeks postoperatively. For concomitant meniscal repair, 4 weeks should be added to these guidelines. After PCL surgery, these intervals are typically increased by 6 to 10 weeks, owing to higher graft demands.

The addition of lateral extraarticular procedures, such as posterolateral reconstruction, requires that intervals be increased by up to 20 weeks. Full return to activity is generally allowed at 6 to 9 months after ACL reconstruction and 12 to 18 months after PCL surgery. It must be emphasized that these protocols are specific to the patient and the procedure and demand that consideration be given to muscle strength, residual muscle atrophy, coordination, endurance, and other variables. Hence, fixed-time estimates for

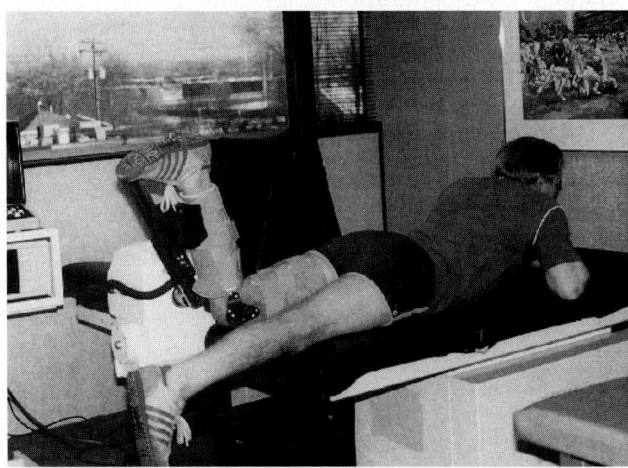

FIG 52–6.
Posterior cruciate ligament surgery requires prone exercise positions with weights and pads placed on the distal tibia.

return to sports should be discouraged. If all other progress determinants are satisfactory, we favor functional bracing for sports until 2 years after surgery.

SPECIFIC PROCEDURE PROTOCOLS

Anterior Cruciate Ligament Reconstruction

Our most common surgical procedure for ACL deficiency is arthroscopic reconstruction using either a patellar tendon or semi-tendonsis autograft. Owing to the bone-tendon-bone construct, fixation can be accomplished with interference screws and, if isometry is true, passive motion can be instituted immediately. When the patient is not performing the range-of-motion exercises, the brace is typically locked at 10 to 30 degrees of flexion for 1 to 2 weeks. The patient is allowed to shower by the third week and to sleep without the brace by the sixth postoperative week. However, the brace should be used for ambulation and exercise for 3 months, and thereafter for exercise only. Usually, a functional brace is fitted at an average of 5 to 6 months, when quadriceps mass has approached that of the nonoperative contralateral limb.

Progressive weightbearing is begun immediately, beginning with partial weightbearing (25% of body weight) and increased by 25% weekly. Spectrum isometrics and proprioceptive neurofacilitation exercises are initiated immediately after surgery. Straight leg raises are encouraged, using up to 10 lbs placed proximally on the tibia. Neuromuscular stimulation is also initiated until a good voluntary quadriceps contraction is present.

The use of patellar glides and tilts is important to maintaining patellar mobility and preventing the patellar entrapment syndrome. Typically, the patient performs these passive and isometric activities a minimum of five times per day. The superoinferior glide motions are considered to be the most important tests.

Functional exercises have proved to be most successful in rehabilitating the quadriceps. Progressive resistive exercises in knee extension are prohibited early, owing to the potential of active quadriceps contraction, which can produce anterior tibial drawer and graft elongation. However, leg-press PREs from 20 degrees of extension to 90 degrees of flexion are allowed early in the rehabilitation protocol.

Our rehabilitation program for hamstring (semi-tendinosus) ACL reconstruction may be more conservative than that used for the bone-tendon-bone construct because of factors discussed above. Initiation of range of motion is not delayed, weightbearing may be delayed until the fourth postoperative week if graft fixation is not ideal.

Posterior Cruciate Ligament Reconstruction

Successful PCL reconstruction is determined as much by proper postoperative care as by meticulous operative technique (see PCL protocol and PCL and PLRI protocol, in Appendix). Consideration must be given to numerous factors. First, the effect of gravity must be minimized by supporting the tibia during postoperative elevation of the limb. PREs are performed prone to minimize posterior tibial sag and its potentially adverse effect on graft healing (Fig 52–6). Strain on the reconstruction is reduced by avoiding active flexion greater than 70 degrees. Generally, passive range of motion is begun immediately from 0 to 40 degrees, unless extra-articular surgery is also performed. In those cases, range of motion is instituted after the third postoperative week.

In contrast to the ACL protocol, progressive weightbearing is delayed to protect the graft from adverse biomechanical forces. Weightbearing is not usually started until 6 weeks postoperatively. A total of 16 weeks on crutches is recommended with PLRI surgery. Knee flexion PREs are deferred 6 months in favor of leg-press PREs and functional exercises.

Associated injuries and reconstructions (e.g., posterolateral and posteromedial) affect the rehabilitative protocol (see PCL and PLRI protocol, in Appendix). Patellofemoral forces must also be considered because of the functional patella baja induced by the preoperative posterior tibial sag. It is essential to avoid exacerbation of patellofemoral chondrosis. The potential for patellar entrapment must be monitored, and patellar mobilization exercises must be carried out in a fashion similar to those described for ACL reconstruction. Isokinetic pads must be placed distally to avoid posterior drawer during the leg-strengthening efforts. Terminal leg presses and gastrocnemius PREs are also indicated.

Bracing is important to PCL rehabilitation. Four-point systems are preferred, with early use of flexion stops and varus and valgus support, especially with associated ligament reconstructions. Return to sports is typically delayed for 12 to 18 months. This is due to the large size of the allografts used, their prolonged revascularization time, and the adverse biomechanical action on the PCL reconstruction.

FAILURE TO PROGRESS

When a patient fails to make the proper progress through the prescribed rehabilitation protocol, it is extremely important that the treatment be reexamined and a more appropriate regimen be instituted (Fig 52–7).

Failure to make gains in muscle strength is generally due to lack of exercise, an improperly applied progressive or resistive exercise program, recurrent knee effusions, or pain which retards progress. Usually, the cause for lack of strength is easily discerned, and the appropriate treatment prescribed. On the other hand, if failure to progress is due to lack of motion, the problem is more difficult to resolve. In fact, it is considered one of the most important problems encountered after knee ligament surgery.[30]

Diagnosis of patellar entrapment is paramount in the treatment algorithm for a stiff knee. If entrapment is not present, the patella can be easily moved superiorly, inferiorly, and from side to side. Loss of motion is then likely due to an overcautious patient or poor physical therapy.

Increasing the frequency of physical therapy and applying more manual exercises will usually result in appropriate increases in motion. If necessary, extension drop-out casts can be used without fear of creating chondral damage or more pain. If the patient fails to progress with the more aggressive physical therapy program, then gentle manipulation under anesthesia can be undertaken.

If the patella is entrapped, as demonstrated by decreased patellar glides medially and laterally, as well as decreased superior and inferior excursion of the patella in the femoral sulcus, then care must be taken to determine its position. When suprapatellar entrapment is present, arthroscopy followed by gentile manipulation usually results in the desired range of motion. However, if infrapatellar contracture is present, with or without suprapatellar entrapment, neither closed manipulation nor increasingly painful physical therapy sessions should be entertained, as both would worsen the problem.

The most common mistake made by the physician and therapist in treating infrapatellar contracture syndrome (IPCS) is to increase the forceful manipulations, thus inducing more pain, quadriceps spasm, and inflammation. These measures often result in further thickening of the scar tissue in the infrapatellar region and loss of motion. Ultimately, the process can lead to patella infera.[53]

When IPCS is present, all forceful physical therapy must cease. The patient should be put strictly on a muscle-strengthening program and oral anti-inflammatory drugs. The knee must be allowed to "cool down" before any surgical or manipulative intervention is used. When the swelling and pain have subsided and the patient can demonstrate a forceful quadriceps contraction, then surgery can be entertained.

Although many patients will regain their motion after this program has been instituted, some will not and thus will require surgery. Rarely can this type of knee problem be treated by arthroscopy or closed manipulation alone. Generally, because of the severe scarring in the infrapatellar area, a miniarthrotomy is required. With this arthrotomy, a lateral retinacular release is performed along with resection of the fibrous portion of the fat pad which impinges in the intercondylar notch and impedes extension. The patellar tendon is also freed from the front of the tibia to prevent infrapatellar migration. If patella infera is already present, a DeLee osteotomy may be necessary (superoanterior relocation of the tibial tubercle). After the surgical release, but prior to any tibial tubercle osteotomy, a manipulation can be performed to achieve full extension. A posterior capsular release is *not necessary*. The only time posterior capsular releases should be considered is when there has been previous surgery at the posterior corners.

After the initial procedure, physical therapy is resumed in the mode similar to that prior to the procedure. That is, no forced manual passive exercises are used and the patient is encouraged to do assisted passive range-of-motion exercises and muscle strengthening. Closed-chain exercises are instituted in preference to open-chain concentric exercises, which can overload the patellofemoral joint. Extension is a priority, and flexion is not stressed. After full extension is achieved and there is no quadriceps lag, the amount of flexion is assessed. If flexion is still less than 130 degrees, the patient can be returned to surgery where an arthroscopy and closed manipulation for flexion will generally restore a near-normal range of motion.

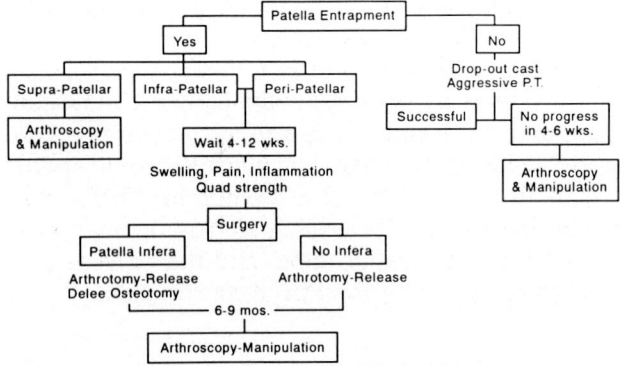

FIG 52–7.
Algorithm designed to treat a patient who fails to make proper progress in the rehabilitation program. P.T. = physical therapy.

SUMMARY

This discussion has emphasized the team approach to knee surgery. The patient, surgeon, and therapist act together to produce the optimal result.

Specific patient factors, such as age and generalized ligamentous laxity, must be considered when selecting a surgical technique and rehabilitation program. The type of surgical procedure and the type of tissue that must be repaired and healed constrain the rehabilitative protocol. The deleterious effects of immobility and disuse, and attempts to circumvent these through controlled early return to function, must be carefully balanced against the need to protect healing musculoskeletal tissues. Biomechanical factors, such as graft type, graft fixation, and specific surgical technique, particularly with ligament reconstructions, also must be considered.

A generic rehabilitation protocol has been introduced with progression through a phasic program, as healing permits. Our recommendations for selected procedures, such as diagnostic arthroscopy, arthroscopic meniscectomy, chondroplasty, meniscal repair, and ACL and PCL reconstructions, have been outlined. We believe that our approach is sound at this time, as it customizes rehabilitation to the specific needs of the individual patient who has undergone a particular surgical procedure. However, more investigation needs to be done in the search for the ideal rehabilitation program following knee surgery.

REFERENCES

1. Akeson WH, Amiel D, LaViolette D: The connective tissue response to immobility: A study of chondroitin-4 and -6 sulfate and dermatan sulfate changes in periarticular connective tissue of control and immobilized knees of dogs, *Clin Orthop* 51:183–197, 1967.
2. Akeson WH, et al.: The connective tissue response to immobility: Biomechanical changes in periarticular connective tissue of the immobilized rabbit knee, *Clin Orthop* 93:356–362, 1973.
3. Akeson WH, et al: Collagen cross-linking alterations in joint contractions: Changes in the reducible cross-links in periarticular connective tissue collagen after nine weeks of immobilization, *Connect Tissue Res* 5:15, 1977.
4. Akeson WH, et al: Effects of immobilization of joints, *Clin Orthop* 219:28–37, 1987.
5. Alm A, et al: The anterior cruciate ligament—a clinical and experimental study on tensile strength, morphology and replacement by patellar ligament, *Acta Chir Scand Suppl* 445:15–24, 1974.
6. Andriacchi T, et al: Ligament injury and repair. In Woo SL, Buckwalter JA, editors: *Injury and repair of the musculoskeletal soft tissues.* Park Ridge, Ill, American Academy of Orthopaedic Surgeons.
7. Arms SW, et al: The biomechanics of anterior cruciate ligament rehabilitation and reconstruction, *Am J Sports Med* 12:8–18, 1984.
8. Arnoczky SP, Warren RF: The microvasculature of the meniscus and its response to injury: An experimental study in the dog, *Am J Sports Med* 11:131–141, 1983.
9. Arnoczky SP, Warren RF, Ashlock MA: Replacement of the anterior cruciate ligament using a patella tendon allograft—an experimental study, *J Bone Joint Surg [AM]* 68:376–385, 1986.
10. Arnoczky SP, Warren RF, Kaplan N: Meniscal remodeling following partial meniscectomy—an experimental study in the dog, *J Arthrosc* 1:247–252, 1985.
11. Arnoczky SP, et al: Meniscal repair using an exogenous fibrin clot—an experimental study in the dog, 32nd Annual Meeting of the Orthopedic Research Society, New Orleans, Feb 1986.
12. Arnoczky SP, et al: Cellular repopulation of deep-frozen meniscal autografts: An experimental study in the dog, 34th Annual Meeting of the Orthopedic Research Society, Atlanta, Feb 1988.
13. Bassett FH II, Beck JL, Weiker G: A modified cast brace: Its use in nonoperative and postoperative management of serious knee ligament injuries, *Am J Sports Med* 8:63–69, 1980.
14. Cabaud HE, Rodkey WG, Feagin JA: Experimental studies of acute anterior cruciate ligament injury and repair, *Am J Sports Med* 7:18–22, 1979.
15. Cabaud HE, Rodkey WG, Fitzwater JE: Medial meniscus repairs: an experimental and morphologic study, *Am J Sports Med* 9:129–134, 1981.
16. Clancy WG Jr, Ray JM: Anterior cruciate ligament autografts. In Jackson DW, Drez D Jr, editors: *The anterior cruciate deficient knee: New concepts in ligament repair,* St Louis, 1987, Mosby.
17. Clancy WG, Jr, et al: Anterior and posterior cruciate ligament reconstruction in Rhesus monkeys: A histological, microangiographic, and biomechanical analysis, *J Bone Joint Surg [Am],* 63:1270–1284, 1981.
18. Coutts RD, moderator: Symposium: The diagnosis and treatment of articular cartilage injuries, *Contemp Orthop* 19:401–431, 1989.
19. Daniel DM, et al: Fixation of soft tissue. In Jackson DW, Drez D Jr, editors: *The anterior cruciate deficient knee: New concepts in ligament repair,* St Louis, Mosby.
20. DeAndrade JR, Grant C, Dixon A: Joint distension and reflex inhibition in the knee, *J Bone Joint Surg [Am]* 47:313–322, 1965.
21. Dickinson A, Bennett KM: Therapeutic exercise, *Clin Sports Med* 4:417–430, 1985.
22. Eriksson G, Haggmark T: Comparison of isometric muscle training and electrical stimulation supplementing isometric muscle training in the recovery after major knee ligament surgery, *Am J Sports Med* 7:169–171, 1979.

23. Evans EB, et al: Experimental immobilization and remobilization of rat knee joints, *J Bone Joint Surg [Am]* 42:737–758, 1960.
24. Finsterbush A, Friedman B: Early changes in immobilized rabbit knee joints: A light and electron microscopy study, *Clin Orthop* 92:305–319, 1973.
25. Finsterbush A, Friedman B: Reversibility of joint changes produced by immobilization in rabbits, *Clin Orthop* 111:290–298, 1975.
26. France EP, et al: The biomechanics of anterior cruciate allografts. In Friedman M, Ferkel R, editors: *Prosthetic ligament reconstruction of the knee,* Philadelphia, 1988, WB Saunders.
27. Fu FH, et al: Loss of knee motion following arthroscopic anterior cruciate ligament reconstruction, Ninth Annual Meeting of the Arthroscopy Association of North America, Orlando, Fl, April 1990.
28. Furukawa T, et al: Biomechanical studies on repair cartilage resurfacing: experimental defects in the rabbit knee, *J Bone Joint Surg [Am]* 62:79–89, 1980.
29. Gelberman RH, et al: The effects of mobilization on the vascularization of healing flexor tendons in dogs, *Clin Orthop* 153:283–289, 1980.
30. Graf B, Uhr F: Complications of intra-articular anterior cruciate reconstructions, *Clin Sports Med* 7:835–848, 1988.
31. Grood ES, et al: Biomechanics of the knee-extension exercise, *J Bone Joint Surg [Am]* 66:725–734, 1984.
32. Haggmark T, Erikson E: Cylinder or mobile cast brace after knee ligament surgery: A clinical analysis and morphologic and enzymatic studies of changes in the quadriceps muscle, *Am J Sports Med* 7:48–56, 1979.
33. Halkjaer-Kristensen J, Ingemann-Hansen T: Wasting of the human quadriceps muscle after knee ligament injuries: Muscle fiber morphology; oxidative and glycolytic enzyme activity; dynamic and static muscle function, *Scand J Rehabil Med Suppl* 13:5–20, 1985.
34. Hall MC: Cartilage changes after experimental immobilization of the knee joint in the young rat, *J Bone Joint Surg [Am]* 45:36–44, 1963.
35. Heatley FW: The meniscus—can it be repaired? An experimental investigation in rabbits, *J Bone Joint Surg [Br]* 62:397–402, 1980.
36. Hallebrandt FA, Houtz SJ, Kirkorian AM: Influence of bimanual exercise on unilateral work capacity, *J Appl Physiol* 2:452–466, 1950.
37. Hallebrandt FA, Waterland JC: Indirect learning: The influence of uni-manual exercise on related muscle groups of the same and the opposite side, *Am J Physiol Med* 41:45–55, 1962.
38. Hirsch EF, Morgan RH: Causal significance to traumatic ossification in tendon insertions, *Arch Surg* 39:824–837, 1939.
39. Kennedy JC, Weinberg HW, Wilson AS: Anatomy and function of the anterior cruciate ligament, *J Bone Joint Surg [Am]* 56:223–235, 1974.
40. Kurosaka M, Yoshiya S, Andrish JT: A biomechanical comparison of different surgical techniques of graft fixation in anterior cruciate ligament reconstruction, *Am J Sports Med* 15:225–229, 1987.
41. Lambert KL: Vascularized patellar tendon graft with rigid internal fixation for anterior cruciate ligament insufficiency, *Clin Orthop* 172:85–89, 1983.
42. Laros GS, Tipton CM, Cooper RR: Influence of physical activity on ligament insertions in the knees of dogs, *J Bone Joint Surg [Am]* 53:275–286, 1971.
43. Mitchell H, Shepard N: Effect of patellar shaving in the rabbit, *J Orthop Res* 5:388–392, 1987.
44. Morrissey MC, et al: The effects of electrical stimulation on the quadriceps during postoperative knee immobilization, *Am J Sports Med* 13:40–45, 1985.
45. Noyes FR, Mangine RE, Barber S: Early knee motion after open and arthroscopic anterior cruciate ligament reconstruction, *Am J Sports Med* 15:149–160, 1987.
46. Noyes FR, et al: Biomechanics of ligament failure: Analysis of immobilization, exercise and reconditioning effects in primates, *J Bone Joint Surg [Am]* 56:1406–1418, 1974.
47. Noyes FR, et al: Intraarticular cruciate reconstruction. I: Perspectives on graft strength, vascularization and immediate motion after replacement, *Clin Orthop* 172:71–77, 1983.
48. Noyes FR, et al: Biomechanical analysis of human ligament grafts used in knee ligament repairs and reconstructions, *J Bone Joint Surg [Am]* 66:344–352, 1984.
49. Paulos LE, Beck CL, Rosenberg TD: Unpublished observations.
50. Paulos LE, Wnorowski DC, Erickson A: Infrapatellar contracture syndrome: Diagnosis, treatment and long term follow up (submitted for publication.)
51. Paulos LE, et al: Knee rehabilitation after anterior cruciate ligament reconstruction and repair, *Am J Sports Med* 9:140–149, 1981.
52. Paulos LE, Payne FC III, Rosenberg TD: Rehabilitation after anterior cruciate ligament surgery. In Jackson DW, Drez D Jr, editors: *The anterior cruciate ligament deficient knee: New concepts in ligament repair,* St Louis, 1987, Mosby.
53. Paulos LE, et al: Infrapatellar contracture syndrome, an unrecognized cause of knee stiffness with patellar entrapment and patella infera, *Am J Sports Med* 15:331–341, 1987.
54. Paulos LE, et al: Analysis of electrical muscle stimulation in rehabilitating the ACL reconstructed knee, Fourth Congress of the European Society of Knee Surgery and Arthroscopy, Stockholm, June 1990.
55. Peacock EE Jr: Comparison of collagenous tissue surrounding normal and immobilized joints, *Surg Forum* 14:440, 1963.
56. Robertson DB, Daniel DM, Biden E: Soft tissue fixation to bone, *Am J Sports Med* 14:398–403, 1986.
57. Salter RB, et al: The biological effect of continuous passive motion on the healing of full-thickness defects in articular cartilage, *J Bone Joint Surg [Am]* 62:1232–1251, 1980.

58. Schmid A, Schmid F: Results after cartilage shaving studied by electron microscopy (abstract), *Am J Sports Med* 15:386–387, 1987.
59. Shelbourne KD, et al: Arthrofibrosis in acute anterior cruciate ligament reconstruction: The effect of timing of reconstruction and rehabilitation, *Am J Sports Med* 19:332–336, 1991.
60. Shino K, et al: Replacement of the anterior cruciate ligament by an allogeneic tendon graft: An experimental study in the dog, *J Bone Joint Surg [Br]* 66:672–681, 1984.
61. Sisk TD, et al: Effect of electrical stimulation on quadriceps strength after reconstructive surgery of the anterior cruciate ligament, *Am J Sports Med* 15:215–220, 1987.
62. Stratford P: Electromyography of the quadriceps femoris muscles in subjects with normal knees and acutely effused knees, *Phys Ther* 62:279–283, 1981.
63. Troyer H: The effect of short-term immobilization on the rabbit knee joint cartilage, *Clin Orthop* 107:249–257, 1975.
64. Webber RJ, Harris M, Hough AJ Jr: Intrinsic repair capabilities of rabbit meniscal fibrocartilage: A cell culture model, 30th Annual Meeting of the Orthopedic Research Society, Atlanta, Feb 1984.
65. Woo SL-Y, et al: Measurement of mechanical properties of ligament substance from a bone-ligament-bone preparation, *J Orthop Res* 1:22, 1983.
66. Woo SL-Y, et al: The connective tissue response to immobility: A correlative study of biomechanical and biochemical measurements of the normal and immobilized rabbit knee, *Arthritis Rheum* 18:257–264, 1975.

53
Knee Braces for Athletic Injuries

GREGORY T. HARDIN, M.D.
BERNARD R. BACH, JR., M.D.

Prophylactic knee brace
Rehabilitative knee braces

Functional knee braces
Summary

Knee injuries in athletics are a major problem facing the sports medicine community. There is no compelling evidence to suggest that the likelihood of sustaining a knee injury is increasing; however, more knee injuries are being identified and treated as a result of improved diagnostic techniques. Successful prevention of knee injuries has not paralleled the substantial advances in diagnosis and treatment of these knee problems.

A brace can be defined as a device that functions to clasp or connect objects so they can resist deforming forces and provide support for ligament reconstruction. A multitude of braces are available, and prior to the seminar report on knee braces by the American Academy of Orthopaedic Surgeons in 1985,[1] limited objective data were available regarding the ability to perform these functions.[1-54]

This chapter classifies braces into three types: prophylactic, rehabilitative, and functional. The goal is for the reader to be familiar with the types of braces, how to evaluate them, and with studies of these braces.

PROPHYLACTIC KNEE BRACE

The two basic types of prophylactic knee braces are designed to prevent or reduce the severity of knee injuries (Figs 53-1 and 53-2). One includes lateral bars with either single-axis, dual-axis, or polycentric hinges (Fig 53-3). A second type uses a plastic shell that encircles the thigh and calf and has polycentric hinges.

Epidemiologic studies regarding the efficacy of prophylactic knee braces must take into consideration many variables. The ideal study should be randomized and prospective. Controls ideally should be simultaneous rather than historical. The *time* at which the study was conducted is critical as prevailing orthopedic attitudes may affect diagnoses or frequency of surgery. For example, in the late 1970s and early 1980s medial collateral ligament (MCL) injuries were treated routinely surgically, which would affect the surgical frequency rate. How was the diagnosis established? Was the diagnosis established by a trainer and confirmed by a physician? Rule changes may negatively impact injury frequency and severity. What role did the playing surface have on injuries? Were practices conducted on artificial or natural surfaces? Shoewear could play a factor, as some authors have noted an increased frequency of foot and ankle injuries. How was an injury defined or classified? Were thigh, lower leg, and foot and ankle injuries assessed? Did the study critically assess a difference in injury frequency and severity as it pertained to MCL injuries, anterior cruciate ligament (ACL) injuries, meniscal injuries, or combined injuries? Were injuries assessed with reference to position-specific factors? Was time missed defined (practice, week, game)? When studying the literature currently available, one must ask these questions to critically determine the strength and deficiencies of the study.

Nowakowski[34] studied 20 patients who had anteroposterior radiographs of the knee prior to applied stress and with 40 lb of valgus stress applied below the knee. A second radiograph was obtained with the patient wearing a variety of lateral-sided braces, hinged in the middle, and offset from the knee. Less medial gaping of the braced knee was noted. This was the first published study evaluating prophylactic braces worn as protection from laterally applied forces.

The Anderson Knee Stabler was developed in

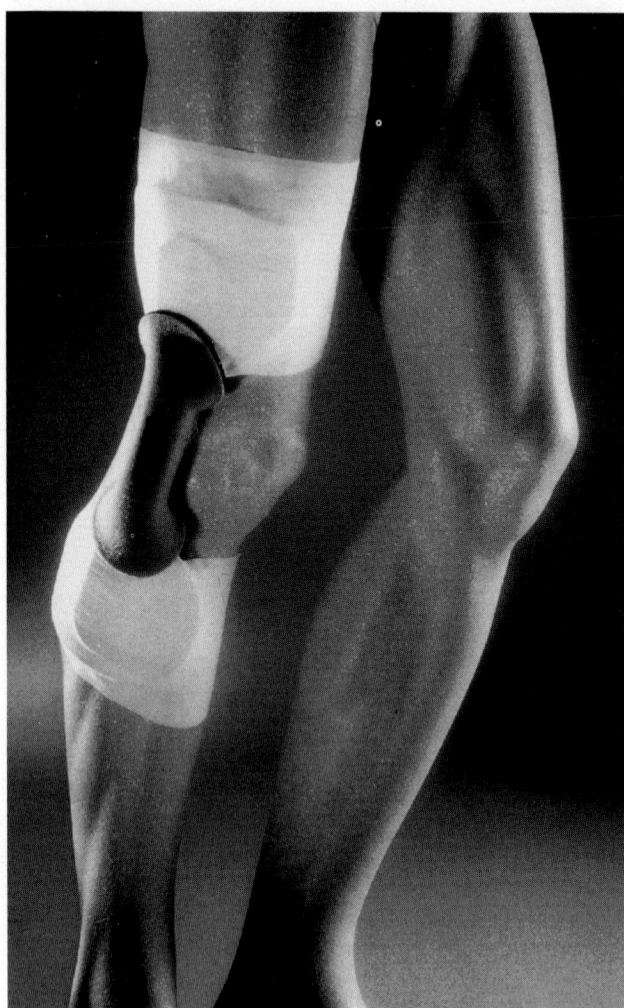

FIG 53-1.
A lateral hinge prophylactic brace produced by OMNI Scientific. (Courtesy of OMNI Scientific, Inc., Concord, Calif.)

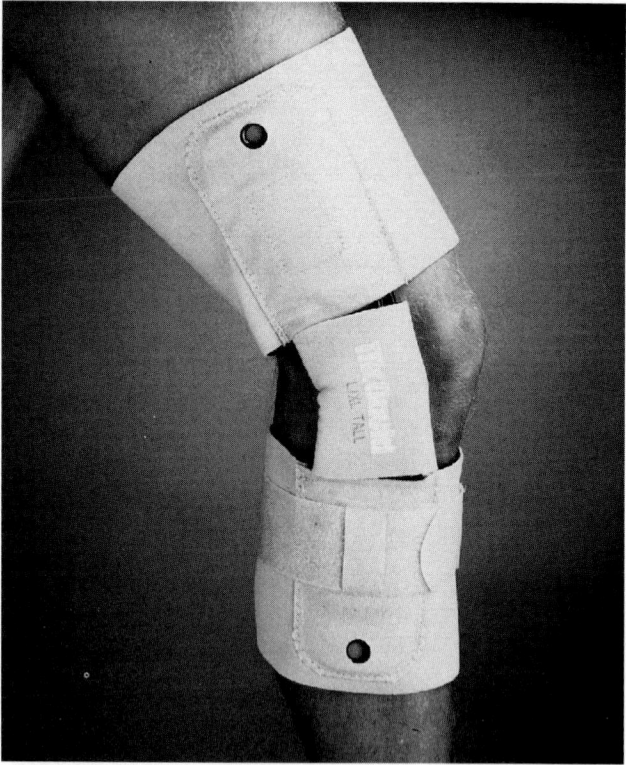

FIG 53-2.
The McDavid lateral hinge prophylactic knee brace. (Courtesy of McDavid Knee Guard, Inc., Chicago.)

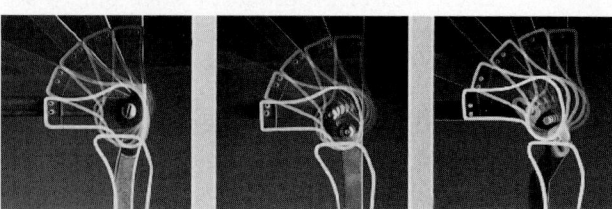

FIG 53-3.
Examples of single-axis, dual-axis, and polycentric hinges are noted from *left to right* (Courtesy of Magnum Orthopaedic, Division of Mueller Sports Medicine, Prairie du Sac, Wisc.)

1978 by George Anderson, head trainer of the Oakland Raiders, to protect MCLs from reinjury.[2] Anderson's colleagues in the professional and college ranks were impressed with the reports of its effectiveness and began using it on their athletes who had sustained MCL injuries. Subsequently, the medical staff of several teams decided that the brace could more importantly be used prophylactically. As the word about the potential to protect the MCL spread, some were not careful to discern between MCL and total knee protection. Considerable controversy remains on how effective these braces are in preventing such injuries (Tables 53-1 and 53-2).

Hewson et al.,[24] Paulos et al.,[35] Rovere et al.,[41] and Teitz et al.,[49] have reported epidemiologic studies that have been nonsupportive in substantiating decreased incidence of MCL, ACL, or combined injuries.

A medical record review was presented by Hewson et al.[24] concerning the University of Arizona intercollegiate football teams over an 8-year period (1977-1985). Exposure to injury was defined as one player at each practice session or game. The nonbraced period was reviewed from 1977 to 1981. Following this, the Anderson Knee Stabler was mandatory for all practices and games for players at greatest risk, including lineman, linebackers, and tight ends, from 1981 to 1985. In the mandatory brace group 28,191 exposures occurred, with 29,293 exposures in the nonbraced group. Information was analyzed by type of injury, severity of injury, player's position, days lost from practice or games, and rate

TABLE 53–1.
Summary of Principal Scientific Investigations of the Anderson Knee Stabler*

Supportive		Nonsupportive	
Hansen et al.[23]	Four-year University of Southern California injury review showed reduction in injuries and surgery for braced players	Hewson et al.[24]	Reduction in injury frequency and severity at University of Arizona due to better care, not braces
McKelvie	Mid-American Conference survey showed significant reduction in injuries and severity with bracing	Rovere et al.[41]	Increase in MCL strains and ACL tears during bracing at Wake Forest
		Teitz et al.[49]	Division I team survey showed braced players had more injuries than nonbraced
Schriner & Schriner[43]	Review of 25 Michigan high schools found 5% injury rate for unbraced players and no injuries for braced	Paulos et al.[35]	Biomechanical testing suggested potential preloading of MCL; now stated as clinically insignificant
Taft et al.[48]	University of North Carolina study, 3 years before bracing (no braces) and 3 years after (100%) braces, showed some injury reduction and significant severity reduction (grade III down 70%).	Baker et al[4]	Biomechanical testing showed reduction in abduction angle using functional brace, but little or no protection with prophylactic braces
Paulos et al.[35]	Braces that increased impact duration protect ACL more than MCL. Most braces provide some degree of protection to the ACL with direct lateral impact	Garrick & Requa[20]	Evaluated six studies finding significant methodologic problems and conflicting results: "Impossible to state with assurance the role of prophylactic knee bracing at this time"
Sitler et al.[44]	Most highly controlled; in a prospective 2-year study of 1,396 West Point cadets, braced defensive players had a significant decrease in number, but not severity, of knee injuries; no difference in foot and ankle injuries	Grace et al.[21]	Two-year high-school study showed four times more knee injuries in the braced group; dramatic increase in foot and ankle injuries in braced group (3 ×)

*ACL = anterior cruciate ligament; MCL = medial collateral ligament.

of knee injury per season per 100 players at risk. The results showed that the number of knee injuries was similar for the braced and nonbraced groups, as well as the type and severity of injury in all categories. Knee bracing did not significantly reduce the number or type of knee injuries or reduce the practice time missed for an entire team or players at risk. Although practice time missed because of third-degree MCL and medial meniscus injuries was significantly lower, this was a result of improved techniques in treating these conditions. The type and severity of injury were similar for braced and nonbraced players at risk: each player faced a 23% chance of knee injury each season, and a 64% chance during a 4-year football career.

Rovere et al.[41] performed a 2-year study including all players on the Wake Forest football team using the Anderson Knee Stabler prophylactically during practice and games. A 2-year nonbrace control period (2 years prior) was also evaluated. Braces were applied with an elastic foam underwrap over the distal thigh and proximal leg, then secured with two neoprene straps, Velcro fasteners, or adhesive tape. The time and mechanism of injury, diagnosis, and treatment were noted. Results showed 24 knee injuries during the control period compared with 29 knee injuries with brace wearing. Grade I MCL sprains accounted for 67% of injuries in the nonbrace period vs. 62% of injuries in the brace period. During the brace period nine knees had surgery compared with five during the control period. There were three ACL repairs during the brace period and one in the nonbrace period. During both periods, offensive team members (especially lineman) had the most knee injuries, and defensive backs the fewest. Brace use did not significantly alter the relative frequency of injuries by player or position. This study concluded that the Anderson Knee Stabler was ineffective for prophylaxis. Knee injuries were more common when braces were worn. As brace wearing was also associated with cramping and added financial expenditures, the authors concluded that they could *not* recommend the use of a prophylactic knee brace without further study.

Teitz et al.[49] used the members of Division I of the National Collegiate Athletic Association (NCAA) as its study population. The authors reviewed statistics from 71 colleges in 1984 and 61 schools in 1985.

TABLE 53–2.
Studies of Prophylactic Braces*

Study	Year	Player Position	Mechanism of Injury	Severity of Injury: Grade	Level of Skill	Total Nonbraced	Total Braced	Conclusion
Hansen et al.[23]	1980–1984	Not specified	Not specified	Not specified	College (University of Southern California)	329	148	Less surgery and injuries for braced players
Taft et al.[48]	1980–1982 Nonbraced 1983–1985 Braced	Not specified	Not specified	Operative vs. nonoperative	College (University of North Carolina)	Not specified	Not specified	Some injury reduction and significant severity reduction (MCL III decreased 70%)
Schriner & Schriner[43]	1984	Not specified	Not specified	Not specified	High school (Michigan)	1,049	197	Nonbraced, 5% injury; braced, 0%
Hewson et al.[24]	1977–1981 Nonbraced 1981–1985 Braced	Offensive lineman, defensive lineman, linebacker, tight end	Not specified	MCL: I,II,III ACL Meniscus	College (University of Arizona)	226	224	No significant reduction in injuries or severity in braced players
Rovere et al.[41]	1981–1982 Nonbraced 1983–1984 Braced	All	76% body contact	MCL: I,II,III ACL Meniscus	College (Wake Forest)	368	374	Increase in ACL and MCL injuries in braced players; offensive linemen injured most in both groups
Teitz et al.[49]	1984–1985	All	Not specified	MCL: I,II,III ACL Meniscus	College (Division I)	3,001	2,387	More injuries in braced running backs and defensive backs than in nonbraced; braces not preventive and may be harmful
Grace et al.[21]	1985–1986	Not specified	Not specified	Time lost (1–21 days)	High school (New Mexico)	250	330	Knee injuries significantly more frequent in braced group; also, more foot and ankle injuries in braced athletes
Sitler et al.[44]	1986–1987	Offense vs. defense	47% direct lateral knee contact (2/3 of MCL injuries)	MCL: I,II,III ACL: partial or complete	College (West Point)	705	691	No difference in severity of injury, but braced players on defense had statistically fewer knee injuries

*ACL = anterior cruciate ligament; MCL = medial collateral ligament.

A total of 6,307 players were analyzed in 1984 and 5,445 players in 1985. Player position; incidence of injury; type, mechanism, and severity of injury; playing surface; level of skill; and prior knee injury were considered contributing factors. Their results showed that in 1984 and 1985 players who wore braces had a significantly higher injury rate than unbraced players. Four different types of prophylactic knee braces were worn and no attempt was made to differentiate between them with data analysis. The severity of injuries did not differ between the two groups. Player position, playing surface, mechanism of injury, or type of brace did not affect the rates of injury. Injuries were more common during contact and at every skill level among those who wore braces. There were also more MCL injuries among players who used braces. The incidence of ACL injury was similar in both groups, but braced players had more meniscal injuries. The severity of injury was assessed by measuring playing time lost and the need for surgery. Surgical rates were similar for both groups. Although the average playing time lost was less for those who used braces, the increased incidence of injury produced an overall time lost that was greater in those using braces. Teitz et al. concluded that prophylactic bracing would not prevent injuries and may in fact be harmful. They did not advise preventive bracing for collegiate football players.[49]

Another study, by Beck et al.,[6] using the KT-1000 knee arthrometer, showed that anterior tibial displacement was unaffected by prophylactic knee bracing. Baker et al.[3] evaluated commercially available athletic braces for their effect on abduction forces applied to a cadaver knee with no instability and with experimentally created medial instability. Under computer control, abduction forces were applied while simultaneous data were obtained from an electrogoniometer and transducers applied to the ACL and superficial MCL at 0, 15, and 30 degrees of flexion. Results showed a reduction in abduction angle using functional braces, whereas prophylactic braces demonstrated little or no protective effect.

Paulos et al.,[37] in a biomechanical study using fresh frozen cadaver knees, measured ligament tension and joint displacement at static, nondestructive valgus forces and at low-rated destructive forces. After nonbraced controls were examined, knees were braced with two different laterally applied preventive braces: the McDavid Knee Guard (see Fig 53-2) and the Anderson Knee Stabler. The effects of lateral bracing were analyzed according to valgus force, joint line opening, and ligament tension. Valgus applied forces, with or without braces, consistently produced MCL disruption at ligament tension surprisingly higher than the ACL and higher than or equal to the posterior cruciate ligament (PCL). In part I of their study, no significant protection could be documented with the two preventive braces used. Also, four potentially adverse affects were noted: MCL preloading, center axis shift, premature joint line contact, and brace slippage.

In part II of their study, brace-induced MCL preload in vivo was negated by joint compressive forces.[38] In summary, Paulos et al.[35, 37, 38] concluded that the majority of prophylactic knee braces presently available are biomechanically inadequate. They believed that before prophylactic knee braces can be categorically recommended, more biomechanical and clinical studies should be initiated. They believed that prophylactic lateral knee bracing could be effective if the proper type of brace is used. They recommended that prophylactic lateral knee bracing not be abandoned, but improved and further evaluated in well-controlled prospective studies.

Scientific investigators supporting the use of prophylactic bracing include Hansen et al.,[23] Schriner and Schriner,[43] Sitler et al.,[44] and Taft et al.[48] These reviews showed reduction in injuries and surgery for braced players.

The study of Hansen et al.[23] involved players on the University of Southern California football team from 1980 to 1984. There were 329 players nonbraced and 148 braced. Neither the criteria for brace usage nor the exposure of those braced or unbraced were defined. No definition of knee injury was given. Only injuries requiring surgical intervention were included. Diagnoses were apparently made by the operating surgeons. These authors concluded that prophylactic bracing was better than no bracing in reducing injuries and surgery.

The University of North Carolina study was reported by Taft et al.[48] This study documented the football team's experience from 1980 through 1982, when no braces were used, and from 1983 through 1985, when all team members were required to wear braces. Injuries were defined as those that "modified or prevented practice for at least one week." MCL injuries were graded by an orthopaedic surgeon as operative or nonoperative. These authors concluded that bracing was helpful in decreasing the severity and frequency of injuries.

Schriner and Schriner[43] reported a survey of 1,246 players from 25 high schools in Michigan during the 1984 season. From 12 of the schools, 197 players volunteered for bracing. Diagnoses were made by physicians as reported by coaches, and only injuries from lateral forces and from hyperextension were analyzed. They found a 5% injury rate for unbraced players, and no injuries for braced players.

Garrick and Requa[20] evaluated six studies (Hansen et al.,[23] Hewson et al.,[24] Rovere et al.,[41] Schriner and Schriner,[43] Taft et al.,[48] and Teitz et al.[49]) designed to determine the effectiveness of prophylactic knee bracing in preventing MCL injury in football. Criteria useful for evaluating studies included the probability of confounding factors, bias in selecting cases and controls, and variations in defining injury and exposure. Cost as well as ethical issues associated with mandated use were discussed. Four of the studies found a reduction in MCL injuries associated with using a brace; two studies reported increases. No consensus arose from these studies, and conflicting results as well as methodologic problems were apparent, which makes it impossible to state with assurance the role of prophylactic knee bracing in football at that time.

Recently, two prospective, randomized studies evaluating prophylactic knee braces resulted in contradictory conclusions.[21,44] Grace et al.[21] evaluated 580 high-school football players over a 2-year period. Two hundred fifty nonbraced athletes were matched according to size, weight, and position with 247 single-hinged and 83 double-hinged braced athletes. The single-hinged prophylactically braced athletes had a significantly higher knee injury rate ($P < .001$). The double-hinged group had a greater number of injuries but this was not statistically significant. Foot and ankle injuries occurred three times more frequently in the braced group ($P < .01$). Different playing surfaces were used and no documentation of prophylactic ankle taping was noted. Their results questioned the efficacy of prophylactic knee braces and called attention to their potential adverse effects on adjacent distal joints.

A study by Sitler et al.[44] from West Point noted a decrease in frequency but not severity of knee injuries. This prospective 2-year study evaluated 1,396 intramural tackle football players whose average age was 19.3 years. Strict definitions of athlete exposure (every athlete participating in a practice or game), identical athletic shoes, and uniform playing surface (natural grass) were involved. Seven hundred five controls and 691 braced (double-hinged single lateral upright) athletes were involved, all undergoing preparticipation physical examination. A significant decrease in frequency and total number of MCL knee injuries was noted in defensive, but not offensive players. Retrospectively, the authors assessed all players for foot and ankle injuries and noted no significant differences between the two groups.

Paulos et al.[36] in 1991 evaluated the effects of six different prophylactic knee braces on ACL ligament strain under valgus loads using a mechanical surrogate limb. Their results indicated that these braces have a beneficial effect in protecting the knee against direct lateral blows, greater for the ACL than the MCL. Brace hinge contact with the lateral joint line of the knee reduced their effectiveness. They concluded that their results should be confirmed clinically, and there is a definite need for improved designs.

Prophylactic knee bracing remains controversial. These braces have not consistently been shown to prevent or reduce the severity of injuries to the ACL or menisci. Several studies have shown a trend toward a reduced incidence of serious MCL injuries, but other studies have shown no change in the incidence of these injuries. With the exception of the West Point study,[44] most studies have overgeneralized from their data and cannot document that prophylactic knee braces are the cause of increased or decreased injuries. Furthermore, if biomechanical data proved clinically applicable, some prophylactic braces may result in an increased incidence of ACL injuries.

The American Academy of Orthopaedic Surgeons in 1985 stated, "Efforts need to be made to eliminate the unsubstantiated claims of currently available prophylactic braces and to curtail the inevitable misuse, unnecessary costs, and medical legal problems."[1] The American Orthopaedic Society for Sports Medicine and the *Journal of Bone and Joint Surgery*, editorial, January 1987, have taken the same position. The American Academy of Pediatrics went even further with its position statement by recommending that prophylactic lateral knee bracing not be considered standard equipment for football players because of lack of efficacy and the potential of actually causing harm.

Additional factors, such as rule changes, including no downfield or below-the-waist blocking, crackback, or high-low double-team blocking, and clipping, have helped to make players aware of the serious knee injuries that result from these techniques.[39] Additional rule changes may help in decreasing the frequency and severity of knee injuries in football. Certain players, particularly offensive lineman, are at marked increased risk of suffering knee injuries. Thus further study and improvements in brace design are warranted.

REHABILITATIVE KNEE BRACES

Rehabilitative knee braces are designed to provide range of motion, either fixed or controlled flexion and extension through predetermined arcs on injured knees treated operatively or nonoperatively. These are for the most part off-the-shelf types of braces, with thigh and calf enclosures, hinges, hinge-brace arms, and straps that encircle the brace components on the thigh and calf (see Fig 53-2). Foot plates are an option that can be used to control tibial rotation and prevent brace migration. The hinges allow the ability to limit motion of the knee to varying degrees. Currently, little information on rehabilitative knee braces exists in the literature.

Cawley et al.[11] performed a biomechanical comparison of eight commonly used rehabilitative knee braces using a mechanical surrogate limb. Most of the braces significantly reduced translations and rotations compared with the unbraced limb under static test conditions. Factors believed to be important in brace design included high overall brace stiffness, hinge design, the use of nonelastic straps which adapt to leg contour better, and finally hinge design, including the presence or absence of joint line contact.

After a repair or reconstruction of certain knee ligaments, it may be necessary to prevent certain knee motions. Stevenson et al.[46] presented data that showed that the knee joint extended approximately 20 degrees more than the setting on the rehabilitative knee brace hinges. Hoffman et al.[26] reported one rehabilitation knee brace to be better than the others in providing stability to static anterior forces. However, this study did not control for tightness of brace application.

Rehabilitative knee braces are more convenient for both the patient and the surgeon. They are easily applied and adjusted, lightweight, and provide easy access to incisions. Caution should be exercised when allowing motion in rehabilitative knee braces, because more knee joint motion than expected can occur and little static anteroposterior control is obtained.

FUNCTIONAL KNEE BRACES

Functional knee braces are designed to provide stability for ACL-unstable or reconstructed knees (Figs 53-4 and 53-8). Although there are many companies that manufacture custom and off-the-shelf ACL orthoses, only a few companies have developed orthoses for PCL insufficiency (Fig 53-9). The two basic construction types have similar design features. Both types utilize unilateral or bilateral hinges and posts; the difference between them is whether they use thigh and calf shell enclosures or straps for suspension (Table 53-3).

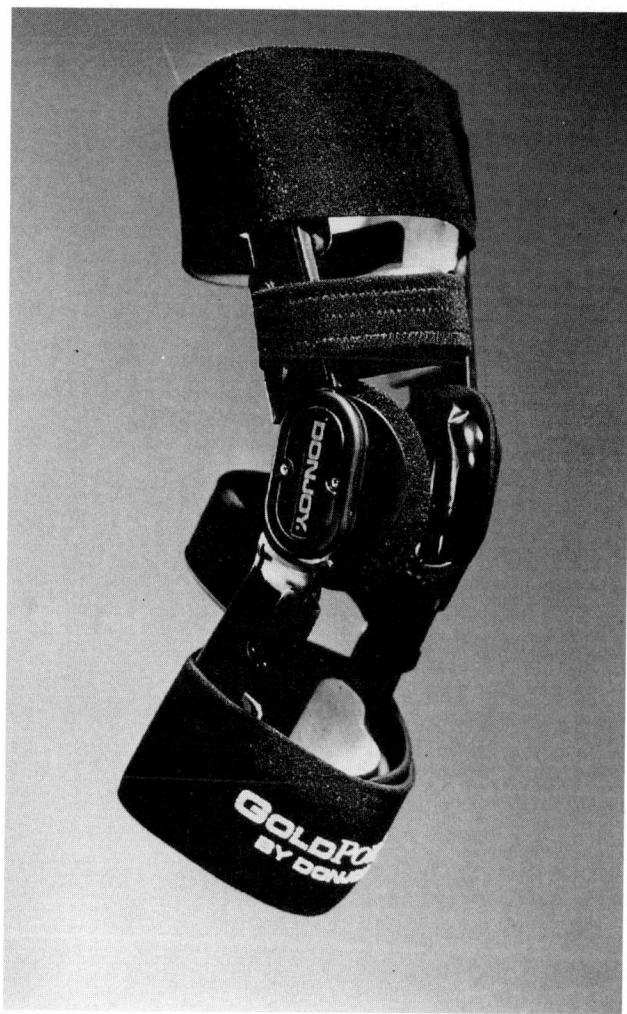

FIG 53-4.
An example of an off-the-shelf anterior cruciate ligament orthosis, the DonJoy Gold Point. (Courtesy of DonJoy, Inc., Carlsbad, Calif.)

ACL injuries are common in athletes and physically active persons. Normal gait patterns at a low cadence rate generally do not pose any difficulty to such patients, but instability and risk of further injury are possible if above-normal cadence or sudden deceleration movements are necessary. Instability is

TABLE 53-3.
Comparison of Functional Knee Braces

Brace	Straps	Shell	Hinge	Weight
Can-Am	X		Polycentric	Moderately heavy
CTi		X	Polycentric	Very light
Feaney	X		Slotted cam	Heavy
Lenox Hill	X		Single pivot	Light
Omni-TS7		X	Polycentric	Moderate
OTI Performer		X	Single pivot	Heavy
Townsend		X	Slotted cam	Moderately light

To determine the effectiveness of functional knee braces, numerous studies have been performed. Beck et al.[6] tested seven functional knee braces on three ACL-deficient knees with the KT-1000 and Stryker knee laxity testers. They found that the hinge, post, and shell types of braces performed consistently better in controlling anterior tibial displacement at low loads. As these forces increased, the effectiveness of the functional knee braces in controlling anterior tibial displacement decreased. Liu et al.[30] evaluated ten functional knee braces on a surrogate knee model and found the post-bilateral hinge-shell models provided the least resistance. None of the braces were capable of controlling displacement at high loads comparable to strenuous activities (i.e., >150–400 N).

Concern that functional knee braces prestrain the ACL and place the patient at additional risk for wear-

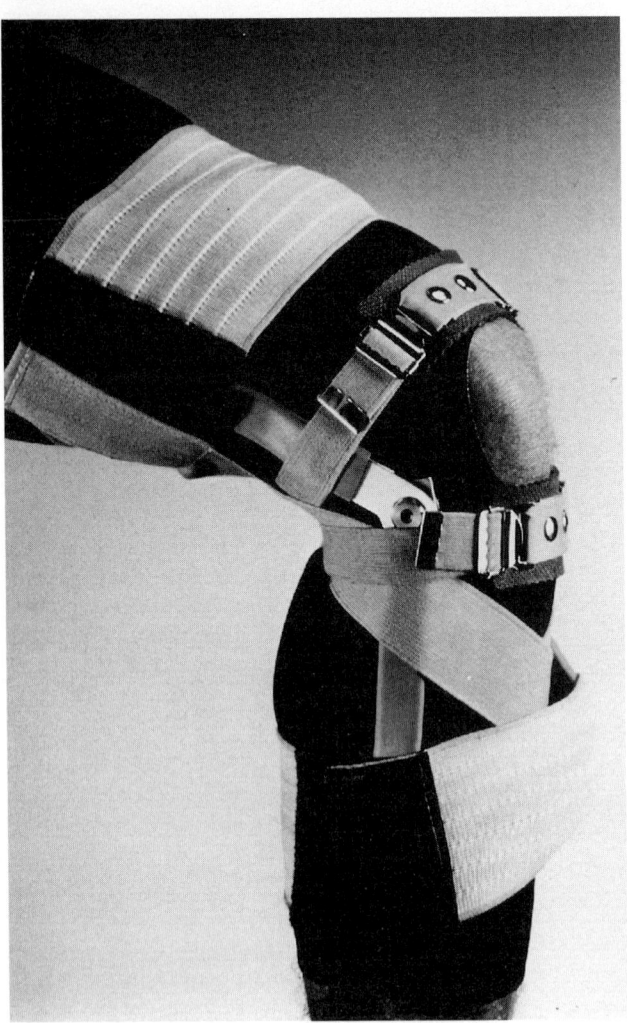

FIG 53–5.
The lightweight custom Lenox Hill anterior cruciate ligament orthosis manufactured by 3M. (Courtesy of 3M Health Care, St. Paul, Minn.)

primarily due to knee subluxation and tibial rotation during the terminal impact of knee extension. The contributing factor for such instability appears to be the increased angular velocity of the knee during fast cadence rates when anatomic deficiencies allow increased impact energy at extension, resulting in anterior displacement and rotation of the tibia relative to the femur.

Braces to improve the stability of the ACL-deficient knee are designed to prevent full extension by mechanical limits to avoid the expected instability. Some braces also incorporate a derotation relief,[51] and one brace[5] is designed on a closed-kinetic-chain concept and attempts to control varus. The designers of this brace believe that the femur displaces anteriorly on the tibia and uses a different axis of rotation with this brace.

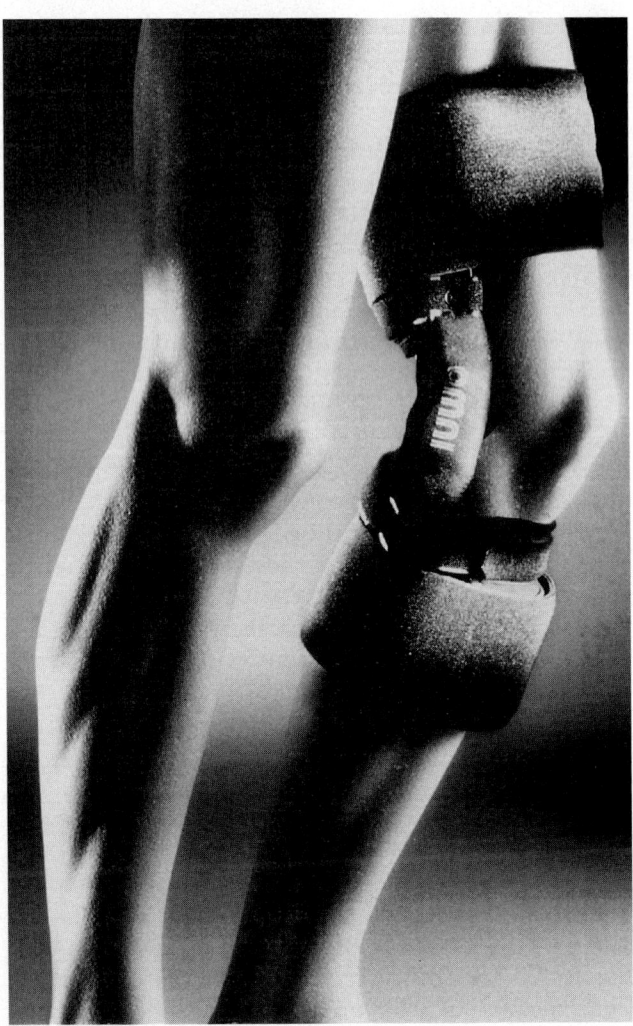

FIG 53–6.
The Omni TS-7 custom brace is another variation of an anterior cruciate ligament orthosis. (Courtesy of OMNI Scientific, Inc., Concord, Calif.)

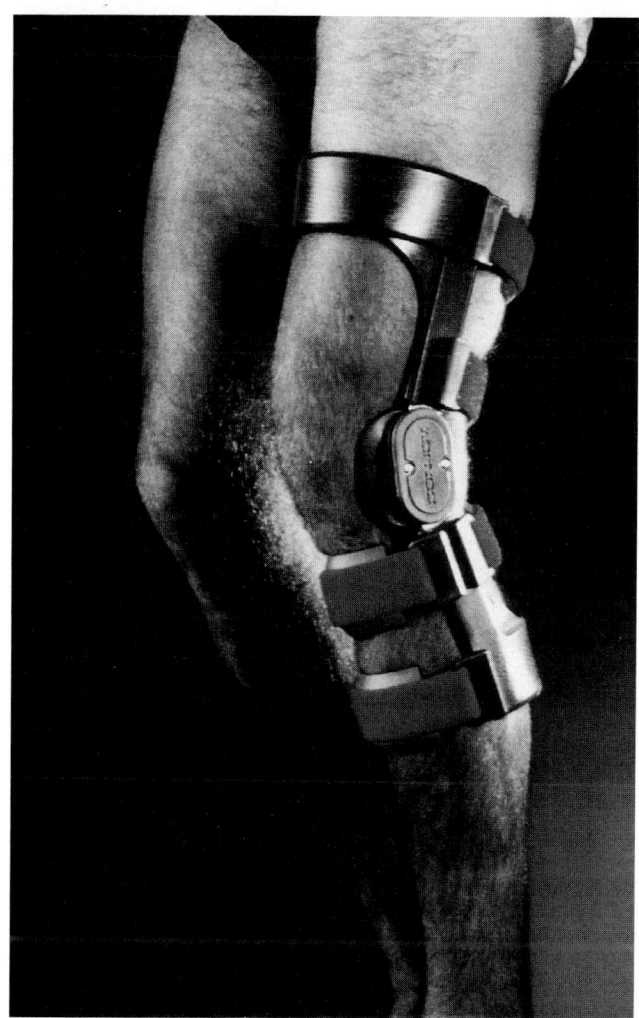

FIG 53–7.
A custom DonJoy ACL orthosis. (Courtesy of DonJoy, Inc., Carlsbad, Calif.)

ing the brace has been evaluated by Beynnon et al.[7] Five patients with normal ACLs underwent diagnostic arthroscopy and had placement of the Hall effect strain transducer (HEST) within the anteromedial band of their ACL. Measurements were performed braced and unbraced. They concluded that for active range of motion, application of a functional knee brace does not increase the normal ACL strain pattern.

Studies of the Lenox Hill brace by Colville et al.[12] demonstrated that the absolute laxity of the deficient knee was unchanged by the brace, but the relative resistance to displacement was increased. Hunter et al.,[27] using the KT-1000, compared the restraining effect of the Lenox Hill and the CTi brace to static loading. Both braces controlled anterior translation at 15 lb, but only the CTi controlled it at 20 lb. Neither brace was effective in controlling anterior tibial translation when higher loading forces were used in the active anterior drawer test.

Branch et al.[9] evaluated the contribution of functional bracing to muscle firing amplitude, duration, and timing which may result in improved dynamic stability. Ten ACL-deficient and five normal controls were evaluated using footswitches and dynamic electromyograms (EMGs). Bracing did not alter the relative EMG activity, nor did it change firing patterns compared with the unbraced situation. All muscles showed a similar reduction in activity suggesting that functional braces do not have a proprioceptive influence.

Cook et al.[14] performed a dynamic analysis of functional knee braces for ACL-deficient athletes. Footswitch, high-speed photography, and force-plate data were recorded with and without their custom-fitted CTi braces. Cutting angle, approach time to cut,

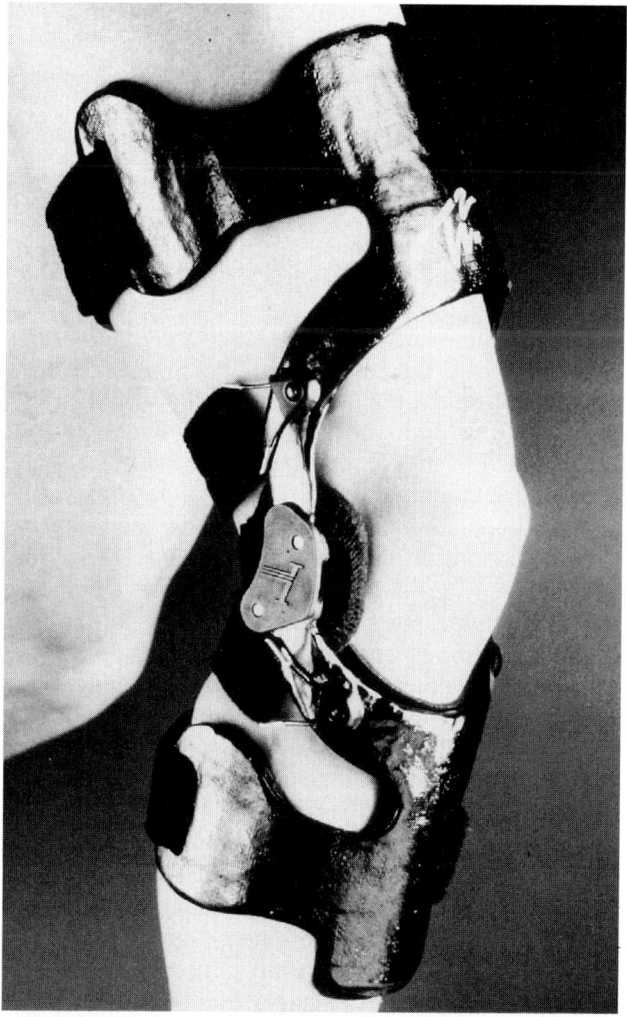

FIG 53–8.
The custom CTi anterior cruciate ligament orthosis. (Courtesy of Innovation Sports, Inc., Irvine, Calif.)

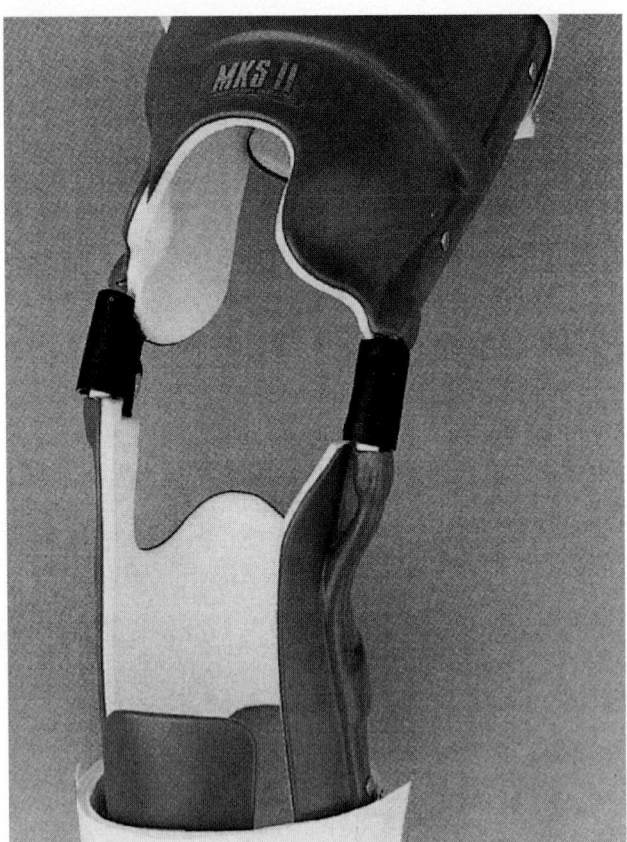

FIG 53–9.
Few posterior cruciate ligament orthoses are available. One example is the custom MKS II brace.

and time on force plate showed no significant differences during brace wear. Athletes who did not achieve 80% of the isokinetic quadriceps torque of the sound limb generated significantly more forces during cutting maneuvers while wearing their braces. Athletes also reported better subjective results while snow- and water-skiing compared to basketball and racquet sports. They noted subjectively fewer subluxation episodes and better performance with the brace. Improvements were even more significant in the quadriceps-deficient patients, suggesting athletes who rehabilitate incompletely may obtain increased benefit from functional knee bracing.

Scott et al.[42] compared the CTi, OTI, and TS7 knee braces in 14 patients with arthroscopically demonstrated ACL-deficient knees. The subjects evaluated the braces and underwent testing with physical examination, KT-1000 arthrometry, and timed running events. All braces reduced subjective symptoms of knee instability, and again a reduction in anterior tibial displacement was seen with all braces at low loads. This reduction decreased, however, as forces increased. A timed figure-eight running event showed no functional advantage of bracing: five subluxation events occurred in four subjects while braced.

Mishra et al.[32] evaluated four functional knee braces and their effect on anterior knee laxity. All braces reduced giving-way episodes and the grade of pivot shift. Brace use decreased anterior displacement on KT-1000 measurements at 89 N, high-load passive anterior displacement, and with quadriceps contraction active displacement. There was no significant effect on functional test results. Interestingly, patients most limited functionally improved with bracing while those minimally affected had diminished performance.

Loubert et al.[31] examined the ability of 14 different functional knee braces to control tibial rotation and translation under rigid mechanical loading conditions on fresh human cadaver legs. They found that braces were more effective at decreasing anteroposterior translation than at decreasing rotation. They were also more effective at decreasing displacement at 60 degrees of knee flexion as opposed to 30 degrees. The authors point out that their model is not a real-life situation and lacks muscular contribution during testing.

In another study, Wojtys et al.[52] evaluated relative restraints of 14 functional knee braces, using six cadaver limbs. Three trends were noted: braces were more effective in decreasing internal and external rotation than anteroposterior translation; they were more effective at decreasing displacement at 60 degrees than at 30 degrees; and they more effectively decreased translation in combined MCL-ACL rather than isolated ACL injuries. The study demonstrated that functional knee braces provide a variable restraining influence that may be beneficial in the control of abnormal knee displacements.

Several studies have evaluated the metabolic costs of knee brace wear.[25, 47, 53] Recently, Highenboten et al.[25] studied four braces in 14 normal subjects undergoing horizontal treadmill running. The braces caused increases in oxygen consumption, heart rate, and ventilation in the 3% to 8% range compared with running without the brace. Subjective exertion was also increased between 9% and 13%. They concluded that these braces cause a consistent increase in metabolic cost, which was related to their weight. These results are consistent with past research on braced ACL-deficient or reconstructed patients.[53]

An increase in intramuscular pressures in the anterior leg compartment has also been associated with functional knee brace wear. Styf et al.[47] evaluated three braces in eight healthy subjects and noted significant increases in anterior tibial muscle pressures regardless of posture. In addition, muscle relaxation pressures during exercise also were increased. The pressure levels reached could decrease muscle blood significantly (40 mm Hg in 9 of 18 subjects) and possibly induce premature muscle fatigue secondary to decreased perfusion.

Recently, patient noncompliance prompted Zvijac et al.[54] to perform a study of the postoperative use of derotation knee braces. Patients underwent arthroscopically assisted ACL reconstruction and at 6 weeks post operation were placed in braced or nonbraced groups. Follow-up between 6 and 30 months, including Lachman, pivot shift, and anterior drawer tests, and KT-1000 measurements, were identical. Range of motion was slightly greater in the nonbraced group but was not statistically significant. The authors concluded that postoperative functional knee bracing is not required, although it may benefit some patients from a psychological standpoint.

Factors to consider when looking at a brace or a study evaluating a brace are the use of extension stops, thigh size, body fat percentage of the subjects, and the effect and type of exercise[22, 45] used for the study. An additional factor is compliance, which may be related to the appearance and comfort of the brace. In athletic competition with conditions of high loading, the ability of the brace to control pathologic anterior laxity is minimal at best. The functional brace may play a role in the overall treatment plan for the ACL-deficient knee even though it does not restore normal stability.

SUMMARY

Three types of knee braces are available. There are two basic types of prophylactic knee braces. One has a lateral bar with single-axis, dual-axis, or polycentric hinges; the other uses a plastic shell that encircles the thigh and calf and has polycentric hinges. Rehabilitative knee braces are essentially off-the-shelf braces that allow protected motion of injured knees treated operatively or nonoperatively. Functional knee braces use hinges and a post, and either a thigh and calf enclosure (shell) or straps for suspension for treatment of ACL-deficient knees.

Prophylactic braces remain controversial, and for the most part have been shown to be ineffective in preventing knee injuries in collegiate and high school players. Biomechanical studies have shown some preloading of the ligaments in vivo, but this had not been demonstrated in vitro. Most studies have design flaws and bias, and therefore no conclusions can be drawn at this time and prophylactic knee bracing cannot be recommended until further prospective and biomechanical studies can demonstrate otherwise.

Rehabilitative braces provide little or no static anteroposterior control of motion, and the hinge setting may not actually affect true joint motion by a factor of 15 to 20 degrees. However, they are useful for the operative and nonoperative treatment of ligamentous knee injuries as long as this is kept in mind.

Functional knee braces alone are not adequate to control the pathologic laxity due to ACL injury with higher loads. Combined with an adequate rehabilitation program and activity modification or surgery, these braces do limit excessive anterior tibial translation under low loads.

Knee bracing remains a complex topic in the field of orthopaedic surgery; however, this need not be so if the orthopaedist remembers the three main types of braces, and their minor variations, and how to assess the data pertaining to clinical, epidemiologic, and biomechanical studies when evaluating these braces.

REFERENCES

1. American Academy of Orthopedic Surgeons: *Knee braces. Seminar report,* St Louis, 1985, Mosby–Year Book.
2. Anderson G, Zeman SC, Rosenfeld RT: The Anderson knee stabler, *Physician Sports Med* 7:125–127, 1979.
3. Baker BE, et al: A biomechanical study of the static stabilizing effect of knee braces on medial stability, *Am J Sports Med* 15:566–570, 1987.
4. Baker BE, et al: The effect of knee braces on lateral impact loading of the knee, *Am J Sports Med* 17:182–186, 1989.
5. Bassett GS, Fleming BW: The Lenox Hill brace and anterolateral rotatory instability, *Am J Sports Med* 11:345–348, 1983.
6. Beck C, et al: Instrumented testing of functional knee braces, *Am J Sports Med* 14:253–256, 1986.
7. Beynnon B, et al: An in-vivo study of the anterior cruciate ligament strain biomechanics during functional knee bracing, 36th Annual Meeting, Orthopaedic Research Society, New Orleans, Feb 5–8, 1990.
8. Biacharski PA, Sommerset JH, Murray DG: A three-dimensional study of kinematics of the human knee, *J Biomech,* 8:375–384, 1975.
9. Branch TP, Hunter R, Donath M: Dynamic EMG analysis of anterior cruciate deficient legs with and without bracing during cutting, *Am J Sports Med* 17:35–41, 1989.
10. Butler DL, Noyes FR, Grood ES: Ligamentous restraints in anterior-posterior drawer in the human knee—A biomechanical study, *J Bone Joint Surg [Am]* 62:259, 1980.
11. Cawley PW, France EP, Paulos LE: Comparison of

rehabilitative knee braces: A biomechanical investigation, *Am J Sports Med* 17:141–146, 1989.
12. Colville MR, Lee CL, Ciullo JV: The Lenox Hill brace—An evaluation of effectiveness in treating knee instability, *Am J Sports Med* 14:257–261, 1986.
13. Cooke C: An analysis of the effect of the rotational, convex, polyaxial, mechanical knee brace on the stability and dynamic range of motion of the knee joint (thesis), Vancouver, University of British Columbia, 1977.
14. Cook F, Tibone JE, Redfern NF: A dynamic analysis of a functional brace for anterior cruciate ligament insufficiency, *Am J Sports Med* 17:519–524, 1989.
15. Curl WW, Mitchell WA: Agility training following anterior cruciate ligament reconstruction, *Clin Orthop* 172:133–136, 1983.
16. D'Ambrosia R: A viscoelastic knee brace for anterior cruciate ligament deficient patients, *Orthopedics* 8:478–481, 1985.
17. Drez D Jr, Millet CW: Knee braces, *Orthopedics* 10:1777–1780, 1987.
18. Drez D Jr, Millet CW: Principles of bracing for the anterior cruciate ligament–deficient knee. Treatment of the anterior cruciate deficient knee, *Clin Sports Med,* 7:827–833, 1988.
19. Flint J: A comparative study of the effectiveness of the Lenox Hill knee brace, the Omni TS-7,1 and Omni TS-7,2 in controlling anterior displacement of the tibia of six ACL injured knees. Martinez, Calif, 1988, Omni Scientific.
20. Garrick JG, Requa RK: Prophylactic knee bracing, *Am J Sports Med* 15:471–476, 1987.
21. Grace TG, et al: Prophylactic knee braces and injury to the lower extremity, *J Bone Joint Surg [Am]* 70:422–427, 1988.
22. Grana WA, Steiner ME, Chillage E: The effect of exercise on A-P knee laxity, *Am J Sports Med* 14:24–29, 1986.
23. Hansen BL, Ward JC, Diehl RC: The preventive use of the Anderson Knee Stabler, *Physician Sports Med* 13:75–81, 1985.
24. Hewson GF, Mendini RA, Wang JB: Prophylactic knee bracing in college football, *Am J Sports Med* 14:262–266, 1986.
25. Highenboten CL, et al: The effects of knee brace wear on perceptual and metabolic variables during horizontal treadmill running, *Am J Sports Med,* 19:639–643, 1991.
26. Hoffman AA, Wyatt RWB, Bourne MH: Knee stability in orthotic knee braces, *Am J Sports Med* 12:371–374, 1984.
27. Hunter R, Branch T, Reynolds P: Controlling anterior tibial displacement under static load—A comparison of two braces, *Orthopedics* 11:1249–1252, 1988.
28. Knutzen KM, Bates BT, Hamill J: Electrogoniometry of post-surgical knee bracing in running, *Am J Phys Med* 62:172–181, 1983.
29. Knutzen KM, Bates BT, Schot P: A biomechanical analysis of two functional knee braces, *Med Sci Sports Exerc* 19:303–309, 1987.
30. Liu SH, Lunsford TR, Vangsness T: Comparison of functional knee braces for control of anterior tibial displacement, 59th Annual Meeting of the American Academy of Orthopaedic Surgeons, Washington, DC, Feb 21, 1992.
31. Loubert PV, et al: A quantitative assessment of the efficacy of fourteen functional knee braces, Orthopedic Research Society, Las Vegas, February 1989.
32. Mishra DK, Daniel DM, Stone ML: The use of functional knee braces in the control of pathologic anterior knee laxity, *Clin Orthop* 241:213–220, 1989.
33. Nicholas JA: Bracing the anterior cruciate ligament deficient knee using the Lenox Hill derotation brace, *Clin Orthop* 172:137–142, 1983.
34. Nowalkowski ED: Alternative methods of knee stabilization in sports: A comparative analysis, *J Can Athletic Therapists Assoc* 5:13–17, 1978.
35. Paulos LE, Drawbert JP, France EP: Lateral knee braces in football: Do they prevent injury? *Physician Sports Med* 14:119–124, 1986.
36. Paulos LE, Cawley PW, France EP: Impact biomechanics of lateral knee bracing, *Am J Sports Med* 19:337–342, 1991.
37. Paulos LE, et al: The biomechanics of lateral knee bracing—Part I: Response of valgus restraints to loading, *Am J Sports Med* 15:419–428, 1987.
38. Paulos LE, et al: The biomechanics of lateral knee bracing—Part II: Impact response of the braced knee, *Am J Sports Med* 15:430–438, 1987.
39. Peterson TR: The cross body block—Major cause of knee injuries, *JAMA* 211:449–452, 1970.
40. Rink PC, Scott RA, Lupo RL: A comparative study of functional bracing in the anterior cruciate deficient knee, *Orthop Rev* 18:719–727, 1989.
41. Rovere GD, Haupt HA, Yates CS: Prophylactic knee bracing in college football, *Am J Sports Med* 15:111–116, 1987.
42. Scott RA, et al: A comparative study of functional bracing in the ACL deficient knee, *Orthop Rev,* 18:719–727, 1989.
43. Schriner JL, Schriner DK: The effectiveness of knee bracing in high school athletes, American Academy of Orthopaedic Surgeons Meeting, San Francisco, Jan 22, 1987.
44. Sitler M, et al: The efficacy of a prophylactic knee brace to reduce knee injuries in football, *Am J Sports Med* 18:310–315, 1990.
45. Skinner HB, Wyatt MI, Stone JA: Exercise-related knee joint laxity, *Am J Sports Med* 14:30–34, 1986.
46. Stevenson DV, et al: Rehabilitative knee braces control of terminal knee extension in the ambulatory patient, *Trans Orthop Res Soc* 34:517, 1988.
47. Styf JR, Nakhostine M, Gershuni DH: Functional knee braces increase intramuscular pressures in the anterior compartment of the leg, *Am J Sports Med* 20:46–49, 1992.

48. Taft TN, Hunter SL, Funderburk CH: Preventative lateral knee bracing in football, 11th Annual Meeting of the American Orthopaedic Society for Sports Medicine, Nashville, July 1985.
49. Teitz CC, et al: Evaluation of prophylactic braces to prevent injury to the knee in collegiate football players; *J Bone Joint Surg [Am]* 69:2–9, 1987.
50. Torzilli PA, et al: In vitro biomechanical evaluation of anterior-posterior motion of the knee, *J Bone Joint Surg [Am]* 64:258–264, 1982.
51. Wojtys EN, Goldstein SA, Matthews LS: A biomechanical evaluation of the Lenox Hill knee brace, *Clin Orthop* 220:179–184, 1987.
52. Wojtys EM, et al: Use of a knee brace for control of tibial translation and rotation, *J Bone Joint Surg [Am]* 72A(9):1323, 1990.
53. Zetterlung AE, Serfass RC, Hunter RE: The effect of wearing the complete Lenox Hill derotation brace on energy expenditure during horizontal treadmill running at 161 meters per minute, *Am J Sports Med* 14:73–76, 1986.
54. Zvijac JE, et al: Functional bracing after ACL reconstruction, 57th Annual Meeting of the American Academy of Orthopaedic Surgeons, New Orleans, 1990.

Appendix

Forms Used in Planning Knee Rehabilitation Program

ACL PROTOCOL
Lonnie Paulos, M.D.

Date													

Activities/Daily Living	Week								Month					
	1	2	3	4	5	6	7	8	3	4	5	6	9	12
Shower without brace	▓	→→												
Sleep without brace	▓	▓	▓	→→										
Break down brace	▓	▓	▓	→→										

Range of Motion	Week								Extension
	1	2	3	4	5	6	7	8	• Lie on stomach and lower leg into extension
Passive									• Sit on firm surface and place 5-10 lbs above knee
Extension/Flexion	0/60	Increase flexion PRN							
Active									**Flexion**
Extension/Flexion	40/90	30/90	20/100	20/110	10/120	0/130	0/140	Full	• Lie on back; use gravity to slide foot down wall • While sitting use gravity and opposite leg to bend knee

Brace Settings	Week								Month					
	1	2	3	4	5	6	7	8	3	4	5	6	9	12
Weight Bearing	▓	50%	100% →→											
Knee Brace ROM Setting	• Brace locked at 10° for 1st 2 weeks post-op • Unlock brace to EXERCISE angles after 2 weeks post-op													
EXERCISE = Ext/Flex	40/90	30/90	20/100	20/110	20/120	20/open	→→→→→→→→→→→→→→→→→→→→→→→→→							
AMBULATION = Ext/Flex	▓	10/10	20/100	20/110	20/120	20/open	→→→→→→		D/C'd for walking at 12th week					

Strength Training	Week								Month					
	1	2	3	4	5	6	7	8	3	4	5	6	9	12
Quad sets, SLR's (brace locked at 40°)	→→→								▓	▓	▓	▓	▓	▓
Electrical stimulation (If poor voluntary quad) (brace locked at 40°)	→→→								▓	▓	▓	▓	▓	▓

See Brace Settings "EXERCISE" for extension/flexion angles														
Hamcurls	▓	→→												
Total Hip (Resistance above knee)	▓	→→→→→→→→→→→→→→→→→→→→→→→→→→→→												
Mini-squat/leg press/toe rise	▓	▓	▓	→→→→→→→→→→→→→→→→→→→→→→→→→→→→→→→→→→→→										

Cycling - Stationary (No brace)	▓	▓	→→→											
Cycling - Outdoor (No brace)	▓	▓	▓	▓	▓	▓	Level ground only			Seated hill climb			Standing hill climbs	

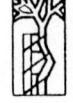

The Orthopedic Specialty Hospital 5848 South 300 East Salt Lake City, Utah 84107 (801) 269-4000

LACL1 3/10/93

Date														

		Week								Month				
Balance - Braced with 20° ext. stop	1	2	3	4	5	6	7	8	3	4	5	6	9	12
Baps/KAT/Sandunes/Rhomberg/Tape touch	▓	▓	━	━	━	━	━	━	━	━	━	━	━	▶
Profitter	▓	▓	▓	▓	▓	━	━	━	━	━	━	━	━	▶
Sport cord lateral agility	▓	▓	━	━	━	━	━	━	━	━	━	━	━	▶

		Week								Month				
Conditioning - Braced with 20° ext. stop	1	2	3	4	5	6	7	8	3	4	5	6	9	12
Cycle with well leg	▶		▓	▓	▓	▓	▓	▓	▓	▓	▓	▓	▓	▓
UBE (upper body conditioning)	━	━	━	━	━	━	━	━	━	━	━	━	━	▶
Walking (100% weight)	▓	▓	━	━	━	━	━	━	━	━	━	━	━	▶
Swimming (refer to pool protocol)	▓	▓	▓	▓	━	━	━	━	━	━	━	━	━	▶
Stairmaster	▓	▓	▓	▓	▓	▓	▓	━	━	━	━	━	━	▶
X-country ski machine	▓	▓	▓	▓	▓	▓	━	━	━	━	━	━	━	▶
Rowing	▓	▓	▓	▓	▓	▓	▓	━	━	━	━	━	━	▶
Run/jog (sports brace must be worn)	▓	▓	▓	▓	▓	▓	▓	▓	▓ As per Dr. Paulos		━	━	━	▶

		Week								Month				
Power Training	1	2	3	4	5	6	7	8	3	4	5	6	9	12
Low repetitions: Leg press/Squats/Hamcurls	▓	▓	▓	▓	▓	▓	▓	▓	20°/90° ━	━	━	━	━	▶
Isokinetics (refer to protocol)	▓	▓	▓	▓	▓	▓	▓	▓	▓	▓	━	━	━	▶

To Return to Sports:

- Minimum of 9 months post-operative
- No swelling
- Complete jog/run program
- Quadriceps strength 85% of opposite knee
- Hamstring strength 90% of opposite knee
- Hop distance 85% of opposite knee
- Range of motion 0° to 140°

ACL PROTOCOL - CRUTCHES
Lonnie Paulos, M.D.

Date														

Activities/Daily Living

	Week								Month					
	1	2	3	4	5	6	7	8	3	4	5	6	9	12
Shower without brace		→→												
Sleep without brace				→→→→→→→→→→→→→→→→→→→→→→→→→→→→→→→→→→→→										
Break down brace				→→→→→→→→→→→→→→→→→→→→→→→→→→→→→→→→→→→→										

Range of Motion

	Week							
	1	2	3	4	5	6	7	8
Passive								
Extension/Flexion	0/60	Increase flexion PRN						
Active								
Extension/Flexion	40/90	30/90	20/100	20/110	10/120	0/130	0/140	Full

Extension
- Lie on stomach and lower leg into extension
- Sit on firm surface and place 5-10 lbs above knee

Flexion
- Lie on back; use gravity to slide foot down wall
- While sitting use gravity and opposite leg to bend knee

Brace Settings

	Week								Month					
	1	2	3	4	5	6	7	8	3	4	5	6	9	12
Weight Bearing						50%	75%	100%	→→→→→→→→→→→→→→→→→→→→→→→→→→→					
Knee Brace ROM Setting	• Brace locked at 10° for 1st 2 weeks post-op • Unlock brace to EXERCISE angles after 2 weeks post-op													
EXERCISE = Ext/Flex	40/90	30/90	20/100	20/110	20/120	20/open	→→→→→→→→→→→→→→→→→→→→→→→→→→→→→→→→→→→→→→							
AMBULATION = Ext/Flex						20/open	→→	D/C'd for walking at 12th week						

Strength Training

	Week								Month					
	1	2	3	4	5	6	7	8	3	4	5	6	9	12
Quad sets, SLR's (brace locked at 40°)	→→													
Electrical stimulation (if poor voluntary quad) (brace locked at 40°)	→→→→→→→→→→→→→→→→→→→→→→→→→→→→→→→→→→													

See Brace Settings "EXERCISE" for extension/flexion angles

Hamcurls		→→												
Total Hip (Resistance above knee)		→→→→→→→→→→→→→→→→→→→→→→→→→→												
Mini-squat/leg press/toe rise					→→→→→→→→→→→→→→→→→→→→→→→→→→→→→→→→→→→→									

| Cycling - Stationary (No brace) | | | | | →→→→→→→→→→→→→→→→→→→→→→→→→→→→→→→→→→→→ | | | | | | | | | |
| Cycling - Outdoor (No brace) | | | | | | | Level ground only | | Seated hill climb | | | Standing hill climbs | | |

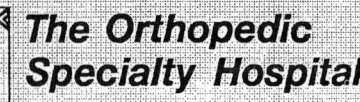

The Orthopedic Specialty Hospital
5848 South 300 East Salt Lake City, Utah 84107 (801) 269-4000

Date														

		Week								Month				
Balance - Braced with 20° ext. stop		1	2	3	4	5	6	7	8	3	4	5	6	9	12
Baps/KAT/Sandunes/Rhomberg/Tape touch															
Profitter															
Sport cord lateral agility															

		Week								Month				
Conditioning - Braced with 20° ext. stop		1	2	3	4	5	6	7	8	3	4	5	6	9	12
Cycle with well leg															
UBE (upper body conditioning)															
Swimming (refer to pool protocol)															
Walking (100% weight)															
Stairmaster															
X-country ski machine															
Rowing															
Run/jog (sports brace must be worn)										As per Dr. Paulos					

		Week								Month				
Power Training		1	2	3	4	5	6	7	8	3	4	5	6	9	12
Low repetitions: Leg press/Squats/Hamcurls										20°/90°					
Isokinetics (refer to protocol)															

To Return to Sports:

- Minimum of 9 months post-operative
- No swelling
- Complete jog/run program
- Quadriceps strength 85% of opposite knee
- Hamstring strength 90% of opposite knee
- Hop distance 85% of opposite knee
- Range of motion 0° to 140°

ACL PATELLAR TENDON AUTOGRAFT
Lonnie Paulos, M.D.

Date														

Activities/Daily Living

	Week								Month					
	1	2	3	4	5	6	7	8	3	4	5	6	9	12
Shower without brace	▓	▓	→	→	→	→	→	→	→	→	→	→	→	→
Sleep without brace	▓	▓	▓	▓	▓	→	→	→	→	→	→	→	→	→
Break down brace	▓	▓	▓	▓	▓	→	→	→	→	→	→	→	→	→

Range of Motion

	Week							
	1	2	3	4	5	6	7	8
Passive								
Extension/Flexion	0/90	0/90	0/100	0/110	0/120	0/130	0/140	Full
Active								
Extension/Flexion	40/90	40/90	30/100	20/110	10/120	0/130	0/140	Full

Extension
- Lie on stomach and lower leg into extension
- Sit on firm surface and place 5-10 lbs above knee

Flexion
- Lie on back; use gravity to slide foot down wall
- While sitting use gravity and opposite leg to bend knee

Brace Settings

	Week								Month					
	1	2	3	4	5	6	7	8	3	4	5	6	9	12
Weight Bearing	▓	50%	100% →	→	→	→	→	→	→	→	→	→	→	→

Knee Brace ROM Setting
- Brace locked at 10° for first 2 weeks post-op
- Unlock brace to exercise angles after 2 weeks post-op

For Exercise														
Extension/Flexion	40/90	40/90	30/100	20/110	20/120	20/open →	→	→	→	→	→	→	→	→
For Ambulation														
Extension/Flexion	▓	10/10	20/100	20/110	20/120	20/open →	→	→	D/C'd for walking at 12th week					

Strength Training

	Week								Month					
	1	2	3	4	5	6	7	8	3	4	5	6	9	12
Quad sets, SLR's (brace locked at 40°)	→	→	→	→	→	→	→	→	▓	▓	▓	▓	▓	▓
Electrical stimulation (brace locked at 40°)	→	→	→	→	→	→	→	→	▓	▓	▓	▓	▓	▓
Hamcurls	▓	→	→	→	→	→	→	→	→	→	→	→	→	→
Total Hip		→	→	→	→	→	→	→						
Mini-squat/leg press/toe rise	▓	▓	→	→	→	→	→	→	→	→	→	→	→	→
Cycling - Stationary	▓	→	→	→	→	→	→	→	→	→	→	→	→	→
Cycling - Outdoor	▓	▓	▓	▓	▓	▓	Level ground only	Level ground only	Seated hill climb	Seated hill climb	Standing hill climbs	Standing hill climbs		

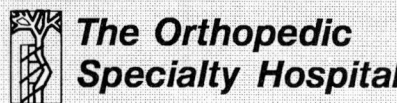

The Orthopedic Specialty Hospital
5848 South 300 East Salt Lake City, Utah 84107   (801) 269-4000

PACLPT1
8/11/92

Date														

Balance/Coordination

	Week								Month					
	1	2	3	4	5	6	7	8	3	4	5	6	9	12
Baps/KAT/Sandunes/ Rhomberg/Tape touch	▒	▒	▒	▒	▒	→	→	→	→	→	→	→	→	→
Profitter	▒	▒	▒	▒	▒	▒	▒	▒	→	→	→	→	→	→
Sport cord lateral agility	▒	▒	▒	▒	▒	▒	▒	▒	→	→	→	→	→	→

Conditioning

	Week								Month					
	1	2	3	4	5	6	7	8	3	4	5	6	9	12
Cycle with well leg	→	→	▒	▒	▒	▒	▒	▒	▒	▒	▒	▒	▒	▒
UBE (upper body conditioning)	→	→	→	→	→	→	→	→	→	→	→	→	→	→
Walking (100% weight)	▒	▒	10° →	→	→	→	→	→	→	→	→	→	→	→
Swimming (refer to pool protocol)	▒	▒	▒	▒	20° →	→	→	→	→	→	→	→	→	→
Stairmaster	▒	▒	▒	▒	▒	▒	20° →	→	→	→	→	→	→	→
X-country ski machine	▒	▒	▒	▒	▒	▒	20° →	→	→	→	→	→	→	→
Rowing	▒	▒	▒	▒	▒	▒	▒	20° →	→	→	→	→	→	→
Run/jog (sports brace must be worn)	▒	▒	▒	▒	▒	▒	▒	▒	▒	▒	▒	20° →	→	→

Power Training

	Week								Month					
	1	2	3	4	5	6	7	8	3	4	5	6	9	12
Low repetitions: Leg press/ Squats/Hamcurls	▒	▒	▒	▒	▒	▒	▒	▒	20°/90° →	→	→	→	→	→
Isokinetics (refer to protocol)	▒	▒	▒	▒	▒	▒	▒	▒	▒	→	→	→		

To Return to Sports:

- Minimum of 9 months post-operative
- No swelling
- Complete jog/run program
- Quadriceps strength 85% of opposite knee
- Hamstring strength 90% of opposite knee
- Hop distance 85% of opposite knee
- Range of motion 0° to 140°

PCL PROTOCOL
Lonnie Paulos, M.D.

Date														

	Week								Month					
Activities/Daily Living	1	2	3	4	5	6	7	8	3	4	5	6	9	12
Shower without brace	▓	▓	▓	───────────────────────────────────►										
Sleep without brace	▓	▓	▓	▓	▓	──────────────────────────────►								
Break down brace	▓	▓	▓	▓	▓	──────────────────────────────►								

	Week								Extension
Range of Motion	1	2	3	4	5	6	7	8	• Lie on stomach and lower leg into extension
Passive									• Sit on firm surface and place 5-10 lbs above knee
Extension/Flexion	15/15	10/50	10/50	0/60	0/70	0/80	0/90	Full	**Flexion**
Active									• Lie on back; use gravity to slide foot down wall
Extension/Flexion	▓	0/30	0/30	0/60	0/70	0/80	0/90	Full	• While sitting use gravity and opposite leg to bend knee

	Week								Month					
Brace Settings	1	2	3	4	5	6	7	8	3	4	5	6	9	12
Weight Bearing	▓	▓	▓	▓	▓	25%	50%	75%	Full ──────────────────────►					
Knee Brace ROM Setting	• Brace locked at 15° for first 4 weeks post-op													
For Ambulation	• Unlock brace to active angles after 4 weeks post-op													
Extension/Flexion						20/100	20/110	20/120	D/C'd for walking at 12ᵗʰ week					

	Week								Month					
Strength Training	1	2	3	4	5	6	7	8	3	4	5	6	9	12
Quad sets, SLR's (Brace locked at 15°)	───────────────────────────────►								▓	▓	▓	▓	▓	▓
Electrical stimulation Quads Only (Brace locked at 15°)		─────────────────────────────►												
Short Arc Quads	▓	0/30 ─────────────────────────►							0/70 ──────────►			Full		
Total Hip	─────────────────►					▓	▓	▓	▓	▓	▓	▓	▓	▓
Mini-squat/leg press/toe rise				──────────────────────────►										
Cycling - Stationary					──────────────────────►									
Cycling - Outdoor	▓	▓	▓	▓	▓	▓	▓	▓	Level ground only			Standing hill climbs		

PPCL1

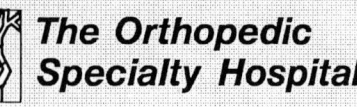

The Orthopedic Specialty Hospital 5848 South 300 East Salt Lake City, Utah 84107 (801) 269-4000

Date														

Balance/Coordination	Week								Month					
	1	2	3	4	5	6	7	8	3	4	5	6	9	12
Baps/KAT/Sandunes/ Rhomberg/Tape touch			→											
Profitter									→					
Sport cord lateral agility									→					

Conditioning	Week								Month					
	1	2	3	4	5	6	7	8	3	4	5	6	9	12
Cycle with well leg				→										
UBE (upper body conditioning)	→													
Swimming (refer to pool protocol)					10° →									
Walking (100% weight)							10° →							
Stairmaster										10° →				
X-country ski machine										10° →				
Rowing										10°/90° →				
Run/jog (sports brace must be worn)												10° →		

Power Training	Week								Month					
	1	2	3	4	5	6	7	8	3	4	5	6	9	12
Low repetitions - leg press/squats									10°/90° →					
Hamcurls												→		
Isokinetics (refer to protocol)												→		

To Return to Sports:

- Minimum of 12 months post-operative
- No swelling
- Complete jog/run program
- Quadriceps strength 100% of opposite knee
- Hamstring strength 80% of opposite knee
- Hop distance 90% of opposite knee
- Range of motion 0° to 140°

PCL and PLRI PROTOCOL
Lonnie Paulos, M.D.

Date

Activities/Daily Living

Activities/Daily Living	Post Operative Week														
	1-3	4	5	6	7	8	9	10	11	12	13	14	15	16	17
Shower without brace				→											→
Sleep without brace								→							→

Range of Motion

Range of Motion	Post Operative Week														
	1-3	4	5	6	7	8	9	10	11	12	13	14	15	16	17
Passive	Cast	DonJoy ROM Splint →												Shields Custom	
Extension/Flexion (prone)	30/30	0/30	0/40	0/50	0/60	0/70	0/80	0/90	0/100	0/110	0/120	0/130	Full	→	
Active															
Extension only (prone)	30/30	0/30	0/40	0/50	0/60	0/70	0/80	0/90	0/100	0/110	0/120	0/130	Full	→	
Patellar tilts, glides		→													→

Brace Setting

Brace Setting	Post Operative Week														
	1-3	4	5	6	7	8	9	10	11	12	13	14	15	16	17
Weight Bearing										25%	50%	75%	100%	Discont. Crutches	
ROM setting for exercise															
Extension/Flexion		20/20	20/20	10/30	10/40	10/50	10/60	10/70	10/80	10/90	Full until 26th week				

N-WT Bearing Conditioning

N-WT Bearing Conditioning	Post Operative Week														
	1-3	4	5	6	7	8	9	10	11	12	13	14	15	16	17
Cycle with well leg	→					→									
UBE (upper body conditioning)	→														→
Swimming (refer to pool protocol)		→													→
Quad sets, SLR's	→				→										
Electric stimulation (quad only)	→								→						
Total hip (no hip extension)	→														→

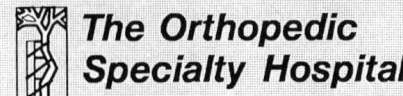

The Orthopedic Specialty Hospital   5848 South 300 East   Salt Lake City, Utah 84107   (801) 269-4000

Date														

Strength Training

	Post Operative Month													
Strength Training	1	2	3	4	5	6	7	8	9	10	11	12	13	14
Knee extension		0/50	0/60	0/70	→									→
Mini-squat/legpress/toe rise					→									→
Hamcurls					→									→

	Post Operative Month													
Balance/Coordination	1	2	3	4	5	6	7	8	9	10	11	12	13	14
Baps/KAT/Sandunes/Rhomberg/Tape touch					→									→
Sport cord lateral agility								→						→
Profitter								→						→

	Post Operative Month													
Power Training	1	2	3	4	5	6	7	8	9	10	11	12	13	14
Low repetitions: Leg press/squats									0/70 →					→
Isokinetics (ext. only - high speed) (low tibial pad placement)									0/70 →					→

	Post Operative Month													
Conditioning	1	2	3	4	5	6	7	8	9	10	11	12	13	14
Cycling - Stationary (no toe clips)(until 6 months)				→										→
Cycling - Outdoor (no toe clips)(until 6 months)							→							→
Walking (100% weight)					→									→
Stairmaster					→									→
X-country ski machine									→					→
Rowing									→					→
Run/jog (DonJoy PCL Brace) (must be worn)													→	→

To Return to Sports:

- Minimum of 15 months post-operative
- No swelling
- Complete jog/run program
- Strength evaluation prior to return to sports
- Range of motion 0° to 140°

54

Nursing Care of the Patient with a Ligament Injury

LINDA L. ALTIZER, R.N., M.S.N.

Treatment decisions
Postoperative nursing care
   Neurovascular assessment of lower extremity
   Postoperative wound drainage
   Leg bracing
   Continuous passive motion
   Electrical muscle stimulation
   Crutch walking
   Pain assessment
   Patient-controlled analgesia
   Psychosocial aspects

Postoperative complications
   Hemarthrosis
   Sepsis
   Thrombophlebitis
   Limitation of motion
   Patellar immobilization
   Incisional binding
Preparation for discharge
Summary

Patients with ligamentous injuries require basic nursing care as well as specific interventions which will vary according to the specific ligament injured and the treatment rendered. Those basic principles of care include managing pain, preventing complications, patient education, meeting the patient's psychosocial needs, and overseeing the coordination of rehabilitation and the preparation of the family and home environment for discharge.

Since one of the most complex and controversial issues regarding knee ligaments is the anterior cruciate ligament (ACL) injury, the primary focus of this chapter is on the nursing care of the patient with an ACL injury. Most of the treatment modalities involved in any knee ligament injury are discussed here as they relate to ACL injury, realizing that some may be used for other knee ligament injuries as well.

TREATMENT DECISIONS

Treatment of an injury to the ACL depends a great deal on the lifestyle of the patient. A person with a sedentary lifestyle or with only slight ligamentous instability will not benefit as much from reconstruction of the ligament as the young, athletic person. The patient's ability to perform activities of daily living—sports, shopping, climbing stairs—as well as the patient's pain and level of functioning, needs to be determined. The patient's motivation is taken into consideration along with his or her age and general state of health. The commitment that the patient has in regaining a knee that is functionally and structurally as near as possible to the preinjury knee must be gauged.

If surgery is indicated, the patient must be informed of how much time he or she will be off from work; of the long, concentrated time that must be spent in rehabilitation; and of the financial and psychological costs of surgery, hospitalization, rehabilitation, bracing, and follow-up care. Surgical candidates usually include those with knee injuries that have not responded to intense rehabilitation, those who are unable to perform activities of daily living, and those who are unwilling to change their athletic activities.

Conservative or nonsurgical treatment of knee ligament injuries includes a muscle-strengthening program, bracing, and avoiding activities that would stress or jeopardize the injured ligament.[20]

POSTOPERATIVE NURSING CARE

Conservative, nonoperative treatment of knee ligament injuries and the postoperative nursing care of the patient who has had a reconstructive procedure depend mainly on the ligament that was injured, the severity of the injury, the type of reconstruction performed, and the rehabilitation philosophy and preferences of the treating orthopaedic surgeon.

This chapter discusses general orthopaedic nursing assessment and care of the patient with a ligamentous injury of the knee, nursing's role in the operation of the equipment and treatment modalities utilized, pain management, patient teaching concepts, and possible complications.

Neurovascular Assessment of Lower Extremity

Neurovascular assessment is one of the most significant assessments that an orthopaedic nurse can perform on a patient with trauma or surgery to an extremity. It is extremely important to perform and document a precise initial neurovascular assessment. The initial assessment can be compared with all further checks to identify a trend of increasing neurovascular functioning, a plateau in neurovascular status, or a decrease in neurovascular function. The criteria used in assessing sensory and motor function and perfusion to an extremity remain constant and therefore facilitate the continuity of nursing assessment and care carried out by various care givers and across shifts of staff. The accurate documentation of neurovascular status should identify a plateau or an upward or a downward trend.

When assessing a patient who has had a knee ligament repair, neurovascular assessments should be performed on the deep peroneal, superficial peroneal, and posterior tibial nerves. The sensory and motor modalities of each are listed in Table 54–1.

The orthopedic nurse must monitor the extremity for motion, sensation, and for evidence of arterial supply and venous return. Palpation of the dorsalis pedis and posterior tibial pulses do not necessarily indicate perfusion to the distal extremity. An assessment of the skin temperature of the leg and the presence or absence of edema should also be documented.

The significance of early detection of signs and symptoms of neurovascular impairment cannot be overemphasized. The orthopedic nurse is responsible for detecting potential impairment of neurovascular status and immediately notifying the physician. Releasing any external wrap or brace that may be causing compression is a temporary action that the nurse may take. [If the arterial supply to the extremity is compromised, the leg should not be elevated above the horizontal level of the patient's heart.]

Neurovascular compromise is rarely seen in the patient who has undergone a postoperative knee ligament repair; however, the consequences of this complication can be irreversible.

Postoperative Wound Drainage

To minimize bleeding postoperatively, ice is applied to the operative area. This has a vasoconstricting effect and assists in hemostasis in the immediate postoperative period.

A wound drainage system or suction device is often used after surgical repair of the ACL.[28] The purpose of keeping the knee joint decompressed of oozing blood is to prevent hemarthrosis which may increase the chances of development of infection.

The nurse maintains an accurate measurement of the drainage as well as a description of the type of drainage obtained in the collection system which is documented on the patient's hospital record (Fig 54–1). The drainage system must be observed for adequate suction capability. Suction is maintained by proper decompression and sealing of the chamber (Fig 54–2). The suction chamber must be secured to the linen or to the patient's clothing when the patient is ambulatory so as not to place undue stress on the drainage tubes or suture line (Fig 54–3). It is also important that the nurse utilize universal precautions when emptying the drainage system or when handling any type of blood or body fluids.

Leg Bracing

Prolonged immobilization and disuse of the supporting structures of the knee can have significant adverse effects.[12] These effects begin immediately after injury and can be irreversible. Ligament healing and maturation require a long time. The ACL repair needs to be protected in order to maintain its integrity.[24] A rehabilitative knee brace is designed to provide controlled early motion of the injured knee whether

TABLE 54–1.

Modalities of the Deep Peroneal, Superficial Peroneal, and Posterior Tibial Nerves

Nerve	Motor	Sensory
Deep peroneal	Extends toes	Web space between great and second toe
Superficial peroneal	Everts foot	Dorsum of foot
Posterior tibial	Inverts foot Flexes toes	Plantar surface of foot and toes

NURSING CARE OF THE PATIENT WITH A LIGAMENT INJURY

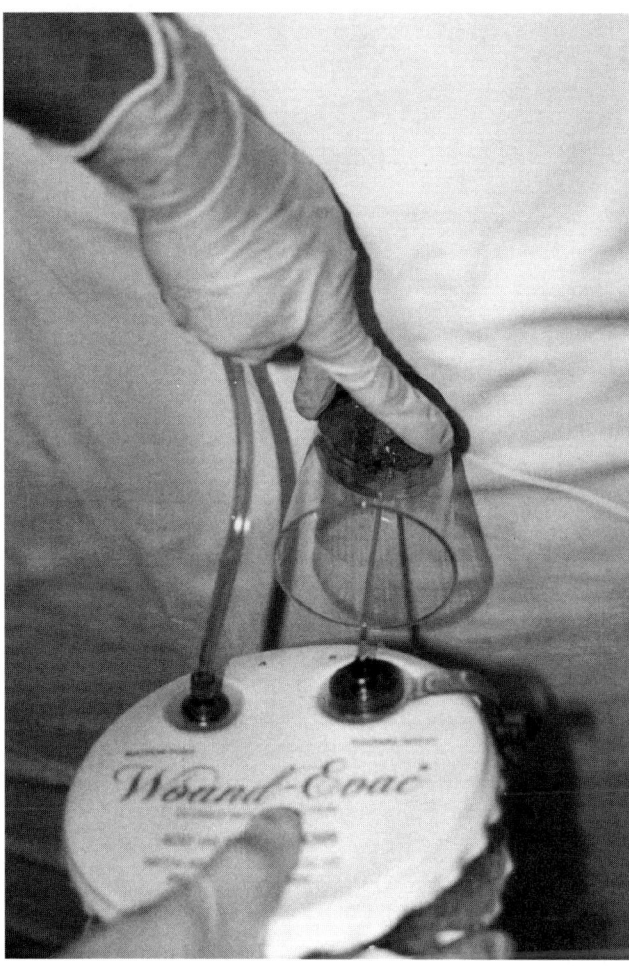

FIG 54–1.
Drainage from the knee is measured and the measurements are accurately documented on the medical record.

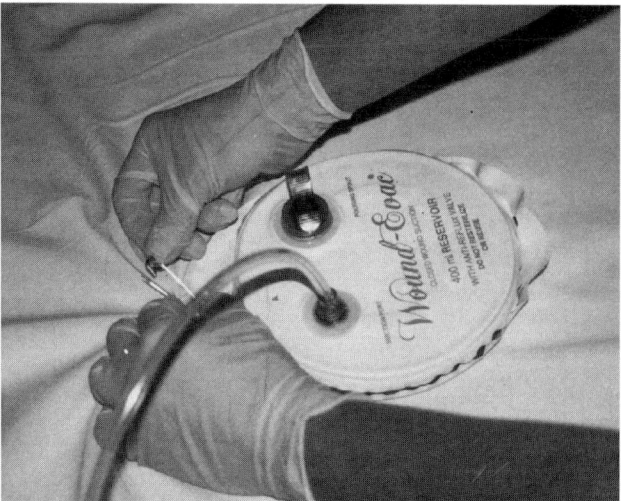

FIG 54–3.
Stabilization of the suction device reduces the risk of stress on the drainage tubing.

treated surgically or conservatively. Postoperative knee braces may be applied in the operating room immediately after surgical repair. It is important that the brace not be repositioned once it is in proper position and stabilized.

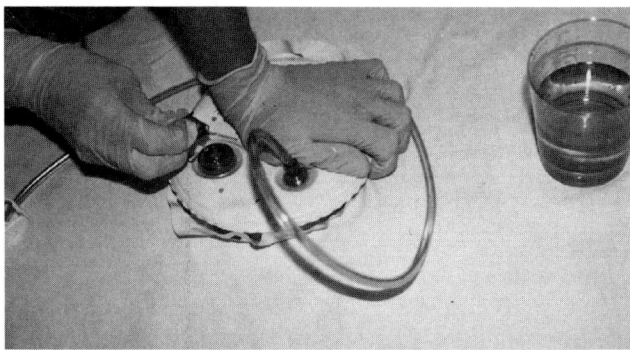

FIG 54–2.
Suction chamber must be adequately decompressed to maintain continuous suction to the operative area.

There are many characteristics of leg braces, but some of the most important features to evaluate are the following:

- Maintenance of position until the position is changed by the therapist or physician.
- Accurate control of knee motion.
- Adjustment to a variety of leg sizes and shapes.
- Comfort—lightweight and not cumbersome.
- Ease of applying and removing.
- Durability.
- Availability.
- Cost.

There are a variety of knee braces used in the orthopaedic community. The nurse should become familiar with the types of braces used most often in his or her facility and become competent in assessing the fit, comfort, flexion and extension settings, and operation of each. It is also important to have a working knowledge of the postoperative regimen of the orthopedic surgeons. There are as many differing philosophies as there are orthopedic surgeons when it comes to how fast and how much to increase range of motion (ROM) on the brace, how to exercise the extremity, how much weight to bear on ambulation of the extremity, what types of pain control to utilize, and what technologies to incorporate postoperatively.

Continuous Passive Motion

Continuous passive motion (CPM) is often part of the routine postoperative treatment of a patient with a knee ligament repair. Salter et al.[27] described the benefits of CPM therapy, including the following:

1. Less postoperative pain
2. Less stiffness
3. Decrease in intraarticular adhesions
4. Increased ROM
5. Facilitation of cartilage nutrition
6. Improvement in rate and quality of cartilage healing
7. Improved orientation and strength of collagen fibers in the graft
8. Improved graft healing
9. Improved blood flow to the extremity
10. Decreased incidence of thrombophlebitis
11. Improved maintenance of normal musculature and skeletal structures

Many surgeons prefer to begin the patient with early knee motion exercises postoperatively. The patient is often placed on a CPM unit the day of surgery. The nurse must coordinate the patient's care to ensure that the operative extremity is maintained in the postoperative brace in proper alignment on the machine. Thigh support when the machine takes the knee through a full arc of motion must be maintained and the knee must be positioned in alignment with the flexion-extension point. With reconstruction of the ACL, the ability to control the thigh with the machine moving the knee into flexion is important in controlling anteroposterior drawer forces on the tibia. An anterior tibial drawer will result if the thigh is not supported in flexion.[22]

Usually the amount of time spent in the CPM varies according to the surgical procedure performed and physician preference. Care should be taken to explain the machine and its method of operation to the patient. The patient's leg should be gently placed in the machine in proper alignment with the knee at the hinged joint of the machine. The foot plate should be adjusted so that the patient's foot is in neutral position and the leg is not rotated. Retaining straps are applied around the extremity. They should be loose enough for several fingers to fit under the strap, yet snug enough to maintain the extremity in position (Fig 54–4).

The usual procedure in CPM therapy is to gradually increase the ROM of the knee by increasing the set amount of flexion and extension of the CPM. The patient may be instructed to start and stop the machine as needed. The nurse should assess the patient's response and tolerance to the therapy and document the findings as well as the degree of extension and flexion, speed, and the amount of time the patient's leg is in CPM. Routine skin care, skin assessment, and neurovascular checks of the opera-

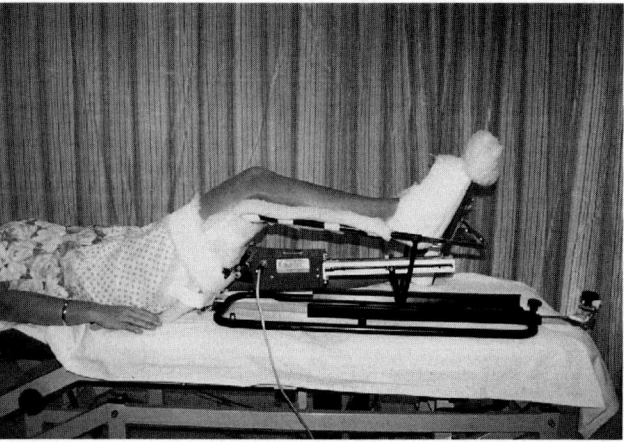

FIG 54–4.
Knee is positioned in the continuous passive motion (CPM) unit with the knee at the flexion-extension hinge and the foot plate in neutral position. Leg straps should secure the leg but be loose enough to allow fingers to slide under the straps.

tive extremity are very important. A flow sheet with space to document machine settings, times of therapy, tolerance, and neurovascular checks may be beneficial and often will increase the consistency and accuracy of nursing documentation.

Any increased effusion or unrelieved pain in the operative knee with extreme points of flexion or extension need to be reported to the physician and may require discontinuing CPM therapy until the knee is assessed by the orthopaedic surgeon.

Electrical Muscle Stimulation

There are varying opinions among orthopaedic surgeons as to whether electrical muscle stimulation (EMS) is beneficial in reducing muscle atrophy and postoperative pain (Fig 54–5). Arvidson and Eriksson,[9] in a study of 38 patients, reported that EMS with a pulse rate of 40 Hz produced some decrease in muscle atrophy in males and a significant decrease in muscle atrophy in females who had undergone ACL reconstruction. If EMS is used, it usually is initiated on the third or fourth postoperative day and continues through 5 to 6 weeks.

Crutch Walking

Crutches are used by patients with knee ligament injuries and by patients who have had surgical repair of a ligamentous injury. In either case the patient may be nonweightbearing or partially weightbearing.

The use of crutches requires upper body strength, balance, and coordination as well as a strong energy reserve and ample practice. The patient can practice shifting body weight in different posi-

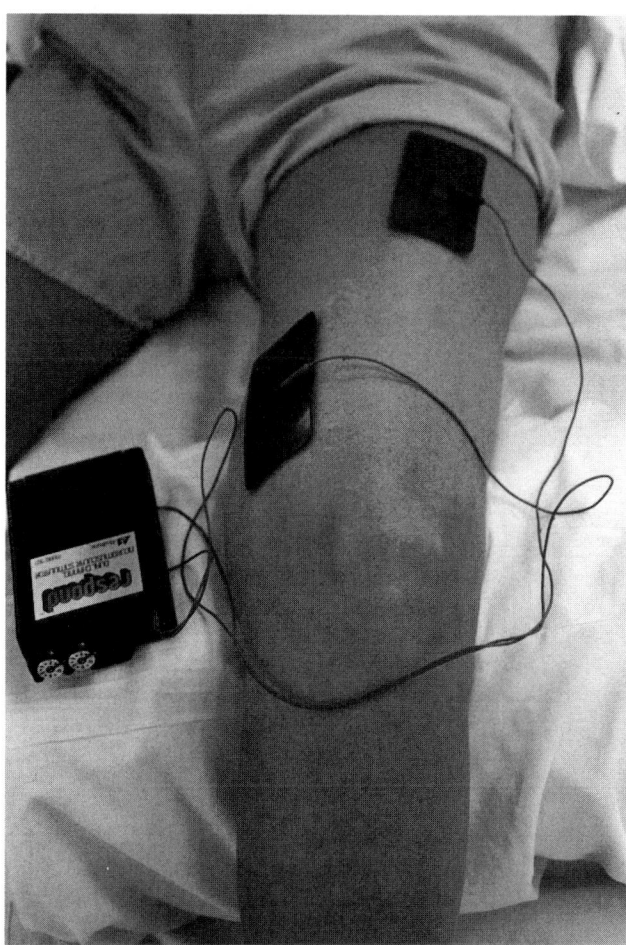

FIG 54–5.
Electrical muscle stimulation may be utilized to decrease muscle atrophy and postoperative pain.

sure of the crosspiece of the crutch in the axilla can cause crutch (compression) paralysis, usually involving the ulnar nerve.

Stair walking should be taught and validated before the patient is discharged home. When ascending stairs, the uninjured leg goes up first. When descending, the injured leg steps down first (Fig 54–8).

Pain Assessment

Pain can be perceived and communicated only by the person experiencing it. These symptoms are relayed to the nurse who in turn assesses the subjective in-

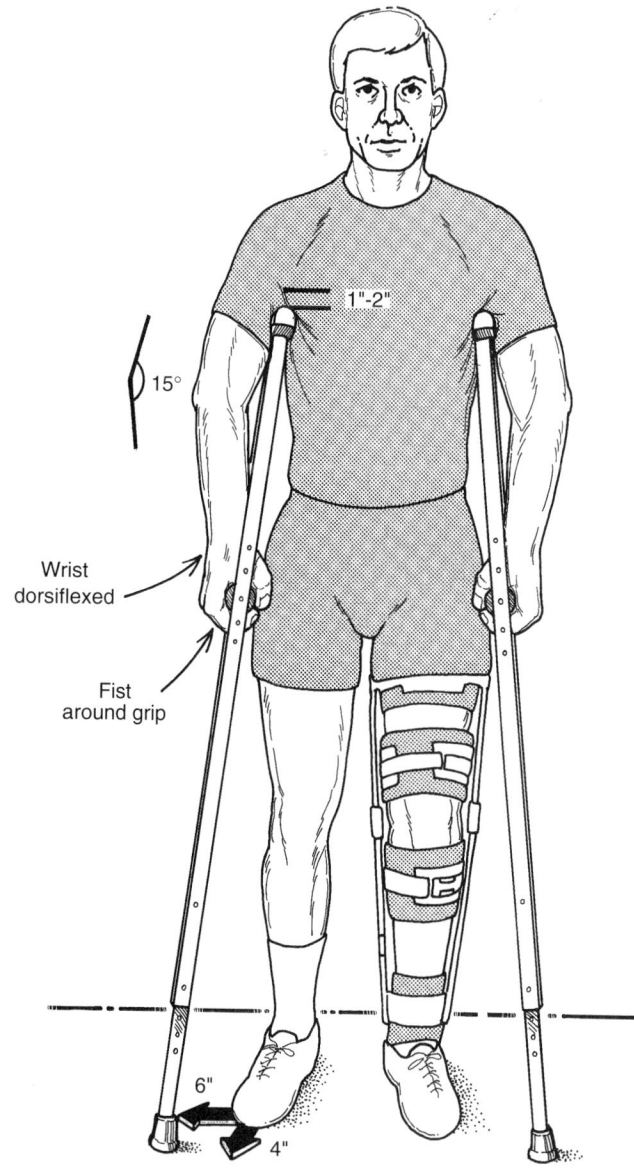

FIG 54–6.
Proper crutch fitting is necessary to facilitate safe ambulation. Pressure for weightbearing is on the hands at the hand grips, not on the axilla.

tions while standing with crutches and resting the back against a wall. When instructing the patient in crutch walking, emphasis must be placed on several points. The first is properly fitting crutches (Fig 54–6). The appropriately measured crutch will have the tip on the floor about 6 in. in front of and about 4 in. lateral to the little toe. There should be a space of two fingerbreadths between the axillary fold and the arm cradle of the crutch, with the handpiece adjusted to allow elbow flexion to 30 degrees. It is important for safety that the patient wear well-fitting, stable, comfortable shoes.

The selection of crutch gait depends on the type of surgery performed, the type of ambulation the patient is allowed, the patient's general physical condition, and arm and trunk strength and tolerance. It is helpful for the patient to learn two different gaits: a slow, stable gait for use in crowded areas and a faster gait when more speed is needed (Fig 54–7).

The patient should be instructed to bear weight on the hands and not to rest on the axillae. The pres-

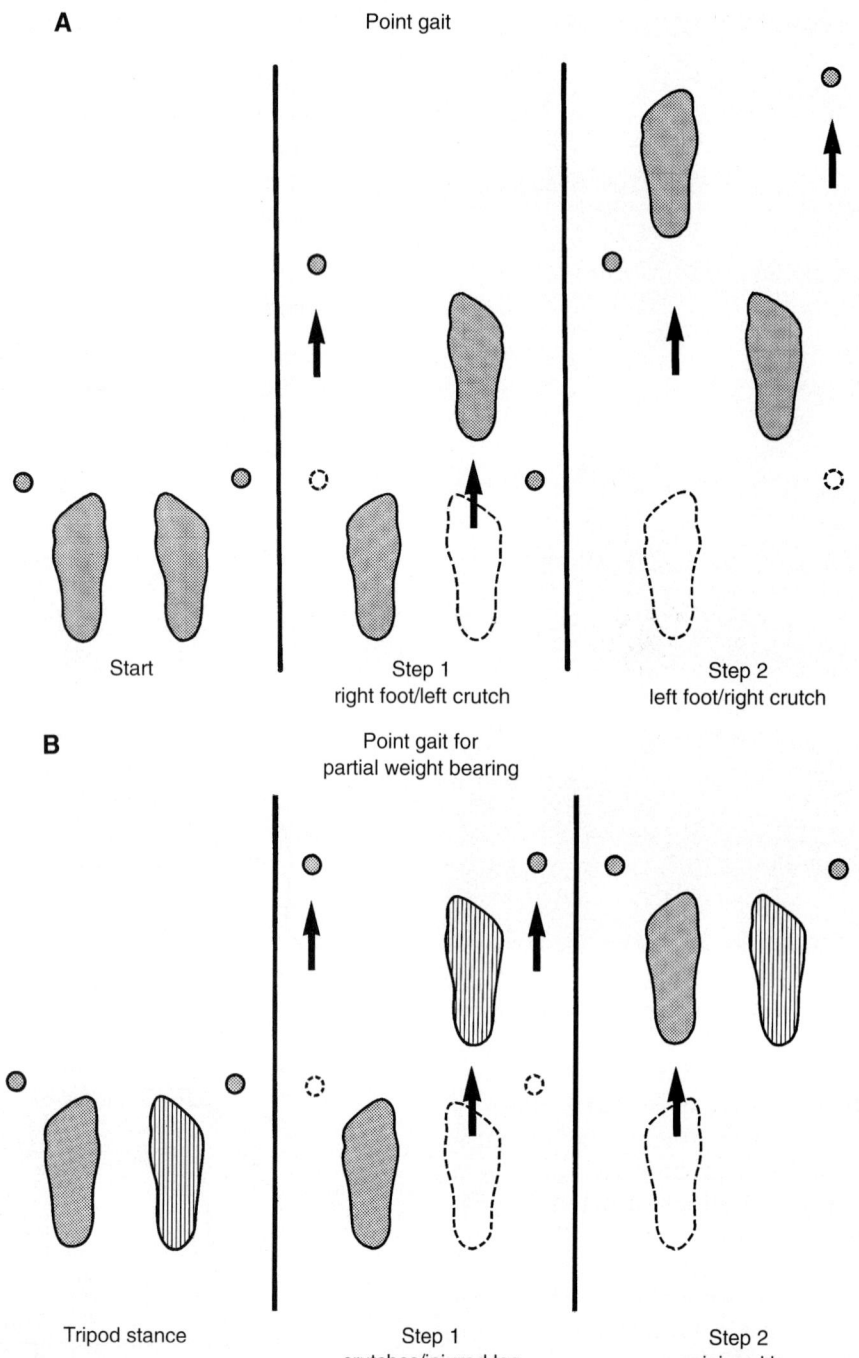

FIG 54–7.
Crutch walking for knee ligament injuries may include instructions for the two-point **(A)** or three-point **(B)** gait, or both.

put, physical findings, and nonverbal characteristics to formulate a plan of care for the patient.

There will inevitably be a reason for the patient to be experiencing pain. McCaffery[19] described the physical findings that the orthopedic nurse should identify, evaluate, and document when assessing the patient in pain:

1. *Occurrence of pain:* What is the perceived reason for this pain? Did an event precipitate this problem?
2. *Intensity:* Is the pain associated with palpation of the affected area? Is it increased or decreased with motion, pressure, contraction, or anxiety? Does the pain increase at a certain time of day?

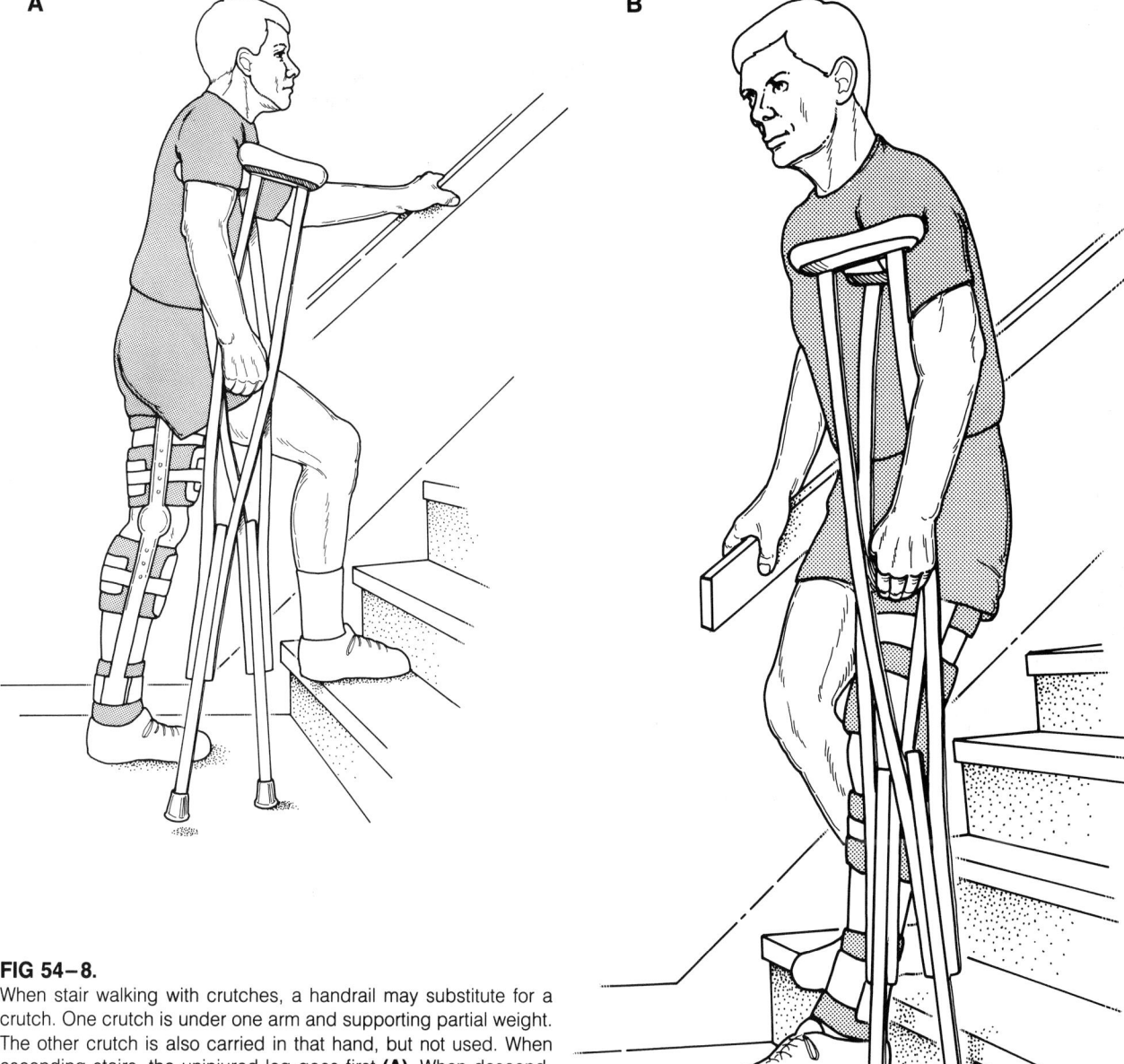

FIG 54–8.
When stair walking with crutches, a handrail may substitute for a crutch. One crutch is under one arm and supporting partial weight. The other crutch is also carried in that hand, but not used. When ascending stairs, the uninjured leg goes first **(A)**. When descending, the injured leg steps down first **(B)**.

3. *Location:* Is the pain over viscera, subcutaneous tissue, periosteum, joints, or is it referred or radicular? Does it radiate?
4. *Duration:* Is the pain intermittent? Does it last for hours, days, months, years?
5. *Pattern:* Is the pain stinging, burning, aching, throbbing, or associated with any particular stimulus?
6. *Past experiences with pain:* Are past injuries remembered as having a significant amount of pain? Does the amount of pain remembered correspond to the type of injury incurred?
7. *Meaning of pain to the patient:* Does the patient feel that he or she will be unable to return to activities that the patient previously enjoyed or even excelled in because of this injury and the pain that represents this injury?

Observations of the patient reveal nonverbal expressions of pain—anguished facial expressions, gestures, holding or rubbing an injured area, moaning or groaning. As the nurse assesses the patient for pain, the subjective input, physical findings, and nonverbal characteristics are evaluated for consistency and congruency. It is not unusual for athletes to try to minimize pain in order to minimize the severity of their injury so that they can return to sports activities as soon as possible.

Patient-Controlled Analgesia

Patient-controlled analgesia (PCA) is a recent method designed to give the patient some control over his or her condition. The method enables the patient to maintain an optimal serum level of analgesic through continual administration. An indwelling peripheral venous catheter provides the method for infusion which is controlled by a microcomputer that has been programmed to administer the drug according to the physician's order. A continual low-dosage of analgesic is usually given with a demand dose so that the patient can self-administer additional pain relief. The demand dose is locked at timed intervals, thus restricting the user to a maximum number of demand doses per hour. Dunwoody[6] compared traditional analgesia with PCA, and confirmed that patient comprehension and cooperation are essential in the selection criteria for use of PCA.

The nurse's role in caring for a patient who is using PCA involves not only the routine assessment and care of the patient receiving analgesia but also a competent knowledge of the PCA setup. This usually includes knowledge of and ability to change a medication cassette (Fig 54–9) and the ability to appropriately reprogram the pump when medication orders are changed by the physician (Fig 54–10). The nurse also plays an important role in educating the patient in the response to analgesia and the procedure for demand doses.

Patients that have had surgical repair of knee ligaments are usually young active persons who are well suited to PCA. The most severe pain will be encountered during the immediate postoperative phase and parenteral narcotics are seldom used beyond 24 to 48 hours. The treating physician may choose to administer intramuscular narcotics instead of PCA. Regardless of the method chosen, pain control is essential. Oral analgesics will typically control pain experienced after the first 48 hours. The nurse's role during the postoperative phase is to evaluate the severity of the patient's pain, attempt to control the pain with analgesics, and evaluate the effectiveness of analgesia. It is imperative that the nurse be aware of the patient's sensitivity to any medication, be knowledgable of

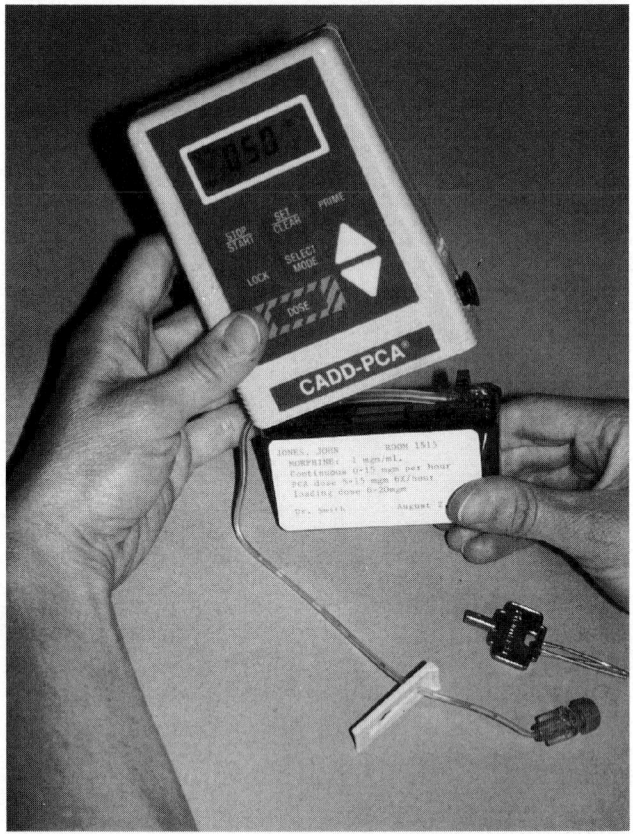

FIG 54–9.
The nurse must be knowledgable in changing the medication cassette or syringe depending on the administration system.

drug incompatibilities, and alert to possible side effects. Table 54–2 summarizes the dosages, contraindications, uses, and effects of some common narcotic analgesics.

Psychosocial Aspects

It is usually difficult for a relatively young, active person to face the possibility of not being able to reach his or her preinjury functional status. The surgical repair of a severe ligamentous injury to the knee may enable the patient to regain normal motion and eventually normal strength in the injured extremity; however, on occasions when the athlete has had to give up a sport due to injury, maladaptive behavior patterns may develop. These patterns may develop if the athlete has to suspend play for a game, a season, or a lifetime. The health care team strives to meet the psychological needs of the patient as well as the physical risk of reinjury. The orthopaedic nurse should be aware of the symptoms of maladaptive behavior.

Pennsylvania State University was the site of a

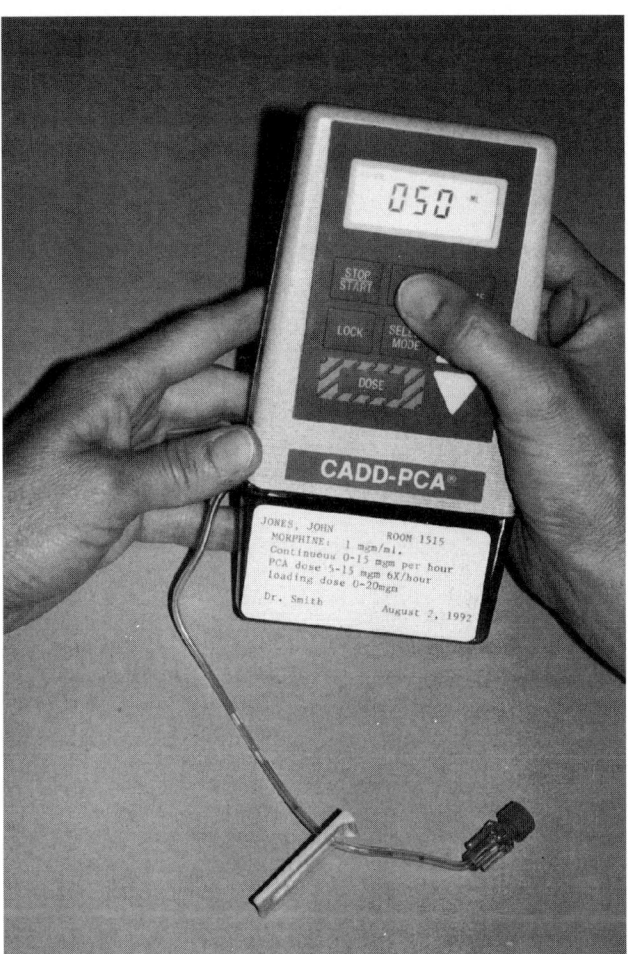

FIG 54–10.
Change in medication order necessitates reprogramming the pump.

12-year study by Whiteside et al.[30], which revealed that knee injuries in athletes accounted for more loss of playing time than any other injury. In a 3-year study of over 42,000 athletes, Chandy and Grana[3] reported that knee injuries were the most common cause of terminating play.

Ogilvie[9a] describes profound psychological trauma in not only the career athlete but also the recreational athlete who has had to relinquish continued athletic activity. He identifies a series of emotional reactions that are observed in such athletes. The first stage is *denial*. This stage leads the injured athlete to doubt the professional judgment of his or her treating physician. According to Ogilvie, the patient displays compulsive behavioral patterns such as continuing to dress in full gear for a game, persisting on sitting on the sidelines and attending practice sessions.

During this acute stage the nurse must realize that the patient's behavior is a normal defense mechanism used when reality is too difficult to confront. The nurse gives emotional support to the patient and lends professional support to the orthopaedist's diagnosis in an attempt to assist the patient into accepting reality.

The second stage is *projection*, as the patient begins to realize the truth about his prognosis. The patient displays resentment, anger, and sometimes open hostility. In an attempt to cope, the patient may try to displace his or her own responsibility for this unpleasant situation. In so doing, the athlete may blame the coach, the trainer, or even someone remotely affiliated with the team. If blame is projected onto someone on the health care team, the other team members must support one another. This support is more readily achieved, if the care providers are aware of projection as an unconscious defense mechanism.

The third stage is *grief*. This stage can continue for long periods of time and is characterized by lethargy, listlessness, lack of caring, and even depression. When a person feels this helpless, he or she tends to pay attention to anyone who offers what appears to be a quick fix. Until this stage is completed, the person is unable to carry on a productive life.

Reintegration is the final stage and is an indication that the patient is prepared to resume responsibility for his or her actions and return to well-integrated functioning. It is during this stage that the health care team collaborates with the patient in developing new goals that are realistic and attainable and provide a new direction in life.

The steps listed here are similar to the stages of dying described by Kübler-Ross.[16] Nursing support has been recognized as a valuable tool in assisting patients through a loss.

There was a time when the nurse was employed mainly in the acute care facility and was concerned with conditions or behaviors that occurred there. During the past several years, however, we are seeing an increased number of nurses in physicians' offices, sports clinics, home health facilities, orthopaedic centers, and so forth. It is important that nurses comprehend the various emotional reactions that patients and their significant others may demonstrate throughout the postoperative phase so that they may participate with the health care team in identifying those reactions and assist the team with the counseling and support needed in the various phases.

POSTOPERATIVE COMPLICATIONS

Complications may arise during management of knee injuries whether the injury is treated surgically or conservatively. Nonoperative management of a knee

TABLE 54–2.

Narcotic Analgesics

Drug	Adult Dosage	Contraindications	Comments
Codeine	*SC:* 15–60 mg qid prn or *PO:* 15–60 mg qid prn	Hypersensitivity Use with caution in patients with pulmonary compromise	May also be used as an antitussive agent; may cause nausea, vomiting and other GI problems
Hydromorphone (Dilaudid)	*Parenteral:* 2 mg q4–6h prn *PO:* 2 mg q4–6h prn *PR suppository:* 3 mg q6h prn	Hypersensitivity Increased ICP Use with caution in pregnancy	May cause CNS, GI or respiratory depression Adjust dose to patient size and severity of pain Not so long-acting as morphine
Levorphanol (Levo-Dromoran)	*Parenteral:* 2 mg q4–6h *PO:* 4 mg q4–6h	Hypersensitivity Acute alcoholism Increased ICP Respiratory depression	Analgesic effect equal to morphine and less than meperidine in far smaller doses than either Cumulative analgesic effect Longer-acting than most (6–8 hrs of pain relief) Less gastric upset than with morphine or meperidine
Meperidine (Demerol)	*Parenteral:* 50–150 mg q3–4h prn *PO:* 50–150 mg q3–4h prn	Hypersensitivity Use with caution in increased ICP, asthma, and pregnancy Use with caution in presence of renal impairment	Injectables are chemically incompatable with barbiturates May cause CNS depression Accumulation may cause neuroexcitability Provides analgesia for 2–4 hr
Methadone (Dolophine)	*Parenteral:* 2.5–10 mg q3–4h prn *PO:* 2.5–10 mg q3–4h prn	Hypersensitivity Patients <18 yr Respiratory compromise CNS depression	Use with caution with monoamine inhibitors Use with caution in acute abdominal conditions Rifampin lowers blood concentrations of methadone
Morphine sulfate	*Parenteral:* 5–15 mg q4–6h *PO:* 5–15 mg q4h *IV:* 2–15 mg diluted, pushed slowly over 5 min *PR suppositories* available *Solution* free of preservatives available for spinal administration	Hypersensitivity Use with caution in CNS depression, asthma, and pregnancy	Analgesic plus sedation effect Duration of action 4–6 hr
Nalbuphine (Nubain)	*Parenteral:* 10 mg q3–6h prn (for approx 70 kg patient)	Hypersensitivity	Analgesic effect equal to morphine Onset of action 2–15 min depending on route of administration Duration of effect 3–6 hr Naloxone may be used to treat overdosage
Opium tincture (Pantapon)	*Parenteral:* 5–20 mg q4–6h prn *PO:* 0.5–1.5 mL q4h prn	Hypersensitivity Bronchial asthma	Use with caution in patients with increased ICP, prostatic obstruction, and myxedema Infrequently used Narcotic antagonists may be used for overdosage
Oxymorphone (Numorphan)	*Parenteral:* 1–1.5 mg q4–6h prn *PR suppositories* available	Hypersensitivity Status asthmaticus Increased ICP	Rapid-acting (5–10 min) Duration of action 3–6 hr Produces mild sedation Causes very little depression of cough reflex

ICP = intracranial pressure.

*Landrum DF: Pharmacological therapeutics. In Hilt N, Cogburn S (eds): *Manual of orthopaedics*, St. Louis, 1980, Mosby–Year Book, pp 553–670. Used by permission.

injury may be followed by instability, joint effusion, and early degenerative joint disease. The same complications, however, may follow surgery.[7]

Hemarthrosis

After knee ligament injury and reconstruction, the operative area tends to ooze large amounts of fluid. As mentioned earlier, a postoperative drain is usually in place to keep the knee joint decompressed of postoperative blood accumulation. Suction drains are left in place until the 24-hour drainage is less than 30 mL. As the discharge tapers, the drain can be removed.[7] If the discharge suddenly increases and obvious hematoma formation occurs, a major vessel may be involved and need to be ligated. This may be accomplished by returning the patient to the operating room, reopening the incision to evacuate the hematoma, and locating and ligating the bleeding vessel. Adequate hemostasis during the initial reconstructive procedure will help prevent hematoma formation.

The role of the nurse is to closely observe the amount of drainage, maintain constant suction of the operative area, and apply ice to the incision postoperatively, which will help to minimize the chances of hematoma formation.

Sepsis

Strict adherence to aseptic technique during the operative procedure is essential with knee ligament reconstruction as it is with any surgical procedure. The circulating and scrub nurses in the operating room are obligated to inform the operating surgeon of any break in aseptic technique by any member of the operating team that may jeopardize the sterility of the procedure. Postoperatively, knee dressings are kept clean and dry. Aseptic technique must be used when changing dressings, and any break in the integrity of the drainage system must be addressed immediately. The nursing assessment at each shift includes inspecting the operative area, evaluating vital signs for temperature elevation, checking for warmth or redness over or near the surgical incision, and evaluating the patient for indications of increased pain in the knee.

Thrombophlebitis

The incidence of thrombophlebitis is increased in patients with certain risk factors. These include obesity, smoking, a previous history of thrombophlebitis, advanced age, and prolonged immobilization of an extremity. The nurse who is caring for a patient with knee ligament repair should be aware of any increased soreness in the gastrocnemius area or any increased sensitivity in this area elicited by dorsiflexing the toes. The nurse assists in the prevention of thrombophlebitis by operating the CPM unit, increasing the ROM, as appropriate. Leg exercises prescribed by the surgeon are encouraged and monitored not only by the physical therapist but also by the nursing staff. Early and frequent ambulation is also part of the team's goal for the patient's noneventful postoperative course.

Limitation of Motion

Limitation of motion is a well-documented complication after ACL reconstruction.[23] One of the major goals of postoperative rehabilitation is to establish early mobilization of the knee joint; however, this goal is complicated by the fact that the repaired or reconstructed ACL must be protected to prevent additional injury and allow it to heal. The dilemma of trying to accomplish early mobilization of the knee joint without disrupting the integrity of the ACL repair has led to the use of the hinged knee brace and the process of CPM. The nurse must have a good working knowledge of both technologies and the principles behind them.

There have been a small number of knees that have developed an extreme inflammatory response postoperatively. This response is manifested by severe pain and erythema, as well as by warmth and swelling in the tissues about the knee. These patients progress slowly and are treated aggressively with ice, compression, elevation, and anti-inflammatory medications. Exercise is deferred to avoid aggravating the condition.[23]

Patellar Immobilization

Scarring around the peripatellar and infrapatellar tissues can occur after an injury or surgical procedure. This scarring can lead to functional limitation of the knee joint. Early mobilization of the knee joint postoperatively will assist in preventing scarring and the resultant limited flexion and extension; however, problems may still occur with patellar immobilization. Patellar mobilization exercises may be ordered which include manually manipulating the patella in various directions (Fig 54–11). Patients can be taught these exercises by demonstration, and learning validated in turn by having the patient demonstrate the maneuver. Teaching can be augmented with illus-

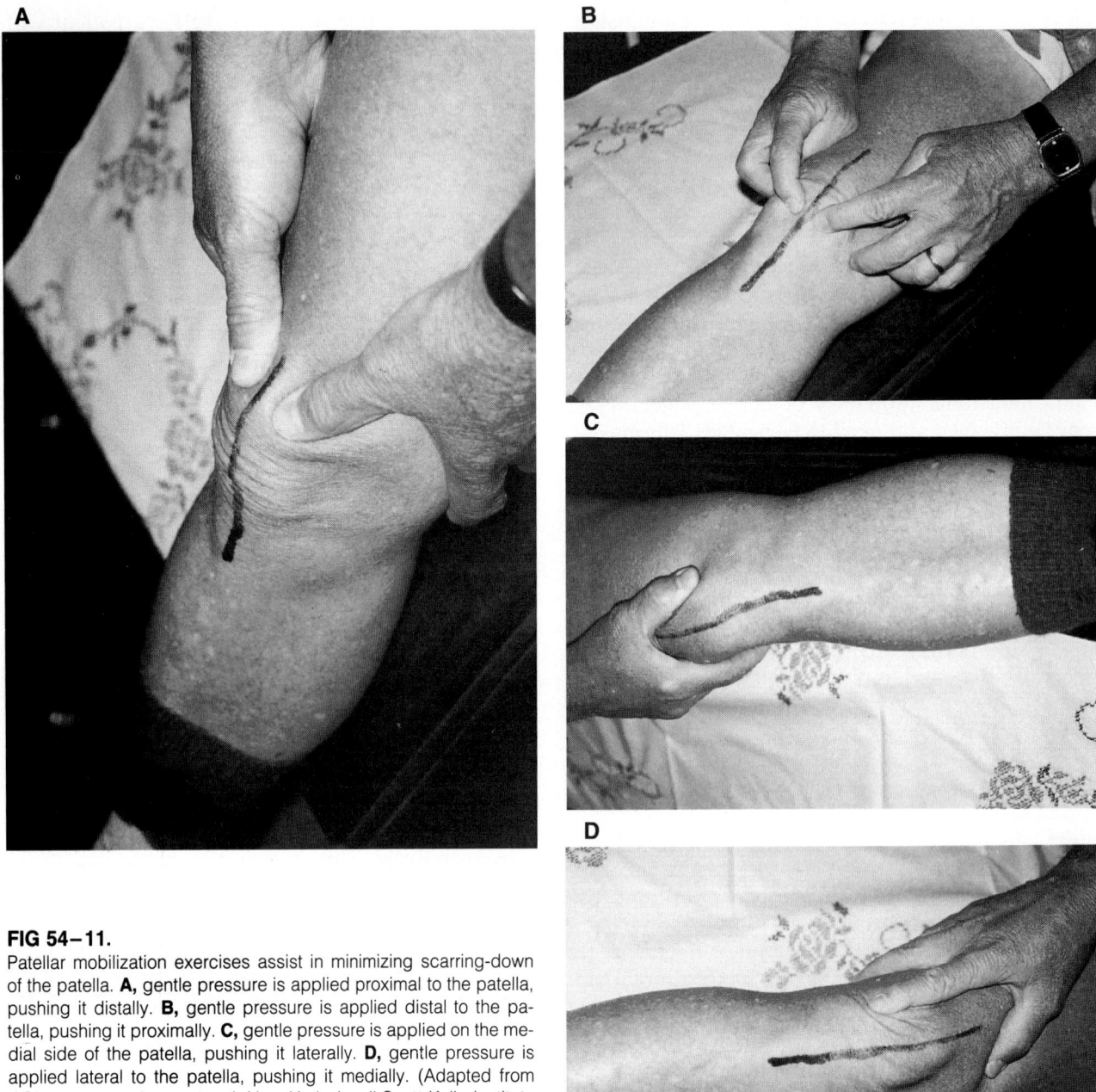

FIG 54–11.
Patellar mobilization exercises assist in minimizing scarring-down of the patella. **A,** gentle pressure is applied proximal to the patella, pushing it distally. **B,** gentle pressure is applied distal to the patella, pushing it proximally. **C,** gentle pressure is applied on the medial side of the patella, pushing it laterally. **D,** gentle pressure is applied lateral to the patella, pushing it medially. (Adapted from *ACL reconstruction protocol*, New York, Insall-Scott-Kelly Institute for Orthopaedics and Sports Medicine, 1990.)

trated teaching pamphlets that can be personalized for the individual patient.

Incisional Binding

Pain and limited motion at the incisional site can occur if the skin incision binds to the underlying tissue. This binding may cause limitation of motion and pain, but some think this can be prevented or minimized by massaging over and around the incision (Fig 54–12). When scar massage is prescribed, the patient is usually instructed to apply natural skin oil or cream to the area and gently massage across and around the incision. Any drainage from the incision or open area in or around the incision is a contraindication to scar manipulation. Massage is done gen-

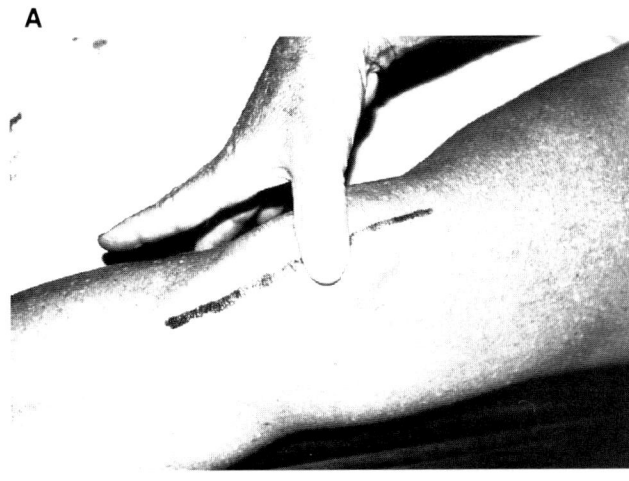

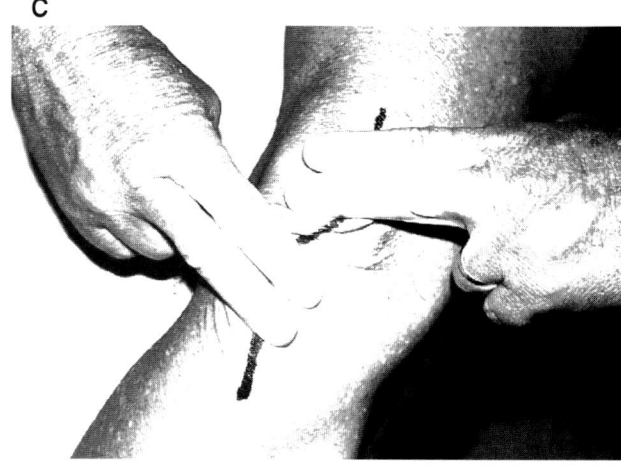

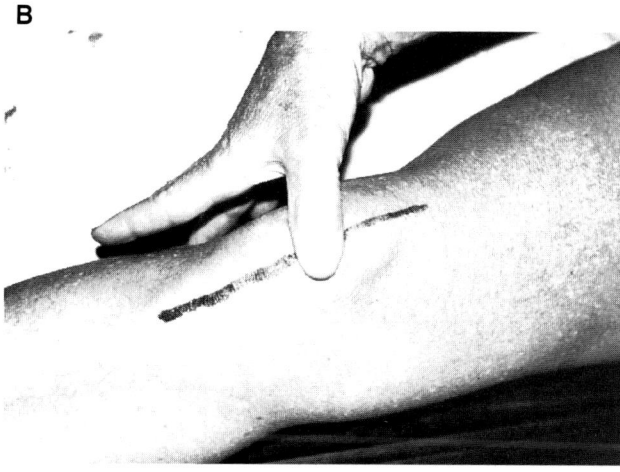

FIG 54-12.
Incisional massage exercises assist in freeing up the subcutaneous tissue and reducing scarring. **A,** transverse friction is achieved by placing a finger on either side of the incision and gliding the fingers in opposite directions, back and forth. **B,** cross-friction laterally across the incision is performed by using the distal portion of the thumb to move the incision from side to side. **C,** crisscross friction can be accomplished using two fingers on each hand to push and pull in a sawing-type motion as firmly as possible. **D,** plucking is performed by picking up an area of the incision or an area close to the incision and pulling it away from the underlying subcutaneous tissue along the incision. (Adapted from *ACL reconstruction protocol*, New York, Insall-Scott-Kelly Institute for Orthopaedics and Sports Medicine, 1990.)

tly initially, progressing to a more forceful manipulation to just below the pain threshold. As with all patient education, a demonstration of the process is helpful to the patient. By a return demonstration the patient validates his or her understanding of the instructions and his or her ability to perform them.

PREPARATION FOR DISCHARGE

Discharge planning begins when it is learned that the patient will be admitted. Planning includes incorporating the patient, family, and significant others in preparing for discharge. Patient and family teaching should be validated and documented. Teaching includes postoperative exercises, including frequency and duration; care of the leg brace; proper ambulation and mobility techniques; and proper operation and care of CPM devices, electrical stimulation equipment, and any other piece of equipment that may be used at home.

The home environment should be prepared to facilitate safe ambulation. Such measures include removing scatter rugs or any other items that may be hazardous and items that obstruct the normal paths inside. It is convenient to have a sleeping area and bathroom facility on one level, even though the patient has learned to ascend and descend stairs prior to discharge.

The patient and family should be instructed to notify the physician if excessive pain develops in the operative area, if the extremity develops severe edema, if the patient develops a fever, or if any questions arise that need answering.

SUMMARY

The importance of correct diagnosis, treatment, and rehabilitation of the patient with a knee ligament injury is well recognized.[15] Rehabilitation of the reconstructed knee is as important as the completeness of the repair. The goals of the first 3 to 4 postoperative months are for the patient to regain a full, normal ROM, maintain mobility of the patella, progress to full weightbearing on the affected extremity, reestablish normal gait, have minimal joint swelling, and be pain-free.

The care of the patient with a knee ligament injury is a challenge for the health care team regardless of whether the injury was treated nonsurgically or with surgical reconstruction. The orthopaedic nurse is one member of that multidisciplinary team. Several team functions overlap, but the goal of the team remains—to facilitate the restoration of maximal function, ROM, and endurance to the injured extremity, and, to restore the patient to a safe level of optimal activity as soon as possible, ensuring the avoidance of reinjury.

REFERENCES

1. *ACL reconstruction protocol,* New York, Insall-Scott-Kelly Institute for Orthopaedics and Sports Medicine, 1990.
2. Burks R, Daniel D, Losse G: The effect of continuous passive motion on anterior cruciate ligament reconstruction stability, *Am J Sports Med* 12:323–327, 1984.
3. Chandy TA, Grana WA: Secondary school athletic injuries in boys and girls: A three-year comparison, *Physician Sports Med* 13:106–111, 1985.
4. Chapman MW: Operative orthopaedics. In Feagin JA, Lambert K, Cunningham R (eds): *Repair and reconstruction of the anterior cruciate ligament,* Philadelphia, 1988, JB Lippincott, pp 1641–1698.
5. Dehne E, Torp RP: Treatment of joint injuries by immediate mobilization. Based upon the spinal adaptation concept, *Clin Orthop* 77:218–232, 1971.
6. Dunwoody C: Patient controlled analgesia: Rationales, attributes and essential factors, *Orthopaedic Nurs* 6:31–35, 1987.
7. Epps CH: *Complications in orthopaedic surgery,* ed 2, Philadelphia, 1986, JB Lippincott, pp 557–564.
8. Farrell J: *Illustrated guide to orthopedic nursing,* ed 3, Philadelphia, 1986, JB Lippincott.
9. Arvidson D, Eriksson E: Counteracting muscle atrophy after ACL injury: Scientific bases for a rehabilitation program. In Feagin, JA Jr, editor: *The crucial ligaments: Diagnosis and treatment of injuries about the knee,* New York, 1988, Churchill Livingstone, pp 451–459.
9a. Ogilvie BC: Counseling patients with career-ending injuries. In Feagin JA (ed): *The crucial ligaments: Diagnosis and treatment of injuries about the knee,* New York, Churchhill Livingstone, 1988, pp 357–366.
10. Hilt N, Cogburn S: *Manual of orthopaedics,* St Louis, 1980, Mosby–Year Book, pp 553–670.
11. Hoberman M, Basmajian JV: Crutch and cane exercises and use. In Basmajian JV, editor: *Therapeutic exercise,* ed 4, Baltimore, 1984, Williams & Wilkins, pp 267–284.
12. Jackson DW, Drez D Jr: *The Anterior Cruciate deficient knee: New concepts in ligament repair,* St Louis, 1987, Mosby–Year Book.
13. Jackson DW, Kurzweil PR: Allographs in knee ligament surgery. In Scott WN, editor: *Ligament and extensor mechanism injuries of the knee: Diagnosis and treatment,* St Louis, 1991, Mosby–Year Book, pp 349–360.
14. Jackson RW: The torn ACL: Natural history of untreated lesions and rationale for selective treatment. In Feagin JA, editor: *The Crucial Ligaments: Diagnosis and treatment of injuries about the knee,* New York, 1988, Churchill Livingstone, pp 341–348.
15. Johnson RJ et al: The treatment of injuries of the anterior cruciate ligament. *J Bone Joint Surg [Br]* 74:140–151, 1992.
16. Kübler-Ross E: *On death and dying,* New York, 1970, Macmillan.
17. Long L, Prophit P: *Understanding/responding: A communication manual for nurses,* Belmont, Mass, 1981, Wadsworth.
18. Lossee GM: Anterior cruciate ligament injuries in downhill skiing: Evaluation, surgical treatment, and rehabilitation, *Top Acute Care Trauma Rehabil* 3:40–72, 1988.
19. McCaffery M, Hart L: Undertreatment of acute pain with narcotics, *Am J Nurs* 76(10):1586–1591.
20. McGinnis GH, Noyes FR: Controversy about treatment of the knee with anterior cruciate ligament laxity, *Clin Orthop* 198:61–76, 1985.
21. Narrow B: *Patient teaching in nursing practice: A patient and family-centered approach,* New York, 1979, John Wiley & Sons.
22. Nelson K: The use of knee braces during rehabilitation, *Clin Sports Med* 789–811, 1990.
23. Noyes FR, Mangine RE, Barber S: Early knee motion after open and arthroscopic anterior cruciate ligament reconstruction, *Am J Sports Med* 15:149, 1987.
23a. Noyes FR, Mangin RE, Barber BS: Early treatment of motion complications after reconstruction of the anterior cruciate ligament, *Clin Orthop* 277:217–228, 1992.
24. O'Donoghue DH: *Treatment of injuries to athletes,* ed 4, Philadelphia, 1984, WB Saunders.
25. Paulos LE: Knee bracing, *Clin Sports Med* 9:763–769, 1990.
26. Rankin SH, Duffy KL: *Patient education: Issues, principles, and guidelines,* Philadelphia, 1983, JB Lippincott.
27. Salter R, et al: Clinical application of basic research on continuous passive motion for disorders and injuries of synovial joints. A preliminary report of a feasibility study, *J Orthop Res* 1:325, 1984.
28. Schoen D: *The nursing process in orthopaedics,* Norwalk, Conn, 1986, Appleton-Century-Crofts.
29. Scott WN, Nisonson B, Nicholas JA: *Principles of sports medicine,* Baltimore, 1984, Williams & Wilkins.
30. Whiteside JA, Fleagle SB, Kalenak A, Weller HW: Man power loss in football: A 12-year study at Pennsylvania State University, *Physician Sports Med* 13:103–114, 1985.

Part XIII

Knee Dislocation

55

Traumatic Dislocation of the Knee

JOHN M. SILISKI, M.D.

Classification and diagnosis
Evaluation
Treatment
  Historical results
Timing
Nonoperative management
Operative techniques
Rehabilitation

Dislocation of the knee (tibia from the femur) has long been recognized as a severe injury. In 1824 Sir Astley Cooper wrote, "Of this I have seen only one instance, and I conclude it, therefore, to be a rare occurrence; and there are scarcely any accidents to which the body is liable which more imperiously demand immediate amputation as these." Developments in vascular surgery now permit salvage of most legs with knee dislocation, although amputation occasionally is still necessary. Associated neurologic injuries can be treated by tendon transfer and newer techniques of nerve grafting. The "orthopedic" aspects of these injuries, including the ligamentous, tendinous, and meniscal disruptions, have only recently been treated by aggressive, acute surgical repair and reconstruction. The surgical treatment of knee dislocation is built on the individual procedures developed to repair isolated soft tissue injuries of the knee.

No single approach to the treatment of knee dislocation has yet been identified as best. Since this injury is relatively uncommon, controlled studies are difficult to do except over a long period, even at large referral centers. In addition, many factors make each knee dislocation unique. There are, however, established principles for evaluation and treatment of knee dislocations with which the knee surgeon should be familiar. This chapter reviews the topic of dislocation of the knee, including the literature and my experience.

CLASSIFICATION AND DIAGNOSIS

Dislocation of the knee may be defined in a pure sense as the knee that by radiograph or clinical examination is grossly dislocated (Fig 55–1,A and B).

It is reasonable to include those knees that are grossly unstable (both cruciate ligaments and at least one collateral ligament complex disrupted), even though the knee is not completely dislocated at the time of evaluation by the orthopaedic surgeon (Fig 55–2,A–C). These knees have the same type of soft tissue injuries and the same neurovascular complications as those that are frankly dislocated. It is presumed that some knee dislocations are reduced by the patient or those assisting the patient prior to arrival at a hospital.

The incidence of knee dislocation varies in available reports, but clearly is low compared with many other orthopaedic injuries: Hoover[7] identified only 14 knee dislocations in 2 million admissions at the Mayo Clinic; Meyers and Harvey[14] reported 53 cases over 10 years at Los Angeles County Hospital; Shields et al.[28] reported 26 cases over 28 years at Massachusetts General Hospital. During the past 8 years, Massachusetts General Hospital has seen five knee dislocations per year, accounting for 1 of every 800 orthopaedic inpatient admissions. The frequency with which this injury is seen depends on the volume of trauma an institution sees and its referral patterns.

Knee dislocations were classified by Kennedy[10] into five types, depending on the position of the tibia in respect to the femur. Green and Allen[5] classified 245 cases collected from several series with the following distribution: 75 (31%) anterior, 61 (25%) posterior, 33 (13%) lateral, 9 (4%) rotatory, 8 (3%) medial, and 59 (20%) unspecified. Classification by direction of tibial displacement is of some use in predicting which structures may have been injured, although specific steps (see Evaluation) must be followed to define the injuries in each case. In general, vascular injuries are more likely to occur in anterior

999

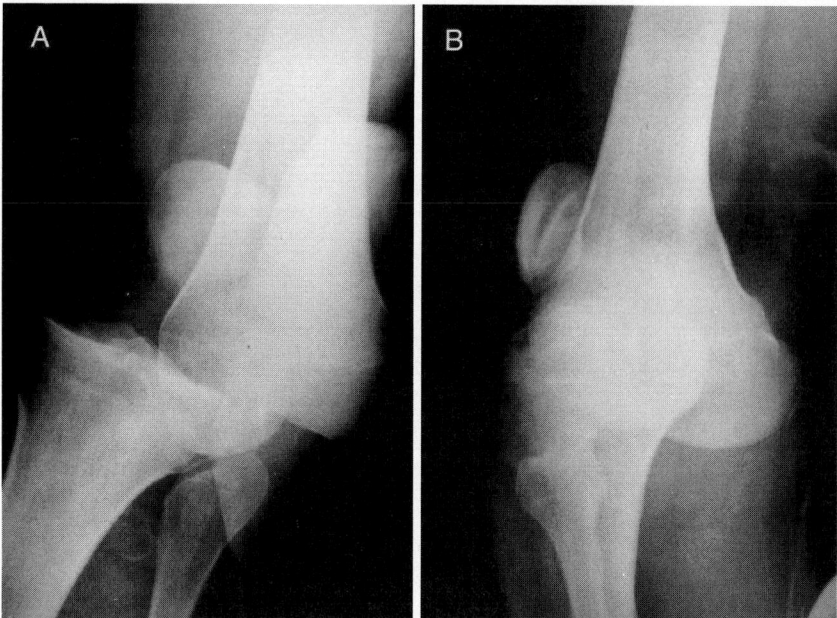

FIG 55-1.
X-ray films in anteroposterior **(A)** and lateral **(B)** views show complete dislocation of the knee.

and posterior dislocations, because the popliteal artery is at risk for traction and direct contusion, respectively. The peroneal nerve is most likely to be injured in medial dislocations that place traction on the nerve. Anterior dislocations probably occur most frequently during hyperextension injuries. Posterior dislocations are the result of direct blows to the upper anterior tibia, which is pushed posteriorly on the femur; although rare, a posterior dislocation can occur with an isolated posterior cruciate ligament (PCL) disruption. Varus and valgus stresses produce medial and lateral dislocations, respectively. Many dislocations have a rotatory component that may be difficult to classify by radiographic examination. The most important aspect of classification, particularly if the surgeon plans to operatively repair the injured structures, is the instability pattern of the knee, which is determined best by examination with the patient under anesthesia.

EVALUATION

Gross dislocation of the knee is unlikely to be missed in the emergency room evaluation. The tibia is clearly malaligned in relationship to the distal femur. What may be difficult to determine on examination is whether there is dislocation, a grossly displaced fracture of the distal femur or proximal tibia, or a fracture-dislocation of the knee, which usually leaves a portion of the tibial plateau with the femur. The knee should be splinted and x-ray films taken in anteroposterior and lateral views to determine the exact diagnosis. If there is any question regarding the integrity of the neurovascular supply to the foot, a closed reduction should be attempted first, using longitudinal traction on the calf. In most cases, knee dislocation can be reduced relatively easily; if a fracture is present, its position will most likely be improved. Reduction of the orthopaedic aspect of the injury will relieve compression that may be present on vessels and nerves, but will do little for a thrombosed or torn popliteal artery. During the process of reduction the knee should be assessed gently for any residual ligaments that are intact. With very rare exceptions, both cruciate ligaments and at least one collateral ligament will be noted to be disrupted.

In the knee that presents itself in a reduced position, massive ligamentous disruption can be misdiagnosed initially, leading to severe consequences if there is vascular injury. Such a knee on visual inspection may not appear grossly abnormal, because the capsular disruption permits bleeding to diffuse into the thigh and calf rather than collect as an effusion within a contained joint space. If the patient is alert and cooperative, localized pain and tenderness may alert the examiner to substantial injury. However, stress tests for ligament instability are needed to diagnose the knee as having been dislocated at the time of the original injury. Without anesthesia, the knee examination must be somewhat limited, but should

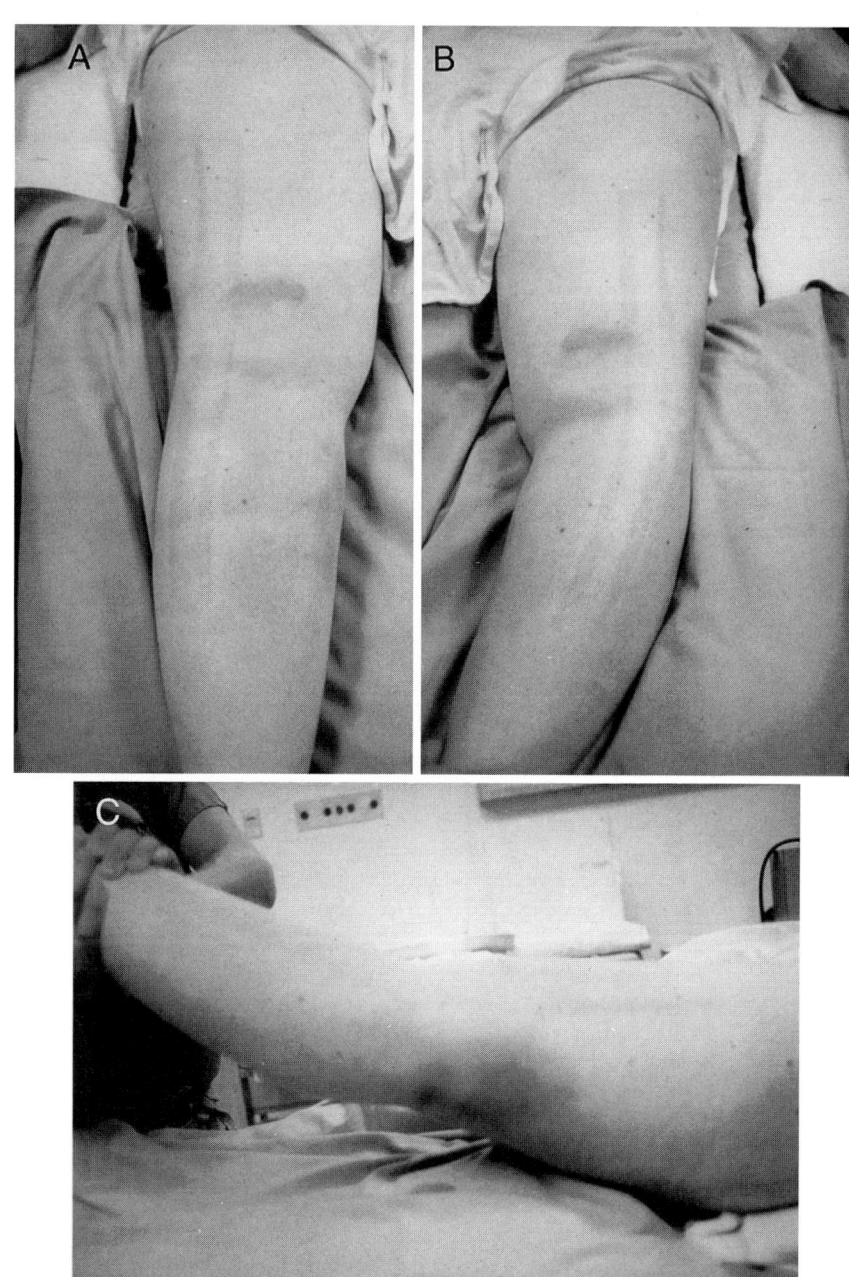

FIG 55–2.
A–C, examination of this injured knee shows gross instability on varus stress and hyperextension. The knee was not originally given the diagnosis of dislocation, but surgical exploration confirmed disruption of both lateral structures.

be performed in the emergency setting to make the diagnosis. Usually the examiner should be able to determine if the knee hyperextends and whether at 20 to 30 degrees of flexion both cruciate ligaments and one or both collateral ligaments are disrupted. It is not necessary to attempt a pivot shift test or stress at 90 degrees or to completely re-dislocate the knee to make the diagnosis of knee dislocation.

Plain films of the knee may be helpful in planning the operative repair. Small flecks of avulsed bone in the intercondylar region suggest avulsion rather than midsubstance tear of the cruciate ligaments (Fig 55–3). Avulsion fragments can also be seen with collateral ligament avulsion (Fig 55–4).

Once the orthopaedic diagnosis of dislocated knee has been made, or even suspected, in the emergency setting, complete and careful neurovascular examination of the lower extremity should be performed. Even if pulses are present and normal in the foot, it is appropriate for a vascular surgeon to ex-

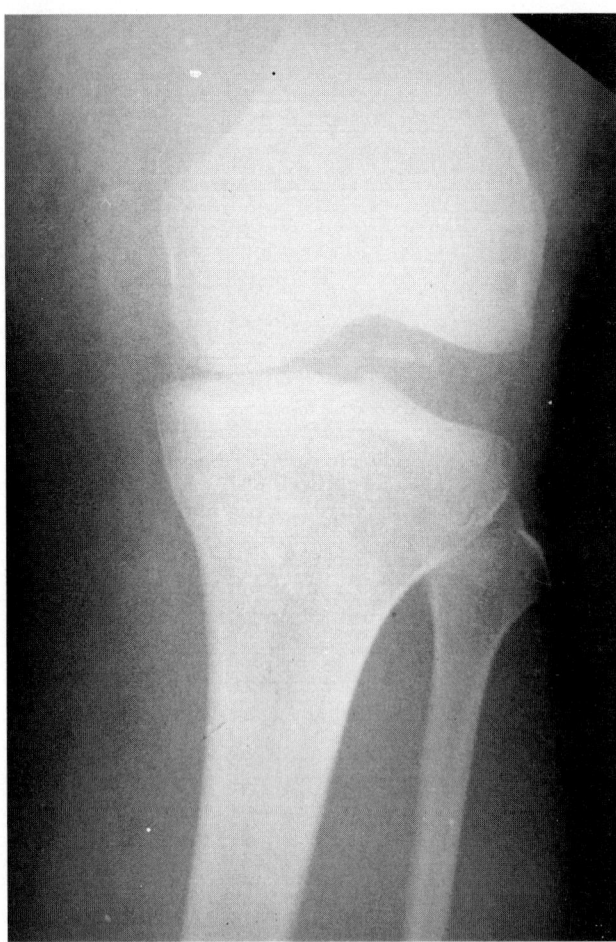

FIG 55–3.
Avulsion fragments in the intercondylar region, found on exploration to represent avulsion of cruciate ligaments from the tibial side of the joint.

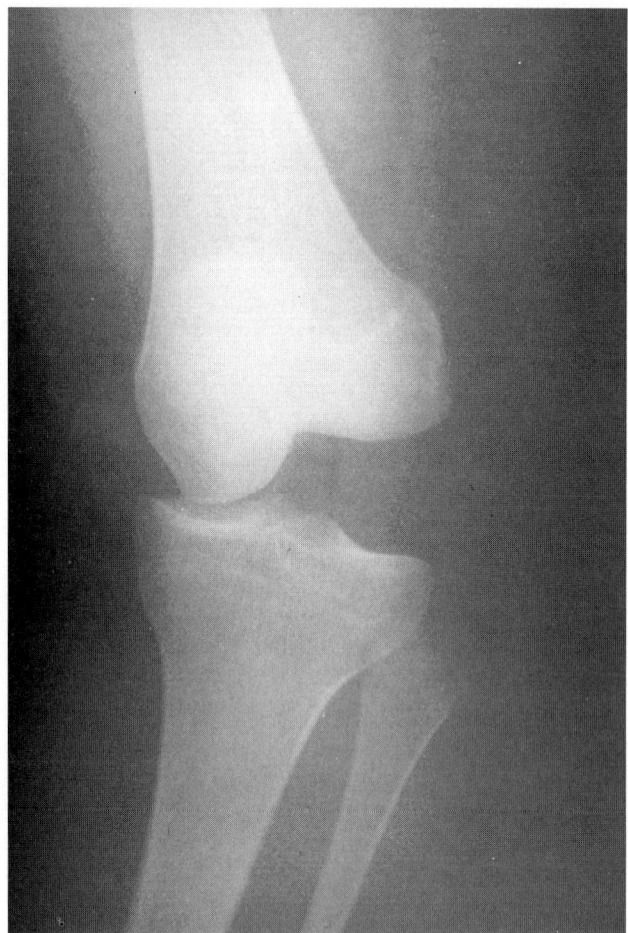

FIG 55–4.
Avulsion fragment on the lateral side of the knee, found on exploration to be an avulsion of the lateral collateral ligament from the fibula.

amine and follow the patient. An arteriogram is not mandatory in every patient with knee dislocation and normal circulation to the foot, but the risk of not obtaining an arteriogram is in missing an intimal tear of the popliteal artery that may subsequently thrombose, which can be limb-threatening and result in emergency surgery. In our institution arteriography is routine in all patients with acute knee dislocation, even when the vascular supply to the foot is clinically normal.

Thorough neurologic examination of the knee is essential at the time of initial evaluation. Any neurologic deficit should be assessed as being either partial or complete for both sensory and motor function. Peroneal nerve palsy is particularly common (25%–40%) in knee dislocations, and approximately half of these palsies are permanent.[28–30] If the palsy is complete, recovery is less likely than if it is only partial. The initial evaluation is therefore of some prognostic value.

TREATMENT

Historical Results

Limb salvage remains a fundamental issue in knee dislocation with popliteal artery injury, which occurs in 20% to 30% of these cases. During World War II, 49.6% of limbs with major arterial injury required amputation.[2] With the development of methods for acute arterial repair, this rate of amputation dropped to 11.1% during the Korean War.[5] In 1969, Shields et al.[28] reported that 5 of 26 knee dislocations required amputation. O'Donnell et al.,[22] also from Massachusetts General Hospital, reported in 1977 that in 9 of 28 legs with arterial injuries associated with knee dislocation and major fractures, amputation was necessary. Saphenous vein grafting of the popliteal artery is not always successful, and the delay from the time of injury to completion of arterial repair may not exceed 6 to 8 hours, the maximum that soft tissues will tolerate.[33] In a more recent series reviewed at Massachusetts General Hospital, 4 of 40 knee dislocations resulted in above-knee amputation, 3 because of arterial injury and 1 because of late infection.[29] Limb salvage remains a major issue in dislocation of the knee.[1, 8, 9, 11, 16, 25, 32]

Peroneal nerve palsies were reported by Shields et al.[28] in 9 of 26 knee dislocations. Sisto and Warren[30] noted 8 palsies in 20 dislocations. Siliski and Plancher[29] reported on 40 dislocations with 16 palsies, of which 8 were permanent. The incidence of peroneal palsy remains fairly constant in reported series. Inasmuch as approximately half of these nerve injuries are permanent, an aggressive approach to nerve grafting may be warranted, especially in the young person whose nerve at the time of ligament repair is noted to be severely damaged and judged unlikely to recover spontaneously. The other options for permanent peroneal nerve palsies have included bracing and tendon transfer as reconstructive procedures.

Closed reduction and cast immobilization was the treatment of choice for the ligamentous aspect of knee dislocation.[17, 20, 23] Shields et al.[28] in 1969 reported results in 26 dislocations treated primarily by closed methods, but without a clear recommendation for nonoperative or operative repair. Meyers and colleagues[14, 15] in 1971 reported a better functional rating in 11 knees that underwent acute repair, compared with 7 treated nonoperatively. Taylor et al.[31] in 1972 reported poorer results in 16 knees treated operatively than in 26 knees treated nonoperatively, 18 of which were rated good results; they advocated nonoperative treatment for the ligamentous aspect of this injury. Sisto and Warren[30] in 1985 reported 16 dislocations that were treated by acute ligament repair: the PCL was avulsed in 14, and the anterior cruciate ligament (ACL) in 10. Of the 13 that had complete ligament repair, 6 had chronic pain, none had major instability, and overall there was minor loss of motion compared with unoperated knees. Based on their results, these authors advocated acute operative repair. They believed that early repair permitted an earlier, more aggressive rehabilitation program for the knee. Roman et al.[26] in 1987 reported on 19 cases; the 14 that underwent acute repair had better stability but less motion, particularly extension. Those knees that were immobilized for more than 6 weeks after operative repair had more limited motion. Shelbourne et al.[27] advocated repair of the posterior and collateral ligament complexes, but not the ACL, pointing out that range of motion may be better after a lesser surgical procedure. Flandry et al.[3] advocated repair of the ACL in knee dislocations only if it had bony avulsion. Although their patients had an acceptable range of motion, over 80% had positive Lachman and pivot shift tests. Other authors have recently advocated acute repair or reconstruction of both cruciate ligaments in dislocations.[4, 12, 18, 19]

Timing

Some aspects of the evaluation and treatment of knee dislocations are clearly emergencies. Closed reduction and neurovascular evaluation should be done immediately, and an arteriogram should be obtained early to rule out an intimal tear of the popliteal artery. If the leg is clinically ischemic, the vascular surgeon may eliminate the arteriogram in the angiography department and proceed directly to the operating room for exploration of the popliteal artery, bypass grafting with saphenous vein, and fasciotomies of the calf. Since repair of the orthopaedic portions of the injury is a major operation by itself, it is prudent to delay ligament repair for a second operation if saphenous vein grafting of the popliteal artery has been performed initially. The vein graft may be disrupted or it may thrombose during the manipulation required for ligament repair. The surgeon should therefore consider the option of leaving the knee splinted until the vascular surgeon is satisfied that the popliteal artery repair is functioning well. An additional reason to delay ligament repair is the associated multiple trauma that many of these patients have. Treatment of life-threatening and limb-threatening injuries takes precedence over knee instability. I have performed "acute" repair of the ligaments and menisci up to 20 days after the injury and have been able to identify all structures well at that time. With further delay after injury, anatomic definition is lost and scar tissue is present, and it is more difficult to reattach avulsed structures and to directly suture together torn capsule and collateral ligaments.

There are two reasons to operate on a dislocated knee emergently, in addition to popliteal artery injury. Open injuries require irrigation and debridement to decrease the risk of infection. If the wound and joint can be cleaned well, immediate surgical repair is warranted, although there is no harm in delaying ligament repair to a second surgery. Irreducible dislocations are uncommon, but can occur as a result of interposition of soft tissues between the tibia and femur.[21, 24] Since substantial surgical dissection is necessary to reduce the joint, it is reasonable to complete the ligament repair at the same time.

Nonoperative Management

If the knee dislocation is to be treated nonoperatively, a few options for immobilization exist. The most straightforward method is to apply a cast with the knee in a slightly flexed position, as recommended by Taylor et al.[31] Immobilization is most frequently for 6 weeks. Rehabilitation can then begin, with a hinged brace.

An external fixator crossing the knee will also provide immobilization, and may be the treatment of choice when there has been an open dislocation or other major soft tissue injury in the lower extremity.

A large Steinmann pin can be drilled across the knee through the intercondylar area to add stability to the closed reduction. The knee will still require full cast immobilization, or the pin will loosen or break prior to removal. This technique is rarely indicated for either the nonoperative or acutely repaired knee dislocation. Olecranonization of the patella, which is done by drilling a large Steinmann pin vertically through the patella and into the tibial eminence, helps to prevent posterior subluxation of the tibia on the femur. Since the pin is not crossing the tibiofemoral joint itself, the forces on the pin are not so great that breakage or loosening is likely. Assisted knee motion can be done with the pin in place. One complication that can occur with this method of supplemental stabilization is infection at the insertion site over the patella. Even though the pin is left subcutaneous, the skin is thin at this site, and wound breakdown can occur.

Operative Techniques

Since access to all parts of the knee is necessary, the patient is best positioned supine. Most of the surgery is performed with the knee flexed. A leg holder may be used to help maintain the knee in flexion.

Arthroscopic evaluation of the knee is contraindicated in knee dislocation. The disrupted capsule will not retain fluid in a closed space, and therefore the surrounding soft tissue may become massively swollen if arthroscopy is attempted. Since the major structures that require repair can be determined by examination for clinical ligament instability, arthroscopy offers little diagnostically. Meniscal tears are usually peripheral detachments that are found and repaired as part of the capsular repair. The numerous structures that need to be repaired require an open surgery, and arthroscopy would be of little benefit in assisting in visualization during surgery.

Before beginning the surgical repair, an examination under anesthesia should be performed. This will demonstrate in most cases ACL and PCL laxity. More important the examination will determine if one or both collateral ligaments are disrupted. The pattern of instability dictates surgical exposure.

If the cruciate ligaments and medial capsular structures are disrupted, a single medial incision is sufficient, starting over the vastus medialis and extending vertically along the medial margin of the patella and patellar tendon. A medial parapatellar arthrotomy can be done, allowing retraction of the extensor mechanism laterally and wide exposure of the interior of the joint. Since the distal end of the femur is exposed, the lateral metaphysis can be reached for tunnels to reattach or reconstruct the ACL. The patellar tendon is easily exposed if a midthird patellar tendon graft is to be used. As well, the hamstring tendons can be harvested medially. The medial meniscus, medial collateral ligament, and medial capsule all can be exposed through this incision.

Often the lateral side of the knee has been disrupted as well, and a second incision is required to repair structures on that side of the knee. The second incision should be made starting over the posterior edge of the lateral femur and extending vertically over the knee and along the anterior edge of the proximal fibula. On making the skin incision, the surgeon will usually encounter disruption of most of the structures on the posterolateral side of the knee, including the iliotibial band, lateral collateral ligament, biceps femoris tendon, popliteus tendon, posterolateral capsule, and lateral meniscus. Every structure on this side of the knee should be systematically identified before beginning the repair. One should not be discouraged by the initial appearance on this side of the joint; in most cases most structures can be satisfactorily repaired. The peroneal nerve is usually located easily in the posterior and inferior regions of the surgical exposure. It should be examined for severe traction injury and consideration of nerve grafting at a later date if the nerve is judged to be permanently injured. The peroneal nerve and the major neurovascular bundle in the popliteal fossa must be protected throughout surgery.

It is reasonable to repair the cruciate ligaments first, then to proceed to the medial or lateral side of the joint. On opening the knee through an anteromedial arthrotomy, the intercondylar notch is explored. Synovium on the cruciate ligaments should be preserved if they have been avulsed and are satisfactory for reattachment to bone. In reports that have documented the type of injury to the cruciate ligaments, more than half of these injuries have been noted to be avulsions rather than midsubstance tears. If the ligament has been avulsed with a fragment of bone, the likelihood of successful reattachment is high, especially with the PCL. Not all cruciate ligament reattachments will be successful, but in the dislocated knee with so many structures injured it is currently reasonable to reattach an avulsed PCL. This can be done using techniques described by Marshall et al.[13] Unless ACL avulsions have a sizeable piece of bone with the free end of the ligament, it is best to acutely reconstruct this ligament. Familiarity with the attachment sites of both cruciate ligaments to the femur and tibia is necessary. The avulsion sites should be taken down to a bleeding surface, with hand instruments or a power burr. It is helpful to have a ligament guide system available that permits easy and safe passage of Kirschner-wires through bone, so that the tips are brought out through the avulsion site on the bone. The Kirschner wires should have small holes drilled in the tips so that sutures can be pulled with the wires out through the bone to be tied over a bony bridge on the cortical surface (Fig 55–5).

Two or four Kirschner wires need to be used for each ligament reattachment site, corresponding to four whipstitch suture ends in the avulsed ligament. The type of suture used depends on the surgeon's preference, although a nonabsorbable heavy (no. 5) suture is recommended. These sutures should be passed as atraumatically as possible in the surface fibers of the cruciate ligament, preserving as much as possible the synovium and vascular supply of the ligament. Usually it is difficult to thread the suture ends from the ligament through the hole in the guide wire. A no. 0 suture can be passed through the guide wire tip and tied into a loop; the end of a whipstitch suture can be placed through this loop to be pulled out through the bone. The guide wire must be pulled out by hand, not on a power drill, or the loop and ligament sutures will become twisted and break. After passage of the sutures, it is best to prepare the rest of the repair, returning to the cruciate ligaments to tie them in place when all structures about the knee are ready to be secured into place. The laxity of the knee is of benefit in exposure of the other portions of the joint.

The site of ligament reattachment that is most difficult is the PCL to the tibia.[6] However, since the knee is so lax, the tibia can be drawn well anterior of the femur, permitting preparation of the avulsion site and the safe passage of Kirschner-wires and sutures on the posterior side of the tibial plateau (Fig 55–6).

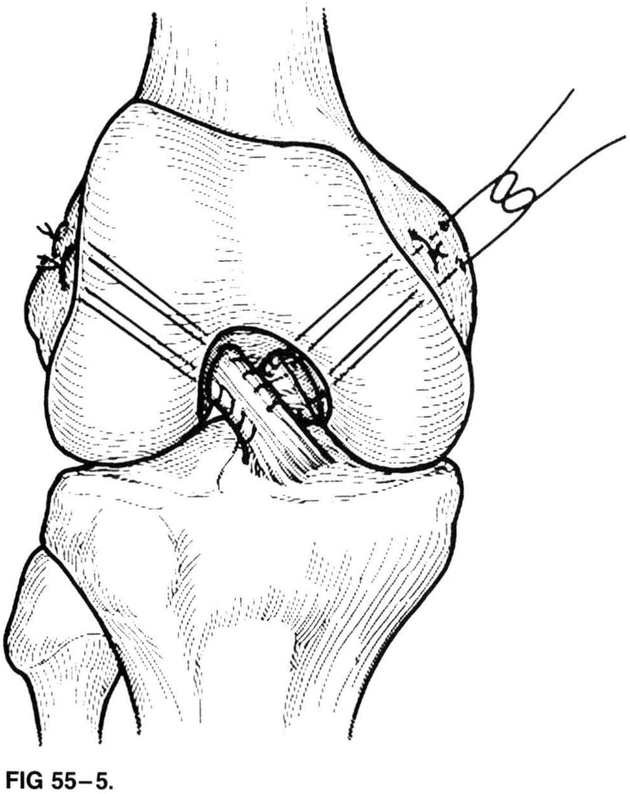

FIG 55–5.
Diagram of reattachment of cruciate ligaments to the femur with sutures passed through small drill holes and tied over bone bridges.

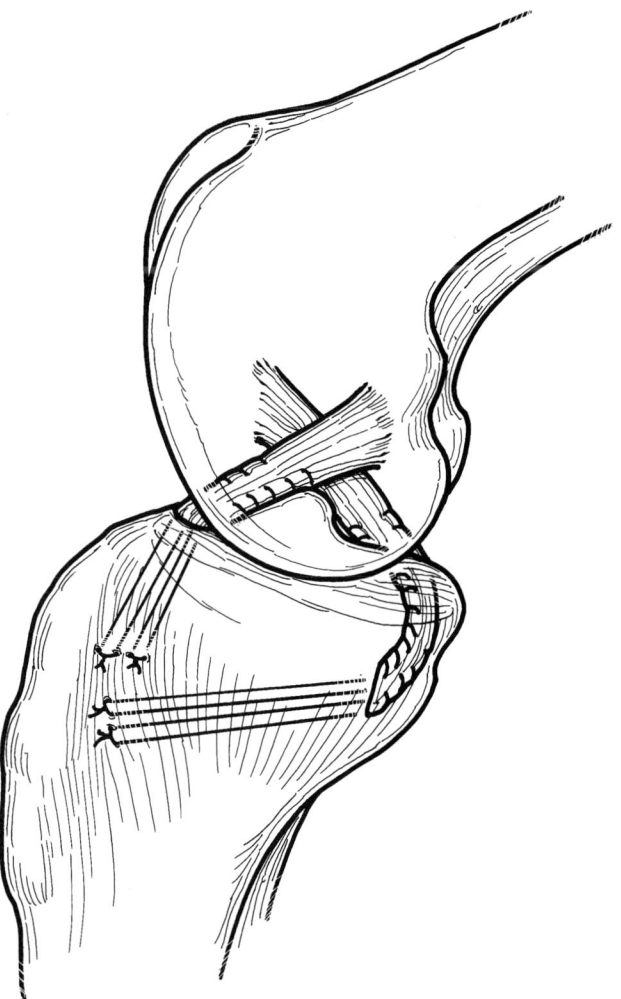

FIG 55–6.
Diagram of cruciate ligament reattachment to the tibia.

Cruciate ligaments torn in midsubstance usually are not repairable. Primary reconstruction is indicated and best done as an intraarticular procedure. Extraarticular reconstruction is not feasible in most cases, because of associated injuries. Using an appropriate guide system, Kirschner-wires are placed in the femur and tibia so that cannulated reamers can be used to drill appropriately sized tunnels for the passage of ligament grafts (Fig 55–7,A and B). Depending on availability and the surgeon's preference, autograft, allograft, synthetic ligaments, or a combination may be used to reconstruct the cruciate ligaments. Allografts have several advantages in the repair of knee dislocation. Surgical time and dissection are reduced. Both cruciate ligaments can be reconstructed from one extensor mechanism allograft. The fixation achieved with patellar tendon–bone block grafts permits early motion and rehabilitation.

The medial side of the joint is usually the easier to repair. The medial collateral ligament most commonly is avulsed from the femur, to which it may be reattached with a staple or screw with a ligament washer. If the medial collateral ligament is torn in midsubstance the repair is more complicated. The surgeon should attempt to identify the superficial and deep layers and directly suture the ends together. This may need to be done simultaneously with suturing of a detached medial meniscus. Portions of the medial capsule that have been avulsed from the tibia may be reattached using staples, screws with ligament washers, or suture anchors. Most medial meniscal tears are detachments and can be repaired by suturing. Sutures should be placed as the capsule and ligament repair progresses so that the meniscal sutures can be tied down at the end of the surgery.

With lateral joint involvement there usually is disruption of the iliotibial band, lateral and posterolateral capsules, lateral meniscus, biceps femoris muscle, popliteus muscle, and lateral collateral and posterior cruciate ligaments (Fig 55–8). The initial step is to identify each structure, determining the best method of repair. The popliteal vessels and tibial nerve can usually be seen posterior to the tibia and should be protected. The repair should start with the posterolateral capsule, which is either torn in its midsubstance or avulsed from the tibia. Direct suturing can be done for tears, and reattachment can be done for avulsions using sutures passed through bone. The repair of the capsule is continued to the lateral and anterolateral sides of the joint; since exposure is better here, avulsions from the tibia can be reattached with staples or screws. If the popliteus tendon has been avulsed from the femur it can be easily reattached. However, when it is torn at the musculotendinous junction, it is usually not repairable. The biceps femoris tendon usually is avulsed from the fibula, sometimes with the lateral collateral ligaments; the tendon can be reattached using a no. 5 suture passed through drill holes in the fibula and tied

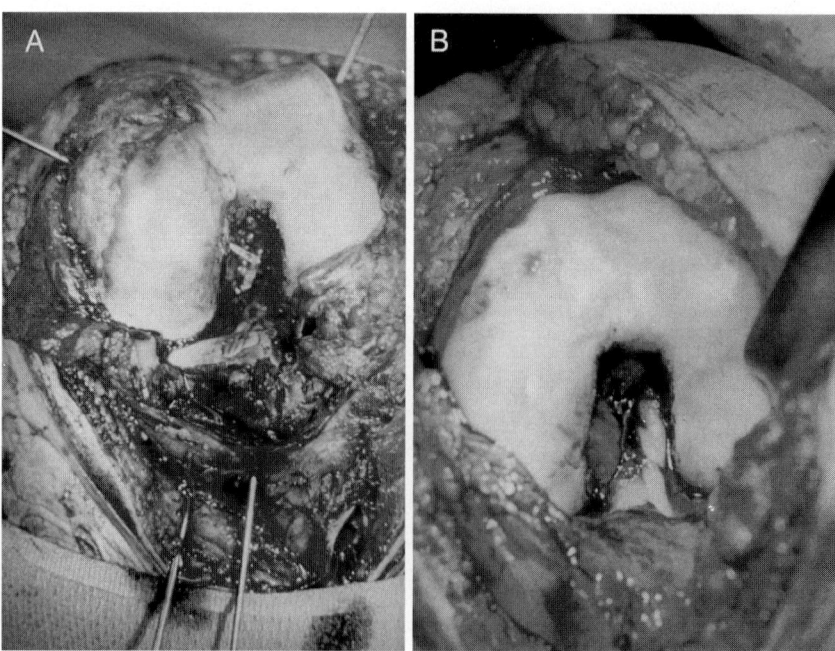

FIG 55–7.
A, intraoperative photograph shows guide wires in the femur and tibia for drilling of interosseous tunnels. **B,** completed intraarticular reconstruction of the cruciate ligaments.

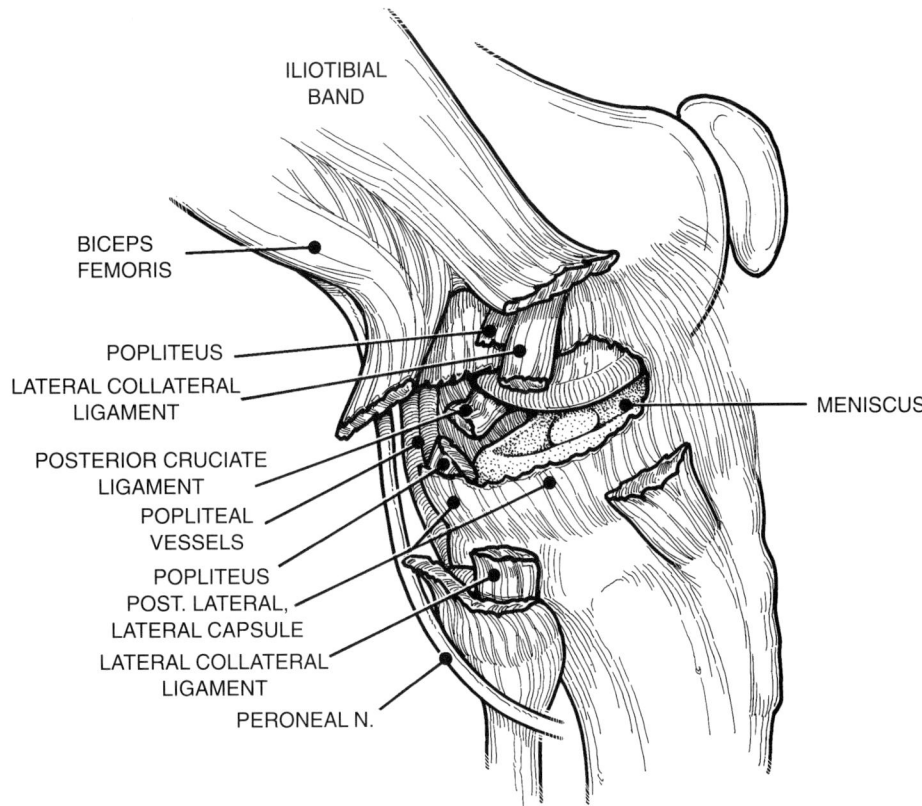

FIG 55-8.
Diagram of structures typically involved on the posterolateral and lateral side of the joint in knee dislocation.

over a bone bridge. The lateral collateral ligament may be avulsed from the femur, in which case it may still be attached to the popliteus. This is very easily reattached to the femoral condyle with either a screw and ligament washer or staple. If the lateral collateral ligament is avulsed from the fibula, it is best reattached by using no. 2 or no. 5 sutures in the ligament passed through drill holes in the bone; when it is torn in midsubstance, whipstitches may be placed in both ends and tied to each other, pulling the stumps into contact. The iliotibial band is commonly avulsed from the tibia at Gerdy's tubercle, and can be reattached with a screw and washer.

Associated fracture of the tibial plateau should be reduced and internally fixed using appropriate techniques and implants. Bone grafting is not usually necessary because these associated fractures typically do not have a depression or impaction component. Exposure of the fracture is accomplished through the two incisions used for the ligament repairs. Because of the soft tissue disruptions, exposure of the fracture is relatively easy. Some coordination of the fracture and ligament repairs needs to be done intraoperatively so that fracture implants do not interfere with the subsequent ligament repair. In general, the fracture lines should be reduced and internally fixed first, and the soft tissue repair done as the second part of the surgery.

REHABILITATION

One of the basic goals of any joint surgery is to begin early motion and functional rehabilitation. The results of reported series on knee dislocations suggest that prolonged immobilization after repair decreases the ultimate range of motion. More than 6 weeks of postoperative immobilization is likely to reduce motion and provide no improvement in stability. The most favorable situation is a repair that at the completion of surgery is judged strong enough for early continuous passive motion, physical therapy, and use of a hinged brace. Early motion may limit the formation of intraarticular adhesions and extraarticular scarring. The surgeon must make a decision intraoperatively as to how aggressive early rehabilitation can be without resulting in pulling apart the numerous structures that have been repaired. Cruciate ligament reconstructions done through osseous tunnels are more secure than ligament reattachments done with sutures. Collateral ligaments reattached to bone with large staples or screws are more secure than midsubstance suturing. Menisci that have no or limited detachments are more secure than those that required suturing of a complete detachment. If a popliteal artery has required grafting, this may add to the indications to proceed slowly with joint motion during the first month after repair. Because there are so many variables, and each dislocation and repair is somewhat different, the surgeon has a wide window in which to work. The timing of initiation of motion after repair of a dislocated knee may range from immediately to 6 weeks postoperatively. Should a knee remain stiff after surgical treatment and therapy, arthroscopic lysis of adhesions with manipulation is necessary.

REFERENCES

1. Cone JB: Vascular injury associated with fracture-dislocations of the lower extremity, *Clin Orthop* 243:30–35, 1989.
2. DeBakey ME, Simeone FA: Battle injuries in World War II, *Ann Surg* 123:534, 1946.
3. Flandry FC, Schwartz MG, Hughston JC: Long term follow-up of operatively treated knee dislocations, 58th Annual Meeting of the American Academy of Orthopaedic Surgeons, Anaheim, Calif, 1991.
4. Frassica FJ, et al: Dislocation of the knee, *Clin Orthop* 263:200–205, 1991.
5. Green NE, Allen BL: Vascular injuries associated with dislocation of the knee, *J Bone Joint Surg [Am]* 59:236–239, 1977.
6. Hughston JC: Acute tears of the posterior cruciate ligament, *J Bone Joint Surg [Am]* 62:438, 1980.
7. Hoover NW: Injury of the popliteal artery associated with fracture and dislocation, *Surg Clin North Am* 41:1099–1112, 1961.
8. Jones RE: Vascular and orthopaedic complications of knee dislocations, *Surg Gynecol Obstet* 149:554, 1979.
9. Kaufman SL, Martin LG: Arterial injuries associated with complete dislocation of the knee, *Radiology* 184:153–155, 1992.
10. Kennedy JC: Complete dislocation of the knee joint, *J Bone Joint Surg [Am]* 45:899–901, 1963.
11. Lefrak EA: Knee dislocation: An illusive cause of critical arterial occlusion, *Arch Surg* 111:1021, 1976.
12. Lipscomb AB, Anderson AF: Surgical reconstruction of both the anterior and posterior cruciate ligaments, *Am J Knee Surg* 3:29–40, 1990.
13. Marshall JL, et al: The anterior cruciate ligament: A technique of repair and reconstruction, *Clin Orthop* 143:97, 1979.
14. Meyers M, Harvey JP: Traumatic dislocation of the knee joint, *J Bone Joint Surg [Am]* 53:16, 1971.
15. Meyers M, Moore T, Harvey JP: Follow-up notes on articles previously published in the journal: Traumatic dislocation of the knee joint, *J Bone Joint Surg [Am]* 57:430, 1975.
16. Miller HH, Welch CS: Quantitative studies on the time factor in arterial injuries, *Ann Surg* 130:428, 1949.
17. Mitchell JI: Dislocation of the knee, *J Bone Joint Surg* 12:640–642, 1930.
18. Montgomery JB: Dislocation of the knee, *Orthop Clin North Am* 18:149, 1987.
19. Moore TM: Fracture-dislocation of the knee, *Clin Orthop* 156:128, 1981.
20. Myles JW: Seven cases of traumatic dislocation of the knee, *Proc R Soc Med* 60:279, 1967.
21. Nystrom M, Samimi S, Ha'Eri GB: Two cases of irreducible knee dislocation occurring simultaneously in two patients and a review of the literature, *Clin Orthop* 277:197–200, 1992.
22. O'Donnell TF, et al: Arterial injuries associated with fractures and/or dislocations of the knee, *J Trauma* 17:775, 1975.
23. O'Donoghue DH: An analysis of end results of surgical treatment of major injuries to the ligaments of the knee, *J Bone Joint Surg [Am]* 37:1, 1955.
24. Quinlan AG, Sharrard WJW: Posterolateral dislocation of the knee with capsular interposition, *J Bone Joint Surg [Br]* 40:660–668, 1958.
25. Reckling FW, Peltier LF: Acute knee dislocations and their complications, *J Trauma* 9:181–190, 1969.
26. Roman PD, Hopson CN, Zenni EJ: Traumatic dislocation of the knee. A report of 30 cases and literature review, *Orthop Rev* 16:33, 1987.
27. Shelbourne KD, et al: Low velocity knee dislocations, *Orthop Rev* 20:995–1004, 1991.
28. Shields L, Mital M, Cave E: Complete dislocation of the knee: Experience at the Massachusetts General Hospital, *J Trauma* 9:192, 1969.
29. Siliski, JM, Plancher K: Dislocation of the knee, Annual meeting of the American Academy of Orthopaedic Surgeons, 1989.
30. Sisto DJ, Warren RF: Complete knee dislocation: A follow-up study of operative treatment, *Clin Orthop* 198:101, 1985.
31. Taylor AR, Arden GP, Rainey HA: Traumatic dislocation of the knee joint, *J Bone Joint Surg [Am]* 57:430, 1972.
32. Welling RE, Kakkasseril J, Cranley JJ: Complete dislocation of the knee with popliteal vascular injury, *J Trauma* 21:450–452, 1981.
33. Wolma FJ: Arterial injuries of the legs associated with fractures and dislocations, *Am J Surg* 140:806, 1980.

56

Dislocation of Proximal Tibiofibular Joint

STUART D. KATCHIS, M.D.
W. NORMAN SCOTT, M.D.

Historical perspective
Surgical anatomy
Classification
Mechanism of injury
Signs and symptoms

Roentgenographic findings
Methods of treatment
Authors' preferred treatment
Prognosis and complications

HISTORICAL PERSPECTIVE

Dislocation of the proximal tibiofibular joint is a rare entity initially described by Nelaton[11] in 1874. The first comprehensive review was by Lyle[9] in 1925, but a literature review in the mid-1970s revealed only 100 reported cases.[12] Although originally described as an isolated injury secondary to major forces (horseback riding and parachuting[8]), many later cases were found associated with major limb trauma.[6] Indeed there are now some reported cases of isolated proximal tibiofibular joint dislocation secondary to relatively minor trauma.[2, 4, 6, 11, 13, 14]

Surgical Anatomy

The embryologic development of the proximal tibiofibular joint has been described by Gray and Gardner[5] in their report of 45 fetal dissections. Cavities representing the joint were seen in a majority of specimens at 15 or more weeks of gestation. In most cases the cavity of the knee joint was separated from that of the proximal tibiofibular joint by a small amount of very loose tissue. Communication between the two joint cavities was documented in one 19-week specimen. Synovial tissue folds were seen to project into the proximal tibiofibular joint at 18 weeks' gestation. By 27 weeks the synovial tissue was well vascularized and separated from the fibrous capsule by a layer of fat. Even in older specimens, separation of the cavities of the knee and proximal tibiofibular joints was by a thin layer of tissue.

The adult proximal tibiofibular joint is an arthrodial joint composed of two facets, a synovial membrane and a joint capsule.[6, 7, 14] It may communicate with the knee joint in as many as 10% of adults.[15] The capsule is thicker and stronger anteriorly than posteriorly. Anteriorly it is reinforced by the three broad bands of the anterior tibiofibular ligament, which run obliquely upward from the fibular head to the lateral tibial condyle, and by an extension of the biceps femoris tendon, which passes anterior to the ligament, also to attach to the lateral tibial condyle. The posterior capsule is supported by the single band of the posterior tibiofibular ligament, which courses obliquely from the posterior fibular head to the posterior aspect of the lateral tibial condyle.[14] The popliteus muscle also crosses the proximal tibiofibular joint and lends posterior support. Superior support is provided by the lateral collateral ligament (LCL) as it passes from its origin on the lateral femoral condyle to its insertion on the head of the fibula. The proximal tibiofibular joint also depends on structures distal to it that bind the tibia and fibula together for stability, namely, the interosseus ligament and the fibrous bands of the inferior tibiofibular joint.[6]

Of note with regard to the surrounding tissues is their relative avascularity, which limits postinjury edema, as well as the close proximity of the common peroneal nerve as it winds around the neck of the fibula. In this position the nerve is subject to injury during joint dislocation, especially in the posterior direction.

The inclination of the proximal tibiofibular joint has long been of interest to those investigating injury there. As early as 1952 Barnett and Napier[1] stated that the plane in which this joint lies may vary from one near horizontal to one steeply inclined to the horizontal. Subsequent authors postulated that the ease with which dislocation occurred may be related to the inclination angle, but were unable to draw specific conclusions from plain radiographs.[6]

It remained until the classic 1974 article by Ogden[12] describing his anatomic dissections and clinical experience before the relationship between the inclination angle and dislocation was further elucidated. Ogden's anatomic observations were based on dissections of 84 specimens (54 cadaver knees, 4 knees from fresh autopsies, and 30 tibiofibular units). He was able to distinguish two basic types of proximal tibiofibular joint: horizontal and oblique (Fig 56–1). Arbitrarily, he determined 20 degrees as the borderline between the two. The inclination angle of most of the joints fell between 10 and 40 degrees, although the range was between 10 and 76 degrees. Ogden found that in the horizontal joints the articular surfaces of the proximal tibiofibular joint were circular and planar and that these articular surfaces were under and behind a projection of the lateral edge of the tibia, which provided some stability by preventing forward displacement of the fibula. The oblique joints were found to have articular surfaces more variable in area and configuration. They were, however, found to be less able to rotate to accommodate torsional forces than the horizontal joints. In light of the rotatory mechanism of injury (see below), Ogden postulated that the oblique joints were more likely to dislocate, and indeed in his clinical series 70% of the injuries occurred through oblique joints.[12]

CLASSIFICATION

Proximal tibiofibular dislocations are primarily due to trauma but may rarely be secondary to disturbances in growth, acute osteomyelitis, complicated fractures of the tibia and fibula, or complications involving amputation stumps.[3] Lyle[9] described four basic types of dislocation: anterior, posterior, upward, and double. The last type referred to simultaneous dislocations to both the proximal and distal tibiofibular joints. Ogden[12] believed this category to be redundant, because all of Lyle's patients with double dislocation had either anterior or upward dislocation of the proximal joint.

In 1974 Ogden[12] modified Lyle's classification system to include subluxation and three categories of dislocation: anterolateral, posteromedial, and superior (Fig 56–2). *Subluxation* was defined as excessive, symptomatic anteroposterior movement without frank dislocation. In his review of 43 patients, Ogden found 10 with subluxation of the proximal tibiofibular joint and 29 with anterolateral, 3 with posteromedial, and 1 with superior dislocation. Patients ranged in age between 8 and 67 years, with the majority of dislocations occurring during the second and third decades of life. The preponderance of anterolateral dislocations is in agreement with other series in

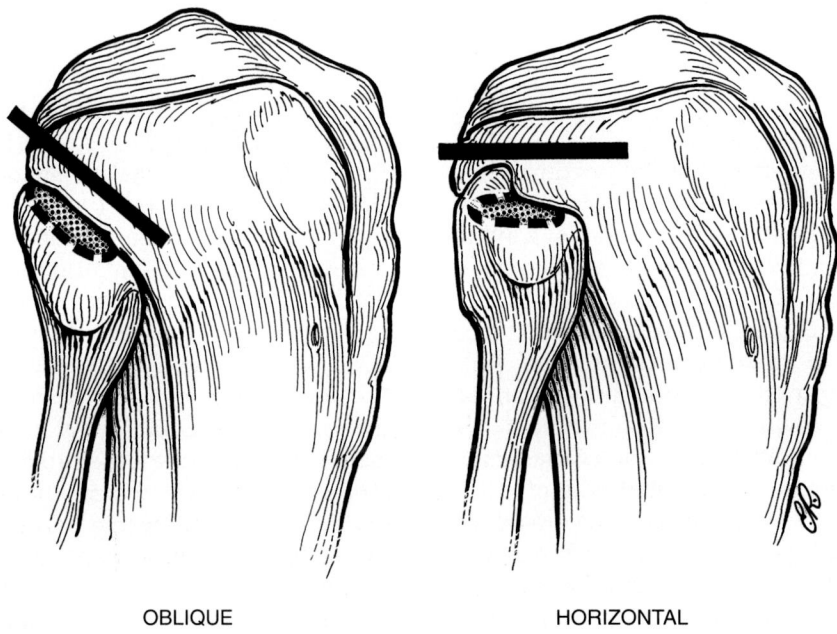

FIG 56–1.
Schematic representation of oblique and horizontal proximal tibiofibular joint, as described by Ogden.

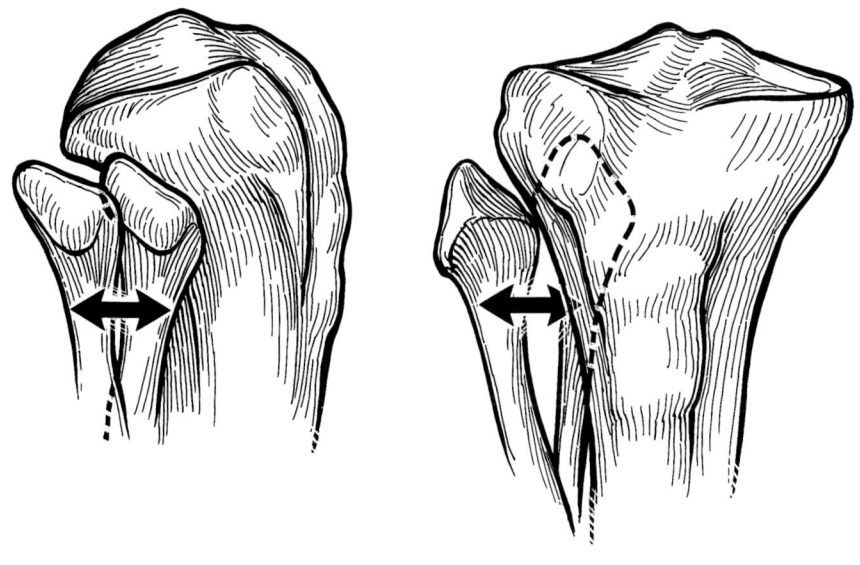

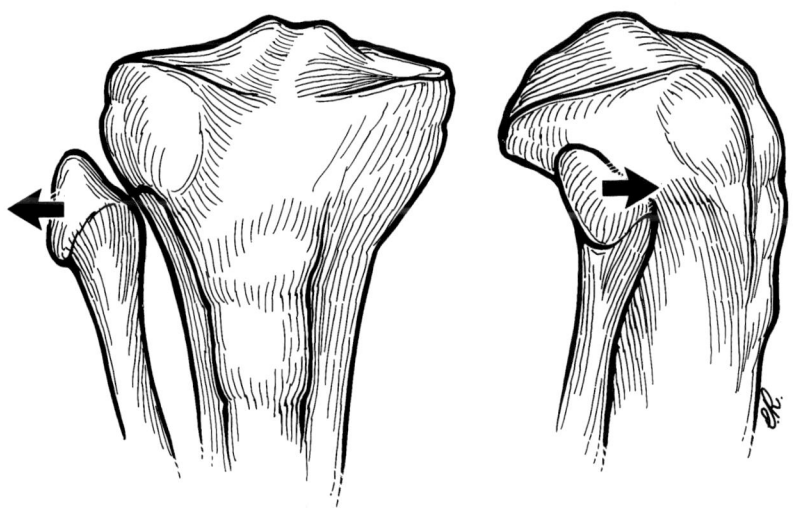

FIG 56–2.
Ogden's classification of proximal tibiofibular disruptions: subluxation, and anterolateral dislocation.

which the incidence of this type was twice that of posteromedial dislocation.[3]

MECHANISM OF INJURY

In isolated dislocations and in most combined injuries the LCL must be relaxed at the time of dislocation. Marshall et al.[10] have stated that the LCL is normally taut only in extension and that it becomes progressively slack as flexion progresses beyond 10 to 30 degrees. The posterior pull of the biceps femoris tendon compensates somewhat for this slack, keeping some tension on the LCL, but much less than in extension.

Anterolateral dislocations are caused by falling on a flexed knee with the leg adducted.[2, 8, 9, 12] There is usually associated inversion of the ankle. When this occurs the ankle mortise must widen to accommodate the talus. When the torque is excessive, diastasis of the distal tibiofibular joint, or less frequently dislocation of the proximal tibiofibular joint, occurs. At the proximal joint the posterior tibiofibular ligament is weakest and tears first. A violent reflex contracture of the peroneal muscles, in response to the ankle inversion, then acts as the deforming force on the fibular head, hinging it on the intact anterior tibiofibular ligament into the anterolateral dislocated position. Once dislocated, the fibular head is stable in the abnormal position.[12] Cadaver dissections have shown that the LCL is taut when the head is dislocated. Ogden[12] has stated that as long as the knee remains in extension with the LCL taut, reduction is difficult, but that by flexing the knee and relaxing the LCL, reduction of the fibular head can be easily achieved. Others have reported more difficulty effecting reduction in this way.[3]

Posteromedial dislocation is thought to result from a direct blow to the knee.[6] Severe injury to the joint capsule as well as the anterior and posterior tibiofibular ligaments allows the biceps femoris tendon to pull the unsupported fibular head posteriorly and medially.

Superior dislocations are essentially dislocations of the entire fibula and are always associated with lateral malleolar injuries and usually with tibial fractures.[12, 14]

SIGNS AND SYMPTOMS

Subluxation of the proximal tibiofibular joint is seen most often in adolescents. Patients complain of locking, buckling, and clicking in the knee.[16] Pain is felt along the lateral side of the knee and leg. Palpation over the fibular head will usually elicit the discomfort. A frequent concomitant finding is generalized joint laxity, and Ehlers-Danlos syndrome has been associated with this condition.[12] The instability is best demonstrated in the supine patient whose knee is flexed to 90 degrees. In this position, with the LCL and the biceps femoris tendon relaxed, the fibular head can be moved anteriorly and laterally. On release it returns with a click to its original position.[6]

Anterolateral dislocations are seen during athletic activity associated with violent twisting motion. Immediately after injury the patient may be unable to bear weight because of lateral knee pain. The fibular head is most easily palpated in its anterolateral position with the knee flexed. There is little swelling, because of the relative avascularity of the surrounding tissues. The fibular head is very tender to palpation, but associated knee effusion is rarely seen. Although movement of the knee is not severely restricted, ankle motion will elicit pain at the dislocation site. Several of Ogden's[12] patients with anterolateral dislocation had other associated skeletal injuries, such as hip fracture-dislocation, open tibia fracture, and fracture-dislocation of the ankle or distal femoral epiphysis. Invariably the dislocation of the proximal tibiofibular joint was missed when accompanied by these severe injuries.[12]

Posteromedial dislocation is the result of direct trauma to the knee, with pain secondary to that trauma. More important, however, is the association of common peroneal nerve injury with these dislocations. Lyle[9] reported an incidence of nerve symptoms in 5% of posteromedial dislocations.

Superior dislocation is extremely rare, and is associated with lateral knee pain and the presence of a lateral mass, which is actually the displaced fibular head.

ROENTGENOGRAPHIC FINDINGS

Radiographic comparison of the injured knee with the uninjured knee is helpful when the diagnosis of proximal tibiofibular joint dislocation is being entertained. In an anteroposterior view of a normal knee an overlap of the fibular head and the lateral aspect of the lateral tibial plateau is seen. In a normal lateral view a small portion of the fibula is visible posterior to the tibia. With anterolateral dislocation, the anteroposterior radiograph shows the entire fibular head lying lateral to the lateral tibial plateau (Fig 56–3). On the lateral view the fibula has moved anteriorly and is entirely overlapped by the tibia. Posteromedial and superior dislocations are also readily appreciated on x-ray films when compared with the contralateral normal knee, although one must always be careful not to overlook these injuries in the face of more dramatic radiographic findings.

METHODS OF TREATMENT

The acutely dislocated proximal tibiofibular joint does not require surgical intervention; closed reduction is almost invariably successful. Good muscle relaxation is essential. Occasionally general anesthesia must be administered. The patient is positioned with the affected knee in 90 degrees of flexion to relax the LCL. Direct pressure is applied to the displaced fibular head in the appropriate direction. Some have advocated strong foot inversion during reduction[12]; others have stated that ankle and foot position during reduction is not important.[14] Reduction, which oc-

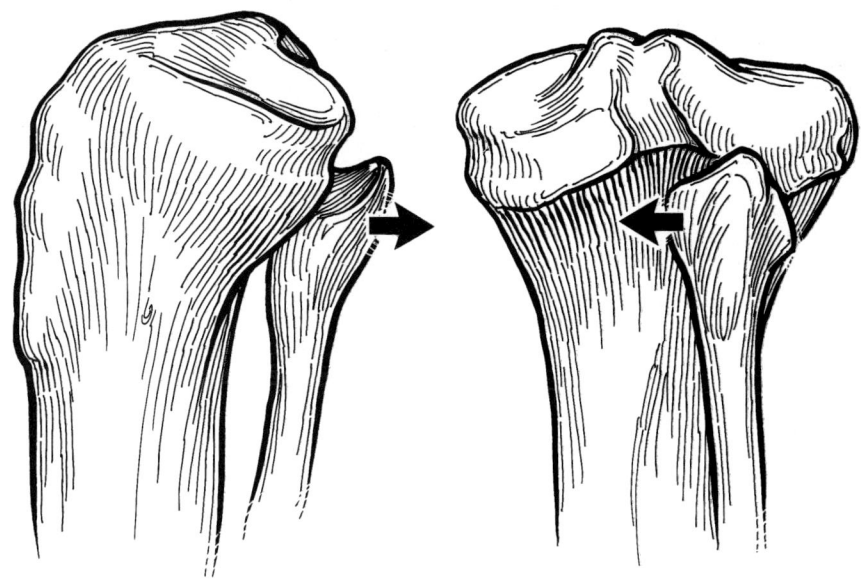

POSTEROMEDIAL

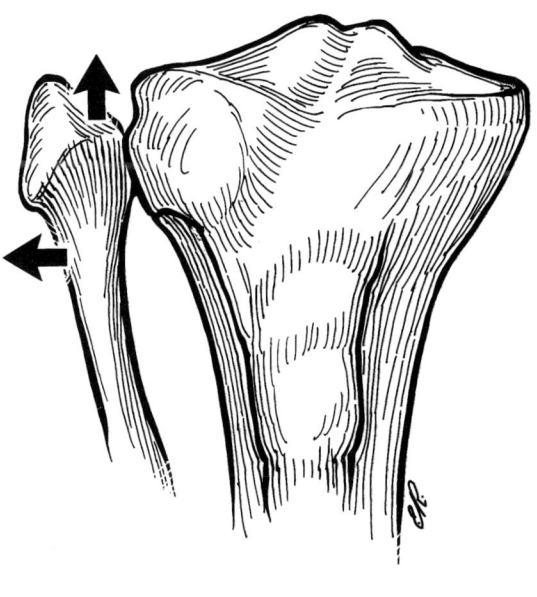

SUPERIOR

FIG 56–2, cont'd.
Ogden's classification of proximal tibiofibular disruptions: posteromedial dislocation and superior dislocation.

curs with an audible "pop," is usually stable. Postreduction immobilization techniques range from soft elastic wraps to short leg casts. Nonweightbearing status is maintained for 2 weeks. Progressive weightbearing is then begun, with return to full athletic activities usually within 6 weeks of the dislocation.

Rarely, closed reduction is unsuccessful or dislocation recurs after reduction. Recurrence is most common after posteromedial or superior dislocations. In such situations open reduction is required. A number of treatment methods have been described, including arthrodesis, proximal fibular resection, and

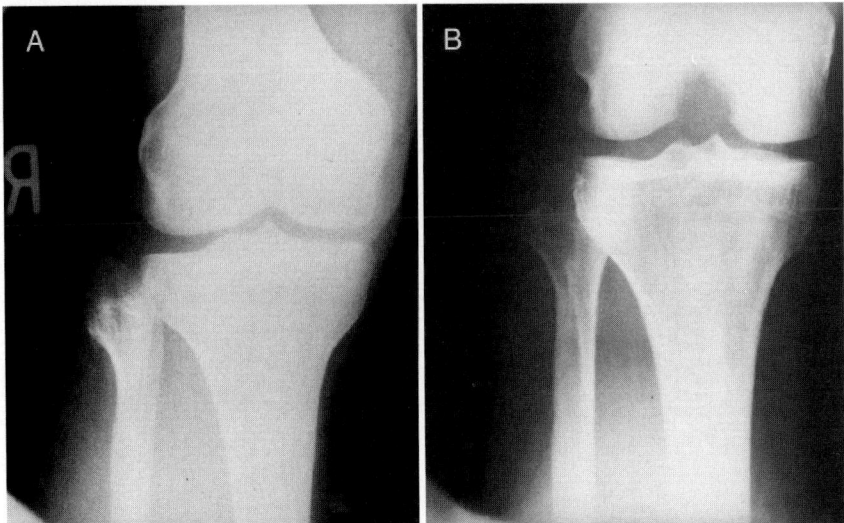

FIG 56-3.
(A) Anteroposterior view of the right knee with anterolateral proximal tibiofibular dislocation. **(B)** after closed reduction.

fixation. Arthrodesis, although advocated by some authors, has recently been condemned because of loosening of the screw and extensive resorption of bone about the screw. Dennis and Rutledge[3] have also warned that arthrodesis might prevent the outward rotation of the fibula that normally accompanies dorsiflexion of the foot, thereby increasing wear and tear on the ankle. They recommended resection of the proximal fibula with adequate margin to protect the common peroneal nerve.[3] Parkes and Zelko[14] have recommended open reduction and internal fixation with smooth Kirschner wires along with anatomic repair of the torn joint capsule and ligaments. The smooth wires are used because they are easier to remove under local anesthesia than the threaded wires. To prevent migration of the wires, nonweightbearing status and joint immobilization are instituted. Fixation is maintained for 6 weeks, at which time the wires are removed and immobilization is discontinued. Progressive weightbearing is then allowed as tolerated to full activity.

AUTHORS' PREFERRED TREATMENT

For acute proximal tibiofibular dislocations we prefer closed reduction, if necessary using general anesthesia. Immobilization is probably not necessary, because most reductions are inherently stable. Should closed reduction fail or redislocation occur, we prefer open reduction and internal fixation, with capsule and ligament repairs as described by Parkes and Zelco.[14] For those patients with symptoms of common peroneal nerve injury or for those in whom fixation has failed, we prefer proximal fibular resection. We do not advocate arthrodesis for any patient, for reasons previously mentioned.

PROGNOSIS AND COMPLICATIONS

In the appropriately treated, acute, isolated dislocation of the proximal tibiofibular joint, the prognosis is good. Common peroneal nerve symptoms are rare and usually transient. Lyle[9] reported nerve palsies in up to 5% of patients. Attention must always be directed to documenting and minimizing nerve symptoms. If necessary, proximal fibular resection should be performed.

In patients with multiple injuries of the lower extremity, the proximal tibiofibular joint should be examined to rule out dislocation. Although rare in this setting, dislocations invariably are unnoticed when associated with other more severe injuries. Neglect may result in joint instability and erosion of the joint surfaces. Treatment in this situation with proximal fibular resection will preserve normal knee and ankle function.[14]

REFERENCES

1. Barnett CH, Napier JR: The axis of rotation of the ankle joint in man: Its influence upon the form of the talus and the mobility of the fibula, J Anat 86:1–9, 1952.
2. Crothers DC, Johnson JTH: Isolated acute dislocation of the proximal tibio-fibular joint. J Bone Joint Surg [Am] 55:181–183, 1973.

3. Dennis JB, Rutledge BA: Bilateral recurrent dislocation of the superior tibio-fibular joint with peroneal nerve palsy, *J Bone Joint Surg [Am]* 40:1146–1148, 1958.
4. Freeman BL: Acute dislocations. In Crenshaw AH, editor: *Campbell's operative orthopaedics,* vol 3, ed 7. St Louis, 1987, Mosby–Year Book.
5. Gray DJ, Gardner E: Prenatal development of the human knee and superior tibiofibular joints, *Am J Anat* 86:235–287, 1950.
6. Harrison R, Hindenach JCR: Dislocations of the upper end of the fibula, *J Bone Joint Surg [Br]* 41:114–120, 1959.
7. Insall JN: Anatomy of the knee, In Insall JN, editor: *Surgery of the knee,* New York, 1984, Churchill Livingstone.
8. Lord DC, Coutts JW: A study of typical parachute injuries occurring in 250,000 jumps at the parachute school, *J Bone Joint Surg* 26:547–577, 1944.
9. Lyle HHM: Traumatic luxation of the head of the fibula, *Ann Surg* 82:635–639, 1925.
10. Marshall JL, Girgis FG, Zelko RR: The biceps femoris tendon and its functional significance, *J Bone Joint Surg [Am]* 54:1444–1450, 1972.
11. Nelaton A: *Elements de pathologie chirurgicale,* ed 2, Paris, 1874, Librairie Germen Ballière.
12. Ogden JA: Subluxation and dislocation of the proximal tibiofibular joint, *J Bone Joint Surg [Am]* 56:145–154, 1974.
13. Owen R: Recurrent dislocation of the superior tibiofibular joint, *J Bone Joint Surg [Br]* 50:342–345, 1968.
14. Parkes JC II, Zelko RR: Isolated acute dislocation of the proximal tibio-fibular joint, *J Bone Joint Surg [Am]* 55:177–180, 1973.
15. Resnick D, et al: Proximal tibio-fibular joint: Anatomic-pathologic-radiologic correlation, *AJR* 131:133–138, 1978.
16. Sijbrandij S: Instability of the proximal tibio-fibular joint, *Acta Orthop Scand* 49:621–626, 1978.

PART XIV

Osteotomy and Primary Total Knee Replacement

57

Osteotomy in Treatment of the Arthritic Knee

WILLIAM L. HEALY, M.D.
RICHARD M. WILK, M.D.

Rationale of osteotomy
Patient selection
  Patient personality
  Age
  Angular deformity
  Range of motion
  Activity level
  Weight
  Rheumatoid arthritis
  Stability
  Bone loss
  Tibiofemoral subluxation
  Lateral thrust
  Patellofemoral pain
  Cosmesis
Preoperative evaluation
  Physical examination
  Radiographic examination
  Physical therapy
  Patient education
  Arthroscopy and joint debridement
  Preoperative surgical planning

Choice of osteotomy
  Medial tibiofemoral osteoarthritis with varus deformity
  Proximal tibial valgus osteotomy (authors' technique)
  Lateral tibiofemoral osteoarthritis with valgus deformity
  Distal femoral varus osteotomy (authors' recommendation)
Complications
  Undercorrection
  Thromboembolic disease
  Peroneal palsy
  Nonunion
  Infection
  Vascular injury
  Internal fixation
  Intraarticular fracture
Results
  Proximal tibial valgus osteotomy
  Proximal tibial varus osteotomy
  Distal femoral varus osteotomy
Total knee arthroplasty following osteotomy
Summary

Surgical treatment of the arthritic knee has improved over the past two decades with advances in total knee arthroplasty. Early success in relieving pain and improving function following total knee arthroplasty is well documented. Long-term success with total knee replacement is now being recognized with many different implants. The authors acknowledge that total knee arthroplasty is the gold standard for surgical treatment of the arthritic knee; however, there is also a role for osteotomy in surgical treatment of the arthritic knee.

Osteotomy of long bones was initially developed to correct alignment deformities following trauma or developmental abnormality. This concept was later expanded to correcting malalignment associated with joints. The concept of performing an osteotomy for treatment of arthritis of the knee was first presented by Gariepy[19] and Jackson and Waugh.[33, 34] Proximal tibial valgus osteotomy was later popularized by Coventry.[8–12, 14] These authors believed that osteoarthritis of the knee usually involved one tibiofemoral compartment predominantly. Furthermore, unicompartmental disease was generally associated with a varus or valgus deformity of the knee.

Tibial osteotomy for osteoarthritis of the knee evolved following the success of intertrochanteric osteotomy for osteoarthritis of the hip.[12] According to Pauwels,[53] pain in the arthritic hip was related to a reduction in the weightbearing surface. In the acetabulum, an area of dense sclerotic bone represented the area of force transmission, which he called the sourcil. In osteotomy of the hip, the unit load crossing the sourcil is reduced by increasing the surface area that transmits the load. Angular, rotatory, and displacement osteotomies of the hip have provided clinical improvement when used for osteoarthritis of the hip.[53, 56]

Several theories have been presented to account for pain in the osteoarthritic knee. One plausible explanation is that pain occurs as a result of microfractures of subchondral bone.[10, 42] Deformity associated with unicompartmental joint space deterioration leads to overload of the affected compartment resulting in subchondral microfractures. It has also been suggested that pain in the arthritic knee is due to increased interosseous pressure in the metaphysis of the proximal tibia.

The pain and dysfunction associated with medial tibiofemoral osteoarthritis and varus deformity are usually ascribed to malalignment and medial impingement. Wagner and co-workers[66-68] have expanded our knowledge of osteotomy with their description of anterior impingement. Anterior impingement occurs as a secondary bony adaptation in the arthritic process of the proximal tibia. Hypertrophic overgrowth in the intercondylar notch of the distal femur also contributes to anterior impingement. Flexion contracture in the arthritic knee is a combination of soft tissue contracture and bony adaptation.[66-68]

RATIONALE OF OSTEOTOMY

The goal of knee osteotomy is to realign the mechanical axis of the limb thereby shifting weightbearing forces from a diseased compartment to a more normal compartment and decreasing medial impingement. In the normal knee, the mechanical axis of weightbearing is defined by a straight line drawn from the center of the femoral head through the center of the knee to the center of the ankle mortise. In the normal knee, approximately 60% of weightbearing forces are transmitted through the medial compartment and approximately 40% through the lateral compartment. The tibiofemoral angle of the lower extremity is determined by the angle created by a line drawn down the longitudinal axis of the femur and a line drawn down the longitudinal axis of the tibia. A normal mechanical axis is a straight line and is defined as 0 degrees. A normal tibiofemoral angle deviates from the straight line with a valgus angle of approximately 5 to 7 degrees (see Fig 57-5).

Unicompartmental joint space deterioration is associated with abnormal lower extremity alignment and abnormal force transmission through the knee. This malalignment may be the result of developmental, traumatic, or inflammatory factors. Varus and valgus malalignment may also be associated with flexion, extension, and rotatory deformities.

As varus or valgus deformity of the knee develops, forces crossing the tibial joint are altered, and the relative contact stress in the medial and lateral compartments changes. In varus knees, contact stress increases in the medial tibiofemoral joint. In valgus knees, contact stress increases in the lateral tibiofemoral joint. As the articular cartilage is exposed to increased stress, normal cartilage metabolism is disrupted. This leads to a cycle of increasing malalignment with increasing deterioration of articular cartilage. In the absence of meniscal lesions, the patient experiences pain when articular deterioration and malalignment reach the point where microfractures of the subchondral bone occur.

Progression of unicompartmental arthritis in the knee and its attendant deformity affect the ligamentous support of the knee. Tensile forces lead to stretching of collateral ligaments on the convex side while compressive forces result in early laxity and late contracture of collateral ligaments on the concave side of the knee. Disruption of normal collateral ligament function contributes further to abnormal force transmission through the knee during gait.

The goal of osteotomy about the knee is to relieve pain. It has been demonstrated that by transferring joint forces from an arthritic compartment to a more normal compartment, pain can be relieved and the arthritic joint space can be preserved. In medial tibiofemoral osteoarthritis with varus deformity, valgus osteotomy of the tibia decreases the excess load in the medial compartment and shifts the transmission of force to the lateral compartment. In lateral tibiofemoral osteoarthritis with valgus deformity, varus osteotomy of the femur decreases the load in the lateral compartment and transfers this load to the medial compartment. In cases of severe anterior impingement, an extension osteotomy of the distal femur will relieve the impingement.

The biomechanics of varus and valgus deformities of the knee differ because of the intrinsic valgus angle at the articulation of the femur with the tibia. These differences must be considered when designing an osteotomy to correct angular deformity. In varus deformity, the tibiofemoral joint line is usually parallel to the floor, even in the presence of medial tibiofemoral bone loss. Tsumura et al.[64] have used computer analysis to demonstrate that proximal tibial valgus osteotomy can effectively transfer load from the medial to the lateral compartment (Figs 57–1 and 57–2).[64]

In valgus deformity of the knee, the tibiofemoral joint line frequently has a valgus or superolateral tilt. While tibial varus osteotomy may realign a valgus limb, it is not able to correct the joint line tilt because the procedure is performed distal to the joint line. Furthermore, Tsumura et al.[64] have demonstrated that load transmission is not effectively transferred from the lateral to the medial compartment following tibial varus osteotomy. In spite of satisfactory realignment, tibial varus osteotomy of the valgus knee transfers load medially only to the lateral portion of the tibial spine.[64] Tibial varus osteotomy is contraindicated in patients with large valgus deformities because the resultant valgus tilt of the joint line leads to increased shear forces and lateral subluxation during gait.[13]

Distal femoral varus osteotomy has been shown to effectively transfer load from an arthritic lateral compartment to a more normal medial compartment.[64] Distal femoral varus osteotomy may correct valgus tilt of the joint line when used to treat lateral tibiofemoral osteoarthritis with valgus deformity.[25] An extension component of distal femoral osteotomy can relieve anterior impingement (Figs 57–3 and 57–4).

PATIENT SELECTION

Optimal results following osteotomy about the knee occur when patients have been selected properly. The ideal patient for knee osteotomy is young and active with unicompartmental osteoarthritis in a stable and mobile knee. It is also essential that the patient be motivated to participate fully in postoperative physical therapy. Early results of osteotomy about the knee for osteoarthritis during the 1960s and 1970s were not as good as the results of osteotomy reported more recently. This discrepancy occurs because of patient selection. In the 1960s osteotomies were performed on patients who would now be treated with total knee arthroplasty. Patient selection is the most critical factor in planning and achieving a successful osteotomy of the knee. The criteria for patient selection are discussed below.

Patient Personality

The personality of the patient is a very important factor when considering osteotomy of the knee. A patient's profession, domestic situation, and expectations will influence outcome. Patient education is essential in osteotomy. Osteotomy is performed early in the course of osteoarthritis at a point when patients can probably still tolerate their discomfort and accept their diminished level of function. Osteotomy is part of the lifelong management of an arthritic knee.

Pain relief following osteotomy is not as dramatic as it is following total knee arthroplasty. Patients cannot compare their postoperative experiences with total knee arthroplasty patients. Osteotomy patients need to understand the natural history of their disease and the goals of osteotomy. This requires a patient who can understand the operation and have confidence in the judgment of the surgeon.

Age

While there are no absolute age limits, it is generally agreed that osteotomy is an operation best suited for younger, more active patients.[48] Insall et al.[29] demonstrated that patients more than 60 years of age had a 52% rate of good results with proximal tibial valgus osteotomy at 9-year follow-up. In the same series, patients who were less than 60 years old at the time of osteotomy had a 74% rate of good results at 7-year follow up.[29] Furthermore, the impressive results from total knee arthroplasty and unicompartmental arthroplasty are more likely to endure a patient's lifetime in those over 60. As the average life span increases, osteotomy may be more often indicated for older patients. Currently, we reserve osteotomy about the knee for patients less than 55 to 60 years of age.

Angular Deformity

In discussing angular deformity, it is important to use a standard reference axis. In this chapter, when discussing angular deformity, we consider deviation from the normal mechanical axis, which is 0 degrees (see Fig 57–5). There are limits of deformity that can be reliably corrected through a proximal tibial or distal femoral osteotomy. When correcting a varus deformity, the results of proximal tibial valgus osteotomy are best when the varus deformity is 10 degrees or less.[1] Varus deformity of more than 15 degrees is frequently associated with lateral subluxation at the tibiofemoral joint and pain at the patellofemoral joint.[17, 30] It has also been suggested that a varus deformity greater than 15 degrees is associated with increased medial bone loss and bicompartment articular cartilage deterioration.[30]

When correcting a valgus deformity associated with lateral tibiofemoral osteoarthritis, correction can be performed through either a varus osteotomy of the proximal tibia or a varus osteotomy of the distal fe-

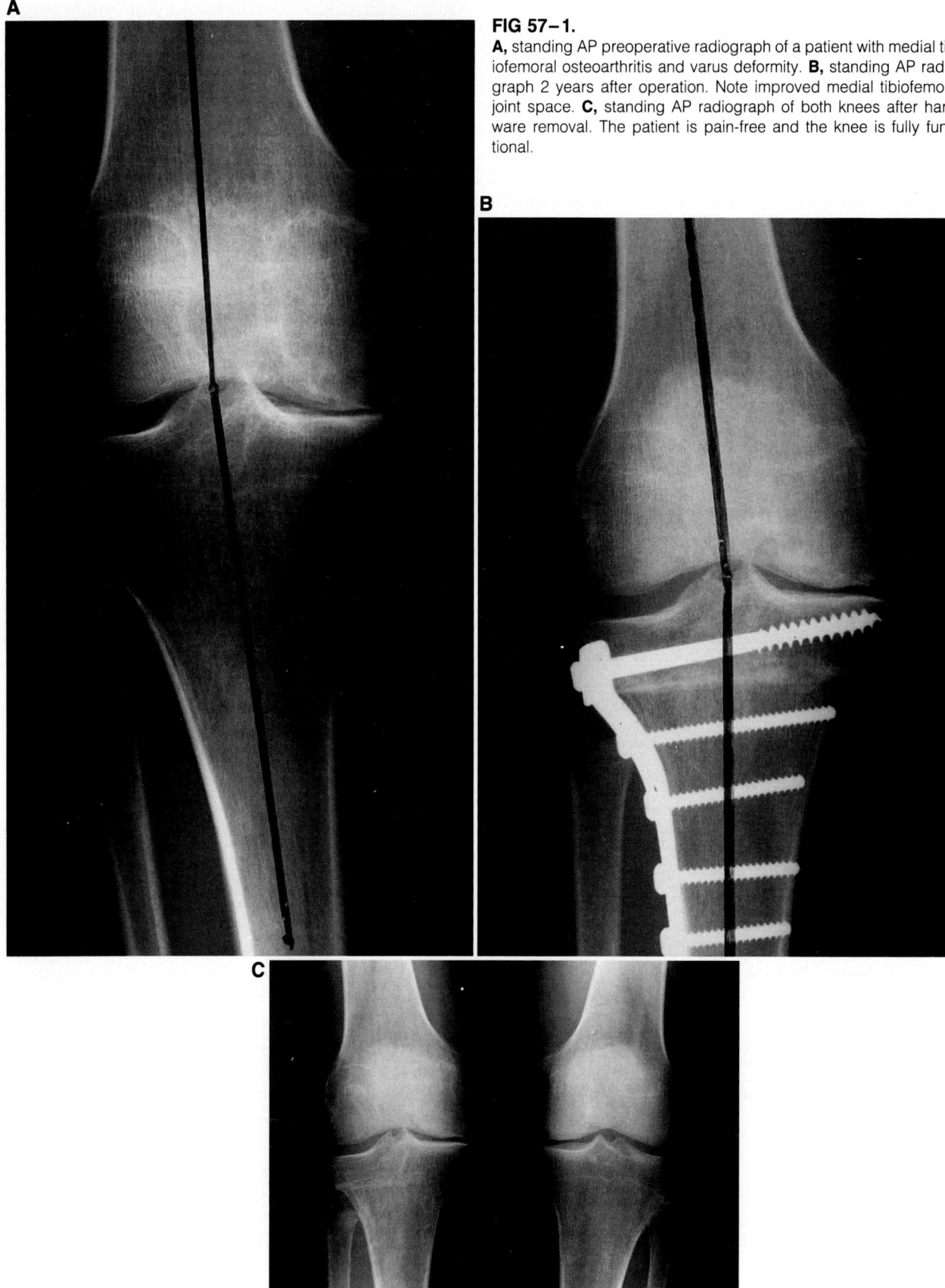

FIG 57–1.
A, standing AP preoperative radiograph of a patient with medial tibiofemoral osteoarthritis and varus deformity. **B,** standing AP radiograph 2 years after operation. Note improved medial tibiofemoral joint space. **C,** standing AP radiograph of both knees after hardware removal. The patient is pain-free and the knee is fully functional.

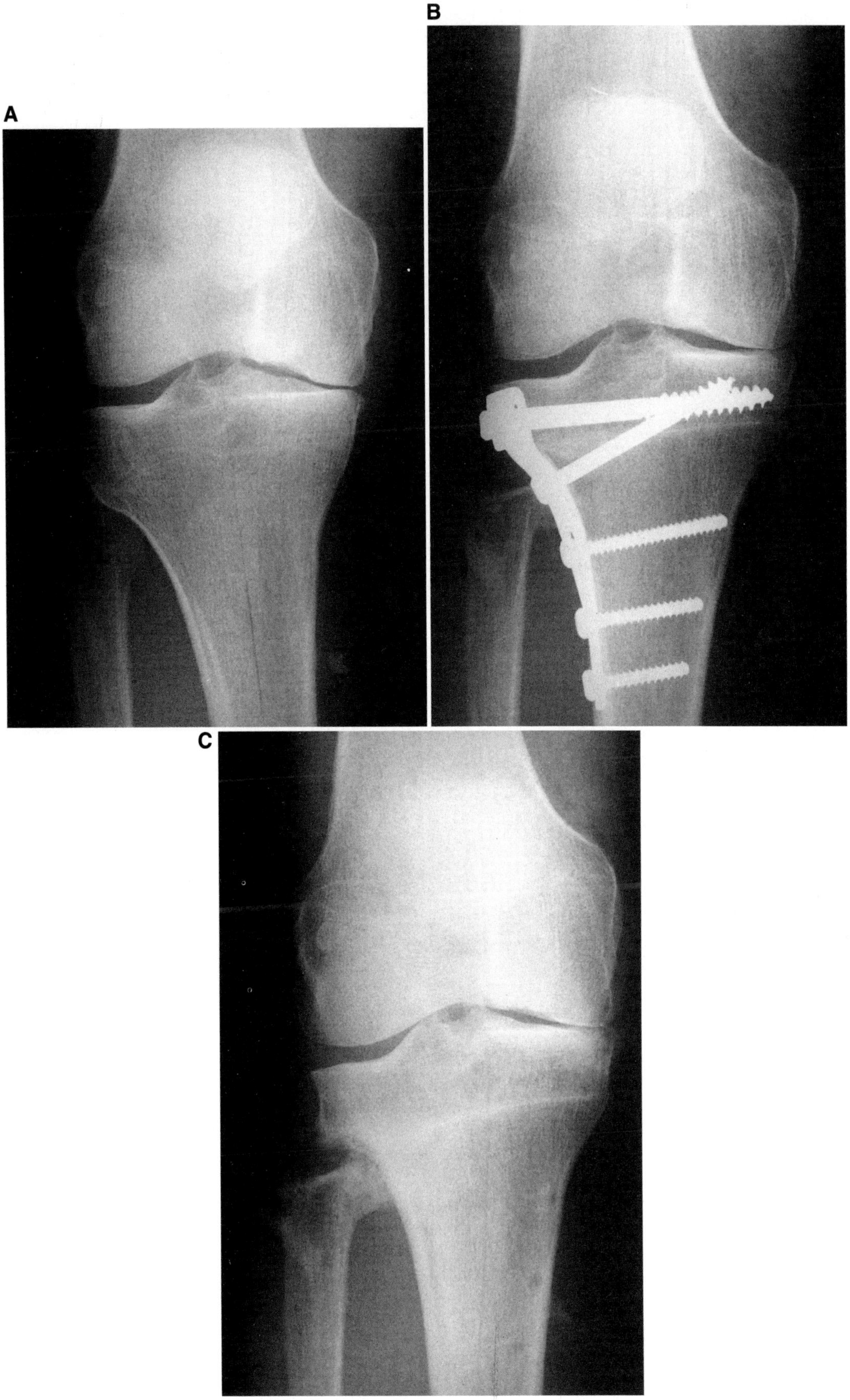

FIG 57-2.
A, standing AP preoperative radiograph of a patient with medial tibiofemoral osteoarthritis and varus deformity. **B,** standing AP radiograph 5 years following operation. **C,** standing AP radiograph 6 years following osteotomy and following hardware removal. The patient is pain-free and the knee is fully functional.

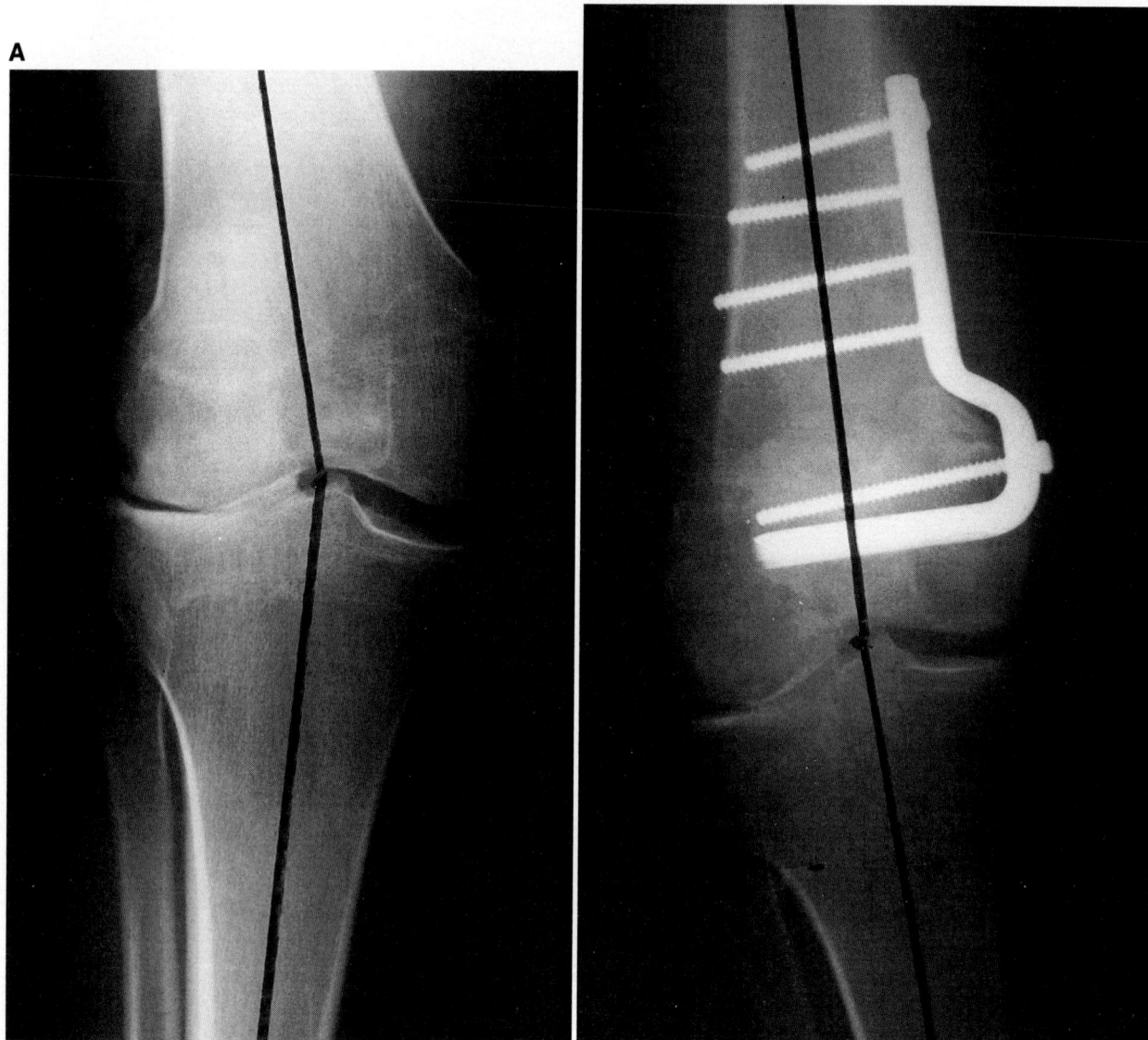

FIG 57–3.
A, standing AP radiograph of a patient with lateral tibiofemoral osteoarthritis and valgus deformity. **B,** standing AP radiograph 3 years following distal femoral varus osteotomy. The patient has no pain, full function, and an improved cosmetic appearance.

mur. Coventry[13] suggests that for small valgus deformities, i.e., up to 6 degrees of valgus, proximal tibial varus osteotomy is satisfactory. However, for patients with greater than 6 degrees of valgus deformity, distal femoral osteotomy is indicated in order to correct the valgus tilt of the tibiofemoral joint line, which may lead to tibiofemoral subluxation and increase shear forces in the joint.[13, 23, 25]

Range of Motion

Adequate range of motion is an important consideration for osteotomy as poor results have been associated with stiff knees. There has not been a controlled study demonstrating an optimal arc of motion for osteotomy. Most authors recommend a 90-degree flexion arc with flexion contractures not exceeding 10 to 15 degrees.[23] In the early arthritic knee, preoperative physical therapy can improve the range of motion by stretching the posterior capsule and the hamstrings to minimize flexion contracture. When a distal femoral osteotomy is the osteotomy of choice, the fixed flexion contracture can be partially addressed by adding an extension component to the osteotomy.[66–68]

Activity Level

Patients who are employed as heavy laborers or who wish to continue participation in athletic activities are better suited for osteotomy than for arthroplasty.

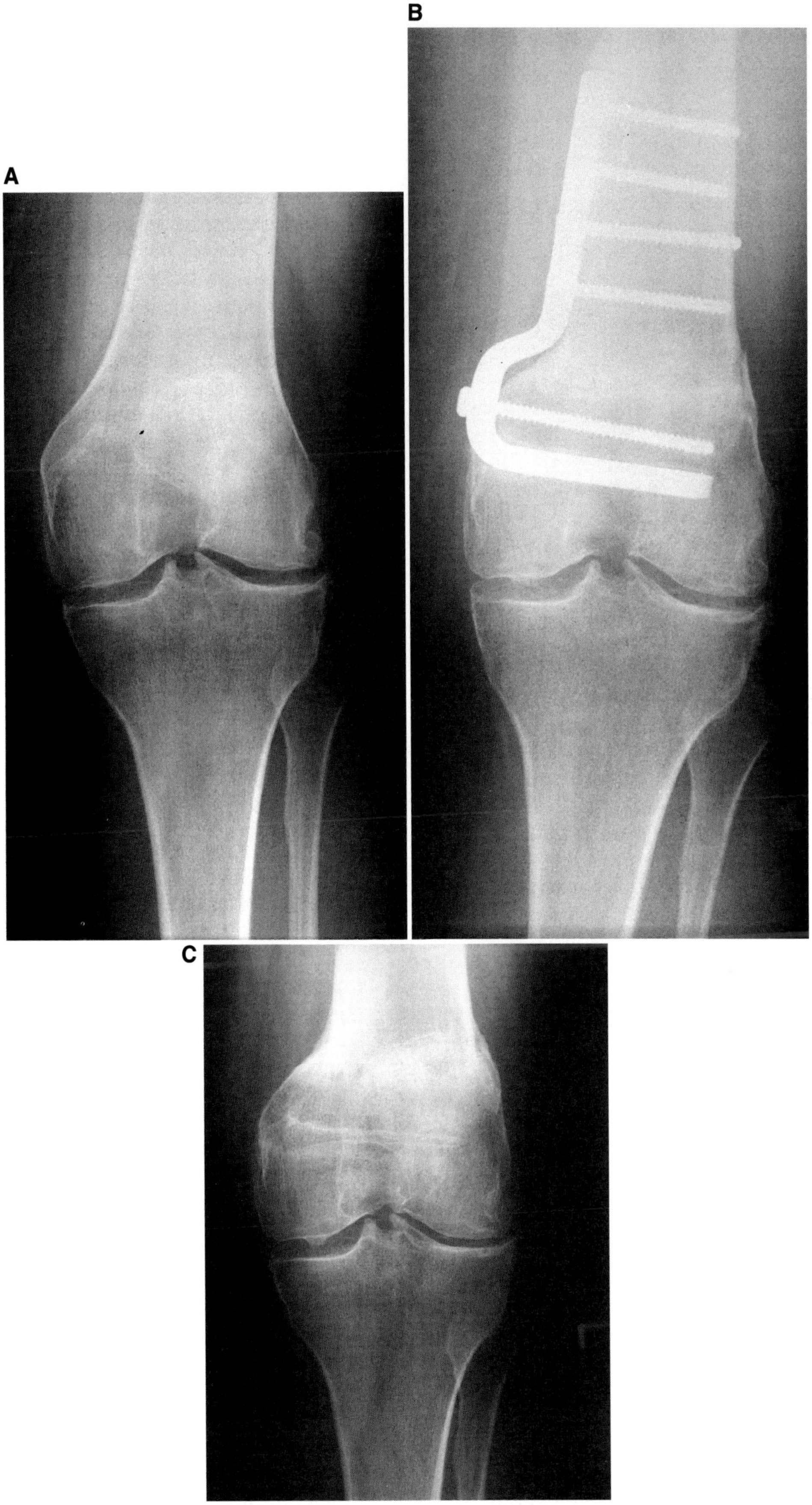

FIG 57–4.
A, standing AP preoperative radiograph of a patient with lateral tibiofemoral osteoarthritis and valgus deformity. **B,** standing AP radiograph 2 years following operation. **C,** standing AP radiograph 5 years following operation and following hardware removal. The patient is pain-free and the knee is fully functional. The patient is pleased with the straightened limb.

Once an osteotomy is healed there is no contraindication to any impact-loading activities. This contrasts with prosthetic arthroplasty of the knee in which impact loading must be minimized.

Weight

Excess body weight is not necessarily a contraindication to osteotomy. In fact, it is a factor that might make a patient a better candidate for osteotomy than for arthroplasty. Excess weight is associated with increased rates of implant loosening and prosthetic failure following total knee arthroplasty or unicompartmental arthroplasty of the knee. However, in offering osteotomy to obese patients, it should be noted that Matthews et al.[48] related obesity to decreased survivorship for osteotomy.

Rheumatoid Arthritis

Osteotomy of the knee for rheumatoid arthritis has not proved to be a predictably successful procedure.[3, 6, 11, 51] Chan and Pollard[6] reported a 75% rate of good results in patients with rheumatoid arthritis in the first 3 years following proximal tibial valgus osteotomy. The results in these patients deteriorated to 41% good results at greater than 3-year follow-up.[6] Coventry[9] reported only 55% good results in a 2- to 9-year follow-up in patients with rheumatoid arthritis. In sharp contrast, total knee arthroplasty in patients with rheumatoid arthritis demonstrated an 85% rate of good results.[31] We do not recommend osteotomy about the knee for rheumatoid arthritis or for other inflammatory conditions associated with severe osteopenia.

Stability

Stability of the knee is required for a successful osteotomy. Realignment of the limb with collateral ligament insufficiency will not improve gait, redistribute weightbearing, relieve pain, or improve function.

With progressive angular deformity of the knee the collateral ligaments are often stretched on the convex side of the deformity and contracted on the concave side. When a corrective osteotomy is performed, weightbearing forces are transferred from the concave to the convex side of the deformity. This generally results in reduction of tension in the previously stretched collateral ligament, thus rendering it functionally lax.

In varus deformity, relative laxity of the medial collateral ligament may occur with loss of medial bone, but usually the ligament is competent. As the varus deformity develops the lateral collateral ligament may be stretched. Correction of the mechanical axis can therefore result in a lax lateral ligamentous complex. In general, this is treated expectantly without compromise of function. In younger patients with severe deformities it can be argued that tightening of the lax lateral ligamentous complex is indicated, but this is not routinely performed by us.

In valgus deformity there is frequently an associated recurvatum with some stretching of the posterior capsule and posterior cruciate ligament. This is generally not a problem following corrective osteotomy. When corrective osteotomy for valgus deformity is performed in the distal femur, obliquity of the joint line is corrected and ligament reconstruction is rarely indicated.

When a patient's knee gives way or shifts because of anterior cruciate ligament insufficiency, osteotomy may be only partially successful. Concomitant anterior cruciate ligament reconstruction and proximal tibial valgus osteotomy may be sufficient to treat both problems. Treatment of only the anterior cruciate ligament insufficiency is likely to fail, as a varus knee with a varus thrust on ambulation is likely to lead to stretching and failure of an anterior cruciate ligament graft. This can be prevented with prior or simultaneous osteotomy.

No long-term studies exist to address the question of concomitant anterior cruciate ligament insufficiency and varus osteoarthritis. We believe that symptom complexes must be separated as clearly as possible into instability or giving way, as opposed to medial joint line pain on weightbearing. In sedentary patients, correction of alignment and relief of medial joint line pain has proved to be a satisfactory treatment in the absence of giving way. When giving way is a significant component of a patient's knee problem, the patient's demands and expected activities should be taken into account.

Bone Loss

A relative contraindication to osteotomy of the proximal tibia is bone loss of the medial or lateral tibial plateau. When medial or lateral compartment bony support is insufficient, congruent weightbearing on both tibial plateaus following osteotomy is not possible. In this situation, tibiofemoral contact will "teeter" on the relatively prominent intercondylar tibial spines.[17, 40] Bone insufficiency may also be associated with instability of the knee.

Tibiofemoral Subluxation

The presence of severe varus or valgus deformity may be associated with lateral or medial subluxation of the tibia, respectively. Subluxation may be associated with bone loss or previous trauma. Lateral tibiofemoral subluxation increases with varus deformities greater than 15 degrees.[30] Subluxation greater than 1 cm is an absolute contraindication to corrective osteotomy and some authors suggest that osteotomy should not be performed if any translation or subluxation is present.[9, 10, 12, 23, 30] Tibiofemoral subluxation and translation can be best documented on single-leg weightbearing radiographs.

Lateral Thrust

Most studies on the biomechanics of osteotomy about the knee have been based on static double-leg and single-leg weightbearing radiographs. Dynamic gait studies have more accurately addressed the issue of varus or lateral thrust of the knee during ambulation. Prodromos et al.[55] measured adductor moments of the knee in patients with unicompartmental medial tibiofemoral osteoarthritis following proximal tibial valgus osteotomy. The term adductor moment was used to describe the amount of lateral or varus thrust of the knee observed during gait. They determined that patients with a high adductor moment had worse results following osteotomy than patients with a low adductor moment. Furthermore, patients with a high adductor moment were more likely to have a recurrent varus deformity following valgus osteotomy. These results were confirmed more recently by Wang et al.[69] At 6 years following osteotomy, 79% of low adductors maintained valgus alignment, while only 29% of knees in the high adductor group maintained valgus postoperative correction.[69] These gait studies suggest that patients with significant lateral thrust may be poor candidates for tibial valgus osteotomy. When osteotomy is chosen for patients in spite of a high adductor moment, overcorrection of the mechanical axis may be helpful.

Patellofemoral Pain

Osteotomy of the proximal tibia or the distal femur is designed to relieve symptoms of medial or lateral tibiofemoral osteoarthritis. Slight degenerative changes of the patellofemoral joint are not a contraindication to angular osteotomy. Following proximal tibial valgus osteotomy with a lateral closing wedge, the mechanics of the patellofemoral joint are changed. The working length of the patellar tendon is decreased and the quadriceps angle (Q angle) is increased. Depending on the size of the lateral closing wedge, the anterior tibial tubercle is effectively elevated. Frequently this will decrease patellofemoral symptoms which, in varus deformity, are commonly due to medial facet articular cartilage changes.

Similarly, following distal femoral varus osteotomy the Q angle is decreased and excess lateral patellofemoral pressure is reduced by the realignment of the patellofemoral mechanism. Sufficient repair of the vastus medialis is essential to prevent patellofemoral pain following distal femoral osteotomy through a medial approach.

Cosmesis

The appearance of the lower extremity following corrective osteotomy may surprise some patients. A discussion with the patient before surgery is essential to address the postoperative alignment of the extremities and the patient's body image. If a patient has a bilateral genu varus or genu valgum, the patient needs to understand that the appearance of the limb will be changed following osteotomy. Cosmesis and patient acceptance is an important consideration in determining how much overcorrection to incorporate into an osteotomy. In our experience, patient acceptance decreases with valgus angles greater than 5 degrees (mechanical axis).

PREOPERATIVE EVALUATION

Careful preoperative planning is essential for a successful osteotomy of the knee. Preoperative considerations include a physical examination of the knee, a radiographic examination of the lower extremity, patient education, physical therapy, consideration of arthroscopy or joint debridement, and preoperative surgical planning.

Physical Examination

A knee joint sufficient for corrective osteotomy must have satisfactory range of motion and joint space congruence that will allow transmission of weightbearing following realignment. The bone must be of sufficient density and strength to transmit weightbearing forces and provide secure fixation of internal fixation devices. Ligamentous stability should be sufficient for the function desired postoperatively. Fixed flexion contractures should be evaluated to determine the contribution to the contracture by posterior capsule contraction and bony adaptation. The physical examination should also document a competent extensor mechanism.

Radiographic Examination

When a lower extremity is in normal alignment, the tibiofemoral joint space is approximately parallel to the ground and the articular condyles of the proximal tibia and the distal femur transmit compressive weightbearing forces evenly and symmetrically across the knee joint. In this case, a standing radiograph which includes the center of the hip, center of the knee, and center of the ankle, demonstrates a normal mechanical axis on a line drawn from the center of the hip through the center of the knee to the center of the ankle. This radiograph is essential for planning an osteotomy of the knee. Varus or valgus angular deformity is determined by drawing lines down the femoral shaft axis and down the tibial shaft axis. In the normal limb, these lines are colinear and intersect at the center of the knee. In a malaligned lower extremity, these lines deviate by their angular deformity at the center of the knee (Fig 57–5). Subluxation of the tibiofemoral joint can create a drawing where the intersection of the tibial shaft axis and the femoral shaft axis is not at the center of the knee joint. During gait the tibiofemoral joint line tilts to a few degrees of varus associated with varus thrust. Single-leg standing radiographs can demonstrate increased dynamic deformities. In addition to a standing radiograph, close-up views of the knee prior to osteotomy include anteroposterior (AP), lateral, tangential (sunrise), and tunnel (intercondylar) views.

The angle of correction for an osteotomy is determined by adding to the absolute deformity of the limb an overcorrection of 2 to 4 degrees. During gait in the normal limb, the weightbearing force vector passes medial to the center of the knee joint. Overcorrection following proximal tibial valgus osteotomy ensures that weightbearing forces will pass lateral to the center of the knee joint.[64] Insall et al.[29] demonstrated that overcorrection resulted in a 77% rate of good results, whereas correction only to the mechanical axis resulted in 60% good results.

Stress radiographs to evaluate ligament integrity on the concave side of the deformity may also evaluate the unaffected joint space under loaded conditions. Computed tomography (CT) scans, bone scans, and magnetic resonance imaging have also been used as preoperative studies in candidates for knee osteotomy. In the majority of cases, we do not recommend these additional imaging studies.

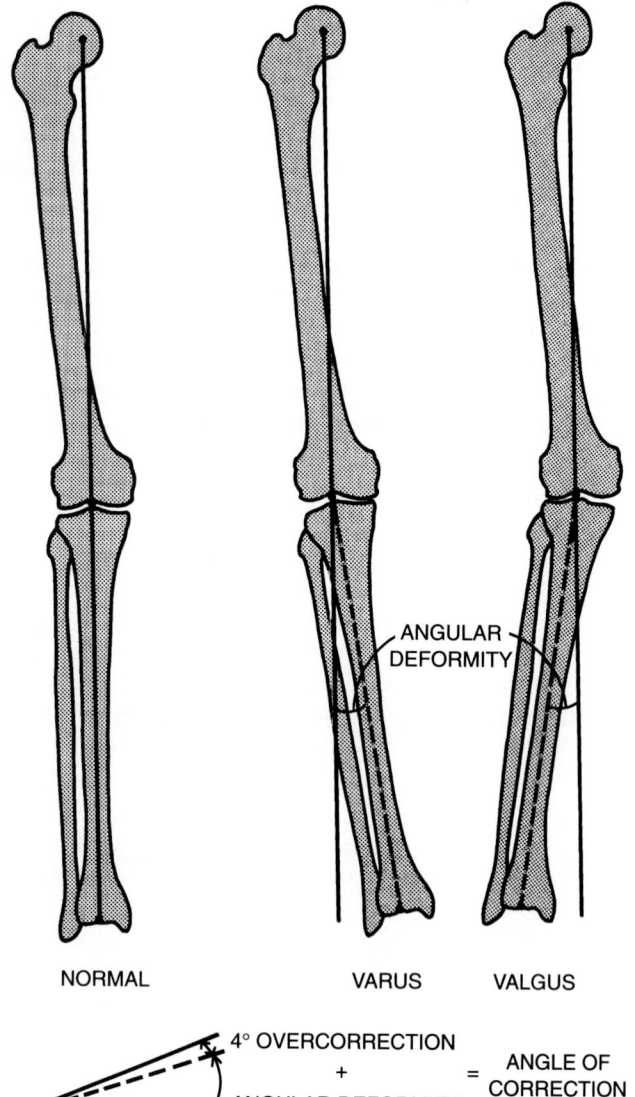

FIG 57–5.
The mechanical axis is a line drawn from the center of the femoral head through the center of the knee to the center of the ankle. The tibiofemoral angle is created by a line drawn down the longitudinal axis of the femur and a line drawn down the longitudinal axis of the tibia. A normal mechanical axis is a straight line (0 degrees). In a normal limb, the tibiofemoral angle deviates from the straight line with a valgus angle of approximately 5 to 7 degrees.

Physical Therapy

Preoperative physical therapy is important in order to increase the strength of the extensor mechanism and decrease the extent of the flexion contracture. Quadriceps strengthening of the arthritic knee allows more rapid rehabilitation postoperatively. Stretching of the soft tissue component of the flexion contracture, including the hamstrings, decreases the contracture to the point where only bony adaptation persists. Preoperative instruction in crutch walking can contribute to faster ambulation following osteotomy.

Patient Education

Educating the patient as to the natural history of the arthritic knee and the goals of osteotomy improve the patient's acceptance of the treatment regimen. It is important that patients are advised not to expect their knee operation to be the same as total knee replacement. Since arthroplasty is more common than osteotomy, patient misconceptions can affect patient outcome. When patients understand their problem and the solution, they are more apt to accept their surgical result.

Arthroscopy and Joint Debridement

The role of preoperative debridement by arthrotomy or arthroscopy in conjunction with osteotomy is controversial. MacIntosh and Welsh[45] reviewed a series of 120 patients who had high tibial osteotomy and an open joint debridement. The long-term results of those patients were no better than the long-term results of patients who had osteotomy alone. Furthermore, 10% of the open debridement group required manipulation under anesthesia to achieve a satisfactory range of motion.[45]

The role of routine preosteotomy arthroscopy has been studied by Keene and Dyreby and coworkers.[37, 38] In short-term and later intermediate-term follow-up of 51 knees, preosteotomy arthroscopy had no significant predictive or therapeutic value.[37, 38]

The advent of arthroscopic debridement of the knee has reduced the role of arthrotomy and debridement to the point of deleting it from surgical treatment of the arthritic knee. However, arthroscopic debridement of the arthritic knee without osteotomy has proved to be efficacious in relieving pain due to osteoarthritis for short periods of time, ranging from 2 to 5 years. Knees benefiting the most from arthroscopic debridement have meniscal abnormalities or loose bodies, without significant angular deformity. In general, patients with sufficient deformity to be good candidates for osteotomy are not ideal candidates for arthroscopic debridement of the arthritic knee. We use arthroscopy in conjunction with osteotomy when patients have mechanical symptoms suggestive of meniscal abnormalities or loose bodies in addition to unicompartmental osteoarthritis associated with deformity.

Preoperative Surgical Planning

Corrective osteotomy is most likely to achieve its goals when the angular correction and the method of fixation are determined preoperatively. One conventional method of determining the size of the proximal tibial lateral wedge to be removed involves removing 1 mm of bone for each 1 degree of angular correction desired. However, this method has severe limitations when different-size tibias are involved. We recommend a method of determining angular deformity from standing radiographs and adding an overcorrection of 2 to 4 degrees (see Fig 57–5). Specific angular wedges can be removed by using guide pins and templates. Recently, cutting jigs have been developed incorporating specific wedge angles.

Computers have provided orthopaedic surgeons with new tools in planning osteotomies of the lower extremity. AP and lateral radiographs and CT scans can be digitized and incorporated into software programs. Surgeons can then generate computer models to simulate the surgical procedure, including bone cuts. Depending on the software, these programs can predict the alignment and the postoperative mechanical axis. Computer templating and instrument systems to decrease surgical error have the potential to improve the technique for corrective osteotomy about the knee in the future.

CHOICE OF OSTEOTOMY

Medial Tibiofemoral Osteoarthritis with Varus Deformity

Several different osteotomy techniques have been described for medial tibiofemoral osteoarthritis associated with varus deformity. Jackson and Waugh[33] in 1961 described a ball-and-socket, or dome, osteotomy distal to the anterior tibial tuberosity. An osteotomy of the proximal third of the fibula was performed through a separate incision. Internal fixation was not used and patients were immobilized in a cylinder cast for 6 to 8 weeks.[32–34]

Gariepy[19] and Coventry[8–12, 14] popularized the technique of laterally based closing wedge osteotomy proximal to the anterior tibial tubercle. They removed the fibular head and reattached the biceps femoris and lateral collateral ligament to the fibular shaft. The osteotomy was stabilized with staples.[8–12, 14, 19] Slocum et al.[58] used a modification of this proximal tibial closing wedge osteotomy which involved leaving a posterior lip of cortex in the proximal tibial segment. The authors believe that this added to the stability of the osteotomy construct. Additionally, they enucleated the fibular head without disturbing the lateral collateral ligament or biceps femoris attachments.[58]

Maquet[46, 47] described a barrel vault, or dome osteotomy, similar to the ball-and-socket osteotomy of Jackson. Maquet's osteotomy, however, was proximal to the tibial tubercle. His osteotomy was stabilized with a Charnley external compression device to allow external motion of the knee. Maquet stated that this barrel vault osteotomy allowed satisfactory correction of larger deformities and was satisfactory for knees with tibiofemoral subluxation[46, 47] (Fig 57–6).

Wagner described an oblique metaphyseal proximal tibial osteotomy just below the tibial tubercle (Fig 57–7). Wagner also described a displacement osteotomy of the proximal tibia for larger varus deformities associated with medial tibiofemoral osteoarthritis[66–68] (Fig 57–8).

In general, varus deformities up to 10 degrees off the mechanical axis can be corrected with a transverse laterally based closing wedge proximal tibial valgus osteotomy. Larger varus deformities of up to 20 degrees off the mechanical axis can be effectively corrected with Wagner's oblique proximal tibial osteotomy. Above 20 degrees, the deformity should be treated with a dome osteotomy of the proximal tibia or a metaphyseal displacement osteotomy of the proximal tibia. The one critical factor associated with

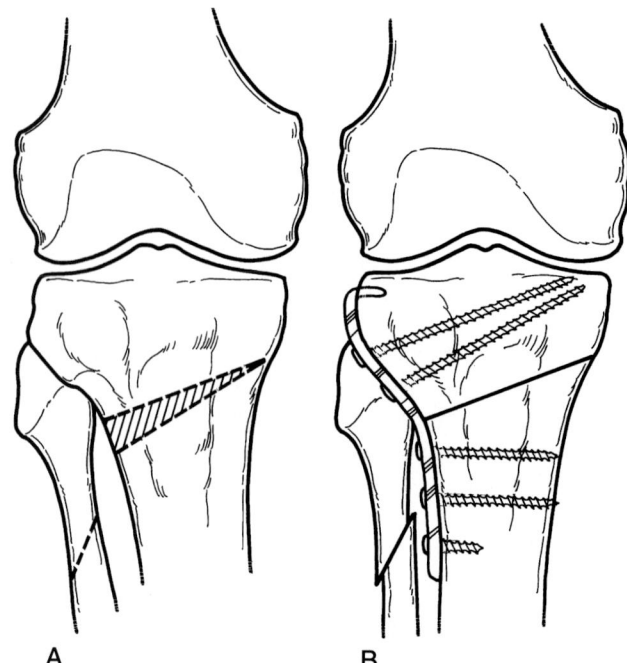

FIG 57–7.
Wagner oblique metaphyseal osteotomy.

all techniques described for osteotomy of the proximal tibia is satisfactory correction of the mechanical axis. Furthermore, most authors recommend some mild overcorrection to satisfactorily unload the arthritic medial tibiofemoral compartment.

Proximal Tibial Valgus Osteotomy (Authors' Technique)

We prefer a proximal tibial valgus osteotomy with removal of a laterally based wedge proximal to the anterior tibial tubercle (Fig 57–9). The desired angle of correction is determined preoperatively from standing radiographs (see Fig 57–5).

The patient is placed in a supine position with a small bolster under the buttock on the operative side to hold the operative leg in a neutral position of rotation. A bolster is also placed on the operating table at the level of the calf to allow for stable positioning of the knee at 90 degrees of flexion. A tourniquet is placed around the thigh to provide for a bloodless field during the procedure.

Transverse and longitudinal skin incisions have been described. Although a transverse incision can give satisfactory exposure, the longitudinal incision has the advantage of allowing distal exposure for the use of internal fixation devices. A midline longitudinal incision has a theoretical advantage in the event that arthroplasty is later necessary. We prefer a lateral curvilinear incision along the arcuate line in the

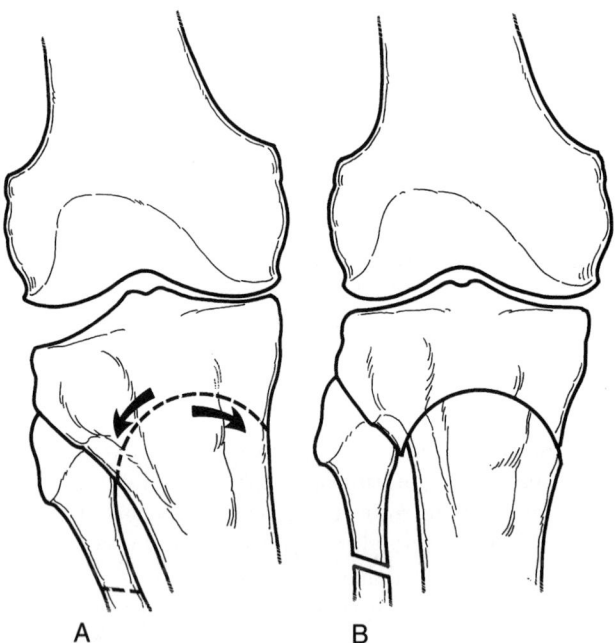

FIG 57–6.
Maquet dome osteotomy. This osteotomy allows for correction of larger deformities.

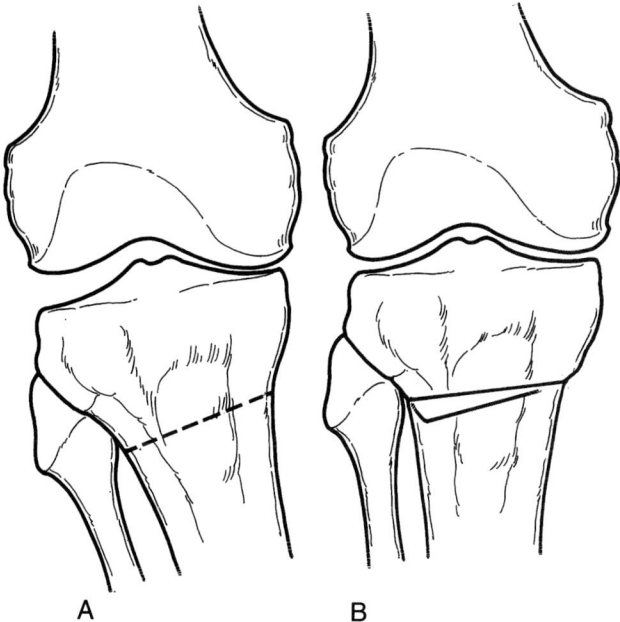

FIG 57–8.
Proximal tibial metaphyseal displacement osteotomy.

proximal tibia. Total knee arthroplasty through a midline incision following this lateral osteotomy incision has not led to problems of skin vascularity.

Following the skin incision, the fascia of the extensor musculature is incised along the arcuate line in the proximal tibia, and the extensor mass is elevated. The elevation of the muscles is more easily performed from distal to proximal. In this manner, the muscle fibers can be followed down to their origin where they are detached with minimal disruption of the muscle mass. The fascial incision is extended posteriorly to allow excision of the fibular head. Removal of a laterally based wedge from the tibia effectively shortens the lateral side of the leg so the fibula must be shortened to achieve satisfactory correction. Fibular shortening may be achieved by osteotomy or ostectomy in the proximal third of the fibula, resection of the fibular head, or partial resection of the fibular head. We recommend partial or total resection of the fibular head, taking care to protect the soft tissue sleeve, incorporating the lateral collateral ligament and the biceps tendon. Osteotomy or ostectomy in the proximal third of the fibula is associated with an increased risk of compartmental syndrome and peroneal nerve injury.

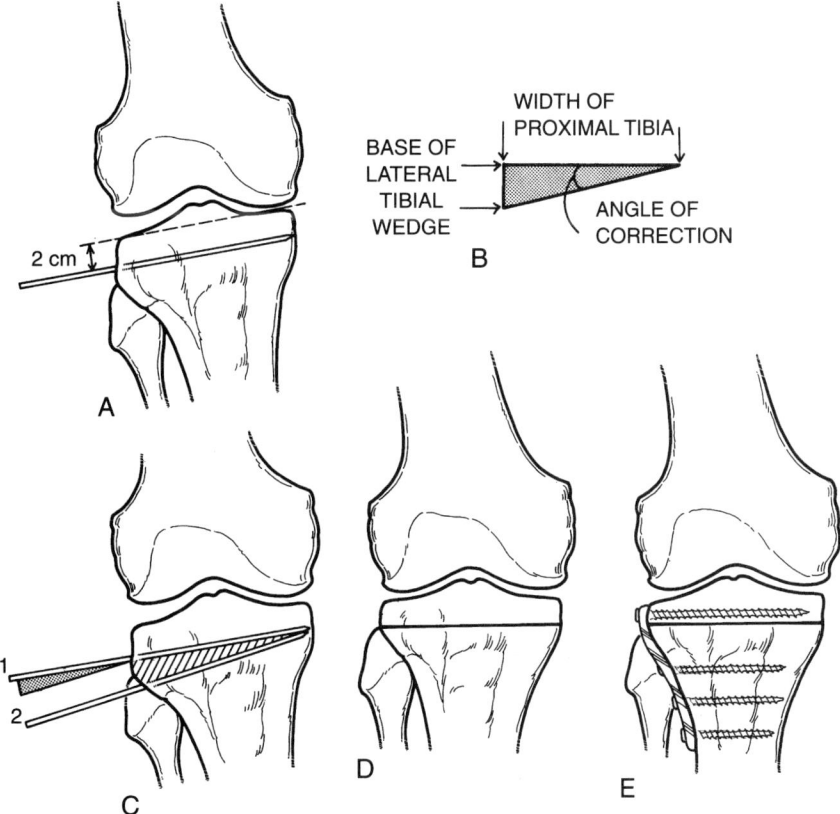

FIG 57–9.
Surgical technique for proximal tibial valgus osteotomy.

When the entire lateral aspect of the proximal tibia is satisfactorily exposed, two ⅛-in. Steinmann pins are placed into the proximal tibia to circumscribe the wedge to be removed. The first guide wire is placed 2 cm distal to the subchondral bone, parallel to the proximal tibia joint line. A template that incorporates the precise desired angle of correction is then cut. A depth gauge is used to measure the width of the proximal tibia at the site of the first guide wire. The exact lateral border of the wedge to be removed can be measured on the template. The point of entry for the second guide wire can then be determined easily and the second pin drilled across the proximal tibia from lateral to medial to converge with the first pin. The specific angled template can also be used to guide the position of the second guide wire across the tibial metaphysis.

The position of the guide wires is checked by fluoroscopy or radiographs. The pin should be parallel in the lateral plane to prevent rotational problems. The wedge is removed using an oscillating saw and osteotomes. The medial cortex of the proximal tibia is perforated but left intact to prevent translation of the osteotomy fragments. It is important to remove all the bone circumscribed by the wedge in order to prevent flexion-extension deformity and overcorrection or undercorrection when the osteotomy wedge is closed.

Once the laterally based wedge is removed, the wedge space is closed by applying valgus stress on the distal tibia. Frequently, a crack of the medial cortex is audible and palpable. We prefer stable internal fixation using an L plate contoured to the lateral aspect of the proximal tibia. The plate is applied with cancellous screws in the proximal fragment and cortical screws in the distal fragment. Stable internal fixation allows early aggressive rehabilitation of the knee. During closure, repair of the extensor muscle mass is essential to prevent extensor weakness and a visible palpable muscle defect. A deep drain helps to avoid compartment syndrome.

After operation, we apply a soft fracture brace with free hinge motion and place the knee in a continuous passive motion (CPM) machine. The surgeon's judgment of the stability of fixation is the most important factor in determining the pace of postoperative physical therapy. CPM has proved to be beneficial in healing articular cartilage lesions, and joint immobilization has shown to be deleterious to articular cartilage. However, immobilization has not been shown to lead to any reduction in range of motion following proximal tibial osteotomy.

Physical therapy begins on the first postoperative day. Patients are allowed toe touching for balance without any significant weightbearing. Range-of-motion and isometric exercises are begun immediately. Weightbearing is allowed 6 weeks following surgery. Quadriceps strengthening is allowed somewhere between 4 and 6 weeks following surgery. Patients are allowed to return to full activity after there is clinical and radiographic evidence of healing of the osteotomy site.

Lateral Tibiofemoral Osteoarthritis with Valgus Deformity

Osteotomy for correction of valgus deformity associated with lateral tibiofemoral osteoarthritis can be performed in the medial aspect of the proximal tibia, the medial aspect of the distal femur, or the lateral aspect of the distal femur. Correction of small valgus deformities up to 6 degrees off the mechanical axis have been successfully performed by Coventry[13] in the medial aspect of the proximal tibia. A medially based wedge is removed, the medial collateral ligament is preserved and repaired, and most patients have had good results for up to 9 years[13] (Fig 57–10).

Larger valgus deformities associated with lateral tibiofemoral osteoarthritis are frequently associated with a valgus tilt of the joint line. This requires an osteotomy proximal to the joint line in order to create a neutral joint line. Opening wedge osteotomy has been described in the lateral aspect of the distal femur (Fig 57–11). Closing wedge osteotomy has been described in the medial aspect of the distal femur through medial and lateral approaches. For larger valgus deformities, distal femoral metaphyseal displacement osteotomy has been described by Wag-

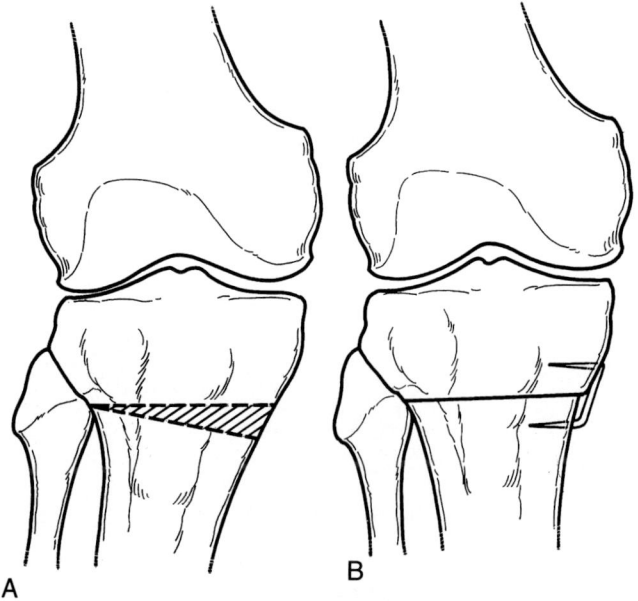

FIG 57–10.
Proximal tibial varus osteotomy.

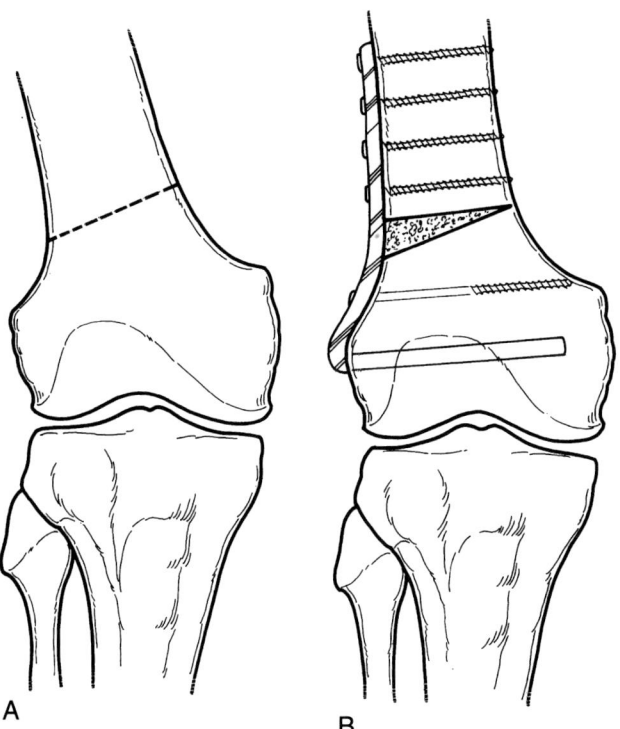

FIG 57–11.
Distal femoral varus osteotomy (lateral approach).

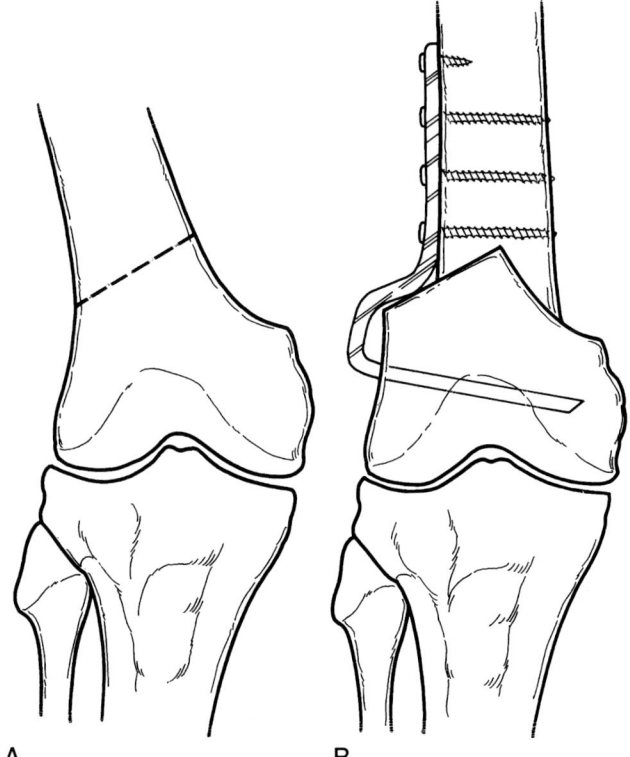

FIG 57–12.
Femoral metaphyseal displacement osteotomy.

ner[66–68] (Fig 57–12). All of these techniques can produce predictably successful results as long as the mechanical axis is satisfactorily corrected.

Aglietti et al.[2] described a V-shaped sagittal-plane distal femoral osteotomy for valgus deformity with lateral joint line pain. The advantage of this osteotomy is that no internal fixation is required.[2] Wagner has emphasized the importance of an extension osteotomy of the distal femur to relieve anterior impingement in the proximal tibia. In some cases, he believes a two-level osteotomy combining proximal tibial valgus osteotomy with an extension supracondylar femoral osteotomy is indicated[66–68] (Fig 57–13).

Intercondylar distal femoral osteotomy, as originally described by Debeyre and Frain,[15] removes a wedge of bone from the mediofemoral condyle as viewed from the coronal plane. This operation is performed for lateral compartment osteoarthritis. In reports by Goutallier and Hernigou and co-workers there were 80% good results after 9 years, but the intercondylar osteotomy was associated with intraarticular stiffness.[20, 26]

Distal Femoral Varus Osteotomy (Authors' Recommendation)

The preoperative radiographic evaluation for distal femoral varus osteotomy is the same as that described for proximal tibial valgus osteotomy. The wedge to be taken from the medial aspect of the distal femur is equal to the sum of the angle of deformity plus 2 to 4 degrees of overcorrection (Fig 57–14).

The distal femur can be approached medially through an anterior longitudinal incision, as in total knee arthroplasty, or more commonly, through a medial longitudinal incision made from the level of the anterior tibial tubercle distally to a point 15 cm proximal to the patella. Dissection is carried out through the subcutaneous tissue, taking care to spare the branches of the anterior femoral cutaneous nerve and the infrapatellar branch of the saphenous nerve.

The fascia of the adductor muscles is exposed. The interval between the vastus medialis and sartorius muscles is developed. The sartorius is retracted posteriorly and the vastus medialis is retracted anteriorly. Care must be taken in the medial approach to the distal femur to protect the posteromedial neurovascular structures. In developing the plane of the vastus medialis, interruption of the posterior perforating arteries is to be expected and bleeding should be controlled. Once the joint capsule is exposed distally, the epicondyle is palpated and the distal aspect of the medial part of the femoral condyle is identified. The joint capsule is not opened. Four ⅛-in. Steinmann pins are used to guide the osteotomy (see Fig 57–14).

The first pin is inserted perpendicular to the shaft

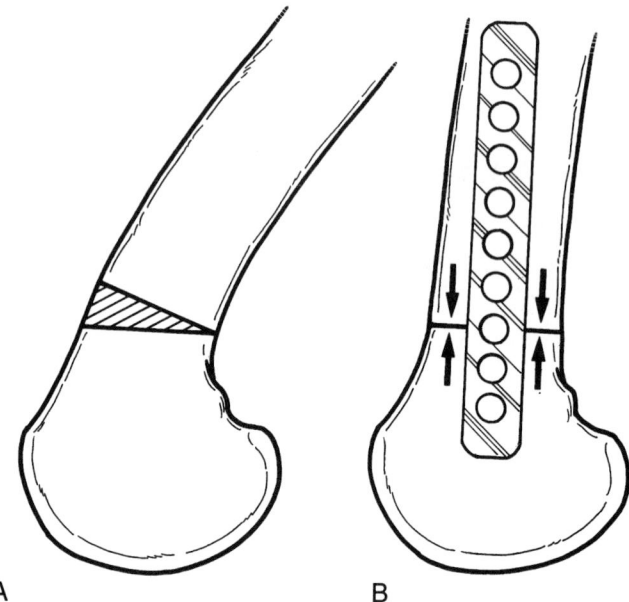

FIG 57–13.
Distal femoral extension osteotomy.

of the femur using a 90-degree osteotomy guide. This pin is parallel to, but does not coincide with, the proximal osteotomy cut. A second guide pin is inserted into the femoral condyle at an angle deviating from that of the first pin by the desired angle of correction. A preformed template incorporates this precise angle and permits positioning of the second pin. A third pin is placed parallel and distal to the second pin. The third pin guides the placement of the seating chisel for the blade plate. A bony bridge of at least 2 cm should be left between the second and third pins as a bony bridge between the osteotomy and the blade plate. A fourth pin may be placed at the site of the proximal osteotomy. The insertion point is determined using the preformed template. A depth gauge is used to determine the width of the distal femur at the site of the second pin and the template is cut to exactly the size and shape of the wedge to be removed. When the template is placed on the medial cortex of the femur, the site of insertion for the fourth pin is determined. The blade plate–seating chisel is inserted before the osteotomy is performed. The position of the guide pins and the seating chisel are checked with fluoroscopy or radiographs.

The medially based wedge is removed from the distal femur using an oscillating saw and an osteotome. The lateral femoral cortex is perforated but not interrupted. Once the wedge has been removed, a varus force is applied to the lower leg and the osteotomy site is closed. The seating chisel is removed and a 90-degree osteotomy blade plate is inserted.

One cortical screw is applied through the plate into the distal fragment. Four cortical screws are applied through the plate, into the proximal fragment. This osteotomy is an extraligamentous procedure and medial or lateral collateral ligament tension should not be affected. Intraoperatively, it should be determined that the knee can be put through a satisfactory range of motion.

In patients with excessive flexion contractures or recurvatum deformities, flexion or extension components can be added to the distal femoral osteotomy. Flexion contracture frequently contributes to the arthritic process as weightbearing is shifted posteriorly onto the femoral condyles, which have smaller radii of curvature. This transmits more force through less surface area and accelerates the arthritic process of articular cartilage deterioration. Wagner has emphasized the importance of flexion-extension correction in addition to varus-valgus correction during distal femoral osteotomy.[66–68]

During closure, repair of the vastus medialis is essential to restore the extensor mechanism and avoid patellofemoral pain. A deep drain is used routinely. Postoperative care is similar to the routine described for proximal tibial osteotomy. If immobilization is required, 90-degree flexion splinting for 4 to 7 days is recommended to maintain extensor mechanism length and prevent quadriceps scarring and contracture.

COMPLICATIONS

The complications of osteotomy are undercorrection, thromboembolic disease, peroneal palsy, nonunion, infection, vascular injury, internal fixation, and intraarticular fracture. A discussion of each follows.

Undercorrection

Insufficient correction of deformity to realign the limb and redistribute weightbearing is the most common complication following osteotomy. Undercorrected knees may show short-term improvement, but deformity and symptoms recur. Undercorrection can be prevented by preoperative planning and careful surgical technique.

Thromboembolic Disease

The reported incidence of deep venous thrombosis following osteotomy about the knee ranges from 1% to 8%. Most studies report rates of less than 3%.[14, 51, 65] The incidence of subclinical deep venous thrombosis following osteotomy has not been stud-

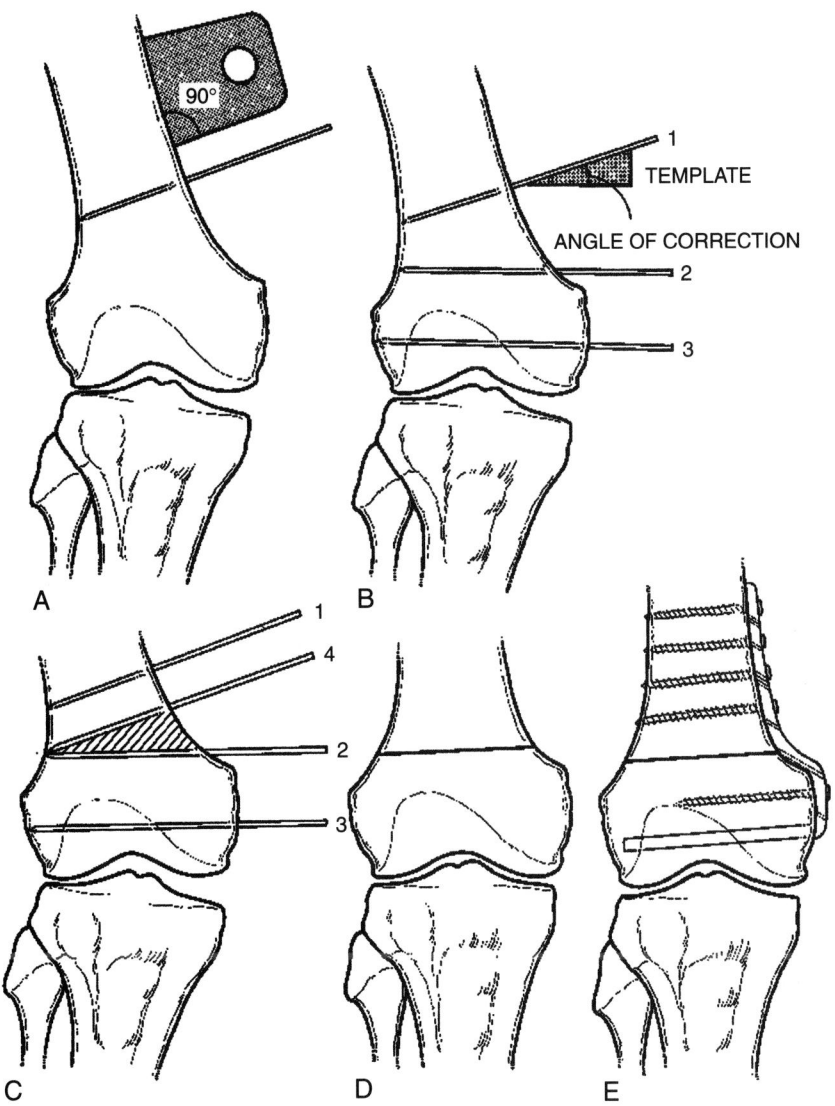

FIG 57–14.
Surgical technique for distal femoral varus osteotomy (medial approach).

ied by venography. Our thromboembolic prophylaxis following osteotomy consists of noninvasive venous monitoring with duplex color flow scan, early motion in CPM, and enteric-coated aspirin. Patients with a history of previous deep venous thrombosis are treated with a low-dose warfarin sodium (Coumadin) anticoagulation program and intermittent calf compression cuffs.

Peroneal Palsy

The incidence of peroneal palsy following a laterally based closing wedge proximal tibial valgus osteotomy has been reported at less than 1%.[12, 14, 29, 65] The peroneal nerve is more likely to be injured in procedures that involve an osteotomy or ostectomy in the proximal third of the fibula.[12] The incidence of peroneal palsy after dome osteotomy of the proximal tibia with osteotomy of the proximal fibula was 15% when the osteotomy was proximal to the tibial tubercle, and 25% when the osteotomy was below the tibial tubercle.[34, 60] Peroneal nerve palsy is also more common when external fixation is used to fix the proximal tibial osteotomy.[34, 41, 44, 45, 51]

Gibson et al.[21] have suggested that replacement of a drain after operation may significantly reduce the incidence of transient peroneal nerve palsy. Prophylactic anterior compartment fasciotomy has been recommended by some surgeons. The literature neither supports nor refutes this procedure. We routinely identify the peroneal nerve during excision of the fibular head.

Nonunion

The reported rate of nonunion following proximal tibial osteotomy ranges from 0% to 3%.[51, 61, 62] The reported nonunion rate is slightly higher following distal femoral osteotomy, occurring in 6% to 7% of cases.[25, 35] Treatment of nonunion following osteotomy consists of bone grafting or bone grafting and compression fixation in cases where plate fixation was not used originally.[5] Routine bone grafting using the resected bone wedge during the initial distal femoral osteotomy or proximal tibial osteotomy is recommended, although there are no data in the literature to support or refute the effectiveness of this technique.

Infection

The incidence of wound infections following osteotomy about the knee is less than 2%. Higher infection rates have been observed in association with arthrotomy and joint debridement,[45] and when external fixation has been used following osteotomy.[10, 41, 51] Routine antibiotic prophylaxis is recommended.

Vascular Injury

Vascular injuries following osteotomy of the proximal tibia or the distal femur are rare. Flexing the knee during the osteotomy can decrease the likelihood of this complication by relaxing the posterior vessels. Special care must be paid to the posteromedial neurovascular structures when performing a distal femoral varus osteotomy through the medial approach.

Internal Fixation

The use of internal fixation during proximal tibial osteotomy can be associated with several problems. Staples, screws, or plates can be applied improperly, resulting in poor fixation, penetration of the articular surface, or fracture. The use of fluoroscopy can help to minimize these problems. The joint space is protected when at least a 2-cm proximal fragment size is maintained in the proximal tibia.

Intraarticular Fracture

Intraarticular fractures of the proximal tibia occur because of poor surgical technique. The reported incidence is 2%. These fractures can occur when an insufficient thickness of proximal bone is maintained or when an osteotomy is not completed across the proximal tibial metaphysis. Careful surgical technique is essential in avoiding intraarticular fractures.

RESULTS

Proximal Tibial Valgus Osteotomy

Since 1958, many authors have reported the results of proximal tibial valgus osteotomy. In general, proximal tibial osteotomy has been demonstrated to be effective for approximately 5 to 7 years. Ritter and Fechtman[55] substantiated this generalization with a survivorship analysis of 78 tibial osteotomies. In their patients, the survival rate for the osteotomy was 80% at 6 years; however, the survival rate dropped to nearly 60% at 7 years.[55]

Morrey[51] reviewed the results of proximal tibial valgus osteotomies reported in 19 publications with a 1- to 10-year follow-up. Of 1,364 patients 76% were rated good or excellent, 19% were rated fair, and 14% had poor results. Seventy-five percent of the patients were satisfied with the outcome of the proximal tibial valgus osteotomy which was performed for medial tibiofemoral osteoarthritis associated with varus deformity.[51]

During the 1960s and 1970s, early series of proximal tibial valgus osteotomies reported good to excellent results in between 60% and 70%. Reports during the 1980s suggested good to excellent results in 85% to 88% at 5 years following proximal tibial valgus osteotomy. The discrepancy is due to the fact that in the early series, total knee arthroplasty was not a predictably successful alternative. In later reports, patients for osteotomy were preselected in that patients with tricompartmental disease were treated with total knee arthroplasty.

Despite 5-year success rates of 80% to 90% for proximal tibial valgus osteotomy, the results deteriorate over time.[12, 26, 29, 51] Insall et al.[29-31] reported 97% good results at 2 years, 85% good results at 5 years, and 63% good results at 9 years. At 9 years, only 37% of these patients were pain-free. Deterioration in these patients was primarily the result of time and not recurrence of deformity. Deterioration in results has also been reported by Coventry and Bowman[14] who noted deterioration from 67% good results at 4 years to 61% good results at 10 years. Aglietti et al.[1] reported a decrease from 88% good results at 4 years to 64% good results at 10 years. Kettlekamp et al.[41] reported deterioration from 81% good results at 3 years to 67% good results at 5 years. Undercorrection of deformity has been associated with less good results, decreased survivorship, and deterioration of good results. These findings emphasize the importance of surgical technique and satisfactory correction of deformity.[27, 38, 48, 52]

In contrast to the reports of Insall et al., Vainionpaa et al.[65] reported that deterioration of results was due to recurrence of deformity. Wang et al.[69] noted the significance of recurrence deformity associated with patients with high adduction moments. For this reason, Wang et al. state that patients with high adductor moments are not good candidates for proximal tibial valgus osteotomy.[69]

In general, patients should be advised that pain can be relieved and function can be improved following proximal tibial valgus osteotomy for medial tibiofemoral osteoarthritis with varus deformity. We cite 80% good results at 5 to 7 years. Patients are advised that the joint space may improve with time following realignment. Theoretically, when weightbearing stress is removed from an arthritic compartment in the knee to a healthier compartment, the arthritic compartment has an opportunity to heal. We emphasize to patients that osteotomy is one of the methods we have to manage an arthritic knee over a lifetime.

Fujisawa et al.[18] have documented improvements in degenerative articular cartilage following proximal tibial valgus osteotomy. They arthroscoped and biopsied degenerative femoral condyles following proximal tibial valgus osteotomy. Six to 12 months following osteotomy, fibrous tissue covered ulcerated areas in the degenerative condyle. Twelve to 18 months following osteotomy, the ulcers were filled in with fibrocartilage, but the condylar surface was still uneven. Two years following osteotomy, a hardened fibrous surface had developed where full-thickness defects had been noted at the time of osteotomy. The biopsies of these areas demonstrated fibrocartilage of type I collagen. This study suggests that osteotomy may not only redistribute forces in a damaged joint but may also permit the opportunity for biologic repair of the joint.[18]

Bergenudd et al.[4] evaluated 19 patients with varus gonarthrosis following proximal tibial valgus osteotomy. Medial femoral condyle biopsies were obtained at the time of osteotomy and at the time of follow-up. Nine knees demonstrated improvement in articular cartilage, eight knees were unchanged, and in two knees the articular cartilage had deteriorated at the time of follow-up. Improvement was associated with new fibrocartilage. There were no signs of normal hyaline cartilage regeneration. Despite statistically significant histologic improvement in the articular cartilage biopsies, the biologic improvement in the joint did not correlate with the clinical or radiographic outcome.[4]

Proximal Tibial Varus Osteotomy

Tibial varus osteotomy can be used for treating small valgus deformities. A report by Shoji and Insall[57] in 1973 presented data on 49 knees treated with varus osteotomy of the proximal tibia for painful valgus deformity of the knee. Fifty-three percent of these had pain relief, 14% had partial pain relief, and 33% had no pain relief with an average follow-up of 31.5 months.[57] In 1987, Coventry[13] presented the results of 31 knees treated with tibial varus osteotomy for painful osteoarthritis of the lateral compartment. With an average follow-up of 9.4 years, 77% of the patients had no pain or only mild occasional pain. In his report, Coventry pointed out the limited role for tibial varus osteotomy.[13]

Distal Femoral Varus Osteotomy

Wagner et al. have published the largest review in the German literature of distal femoral osteotomies which demonstrated very good results.[66-68] In North America, Johnson and Bodell[35] have reported their experience with distal femoral varus osteotomy at the Mayo Clinic. They were not encouraged by the procedure because only 46% of their patients had satisfactory results. However, they correctly noted the importance of mechanical realignment of the valgus knee and their results were compromised because the osteotomies were performed by different surgeons who used different methods of fixation.[35]

In 1988, Healy et al.[25] reported the results of 23 distal femoral osteotomies with an average follow-up of 4 years. Overall, 83% of the patients had good or excellent results. When they looked at patients specifically with osteoarthritis, 93% of the patients had a good or excellent result.[25] Also in 1988, McDermott et al.[49] reported on 24 patients following distal femoral varus osteotomy for arthritis of the lateral compartment of the knee with valgus deformity. At an average follow-up of 4 years, 22 (92%) of their patients were improved.[49] Neither Healy et al. nor McDermott et al. commented on deterioration rates for distal femoral varus osteotomy.

TOTAL KNEE ARTHROPLASTY FOLLOWING OSTEOTOMY

There have been several reports addressing the issue of total knee arthroplasty following proximal tibial valgus osteotomy. Staeheli et al.[59] reported on 35 patients following total knee arthroplasty for failed proximal tibial osteotomy. Thirty-one (89%) patients had an excellent or good result. Furthermore, the patients demonstrated a similar rate of intraoperative and postoperative complications as compared with studies of primary total knee replacements. Satisfactory alignment was achieved in 95% of the patients following osteotomy and the authors believed that the results were similar to the results obtained in patients who had not had a prior osteotomy.[59]

In 1987, Katz et al.[36] reviewed 21 patients who had a minimally constrained total knee arthroplasty following a failed proximal tibial osteotomy. These 21 patients were compared with a cohort of 21 patients who underwent a primary total knee arthroplasty without having had a prior osteotomy. The cohort group was matched according to age, sex, type of prosthesis, and length of follow-up. These patients had an average follow-up of almost 3 years. A good or excellent result was obtained in 81% of the failed osteotomy group (17/21) compared with 100% (21/21) of the primary arthroplasty group. The authors described several technical difficulties in exposing the proximal tibia. The average operative time was 35 minutes longer in the osteotomy group.[36]

In 1992, Mont et al.[50] reported the results of total knee arthroplasty after failed high tibial osteotomy in 80 patients. The patients were compared with a matched control group. Fifty-one (64%) of the failed osteotomy total knee arthroplasty patients had good or excellent results, while 71 patients (89%) in the matched control group with total knee arthroplasty had good or excellent results. This difference was statistically significant. Analysis of the patients with failed osteotomies suggested six factors associated with a worse clinical outcome: multiple surgeries prior to high tibial osteotomy, Workers' Compensation, reflex sympathetic dystrophy, no period of pain relief following osteotomy, early onset of pain after osteotomy, and occupation as a laborer.[50]

Windsor et al.[70] discussed the technical aspects of total knee arthroplasty following failed proximal tibial osteotomy. They presented a prospective review of 45 patients who were treated with total knee arthroplasty because of severe pain following a proximal tibial osteotomy. Thirty-six (80%) patients had a

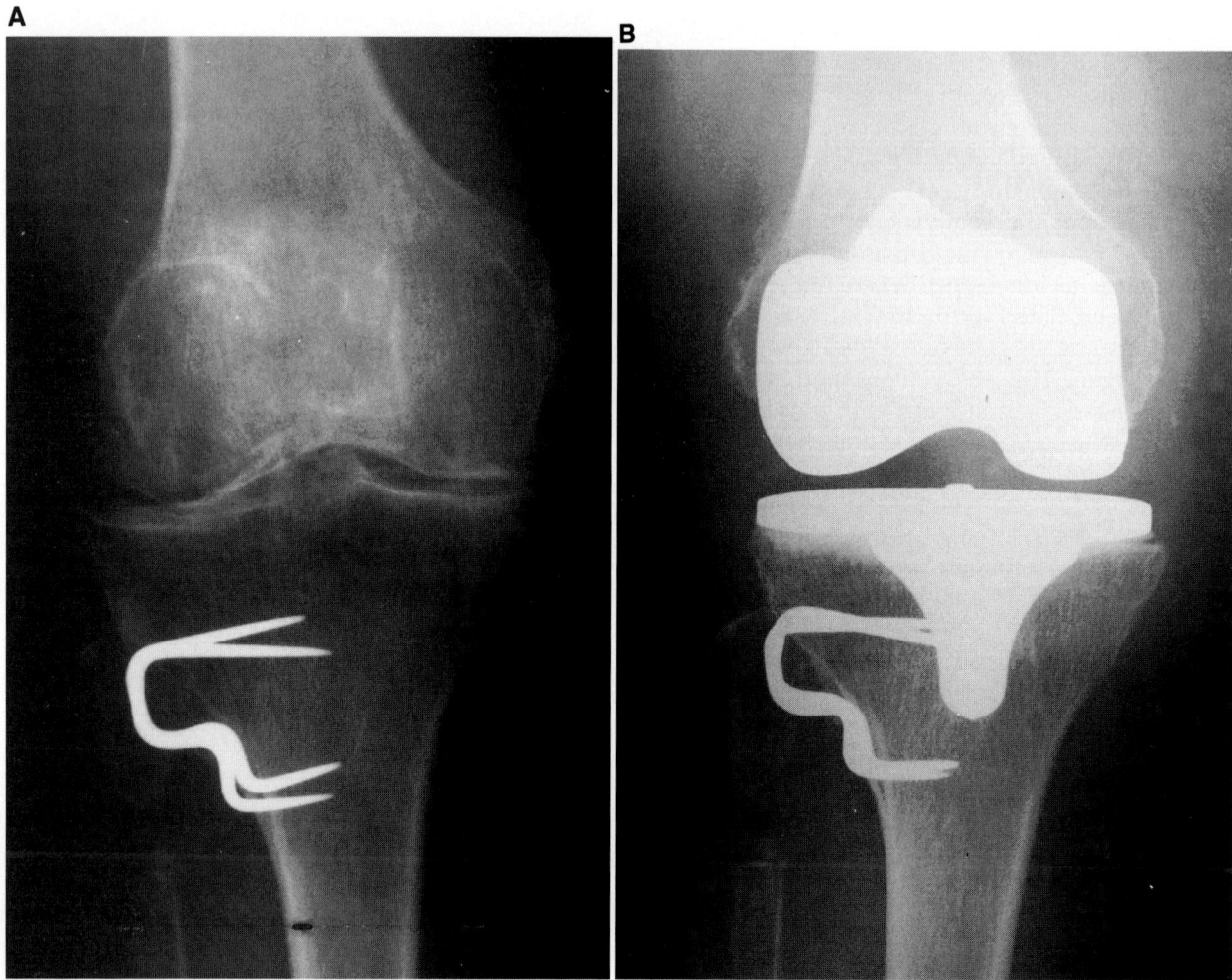

FIG 57–15.
A, standing AP radiograph of a 70-year-old patient 15 years following proximal tibial valgus osteotomy. The patient complains of tricompartmental knee pain. **B,** 3 years status post total knee arthroplasty, the patient is pain-free and the knee is fully functional.

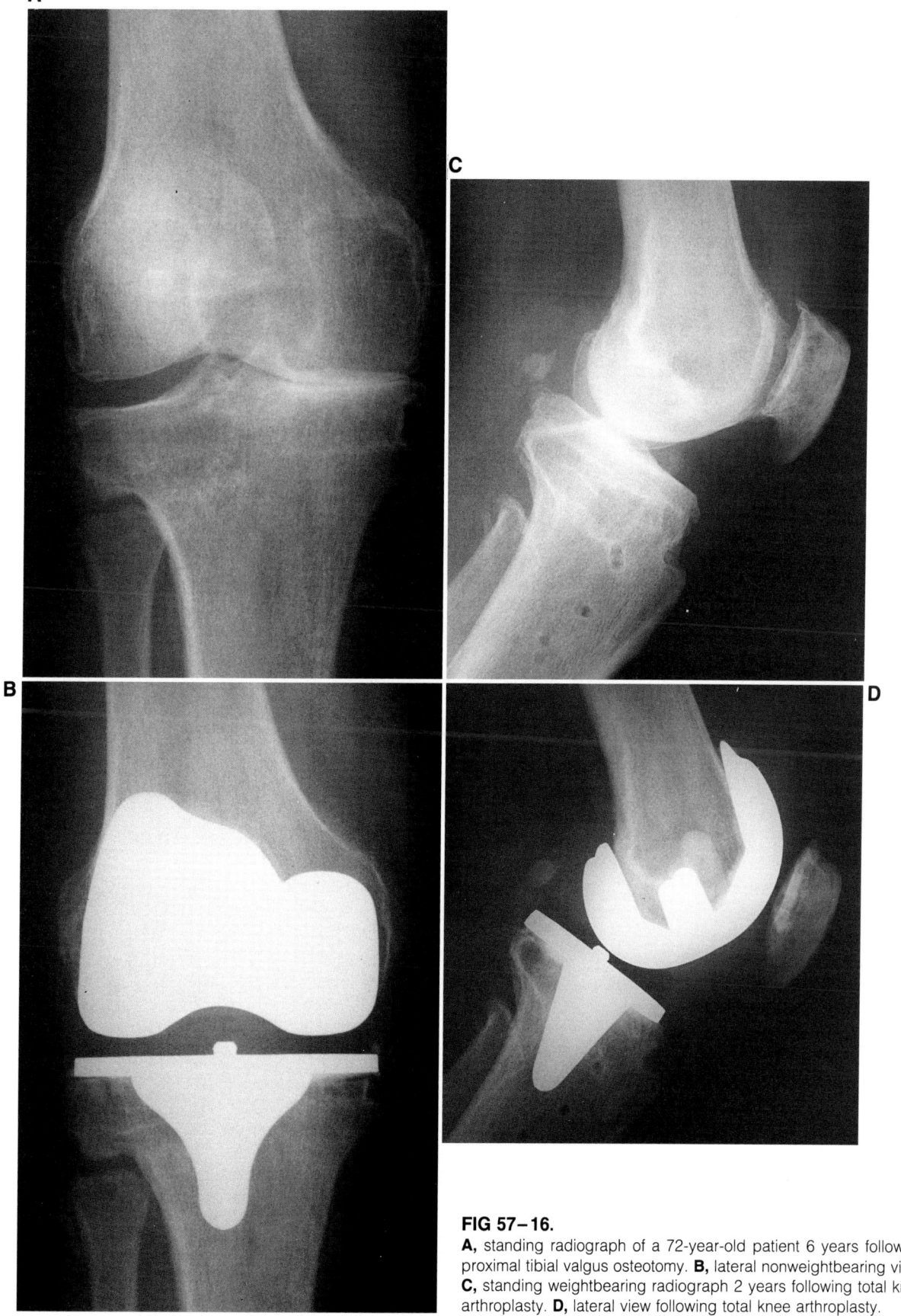

FIG 57–16.
A, standing radiograph of a 72-year-old patient 6 years following proximal tibial valgus osteotomy. **B,** lateral nonweightbearing view. **C,** standing weightbearing radiograph 2 years following total knee arthroplasty. **D,** lateral view following total knee arthroplasty.

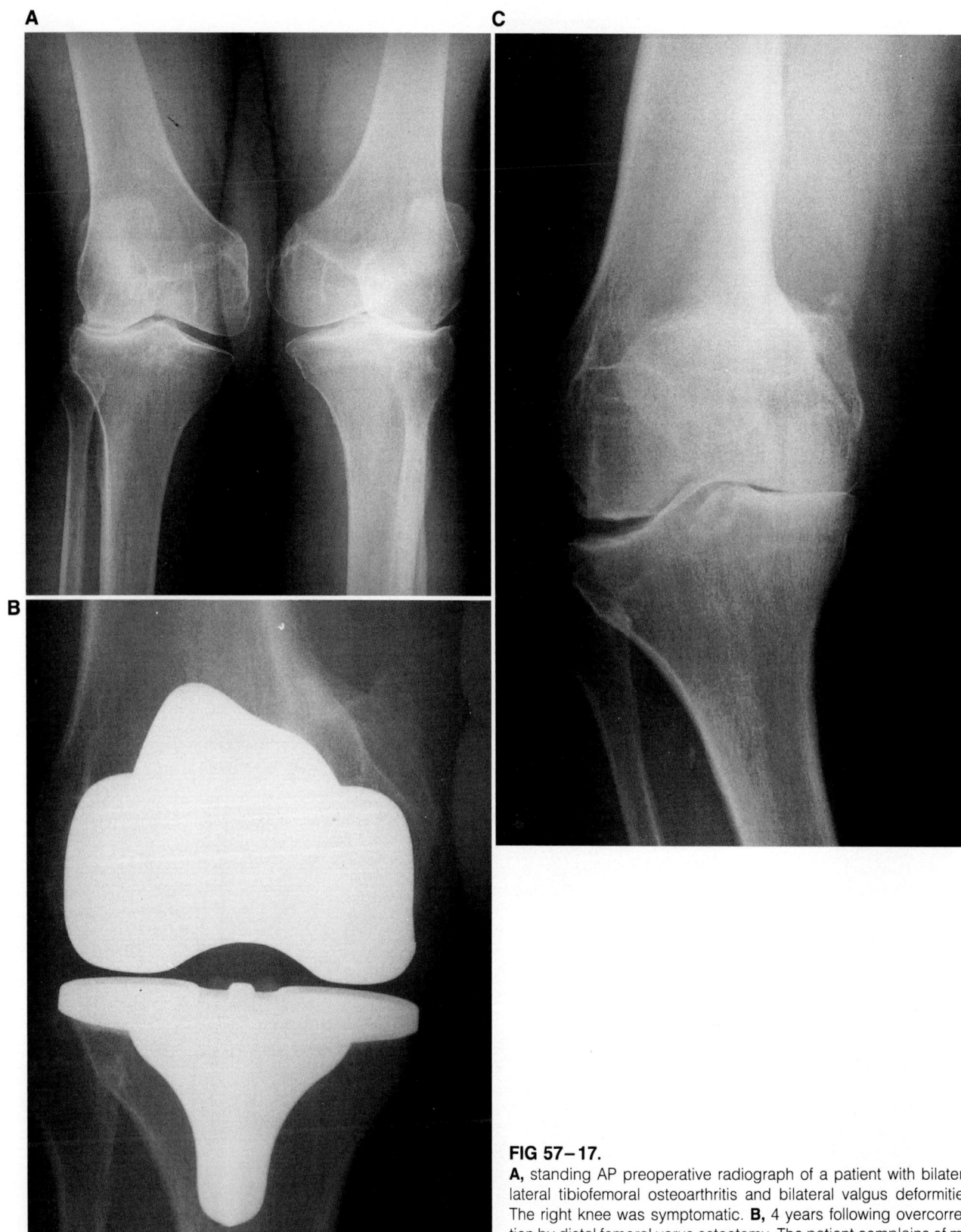

FIG 57–17.
A, standing AP preoperative radiograph of a patient with bilateral lateral tibiofemoral osteoarthritis and bilateral valgus deformities. The right knee was symptomatic. **B**, 4 years following overcorrection by distal femoral varus osteotomy. The patient complains of medial joint line pain and varus deformity. **C**, 2 years following total knee arthroplasty. The knee is pain-free and stable with full motion.

good or excellent result with two (4%) fair and seven (16%) poor results after a minimum 2-year follow-up. The results in these patients were comparable to those seen in revision total knee arthroplasty at the same institution. The results of total knee arthroplasty following osteotomy were significantly less favorable than the results seen in primary total knee arthroplasty without prior osteotomy.[70]

In considering total knee arthroplasty following failed proximal tibial osteotomy, preoperative planning is essential. The surgeon must assess internal fixation devices used for the osteotomy. If they will interfere with implantation of the total knee prosthesis, they must be removed. The location of the osteotomy incision must be considered in planning a total knee arthroplasty incision. Intraoperatively, the length of the patella tendon must be carefully considered. Lateral closing wedge osteotomies can reduce the patellar tendon length which may make exposure of the lateral compartment more difficult. The surgeon must be prepared for an osteotomy of the tibial tubercle if necessary. Bony insufficiency of the lateral tibial plateau following proximal tibial valgus osteotomy should be expected. This may be addressed by an increased resection of bone in the medial proximal tibia. It may also necessitate bone grafting or incorporation of metal spacers in the lateral compartment. The design of the tibial component must be carefully considered preoperatively. If a large correction in the proximal tibia was achieved, the center of the tibial articular surface may be above the lateral cortex of the tibial shaft. In this case, insertion of a central tibial peg or pin may abut the lateral cortex of the tibia. Careful evaluation of preoperative radiographs with component templates may help avoid this problem (Figs 57–15 and 57–16).

To date, there are no reported studies on total knee arthroplasty following distal femoral varus osteotomy. In our experience, care must be taken to avoid excess resection of the lateral femoral condylar bone which would unnecessarily raise the tibiofemoral joint line. Ligamentous stability has not been a problem in these cases. Furthermore, a midline incision for total knee arthroplasty following medial or lateral incisions for femoral osteotomy have not led to problems of skin vascularity (Fig 57–17).

SUMMARY

Osteotomy of the arthritic knee has been scrutinized in the recent orthopaedic surgery literature. Appropriately, osteotomy is measured against total knee arthroplasty, which represents the gold standard for surgical treatment of the arthritic knee. Improvements in osteotomy about the knee include better patient selection criteria and improved surgical techniques. These do not appear to have improved the short-term results, but they may improve the long-term results.

Medial tibiofemoral osteoarthritis associated with a varus deformity can be treated effectively with proximal tibial valgus osteotomy. Eighty percent of properly selected patients can expect good to excellent results for approximately 6 years. Lateral tibiofemoral osteoarthritis associated with a valgus deformity can be treated effectively with distal femoral varus osteotomy. Both medial and lateral approaches to the distal femur provide satisfactory results. Ninety percent of properly selected patients can expect good to excellent results for 4 years or more.

As in all reconstructive surgical procedures, appropriate patient selection, preoperative planning, and careful surgical technique optimize clinical results and minimize complications.

Acknowledgment

Ms. Bebe Dominick and Ms. Lesley Roumeliotis assisted in the preparation of this chapter.

REFERENCES

1. Aglietti P, et al: Tibial osteotomy for the varus osteoarthritic knee, *Clin Orthop* 176:239–251, 1983.
2. Aglietti P, et al: Correction of valgus knee deformity with a supracondylar V osteotomy, *Clin Orthop* 217:214, 1987.
3. Ahlberg A, Scham S, Unander-Scharin L: Osteotomy in degenerative and rheumatoid arthritis of the knee joint, *Acta Orthop Scand* 39:379–388, 1968.
4. Bergenudd H, et al: The articular cartilage after osteotomy for medial gonarthrosis, *Acta Orthop Scand* 63:413–416, 1992.
5. Cameron HV: Repair of nonunion of supracondylar femoral osteotomy, *Orthop Rev* 21:349–350, 1992.
6. Chan RN, Pollard JP: High tibial osteotomy for rheumatoid arthritis of the knee. A one to six year follow up study, *Acta Orthop Scand* 49:78–84, 1978.
7. Conrad EU, Soudry M, Insall JN: Supracondylar femoral osteotomy for valgus knee deformities, *Orthop Trans* 9:25–26, 1985.
8. Coventry MB: Osteotomy of the upper portion of the tibia for degenerative arthritis of the knee. A preliminary report, *J Bone Joint Surg [Am]* 47:984–990, 1965.
9. Coventry MB. Osteotomy about the knee for degenerative and rheumatoid arthritis, *J Bone Joint Surg [Am]* 55:23–48, 1973.
10. Coventry MB: Upper tibial osteotomy for gonarthrosis. The evolution of the operation in the last 18 years and

long term results, *Orthop Clin North Am* 10:191–210, 1979.
11. Coventry MB: Upper tibial osteotomy, *Clin Orthop* 182:46–52, 1984.
12. Coventry MB: Upper tibial osteotomy for osteoarthritis, *J Bone Joint Surg [Am]* 67:1136–1140, 1985.
13. Coventry MB. Proximal tibial varus osteotomy for osteoarthritis of the lateral compartment of the knee, *J Bone Joint Surg [Am]* 69:32–38, 1987.
14. Coventry MB, Bowman PW: Long-term results of upper tibial osteotomy for degenerative arthritis of the knee, *Acta Orthop Belg* 48:139–156, 1982.
15. Debeyre J, Frain P: Technique d'oséotomie intercondylienne du fémur pour corriger les déviations arthritiques du genou, *Ann Chir* 21:548, 1967.
16. Dugdale TW, Noyes FR, Styer D: Preoperative planning for high tibial osteotomy, *Clin Orthop* 274:248–264, 1992.
17. Engel GM, Lippert FG III: Valgus tibial osteotomy. Avoiding the pitfalls, *Clin Orthop* 160:137–143, 1981.
18. Fujisawa Y, Masuhara K, Shiomi S: The effect of high tibial osteotomy on osteoarthritis of the knee. An arthroscopic study of 54 knee joints, *Orthop Clin North Am* 10:585–608, 1979.
19. Gariepy R, cited by Morrey BF: Upper tibial osteotomy. Analysis of prognostic features: A review, *Adv Orthop Surg* 9:213–222, 1986.
20. Goutallier D, Hernigou P, Lenoble E: Debeyre intercondylar femoral osteotomy for severe lateral compartment osteoarthritis of the knee with laxity: A clinical and radiological study of 55 knees treated more than 5 years ago, *Fr J Orthop Surg* 2:573, 1988.
21. Gibson MJ, et al: Weakness of the foot dorsiflexion and changes in compartment pressures after tibial osteotomy, *J Bone Joint Surg [Br]* 68:471–475, 1986.
22. Harding ML: A fresh appraisal of tibial osteotomy for osteoarthritis of the knee, *Clin Orthop* 114:223–234, 1976.
23. Healy WL, Barber TC: The role of osteotomy in the treatment of osteoarthritis of the knee, *Am J Knee Surg* 3:97–109, 1990.
24. Healy WL, Riley LH Jr: High tibial valgus osteotomy. A clinical review, *Clin Orthop* 209:227–233, 1986.
25. Healy WL, et al: Distal femoral varus osteotomy, *J Bone Joint Surg [Am]* 70:102–109, 1988.
26. Hernigou P, et al: Proximal tibial osteotomy for osteoarthritis with varus deformity. A ten to thirteen year follow up study, *J Bone Joint Surg [Am]* 69:332–354, 1987.
27. Holden DL, et al: Proximal tibial osteotomy in patients who are fifty years old or less: A long term follow up study, *J Bone Joint Surg [Am]* 70:977, 1988.
28. Hofmann AA, Wyatt RW, Jones RE: Combined Coventry-Maquet procedure for two-compartment degenerative arthritis, *Clin Orthop* 190:186–191, 1984.
29. Insall JN, Joseph DM, Msika C: High tibial osteotomy for varus gonarthrosis. A long-term follow up study, *J Bone Joint Surg [Am]* 66:1040–1048, 1984.
30. Insall J, Shoji H, Mayer V: High tibial osteotomy. A five-year evaluation, *J Bone Joint Surg [Am]* 56:1397–1405, 1974.
31. Insall JN, et al: The total condylar knee prosthesis in gonarthrosis. A five to nine year follow up of the first one hundred consecutive replacements, *J Bone Joint Surg [Am]* 65:619–628, 1983.
32. Jackson JP: Osteotomy for osteoarthritis of the knee. Proceedings and reports of councils and associations: The Sheffield Regional Orthopaedic Club, *J Bone Joint Surg [Br]* 40:826, 1958.
33. Jackson JP, Waugh W: Tibial osteotomy for osteoarthritis of the knee, *J Bone Joint Surg [Br]* 43:746–751, 1961.
34. Jackson JP, Waugh W: The technique and complications of upper tibial osteotomy. A review of 226 operations, *J Bone Joint Surg [Br]* 56:236–245, 1974.
35. Johnson EW Jr, Bodell LS: Corrective supracondylar osteotomy for painful genu valgum, *Mayo Clin Proc* 56:87–92, 1981.
36. Katz MM, et al: Results of total knee arthroplasty after failed proximal tibial osteotomy for osteoarthritis, *J Bone Joint Surg [Am]* 69:225–233, 1987.
37. Keene JS, Dyreby JR Jr: High tibial osteotomy in the treatment of osteoarthritis of the knee. The role of preoperative arthroscopy, *J Bone Joint Surg [Am]* 65:36–42, 1983.
38. Keene JS, et al: Evaluation of patient for high tibial osteotomy, *Clin Orthop* 243:157, 1989.
39. Kettlekamp DB, Chao EY: A method for quantitative analysis of medial and lateral compression forces at the knee during standing, *Clin Orthop* 83:202–213, 1972.
40. Kettlekamp DB, Leach RE, Nasca R: Pitfalls of proximal tibial osteotomy, *Clin Orthop* 106:232–241, 1975.
41. Kettlekamp DB, et al: Results of proximal tibial osteotomy. The effects of tibiofemoral angle, stance-phase flexion-extension, and medial-plateau force, *J Bone Joint Surg [Am]* 58:952–960, 1976.
42. Koshino T, Ranawat NS: Healing process of osteoarthritis in the knee after high tibial osteotomy: Through observation of strontium-85 scintimetry, *Clin Orthop* 82:149, 1972.
43. Koshino T, et al: High tibial osteotomy with fixation by a blade plate for medial compartment osteoarthritis of the knee, *Orthop Clin North Am* 20:227, 1989.
44. Lemaire R: Étude comparative de deux séries d'ostéotomies tibialis avec fixation par lameplaque ou par cadre de compression, *Acta Orthop Belg* 1982; 48:157–171.
45. MacIntosh DL, Welsh RP: Joint debridement—a complement to high tibial osteotomy in the treatment of degenerative arthritis of the knee, *J Bone Joint Surg [Am]* 59:1094–1097, 1977.
46. Maquet PGJ: Biomechanical treatment of osteoarthritis of the knee. In Maquet PGJ, editor: *Biomechanics of the knee. With application to the pathogenesis and the surgical treatment of osteoarthritis,* New York, 1976, Springer-Verlag, pp 145–180.
47. Maquet PGJ: *Biomechanics of the knee. With applica-*

tion to the pathogenesis and the surgical treatment of osteoarthritis, ed 2, New York, 1983, Springer-Verlag.
48. Matthews LS, et al: Proximal tibial osteotomy: Factors that influence the duration of satisfactory function, Clin Orthop 229:193, 1988.
49. McDermott AG, et al: Distal femoral varus osteotomy for valgus deformity of the knee, J Bone Joint Surg [Am] 70:110–116, 1988.
50. Mont MA, et al: Total knee arthroplasty after failed high tibial osteotomy: Long term follow-up and results. A comparison to a matched control group, Association of Arthritic Hip and Knee Surgeons, Dallas, November 1992, no. 27.
51. Morrey BF: Upper tibial osteotomy. Analysis of prognostic features: A review. Adv Orthop Surg 9:213–222, 1986.
52. Pachelli AF, Kaufman EE: Long-term results of valgus tibial osteotomy, Orthopedics 10:1415–1418, 1987.
53. Pauwels F: Atlas: The biomechanics of the normal and diseased hip, New York, 1976, Springer-Verlag.
54. Prodromos CC, Andriacchi TP, Galante JO: A relationship between gait and clinical changes following high tibial osteotomy. J Bone Joint Surg [Am] 67:1188–1194, 1985.
55. Ritter MA, Fechtman RA: Proximal tibial osteotomy: A survivorship analysis, J Arthroplasty 3:309, 1988.
56. Schatzker J: The intertrochanteric osteotomy, New York, 1984, Springer-Verlag.
57. Shoji H, Insall J: High tibial osteotomy for osteoarthritis of the knee with valgus deformity, J Bone Joint Surg [Am] 55:963–973, 1973.
58. Slocum DB, et al: High tibial osteotomy, Clin Orthop 104:239, 1974.
59. Staeheli JW, Cass JR, Morrey BF: Condylar total knee arthroplasty after failed proximal tibial osteotomy, J Bone Joint Surg [Am] 69:28–31, 1987.
60. Sundaram NA, Hallett JP, Sullivan MF: Dome osteotomy of the tibia for osteoarthritis of the knee, J Bone Joint Surg [Br] 68:782–786, 1986.
61. Tjornstrand B, Hagstedt B, Persson BM: Results of surgical treatment for non-union after high tibial osteotomy in osteoarthritis of the knee, J Bone Joint Surg [Am] 60:973–977, 1978.
62. Tjornstrand BA, Egund N, Hagstedt BV: High tibial osteotomy. A seven-year clinical and radiographic follow-up, Clin Orthop 160:124–136, 1981.
63. Torgerson WR Jr, et al: Tibial osteotomy for the treatment of degenerative arthritis of the knee, Clin Orthop 101:46, 1974.
64. Tsumura H, et al, cited by Coventry MB: Proximal tibial varus osteotomy for osteoarthritis of the lateral compartment of the knee, J Bone Joint Surg [Am] 69:32–38, 1987.
65. Vainionpaa S, et al: Tibial osteotomy for osteoarthritis of the knee. A five to ten year follow up study, J Bone Joint Surg [Am] 63:938–946, 1981.
66. Wagner H, Zeiler G, Baur W: Indikation, Technik und Ergebnisse der supra- und infracondylaren Osteotomie bei der Kniegelenkarthrose, Orthopade 14:172–192, 1985.
67. Wagner H: Principles of corrective osteotomies in osteoarthrosis of the knee, Orthopade 6:145–177, 1977.
68. Wagner H: Principles of corrective osteotomy in osteoarthritis of the knee. Prog Orthop Surg 4:75–102, 1980.
69. Wang J, et al: The influence of walking mechanics and time on the results of proximal tibial osteotomy, J Bone Joint Surg [Am] 72:905–909, 1990.
70. Windsor R, Insall JN, Vince KG: Technical considerations of total knee arthroplasty after proximal tibial osteotomy, J Bone Joint Surg [Am] 70:547–555, 1988.

58
Evolution of Total Knee Arthroplasty

KELLY G. VINCE, M.D.

Hinges
   Lessons from hinges
   Early failures
   Later experience with conventional hinges
      Hinges abandoned
   Rotationally nonconstrained hinges
Acrylic and metallic interpositional arthroplasties
Mold arthroplasty
Townley's development of knee arthroplasty
   Townley's original sketches
   Tibial articular plate hemiarthroplasty
   Townley anatomic knee replacement
   Porous anatomic total knee replacement
Unicondylar knee prosthesis
   Gunston polycentric
   Marmor modular knee
   Laskin unicondylar and unicompartmental replacement experience
   Hospital for special surgery and unicondylar replacement
   Boston and Brigham unicompartmental arthroplasty
Development of bicondylar knees
   Problems with early bicondylar knees
      Geometric-kinematic conflict
      UCI Prosthesis: Inadequate polyethylene thickness
   Preserving cruciate ligaments in total knee arthroplasty
Tricompartmental total knee arthroplasty
   Patellar resurfacing
   Kinematic conflict and development of modern total knee replacement
   Early posterior cruciate ligament controversy
   Freeman-Swanson prosthesis
  Hospital for special surgery pedigree
   Duocondylar prosthesis
   Duopatellar prosthesis
   Total condylar prosthesis
   Posterior-stabilized prosthesis
   Stabilocondylar prosthesis
   Parallel evolution
   Contemporary cruciate-retaining prostheses
      Cruciate condylar prosthesis
      Kinematic prosthesis
   Posterior cruciate ligament controversy: Update
The Future: Convergence of Ideas?
   Three principles of knee arthroplasty
      Fixation: Preserving proximal tibial bone
      Kinematics: Maintaining level of joint line
      Wear: Maintaining minimal polyethylene thickness
   New arguments and data
      Motion and posterior cruciate ligament
      Loosening
      Correction of deformity
      More normal knee
      Is the Spine and Cam Mechanism Always Necessary?
      Posterior cruciate ligament in osteoarthritis
      Destructive wear
Conclusion

There are many facets to the development of successful contemporary knee arthroplasties. They range from the people who contributed their ideas and experiences, to the materials and expectations of the time. Making knee replacements work has meant solving problems that may have surfaced at different times, but which have always been related. Relieving pain and restoring motion have been the goals of this surgery since its inception. Fixation, deformity, and stability are issues that recur in the development of surgical technique. Some paths, such as the pursuit of a durable linked constrained prosthesis, had to be abandoned entirely after decades of effort. Other issues, such as fixation and the role of the cruciate ligament, are still being debated.

This history focuses on the kinematics of knee replacement and how surgeons and engineers have tried to make implantable devices that would enable the knee to "work" as much like a human knee as possible. The early approaches were markedly divergent. By comparison, current beliefs have become very similar. And there are indications that ideas will converge even more in the near future. There are many lessons in this story, no matter how arcane the particular device, that pertain to today's problems.

Our chronology starts with the earliest attempts at reconstructing the arthritic or ankylosed joint by the interposition of biologic or synthetic membranes. Initiated in the 19th century, this concept persisted until the middle of this century. In the 1950s metal was introduced into arthroplasty surgery and was applied in two divergent modes—hinge reconstruction and the continued development of interpositional arthroplasty.

MEMBRANE INTERPOSITIONAL ARTHROPLASTY: EARLIEST ATTEMPTS AT KNEE ARTHROPLASTY

Potter et al. in 1972 assembled a succinct history of early arthroplasty surgery.[127] The concept of interposition focused on the loss of articular cartilage as the central problem in arthritis. Early efforts were directed at the temporomandibular joint (TMJ). The problem was simple and compelling: when the TMJ was diseased and immobile, the patient could not eat. Verneuil[178] interposed soft tissue between the bones of a TMJ in 1860 and then applied the technique to the knee in 1863, using joint capsule.[178] Ollier[124] in 1886 proposed muscle interposition to prevent reankylosis of the knee and Helferich[59] in 1894 reported using muscle successfully in the TMJ. Gluck[48] later covered bone ends with skin, but with poor results.

Other membrane arthroplasties included fat and fascia[4, 120] and chromicized pig's bladder.[9] Henderson,[61] in 1918, published the results of four of his own cases with these primitive arthroplasties and reviewed 117 knee arthroplasties from other hospitals. He decided that only 18 of the 121 operations could be considered successful.[61] Campbell[23] used fascial flaps, chromicized pig's bladder, and free fasciae latae, but only 5 of 24 achieved useful motion.

After World War II there was renewed interest in fascial knee arthroplasty. Miller and Friedman[117] reviewed 37 fascial arthroplasties performed for ankylosis at the State University of Iowa from 1917 to 1947. They thought that the modest increases in mobility were of value in selected cases.[117] Speed and Trout[159] reported good results in 65% of the cases they reviewed. Samson[141] described 26 of 50 fascial arthroplasties as stable and painless with 45 to 90 degrees of motion.

At different times, cutis,[20] cellophane,[116] nylon,[93] and fluon[161] were interposed between the femur and tibia. The most recent report on fascial arthroplasties originates in Japan. Koga and colleagues[92] evaluated 25 interposition arthroplasties of the knee using chromicized fascia lata that had been performed between 1951 and 1975. Ten patients had occasional pain after heavy labor and 13 had more than 60 degrees of motion. Twelve had 45 degrees of motion or less. Are these results any different than those of resection arthroplasty, which we occasionally still see after incurably infected knee replacements?

In contrast to what some surgeons were writing about interpositional arthroplasties, Shiers concluded that "these results are not good—they are bad."[150] Despite the limitations of membranous interpositional arthroplasties, they represented nonetheless an anatomic orientation to arthritis, an attempt to replace damaged articular cartilage, but without the capacity to correct deformity or reestablish stability. That was to be accomplished for the first time with hinges.

HINGES

> Replacement surgery at the knee joint is still at a pioneering stage, and it would be presumptuous to evaluate the method at this early date. It is possible by prosthetic reconstruction to meet the requirements of mobilization of the knee joint. Moreover, recovery is relatively painless. Whether the body will tolerate such a large metallic prosthesis is not known. There is little doubt, however, that in this new era of the utilization of foreign substances in the body, investigation into this method of mobilizing the knee joint will be continued.[100]

The other approach, far more mechanical in nature than interpositional arthroplasty, was characterized by complete replacement of knee anatomy with a hinge, or technically, a linked device featuring some type of axle that permitted rotation in the sagittal plane only and that did not require ligaments for stability. This radical treatment provided the means for correcting deformity and reestablishing stability. Hinges produced, at least for a short time, strikingly good results in very bad knees. The hinge did not, however, duplicate complex knee function. It was a mechanical approach in the extreme.

Lessons From Hinges

There are lessons to learn from the literature on hinge arthroplasties:

1. Early failure does not necessarily mean that the entire concept is unworkable. Some of the first linked implants failed quickly.[90, 191] Later versions worked well for a short time in patients whose activity was limited.

2. Work on hinged replacements extended over more than 30 years with many innovations that were supposed to make them work better and longer: cement fixation, offset axis, and finally rotational freedom. The basic concept of constraint had to be abandoned before modern condylar replacements could be used to realign and stabilize arthritic knees.

3. Contemporary expectations color our conclusions. Some of the results of the hinge (and membranous interpositional) reconstructions were regarded as excellent by the criteria of the day. These results would not compare favourably with our present expectations of an "excellent result."

4. Short-term studies must be viewed critically. After all, the hinge outperformed many other designs within 2 years of surgery.

5. Information on implants is necessary from developers and independent surgeons. The developers have had the longest experience with the device and should be among the first to recognize, and make known, shortcomings in design. Many surgeons who wrote about hinge arthroplasties cautioned that it was a last resort for the severely disabled patient and that failure would yield an arthrodesis at best. Despite the enthusiastic literature of the design attributes and clinical results (always with an explanation for the failures) with hinges, the ultimate condemnation of these devices usually came from independent surgeons.

Early Failures

MacAusland[100] gave Judet and associates[90] credit in 1947 for being the first to attempt "total replacement of the knee joint" (distinct from interpositional arthroplasty). They had implanted an acrylic prosthesis with a femoral and tibial part. It unfortunately had to be removed owing to early complications. Majnoni d'Intignano[103] pioneered another acrylic prosthesis in 1950. Although he described one good result 1 year after surgery, there was later evidence that it had became stiff and had failed. These devices were never implanted in any numbers by the designers or any other surgeons.[103]

Walldius: 1951

Walldius[191] initially developed an acrylic hinge arthroplasty which he implanted in Scandinavia. The hinge concept enabled him to correct deformity and stabilize the badly arthritic knee. While the acrylic version was unsuccessful, a metal-on-metal device was eventually implanted in large numbers by him and others over the next several decades.[10, 47, 55, 57, 85, 87, 192–194, 196] By 1968 he had inserted the metallic prosthesis in 93 knees, using cement in rare cases where there was gross deformity. Arthrodesis was the preferred salvage operation.[194]

Shiers: 1953

No arthroplasty may be considered successful until it has stood up to at least ten years of normal use; therefore to lay down indications for operation at this stage would be presumptuous. It is merely suggested that if an arthrodesis of the knee be contemplated for instability due to injury, or from pain from osteoarthritis, this method be given a trial. Should it fail, arthrodesis can easily be performed—the bone ends are already prepared.[150]

This may in fact have been the first successful hinge arthroplasty, bearing in mind that Walldius abandoned his early acrylic implants. The Shiers hinge was rudimentary; it was implanted in the medullary canal without cement and the smaller sizes served as elbow replacements. Shiers wrote that the implant was a last resort before arthrodesis. He preserved the collateral ligaments and did not conceive of the operation specifically to stabilize the deformed knee. His 1954 report described 5 years of development (ostensibly beginning in 1949) and two cases with good function within a year of surgery.[150]

In 1960 Shiers[195] described his experience with 28 operations in 17 patients. The original implant was stainless steel. It was later made of molybdenum bearing stainless steel for strength. Vitallium, it was concluded, was simply too expensive. Shiers reported breakage in seven knees from 4 to 40 months after implantation.[151] While the original implants were press-fitted into the medullary canal, Shiers later adopted cement fixation to prevent implants from sinking into the bone.[194]

Arden[7] described 192 cemented Shiers hinge arthroplasties, of which only 9 were not implanted in patients with inflammatory arthropathy. Defining a good result as flexion from 60 to 90 degrees with occasional pain, he reported that 80% of the knees were good or excellent. The follow-up was limited to 1 year.

MacAusland: 1956

MacAusland[100] described one case of a profoundly debilitated patient with polyarthritis in whom he implanted his vitallium hinge prosthesis in 1956. Fixation came from stems with flanges that were perforated for ingrowth (with large holes in the fashion of the fenestrations in Austin Moore hip arthroplasties) and teeth on the posterior side of the compartments to grip the cortical bone. It was an unwieldy device in appearance, with long flaps of metal that hung over the edge of the bone for fixation. No cement was used and no follow-up was given beyond describing that the wound had healed and motion improved.[100]

Young: 1958

Young[206] in 1963 described the first implantation of his vitallium-designed hinge at the Mayo Clinic 5 years earlier. His paper includes an excellent summary of existing hinge designs and the failure of interpositional arthroplasties that spawned these devices. The Young hinge had a 15-degree valgus angle and was held together with a bolt, locknut, and washer. The femoral rod was curved to prevent perforation of the femoral cortex and spikes were included on the "shoulders" of each part of the prosthesis to resist rotation. Screws prevented distraction and no methacrylate was used. He reported eight cases over 5 years: only two patients were improved; the others ended up with fusions and infections.[206] Much better results with the Young prosthesis were reported in 1973 from West Germany, in 52 knees. Many of these had been implanted with McKeever patellar resurfacings.[57]

Guepar: 1971

As late as 1970[114] several surgeons in Paris embarked on the design of a new hinge arthroplasty—GUEPAR. They identified shortcomings in the Walldius, Young, and Shiers devices, which they translated into a device with (1) minimal bone resection, (2) flexion not limited by the parts, (3) tibial rolling under the femur in flexion, (4) a metallic trochlea for patellar articulation, (5) a silastin dampening on the extension stop, and (6) valgus alignment with right and left implants. The group used this device exclusively and implanted 112 of them by March 1972. They listed 7 failures, but did not think that any of the complications "could be ascribed to the prosthesis itself." They experienced no cases of loosening.[114]

By 1976 they reported a minimum 2-year follow-up of 103 GUEPAR arthroplasties with six cases of aseptic loosening, all of which had occurred by 1 year. They had not observed loosening in those patients they observed for longer than 2 years and felt that, while longer observation was necessary, these results represented a stable situation.[30]

In 1976, they acknowledged "theoretical drawbacks" to the hinge concept, but believed that the GUEPAR had given excellent results. The infection rate was 6.6% and they had begun to limit the device to either very old patients or grossly dislocated knees.[30] Perservering with the concept of hinged arthroplasty, they introduced the GUEPAR II with shorter stems. The second device was initially cemented, but the designers attributed the accumulating failures (15% at 5 years) to the inadequacy of the cement. They began implanting the GUEPAR II without cement.[31]

Having used 112 GUEPAR replacements from 1972 to 1975, Jones and colleagues at The Hospital for Special Surgery in New York reported the results of 108 arthroplasties at 1 to 13 years.[86] This was a sequel to their comparison of four models of knee arthroplasty in which the GUEPAR provided the best results at 2 years despite the fact that it had been selected for the worst knees.[82] Their patients had an 11% infection rate with 27% having radiographic evidence of loosening. The functional results had been declining as time advanced. Patellar subluxation and dislocation complicated 49% of reconstructions. The authors concluded that the GUEPAR hinge should be used judiciously, and only for knees with severe deformity.[86]

Herbert Prosthesis

One of the most vulnerable hinges was the Herbert prosthesis. In a lengthy 1973 article, only a single paragraph described the 2.5-year follow-up of 25 cases.[62] No failures were described; it was other surgeons who later reported the extremely high rate at which the device broke.[123, 135]

Later Experience With Conventional Hinges

Volume 94 of *Clinical Orthopaedics and Related Research* (1973) contains many articles on knee arthroplasties, mainly Walldius hinges. Many reports described favorable experiences by independent surgeons.[10, 47, 55, 57, 85, 87] None proposed that the operation be abandoned. There was a debate over cement fixation, and whether the "painless subsidence of the uncemented Walldius" was preferable to the painful loosening that occurred in cemented hinges. This was, however, just about the last time that these devices were held in any esteem.

The "new" implants, such as the geometric and Freeman-Swanson, were described a year later. Because they were "smaller, used less cement and less bone was removed," there would be fewer complications.[7] There was little hope that they could be used for knees with gross deformity or which were badly damaged. Condylar-type resurfacing arthroplasty in deformed joints awaited the development of techniques for ligament releases.

Hinges Abandoned

The future was apparent. Young[207] wrote in 1971 that, in his experience, none of the modified Walldius or Young hinged prostheses had survived 10 years. Hui and Fitzgerald[66] reported a 23% incidence of major complications in 77 hinged arthroplasties, prominently infection (11.7%). They concluded that "whenever possible, a moderately constrained replacement arthroplasty should be considered."[66] Eventually, the only discussion of hinges was for revision surgery. Bargar and colleagues[11] found that the GUEPAR and Herbert prostheses they had used in difficult situations ultimately resulted in a high incidence of failures and did not solve the problem of the patient with a failed knee arthroplasty. "There is *no* indication for hinge prosthesis in revision surgery," wrote Insall and Dethmers in 1982.[75] The hinges had been condemned and abandoned, but generally in studies from independent investigators.

Rotationally Nonconstrained Hinges

The last gasp of linked, constrained devices were the rotating hinges. The idea that rotation was the most damaging mode of constraint motivated the development of the spherocentric, the Noiles hinged knee prosthesis, and the kinematic rotating hinge. None were successful.

Spherocentric: 1973

Matthews and colleagues[112] formulated nine design criteria for knee arthroplasty in 1973, which guided the development of the spherocentric prosthesis (Fig 58–1). This constrained device did not permit translational motion or varus or valgus instability with the knee fully extended. The first publication contained no clinical results.[112] In 1979 Kaufer and Matthews[91] reported the results of 134 consecutive spherocentric arthroplasties (of which 21 were revisions and 3 were for failed arthrodesis) at 1 to 5 years. They noted subsidence in 10 (7.7%), 5 of which were revised.[91] A report followed on 84 spherocentric knee arthroplasties that had been implanted at the University of Michigan from December 1973 to February 1977. Only patients with large deformities were selected for the prosthesis, and they were evaluated at 24 to 73 months after surgery. Eight knees in this group had loosened during the study.[111] The final evaluation of the spherocentric prosthesis was published by the same surgeons in 1986. At an average of 8 years following surgery, 9 (11%) of the previously reported 84 spherocentric replacements had loosened. The design has been abandoned.[113]

Noiles Hinge: 1978

The Noiles hinge allowed 40 degrees of rotation—a generous amount but not in any way resembling normal knee function. This was purported to reduce stresses at the interface. The developers described the device as "semi-constrained," a term which should not be used for any linked prosthesis. The implant was comprised of a cemented femoral stem that articulated through a hinge pin with an uncemented tibial stem, which fit into a polyethylene sleeve that was cemented into the tibia (Fig 58–2). Reports by the originators of the design were favorable.[1, 2, 63] Shindell and associates[152] denounced the design and the claims of prior published reports in 1986. They compared their 10 of 18 implants that required revision by an average of 32 months, with the developers' report of 1 failure in 87 implants at an average follow-up of 33 months. Several important principles emerge from this experience. The objectivity of developers is often questioned, as are the skills of independent surgeons who cannot duplicate excellent results. In addition, selection of patients is paramount. Shindell and associates interpreted the literature to say that the device was indicated for anticipated heavy use, gross ligamentous laxity, and severe varus or valgus malalignment, but not limited to revision surgery.[152]

Kinematic Rotating Hinge: 1978

The kinematic rotating hinge was devised by a group of experienced engineers and surgeons to reconstruct the badly damaged knee—to substitute for bone loss and absent ligaments. Acutely aware of the limitations of fixed-axis hinges, the group evaluated the advantages of rotational nonconstraint. Twenty-two of these hinges, each made up of seven mobile parts, were implanted in Boston between November 1978 and October 1980 (Fig 58–3). They were evaluated in 1982 at 5 to 24 months following surgery, an interval that the investigators cautioned is too short to allow reasonable conclusions.[190] The developers have since declared that the implant is not viable, conclusions that were also reached by Rand and associates at the Mayo Clinic.[132] While other surgeons unassociated with the developers contend that this device can yield "a high percentage of satisfactory clinical" results in highly selected patients at a minimum 25-month follow-up,[149] the device has largely been abandoned.

Conclusion

Thirty years of arthroplasty development was devoted to making the linked constrained device work. While techniques of ligament releases paved the way for condylar resurfacing of the severely deformed knee, there are still situations where the majority of surgeons seek an intrinsically constrained, though nonlinked device. The essence of the problem is the

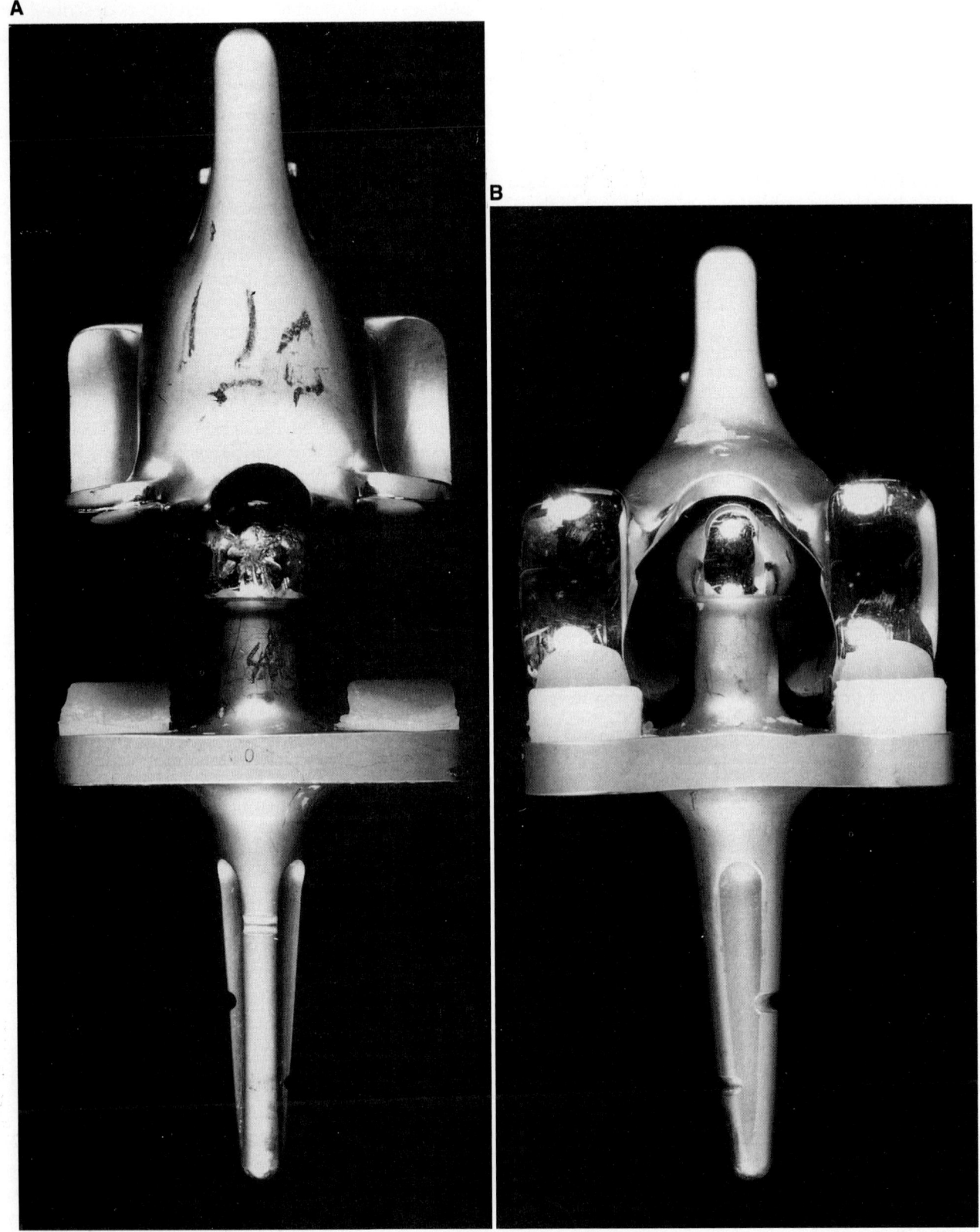

FIG 58–1.
Spherocentric arthroplasty. **A,** frontal view with components distracted. In normal position, the ball would be obscured by its housing. There is no patellar resurfacing **B,** viewed from behind, the ball is visible in its housing. This opening is necessary to allow flexion.

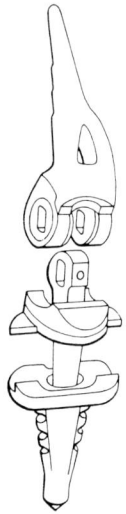

FIG 58-2.
The Noiles total knee prosthesis is a semiconstrained hinged device with three major components. A femoral component is cemented into the femoral canal with methacrylate. The tibial stem is inserted into a cemented tibial sleeve and is joined to the femoral component by a hinge. This design theoretically allows a 20-degree arc of motion in both the medial and lateral direction with decreased axial loading. (From Shindell R, et al: *J Bone Joint Surg [Am]* 68:579, 1986. Used by permission.)

patient with intrinsic failure of the medial collateral ligament.

We have followed the development of hinged arthroplasties from beginning to end. However, in doing so, we have passed over the story of condylar-type replacements, a story that eventually led to successful implants.

ACRYLIC AND METALLIC INTERPOSITIONAL ARTHROPLASTIES

The development of modern condylar arthroplasties resumes with the interpositional arthroplasties: the McKeever and MacIntosh implants, developed independently in Los Angeles and Toronto. MacIntosh[101, 102] first used an acrylic implant and then converted to chrome cobalt (Fig 58–4). McKeever[116] used metal from the outset. Fixation was not part of the agenda in these early attempts to resurface the knee. McKeever believed that fixation was simply not feasible and that "an endoprosthesis must be self retaining. It must be so designed and inserted that the normal forces existing in the joint in action hold it in place. Any screw, pin, flange or other retention device that functions as anything more than a guide to alignment or to retention of the prosthesis when the joint is at rest must eventually give way as a result of cyclic stress."[116]

McKeever: 1960

The McKeever and MacIntosh arthroplasties were single components lying on the tibial surface. The MacIntosh implant came in several sizes and thicknesses, whereas the McKeever implant was one shape but came in several thicknesses. It had a superficial crosshatched pattern on the distal surface that amounted to little more than surface roughness, as opposed to the T-shaped fins on the McKeever device.[127]

The metal interpositional arthroplasties provided some of the first good results with nonhinged knee implants. MacIntosh[101] used them mainly in advanced rheumatoid arthritis. These knees were badly destroyed, the patients had limited activity levels, and arthrodesis was out of the question because of polyarticular involvement. Of 58 knees, 51 received arthroplasties on both condyles. There were 8 failures.[101] In 1967 he reported the results of 103 cases with a minimum follow-up of 6 months. Seventy two were graded as good, 5 fair, and 26 poor.[102]

A detailed and thoughtful compilation of McKeever's notes was assembled posthumously by Dr. Robert B Elliott of Houston Texas, following Dr McKeever's untimely death in an automobile accident. The paper includes several insightful case studies, but no formal clinical data.[116]

Other surgeons have reported their experience with McKeever's device. Henderson and Peterson[60] treated 21 knees in 15 patients, including profoundly contracted joints in bedridden patients. They concluded in 1969 that the device had a place in treating the rheumatoid knee, but that results were better if the patients were ambulatory to a degree, did not have severe osteoporosis, and if flexion contractures were limited to less than 30 degrees.[60]

Potter and associates,[127] at the Robert Brigham Hospital in Boston, performed 142 interpositional arthroplasties in 119 patients. They published a comprehensive history of knee arthroplasty surgery, and a detailed analysis of their experience with both the McKeever and MacIntosh devices. They found surprisingly good results, using an early scoring system. Patients with osteoarthritis did particularly well up to 9 years after surgery.[127]

In New York, Ranawat et al.[130] reported on a 6-month to 4-year follow-up of MacIntosh arthroplasties from The Hospital for Special Surgery. All patients had rheumatoid arthritis and were treated concurrently with synovectomy. While results were good, the authors considered the implant suitable only for moderate deformities (less than 20 degrees) with good motion. They predicted that condylar re-

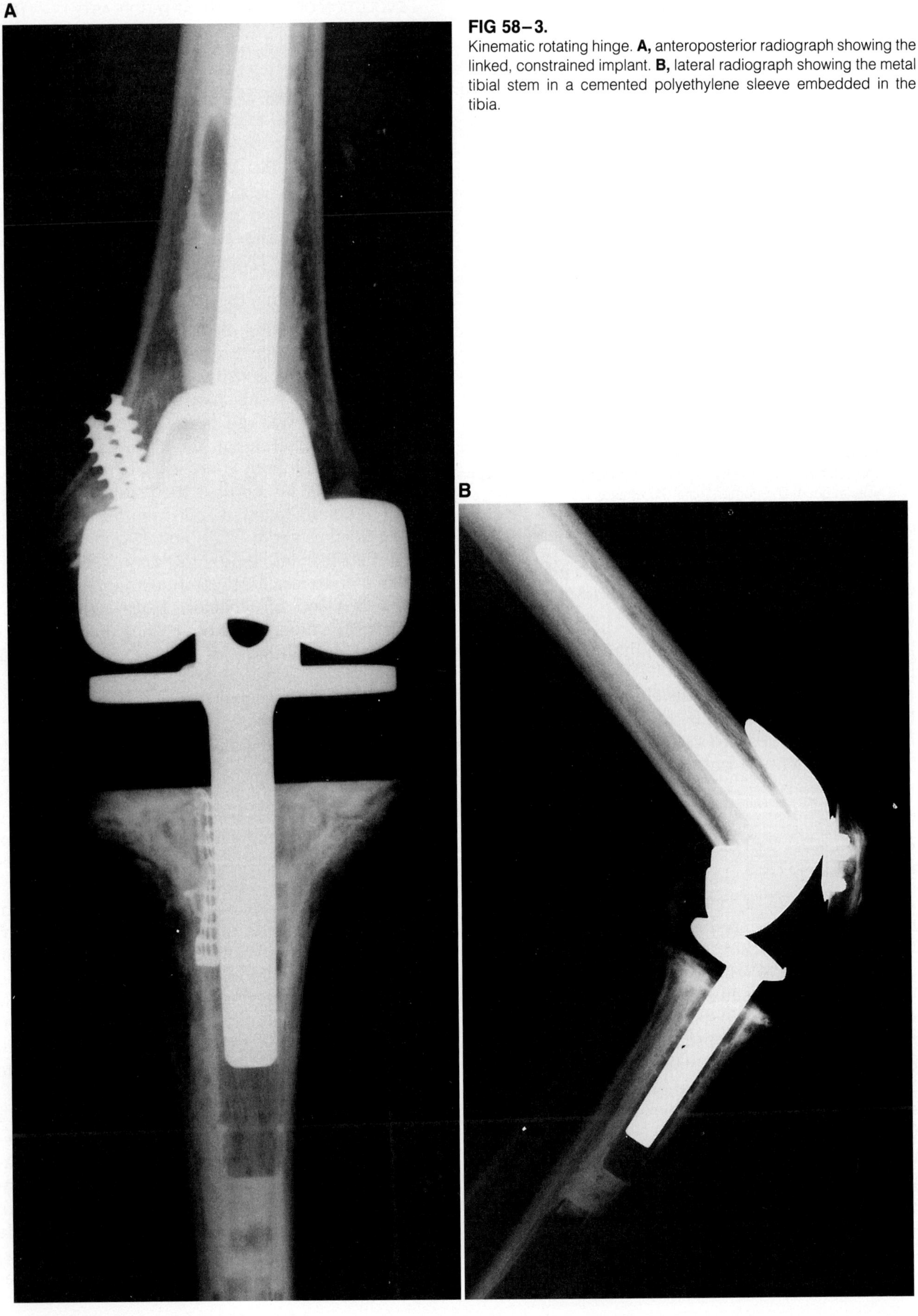

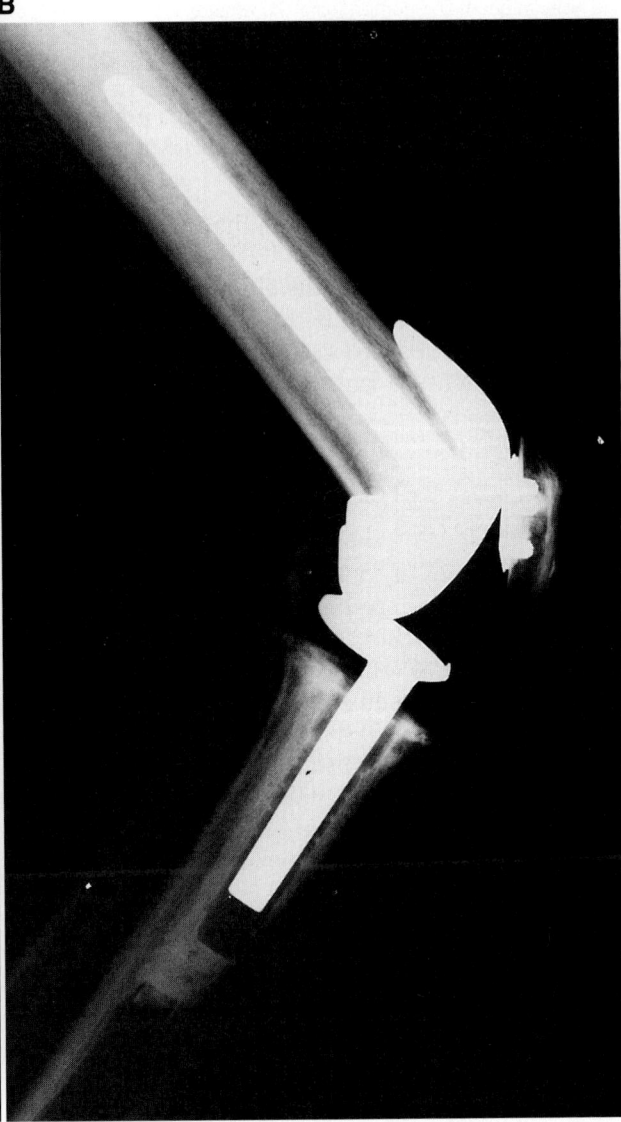

FIG 58–3.
Kinematic rotating hinge. **A,** anteroposterior radiograph showing the linked, constrained implant. **B,** lateral radiograph showing the metal tibial stem in a cemented polyethylene sleeve embedded in the tibia.

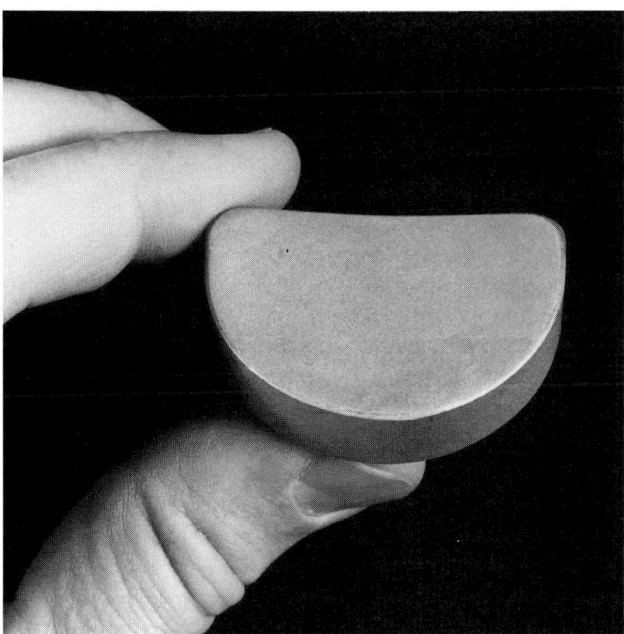

FIG 58–4.
MacIntosh interpositional arthroplasty. This was originally introduced as an acrylic implant. It was interposed between the tibia and femur, without fixation. The undersurface had a superficial grid compared with the similar McKeever, which had fins to maintain its position.

placements of both the tibia and femur would relieve pain better.[130]

Although these devices seem like true antiques, two long-term studies of McKeever implants were reported from Boston as late as 1985. Observing good bone quality in their patients in whom they had performed total knee replacements after years of implantation, these surgeons concluded there was a limited place for the arthroplasty: in the very young, active patient with posttraumatic arthritis.[33, 146]

MOLD ARTHROPLASTY

One of the earliest uses of metal in knee arthroplasty came from Willis Campbell in 1940.[24] He applied a contoured vitallium plate on the femoral condyles of two patients whose knees were ankylosed following acute pyogenic arthritis. The fixation was limited to two triangular flanges that hooked into the posterior femoral condyles and one screw that was placed anteriorly. Motion was poor after this hemiarthroplasty, and Campbell abandoned the technique.

Smith-Petersen used metal for knee arthroplasty as early as 1942 when he implanted mold arthroplasties in the first of a series of 18 knees that were eventually reported by Aufranc and Jones in 1958.[8] Three different designs were used. The first was unique: one fin in the intercondylar region projected superiorly into the femur and another inferiorly into the tibia. The surfaces covering the condyles were hollowed slightly to conform to the articular surface. A second design lacked the fins and had more of a femoral trochlea. Despite the optimism that Jones and Aufranc reported initially,[8] Jones later described disappointing results.[89] Jones later collaborated with Aufranc to develop an anatomically shaped surface replacement for the femur with a medullary stem. This became the MGH (Massachusetts General Hospital) mold arthroplasty that was implanted in relatively large numbers.[88, 89, 176] Jones described the evolution of these devices in an entertaining and informative article in 1969.[88] By that time femoral mold arthroplasties of one design or other had been implanted in 83 knees of 65 patients, all with profoundly diseased joints.

Turner and associates[175] described the results in 68 patients from the University of Pennsylvania that had received either vitallium femoral mold or McKeever interpositional arthroplasties. Four had both. All patients had rheumatoid arthritis. Noting 47 complications in 38 of the 68 operations, the authors concluded that "the failure of these procedures to produce consistently striking improvement and the impressive incidence of complications are great cause for concern."[175]

Mold arthroplasty enjoyed some success in the United Kingdom for a little more than a decade beginning in 1955. Sixty operations using a nonstemmed stainless steel femoral mold were evaluated by Platt in 1969.[126] Each was a minimum of 10 years after surgery. The results would not be acceptable by contemporary standards: 13 had ankylosed, 5 had fused, and 2 were amputated. These were, of course, profoundly arthritic joints.[126]

Murray and Barranco[122] described their experience with 59 knees in 43 patients, all of whom had severe disease. Like many of these early series, a transverse incision and removal of the tibial tubercle were used for exposure. Infection occurred in 3 (5%) patients, necessitating removal of the prosthesis in two cases. They reported no cases of symptomatic loosening. When they published their report, femoral hemiarthroplasty had already fallen out of favor, but the authors felt that there were still features of the procedure that could be successfully adapted to knee arthroplasty designs.[122]

TOWNLEY'S DEVELOPMENT OF KNEE ARTHROPLASTY

The story of modern knee arthroplasties can be told twice, or probably numerous times. The path from interpositional arthroplasties to mold-type replacements inevitably comes to Charles Townley and the ideas he has espoused consistently through a long and continuing career. His experience alone is one, nearly complete, story of knee prosthesis development.

Townley's Original Sketches: 1940s

Townley's designs were based on replicating natural knee function as closely as possible. It may be said that, inspired by the Smith-Petersen metal mold arthroplasty of the hip, he conceived a modern condylar-type arthroplasty even before the means or materials were available to produce one. Townley sketched his original ideas (Fig 58–5) in the late 1940s, about the time he completed an orthopaedic residency at Henry Ford Hospital in Detroit. These sketches depict a total resurfacing knee arthroplasty of the condylar type that preserved all ligaments and resurfaced the anterior femoral trochlea.[172] It was originally conceived as a metal-on-metal articulation but was abandoned in the planning stages because of concerns over corrosion and wear.

Tibial Articular Plate Hemiarthroplasty: 1951

The (metal) articular plate replacement arthroplasty was devised in 1951 and implanted from 1953 until the mid-1960s. This thin bicondylar stainless steel plate was secured exclusively with screws (Fig 58–6). By 1964, 39 had been implanted, and 19 had been followed for more than 2 years. Fourteen implants were described as causing minimal or no pain and 2 had "good" motion but moderate pain. Three were described as poor, 2 of which were complete failures in patients with rheumatoid arthritis. One plate, in an unstable knee, broke.[166, 173]

Townley Anatomic Knee Replacement

Twenty years' experience implanting 150 plate resurfacing hemiarthroplasties[170] led to the development of the anatomic total knee arthroplasty in 1972. It was made possible by the development of a suitable material to mate with the metal tibial component. The breakthrough, in Townley's words, came with Charnley's introduction of high-density polyethylene for the hip in the late 1960s. Until September 1972, when the first anatomic total knee arthroplasty became available, manufacturers had told him that the design was "too radical" or required the implantation of "too much metal."

The anatomic total knee was so named because of its dedication in function and appearance to normal anatomy. It was distinguished by retention of both cruciate ligaments and other technical features:

Thinnest possible implants
Total resurfacing including patellar articulation
Normal rotatory and anteroposterior excursion
Normal polycentric femoral surface contouring
Accurate implant sizing
Anatomic implant positioning
Preservation of all available ligaments
Anatomic multiplaned alignment of joint and implants

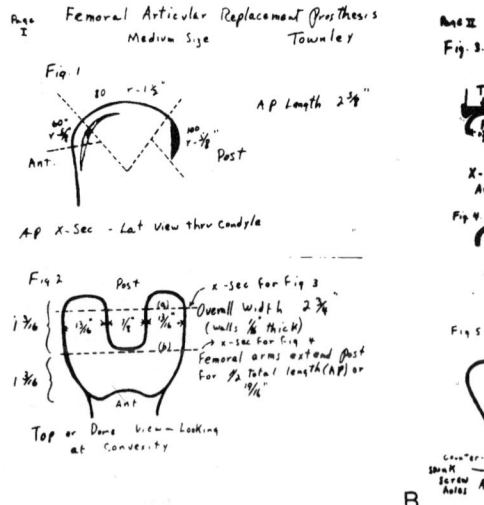

FIG 58–5.
Townley's sketch of his original total knee replacement. (From Townley CO: *Clin Orthop* 236:8–22, 1988. Used by permission.)

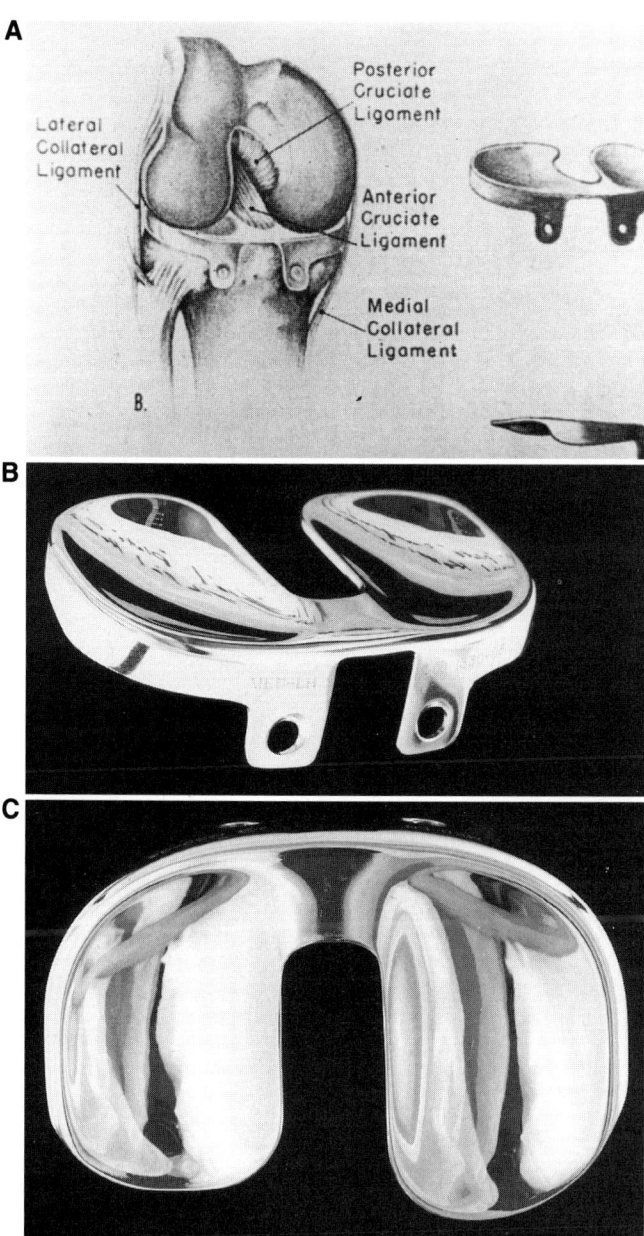

FIG 58–6.
Townley tibial articular plate resurfacing. **A,** sketch of implanted tibial articular plate resurfacing. (From Townley CO: *Clin Orthop* 36:77–85, 1964. Used by permission.) **B,** oblique view showing the thin implant with two screw holes in anterior flanges. This was the only means of fixation. **C,** top view showing cutout for cruciate ligaments and the symmetric shape.

The implant is described in a 1973 product monograph[166] (Fig 58–7). By 1974 50 had been implanted.[173] No data were available at that time. In 1983 Townley[167] reported on 438 anatomic total knee replacements at a minimum of 2 years post surgery. By 1985, he had done over 700 anatomic knee replacements and reviewed 532 at 1.5 to 11 years. Excluding nine knees with infection, ten had tibial implant loosening, four had dislodged the patellar implant, and three suffered residual ligament imbalance. Two patients dislocated their patellae and ruptured the patellar tendon.[170]

Porous Anatomic Total Knee Replacement: 1982

From September 1982 to August 1984, Townley implanted 89 porous-coated versions of the anatomic knee. Sixty-six of them were available from 4 months to 2 years after surgery, with salutary early results.[169, 171] A unicompartmental replacement became part of the anatomic knee replacement system in 1981.[168] Medial and lateral unicompartmental replacements were paired with a standard tricompartmental femoral component for a total knee replacement that preserved both cruciate ligaments.[174]

Townley's involvement extends from the 1940s (before the earliest hinge) through the development of successful tricompartmental condylar designs and into the era of uncemented knee replacements. He was the earliest, if not the first, to design and implant a one-piece bicompartmental tibial resurfacing prosthesis (tibial plate hemiarthroplasty), and to design and implant a full resurfacing anatomically contoured femoral component for total bi- or tricompartmental replacement.

UNICONDYLAR KNEE PROSTHESIS

The term *unicondylar* knee replacement refers to a device with two components that resurface the tibiofemoral articulation (but not the patellofemoral articulation). Two may be used to treat the medial and lateral compartments. This is the generic description, distinct from a specific implant from The Hospital for Special Surgery, called the unicondylar (see below). Unicondylar replacements were originally conceived as implants that preserved both cruciate ligaments. Later, bicompartmental and tricompartmental designs were introduced that were favored except in situations where articular cartilage damage was restricted to a single compartment. The term *unicompartmental* refers to the philosophy of resurfacing only the medial or lateral compartment, with unicondylar implants. The terms have been used interchangeably, now that bicondylar resurfacing with unicondylar components has fallen out of favor.

Gunston Polycentric: 1969

Solid fixation with polymethyl methacrylate promised better pain relief. This concept was inspired by

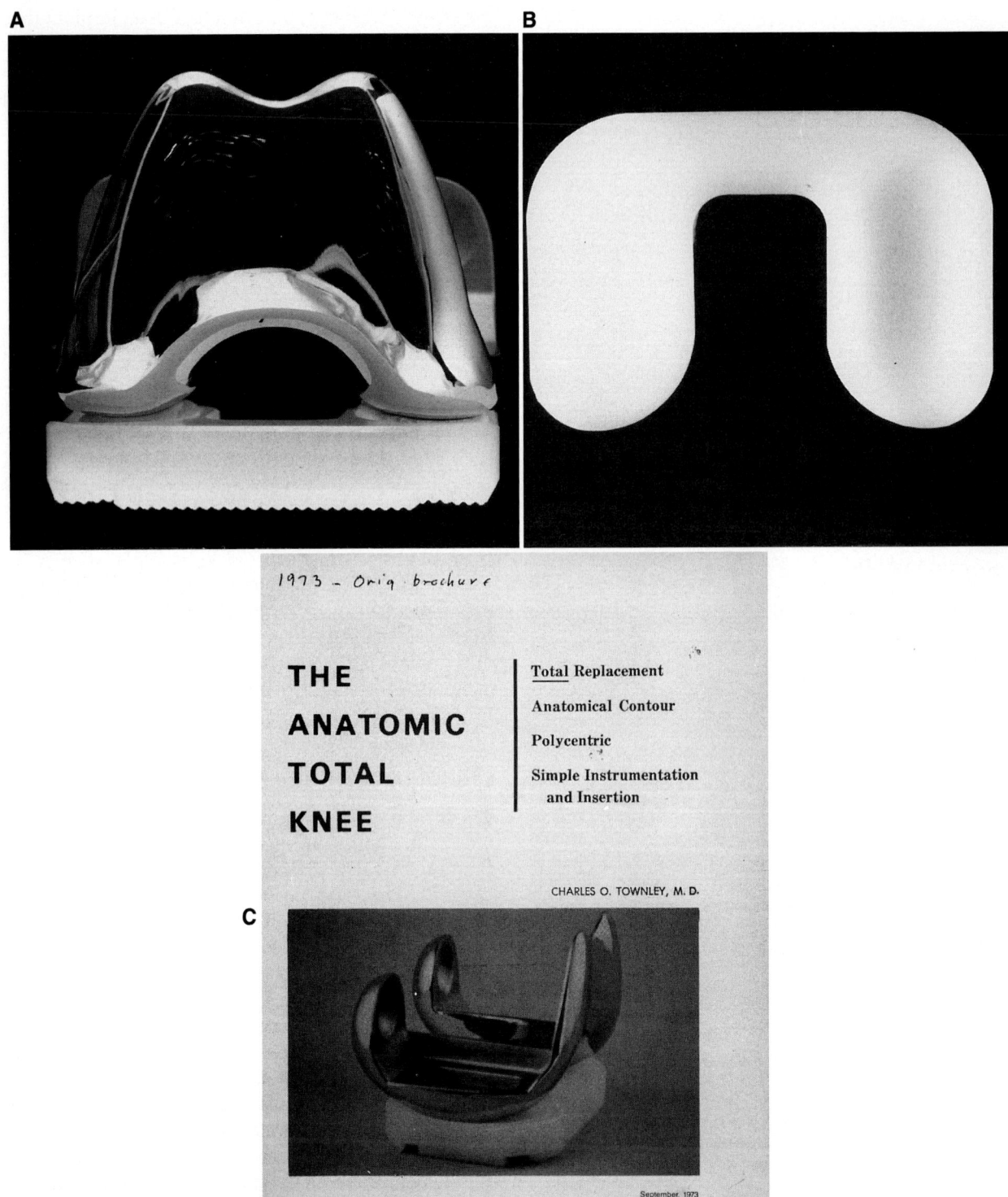

FIG 58–7.
Cemented anatomic total knee arthroplasty. **A,** articulated replacement from the front with all-polyethylene tibial component. There was no keel to intrude into the tibia for fixation. **B,** tibial component from above showing large cutout to allow retention of both cruciate ligaments. Dished tibial contours are apparent. **C,** first brochure describing the anatomic total knee arthroplasty, September 1973.

Charnley and implemented by Gunston with the polycentric prosthesis, a unicondylar design. Gunston, having worked with Charnley, also emphasized that the knee does not rotate about a single axis like a hinge, but that the femoral condyles roll and glide on the tibia (Fig 58–8). This concept, referred to as "femoral rollback" and "multiple instant centers of rotation," resulted in 1969 in the polycentric knee prosthesis. Effective and surprisingly durable, the polycentric design focused narrowly on kinematics with little concern for the problems of fixation and wear, which proved to be its undoing.[54]

Marmor Modular Knee

Leonard Marmor performed his first Marmor modular knee replacement on October 19, 1972.[105] The concept was to resurface the destroyed articular surface of the joint and to depend entirely on the patient's ligaments for stability. Unlike the Gunston polycentric, the Marmor modular knee had no groove or track in the polyethylene component for the metal femoral condyle to ride in. Whereas Gunston had identified the multiple instant centers of rotation in the sagittal plane, he had not incorporated rotation between the tibia and femur into his design. The Marmor knee, while identified in later years as a "unicompartmental" replacement, was originally used as a modular design to resurface either or both condyles as the pathologic conditions dictated.[104] Reporting the minimum 2-year results in 1976, Marmor described double-compartment replacements in 65 rheumatoid patients and 20 of 34 osteoarthritic knees. The implants were also used in hemophilic arthropathy, posttraumatic arthritis, and rheumatoid patients with ankylosis. The results, especially in the early 1970s, for correction of deformity and restoration of motion were admirable. At 2 years loosening was reported in one patient, who had had a varus deformity of 20 degrees.[104] Marmor refined and continues to implant the modular design.[106, 107] By 1985 the modular system was reserved for unicompartmental replacements.[108] Standard condylar designs were favored for tricompartmental disease, especially in the presence of deformity.

Marmor's subsequent report of unicompartmental replacements in 60 cases over a minimum of 10 years documented solid clinical performance.[108] The report detailed individual cases, successful or not. One lesson learned was the importance of adequate polyethylene thickness. Marmor noted a greater frequency of destructive wear and loosening with tibial components thinner than 9 mm. This is an example of a developing surgeon refining the design and bringing problems to light.

Laskin Unicondylar and Unicompartmental Replacement Experience

In two separate institutions in New York, the modular (unicondylar) replacement had a different fate. Laskin[94] described a good experience in 1976, with double-compartment (medial and lateral) modular-type implants in 58 osteoarthritic and 31 rheumatoid patients. At 2 years after these double-modular arthroplasties there was a general improvement in function, with good pain relief and no cases of loosening that required revision.[94] By 1978, Laskin[95] had abandoned the unicompartmental replacement for the medial side of the knee after reviewing the results at a minimum of 2 years. Disease in the lateral compartment, which was difficult to evaluate at surgery and may have been exacerbated by overcorrection of varus deformity, led to 4 of 34 (12%) patients requiring operation for lateral compartment pain. Wear debris from the unicompartmental replacement was observed in the articular cartilage of the other compartment at revision. Two patients had patellofemoral pain and more than half of the patients had settling of the components greater than 1 mm. Disenchantment with the unicondylar type of replacement in New York coincided with the introduction of promising bicondylar arthroplasties.

Hospital for Special Surgery and Unicondylar Replacement

Unicondylar replacements did not fare well in New York with Laskin or at The Hospital for Special Surgery. In 1976, Insall et al.[83] reported their experience with 24 knees at 2 to 4 years. The implant was called the unicondylar and yielded disappointing results. The lateral compartment was replaced in 5 and the medial in 19 knees. Three (16%) of the medial replacements were rated as fair and 5 as poor (26%). Three prostheses were removed. This study has been criticized by proponents of unicompartmental replacement because (1) patellectomy either had been done prior to arthroplasty or was done concurrently in 15 (62%) knees (3 lateral and 12 medial) and (2) overcorrection of varus deformity may have accelerated disease in the opposite compartment.

A later paper from Insall and Aglietti[74] confirmed their original observations, this time in 32 unicondylar replacements followed from 5 to 7 years. One was rated excellent, 10 were poor, and 7 had been con-

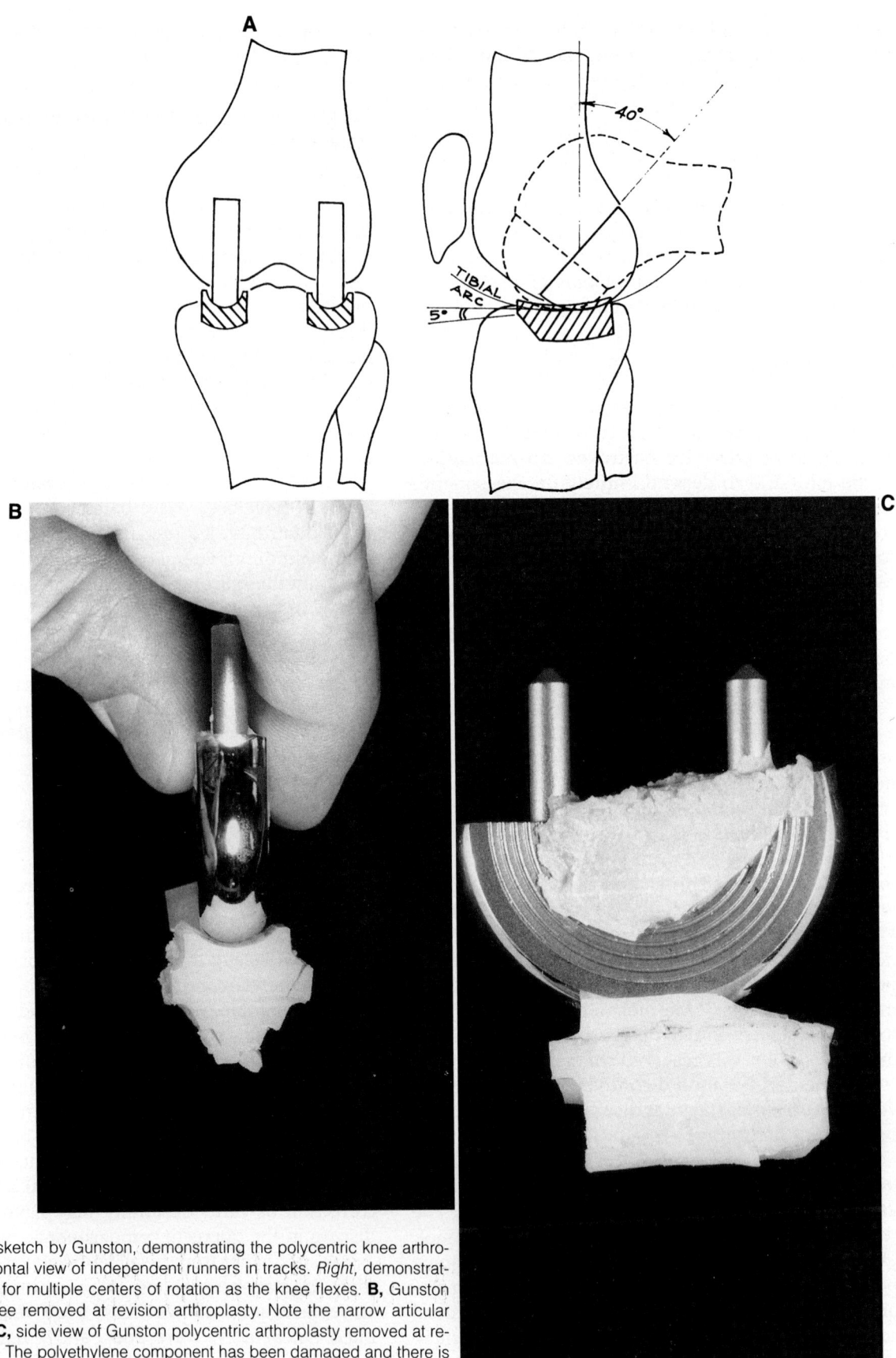

FIG 58–8.
A, schematic sketch by Gunston, demonstrating the polycentric knee arthroplasty. *Left,* frontal view of independent runners in tracks. *Right,* demonstrating provisions for multiple centers of rotation as the knee flexes. **B,** Gunston polycentric knee removed at revision arthroplasty. Note the narrow articular contact area. **C,** side view of Gunston polycentric arthroplasty removed at revision surgery. The polyethylene component has been damaged and there is methacrylate cement remaining on the femoral component. While the femoral component is circular in cross section, the runner is flat from anterior to posterior.

verted to total condylar–type replacements.[74] Further work at The Hospital for Special Surgery focused on total knee arthroplasties.

Boston and Brigham Unicompartmental Arthroplasty

The unicompartmental arthroplasty, still implanted on the West Coast by Marmor, is still regarded favorably in Boston.[163] Acknowledging a failure rate of about 1% per year, Scott and Santore,[144] based on their first 100 unicondylar replacements at 2 to 6 years, detailed factors leading to poor results. Most of their cases (88 knees) were medial compartment implants, which they did not believe were inferior to those in the lateral compartment. Citing preservation of the cruciate ligaments, patellofemoral joint, and opposite compartment, the authors believed that unicondylar arthroplasty was an attractive treatment for unicompartmental disease in the elderly patient. They remained strong advocates of high tibial osteotomy for the younger more active patient with varus deformity.[144]

Controversy persists as to whether the unicondylar replacement is a conservative operation that preserves bone. The failure rate appears to be marginally higher than total knee arthroplasty with cement fixation and considerably higher for uncemented unicompartmental replacements.[16] Some failures require extensive reconstruction at revision surgery.[56] One characteristic of the unicompartmental replacement is the necessity of maintaining the joint line at its anatomic level. To accommodate a minimum polyethylene thickness, this means that a relatively deep tibial resection is required.

Barrett and Scott,[15] from Boston, described 29 unicompartmental replacements that were revised. Only one could be revised to another unicompartmental replacement and 9 of 29 (31%) had bone defects requiring reconstruction. Three (10.3%) revisions failed owing to tibial component loosening.[15] Padgett et al.[125] from The Hospital for Special Surgery reported on revision of 21 failed unicondylar cases. They emphasized that reconstruction of tibial and femoral defects will often be required. The point is clear from both advocates and opponents of unicompartmental replacement: these are not necessarily simple operations to revise.[125]

DEVELOPMENT OF BICONDYLAR KNEES

Problems With Early Bicondylar Knees

Geometric-Kinematic Conflict

The Mayo Clinic, reasonably close to Winnipeg, where Gunston had returned to practice (and reputedly to manufacture polycentric knees in his garage), adapted his polycentric design[155] and reported their 10-year results in 1984.[97] Concurrently, Coventry[28] and others at the Mayo Clinic introduced the geometric knee replacement. Its single-piece tibial component facilitated surgery. Looking back, there was scant discussion of the cruciate ligaments in the literature on the geometric prosthesis (References 28, 67, 71, 98, 133, 134, 154, 164, 197) or its contemporaries. The conforming mechanical articulation between tibia and femur enhanced its stability, but was problematic when the cruciate ligaments were retained (Fig 58–9). This problem, later known as "kinematic conflict,"[73] explained in part why the geometric replacement was less serviceable than its predecessor, the polycentric design.[29]

It might seem that the biologic philosophy behind the polycentric design had proved superior to the mechanical thinking behind the geometric replacement—wanting greater stability from more conforming implants. The issue is not the triumph of biologic over mechanical thinking at this point, but rather inadequate design in the geometric implant. The design agenda was mixed; the prosthetic articular surfaces were not compatible with the kinematics of the cruciate ligaments. Kinematic conflict notwithstanding, the legacy of the geometric prosthesis remains the importance of alignment. Lotke and Ecker,[98] studying this implant, published their landmark paper linking valgus alignment to durable fixation.

UCI Prosthesis: Inadequate Polyethylene Thickness

The UCI (University of California at Irvine) prosthesis was a contemporary of the geomedic implant, both early bicondylar resurfacing arthroplasties (without patellofemoral resurfacing). Rotational freedom was possible between the tibia and femur owing to the circular track on the tibial component[32, 34, 58, 195] (Fig 58–10). Until 1978, when Ducheyne and colleagues[32] published their experience with 100 UCI arthroplasties, component failure was not a prominent topic in the literature. These authors found that 7 UCI replacements had failed within a mean of 20 months after surgery. Furthermore, the

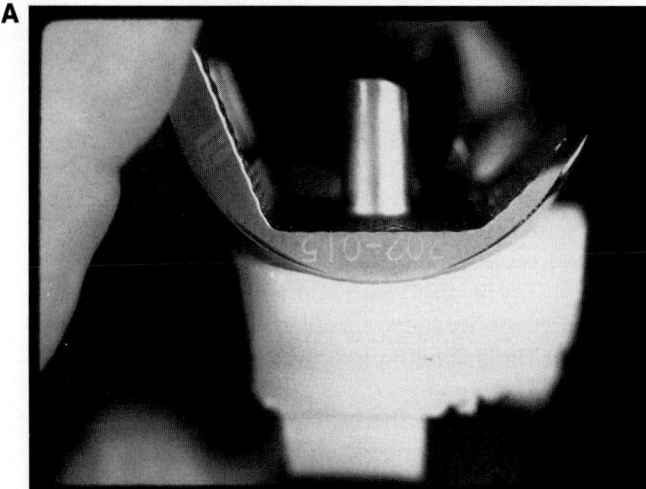
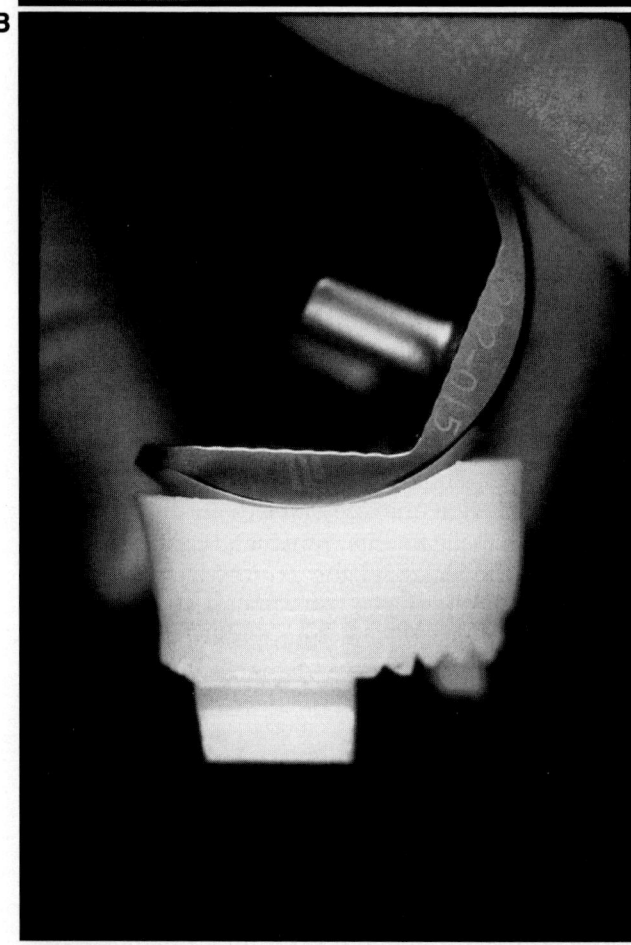

FIG 58–9.
Geometric prosthesis. **A,** side view in extension. As there was no provision for patellofemoral resurfacing, the femoral runners seen in the back of the prosthesis are the posterior femoral condyles. **B,** side view in flexion demonstrates the conformity between the tibial and femoral articular surfaces. When the posterior cruciate ligament is retained and tries to duplicate femoral rollback, this conforming articulation binds. This phenomenon is called kinematic conflict.

cause of each of the failed components had been the 5-mm thickness of polyethylene. The sequence of events that these surgeons postulated was: implantation of the tibial component with medial or lateral tilt, lack of firm skeletal stabilization, continual microtrabecular fractures, change in alignment of the extremity, and permanent deformation of the plastic component. Marmor had already cautioned against the inadequacies of thin polyethylene—a mistake that was to be repeated with the PCA (porous-coated anatomic) prosthesis,[204] in which it was hoped that metal backing would permit the use of thinner polyethylene.

Preserving Cruciate Ligaments in Total Knee Arthroplasty

Townley: 1972; and Cloutier: 1975

The ultimate cruciate conservationists were Townley,[170] whose anatomic knee was discussed above, and Cloutier[25, 26] of Montreal (Cloutier arthroplasty) both of whom supported designs that retained the anterior (ACL) and posterior (PCL) cruciate ligaments. These "biologically minded" surgeons wanted stability from the ligaments exclusively: no constraint, no loosening. The mechanically inclined surgeon, by comparison, wants full control of kinematics: no binding, no conflict. The idea of conserving both cruciate ligaments faded when bicondylar arthroplasties superseded modular implants (bicompartmental unicondylar replacements). There was a new emphasis on structure and fixation, a preference for a larger tibial component that would be less likely to break or loosen. These could not easily be implanted while leaving the tibial spines intact.

Cloutier's nonconstrained resurfacing prosthesis was introduced in 1975. It had right and left femoral components and separate polyethylene tibial articulations that snapped into a metal tray at the time of surgery (Fig 58–11). While the device had an anterior femoral flange, patellar resurfacing was not initially part of the procedure. The preliminary results were published in 1983[25] and by 1991, 61 knees could be evaluated at 10 to 13 years after surgery. All were fixed with cement. The ACL and PCL were intact in 28 knees and absent in 24. Of the former group, 26 of 28 knees (93%) had good or excellent results with 1 revision required for infection. When the ligament was absent, only 15 of 24 (62.5%) had good or excellent results and 6 required revision for infection, loosening, or instability. Seventy-five porous-coated implants had a significantly higher failure rate within 4 years.[26]

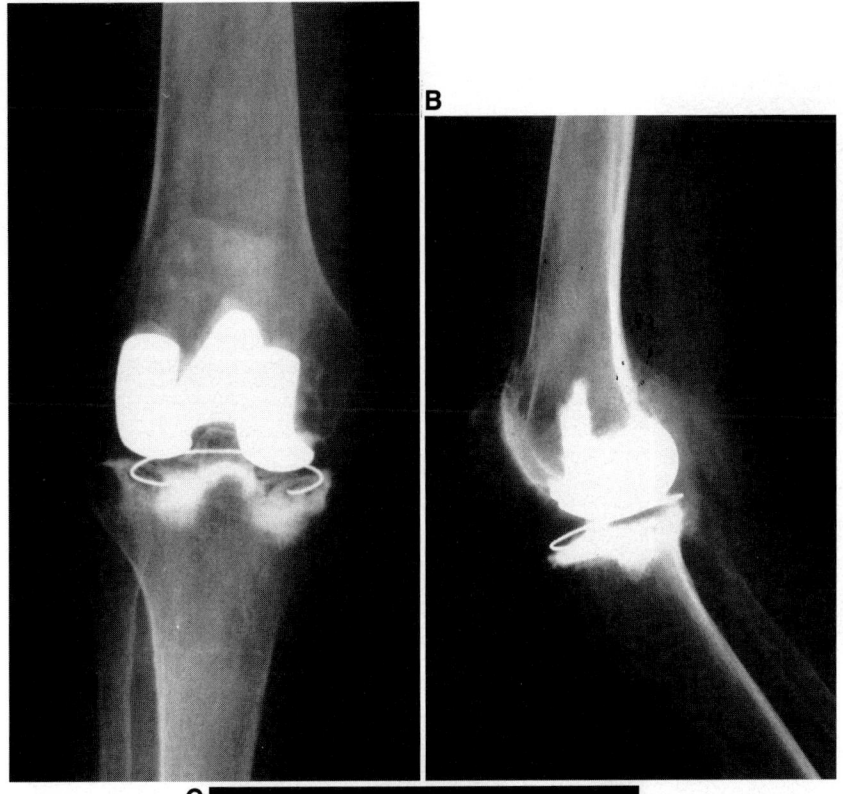
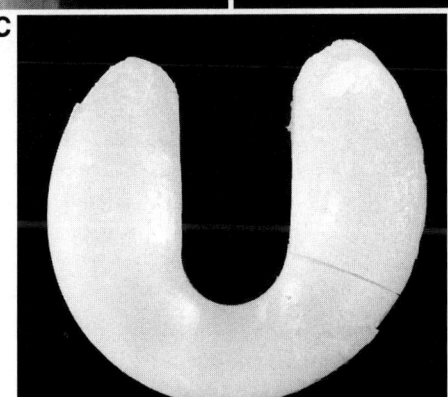
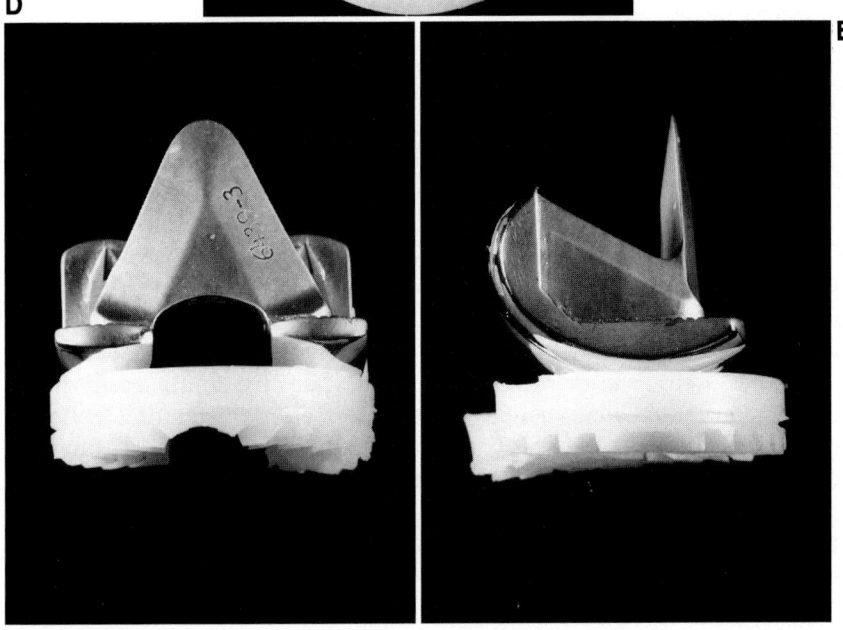

FIG 58–10.
UCI (University of California at Irvine) knee arthroplasty. **A,** Anteroposterior radiograph. The triangular eminence on the femoral component is for fixation; there is no resurfacing of the patellofemoral articulation. **B,** lateral radiograph of the cemented UCI arthroplasty. The all-polyethylene tibial component was subject to breakage when manufactured in thin sizes. **C,** retrieved polyethylene component from UCI arthroplasty. Note the semicircular articular surface. This implant has broken (note crack). **D,** frontal view of UCI arthroplasty. Again, the triangular flange is for fixation of the femoral component, not patellofemoral resurfacing. **E,** side view of UCI knee prosthesis. Anterior is to the right. Note deformity of tibial component—a prelude to breakage and loosening.

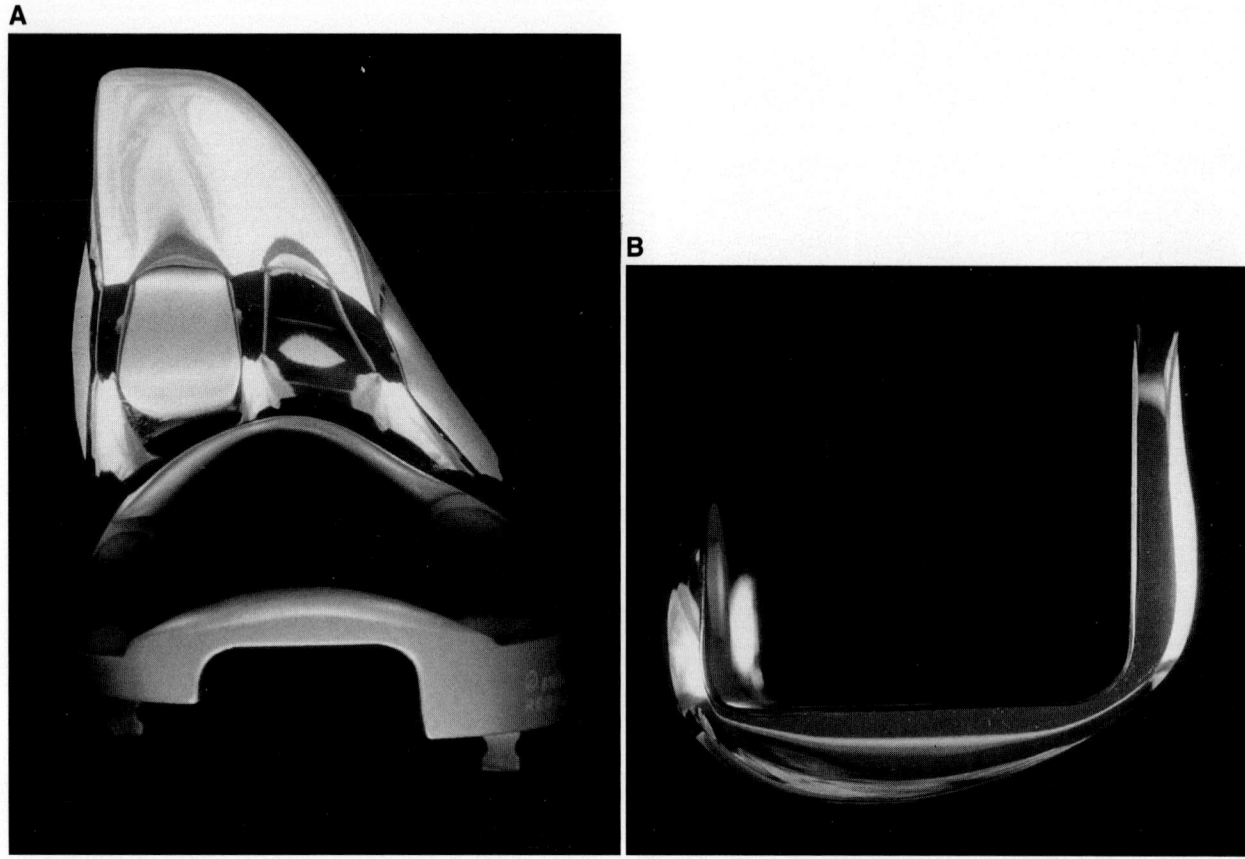

FIG 58–11.
Cloutier nonconstrained knee arthroplasty. **A,** frontal view shows the right-sided femoral component and the metal backing for the tibial component. Polyethylene inserts were inserted at the time of surgery. **B,** side view of the femoral component. There is a femoral flange, but initially the patella was not resurfaced.

TRICOMPARTMENTAL TOTAL KNEE ARTHROPLASTY

The development of true tricompartmental resurfacing knee arthroplasties revolved around the patellofemoral joint and how to deal with the cruciate ligaments. The problems to be solved, as ever, were fixation and stability.

Patellar Resurfacing

Early patellar resurfacing was not in the context of knee arthroplasty. McKeever[115] applied a metal button to the patella in cases of severe chondromalacia. Aglietti, Insall, and colleagues[3, 80] described their work in the development of metal and plastic versions to be used alone or with total knee arthroplasties respectively. Worrell[191–201] described some success with patellar resurfacing and Blazina et al.[18] developed a two-piece patellofemoral resurfacing arthroplasty.

Kinematic Conflict and Development of Modern Total Knee Replacement

Kinematic conflict marked the point when the cruciate ligament became an issue in knee arthroplasty surgery. This was the great divorce: you implanted either a cruciate-sacrificing or a cruciate-retaining device. The concept describes the inability of the knee to serve two masters. Either the articular geometry of the implants (inevitably different from the human knee) must be free to determine how the components will move with respect to one another, or anatomic structures such as the PCL must be allowed to pull the femur across the surface of the tibia. When the knee flexes, the point where the femur contacts the tibia usually moves posteriorly—femoral rollback. While rollback in the normal knee results from both cruciate ligaments working as a four-bar linkage[120, 121] (Fig 58–12) in concert with the individual's articular geometry, the PCL is the major player in knee arthroplasties. If the PCL induces femoral roll-

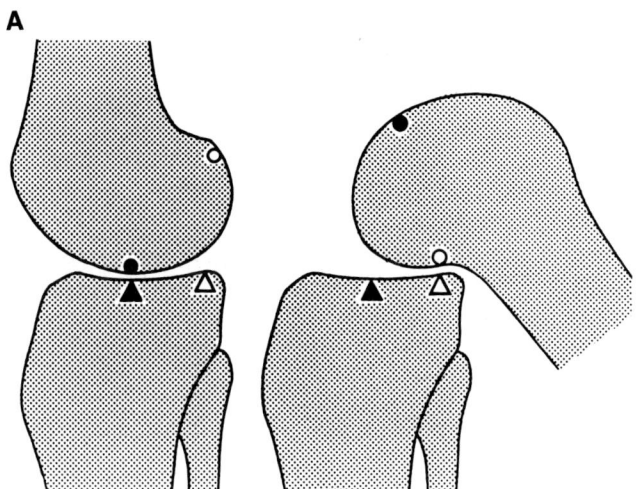
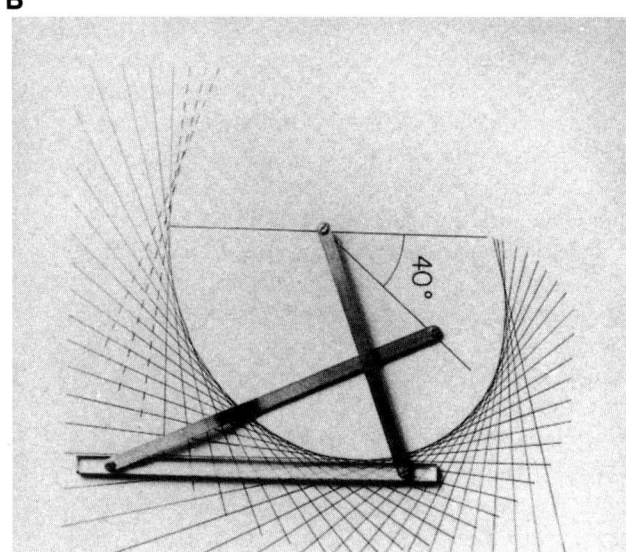

FIG 58–12.
A, schematic showing the effect of femoral rollback. **B,** the four-bar linkage that defines the intimate relationship between both cruciate ligaments and the articular surface. This functional relationship is difficult to duplicate with knee prostheses. (From Muller W: *The knee. Form, function and ligament reconstruction*, New York, 1983, Springer-Verlag. Used by permission.)

back, but the dished or conforming articulation does not permit it, the knee will bind. A knee with kinematic conflict is tight posteriorly, flexes poorly, and may apply sufficient pressure to the posterior tibial component to loosen it.

Early Posterior Cruciate Ligament Controversy

The early arguments favoring cruciate retention claimed that the PCL must provide stability in response to the loosening that had been seen with hinged arthroplasties. Some surgeons believed that virtually any conformity in the articulation could lead to loosening.[145, 156] Most advocates of cruciate retention were content to conserve the PCL alone, probably because the ACL was technically difficult to retain.

Freeman-Swanson Prosthesis

The Freeman-Swanson prosthesis, first implanted in March 1970, has been characterized as a "roller in a trough." The prosthesis was implanted only after resection of both cruciate ligaments, although this point was not mentioned in the original case report where the prosthesis had been implanted in a patient with rheumatoid arthritis.[42] From April 1970 to August 1972, sixty-nine operations had been performed with the Freeman-Swanson prosthesis. In the first published series,[41] several goals of the design were defined:

1. A salvage procedure should be readily available, in this case arthrodesis.
2. Loosening should be minimized, requiring an incomplete constraint (i.e., not a hinge).
3. Friction should be minimized by the use of metal against polyethylene.
4. The hyperextension stop should be progressive and not sudden.
5. The prosthesis should be fitted by a means that spreads the loads over a maximal area, requiring large bone surfaces and the use of acrylic cement.
6. Production of wear debris should be minimized,[40] meaning that bearing surfaces should be large and close production tolerances maintained.
7. Debris that is produced should be as innocuous as possible, indicating a preference for polyethylene.
8. The possibility of infection should be minimized by having a compact prosthesis with minimal dead space.
9. The consequences of infection should be minimized, so intramedullary stems should be avoided.
10. Standard surgical procedure is required.
11. The prosthesis should allow 5 degrees of hyperextension and at least 90 degrees of flexion.
12. Some freedom of rotation and abduction and adduction is necessary.

13. Excessive movements in any direction should be resisted by force systems which include the soft tissue and do not loosen the components.
14. It is unwise to depend on the cruciate ligaments given their condition in the arthritic knee.
15. The prosthesis should permit removal of the intercondylar tissue in the knee and restore cruciate function (mechanically).
16. The tibiofemoral joint should accommodate the patella or provide for patellectomy.
17. The cost of the prosthesis should be minimized.[41]

By 1977 a multicenter report was published on 71 knees that were severely deformed. Despite the severity of the pathologic changes, and the sacrifice of both cruciate ligaments, only 3 knees required revision after a minimum 2-year follow-up.[39] Several other reports document the experience with the implant, which eventually came to resemble the total condylar prosthesis.[12, 44–46, 119]

Goldberg and associates[49] at Case Western Reserve reported the results of 70 Freeman-Swanson arthroplasties. They had originally adopted the implant because of its ease of insertion and the fact that the cruciate ligaments were not necessary for the reconstruction. They indicated several important shortcomings with the design: instability, abnormal insertion, loosening, patellofemoral abnormalities, and production of cement debris. Their patients experienced an overall reoperation rate of 28.5%.[49] Burstein[22] has indicated that this type of design may be subject to loosening because of "edge loading," which results from the flat articulation when viewed from the front. Despite its shortcomings, the implant demonstrated that a resurfacing knee arthroplasty was feasible without cruciate ligaments.

HOSPITAL FOR SPECIAL SURGERY PEDIGREE

There was coherent development of ideas and prostheses at The Hospital for Special Surgery, from the late 1960s through the 1980s. There was experience with a variety of implants, from the GUEPAR hinge to the unicondylar replacement. Based on this experience, the surgeons at The Hospital for Special Surgery developed a preference for cruciate-sacrificing and then cruciate-substituting implants.

The era that was dominated by debate over the cruciate ligament produced some remarkable knee replacements. The paper "A Comparison of Four Models of Total Knee Replacement Prostheses" exemplifies the thinking and challenges of the time.[82] In it, Insall, and colleagues from The Hospital for Special Surgery reflected on their experience with the GUEPAR (hinge), the geomedic (conforming resurfacing arthroplasty), the unicondylar, and the duocondylar (a cruciate-retaining arthroplasty without patellofemoral resurfacing) arthroplasties. The prostheses were implanted according to the preference of the surgeon, based on the deformity and type of arthritis in the knee. Ironically, the best results 2 years after surgery were with the GUEPAR hinge, despite the fact that it had been implanted in the worst knees. Fortunately, recognizing the impending problems with hinges, these surgeons endeavored to improve tibial fixation, and deal with patellofemoral pain in condylar designs.

Duocondylar Prosthesis

The duocondylar prosthesis, effectively two unicondylar replacements that have been joined together, was evaluated in 1973 and 1976 by surgeons from The Hospital for Special Surgery. Crediting Gunston with the development of condylar knee replacements that rely on ligaments for stability, Ranawat et al.[129] listed the duocondylar implant among others that modified the polycentric: the geometric, Freeman-Swanson, and UCI. The implant did not provide patellofemoral resurfacing. Twenty arthroplasties had been followed for a short duration by 1973, without failures. By 1976, 94 knees were reported, with pain-free, unlimited walking ability without external aids possible in 27.9% of cases. The shortcomings of the implant were: (1) patellofemoral symptoms; (2) poor fixation of the tibial component; (3) instability of the knee, due either to improper patient selection or improper technique with under- or overcorrection of the deformity; (4) excessive scar tissue formation with soft tissue impingement and limited motion; and (5) hypoesthesia following section of the infrapatellar branch of the saphenous nerve.[129]

Duopatellar Prosthesis

This design group at The Hospital for Special Surgery developed one of each type of prosthesis—the duopatellar[146, 162] (retaining the PCL, yet less conforming than the geomedic) and the total condylar (a cruciate-sacrificing tricompartmental device).[131, 187] The duopatellar prosthesis was effectively a duocondylar replacement[129, 157] with patellofemoral resurfacing. The goal of the design was to retain both cruciate ligaments and improve motion by reducing the conformity between joint surfaces. After an average of 2.2 years there were two failures in 53 knees reported by Inglis and Lane.[72]

The duopatellar prosthesis was used extensively in Boston, where the revision rate for the first 747 duopatellar arthroplasties (some of which probably had two separate tibial components) at 2 to 5 years was 2.8%. By 1982, Richard Scott[143] was able to report on the first 100 duopatellar replacements that used a one-piece flat (front-to-back) all-plastic tibial component. After a minimum of 2 years there had been two reoperations, both to insert a patellar button.[146]

Total Condylar Prosthesis

The total condylar prosthesis was influenced, as acknowledged in the "four-design" paper,[82] by the Freeman-Swanson design, which sacrificed both cruciate ligaments. Its development, including mechanical testing by independent laboratories,[182] has been documented extensively.[131, 182, 186, 187] It established a gold standard for long-term results in knee arthroplasty surgery.

The total condylar prosthesis remained essentially the same through almost 15 years of use.[78, 83] Some versions featured metal-backed tibial components; others had a posterior slope built into the tibia (Fig 58–13). The published results proved exceedingly good, even in the early series, when the implant was available in a limited range of sizes and without full understanding of the techniques for ligament balance. Rudimentary cement technique was in use and the tibial components were made exclusively of polyethylene. Loosening, in the few cases where it occurred, resulted primarily from malalignment.[76, 186] By 10 to 12 years only 6 cases of 112 had required revision surgery.[186] The experience at independent institutions confirmed the results of Insall and Ranawat.[50, 142, 182, 198]

Posterior-Stabilized Prosthesis

The first attempt to create posterior stabilization was the ill-fated total condylar type II prosthesis.[79] Within 1 to 2½ years, 4 of 105 knees had loosened, presumably because of a hyperextension stop in the prosthesis. The design was abandoned. While the results with the total condylar prosthesis had been good, there was concern that motion was limited because femoral rollback was not duplicated once the PCL had been sectioned. The spine and cam mechanism was also expected to prevent posterior tibial dislocation, something that had occurred in knees with prior patellectomy. A spine and cam mechanism was successfully added to the total condylar prosthesis by 1978,[77, 147, 179, 184] creating the posterior-stabilized knee prosthesis (Fig 58–14). It conferred no varus-valgus stability in any position of flexion and did not even engage until about 70 degrees of flexion. The entire experience with the Insall-Burstein posterior-stabilized knee prosthesis has been documented, including literature from the developers of the implant and independent surgeons.[147, 179] Most recently, extended follow-up has demonstrated that while the spine and cam mechanism stabilizes the knee as intended, it does not result in loosening.[148, 160]

Stabilocondylar Prosthesis

The stabilocondylar prosthesis was developed after the total condylar, as a device that would stabilize the knee that lacked collateral ligaments.[189] This was achieved with a relatively large central post on the tibial component that fit into an intercondylar notch in the femoral component. By design it gave varus-valgus as well as anteroposterior stability. The early prototypes included a thin-diameter retaining pin, eventually discarded, to prevent the components from distracting (Fig 58–15). Without the pin, this implant evolved into what is recognized as the total condylar III prosthesis. This prosthesis has been remarkably effective in the unstable knee in low-demand patients. Fixation was originally achieved with fully cemented, small-diameter, intramedullary stems.[139] The constrained condylar implant, very similar to the total condylar III, became a modular device with press-fitted medullary stems for fixation (Fig 58–16).

Parallel Evolution

As the principles of knee arthroplasty became apparent, most designs matured along similar lines. Freeman's cruciate-sacrificing ICLH evolved dramatically through several stages until it bore a strong resemblance to the tricompartmental total condylar.[45] Others shared the conviction that the roller in a trough was unstable to medial and lateral translational forces, and that an intercondylar eminence was required in knee arthroplasty.[36] A parallel evolution occurred with the geomedic,[28] which ran through four stages (Mark I–IV) that culminated in the anametric design[99] (Fig 58–17).

Contemporary Cruciate-Retaining Prostheses

Cruciate Condylar Prosthesis

Meanwhile, the duopatellar prosthesis had led to the development of the cruciate condylar prosthetic knee. It was in many ways similar to the total con-

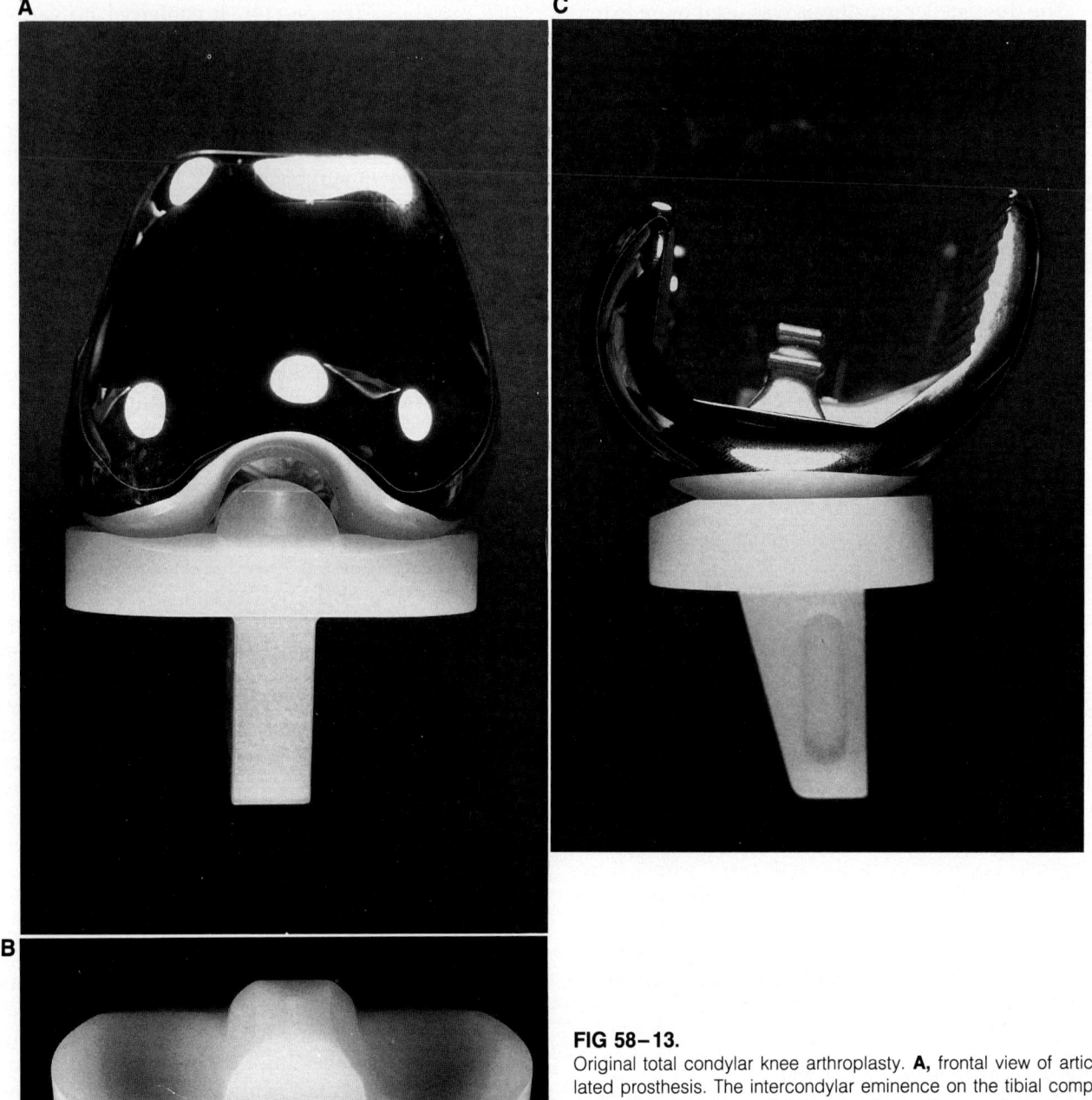

FIG 58–13.
Original total condylar knee arthroplasty. **A,** frontal view of articulated prosthesis. The intercondylar eminence on the tibial component was added for medial lateral stability. The rounded condyles, when viewed from the front, establish a contact in the middle of the hemiplateau eliminating the effect of "edge loading." **B,** the all-polyethylene tibial component, showing the dished articular surface, which is less conforming than the geomedic. This is the "uphill" principle of ligament stability. As the femoral condyles try to escape from the plateau, they must ride uphill, tightening the collateral ligaments. **C,** lateral view showing the decreasing curvature of the posterior articular surface and the keel which was credited with low loosening rates at 10 years in implants with valgus alignment. (From Vince KG, Insall JN: The total condylar knee arthroplasty. In Laskin RS, editor: *Total knee arthroplasty,* New York, 1991, Springer-Verlag. Used by permission.)

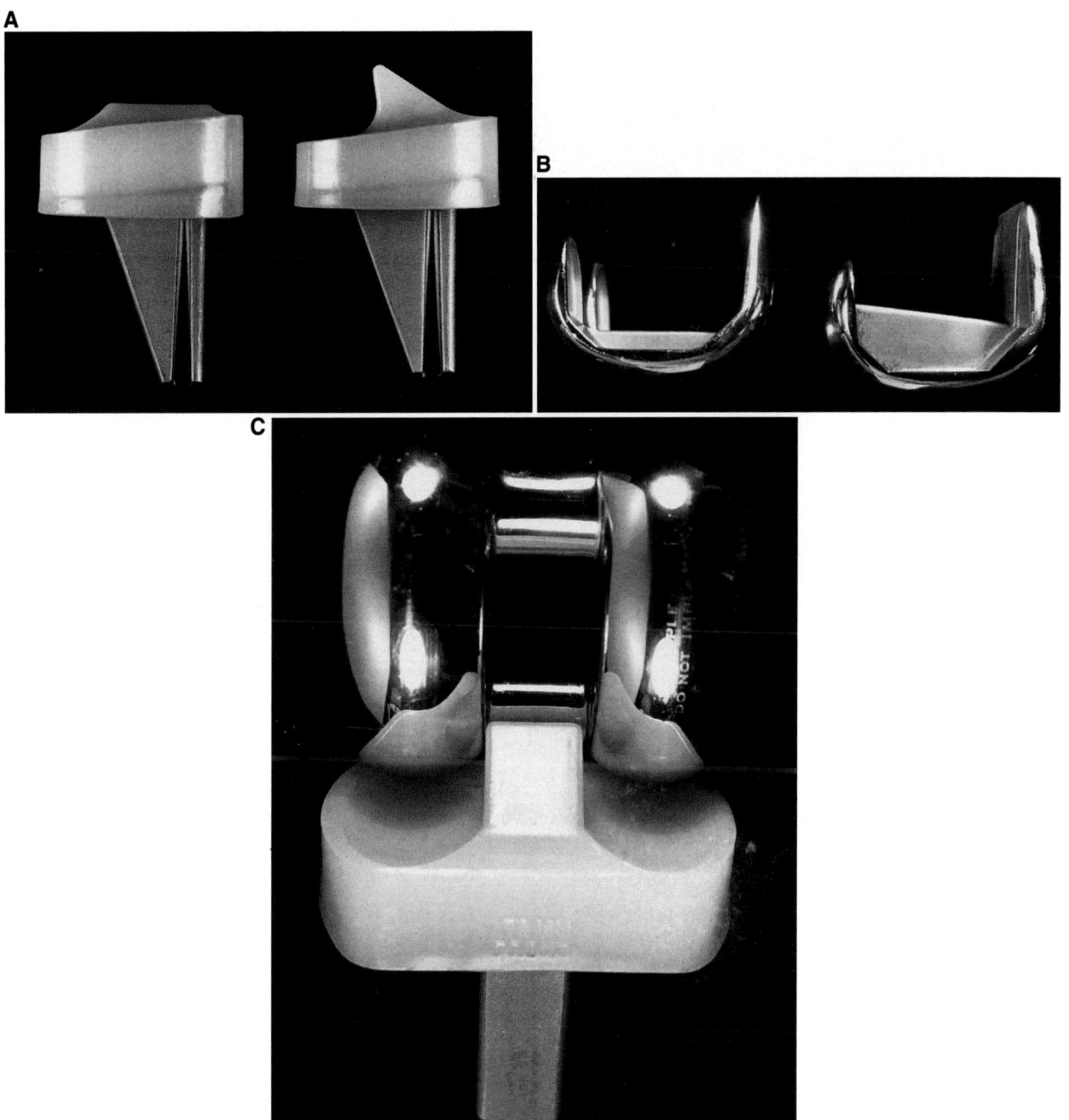

FIG 58-14.
The posterior stabilized knee arthroplasty. **A,** *left,* a metal-backed total condylar knee prosthesis. *Right,* a spine has been added to the total condylar tibial component creating the posterior stabilized prosthesis. **B,** *left,* the total condylar femoral component viewed from the side. *Right,* the larger housing on the posterior-stabilized femoral component accommodates a cam that articulates with the tibial spine. **C,** articulated, flexed posterior-stabilized knee arthroplasty viewed from the front. The femoral cam engages the tibial spine in this position only. The mechanism confers no varus or valgus stability.

dylar but designed for retention of the PCL. Ritter et al. implanted cruciate condylar knee prostheses and reported excellent function and durability at 5[137] and 10 years.[138] Using revision surgery as a criterion for failure, survivorship analysis predicted a 94.7% success rate at 10 years. If two other criteria, radiolucencies in all zones exceeding 2-mm thickness or pain and a knee score of less than 20 points, were included, the success rate dropped to 81%.

The 5-year results were confirmed by Bourne et

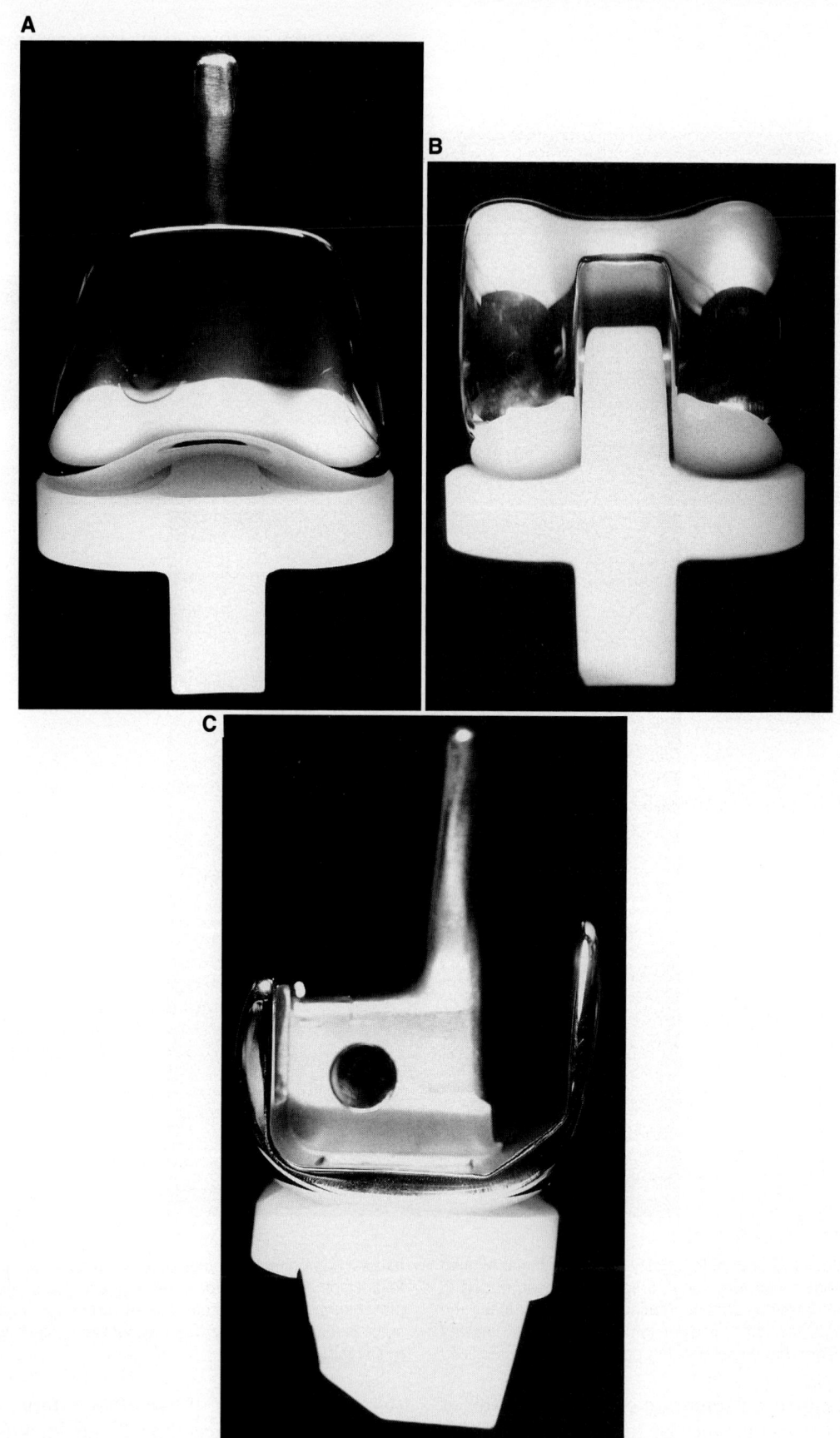

FIG 58–15.
Stabilocondylar knee arthroplasty. **A,** frontal view of articulated prosthesis. The joint geometry resembles the total condylar prosthesis. **B,** the flexed arthroplasty viewed from the front shows the prominent tibial spine that fits between the femoral condyles, conferring varus-valgus and anteroposterior stability. **C,** side view showing the pin that was originally used in some prototypes to prevent the components from disarticulating.

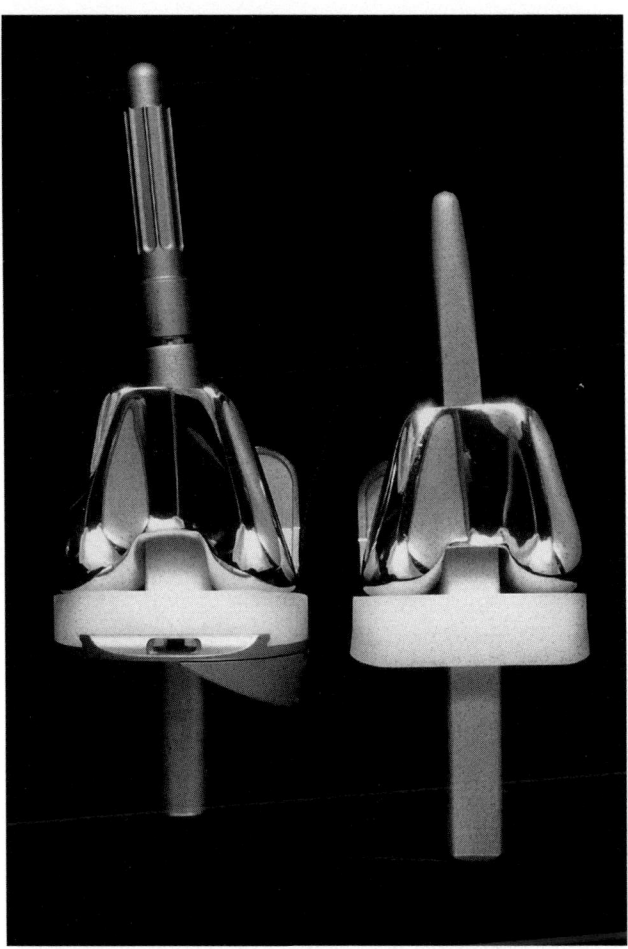

FIG 58–16.
Nonlinked constrained knee arthroplasty. Both of these devices gain varus-valgus stability by the larger tibial spine fitting into the large intercondylar housing in the femoral component. *Left,* a contemporary modular constrained condylar implant. *Right,* a conventional total condylar III implant with fixed, small-diameter stems, which were cemented into the medullary canal.

al. at the Mayo Clinic. Having studied 189 consecutive PCL condylar knee arthroplasties at 5 years, they had a revision rate of 1.6% and a reoperation rate of 3.7%.[19]

Kinematic Prosthesis

Walker left New York for Boston and worked with surgeons dedicated to the preservation of the PCL. The Kinematic design evolved from the duopatellar.[37] Wright and associates,[203] in 1990, reported on 192 kinematic arthroplasties at 5 to 9 years after surgery. As with the total condylar prosthesis, these results were excellent. Complications included loose patellar components in five knees, one fracture of the tibial tray with loosening of the patellar component, one fracture of the patellar component, and one dislocation of the patellar component.[202]

Posterior Cruciate Ligament Controversy: Update

Some, but not all, of the original arguments on both sides of the PCL debate remain pertinent[6, 38, 43, 156] (Table 58–1). For example, the increase in coverage of the tibial plateau that is possible when the posterior cutout for the PCL on the tibial component is eliminated, has proved of no consequence. Considering surgical technique, the PCL does not have to be sacrificed to fully expose the knee. Much of the original debate on the PCL proved nonsubstantive: both designs yielded superb results because collateral ligament balance and alignment proved to be so much more important.

Fred Ewald summarized the controversy in his 1991 presidential address to the Knee Society with a broad comparison of the published literature.[35] His synthesis of the literature indicates how the sundry arguments have been reduced to two concerns: (1) conformity in cruciate-sacrificing designs may lead to loosening (not yet demonstrated in 10- to 15-year follow-ups); (2) flatter (and often thinner) tibial components of the cruciate-retaining prostheses may fail by wear and breakage.[35]

THE FUTURE: CONVERGENCE OF IDEAS?

Three Principles of Knee Arthroplasty

Where did the debate on the PCL lead, beyond providing lively discussion for the better part of two de-

TABLE 58–1.
Posterior Cruciate Ligament Debate: The Original Arguments

Cruciate retention: Anatomic Laws, Duocondylar
Advantages
  Keep normal anatomy
  Recoil from hinges and constraint
  Need ligament to take shear
  Need femoral rollback for motion
  Cruciates assist collaterals for varus-valgus stability
Disadvantages
  Seesaw effect causing rocking
  Ligament deficiency results in instability
  Increased wear from increased point contact
Cruciate Sacrifice: Mechanical Laws, Total Condylar
Advantages
  Fixation improved by full coverage
  Easier to correct deformity
  Simpler technique
  Easier exposure (cement removal)
  Improved mobility for stiff knee
Disadvantages
  Posterior subluxation if gaps not balanced
  Increased bone-cement interface stress
  Limited flexion

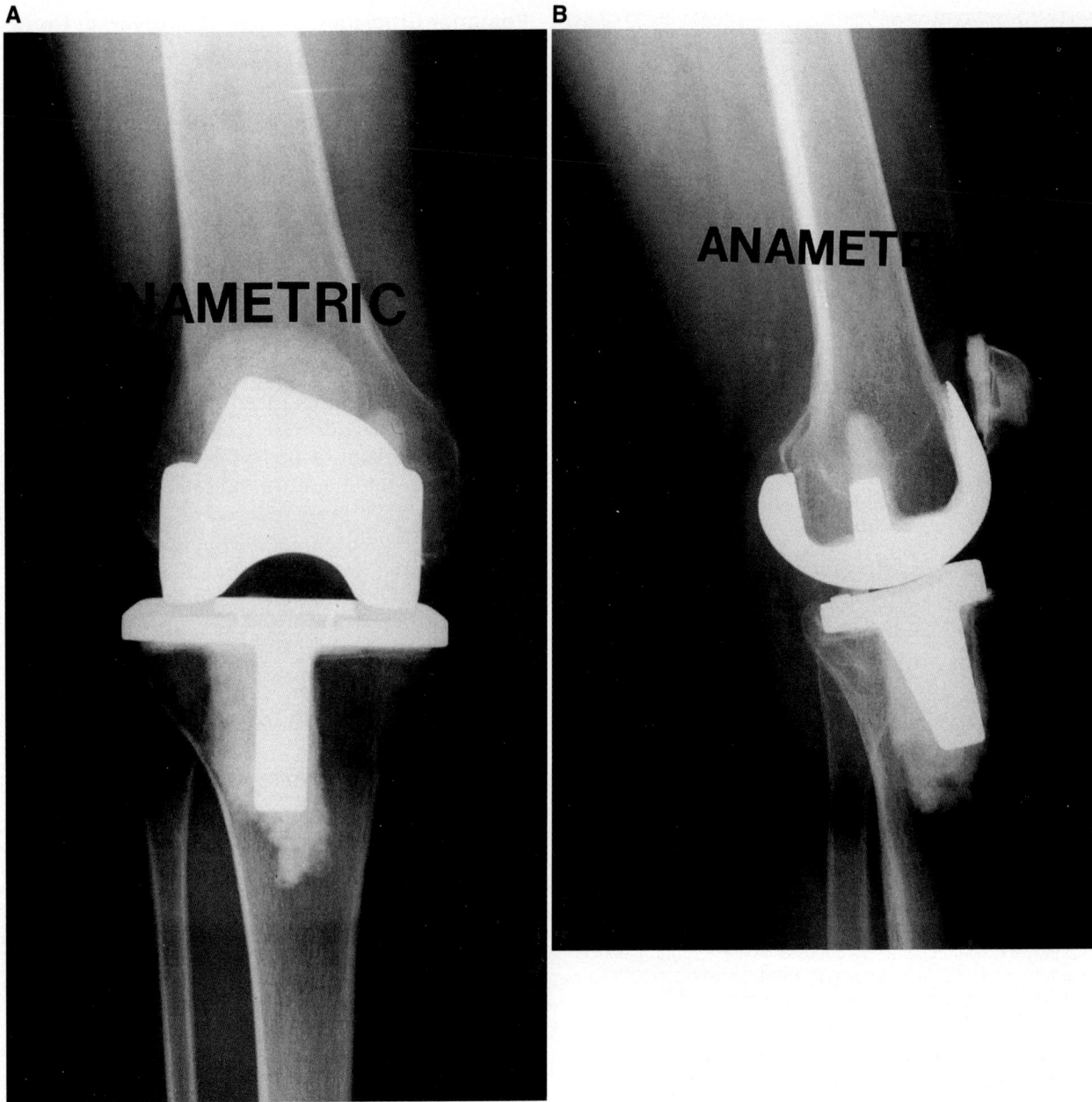

FIG 58–17.
Anametric total knee replacement. **A,** anteroposterior radiograph showing tricompartmental bicondylar arthroplasty with provisions for patellofemoral resurfacing. A metal-backed tibial tray is cemented in place. **B,** lateral radiograph showing cemented all-polyethylene patellar component and surface geometry resembling total condylar arthroplasty.

cades? Three principles define the central problems of knee arthroplasty surgery: fixation, kinematics, and wear.[180, 181] The corresponding design problems in total knee replacement are (1) to preserve proximal tibia, (2) maintain the joint line, and (3) maintain a minimum of polyethylene thickness.

Fixation: Preserving Proximal Tibial Bone
This was one of the first, widely accepted principles in the debate on tibial component loosening. The subchondral bone is regarded as the strongest in the proximal tibia. Proceeding distally, the size and surface area of the tibia diminish, as does its strength. The data come from the laboratory[68–70, 158] and common sense. No good clinical study has shown a higher incidence of tibial component loosening when additional bone is resected, mainly because excessive resection and a varus tibial cut are difficult variables to separate.

Kinematics: Maintaining the Level of the Joint Line

The level of the joint line must be maintained within certain tolerances if the arthroplasty is to function well. A knee that bends at a higher level than normal has collateral[110] and cruciate ligaments that no longer function properly. The knee will be stiff. While cruciate sacrifice increases the latitude for repositioning the joint line,[185] patellar function will eventually be compromised.

Wear: Maintaining Minimal Polyethylene Thickness

Wear has long been a concern in the design of total joint replacements.[188, 204] Thin components, especially those made of polyethylene, are susceptible to wear and breakage. This was predicted by engineers[13, 14] and confirmed with both Marmor modular[104–109] and UCI arthroplasties.[32, 34, 58, 195]

These problems are intimately related. If proximal tibial bone is to be preserved, then either a thinner, vulnerable tibial component will be required, or a thicker component will require resection of additional bone. When the bone comes off the distal femur, the joint line is elevated. If the distal femur and joint line are maintained, then either more bone has to be removed from the proximal tibia or a thinner component is necessary. Only two of three conditions can be satisfied. How one resolves this triad distinguishes those who favor an anatomic strategy from those with a mechanical philosophy. The more anatomically oriented, cruciate-retaining prostheses have recently experienced problems related to the limits of thin polyethylene.

New Arguments and Data

As new arguments and data emerge, much of the old PCL debate becomes irrelevant. Perhaps unwittingly, surgeons who have traditionally been on different sides of the PCL debate are expressing compatible ideas.

Motion and the Posterior Cruciate Ligament

Without a PCL, there could be no rollback and without rollback, motion would inevitably be limited. Was not the total condylar prosthesis limited to a mean flexion of 95 degrees?[81, 84, 182, 186] Not so simple. The original total condylar, produced with one size of femoral component and only three tibial thicknesses, was implanted without instruments and prior to the advent of alignment and ligament release techniques. It did flex poorly. The total condylar of the 1980s, with modern techniques and instruments, a full complement of implant sizes, and contemporary physical therapy, yielded much better results—an average of 109 degrees in one study.[128]

The most flexion reported for any total knee arthroplasty comes from Yoshino and Shoji.[205] They used a device modeled on the total condylar prosthesis, with provisions for cruciate retention. In their patients, however, they sacrificed the PCL and observed an average motion of 129 degrees.[205] They attributed these results to restoring the suprapatellar pouch and accurately balancing the flexion and extension gap tension.[153]

Loosening

Loosening is not increased after cruciate sacrifice.[160] Recent data from the sophisticated radiographic technique called Roentgen stereogrammetry (RSA) indicate that rollback in a cruciate-*retaining* device may be responsible for increased micromotion as the result of eccentric loads on the tibia.[73, 140] By alternately loading the plateau anteriorly and then posteriorly, the tibial component may cyclically tilt and loosen. While full femoral rollback in cruciate-retaining arthroplasties was once considered desirable, many surgeons now prefer that it be limited because of tilting and the wear that occurs on the thin posterior tibial surface.

While rollback occurs in a posterior stabilized implant, the joint reaction force that is applied to the posterior plateau is balanced by the anteriorly directed vector of the femoral cam against the tibial spine. This has been the explanation for no increased rate of loosening over the total condylar design despite the spine and cam mechanism.[22, 77, 148, 160, 179, 183]

Correction of Deformity

It is easier to correct severe deformity if you sacrifice the PCL. Laskin et al.,[96] with an extensive experience of both cruciate-retaining and -sacrificing designs, concluded that they could more reliably correct flexion contractures and varus deformities exceeding 15 degrees after sacrificing and substituting for the PCL. The results in milder deformities were not different.

More Normal Knee

Just what does this mean? The gait laboratory data comparing cruciate retention and sacrifice in knee arthroplasty make dense reading. The techniques of gait analysis and the interpretation of data are difficult to master. Because of the difficulty in performing the studies, there are generally few experimental subjects. Some studies have concluded that cruciate retention yields knees that work and feel more like the normal knee. This makes sense, but is it truly for mechanical reasons? Or is it because the PCL contributes proprioception to the joint?[6, 38]

Is the Spine and Cam Mechanism Always Necessary?

Sometimes the posterior-stabilized prosthesis seems like too much implant for the relatively nondeformed knee. There are reasons to avoid a posterior-stabilized prosthesis in relatively undeformed knees. Posterior-stabilized arthroplasties require removal of a relatively large piece of bone from between the femoral condyles. It is difficult to include a spine and cam mechanism without compromising the patellofemoral articulation. The leading edge of the femoral trochlea must end rather sharply so as not to impinge on the tibial spine, and this edge has been the site where scar tissue on the deep surface of the quadriceps tendon catches and "clunks."[65] In this trend of convergence, some surgeons select implants based on the pathologic changes at hand, not because of a uniform commitment to one way of dealing with the PCL. The biologic philosophy becomes appealing, even to mechanically minded surgeons, in the appropriate setting.

Posterior Cruciate Ligament in Osteoarthritis

Normal tension of the PCL, owing to arthritic scarring or because the articular geometry of the implant differs from normal anatomy, can be difficult to reproduce at arthroplasty. Using strain gauges intraoperatively, Corces and colleagues[27] quantified this difficulty, thinking that it was nearly impossible to produce an arthroplasty with tension in the PCL comparable to what existed prior to surgery. If the ligament remains tight, the arthroplasty cannot be expected to flex fully and reproduce the function that the surgeon and patient expect.[136]

Alexiades and colleagues[5] contend that the PCL is abnormal in arthritis. They examined PCLs that had been excised at surgery, demonstrating distinct and not surprising degenerative changes. The study lacked controls (which is the basis for new work in progress) and is countered by the challenge that the medial collateral ligament is abnormal in the arthritic varus knee and yet remains important to good function even if released.

The surgical technique that has become common in PCL-retaining knee arthroplasties is to lengthen, release, or "recess" the ligament.[136] This would seem to further alter the mechanics of the cruciate system from the normal knee, rendering the arthroplasty kinematically more similar to the total condylar, cruciate-sacrificing design.

Many "cruciate-retaining" knee systems have introduced polyethylene inserts with increased conformity to cope with an incompetent or released PCL. These condylar knee arthroplasties, without posterior stabilization, function like the original total condylar prosthesis—a cruciate-sacrificing arthroplasty that depended on slightly increased conformity for stability.

Destructive Wear

Reenter the problem of destructive wear. Noncemented, porous ingrowth technology was introduced amid conviction by some that any conformity in the tibial femoral articulation would jeopardize the interface. Wanting to maximize initial fixation and heighten the probability of bone ingrowth, flat tibial components were favored. If we review the three principles (see above), we see that this approach was bound to create problems. Preservation of strong proximal tibial bone remained important. The cruciate ligament was integral to the design, and the level of the joint line had to be preserved. The tibial components that had already been made flat were now also made thin. Metal backing did not render thin polyethylene durable.

Is there a way to have conformity, for superior wear characteristics with full mobility, to satisfy the kinematic requirements of a retained PCL? This is the proposition of the mobile bearing implants. The tibiofemoral and patellofemoral articulations conform, while the meniscal (or patellar) bearing implant moves with respect to the base plate.[21, 51-53, 118] It is, however, possible for these bearings to dislocate[17] and the theoretical problem of wear debris originating from the interface between bearing and base plate has not been resolved.

Wear has become the prime issue in knee arthroplasty surgery, first with the failure of metal-backed patellar buttons, and then with destructive wear complicating a large series of uncemented tibial inserts.[204] The magnitude of the problem surpasses what Ewald hinted at in 1991.

CONCLUSION

Hinges and McKeevers, geomedics and polycentrics, total condylars and duopatellars, posterior-stabilized and kinematic arthroplasties—these implants represent the extremes of debates that have waged for decades and they confirm the dichotomy between mechanical and biologic thinking. As understanding becomes more complete, opinions are clearly converging.

The challenge to duplicate with manufactured

parts the relationship between articular geometry and ligamentous stability that is programmed genetically and that is structurally evident at 7 weeks' gestation is prodigious.[120] To duplicate in less than 2 hours of surgery the relationship between parts that evolves in utero and through childhood and adolescence is daunting. Resolving fixation, kinematics, and wear is not simple. Nor is it completely biologic or mechanical.

REFERENCES

1. Accardo NJ Jr. Noiles knee replacement procedure. A six year experience, *Orthop Trans* 6:436–437, 1982.
2. Accardo NJ, et al. Noiles total knee replacement procedure, *Orthopedics* 2:37–45, 1979.
3. Aglietti P, et al: A new patellar prosthesis, *Clin Orthop* 107:175–187, 1975.
4. Albee FH: Original features in arthroplasty of the knee with improved prognosis, *Surg Gynecol Obstet* 47:312, 1928.
5. Alexiades M, et al: A histologic study of the posterior cruciate ligament in the arthritic knee, *Am J Knee Surg* 2:153–159, 1989.
6. Andriacchi TP, Galante JO: Retention of the posterior cruciate in total knee arthroplasty, *J Arthroplasty* (suppl)S13–S19, 1988.
7. Arden GP: Total knee replacement, *Clin Orthop* 94:92–103, 1973.
8. Aufranc OE, Jones WN: Mold arthroplasty of the knee (abstract). *J Bone Joint Surg [Am]* 40:1431, 1958.
9. Baer WS: Arthroplasty with the aid of animal membrane, *Am J Orthop Surg* 16:1–29, 171–199, 1918.
10. Bain AM: Replacement of the knee joint with the Walldius prosthesis using cement fixation, *Clin Orthop* 94:65–71, 1973.
11. Bargar WL, Cracchiolo A III, Amstutz HC: Results with the constrained total knee prosthesis in treating severely disabled patients and patients with failed total knee replacements, *J Bone J Surg [Am]* 62:504–514, 1980.
12. Bargren JH, et al: ICLH: knee. Two- to four-year review, *Clin Orthop* 120:65, 1976.
13. Bartel DL, Bicknell VL, Wright TM: The effect of conformity, thickness and material on stresses in ultra-high molecular weight components for total joint replacement, *J Bone J Surg [Am]* 68:1041–1051, 1986.
14. Bartel DL, et al: The effect of conformity and plastic thickness on contact stresses in metal-backed plastic implants, *J Biomech Eng* 107:193–199, 1985.
15. Barrett WP, Scott RD: Revision of failed unicondylar unicompartmental knee arthroplasty, *J Bone Joint Surg [Am]* 69:1328–1335, 1987.
16. Bernasek TL, Rand JA, Bryan RS: Unicompartmental porous coated anatomic total knee arthroplasty, *Clin Orthop* 236:52–59, 1988.
17. Bert JM: Dislocation/subluxation of meniscal bearing elements after New Jersey low-contact stress total knee arthroplasty, *Clin Orthop* 254:211–215, 1990.
18. Blazina M, et al: Patellofemoral replacement, *Clin Orthop* 144:98–102, 1979.
19. Bourne MH, Rand JA, Ilstrup DM: Posterior cruciate condylar total knee arthroplasty: Five year results, *Clin Orthop* 234:129–136, 1988.
20. Brown JE, McGaw WH, Shaw DT. Use of cutis as an interposing membrane in arthroplasty of the knee, *J Bone Joint Surg* 40:1003, 1958.
21. Buechal FF, Pappas MJ: Long term survivorship analysis of cruciate-sparing versus cruciate sacrificing knee prostheses using meniscal bearing implants, *Clin Orthop* 260:162–169, 1990.
22. Burstein AH: Biomechanics of the knee. In Insall JN, editor: *Surgery of the knee*, New York, 1984, Churchill Livingstone, p 21.
23. Campbell WC: Arthroplasty of the knee: Report of cases, *Am J Orthop Surg* 19:430–434, 1921.
24. Campbell WC: Femoral mold arthroplasty, *Am J Surg* 47:639, 1940.
25. Cloutier JM: Results of total knee arthroplasty with a non-constrained prosthesis, *J Bone Joint Surg [Am]* 65:7, 1983.
26. Cloutier JM: Long term results after nonconstrained total knee arthroplasty, *Clin Orthop* 273:63–65, 1991.
27. Corces A, Lotke PA, Williams JL. Strain characteristics of the posterior cruciate ligament in total knee replacement, *Orthop Trans* 13:527, 1989.
28. Coventry MB: Two-part total knee arthroplasty: Evolution and present status, *Clin Orthop* 145:29–36, 1979.
29. Cracchiolo A, et al: A prospective comparative clinical analysis of the first generation knee, *Orthopedics* 145:37–46, 1979.
30. Deburge A, GUEPAR: GUEPAR hinge prosthesis: Complications and results with two years' follow-up, *Clin Orthop* 120:47–53, 1976.
31. Deburge A, et al: Current status of a hinge prosthesis (GUEPAR), *Clin Orthop* 145:91–93, 1979.
32. Ducheyne P, Kagan A, Lacey JA: Failure of total knee arthroplasty due to loosening and deformation of the tibial component, *J Bone Joint Surg [Am]* 60:384–391, 1978.
33. Emerson RH, Potter T: The use of the McKeever metallic hemiarthroplasty for unicompartmental arthritis, *J Bone Joint Surg [Am]* 67:208–212, 1985.
34. Evanski PM, et al: UCI knee replacement, *Clin Orthop* 120:33–38, 1976.
35. Ewald FC: The second decade, *Am J Knee Surg* 4:107–109, 1991.
36. Ewald FC, et al: The importance of intercondylar stability in knee arthroplasty, *J Bone Joint Surg [Am]* 57:1033, 1975.
37. Ewald FC, et al: Kinematic total knee replacement, *J Bone Joint Surg [Am]* 66:1032–1040, 1984.
38. Freeman MAR, Railton GT: Should the posterior cruciate ligament be retained or resected in condylar

nonmeniscal knee arthroplasty?, *J Arthroplasty* (suppl) S3–S12, 1988.
39. Freeman MAR, Sculco T, Todd RC: Replacement of the severely damaged arthritic knee by the ICLH (Freeman-Swanson arthroplasty), *J Bone Joint Surg [Br]* 59:64–71, 1977.
40. Freeman MAR, Swanson SAV, Heath JC: Study of the wear of particles produced from cobalt-chromium molybdenum manganese total joint replacement, *Ann Rheum Dis* 29(suppl):28, 1969.
41. Freeman MAR, Swanson SAV, Todd RC: Total replacement of the knee using the Freeman-Swanson knee prosthesis, *Clin Orthop* 94:153–170, 1973.
42. Freeman MAR, Swanson SAV, Zahin A: Total replacement of the knee using a metal-polyethylene two-part prosthesis, *Proc R Soc Med* 65:374, 1972.
43. Freeman MAR, et al: Excision of the cruciate ligaments in total knee replacement, *Clin Orthop* 126:209–212, 1977.
44. Freeman MAR, et al: ICLH arthroplasty of the knee, 1968–1977. *J Bone Joint Surg [Br]* 60B:339–344, 1978.
45. Freeman MAR, et al: Cementless fixation of ICLH tibial component, *Orthop Clin North Am* 13:141–145, 1982.
46. Freeman MAR, et al: Knee arthroplasty at the London Hospital: 1975–1984, *Clin Orthop* 205:12–20, 1986.
47. Freeman PA: Walldius arthroplasty: A review of 80 cases, *Clin Orthop* 94:85–91, 1973.
48. Gluck T: Referat uber dic, *Arch Klinische* 41:186, 1891.
49. Goldberg VM, Henderson BT: The Freeman-Swanson ICLH total knee arthroplasty. Complications and problems, *J Bone Joint Surg [Am]* 62:1338–1344, 1980.
50. Goldberg VM, et al: Use of a total condylar knee prosthesis for treatment of osteoarthritis and rheumatoid arthritis, *J Bone Joint Surg [Am]* 70:802–811, 1988.
51. Goodfellow J, O'Connor J: The mechanics of the knee and prosthesis design, *J Bone Joint Surg [Br]* 60:358–369, 1978.
52. Goodfellow J, O'Connor J: Clinical results of the Oxford knee. Surface arthroplasty of the tibiofemoral joint with a meniscal bearing prosthesis, *Clin Orthop* 205:21–42, 1986.
53. Goodfellow J, O'Connor J, Perry N: Fixation of the tibial components of the Oxford knee, *Orthop Clin North Am* 13:65–87, 1982.
54. Gunston FH: Polycentric knee arthroplasty: Prosthetic simulation of normal knee movement, *J Bone Joint Surg [Br]* 52:272–277, 1971.
55. Haberman ET, Deutsch SD, Rovere GD: Knee arthroplasty with the use of the Walldius total knee prosthesis, *Clin Orthop* 94:72–84, 1973.
56. Haines JF, Noble J: Revision arthroplasty of the knee: Two problem knees, *J R Coll Surg Edinb* 31:255–257, 1986.
57. Hanslik L: First experience on knee joint replacement using the young hinged prosthesis combined with a modification on the McKeever patella prosthesis, *Clin Orthop* 94:115, 1973.
58. Hamilton LR: UCI total knee replacement. A follow-up study, *J Bone Joint Surg [Am]* 64:740–744, 1982.
59. Helferich: Ein neues Operation: Verfahren zur Heilung der knöchern Kiefergelenksankylose, *Arch Klin Chir* 48:864, 1894.
60. Henderson ED, Peterson CA: Experience with the use of the MacIntosh prosthesis in knees of patients with rheumatoid arthritis. *South Med J* 62:1311–1315, 1969.
61. Henderson MS: What are the real results of arthroplasty? *Am J Orthop Surg* 16:30–33, 1918.
62. Herbert JJ, Herbert AH: A new total knee prosthesis, *Clin Orthop* 94:202–210, 1973.
63. Holt EP Jr: Use of the Noiles knee prosthesis in advanced disease, *Orthop Trans* 5:467, 1981.
64. Hood RW, et al: Retrieval analysis of 70 total condylar knee prostheses, *Orthop Trans* 5:319, 1981.
65. Hozack WJ, et al: The patellar clunk syndrome. A complication of posterior stabilized total knee arthroplasty, *Clin Orthop* 241:203–208, 1989.
66. Hui FC, Fitzgerald RH Jr: Hinged total knee arthroplasty, *J Bone Joint Surg [Am]* 62:513–519, 1980.
67. Hunter JA, et al: The geometric knee replacement in polyarthritis, *J Bone Joint Surg [Br]* 64:95–98, 1982.
68. Hvid I: Mechanical strength of trabecular bone at the knee, *Dan Med Bull* 35:345–369, 1988.
69. Hvid I: Trabecular bone strength at the knee, *Clin Orthop* 227:210–221, 1988.
70. Hvid I, Hansen SL: Trabecular bone strength patterns at the proximal tibial epiphysis, *J Orthop Res* 3:464, 1985.
71. Ilstrup DM, Coventry MB, Skolnick MD: A statistical evaluation of geometric total knee arthroplasties, *Clin Orthop* 120:27–31, 1976.
72. Inglis AE, Lane LB: Total knee replacement using the duo-patella prosthesis, *Orthop Trans* 2:202, 1978.
73. Insall JN: Total knee replacement. In Insall JN (ed): *Surgery of the knee,* New York, 1984, Churchill Livingstone, pp 587–696.
74. Insall JN, Aglietti P: A five to seven year follow-up of unicondylar arthroplasty, *J Bone Joint Surg [Am]* 62:1329–1337, 1980.
75. Insall JN, Dethmers DA: Revision of total knee arthroplasty, *Clin Orthop* 170:123–130, 1982.
76. Insall JN, Kelly M: The total condylar prosthesis, *Clin Orthop* 205:43–48, 1985.
77. Insall JN, Lachiewicz PF, Burstein AH: The posterior stabilized condylar prosthesis: A modification of the total condylar design, *J Bone Joint Surg [Am]* 64:1317, 1982.
78. Insall JN, Scott WN, Ranawat CS: The total condylar knee prosthesis, *J Bone Joint Surg [Am]* 61:173–180, 1979.
79. Insall JN, Tria AJ: The total condylar prosthesis type II, *Orthop Trans* 4:300, 1980.
80. Insall JN, Tria AJ, Aglietti P: Resurfacing of the patella, *J Bone Joint Surg [Am]* 62:933–936, 1980.

81. Insall JN, Tria AJ, Scott WN: The total condylar knee prosthesis: The first five years, *Clin Orthop* 145:68-77, 1979.
82. Insall JN, et al: A comparison of four models of total knee replacement prostheses, *J Bone Joint Surg [Am]* 58:754, 1976.
83. Insall JN, et al: Total condylar knee replacement. Preliminary report, *Clin Orthop* 120:149, 1976.
84. Insall JN, et al: The total condylar knee prosthesis in gonarthrosis, *J Bone Joint Surg [Am]* 65:619-628, 1983.
85. Jackson JP, Elson RA: Evaluation of the Walldius and other prostheses for knee arthroplasty, *Clin Orthop* 94:104-114, 1973.
86. Jones EC, et al: GUEPAR knee arthroplasty results and late complications, *Clin Orthop* 140:145-152, 1979.
87. Jones GB: Total knee replacement—The Walldius hinge, *Clin Orthop* 94:50-57, 1973.
88. Jones WN: Mold arthroplasty of the knee joint, *Clin Orthop* 66:82-89, 1969.
89. Jones WN, Aufranc OE, Kermond WL: Mold arthroplasty of the knee, *J Bone Joint Surg [Am]* 49:1022, 1967.
90. Judet J, et al: Essais de prosthèses ostéoarticulaire, *Presse Med* 55:302, 1947.
91. Kaufer H, Matthews LS: The spherocentric knee, *Clin Orthop* 145:110-116, 1979.
92. Koga Y, Kono S, Mabuchi K: A long term follow-up of resection interposition arthroplasty of the knee using chromicised fascia lata, *Int Orthop* 12:9-15, 1988.
93. Kuhns JG: Nylon membrane arthroplasty of the knee in chronic arthritis, *J Bone Joint Surg* 46:448, 1964.
94. Laskin RS: Modular total knee-replacement arthroplasty, *J Bone Joint Surg [Am]* 58:766-772, 1976.
95. Laskin RS: Unicompartmental tibiofemoral resurfacing arthroplasty, *J Bone Joint Surg [Am]* 60:182-185, 1978.
96. Laskin RS, et al: The posterior stabilized total knee prosthesis in the knee with a severe fixed deformity, *Am J Knee Surg* 1:199-203, 1989.
97. Lewallen DG, Bryan RS, Peterson LFA: Polycentric total knee arthroplasty: A ten year follow-up study, *J Bone Joint Surg [Am]* 66:1211-1218, 1984.
98. Lotke PA, Ecker ML: Influence of positioning of prosthesis in total knee replacement, *J Bone Joint Surg [Am]* 59:77-79, 1977.
99. Ma SM, Finerman GAM: Anametric total knee arthroplasty, *Orthop Clin North Am* 13:45-54, 1982.
100. MacAusland WR: Total joint replacement of the knee joint by a prosthesis, *Surg Gynecol Obstet* 104:579-583, 1956.
101. MacIntosh DL: Arthroplasty of the knee in rheumatoid arthritis (abstract), *J Bone Joint Surg* 48:179, 1966.
102. MacIntosh DL: Arthroplasty of the knee in rheumatoid arthritis using the hemiarthroplasty prosthesis. In Chapcal G, editor: *Synovectomy and arthroplasty in rheumatoid arthritis (Second International Symposium Jan 27-29, 1967),* Stuttgart, 1967, Georg Thieme, p 131.
103. Majnoni d'Intignano JM: Articulations totales en résine acrylique, *Rev Chir Orthop Paris* 36:535, 1950.
104. Marmor L: The modular knee, *Clin Orthop* 97:242, 1973.
105. Marmor L: The modular (Marmor) knee: Case report with a minimum follow-up of 2 years, *Clin Orthop* 120:86-94, 1976.
106. Marmor L: Marmor modular knee in unicompartmental disease, *J Bone Joint Surg [Am]* 61:347-353, 1979.
107. Marmor L: The Marmor knee replacement, *Orthop Clin North Am* 13:55-65, 1982.
108. Marmor L: Unicompartment and total knee replacement, *Clin Orthop* 192:75-81, 1985.
109. Marmor L: Unicompartmental arthroplasty of the knee with a minimum ten year follow-up period, *Clin Orthop* 228:171-177, 1988.
110. Matsen FA, Laskin RS, Sidles: The effect of joint line position in total knee replacement, 54th Annual Meeting of the American Academy of Orthopaedic Surgeons, San Francisco, 22, 1987.
111. Matthews LS, Kaufer H: The spherocentric knee: A perspective on seven years of clinical experience, *Orthop Clin North Am* 13:173-186, 1982.
112. Matthews LS, Sonstegard DA, Kaufer H: The spherocentric knee, *Clin Orthop* 94:234-241, 1973.
113. Matthews LS, et al: Spherocentric arthroplasty of the knee: Long term and final follow-up evaluation, *Clin Orthop* 205:58-66, 1986.
114. Mazas FB, GUEPAR: GUEPAR total knee prosthesis, *Clin Orthop* 94:211-221, 1973.
115. McKeever DC: Patellar prosthesis, *J Bone Joint Surg [Am]* 37:1074-1084, 1955.
116. McKeever DC: Tibial plateau prosthesis, *Clin Orthop* 18:86-95, 1960.
117. Miller A, Friedman B: Fascial arthroplasty of the knee, *J Bone Joint Surg [Am]* 34:55-63, 1952.
118. Minns RJ: The Minns mensical knee prosthesis: Biomechanical aspects of the surgical procedure and a review of the first 165 cases, *Arch Orthop Trauma Surg* 108:231-235, 1989.
119. Moreland JR, Thomas RJ, Freeman MAR: ICLH replacement of the knee: 1977 and 1978, *Clin Orthop* 145:47-59, 1979.
120. Muller W: *The knee. Form, function and ligament reconstruction,* New York, 1983, Springer-Verlag.
121. Murphy JB: Arthroplasty, *Ann Surg* 57:593-647, 1913.
122. Murray DG, Barranco S: Femoral condylar hemiarthroplasty of the knee, *Clin Orthop* 101:68-73, 1974.
123. Murray DG, et al: Herbert total knee prosthesis, *J Bone Joint Surg [Am]* 59:1026, 1977.
124. Ollier L: Des résections orthopédiques dans le traitement des ankyloses osseuses de la hanche et du genou, *Congrès Française Chirurgie,* 1886.
125. Padgett DE, Stern SH, Insall JN: Revision total knee arthroplasty for failed unicompartmental replacement, *J Bone Joint Surg [Am]* 73:186-190, 1991.

126. Platt G: Arthroplasty of the knee in rheumatoid arthritis, *J Bone Joint Surg* 18:86, 1960.
127. Potter TA, Weinfeld MS, Thomas WH: Arthroplasty of the knee in rheumatoid and osteoarthritis: A follow-up after implantation of the McKeever and MacIntosh prostheses, *J Bone Joint Surg [Am]* 54:1–24, 1972.
128. Ranawat CS, Hansraj KK: Effect of posterior cruciate sacrifice on durability of the cement bone interface: A nine year survivorship study of 100 total condylar knee arthroplasties, *Orthop Clin North Am* 20:63–70, 1989.
129. Ranawat CS, Insall JN, Shine J: Duo-condylar knee arthroplasty: Hospital for Special Surgery design, *Clin Orthop* 120:76–82, 1976.
130. Ranawat CS, Jordan L, Straub LR: MacIntosh hemiarthroplasty in RA, *Acta Orthop Belg* 39:102–112, 1973.
131. Ranawat CS, Sculco JP: History of the development of total knee prosthesis at the Hospital for Special Surgery. In Ranawat CS, editor: *Total condylar knee arthroplasty. Technique, results and complications,* New York, 1985, Springer-Verlag, pp 3–6.
132. Rand JA, Chao EY, Stauffer RN: Kinematic rotating-hinge total knee arthroplasty, *J Bone Joint Surg [Am]* 69:489–497, 1987.
133. Riley D, Hungerford DS: Geometric total knee replacement for treatment of the rheumatoid knee, *J Bone Joint Surg [Am]* 60:523–527, 1978.
134. Riley D, Woodyard JL: Long-term results of geomedic total knee replacement, *J Bone Joint Surg [Br]* 67:548–550, 1985.
135. Ritter MA: The Herbert total knee replacement, *Clin Orthop* 219:237, 1977.
136. Ritter MA, Faris PM, Keating ME: Posterior cruciate ligament balancing during total knee arthroplasty, *J Arthroplasty* 3:323–326, 1988.
137. Ritter MA, et al: The posterior cruciate condylar total knee prosthesis: A five year follow-up study, *Clin Orthop* 184:264–269, 1984.
138. Ritter MA, et al: Long term survival analysis of the posterior cruciate condylar total knee: A ten year evaluation, *J Arthroplasty* 4:293–296, 1989.
139. Rosenberg AG, Verner JJ, Galante JO: Clinical results of total knee revision using the total condylar III prosthesis, *Clin Orthop* 273:83–90, 1991.
140. Ryd L: Micromotion in knee arthroplasty: Roentgen stereophotogrammetric analysis of tibial component fixation, *Acta Orthop Scand Suppl* 220:57, 1986.
141. Samson JE: Arthroplasty of the knee joint, *J Bone Joint Surg [Br]* 31:50–52, 1949.
142. Schurman JR, Borden LS, Wilde AH: Long term results of total condylar knee prosthesis, 54th Annual Meeting of the American Academy of Orthopaedic Surgeons, San Francisco, 1987.
143. Scott RD: Duopatellar total knee replacement: The Brigham experience, *Orthop Clin North Am* 13:89–102, 1982.
144. Scott RD, Santore RF: Unicondylar unicompartmental replacement for osteoarthritis of the knee, *J Bone Joint Surg [Am]* 63:536–544, 1981.
145. Scott RD, Volatile TB: Twelve years' experience with posterior cruciate–retaining total knee arthroplasty, *Clin Orthop* 205:100–107, 1986.
146. Scott RD, et al: McKeever metallic hemiarthroplasty of the knee in unicompartmental degenerative arthritis, *J Bone Joint Surg [Am]* 67:203–212, 1985.
147. Scott WN, Rubinstein M: Posterior stabilized knee arthroplasty: Six-year experience, *Clin Orthop* 205:138–145, 1986.
148. Scuderi GR, et al: Survivorship of cemented knee replacements, *J Bone Joint Surg [Br]* 71:798–803, 1989.
149. Shaw JA, Balcom W, Greer RB: Total knee arthroplasty using the kinematic rotating hinge prosthesis, *Orthopedics* 12:647–654, 1980.
150. Shiers LG: Arthroplasty of the knee: Preliminary report of a new method, *J Bone Joint Surg [Br]* 36:553, 1954.
151. Shiers LG: Arthroplasty of the knee: Interim report of a new method, *J Bone Joint Surg [Br]* 42:31, 1960.
152. Shindell R, et al: Evaluation of the Noiles hinged knee prosthesis, *J Bone Joint Surg [Am]* 68:579–585, 1986.
153. Shoji H, Yoshino S, Komagamine M: Improved range of motion with the Y/S total knee arthroplasty system, *Clin Orthop* 218:150–163, 1987.
154. Skolnick MD, Coventry MB, Ilstrup DM: Geometric total knee arthroplasty: A two year follow-up study, *J Bone Joint Surg [Am]* 58:749–753, 1976.
155. Skolnick MD, et al: Polycentric total knee arthroplasty: A two year follow-up study, *J Bone Joint Surg [Am]* 58:743–748, 1976.
156. Sledge CB, Walker PS: Total knee replacement in rheumatoid arthritis. In Insall JN, editor: *Surgery of the knee,* New York, 1984, Churchill-Livingstone, pp 697–715.
157. Sledge CB, et al: Two year follow-up of the duocondylar total knee replacement, *Orthop Trans* 2:193, 1978.
158. Sneppen O, et al: Mechanical testing of trabecular bone in knee replacement: Development of a osteopenetrometer, *Int Orthop* 5:251–256, 1981.
159. Speed JS, Trout PC: Arthroplasty of the knee. A follow-up study, *J Bone Joint Surg [Br]* 31:53–60, 1949.
160. Stern SH, Insall JN: Posterior stabilized prosthesis. Results after follow-up of nine to twelve years, *J Bone Joint Surg [Am]* 74:980–986, 1992.
161. Taylor FW: Fluon arthroplasty of the knee (abstract), *J Bone Joint Surg* 45:617, 1963.
162. Thomas WH, et al: Duopatellar total knee arthroplasty, *Orthop Trans* 4:329, 1980.
163. Thornhill T: Unicompartmental knee arthroplasty, *Clin Orthop* 205:121–131, 1986.
164. Torisu T, Morita H: Roentgenographic evaluation of geometric total knee arthroplasty with a six year aver-

age follow-up period, *Clin Orthop* 202:125–134, 1986.
165. Townley CO: Articular plate replacement arthroplasty for the knee joint, *Clin Orthop* 36:77–85, 1964.
166. Townley CO: *The anatomic total knee,* Port Huron, Mich, 1973, Acorn Press.
167. Townley CO: The anatomic total knee: Rationale, surgical technique and long term results, *Orthop Trans* 7:531, 1983.
168. Townley CO: Anatomic unicompartmental knee replacement: Rationale and early results, *Orthop Trans* 7:545–546, 1983.
169. Townley CO: The anatomic total knee: Instrumentation and alignment technique. The knee, In Dorr LD, editor: *Papers of the First Scientific Meeting of the Knee Society,* Baltimore, 1984, University Park Press, pp 39–52.
170. Townley CO: The anatomic total knee resurfacing arthroplasty, *Clin Orthop* 192:82–96, 1985.
171. Townley CO: Anatomic total knee replacement using porous-coated implants without cement fixation, *Tech Orthop* 4:59–68, 1987.
172. Townley CO: Total knee arthroplasty: A personal retrospective and prospective review, *Clin Orthop* 236:8–22, 1988.
173. Townley CO, Hill L: Total knee replacement, *Am J Nursing* 74:1612–1617, 1974.
174. Townley CO, Jerry GJ, Nebel EJ: Unicompartmental knee replacement with the use of a full resurfacing femoral component, Annual Meeting of the Knee Society, Las Vegas, Feb 1988.
175. Turner RA, et al: Arthroplasty of the knee with tibial and/or femoral metallic implants, *Arthritis Rheum* 1:15, 1972.
176. Turner RH, Aufranc OE: Femoral stem replacement arthroplasty of the knee, *Surg Clin North Am* 49:917, 1969.
177. Verneuil AS: De la création d'une fausse articulation par section ou résection partielle de l'os maxillaire inférieur, comme moyen de remédier à l'ankylose vraie ou fausse de la mâchoire inférieure, *Arch Gen Med* 15:174–195, 1860.
178. Verneuil AS: Affection articular du genou, *Arch Med* 1863.
179. Vince KG: The posterior stabilized knee arthroplasty. In Laskin RS, editor: *Total knee arthroplasty,* New York, 1991, Springer-Verlag.
180. Vince KG: Principles of condylar knee arthroplasty-issues evolving, *Instr Course Lect* 42:315–324, 1993.
181. Vince KG, Dorr LD: Surgical technique of total knee arthroplasty: Principles and controversy, *Tech Orthop* 1:69–82, 1987.
182. Vince KG, Insall JN: The total condylar knee arthroplasty. In Laskin RS, editor: *Total knee arthroplasty,* New York, 1991, Springer-Verlag.
183. Vince KG, Insall JN, Kelly MA: Posterior stabilized and total condylar knee arthroplasties: Comparative long term survivorship analysis. Accepted for presentation at the 55th Annual Meeting of the American Academy of Orthopaedic Surgeons, Atlanta, 1988.
184. Vince KG, Kelly MA, Insall JN: The posterior stabilized knee arthroplasty: Results at seven to eight years and survivorship analysis, Annual Meeting of the Western Orthopaedic Association, Colorado Springs, 1987.
185. Vince KG, et al: Long term assessment of joint line position and motion in a cruciate sacrificing knee arthroplasty, *Orthop Trans* 12:710, 1988.
186. Vince KG, et al: Total condylar knee prosthesis: 10–12 year follow-up and survivorship analysis, *J Bone Joint Surg [Br]* 71:793–797, 1989.
187. Walker PS: The total condylar knee and its evolution. In Ranawat CS, editor: *Total condylar knee arthroplasty. Technique, results and complications,* New York, 1985, Springer-Verlag, 1985, p 7.
188. Walker PS, Bullough PG: The effects of friction and wear in artificial joints, *Orthop Clin North Am* 4:275–293, 1973.
189. Walker PS, Shoji H: Development of a stabilizing knee prosthesis employing physiological principles, *Clin Orthop* 94:222–233, 1973.
190. Walker PS, et al: The kinematic rotating hinge: Biomechanics and clinical application, *Orthop Clin North Am* 13:187–199, 1982.
191. Walldius B: Arthroplasty of the knee using an acrylic prosthesis, *Acta Orthop Scand* 23:121, 1953.
192. Walldius B: Arthroplasty of the knee using an endoprosthesis, *Acta Orthop Scand* 24:1, 1957.
193. Walldius B: Arthroplasty of the knee using an Endoprosthesis, *Acta Orthop Scand* 30:137, 1960.
194. Walldius B: Prosthetic replacement of the knee joint (abstract), *J Bone Joint Surg [Br]* 50:221, 1968.
195. Waugh J, et al: UCI knee replacement, *Clin Orthop* 120:33–38, 1976.
196. Wilson FC, Venters GC: Results of knee replacement with the Walldius prosthesis, *Clin Orthop* 120:39–46, 1976.
197. Wilson FC, Fajgenbaum DM, Venters GL: Results of knee replacement with the Walldius and geometric prostheses: A comparative study, *J Bone Joint Surg [Am]* 62:497–503, 1980.
198. Windsor RL, et al: Long term results after total condylar knee replacement, *Orthop Trans* 7:415, 1983.
199. Worrell RV: A comparison of patellectomy with prosthestic replacement of the patella, *Clin Orthop* 111:284–289, 1975.
200. Worrell RV: Prosthetic resurfacing of the patella, *Clin Orthop* 144:91–97, 1979.
201. Worrell RV: Resurfacing of the patella in young adults, *Orthop Clin North Am* 17:303–309, 1986.
202. Wright J, et al: Total knee arthroplasty with the kinematic prosthesis. Results after five to nine years: A follow-up note, *J Bone Joint Surg* 72:1003–1009, 1990.
203. Wright TM, Hood RW, Burstein AH: Analysis of material failures, *Orthop Clin North Am* 13:33, 1982.

204. Wright TM, et al: Wear of polyethylene in total joint replacements: Observations from retrieved PCA knee implants, *Clin Orthop* 276:126–134, 1992.
205. Yoshino S, Shoji H: Yoshino-Shoji total knee system: Its features and postoperative results. In Niwa S, Paul JP, Yamamoto S, editors: *Total knee replacement,* Tokyo, 1987, Springer-Verlag pp 221–225.
206. Young HH: Use of a hinged vitallium prosthesis for arthroplasty of the knee: A preliminary report, *J Bone Joint Surg [Am]* 45:1627, 1963.
207. Young HH: Use of a hinged vitallium prosthesis (Young type) for arthroplasty of the knee, *J Bone Joint Surg [Am]* 53:1658, 1971.

59

Biomechanical Aspects of Knee Replacement Designs

LEO A. WHITESIDE, M.D.
RYUJI NAGAMINE, M.D.

Kinematics
   Tibia-femor
   Posterior-stabilized total knee replacement
   Patella
Wear

Fixation
   Femoral component
   Tibial component
   Strength of components
   Design of revision components

The mechanical demands of the knee joint are so high that a completely satisfactory design has not yet been developed for use with currently available materials. An ideal knee must be able to extend fully and achieve excellent mediolateral stability in this fully extended position. It must flex well beyond 90 degrees while maintaining mediolateral and anteroposterior stability. Because the ligaments are arranged in the knee so that rolling and sliding occur simultaneously, it is especially difficult to achieve a durable wear-resistant articular surface.

Normal kinematics of the knee cause major problems in fixation of the implants because the loads are very high, and their points of application shift throughout the gait cycle. Traditionally, long-term fixation of the implants and maintenance of the bone stock have been major clinical problems. Poorly fixed implants that migrate into bone cause severe bone loss, yet rigid fixation of the implants can stress-relieve periarticular bone stock and also cause loss of bone.

An articular surface design that allows ligaments to function at an optimal length throughout a satisfactory range of motion is difficult to achieve in nature, and has not yet been accomplished with artificial components. Highly mobile menisci, which follow the complex surface contours of the femur and tibia, and also flex to maximize articular surface contact, are responsible for the large surface area of contact, low wear, and stable articulation through the large range of motion found in the normal knee. The joint surfaces and the collateral ligaments interact with two complex cruciate ligaments to produce the normal knee's high degree of flexibility in the anteroposterior direction and stability in the mediolateral direction. Materials and designs that duplicate this interaction are not available. To compound the problem, knee anatomy, though roughly similar, is highly variable in detail among individuals. The knee's flexibility and degree of laxity at different angles of flexion varies greatly among individual, normal people. It is clear that compromise must be accepted in the design of total knee arthroplasty. Patellar mechanics may seem simple and straightforward on the surface, but this is a common misunderstanding among those who design for and operate on the arthritic knee. In reality, patellofemoral kinematics also present a challenge for engineers and orthopaedic surgeons. The patellofemoral joint is not inherently stable, and relies on balanced dynamic forces for stable tracking. The shifting load pattern and precarious balance between the medial and lateral and proximal and distal restraints on patellar motion still make the patella the most common source of complications in many clinical series of knee arthroplasty.

Developing a knee replacement system that solves the basic problems of the primary knee arthroplasty and also provides the capabilities of extensive reconstruction necessary in revision arthroplasty must be an evolutionary process. Many ideas that seem to work on the drawing board and in early clinical series have not become long-term successes. Although many of the basic problems have been solved through compromise, refinements of the art and science of total knee arthroplasty (TKA) will add tremendously to the capabilities of reconstructing the severely arthritic knee.

KINEMATICS

Tibia-Femur

Normally the knee becomes stable in full extension through a complex process of ligament tightening and joint surface congruity.[49] When the knee bends the capsular ligaments relax and allow rotational and varus-valgus laxity. This laxity increases steadily throughout the flexion arc up to 150 degrees.[17] As the knee flexes and extends, the joint surfaces and ligaments interact in a complex manner so the surfaces are positioned throughout the arc of flexion by tension in the ligaments. High surface contact area is maintained by the mobile menisci so compressive stress is minimized. The menisci also stabilize the knee against shear, rotational, and varus-valgus loads.[49, 51, 58] These important stabilizing and load-transmitting effects of the menisci have been the most difficult features of the knee to duplicate in total replacement arthroplasty.

Kinematic characteristics vary greatly from one knee to another. The degree of laxity at various degrees of flexion, and the positioning of the tibia on the femur are virtually unique for each knee. This makes it especially difficult to duplicate functions of the normal articular surfaces with a total knee replacement arthroplasty. Ideally, the implants should have a "spacer effect" and adjust the knee ligaments to proper tightness throughout its full functional range of motion. It should not impose an "arbitrary axis for rotation, flexion, etc."[23] However, eliminating rollback allows the articular surface to be designed with a large surface contact area, so it has advantages in terms of wear. Substituting for the posterior cruciate ligament (PCL) achieves stability and provides built-in rollback, but it applies higher shear stresses to the bone-implant interfaces. Improvements in fixation technique have eliminated much of the concern for fixation related to the use of PCL-substituting designs, so each of these design categories (PCL-retaining, PCL-sacrificing, PCL-substituting) is feasible, and should be available to solve the variety of problems presented by the surgical procedure.

How to handle the PCL—whether to preserve it, sacrifice it, or substitute for it—is a topic of active debate and investigation. If the PCL is preserved, the articular surfaces must be designed to allow rollback of the femur on the tibia. This has some advantages in knee function. The mechanical advantage of the posterior position of the femoral component on the tibia can be clearly demonstrated by laboratory and clinical studies.[2, 19] However, the PCL does not always function normally even if it is preserved, and when it does function and the femur rolls posteriorly on the tibial surface, the wear rate may be increased. If the PCL is sacrificed, rollback does not occur and the tibia can sag posteriorly. This decreases the effectiveness of the quadriceps and adversely affects knee kinematics in stair climbing.[2, 19]

Using a rotationally constrained articular surface that guides the knee into the normal "screw-home pattern" seems to produce a normal rotational pattern of the femur and tibia in TKA.[27] However, using a rotationally unconstrained surface likewise produces a near-normal screw-home pattern if the collateral ligaments are correctly balanced in extension,[67] so it is clear that the ligaments are capable of guiding the position of the articular surfaces. Designing the knee for rotational constraint in full extension is a precarious undertaking. Since the ligaments must guide the tibia into its final rotational position at full extension, and since all knees are somewhat different in this regard, it would be difficult to design a knee with only one rotational position that results in good contact surface area. It seems that a compromise is necessary to achieve a large articular surface in full extension to prevent wear and at the same time allow the tibia rotational freedom to accommodate the variability of knee kinematics dictated by the ligaments.

Adjustable posterior slope has been advocated to improve knee flexion. While it may increase flexion, this compromise in design causes other problems in knee kinematics. It increases anteroposterior laxity in flexion by shortening the distance between the femoral and tibial attachments of the PCL, and it eliminates rollback. In fact, when the knee is flexed, the contact point of the femur on the tibia may be anterior to the normal position in extension. This posterior positioning of the tibia in flexed positions may weaken extension by placing the tibia in a disadvantageous position for the quadriceps to exert full torque at the knee joint.[39] It also allows unconstrained anteroposterior sliding of the femur on the tibial surface and creates severe wear conditions.

Numerous femoral and tibial design characteristics are available, but no design-specific patterns of motion have been found during walking. Flexion during the stance phase does not appear to vary among the implants, which suggests that most knee replacements perform in a similar manner during the weightbearing cycle of the walking gait.[43] However, articular design has great potential to affect knee kinematics in stair climbing[3] and the ability of the knee to flex past 110 degrees. An articular surface geometry that restricts posterior rollback is likely to inhibit flexion of the knee. Rollback onto an up-sloping posterior articular surface tightens the PCL and the collateral ligaments (Fig 59–1). This produces a knee that is significantly tighter in flexion than a normal knee, and prevents the knee from gaining normal flexibility.[4] Changes in femoral and tibial component design offer a mechanism for improving flexibility of the knee without compromising stability of the knee or quadriceps efficiency. It is clear that increasing ligamentous tension after 100 degrees of flexion is detrimental to knee flexibility, so decreasing the radius of the posterior femoral condyle should eliminate femoral rollback at high knee flexion angles and diminish the tensioning effect of rollback on ligamentous structures of the knee (Fig 59–2). Sloping the tibial surface posteriorly seems to be necessary to avoid the phenomenon of rolling up onto a higher articular surface and thus overtensioning the knee ligaments in deep flexion.

During normal gait the knee is exposed to torsional anteroposterior shear and axial loads. Although the shear and torsional loads have been discussed extensively and implicated in component loosening, it has been apparent for some time that axial loading is the primary force to be dealt with in fixation.[11] Normal gait produces loads that are higher on the medial side of the knee than on the lateral side even when the knee is correctly aligned at a 5- to 7-degree valgus angle.[29] That is because the line connecting the foot to the center of gravity of the body passes medial to the knee when the mechanical axis of the knee is a straight line (Fig 59–3). Not only is the loading primarily medial in normal gait, but tensioning of the lateral collateral ligament normally occurs during the stance phase. This suggests that slight lateral liftoff is a part of normal, level walking. In the process of making sharp turns and rapidly going up- and downstairs, this lateral liftoff is more pronounced.[29] These kinematic characteristics of the normal knee cause joint surface loading that must be accommodated in the design of the arthroplasty surface.

Posterior-Stabilized Total Knee Replacement

Posterior cruciate ligament laxity is the only type of ligamentous deficiency that requires substitution with a mechanical structure in the implant. A knee

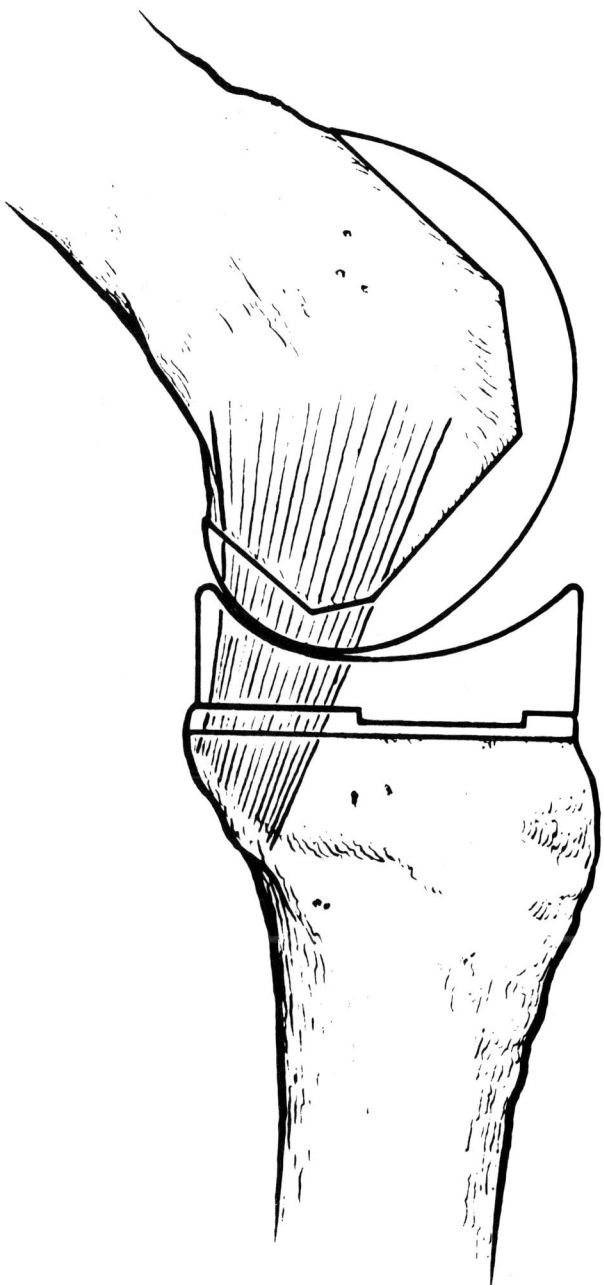

FIG 59–1.
Although a deeply dished tibial component provides a large area of contact in full extension, a functioning posterior cruciate ligament (PCL) causes the femur to roll back onto this upward slope, which tightens the PCL and restricts knee flexion.

that is unstable posteriorly cannot be stabilized by tightening the capsular sleeve of the knee, but posterior stability can be readily achieved by a stabilizing post. Besides posterior stability, an additional feature created by the posterior-stabilizing mechanism is posterior rollback of the femur on the tibia. The tibia is held forward and maintains quadriceps efficiency. The forward position of the tibia in flexion also pre-

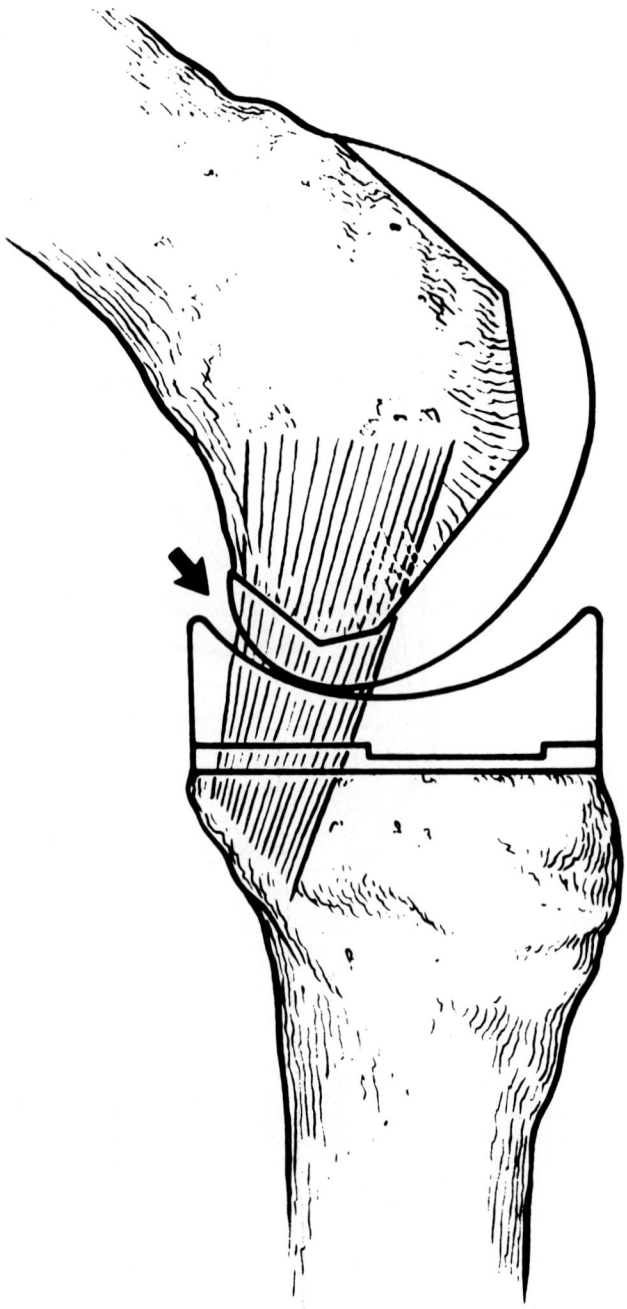

FIG 59–2.
A smaller radius of curvature in the posterior femoral condyle provides more room for knee flexion (arrow).

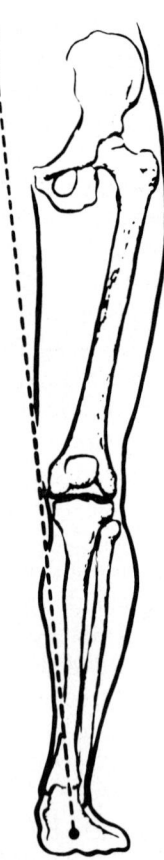

FIG 59–3.
Normally, in one-legged stance, the ground reaction line (between the foot and center of gravity of the body) lies medial to the center of the knee. Thus the medial condyles are more heavily loaded than the lateral condyles.

vents subluxation of the tibia into the posterior femoral recess and may therefore improve knee flexion. Anterior positioning of the tibia requires special design features of the articular surface of the tibia to ensure adequate contact area in flexion and extension, and also to avoid impingement of the anterior edge of the tibial component against the patellar tendon. Design of the stabilizing post is a crucial issue (Fig 59–4). It must restrict posterior displacement of the tibia but not hold the tibia in a posterior position in full extension. It also must be far enough forward on the tibia so it does not cause excessive rollback of the femur in flexion. The polyethylene post and metal stabilizing bar create an articular surface that may produce rapid breakdown of the polyethylene surface, so the contact surface area must be maximized. Impingement of the post against the patella in deep flexion can be a cause of wear, pain, and restricted range of motion, but if the post is not tall enough, posterior dislocation can occur at low flexion angles. Posterior extension of the polyethylene post is necessary to prevent medial or lateral displacement of the post around either femoral condyle when the force is flexed beyond 90 degrees.[31]

Special cases of enhanced varus-valgus stabilizing characteristics have been used over the years. An elongated polyethylene column, tightly fitted between the femoral condyles, can give mediolateral stability to the knee and confer a feeling of stability at the operative table. However, this relatively short post must resist high loads applied to a long lever

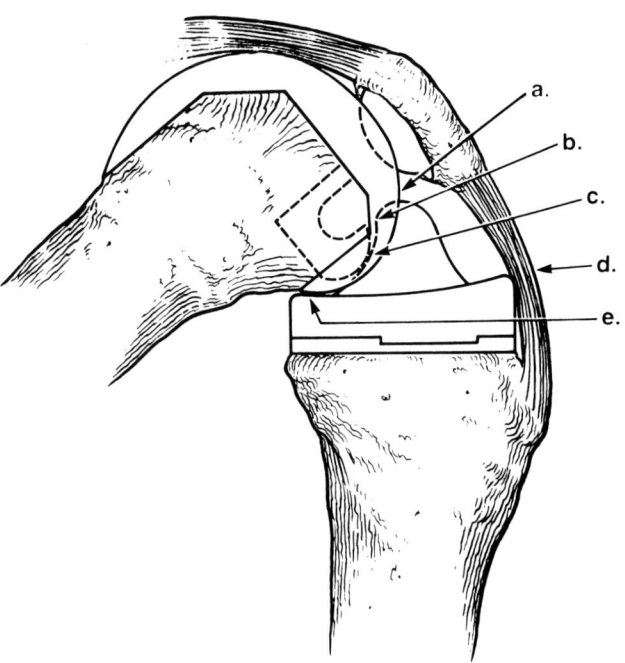

FIG 59–4.
Design of the posterior-stabilized knee. *a.* Impingement against the patella in deep flexion requires that the post be short enough to clear the patella. *b.* The post must be tall enough to prevent dislocation when the knee is flexed from 0 to 130 degrees. *c.* The articular surface should be large. *d.* Excessive rollback must be avoided to prevent patellar tendon impingement. *e.* The post and posterior condyles must be designed so the femoral and tibial surfaces maintain contact in deep flexion.

arm (Fig 59–5). It is not surprising that cold flow and loss of stability occur as time passes.[21]

Patella

Normally the patella is guided throughout its pathway by the lateral facet articulating smoothly with the lateral femoral condylar surface.[56] It must move slightly medially from a resting position in full extension to engage the patellar groove in early flexion. Then, as the knee flexes, the patella shifts laterally and tilts slightly toward the lateral side. As the knee flexes to 110 degrees, the medial patellar facet enters the intercondylar notch and the patella tilts medially. Slight external rotation of the patella occurs as the knee flexes.[56] Although the medial and lateral soft tissue constraints maintain patellar stability, patellar kinematics are mostly dictated by the shape of the joint surfaces. Since the lateral patellar facet is broad and the medial facet is narrow, the prominence of the patella is located medially, and the patella sits laterally on the femur. The lateral edge of the patella closely follows the lateral edge of the femoral condyle, and as the knee flexes past 90 degrees the medial femoral

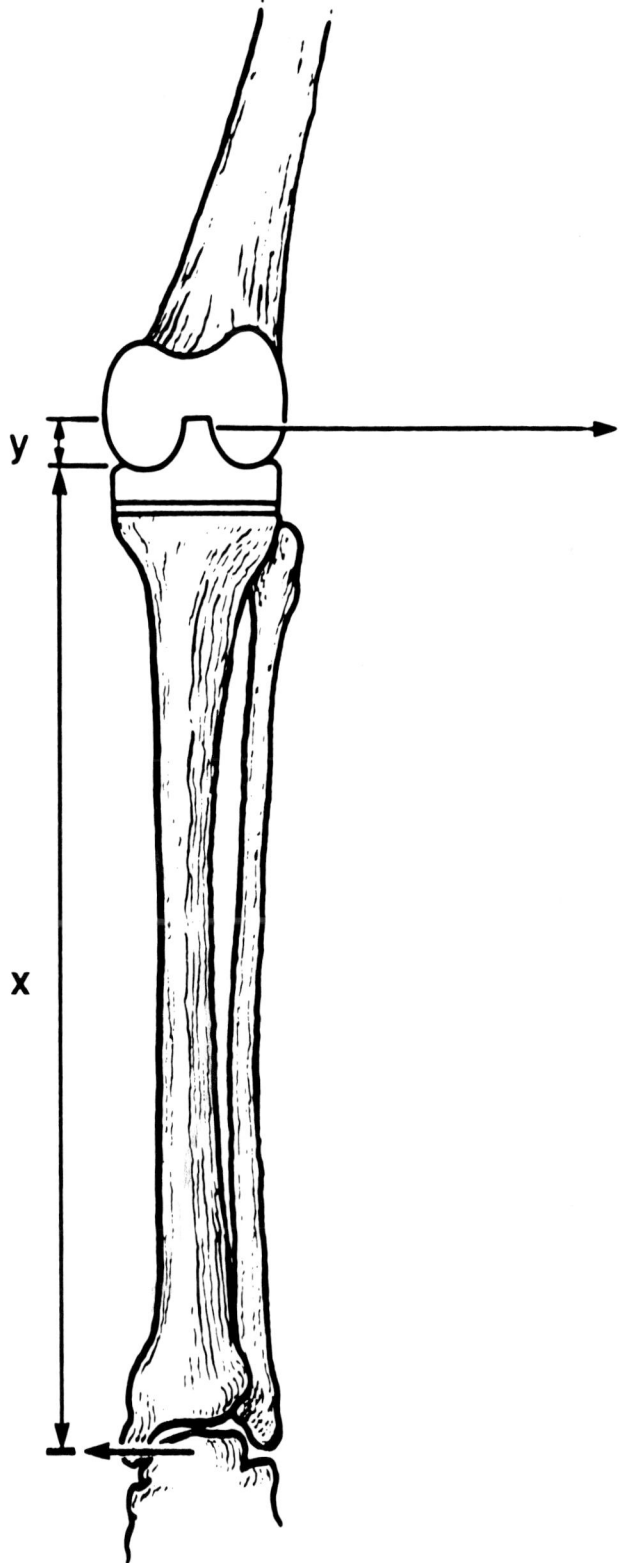

FIG 59–5.
The short polyethylene post *(y)* produces a large force when the long tibia *(x)* is acted on by a small force. It is difficult to achieve varus-valgus stability with a polyethylene post on the tibial component.

condylar surface is uncovered by the patella (Fig 59–6). The articular contact surface area moves proximally as the knee flexes and distally as the knee extends. In full extension the inferior edge of the patella articulates with the upper edge of the patellar groove (Fig 59–7). When the knee is flexed to approximately 45 degrees (Fig 59–8), the load-bearing surface is located in the middle third of the patella, and when the knee is flexed past 100 degrees, the load-bearing surface is located at the superior pole (Fig 59–9). The patella tilts in the anteroposterior plane as the knee flexes, and this enhances the shift from distal to proximal on the surface of the patella as the knee flexes.[56] In deep flexion the inferior pole of the patella is lifted away from the distal femoral surface and only the upper pole of the patella contacts the femoral articular surface. In this position the

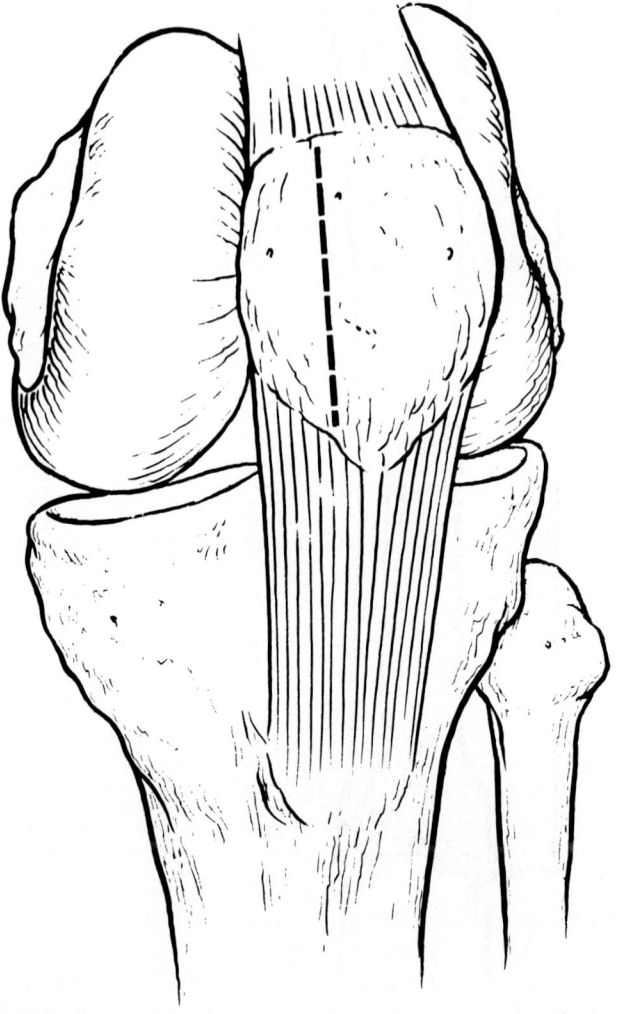

FIG 59–6.
The *dashed line* separates the medial from the lateral facet. Since the lateral is much wider than the medial facet, the patella sits laterally on the surface of the femur.

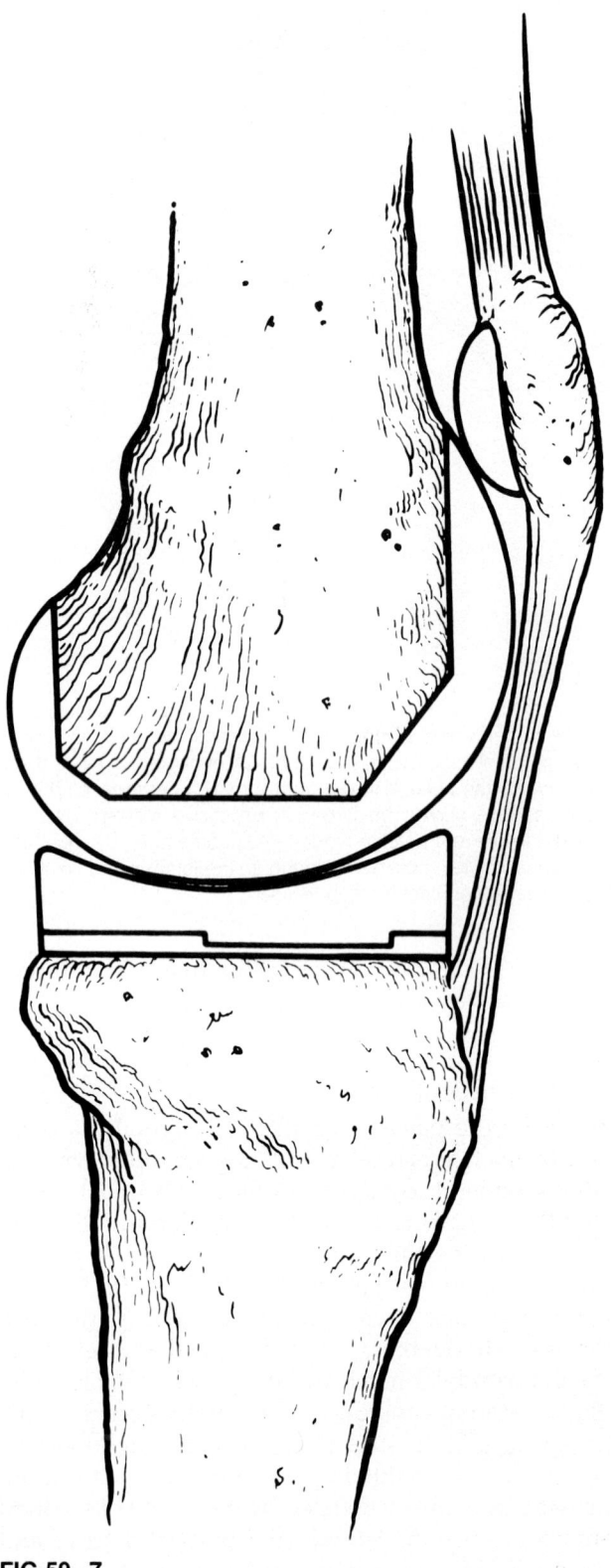

FIG 59–7.
In the normal knee and after total knee replacement, the inferior pole of the patella articulates in full extension.

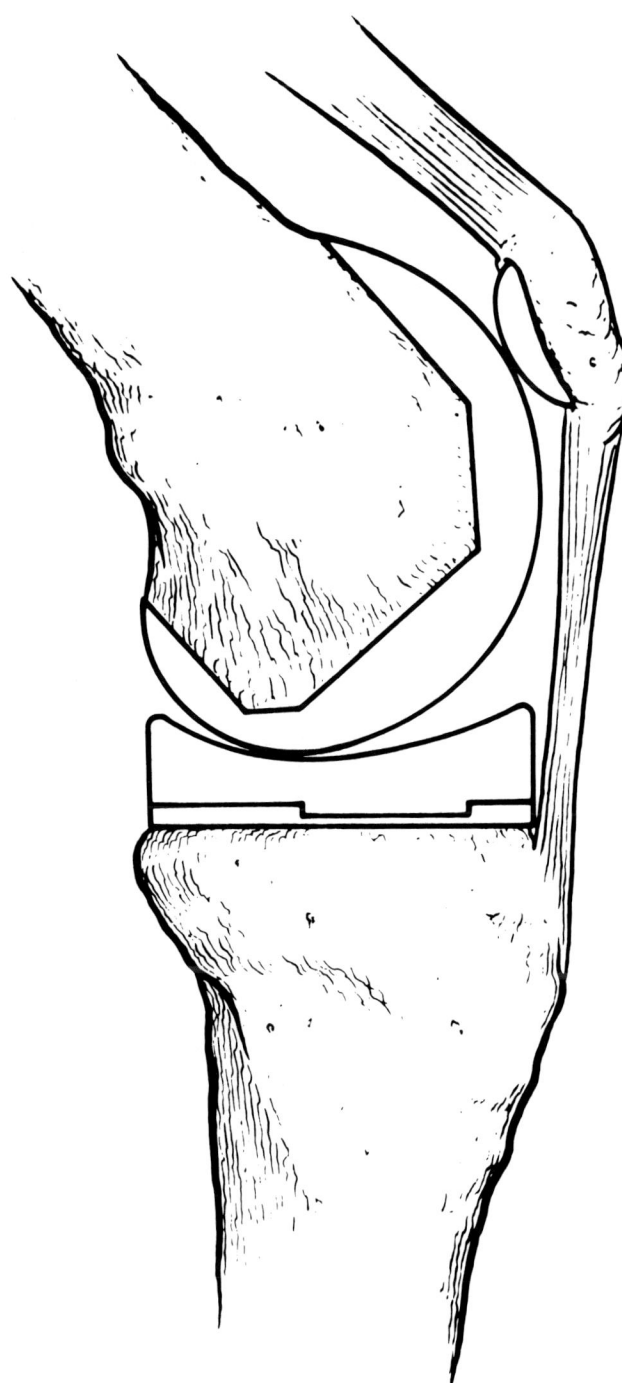

FIG 59–8.
At 45 degrees of flexion the middle of the patella articulates with the femoral surface.

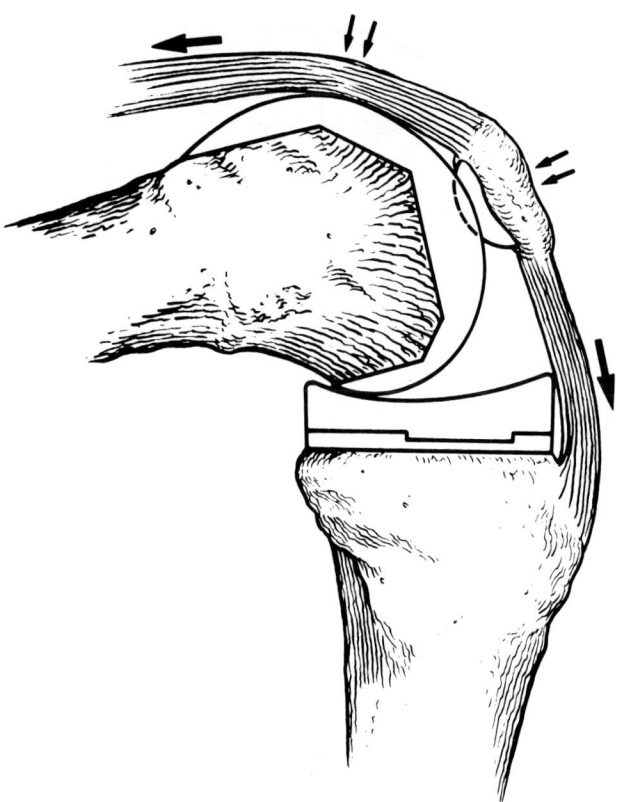

FIG 59–9.
When the knee flexes to 90 degrees, the upper pole of the patella articulates with the femoral surface. Tensile loads in the quadriceps and patellar tendons generate compressive loads. If the patella is well-positioned, much of this compressive load is transferred through the quadriceps to the femoral surface.

quadriceps tendon is firmly compressed against the anterior femur in the patellar groove. At no time is the quadriceps tendon tented across a sharp angle.

The patella is subjected to high compressive and tensile loads.[18, 42] Patellofemoral joint reaction forces as high as 7.6 times body weight occur with deep knee bends. When body weight is 85 kg, the resultant compressive load at the patella is 650 kg. Stair climbing and rising from a chair result in patellofemoral forces of 3.3 times body weight.[42] Because of these extreme mechanical conditions, cold flow and longitudinal elongation of the patellar component are common. Slight changes in the Q (quadriceps) angle resulting from misplacement of the patella on the surface of the femur cause abnormal lateralizing stresses on the patella, a slight shift in patellar position, and drastic increases in contact stresses due to loss of congruity of joint surface contact.[1]

Altering the patellar position also alters the tension in the medial and lateral retinacular structures and may alter the precarious balance of the soft tissue constraints of the patella.[22] Normally the patellar ridge articulates with the patellar groove of the femur, and this positions the patella so that the medial and lateral retinacula are tensioned normally (Fig 59–10). A medialized dome that places the thickest area of the patella medially, as in the normal anatomic patella, allows the patella to assume its normal lateral-

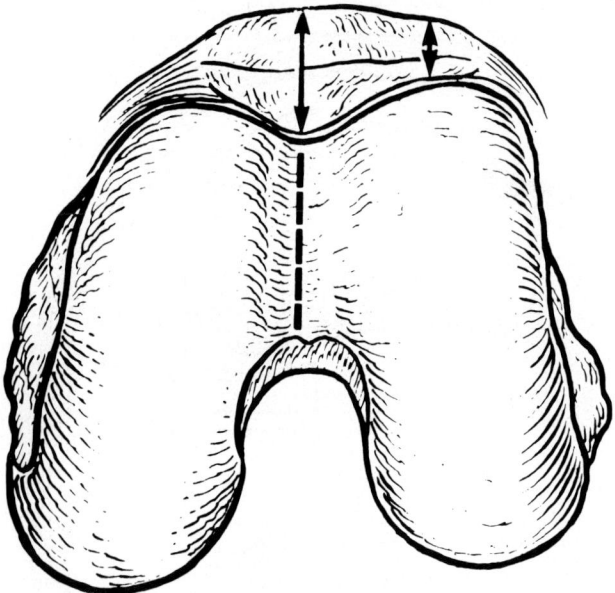

FIG 59–10.
Normal patellar position. Articulation of the lateral patellar facet maintains mediolateral position. Medial and lateral thickness maintain normal patellar tilt.

ized position on the femur and to maintain its normal lateral thickness.[71] Medial and lateral retinacular structures are allowed to function at normal tension (Fig 59–11). Centralization of the arthroplasty surface between the medial and lateral margins of the patella results in medialization of the bony architecture of the patella which increases the angle between the quadriceps and the patellar tendon and causes higher than normal lateralizing forces on the patella (Fig 59–12). This medialization also results in abnormal tensioning of the lateral quadriceps mechanism, which may laterally tilt or subluxate the patella.[71] Concave patellar surface designs are made to fit against the anterior surface of the femur and maintain area contact throughout range of motion. However, the normal cam-like action of the femur against the patella shifts the weightbearing surface from distal to proximal on the patella as the knee flexes. Normally, patellar shape accommodates distal-to-proximal tracking, and allows the patella to assume a low profile in deep knee flexion so that the quadriceps tendon lies against the anterior surface of the femur and bears some of the compressive load generated by contraction of the quadriceps. The concave or saddle shape of the patellar articular surface allows broad surface contact of the patella against the femur over a short arc of flexion only. During the rest of the flexion arc, either the inferior pole or superior pole of the patella articulates with the femur and tents the quadriceps mechanism (Fig 59–13). This may restrict deep knee flexion and cause excessive compressive loads on the patella. The dome shape allows normal distal-to-proximal tracking of the compressive load-bearing area and allows the patella to assume a less prominent (low-profile) position at the extremes of flexion and extension. This helps the patella seat in its

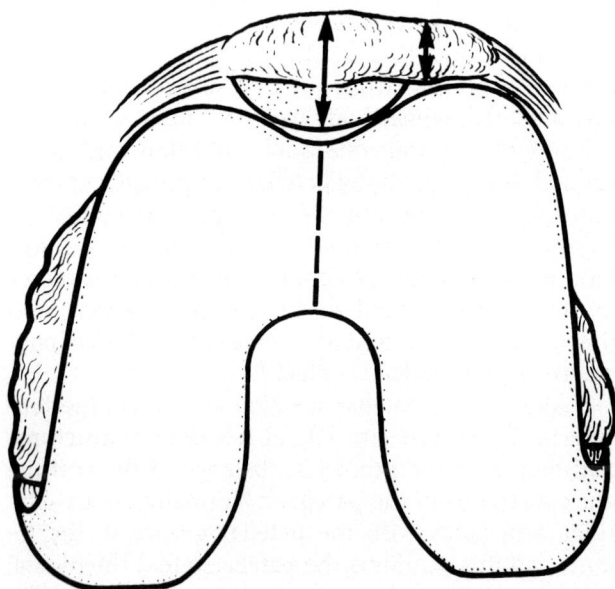

FIG 59–11.
A medialized dome that restores the thickness of the patella also reestablishes normal mediolateral patellar position and tilt if the femoral component is also correctly designed.

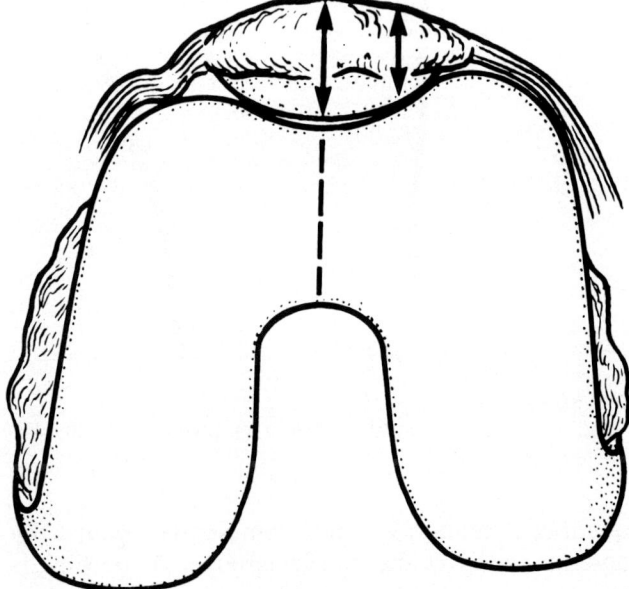

FIG 59–12.
Centralization of a full-dome patellar component shifts the patella medially. This tightens the lateral and loosens the medial retinaculum, which causes medial patellar tilt.

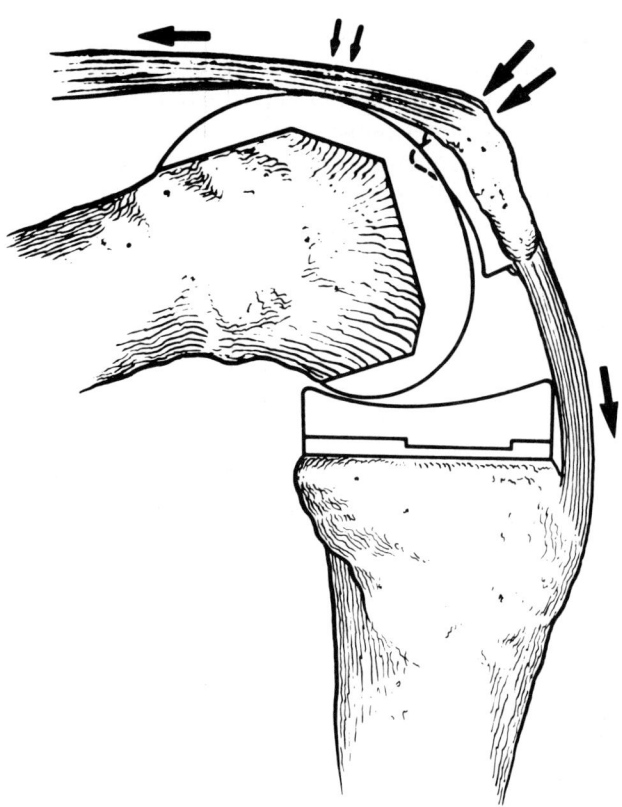

FIG 59–13.
The concave patella presents a thicker-than-normal proximal pole to the articular surface of the femur in full flexion. This tents the quadriceps tendon at the proximal pole of the patella.

groove and avoids tenting of the quadriceps mechanism.

Design of the patellar groove is an essential part of correct patellar mechanics. To adequately support the patella through full range of motion of the knee, the patellar groove must extend well around the curvature of the femur so that the proximal pole of the patella will be supported fully with the knee flexed at 140 to 150 degrees. The patellar groove must also be deep enough to accommodate the patellar dome and avoid displacing the patella anteriorly throughout the entire range of motion of the knee. In most knee replacement designs, this requires resection of a trough in the anterior surface of the femur to adequately recess the patellar groove portion of the femoral component.

The shape of the lateral and medial surfaces of the anterior portion of the femoral component also are important aspects of patellar tracking. An elevated lateral patellar flange and deepened patellar groove are important for stable patellar tracking during the early portion of the flexion arc.[71] Elevating the medial femoral surface to match the height of the lateral femoral flange tightens the medial retinaculum and also may tilt the patella laterally. It is likely that this abnormal kinematic feature would restrict knee flexion or result in abnormal patellar tracking.

WEAR

The kinematic characteristics of the knee produce interactions at the bearing surface to create an especially difficult series of problems with flexibility and wear. Many articular surface features that improve kinematics adversely affect wear conditions, and the reverse is also true. To accommodate the ligaments and maintain correct tension throughout the range of motion, the ligaments must be tensioned much as they are in the normal knee. This produces a joint with a shifting load-bearing area and a combination of rolling and sliding at the articular surface.[69] Although a large surface area contact can be designed in a portion of the arc of knee flexion, at other flexion angles the surface area contact must be much smaller than optimal. A knee that is highly conforming in full extension develops point contact or line contact as the knee flexes past 20 degrees. The posterior lip that is necessary to maintain a large contact area in full extension impinges on the posterior femoral condyles as the knee flexes and restricts range of motion of the knee. A partially conforming articular surface in full extension severely compromises the load-bearing contact surface area, and allows sliding to occur at the interface. This sliding mechanism creates "plowing" as the condylar surface area travels across the soft polyethylene (Fig 59–14). High tensile and shear stresses exist in the subsurface portion of the polyethylene and create a severe mechanical environment.[12] Pitting and delamination result from coalescence of subsurface cracks. On the other hand, highly conforming articular surfaces force the polyethylene structure to constrain the movement of the femoral component. This leads to failure of the structural integrity of the polyethylene and results in deformation due to cold flow of the polymer material.[60]

Wear, deformation, and cold flow of the polyethylene are all closely related to the thickness of the polyethylene implant.[70] Axial load-bearing creates stresses in the polyethylene that are transmitted through its substance into the material below. Because the polyethylene is thin and the counter-stresses from the undersurface are concentrated, areas of very high compressive, shear, and tensile stresses exist in the polyethylene between the femoral component and the underlying support of the polyethylene. These concentrated stresses increase surface wear and pitting and also magnify the tendency for polyethylene cold flow and bending. Metal-

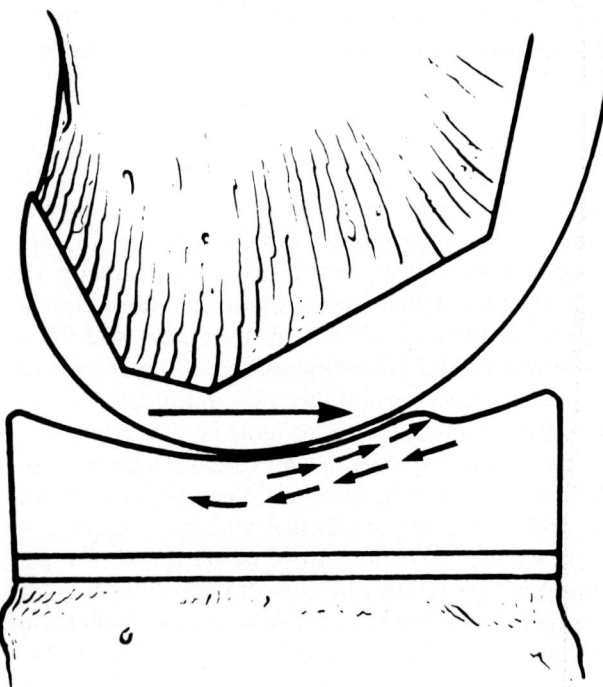

FIG 59-14.
Sliding of the femoral surface on the tibial polyethylene causes a "plowing" phenomenon resulting in subsurface shear stresses.

implants are retrieved during knee revision for unrelated problems such as patellar wear. However, even with Ortholoc I components characterized by linear contact, rotational nonconstraint, and minimal constraint to anteroposterior travel, severe cold flow and catastrophic failure of the polyethylene are rarely seen in this implant. This absence of cold flow and relative durability of this polyethylene-metal construct can be attributed to metal support and peripheral capture of the polyethylene, which prevents cold flow, subsurface wear, and bending of the polyethylene component.

Wear along the mediolateral edges of the contact area between the femoral and tibial components is a phenomenon that is not immediately apparent in design considerations of TKA. Kinematic studies suggest that the lateral side of the knee is often totally unweighted during the stance phase, even in a well-aligned knee, and that the femoral surface can rock

backing the undersurface of the polyethylene diminishes the tendency to cold flow if the polyethylene is captured peripherally.[47] In some knee components linear progression of cold flow with increasing load is found for polyethylene implants thinner than 9 mm if the polyethylene is not backed by a metal shell. As time passes, cold flow and then brittle failure of the polyethylene becomes an important mechanism for clinical failure of the implant.[47]

Meniscal bearing surfaces that slide with the femoral condylar surface resolve some of the dilemmas created by kinematic demands and wear problems in the knee. A large surface area can be maintained while knee flexibility is enhanced by allowing the articular surface of the tibia to follow the femoral surface as it is guided by the ligaments[6] (Fig 59-15). A very low wear rate and polyethylene deformation have been reported in this mechanical construct.[6] However, contact between the undersurface of the polyethylene and the edge of the metal tray may damage the polyethylene.

Small areas of contact, combined with complete freedom to rotate and slide from front to back at the articular interface, could be expected to produce especially severe surface wear[44] (Fig 59-16). The Ortholoc I total knee replacement is an example of this design configuration. After 5 to 10 years of service, severe surface damage is routinely found when these

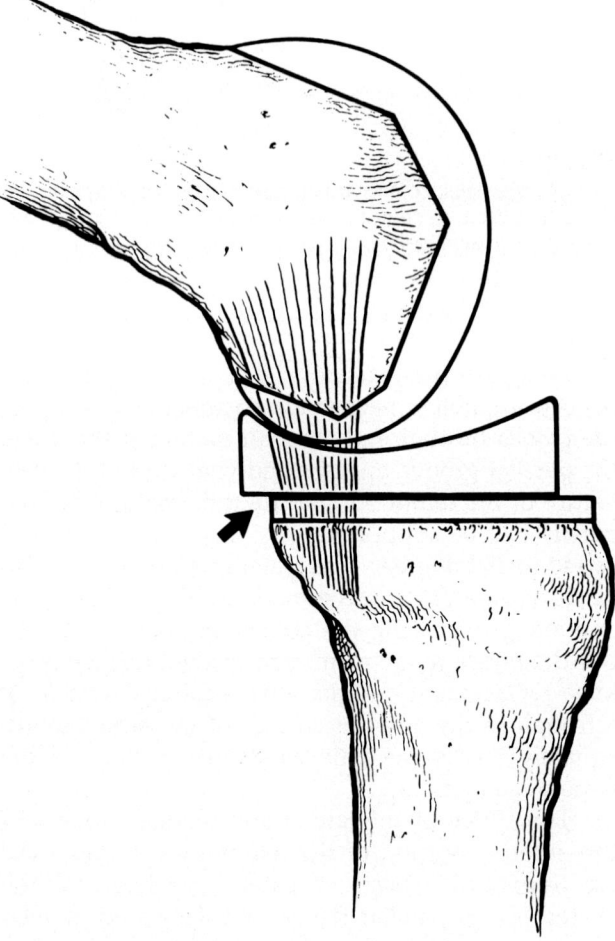

FIG 59-15.
A meniscal bearing surface helps prevent stresses on the upper surface, but may increase stresses on the undersurface of the polyethylene by allowing it to slide over the edge of the metal tray.

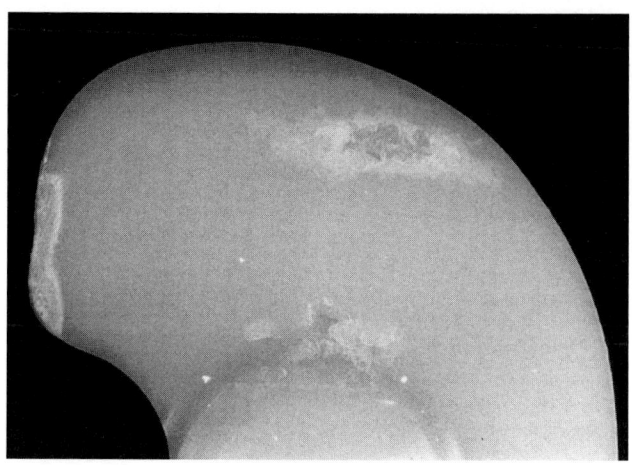

FIG 59–16.
Polyethylene surface in knee arthroplasty with linear contact and minimal constraint to sliding motions. Pitting and delamination have destroyed the surface, but peripheral capture of the polyethylene has prevented cold flow and destruction of the implant.

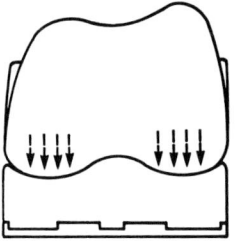 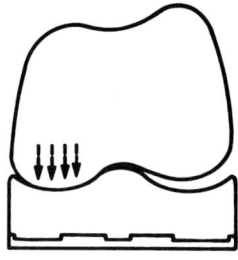

FIG 59–18.
A single radius of curvature on each femoral condyle also achieves a large contact area, but tilting does not cause edge-loading, and contact stresses remain moderate.

into a varus position during the stance phase and load the implant heavily along the medial edge.[26] If, on the anteroposterior view, the implant has a single large radius of curvature or other mechanism that prevents smooth tilting of the implant onto one condyle, extreme wear would be expected in the polyethylene under the medial femoral edge (Fig 59–17). On the other hand, if the surface were designed with a single radius on the medial femoral condyle and a separate single radius on the lateral femoral condyle with matching radii on the tibial component, then slight tilting could occur without edge loading of the implant (Fig 59–18). This should allow smoother functioning of the joint in full extension. Retrieval specimens of the Ortholoc II design have been found to have an improved wear pattern over the Ortholoc I, but also provide an example of edge wear caused by flat contours in the mediolateral plane (Fig 59–19). Minimal cold flow is seen over a large surface area representing the footprint of the femoral component in full extension. However, implants that have been in service for several years in active patients consistently have medial edge wear and cold flow of the intercondylar post—a pattern predicted for flat condylar surfaces. Designs such as the total condylar knee replacement, while restricted in some regards, have an advantage in wear because they avoid edge loading (Fig 59–20).

Patellar wear has been the source of many lessons in implant design. Patellar kinematics dictate a shifting position of load application and an obligatory cam-like action of the anterior femur against the patellar surface. This produces a shifting surface contact area. Despite high loads, the polyethylene must be thin because of anatomic constraints. When enough bone is removed to attach an implant without thickening the articular surface, only 8 to 10 mm of overall thickness of implant can be used to fill the resulting gap. To accommodate the shifting load-bearing surface of the patella, a dome shape appears to be the only design that consistently results in successful patellar tracking. The edges of the dome be-

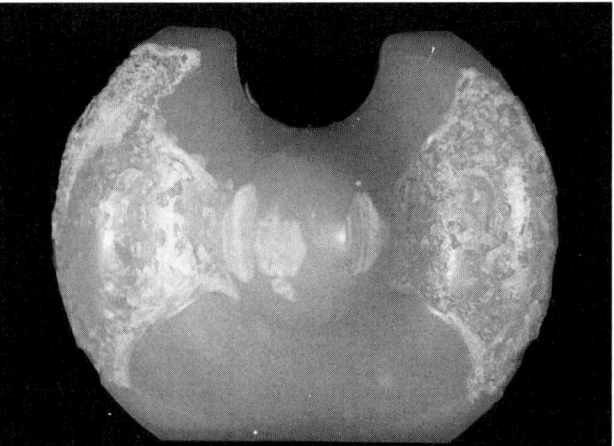

FIG 59–19.
Wear caused by a femoral condyle with a large-radius (flat) distal surface with small radii on either side. Severe wear is present where the medial edge of the femoral component contacted the polyethylene, and cold flow is present where the tibial eminence was impacted.

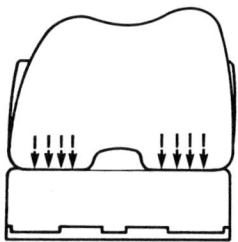 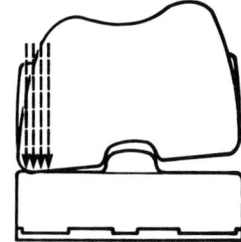

FIG 59–17.
Flat articular surfaces allow large contact areas, but slight tilt causes edge-loading and high contact stress.

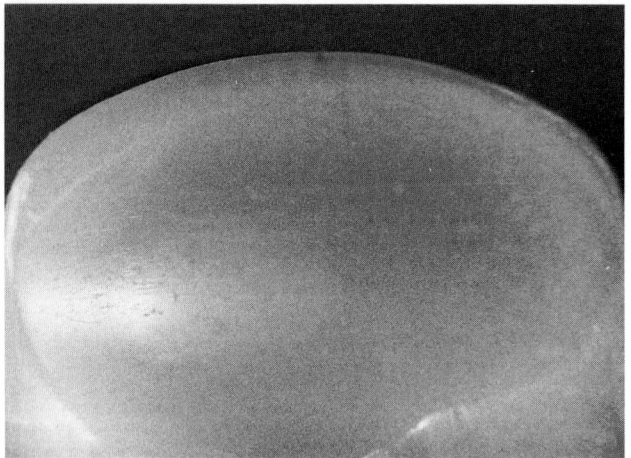

FIG 59–20.
A total condylar tibial component taken from a patient with persistent valgus deformity. Although lateral condylar cold flow occurred, there was little surface damage because the surface area contact was maintained by a single radius of curvature on the lateral femoral condyle.

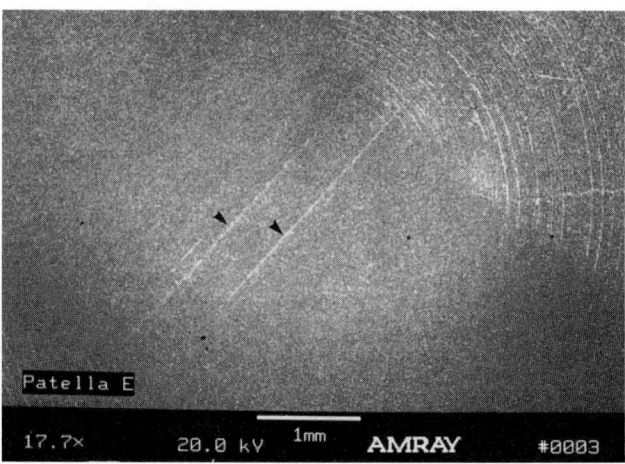

FIG 59–21.
The top of the dome had mostly polishing and cold flow with only minor scratching in the cobalt-chromium test group. (Original magnification ×17.1.) (From Milliano BA, Whiteside LA: *Clin Orthop* 273:209, 1991. Used by permission.)

come dangerously thin, and adding metal backing has produced some disastrous compromises. Metal structures that penetrate the polyethylene surface cause thinning of the polyethylene to a point that the yield stress of the polyethylene is exceeded and cold flow and rapid wear cause early failure of the implants.[31] However, metal backing of implants that are designed to avoid penetration of the polyethylene by the metal have had an excellent track record in TKA.[15]

The architecture of the patella makes resurfacing the lateral facet difficult or impossible without changing the thickness and altering the tension of the soft tissue envelope. A recessed polyethylene dome that leaves the lateral facet to articulate with a smooth femoral condylar surface of the implant has successfully eradicated pain at the patellofemoral joint in TKA and has resulted in very low failure rate. Addition of metal backing to this design has not resulted in an increasing failure rate due to wear.[15]

Articular surface materials as well as design are important factors in wear. Increasing surface hardness has consistently increased wear and precipitated disintegration of the polyethylene.[9, 70] The metal surface also plays an important part in wear at the articular interface. Substituting a titanium component for the standard polished cobalt-chromium surface consistently results in significantly greater wear of both the polyethylene and the metal[33] (Figs 59–21 and 59–22), and ion implantation of the titanium surface only marginally improves its wear characteristics.[33] Metal surfaces themselves are worn by inclusions in the polyethylene. Even polished cobalt-chromium femoral components are found to have abrasive wear after a few months of active use.

FIXATION

Femoral Component

Although fixation of the femoral component has not been as large a problem as fixation of the tibial component, it offers major challenges in design. Ideal loading conditions for cement or porous coating are always compressive with minimal shear and tensile loading. The cuplike shape of the femoral component causes problems because fixation of the surface re-

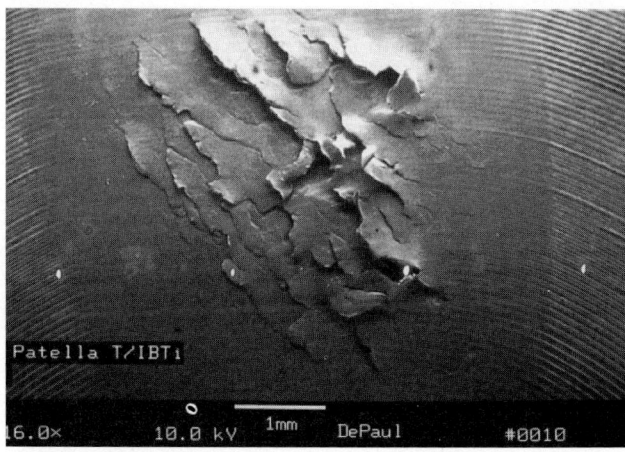

FIG 59–22.
Extreme cold flow and delamination in four of the six patellae tested against ion-implanted titanium. This form of wear was exclusive to this test group. (Original magnification, ×16). (From Milliano BA, Whiteside LA: *Clin Orthop* 273:212, 1991. Used by permission.)

sults in distal bone stress relief and shear loading of the point of attachment to the anterior and posterior flange surfaces[40, 59] (Fig 59–23).

Osteopenia around the distal portion of the bone-cement interface is a common finding with cemented total knee replacements when the anterior and posterior flange surfaces are tightly adherent to the bone.[35] This is predictable in the light of well-documented studies of fixation of the femoral component.[59] Transfer of the axial load of the femur into the anterior and posterior flanges must relieve the distal bone of compressive loading. The resulting stress-relief osteopenia is of no consequence unless the implant loosens. Then severe bone loss is expected, and revision is likely to require extensive substitution of bone to reconstruct the distal femur and replace the joint surface in the correct position relative to the ligament attachments on the femur. A similar phenomenon is seen when the anterior and posterior surfaces of the femoral component are porous-coated. The porous coating accepts the axial load-bearing as shear stresses in the anterior and posterior flanges, so the load bypasses the distal femo-

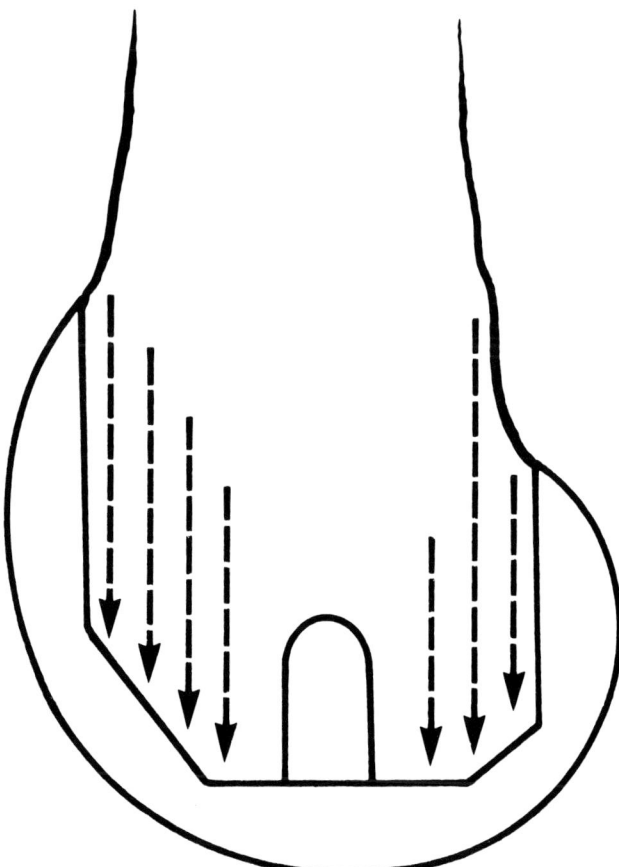

FIG 59–24.
Smooth anterior and posterior flange surfaces and smooth pegs allow distal femoral load-bearing.

ral bone as in cemented components. If porous-coated pegs are added to this system, more severe stress relief occurs in the distal surface of the femur since much of the compressive load will be transferred to the rigid pegs, leaving the distal surface almost completely unloaded (see Fig 59–23). Revision is especially difficult in these cases because the pegs are encased in firm cancellous bone while the rest of the distal femur is osteoporotic.

Smooth anterior and posterior surfaces of the femoral component consistently result in distal femoral bone hypertrophy[68] (Fig 59–24). However, the presence of a smooth surface invites fibrous tissue ingrowth which can conduct wear debris and result in cyst formation and bone loss. It is also theoretically possible that bone loss due to stress relief of these anterior and posterior surfaces could occur.[13] Progressive widening of gaps on the anterior and posterior flange surfaces does not occur although a thin fibrous tissue membrane occasionally develops between the posterior flange surface and bone. However, in cases of severe wear, as in patellar failure,

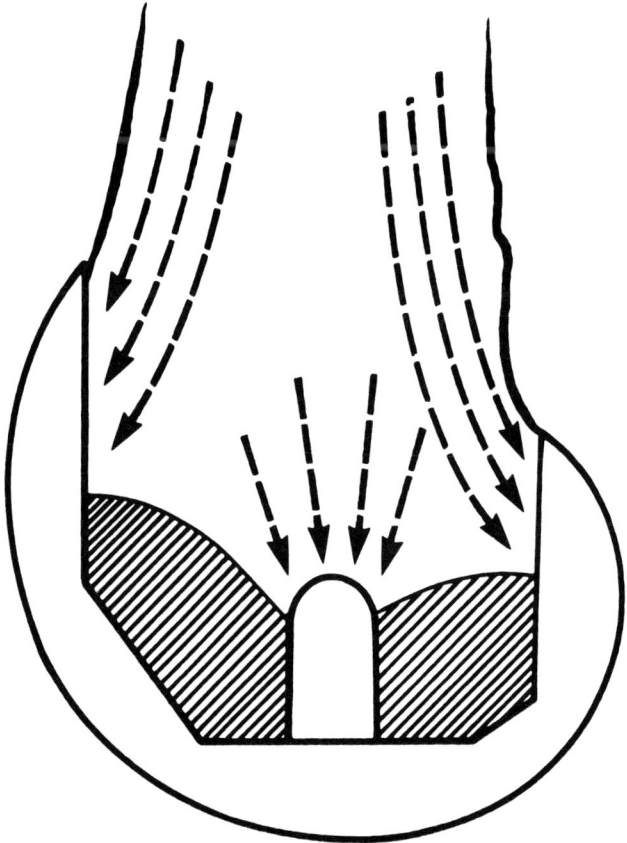

FIG 59–23.
Fixation of the femoral component to the anterior and posterior inner surfaces and to the pegs results in distal stress relief.

posterior cyst formation is common. It is likely that this fibrous tissue membrane between bone and porous coating is quiescent until invaded by particulate debris, which stimulates an inflammatory response.

Compressive loading of the anterior surface of the femur by the patella may be one of the important mechanisms of maintaining anterior femoral bone stock.[5, 16] However, severe anterior distal bone loss after total knee replacement is seen only when anterior and posterior porous-coated or cemented flange surfaces are used. The bone still receives adequate compressive loading to maintain integrity even in the absence of patellar loading after total knee replacement as long as axial load-bearing in this distal femoral bone is not eliminated by femoral component design.

Tibial Component

Tibial component fixation follows the same principles whether cemented or cementless fixation is used. Compressive load-bearing, broad surface coverage, and protection with a central stem are essential in the design for fixation of this implant.[8, 61, 62] Bone quality in the upper tibia after resection is nonuniform, and some areas are consistently weak.[25, 28] Eccentric loading of the upper surface of the tibia results in repetitive side-to-side and front-to-back shifts of the loaded area on the upper surface of the tibia.[30, 34, 52] Compressive failure of cancellous bone is the most common mode of failure of cemented or cementless joint replacements.[11] High compressive loads under the implant are present with moderate activity in the absence of a central stabilizing stem.[11, 32, 38] The use of a stem on the tibial component can decrease these loads to an acceptable level[11, 38, 63] (Fig 59–25). Although stem fixation is an important consideration in stabilization of the tibial component, cementing a rigid stem in the diaphyseal portion of the tibia results in drastic proximal stress relief.[37] A smooth stem that engages the diaphyseal cortex of the tibia and achieves contact with cortical-cancellous bone gives excellent resistance to liftoff and sinking of the tibial component.[50, 72] The stem also adds the benefit of resistance to shear stresses. Fixation of the tibial component without metal backing to distribute the loads into the tibial bone does not give adequate support to the polyethylene, and allows high levels of micromotion between the cement and the upper tibial surface.[7] The flexible polyethylene does not provide adequate rigidity for the junction between the stem and tibial articular surface, so the inevitable eccentric load eventually overloads the cancellous trabeculae, and deformation of the polyethylene occurs[37] (Fig 59–26).

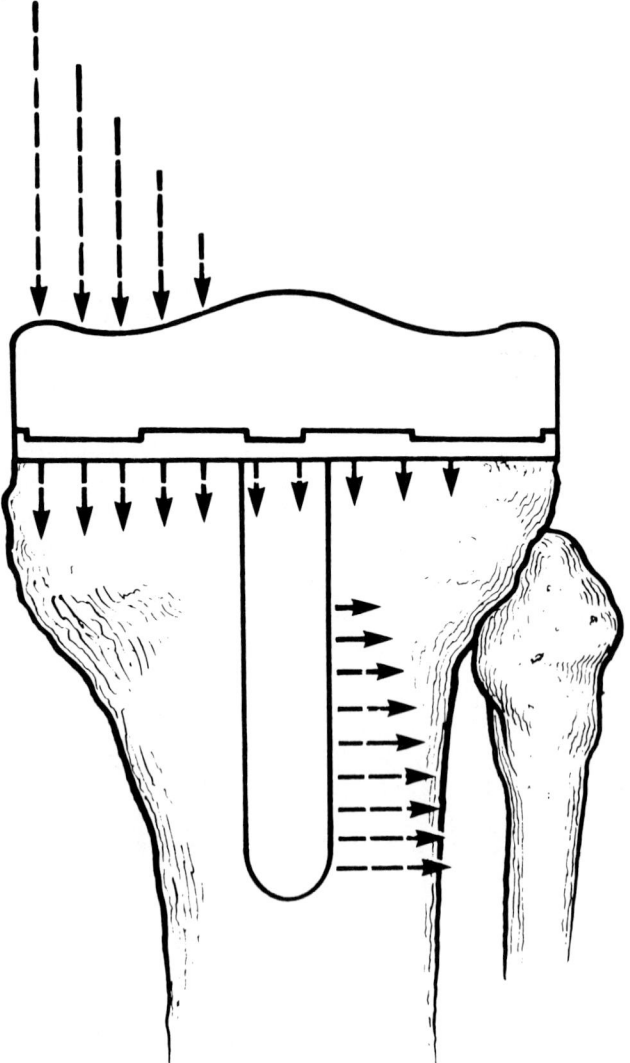

FIG 59–25.
Rigid metal tray and stems support the polyethylene effectively. The stem helps mitigate eccentric loads, and a large surface area is compressed by the tray.

Cemented fixation of the tibial component gives the most rigid fixation available when tested immediately after implantation.[14] Fibrous tissue gradually develops between the cancellous bone and cement, however, so almost all cemented tibial components have radiographically demonstrable motion between cement and bone measuring from 500 to 2,000 μm.[24, 46] Metal-backing the tibial tray greatly diminishes the peak stresses between the arthroplasty surfaces and the cancellous bone, and clinical results suggest that long-term survivorship is closely related to this feature.[41]

Cementless fixation of the tibial component with porous stems and pegs has produced adverse bone remodeling and mechanical failure of implants,[10, 54, 55] but the combination of smooth pegs

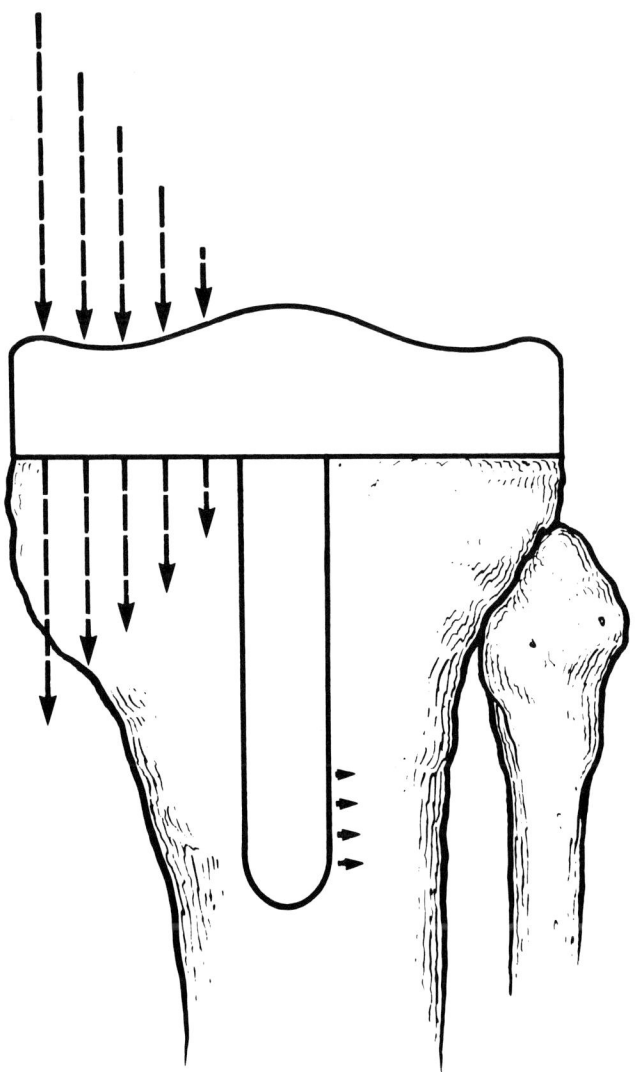

FIG 59–26.
A polyethylene component without rigid metal backing and stem fixation offers inadequate resistance to eccentric loads. Because of its flexibility the stem bears little load, and the load is transferred directly to small areas of bone.

and stems and a porous coating on the undersurface of the implant has been a highly successful means of fixing the tibial component.[65] Use of screws through the tibial component has resulted in a major improvement in the initial rigidity of fixation,[36, 53, 57] but has not yet produced a dramatic improvement in clinical results.[66] Several reports suggest, however, that pain relief and migration of the implant may be significantly improved clinically using this method of fixation.[45, 66] Potential complications of the use of screws include wear debris and upward penetration of the screws into the polyethylene portion of the tibial component. Although this has been reported,[20] inadequate tibial polyethylene-to-metal fixation is likely to cause wear debris generation and pumping of joint fluid into the screw well. Also, placement of the screw wells in the central weightbearing area of the tibia and using two screws instead of four allows penetration of the polyethylene into the screw holes and also fails to fix the tibial component adequately to the upper surface of the tibia.

STRENGTH OF COMPONENTS

The strength of the tibial tray is an important consideration. Polyethylene tibial components generally do not offer adequate strength,[63] and deformation is a major cause of failure. For wear purposes, it is necessary to maintain at least 6 mm, and preferably 8 mm, of polyethylene in the weightbearing area, so maintaining a thin metal tray is an important aspect of tibial component design. Placement of screw holes near the periphery of the tibial tray, and avoiding notches near the center of the implant help prevent stress risers that cause tray fracture. A minimum thickness of 2 to 3 mm is necessary for the usual titanium structure. The addition of struts to add rigidity to the tray and prevent fatigue failure is one of the effective ways of achieving adequate mechanical properties without excessive thickness of metal.

Fracture of metal components in TKA is an unusual problem associated with newer designs developed to conserve bone. Although occasional fractures of metal tibial components have been reported, fracture of the femoral component is rare and is not generally considered to be a significant problem in cemented TKA. However, loads in cementless femoral components differ from those in cemented TKA, and these differences in the location and direction of load application focus high stresses on critical cross-sectional dimensions. Porous coating decreases the strength of metallic implants because the dimensions of the metal substrate are decreased to accommodate it, especially at corners and junction areas where the metal may already be at minimum thickness. The sintering process can also lower the strength of the base metal and thus weaken the implant. Stress concentrations (or the notch effect) caused by the porous coating can also be important in weakening the implant if the porous surface is loaded in tension.

Cementless fixation results in stresses that can cause failure of the femoral component when a mechanical environment exposes the porous inner surface to tensile loads. Although the inner or nonarticulating surface of the femoral component generally is not considered to be the site of significant tensile stresses, the cementless technique has been found to apply tensile stresses to the inner surface of the femoral component by loading the bevel surfaces. This unexpected loading mechanism tends to spread or "open" the femoral component, applying a bending

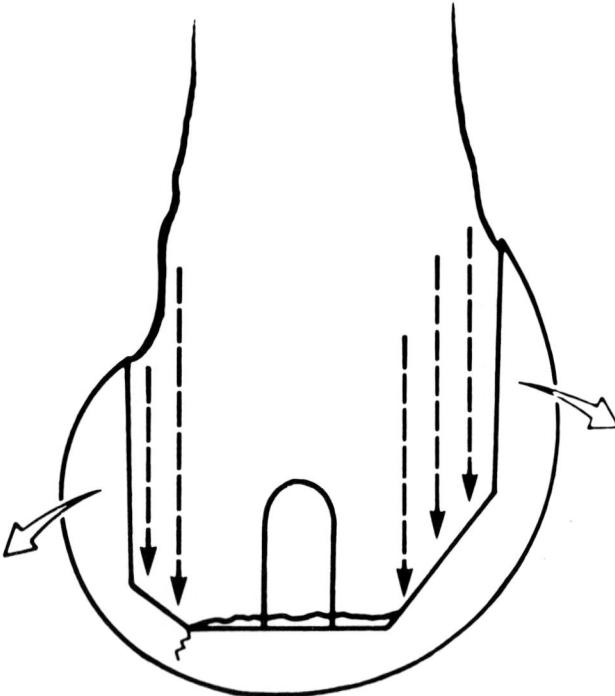

FIG 59–27.
Distal load transfer to the anterior and posterior bevel surfaces can apply a bending load to the femoral component if the distal surface is not seated. This can fracture the implant.

moment in the component so that tensile stresses occur along the distal inner surface (Fig 59–27).

DESIGN OF REVISION COMPONENTS

Revision components must be designed to reestablish ligamentous stability of the knee in flexion and extension and to achieve reliable fixation without further loss of bone stock. Often the distal femoral and proximal tibial bone stock is not adequate support without anchoring the implant into the diaphysis. Problems with bone loss caused by stress-relief osteoporosis preclude the use of porous-coated stems in these difficult cases. However, smooth-surfaced cylindrical stems that press-fit into the diaphyseal cortical bone allow the surfaces of the femur and tibia to bear an attenuated axial load as the stem helps dissipate the eccentric loading and prevent liftoff and other toggle phenomena at the bone-prosthesis interface. Whether the distal femur and proximal tibia are cemented or reconstructed with cementless techniques, the reliability of smooth cylindrical stems has been shown in clinical series.[48, 64]

Joint line positioning in revision arthroplasty is a necessary part of revision implant design. In most cases the distal femoral surface has been severely damaged and the posterior femoral condyles are at least partially absent. Nevertheless, the medial and lateral collateral ligament attachments are almost always intact. So placing the articular surfaces distally and posteriorly near their normal anatomic locations and restoring a smooth articular curvature are enough to regain adequate stability in flexion and extension. Bone stock deficiency on the tibial side as well as overall ligamentous laxity dictates the need for a thick articular component. Implants up to 35 mm in height are sometimes necessary.

Although bone stock is occasionally sufficient to allow repeated use of cement in revision arthroplasty, more often the bone stock deficiency is severe enough to require bone grafting. In cases of moderate bone stock deficiency, wedges and custom buildup implants can be fabricated at the operative table to reliably seat on the host bone and achieve immediate stable fixation. Polymethyl methacrylate cement fixation of these accessories to the tibial and femoral components has proved to be a reliable and effective means of building the composite implant. Laboratory tests show excellent rigidity of fixation and fatigue strength.

Techniques are now available to allow severe bony and ligamentous defects to be reconstructed with bone-conserving techniques. Cemented hinges and implants that link together to substitute for ligamentous stability are no longer necessary to solve the most challenging revision knee problems.

Acknowledgment

D. J. Van Loon provided editorial assistance in the preparation of this manuscript.

REFERENCES

1. Ahmed AM, et al: The effect of quadriceps tension characteristics on the patellar tracking pattern, *Trans Orthop Res Soc* 13:280, 1988.
2. Andriacchi TP, Galante JO: Retention of the posterior cruciate in total knee arthroplasty, *J Arthroplasty Suppl* 1988; S13–S19.
3. Andriacchi TP, Galante JO, Fermier RW: The influence of total knee replacement design on walking and stair-climbing, *J Bone Joint Surg [Am]* 64:1328–1335, 1982.
4. Andriacchi TP, Stanwyck T, Galante JO: Knee biomechanics and total knee replacement, *J Arthroplasty* 1:211–219, 1986.
5. Angelides M, et al: Effect of total knee arthroplasty on distal femur stresses, *Trans Orthop Res Soc* 13:475, 1988.
6. Argenson JN, O'Connor JJ: Polyethylene wear in me-

niscal knee replacement, *J Bone Joint Surg [Br]* 74:228–232, 1992.
7. Askew MJ, Lewis JL, Keer LM: The effect of post geometry, material and location on interface stress levels in tibial components of total knee, *Trans Orthop Res Soc* 25:97, 1979.
8. Bargren J, Blaha J, Freeman M: Alignment in total knee arthroplasty, *Clin Orthop* 173:178–183, 1983.
9. Bartel DL, Bicknell V, Wright T: The effect of conformity, thickness, and material on stresses in ultra-high molecular weight components for total joint replacement, *J Bone Joint Surg [Am]* 63:1041–1051, 1986.
10. Bartel DL, Santavicca EA, Burstein AH: The effects of pegs and trays on stresses associated with knee prosthesis, *Trans Orthop Res Soc* 26:165, 1980.
11. Bartel DL, et al: Performance of the tibial component in total knee replacement, *J Bone Joint Surg [Am]* 64:1026–1033, 1982.
12. Blunn GW, et al: The dominance of cyclic sliding in producing wear in total knee replacements, *Clin Orthop* 273:253–260, 1991.
13. Bobyn JD, et al: Biologic fixation and bone modeling with an unconstrained canine total knee prosthesis, *Clin Orthop* 166:301–312, 1982.
14. Branson PJ, et al: Rigidity of initial fixation with uncemented tibial knee implants, *J Arthroplasty* 4:21–26, 1989.
15. Cameron HU: Comparison between patellar resurfacing with an inset plastic button and patelloplasty, *Can J Surg* 34:49–53, 1991.
16. Cameron H, Cameron G: Stress-relief osteoporosis of the anterior femoral condyles in total knee replacement (a study of 185 patients), *Orthop Rev* 16:22, 1987.
17. Crowninshield R, Pope MH, Johnson RJ: An analytical model of the knee, *J Biomech* 9:397–405, 1976.
18. Denham R, Bishop R: Mechanics of the knee and problems in reconstructive surgery, *J Bone Joint Surg [Br]* 60:345–352, 1978.
19. Dorr LD, et al: Functional comparison of posterior cruciate-retained versus cruciate-sacrificed total knee arthroplasty, *Clin Orthop* 236:36–43, 1988.
20. Engh GA, et al: Analysis of polyethylene wear in metal backed knee arthroplasty, Fifty-eighth Annual American Academy of Orthopaedic Surgeons Meeting, Anaheim, Calif, March 7–12, 1991.
21. Gebhard JS, Kilgus DJ: Dislocation of a posterior stabilized total knee prosthesis—A report of two cases, *Clin Orthop* 254:225–229, 1990.
22. Gomes LS, Bechtold JE, Gustilo R: Patellar prosthesis positioning in total knee arthroplasty, *Clin Orthop* 236:72–81, 1988.
23. Goodfellow J, O'Conner J: The mechanics of the knee and prosthesis design, *J Bone Joint Surg [Br]* 60:358–369, 1978.
24. Green D, et al: Biplane radiographic measurements of reversible displacement (including clinical loosening) and migration, *J Bone Joint Surg [Am]* 65:1134–1143, 1983.
25. Harada Y, Wevers HW, Cooke TDV: Distribution of bone strength in the proximal tibia, *J Arthroplasty* 3:167–175, 1988.
26. Harrington IJ: A bioengineering analysis of force actions at the knee in normal and pathological gait, *Biomed Eng* 11(5):167–172, 1976.
27. Hungerford DS, Haynes DW, Kenna RV: Rotational characteristics of total knee replacements under load, *Trans Orthop Res Soc* 7:126, 1982.
28. Hvid I: Trabecular bone strength at the knee, *Clin Orthop* 227:210–221, 1988.
29. Johnson F, Leitl S, Waugh W: The distribution of load across the knee: A comparison of static and dynamic measurements, *J Bone Joint Surg [Br]* 62:346–349, 1980.
30. Kostuik JP, et al: A study of weight transmission through the knee joint with applied varus and valgus loads, *Clin Orthop* 108:95–98, 1975.
31. Lombardi AV, et al: Fracture dislocation of the polyethylene in metal-backed patellar components in total knee arthroplasty, *J Bone Joint Surg [Am]* 70:675–679, 1988.
32. Miegel RE, et al: A compliant interface for total knee arthroplasty, *J Orthop Res* 4:486–493, 1986.
33. Milliano MT, Whiteside LA: Articular surface material effect on metal-backed patellar components: A microscopic evaluation, *Clin Orthop* 273:204–214, 1991.
34. Minns RJ: Forces at the knee joint: Anatomical considerations, *J Biomech* 14:633–643, 1981.
35. Mintzer CM, et al: Bone loss in the distal anterior femur after total knee arthroplasty, *Clin Orthop* 260:135–143, 1990.
36. Miura H, et al: Effects of screws and a sleeve on initial fixation in uncemented total knee tibial components, *Clin Orthop* 259:160–168, 1990.
37. Murase K, et al: An analysis of tibial component design in total knee arthroplasty, *J Biomech* 16:13–22, 1982.
38. Murrish D, Hillberry B, Heck D: Strain distribution in the proximal tibia with and without tibial prostheses: A Fem Study, *Trans Orthop Res Soc* 10:122, 1985.
39. Nilsson KG, Karrholm J, Gadegaard P: Abnormal kinematics of the artificial knee: Roentgen stereophotogrammetric analysis of 10 Miller-Galante and 5 New Jersey LCS knees, *Acta Orthop Scand* 62:440–446, 1991.
40. Orr TE, et al: Computer predictions of bone remodeling around porous-coated implants, *J Arthroplasty* 5:191–200, 1990.
41. Rand JA, Ilstrup DM: Survivorship analysis of total knee arthroplasty, *J Bone Joint Surg [Am]* 73:397–409, 1991.
42. Reilly D, Martens M: Experimental analysis of the quadriceps muscle force and patello-femoral joint reaction force for various activities, *Acta Orthop Scand* 43:126–137, 1972.
43. Rittman N, et al: Analysis of patterns of knee motion walking for four types of total knee implants, *Clin Orthop* 155:111–117, 1981.
44. Rose R, et al: On the true wear rate of ultra-high mo-

lecular weight polyethylene in the total knee prosthesis, *J Biomed Mater Res* 18:207–224, 1984.
45. Ryd L: The role of Roentgen stereophotogrammatric analysis (RSA) in knee surgery, *Am J Knee Surg* 5:44–54, 1992.
46. Ryd L, et al: Micromotion of conventionally cemented all-polyethylene tibial components in total knee replacements, *Arch Orthop Trauma Surg* 106:82–88, 1987.
47. Ryd L, et al: Cold flow reduced by metal backing, *Acta Orthop Scand* 61:21–25, 1990.
48. Samuelson KM: Bone grafting and noncemented revision arthroplasty of the knee, *Clin Orthop* 226:93, 1988.
49. Seale KS, et al: The effect of meniscectomy on knee stability, *Trans Orthop Res Soc* 28:124, 1982.
50. Shimagaki H, et al: Stability of initial fixation of the tibial component in cementless total knee arthroplasty, *J Orthop Res* 8:64–71, 1990.
51. Shoemaker SC, Markolf KL: The role of the meniscus in the anterior-posterior stability of the loaded anterior cruciate–deficient knee, *J Bone Joint Surg [Am]* 68:71–79, 1986.
52. Soudry M, et al: Effects of total knee replacement design on femoral-tibial contact conditions, *J Arthroplasty* 1:35–45, 1986.
53. Strickland AB, et al: The initial fixation of porous coated tibial components evaluated by the study of rigid body motion under static load, *Trans Orthop Res Soc* 13:476, 1988.
54. Stulberg BN, et al: A new model to assess tibial fixation in knee arthroplasty—I. *Clin Orthop* 263:288–302, 1991.
55. Stulberg BN, et al: A new model to assess tibial fixation—II. *Clin Orthop* 263:303–309, 1991.
56. Van Kampen A, Huiskes R: The three-dimensional tracking pattern of the human patella, *J Orthop Res* 8:372–382, 1990.
57. Volz R, et al: The mechanical stability of various noncemented tibial components, *Clin Orthop* 226:38–42, 1988.
58. Walker PS, Erkman MJ: The role of the menisci in force transmission across the knee, *Clin Orthop* 109:184–192, 1975.
59. Walker PS, Granholm J, Lowrey R: The fixation of femoral components of condylar knee prosthesis, *Eng Med* 11:135–140, 1982.
60. Walker PS, Hsieh H: Conformity in condylar replacement knee prostheses, *J Bone Joint Surg [Br]* 59:222–228, 1977.
61. Walker PS, Hsu HP, Zimmerman RA: A comparative study of uncemented tibial components, *J Arthroplasty* 5:245–253, 1990.
62. Walker PS, Reilly D, Ben-Dove M: Load transfer in the upper tibia before and after tibial component attachment, *Trans ORS* 26:164, 1980.
63. Walker PS, et al: Fixation of tibial components of knee prostheses, *J Bone Joint Surg [Am]* 63:258–267, 1981.
64. Whiteside LA: Cementless reconstruction of massive tibial bone loss in revision total knee arthroplasty, *Clin Orthop* 248:80–86, 1989.
65. Whiteside LA: Clinical results of the Whiteside Ortholoc total knee replacement, *Orthop Clinics North Am* 20:113–124, 1989.
66. Whiteside LA: The effect of patient age, gender, and tibial component fixation on pain relief after cementless total knee arthroplasty, *Clin Orthop* 271:21–27, 1991.
67. Whiteside LA, Kasselt MR, Haynes DW: Varus-valgus and rotational stability in rotationally unconstrained total knee arthroplasty, *Clin Orthop* 219:147–157, 1987.
68. Whiteside LA, Pafford J: Load transfer characteristics of noncemented total knee replacement, *Clin Orthop* 239:168–177, 1989.
69. Wongchaisuwat C, Hemami H, Buchner H: Control of sliding and rolling at natural joints, *J Biomech Eng* 106:368–375, 1984.
70. Wright TM, Bartel DL: The problem of surface damage in polyethylene total knee components, *Clin Orthop* 205:67–73, 1986.
71. Yoshii I, Whiteside LA, Anouchi YS: The effect of patellar button placement and femoral component design on patellar tracking in total knee arthroplasty, *Clin Orthop* 275:211–219, 1992.
72. Yoshii I, et al: The effect of central stem and stem length on micromovement of the tibial tray, *J Arthroplasty* 7(suppl):433–438.

60

Unicompartmental Knee Replacement

C. LOWRY BARNES, M.D.
RICHARD D. SCOTT, M.D.

Historical perspective
Surgical options
Patient selection
Operative procedure
    Component positioning
    Component sizing

Implant design
Rehabilitation
Future developments

HISTORICAL PERSPECTIVE

The status of unicompartmental knee replacement remains uncertain although debated for more than 20 years.[14, 30] Laskin,[15] in 1978, reported poor results in patients with unicompartmental replacement of the medial compartment. Similar reports from The Hospital for Special Surgery in New York City described poor results with medial compartmental replacement but better results with lateral compartment arthroplasty in both short-term and long-term follow-up.[8, 9]

More favorable results have since been reported. Marmor,[19] in a 10- to 13-year follow-up of his original design, reported 70% satisfactory results in medial compartment replacement, with failures being secondary to improper patient selection and technical problems. Similar good long-term results in isolated lateral compartment replacement have been reported by Marmor.[18] Other authors have also reported good results at 3 to 5 years' follow-up.[1, 25] Eight- to 12-year follow-up of a series of 100 knees has demonstrated survivorship of the components in 90% of patients at 9 years, 85% at 10 years, and 82% at 11 years[27] (Fig 60–1). The early results using metal-backed tibial components with improved patient selection were extremely encouraging[13] but have been marred somewhat with longer follow-up showing accelerated wear in 6-mm tibial components (Fig 60–2). Three hundred ten knees followed up for 2 to 9 years had five failures due to polyethylene wear and ten others due to loosening, patellofemoral symptoms, or secondary degeneration of the opposite compartment (a 5% revision rate at an average 4-year follow-up).[31]

SURGICAL OPTIONS

The concept of unicompartmental replacement has potential advantages when compared with proximal tibial osteotomy or total knee arthroplasty. Although proximal tibial osteotomy is preferred in the young, active patient with medial compartment arthritis, the advantages of unicompartmental replacement are realized in the elderly, more sedentary patient.[5, 29] Compared with osteotomy, unicompartmental replacement has fewer perioperative complications and a higher success rate in the early postoperative period.[5, 7, 25] Recently, Ivarsson and Gillquist[10] have reported a marked difference in the rehabilitation course after the two operations. Objective measurements of muscle torque showed that results were better in patients 6 months after a unicompartmental replacement as compared with patients 1 year after a proximal tibial osteotomy. In the arthroplasty group, there was also an increased duration of single-limb support and maximal gait velocity. Patients who need bilateral surgery also do much better from a rehabilitation standpoint because their surgery may be performed simultaneously or staged during the same hospital admission. Osteotomy, on the other hand, may require 3 to 6 months between operations and a recovery period of 1 year or more.[14]

Unicompartmental arthroplasty, as compared to tricompartmental arthroplasty, has the advantage of preserving both cruciate ligaments, the patellofemoral joint, and the opposite compartment, therefore preserving nearly normal knee kinematics.[14, 30] In a review of patients with unicompartmental replace-

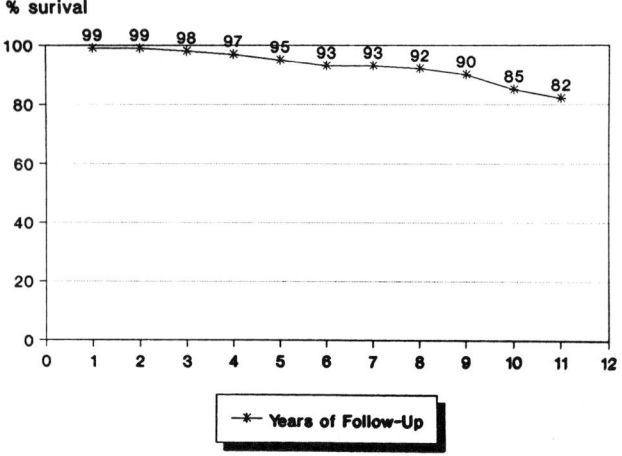

FIG 60–1.
A survivorship curve for unicompartmental arthroplasty showing a tendency for an accelerated failure rate after 10 years. (From Scott RD, et al: *Clin Orthop* 271:98, 1991. Used by permission.)

ment on one side and a bicompartmental or tricompartmental replacement on the other, a majority of the patients preferred the side with unicompartmental replacement, believing it to be closer to normal.[16] Patients with unicompartmental replacement have better range of motion and ambulatory function than patients with tricompartmental replacement.[23]

Another theoretic advantage of unicompartmental replacement is easier revision surgery secondary to retained bone stock.[11] This theoretic advantage,

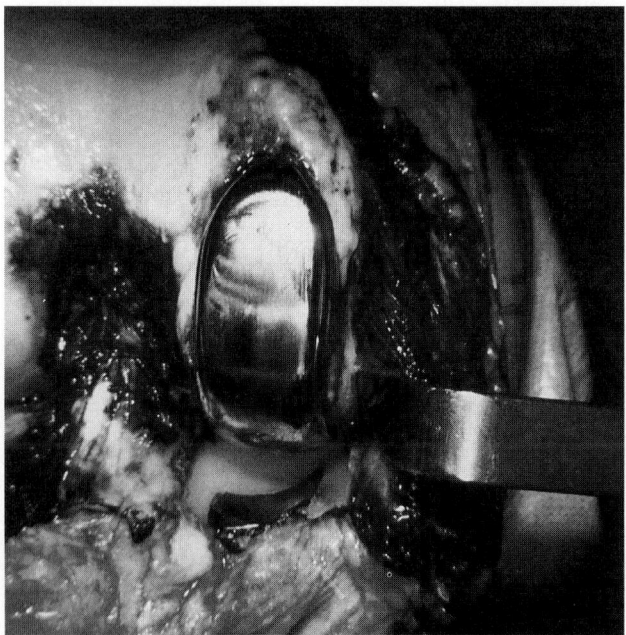

FIG 60–2.
An intraoperative photograph showing wear-through of the tibial polyethylene exposing the metal backing with resultant metal synovitis.

however, has not been proved in two reviews of revision of unicompartmental arthroplasty patients.[2, 20] There was often deficiency of bone in the femoral condyle or tibial plateau which required augmentation with special components or bone graft. The results were also no better than revisions of standard total knee arthroplasty procedures. Modern unicompartmental components with refined surgical techniques are more conservative in replacement of both the femoral and tibial sides and should lead to decreased difficulty in revision surgery[24] (Fig 60–3).

Excellent long-term results have been reported for tricompartmental replacement with or without cruciate sacrifice, and survivorship analyses have been better than 90% at 10 years.[21, 22, 28] As noted, unicompartmental replacements with an early design have a survivorship of only 85% at 10 years.[27] However, improved surgical technique as well as more rigid patient selection should lead to more lasting results competitive with tricompartmental arthroplasty at 10 years.

PATIENT SELECTION

The ideal candidate for unicompartmental replacement is an osteoarthritic patient with unicompartmental disease, a physiologic age greater than 60 years, and a relatively low level of activity. In addition, there should be no inflammatory component to the disease process, often indicated by an effusion or significant pain at rest.[14, 30] Ideally, preoperative motion should be greater than 90 degrees with a flexion contracture of less than 15 degrees. These selection criteria are meant to be guidelines and certain patients may still be good candidates for the procedure even if they fall outside one or more of the criteria listed. Subluxation and greater than 10 degrees of varus or 15 degrees of valgus angular deformity are also relative contraindications to unicompartmental replacement. Unicompartmental metallic interpositional arthroplasty may occasionally be indicated when osteotomy is not appropriate and the patient is too heavy, young, or active for total knee replacement.[6, 26]

Although the patient may appear to be an ideal candidate for unicompartmental replacement by the above criteria, the ultimate decision is made at the time of surgery.[25] An absent anterior cruciate ligament is a relative contraindication to unicompartmental replacement because subluxation resulting in involvement of the opposite compartment may ensue. The opposite compartment as well as the patellofemoral joint must be thoroughly examined for evidence of arthritic involvement. While areas of mild

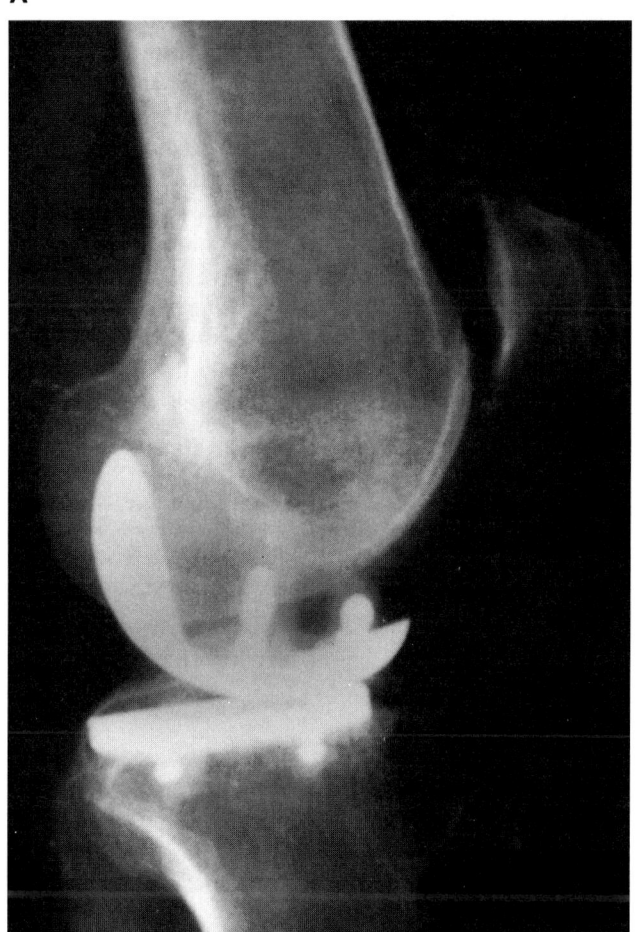 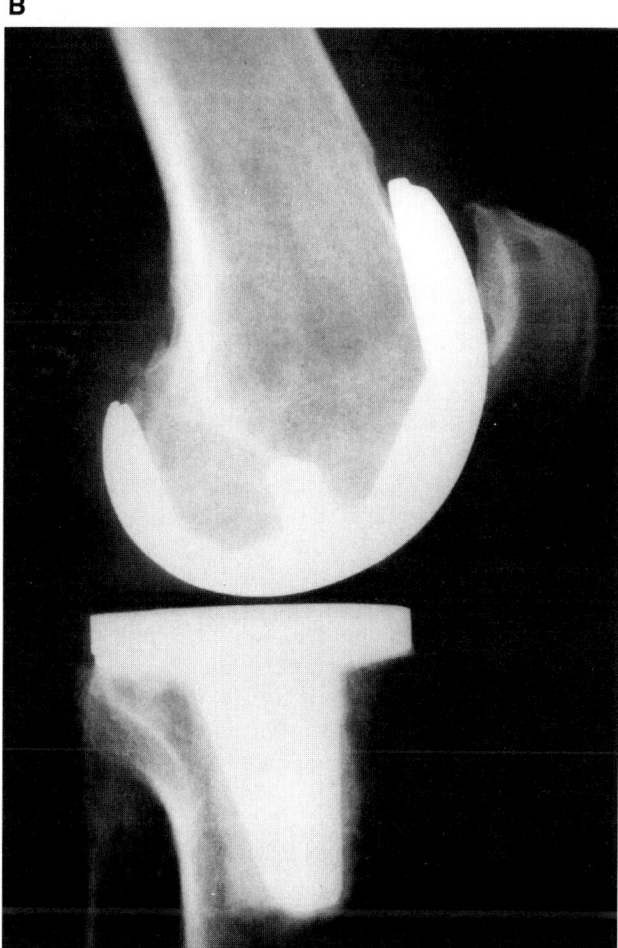

FIG 60-3.
A, Preoperative radiograph of a failed metal-backed tibial component. **B,** postrevision radiograph showing the utilization of primary prosthetic components including a cementless ingrowth femoral component.

chondromalacia may be accepted in the opposite compartment, eburnated bone is a definite contraindication. Significant chondromalacia may be accepted in the patellofemoral joint, but not in association with eburnated bone. If an inflammatory process consisting of synovial proliferation or crystal deposit including chondrocalcinosis is noted at the time of arthrotomy, unicompartmental arthroplasty should probably be abandoned in favor of tricompartmental replacement.

OPERATIVE PROCEDURE

A longitudinal skin incision is made medial to the midline of the patella, although some surgeons recommend a lateral parapatellar incision for lateral compartment replacement.[12] Without disturbing the vastus medialis, a medial parapatellar capsulotomy is performed to allow eversion of the patella during knee flexion.

For replacement of the medial compartment, the coronary ligament is incised at the anterior horn of the medial meniscus. A periosteal sleeve is then raised from the anteromedial aspect of the tibia. Laterally, the dissection is carried to the infrapatellar bursa, protecting the coronary ligament to avoid detachment of the anterior horn of the lateral meniscus. Similarly, the medial aspect of the coronary ligament is protected during lateral compartment replacement, and an anterolateral periosteal sleeve is raised from the lateral aspect of the tibial plateau to Gerdy's tubercle.

All three compartments are thoroughly inspected following adequate exposure, and a decision is made as to the number of compartments to be replaced.

In an osteoarthritic knee with isolated medial compartment involvement and a varus deformity, peripheral osteophytes form at the medial aspect of the femoral condyle and the tibial plateau. Passive correction of the varus deformity may be prevented by

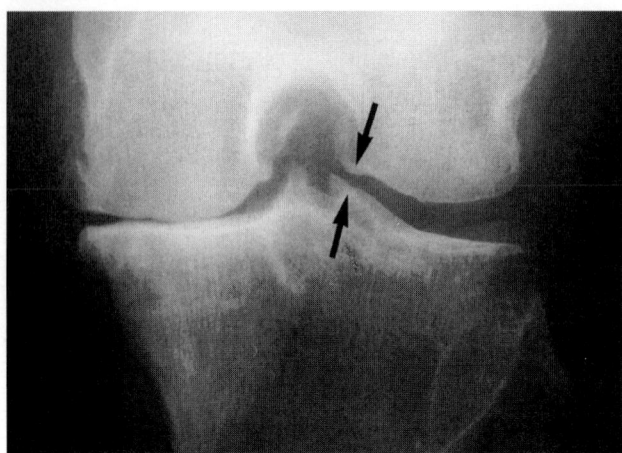

FIG 60-4.
Intercondylar osteophytes and erosion of the medial aspect of the lateral femoral condyle due to tibial spine impingement.

relative shortening of the capsule and medial collateral ligament as they are tented over these osteophytes. Removal of the peripheral osteophytes usually allows passive correction of the varus deformity. A formal medial release is rarely necessary as this would imply a more severe varus deformity requiring bicompartmental or tricompartmental replacement.

Patients who have moderate medial compartment arthritis may develop intercondylar "kissing osteophytes" as the lateral tibial spine impinges on the intercondylar aspect of the lateral femoral condyle (Fig 60-4). If these osteophytes are not removed at the time of unicompartmental replacement, intercondylar impingement can persist and produce pain with weightbearing. If the kissing lesion is large, bicompartmental or tricompartmental arthroplasty may be necessary.

Patients with lateral compartment osteoarthritis do not usually develop tibial subluxation unless the deformity is so severe that unicompartmental replacement is not indicated. The medial capsule and the medial collateral ligament stretch as the valgus deformity develops, and the knee cannot be adequately balanced by unicompartmental arthroplasty.

Component Positioning

The femoral component should be placed centrally in the mediolateral dimension of the femoral condyle after osteophyte removal. If the femoral component is placed too near the midline in a medial unicompartmental arthroplasty, impingement can occur in one of two ways depending upon tibial component design. If the tibial component used provides no mediolateral constraint, impingement can occur between the femoral component and the medial tibial spine. If, on the other hand, the femoral component is matched with a tibial component designed to provide mediolateral constraint, the tibia will move laterally on the femur when the components articulate, leading to impingement between the lateral tibial spine and the lateral femoral condyle.[24, 25]

The tibial component should be placed so that its articular surface is parallel to the femoral component in full extension and in line with the femoral component in the mediolateral direction. The rotation of the tibial component cannot be judged with the patella everted and the knee flexed because this position allows the quadriceps to externally rotate and laterally subluxate the tibia on the femur. Proper congruence of the components should be judged by observing the tracking of the components with flexion and extension while the patella is located in the trochlear groove. Viewed from the front, the tibial resection should be 85 to 95 degrees in relation to the longitudinal axis of the tibia. Viewed from the side, there should be between 0 and 10 degrees of posterior slope, with 3 to 5 degrees of posterior slope usually appropriate.

Component Sizing

The size of the femoral component should reproduce the anteroposterior dimension of the femoral condyle. In borderline cases, it is best to use the larger component as this provides better capping of the bone to resist loosening or subsidence. The posterior condylar bone should be resected to at least the thickness of the femoral implant. To avoid tightness in flexion, it is better to resect too much of the posterior condyle than too little. The anterior weightbearing margin of the femoral condyle is usually well defined by the junction between the eburnated bone on the femoral condyle and the remaining intact cartilage of the trochlear groove. The femoral component should extend far enough anteriorly to cover the full weightbearing surface in contact with the tibia in full extension. The leading edge of the femoral component should also be countersunk flush with the cartilage to avoid interference with patellar tracking.

Ideally, the proper thickness of the tibial component should restore the tibial plateau to its normal height. With appropriate medial peripheral osteophyte removal, correction of the varus deformity should not require thicker tibial components. After medial unicompartmental replacement, the medial joint space should open 1 to 2 mm with application of a valgus stress in full extension. Likewise, the lateral joint space should open 1 to 2 mm with application of varus stress in full extension following lateral compartment replacement. If the components are too tight, the tibia might subluxate toward the opposite compartment and produce excessive pressure and wear.

IMPLANT DESIGN

Experience of the past 20 years has led to a better understanding of the ideal design features of unicompartmental arthroplasty. Many of the early femoral components were narrow in the mediolateral dimension and had a high incidence of subsidence into the femoral condylar bone. The ideal component should be wide enough to maximally cap the resurfaced condyle and adequately distribute the weightbearing forces. Therefore, multiple sizes of femoral components should be available. Revision studies have shown that the condyle should not be deeply invaded with fixation devices. As long as there are two lugs or a fin to control rotation, relatively small fixation lugs appear to be sufficient. The posterior condyle of the component should completely cap the posterior condyle of the femur to allow full range of motion without impingement.

Although it would be preferable to resurface the femoral subchondral bone without any distal condylar resection, this would require sacrifice of more tibial bone stock to accommodate adequately thick components. The ideal compromise is probably to resect 2 to 4 mm of distal femoral condyle, retaining some subchondral bone for prosthetic fixation while conserving enough distal femur to allow easy conversion to a standard bicompartmental arthroplasty. Similarly, sacrificing 2 to 4 mm from the femur preserves 2 to 4 mm of tibial bone stock which should make revision correspondingly easier on the tibial side (Fig 60–5).

The topography of the component articulation must also represent a compromise. A flat surface-to-flat surface articulation would be ideal to improve metal-to-plastic contact. Technically, however, this would be too difficult to properly align and prevent edge contact throughout the range of motion. A femoral articulating surface with a small convex radius of curvature articulating with a flat tibial surface would lead to too much point contact. A small convex femoral radius of curvature articulating with a small concave radius of curvature on the tibia would create too much constraint. A compromise might consist of a femoral component with a large convex radius of curvature and a tibial component with a similar large concave radius to allow adequate metal-to-plastic contact without too much constraint. The an-

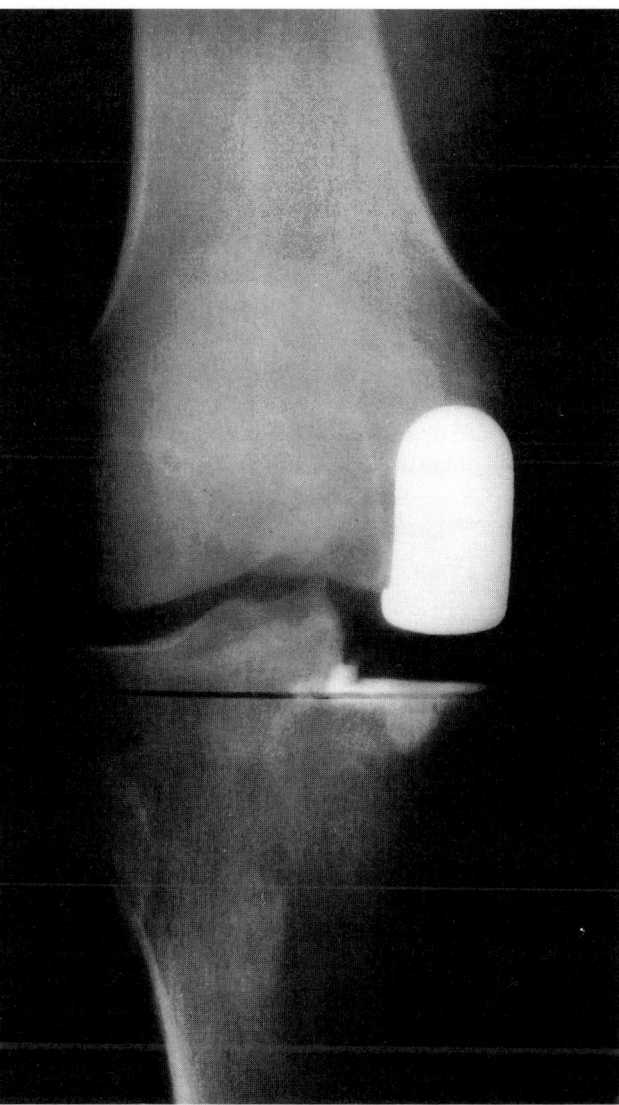

FIG 60–5.
Postoperative radiograph demonstrating conservative femoral and tibial resection and the use of an all-polyethylene tibial component.

teroposterior topography of the tibial component can also provide some anterior and posterior concavity to help guide the femoral component to properly articulate with the central 50% of the tibial component surface.

A tibial component with an anatomic shape to its undersurface will maximize contact between the prosthesis and the bone, widely distributing the forces to resist loosening and subsidence. This requires right and left components with asymmetric shapes and multiple sizes.

Controversy remains as to whether or not the tibial component should have a metal backing. Metal backing was initially introduced to more uniformly distribute the weightbearing forces on the cut surface of the tibia. Although early results were better with metal-backed tibial components, this may have been secondary to better patient selection and improved operative techniques.[13, 31] As noted previously, failures secondary to polyethylene wear have been seen in 6-mm-thick metal-backed tibial components. Wear was most likely in areas where the polyethylene was 2 mm thick with an underlying sharp angle to the metal base. These problems were similarly described in metal-backed patellar components.[3, 17] With metal backing, the tibial component must have at least 6 mm of polyethylene (a composite thickness of 8–10 mm) to minimize early wear. Since this requires more bone sacrifice, there may be a trend back to all-polyethylene tibial components (see Fig 60–5).

REHABILITATION

Postoperative rehabilitation following cemented unicondylar arthroplasty is similar to that of standard cemented total knee arthroplasty. Often, however, rehabilitation goals are met sooner, and patients have less pain, swelling, and blood loss.[16] At the time of capsule closure, a note is made of the patient's flexion with gravity as this should be the limit of expectation in the early postoperative period.

Patients without contraindications to anticoagulation are given warfarin (Coumadin) the night prior to surgery, and warfarin and compression stockings are used postoperatively for prophylaxis against thromboembolic disease. The continuous passive motion (CPM) machine is begun in the recovery room with flexion to 30 to 40 degrees following a general anesthetic and to 70 to 90 degrees if a long-acting spinal or epidural anesthetic has been administered. The CPM is advanced 10 to 20 degrees per day as tolerated until 90 degrees of flexion is achieved and maintained. The CPM is used during the day and a knee immobilizer is applied at night to prevent development of a flexion contracture. Quadriceps setting exercises, straight leg raises, and bed-to-chair transfers are begun on the second postoperative day. By the third day, the patient walks with a walker or crutches at 50% weightbearing. A knee immobilizer is used when walking until the patient can easily perform straight leg raises. Patients remain at protected weightbearing with a walker or crutches until 6 weeks after surgery. At that time, they graduate to a cane outdoors and may walk without support for short walks indoors. The cane is discontinued at 3 months.

FUTURE DEVELOPMENTS

Although there is current interest in the use of non-cemented knee prostheses, the role of uncemented unicompartmental arthroplasty is uncertain. Cementless unicompartmental arthroplasty loses some appeal because more bone resection may be necessary on the femoral side to provide a cancellous bone interface for ingrowth, or on the tibial side to allow for metal backing. Additionally, failure rates have been higher on both the femoral and tibial sides in early reports of cementless unicompartmental replacement.[4]

The future role of cemented unicompartmental arthroplasty also remains uncertain. Proximal tibial osteotomy continues to be the treatment of choice in the young, heavy, active patient with medial compartment osteoarthritis. The same knee in a very elderly patient with a life expectancy of less than 10 years might best be treated with tricompartmental arthroplasty as the definitive procedure. Unicompartmental arthroplasty emerges as a conservative first arthroplasty for selected osteoarthritic patients with greater than 15 years of life expectancy. Both cruciates and bone stock are preserved permitting a higher postoperative functional level and easier revision procedure as long as conservative operative techniques have been utilized. The number of candidates for unicompartmental replacement will remain limited to somewhere between 5% and 25% of osteoarthritic knees depending on the selection criteria, the rigidity by which they are followed, and the experience and enthusiasm of the operating surgeon.

REFERENCES

1. Bae KK, Guhl JF, Keane SP: Unicompartmental knee arthroplasty for single compartment disease, Clin Orthop 176:233, 1983.
2. Barrett WP, Scott RD: Revision of failed unicondylar arthroplasty, J Bone Joint Surg [Am] 69:1328, 1987.
3. Bayley JC, et al: Failure of the metal-backed patellar component after total knee replacement, J Bone Joint Surg [Am] 70:668, 1988.
4. Bernasek TL, Rand JA, Bryan RS: Unicompartmental porous coated anatomic total knee arthroplasty, Clin Orthop 236:52, 1988.
5. Broughton NS, Newman JH, Bailey RA: Unicompartmental replacement and high tibial osteotomy for osteoarthritis of the knee, J Bone Joint Surg [Br] 68:447, 1986.
6. Emerson RH, Potter T: The use of the metallic McKeever hemiarthroplasty for unicompartmental arthritis, J Bone Joint Surg [Am] 67:208, 1985.

7. Inglis G: Unicompartmental arthroplasty of the knee, *J Bone Joint Surg [Br]* 66:682, 1984.
8. Insall J, Aglietti P: A five to seven-year follow-up of unicondylar arthroplasty, *J Bone Joint Surg [Am]* 62:1329, 1980.
9. Insall JN, Walker PS: Unicondylar knee replacement, *Clin Orthop* 120:83, 1976.
10. Ivarsson I, Gillquist J: Rehabilitation after high tibial osteotomy and unicompartmental arthroplasty, *Clin Orthop* 266:139, 1991.
11. Jones WH, et al: Unicompartmental knee arthroplasty using polycentric and geometric hemicomponents, *J Bone Joint Surg [Am]* 63:946, 1981.
12. Keblish PA: Valgus deformity in total knee replacement. The lateral retinacular approach, *Orthop Trans* 9:28, 1985.
13. Kozinn SC, Marx C, Scott RD: Unicompartmental knee arthroplasty, *J Arthroplasty* 4:51, 1989.
14. Kozinn SC, Scott RD: Current concepts review, Unicompartmental knee arthroplasty, *J Bone Joint Surg [Am]* 71:145, 1989.
15. Laskin RS: Unicompartmental tibiofemoral resurfacing arthroplasty, *J Bone Joint Surg [Am]* 60:182, 1978.
16. Laurencin CT, et al: Unicompartmental versus total knee arthroplasty in the same patient: A comparative study, *Clin Orthop* 273:151–156, 1991.
17. Lombardi AV Jr, et al: Fracture/dissociation of the polyethylene in metal-backed patellar components in total knee arthroplasty, *J Bone Joint Surg [Am]* 70:675, 1988.
18. Marmor L: Lateral compartment arthroplasty of the knee, *Clin Orthop* 186:115, 1984.
19. Marmor L: Unicompartmental knee arthroplasty, Ten to thirteen year follow-up study, *Clin Orthop* 226:14, 1987.
20. Padgett DE, Stern SH, Insall JN: Revision total knee arthroplasty for failed unicompartmental replacement, *J Bone Joint Surg [Am]* 73:186, 1991.
21. Ranawat CS, Oheneba BA: Survivorship analysis and results of total condylar knee arthroplasty, *Clin Orthop* 226:6, 1988.
22. Rand JA, Ilstrup DM: Survivorship analysis of total knee arthroplasty. Cumulative rates of survival of 9200 total knee arthroplasties, *J Bone Joint Surg [Am]* 73:397, 1991.
23. Rougraff BT, Heck DA, Gibson AE: A comparison of tricompartmental and unicompartmental arthroplasty for the treatment of gonarthrosis, *Clin Orthop* 273:157–164, 1991.
24. Scott RD: Robert Brigham unicondylar knee surgical techniques, *Orthopedics* 5:15, 1990.
25. Scott RD, Santore R: Unicondylar unicompartmental replacement for osteoarthritis of the knee, *J Bone Joint Surg [Am]* 63:536, 1981.
26. Scott RD, et al: McKeever metallic hemiarthroplasty of the knee in unicompartmental degenerative arthritis, *J Bone Joint Surg [Am]* 67:203, 1985.
27. Scott RD, et al: Unicompartmental knee arthroplasty, eight to twelve year follow-up with survivorship analysis, *Clin Orthop* 271:96–100, 1991.
28. Scuderi GR, et al: Survivorship of cemented knee replacement, *J Bone Joint Surg [Br]* 71:798, 1989.
29. Thornhill TS: Unicompartmental knee arthroplasty, *Clin Orthop* 205:121, 1986.
30. Thornhill TS, Scott RD: Unicompartmental total knee arthroplasty, *Orthop Clin North Am* 20:245, 1989.
31. Thornhill TS, et al: Metal-backed unicompartmental knee replacement, 58th Annual Meeting of the American Academy of Orthopaedic Surgeons, Anaheim, Calif, March 11, 1991.

61

Cementless Total Knee Arthroplasty

MATTHEW J. KRAAY, M.D.
VICTOR M. GOLDBERG, M.D.

Biologic and surgical considerations of porous ingrowth fixation
Implant design considerations
Implant retrieval studies

Clinical results
Complications
Results at University Hospitals of Cleveland

Aseptic loosening of early cemented total joint prostheses and the perception of polymethyl methacrylate as the weak link in this method of fixation stimulated investigation into alternative methods of implant fixation to the underlying bone. The potential for biologic fixation by bone ingrowth into porous-surfaced implants has subsequently been studied extensively. Animal and human investigations have demonstrated that under the appropriate circumstances, stable fixation by tissue ingrowth into porous implants is possible.

Improvements in cemented total knee arthroplasty designs and surgical techniques have significantly reduced the incidence of fixation-related failure. Similar improvements in uncemented total knee replacement (TKR) design, surgical technique, and patient selection have also resulted in improved results with uncemented fixation. As a result, considerable interest regarding the potential for permanent biologic fixation and the clinical use of uncemented total knee arthroplasty has continued. This chapter reviews the basic science, design considerations, and clinical results of uncemented total knee arthroplasty.

BIOLOGIC AND SURGICAL CONSIDERATIONS OF POROUS INGROWTH FIXATION

The basic science and historical development of biologic fixation with porous-coated implants has been well summarized.[22,49,50] Biologic bone ingrowth fixation is a complex process requiring an appropriate porous surface structure for allowing bone ingrowth, adequate osteogenic potential, close proximity of the implant to bone, and limitation of motion across the developing bone-implant interface.

The structural requirements of porous-coated implants have been extensively studied. Pore size and internal porosity are important design and manufacturing factors that can significantly influence the extent and depth of bone ingrowth into porous structures. Although bone ingrowth can occur into surfaces with pore sizes as small as 50 μm under ideal situations, clinical and experimental investigation suggests that more rapid, predictable, and secure fixation occurs into surfaces with pore sizes in the 100- to 500-μm range.[7,8]

The size of attachment between individual particles of the coating, or particle interconnectivity, is an important determinant of the structural integrity of the coating, the bond with the underlying substrate, and ultimately of the ingrowth of bone into the implant. Although increased particle interconnectivity provides for a stronger connection between the individual particles of the porous structure, this may result in a decrease in the volume fraction of porosity available for tissue ingrowth. The depth and extent of bone ingrowth could also be adversely affected in this situation. Decreased particle interconnectivity can potentially compromise the strength of attachment between the individual elements of the porous structure, resulting in mechanical failure. This has been observed clinically as "shedding" of beads from certain types of porous surfaces. Porous surfaces formed by sintering of multiple small metallic beads may be at a disadvantage regarding this balance between porosity and strength in comparison to the more open-structured fibermetal surfaces.

The biologic requirements for successful bone ingrowth are difficult to quantify. In certain conditions, such as avascular necrosis, metabolic bone disease, and following irradiation, the cellular and nutritional prerequisites necessary for this process may be insufficient for bone ingrowth. Many medications, including corticosteroids, nonsteroidal anti-inflammatory drugs, warfarin, and a variety of immunosuppressive medications may adversely affect bone ingrowth. Depending on severity, alterations in bone metabolism associated with the aging process may also compromise bone ingrowth. Although the absolute minimum potential for ingrowth is uncertain, patients with the above risk factors for ingrowth failure should be carefully considered for uncemented fixation.

Close apposition of bone to the porous surface is a necessary requirement for bone ingrowth. Although unloaded porous-coated implants in animal models have demonstrated that gaps of 1.5 to 2.0 mm can be bridged by bone, this may take as long as 12 weeks to occur.[8] Whether gaps between bone and porous surfaces of this magnitude can be bridged by bone in physiologically loaded human joint replacements is uncertain. Bone ingrowth into porous-coated canine acetabular components has been shown to be decreased significantly in the presence of 0.5- to 1.0-mm gaps.[29] Meticulous surgical technique and instrumentation capable of accurately preparing the bone surfaces are critical in providing close apposition to porous-surfaced implants.

Bone ingrowth into porous-coated implants requires that interface motion be minimal until ingrowth is established. Retrieval studies have suggested that the critical ingrowth occurs during the 4- to 6-week healing phase following implantation,[9] although additional ingrowth and remodeling may continue for up to 27 months after implantation.[23] Motion across the bone-implant interface exceeding 150 μm has been experimentally demonstrated to inhibit bone ingrowth and result in ingrowth of fibrous tissue.[39]

The initial implant stability is determined by several factors, one of the most important of which is implant design. The conforming surface geometry of nearly all uncemented femoral components provides for excellent stability resulting in reliable bone ingrowth seen clinically and on evaluation of retrieved specimens. Resistance of uncemented tibial components to micromotion induced by physiologic loads can vary dramatically.

Tibial component stability is determined primarily by the effectiveness of various design features, such as stems, keels, pegs, and screws, in resisting interface motion. Accuracy of surface preparation and resultant implant fit, as well as bone quality, can affect the initial stability of both the femoral and tibial components. The magnitude of implant loading can also affect the degree of micromotion across the bone-implant interface. Protected weightbearing during the healing phase following implantation is a simple way of accomplishing this and is recommended by most authors. Significant implant malalignment or soft tissue imbalance results in eccentric loading and a tendency for liftoff of the opposite side of the component and should be avoided. Seemingly minor malalignment as small as 5 degrees has been demonstrated to result in alterations in tibial load distribu-

A
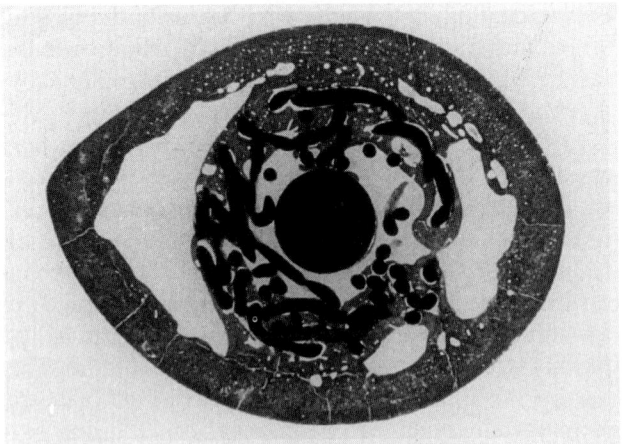

B
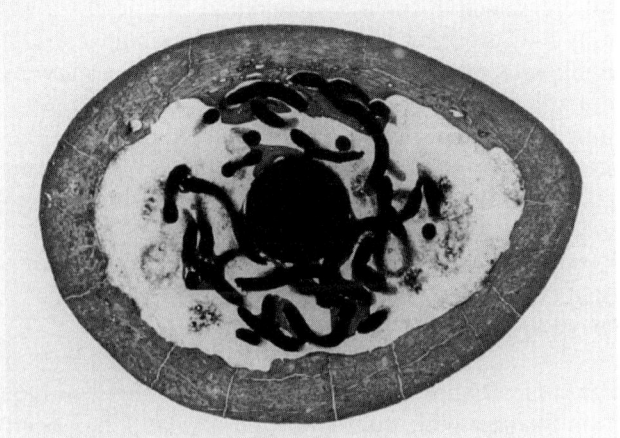

FIG 61–1.
A, Cross section of a plasma-sprayed TCP/hydroxyapatite-coated porous titanium intramedullary implant at 24 weeks' post implantation in the distal femur of a rabbit. Note the extent of ingrowth into the porous surface. **B,** bone ingrowth into an identical implant without TCP/hydroxyapatite in the contralateral femur at 24 weeks. (Courtesy of Sharon Stevenson, D.V.M., Ph.D.)

tion of up to 40% in cemented TKRs.[27] Intramedullary instrumentation, especially of the femur, has been shown to improve the accuracy of implant alignment and its use is recommended by some authors.[17]

Recent investigation of bioactive ceramics may prove to be useful in enhancing bone ingrowth fixation of total knee prostheses (Fig 61–1,A and B). Soballe et al.[48] compared the interface properties of titanium and porous hydroxyapatite (HA)-coated implants subjected to stable (unloaded) and unstable mechanical conditions. The situation of implant instability was simulated by an implanted dynamic loading device which produced controlled motions of 500 μm. Under stable conditions, the shear strength of HA-coated implants was 250% stronger than titanium porous-coated implants and had five times as much bone ingrowth as the titanium implants. Although there was no difference in the amount of bone ingrowth between the two types of implants under unstable conditions, the shear strength of the HA-coated implants was five times greater than that of unstable titanium implants. Gap healing was significantly improved with stable HA implants, but neither implant showed any appreciable gap healing in an unstable situation.

IMPLANT DESIGN CONSIDERATIONS

Retrieval analysis has suggested that bone ingrowth into uncemented, porous-coated tibial components is limited.[10, 12, 22, 54] The implant stability inherent in the design of the tibial component is an important determinant of interface micromotion, and ultimately, quality of biologic fixation.[39] Clinical and retrieval studies suggest that bone ingrowth fixation of uncemented porous-coated femoral components occurs reliably and is probably related to the generally good bone quality of the distal femur and intrinsic stability of the femoral component. As a result, design efforts have been directed almost entirely toward optimizing the stability of the uncemented tibial component.

Several studies have documented the theoretic advantages of metal backing and maximal cortical coverage of cemented tibial components with respect to load transfer and interface micromotion.[5, 32, 57] Tibial component fixation without cement requires some type of supplemental fixation to initially minimize micromotion across the bone-prosthesis interface to levels compatible with bone ingrowth. Shear loads, axial compressive loads, and tension generated by eccentrically applied axial loads can be resisted by a variety of configurations of central or peripheral stems, screws, pegs, or keels. Most currently available uncemented tibial components use a combination of these in attempting to provide adequate initial fixation. Both clinical and laboratory investigations show that certain of these design features are superior to others in providing sufficient implant stability for bone ingrowth to occur. Bone quality itself has been shown to significantly affect tibial component micromotion.[31, 36]

Considerable laboratory data exist supporting the use of screws to provide initial stability of uncemented tibial components. Using foam proximal tibia models with simulated properties of "good quality" and "bad quality" bone, Lee et al.[31] investigated the effects of various combinations of stems and 6.5-mm cancellous screws using an idealized tibial component subjected to cyclic loading. Maximal fixation was obtained with the use of four peripherally placed screws. Although use of a central stem in conjunction with screw fixation had an insignificant effect on implant stability in good-quality bone, it did appear to have a significant effect on stability in poor-quality bone. Similar results have been reported by Yoshii et al.[60]

Using similar methods with an idealized uncemented tibial component and urethane foam bone models, Dempsey et al.[14] demonstrated improved stability with the use of four 6.5-mm cancellous screws in comparison to anchorage systems with four short pegs or a single central peg. Several other investigations using cadaver tibiae have demonstrated significant reduction in implant micromotion to levels compatible with bone ingrowth with the use of four peripherally placed screws.[36, 51, 55] The pullout strength of 6.5-mm cancellous screws has been demonstrated to be twice that of 3.8-mm screws, and the former should provide increased resistance to component liftoff under conditions of eccentric loading.[18]

Walker et al.[56] investigated the effects of various peg and stem configurations in an idealized uncemented tibial component using rigid foam models. Components with central stems and bladed stems performed best with regard to load transfer and micromotion under conditions of offset loading. Configurations with four short peripherally placed pegs or a central peg with blades performed best under shear and torsional loading. Idealized implant designs with two pegs proved to be inferior under all loading situations. Three commercially available tibial components incorporating these design features have been evaluated in vitro under a variety of eccentric loading conditions by Shimagaki et al.[47] For all loading situations, performance with regard to micromotion was superior with the component with a central stem and six small peripheral pegs and inferior with the component with two small posteriorly sloped pegs.

The influence of fixation peg design on implant stability subjected to shear loads has been studied by Giori et al.[19] Peg configurations of various size, aspect ratio, and number were evaluated in urethane foam blocks having mechanical properties similar to that of cancellous bone. Multiple spaced small pegs were more effective in minimizing shear displacement and in resisting shear load per unit of peg volume. The results of this study also suggested that multiple small pegs provide for more uniform distribution of stresses to the underlying material than occurs with fewer large pegs. This may have implications regarding long-term bone remodeling changes which have been a concern with uncemented total joint replacements.

Recent finite element and interface optimization analysis has suggested that multiple conical porous-coated pegs may provide for improved stability and bone apposition in comparison to cylindric pegs.[25] This design concept of multiple conical fixation pegs has been examined in animal implantation studies and in vitro mechanical testing of an experimental tibial component.[21, 34] Stability under torsional, shear, and symmetric and asymmetric axial loading situations was significantly greater than with conventional uncemented implants tested, and approached that of cemented tibial components.

Another finite element analysis has suggested that although an initial interference fit between a peg and the surrounding cancellous bone may promote ingrowth into the peg, it may also relieve stresses in the bone under the tibial tray and inhibit ingrowth into this surface.[13] These results appear to be consistent with observed patterns of tissue ingrowth from many retrieved tibial components.

Roentgen stereophotogrammetric analysis (RSA) has provided some interesting in vivo information regarding tibial implant design and stability. Significant inducible displacements and subsidence over time have been noted for many different tibial component designs.[46] With several of these, inducible displacement was incompatible with bone ingrowth. This appears to correlate with in vitro and clinical data with certain of these designs that have had problems with implant loosening. As suggested by in vitro studies, which predict improved stability with a design incorporating four peripheral pegs and four screws, no subsidence and inducible displacement compatible with bone ingrowth were noted by RSA of the Miller-Galante (Zimmer, Warsaw, Ind.) prosthesis.[46] This technique may prove to be a useful method of in vivo evaluation of prosthesis design in the future.

Problems with failure of metal-backed porous-coated patellar components have been well documented[2, 3, 33, 41, 44, 45, 53] and are related to both implant design and mode of fixation. While there appears to be some theoretic advantage to metal backing of patellar components,[20] clinical failures with a wide variety of metal-backed patellar components raise serious questions as to whether these design objectives can be successfully met.

A basic knowledge of the loading situation of the patellofemoral joint is necessary to understand the problems with metal-backed patellar component designs. Patellofemoral joint reaction forces have been estimated to exceed seven times body weight for certain activities involving marked knee flexion.[42] Study of normal patellofemoral kinematics has shown that the location of patellofemoral contact changes in a distal to proximal fashion as the degree of knee flexion increases. Activities involving knee flexion consequently result in significant eccentric loading of the patella. As the eccentricity of loading increases, an increasing component of the patellofemoral joint reaction force resolves as a shear force on a dome-shaped patellar prosthesis (Fig 61–2). Several other factors related to surgical technique can result in eccentric loading of the patellar component. Problems with patellar tracking secondary to limb or component malalignment or soft tissue balance can contribute to eccentric loading of the patellar component. Patellar tilt due to asymmetric resection or changes in the joint line position can have similar effects. Certain patient

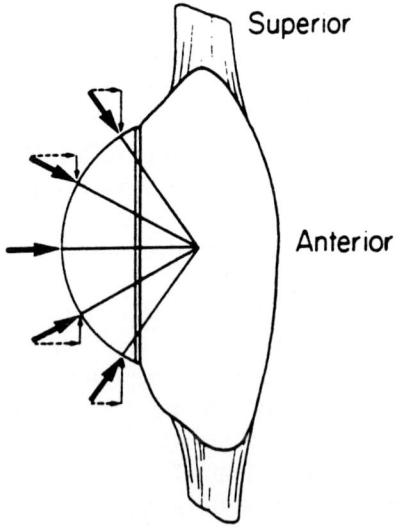

FIG 61–2.
As the eccentricity of patellar loading on a dome-shaped patella increases, an increasing component of the patellofemoral joint reaction force resolves as a shear force. (From Rosenberg AG, et al: *Clin Orthop* 236:106, 1989. Used by permission.)

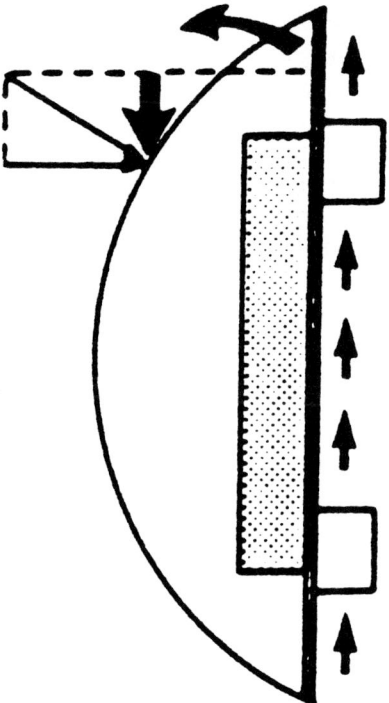

FIG 61–3.
Shear forces resulting from eccentric loading of a dome-shaped patellar component must be balanced within the component or at the implant-bone interface. (From Rosenberg AG, et al: *Clin Orthop* 236:106, 1989. Used by permission.)

factors such as body weight, activity level, and postoperative range of motion have been clinically associated with metal-backed patellar component failures, presumably because of shear component overloading.

The effect of eccentric loading on a domed-shaped patellar component is responsible for many of the problems observed with metal-backed patellar components (Fig 61–3). Three general mechanisms of uncemented patellar component failure have been identified[45] (Fig 61–4). In situations associated with lack of ingrowth into the metal base plate, failure of fixation pegs at their junction can result from the shear loads transmitted across the interface. Delamination or dissociation of the polyethylene from the underlying metal base can occur if the moments induced by these shear forces are not effectively balanced internally by the design of the metal-polyethylene interface. Failure can also occur as a result of local wear over a point of stress concentration or minimal material thickness associated with the underlying metal backing. A definite relationship between polyethylene wear, polyethylene thickness, and articular congruence has been demonstrated and a minimal polyethylene thickness of 8 mm has been recommended for low-conformity articulations such as the tibial component.[4] This may be even more critical when considering the relatively high loads and small contact areas of the patellofemoral joint.[53] The limitations imposed by component size and compromise of patellar polyethylene thickness by the underlying metal backing make the development of a reliable metal-backed patellar component uncertain. Modified dome components having improved patellofemoral congruity may allow for normalization of patellofemoral loads and minimization of shear forces on the patellar component and make metal backing feasible.[26] Considering the serious and increasing complications associated with both cemented and uncemented metal-backed patellar components, we do not recommend their continued use at this time.

IMPLANT RETRIEVAL STUDIES

Implant retrieval studies have demonstrated widely varying results with respect to the degree of bony ingrowth into uncemented total knee prostheses. Interpretation of retrieval data can be misleading when implants are obtained at the time of revision for loosening or for other conditions, such as infection or implant malalignment, which may adversely influence the quantity and quality of bone ingrowth. Patients

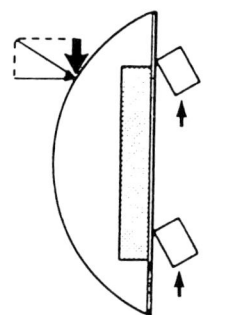 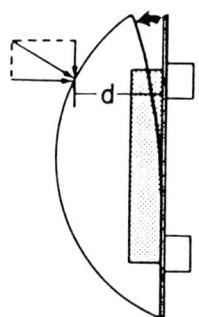 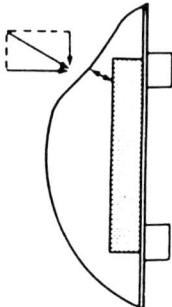

FIG 61–4.
Three general mechanisms of patellar component failure as a result of the shear forces generated by eccentric loads on a dome-shaped patella. (From Rosenberg AG, et al: *Clin Orthop* 236:106, 1989. Used by permission.)

with persistent pain of uncertain cause may indeed have loosening which is unrecognized using current criteria. Histologic characterizations of biologic fixation achieved in asymptomatic, well-functioning porous ingrowth total knee prostheses are rare. Estimation of the extent of bone ingrowth is also dependent on the analytic technique utilized and is subject to sampling error.

Cook et al.[12] reported the histologic and radiographic findings in 85 total knee components removed from 45 patients for reasons other than clinically or radiographically suspected loosening. Retrieved specimens were of five different designs and were submitted for evaluation by many surgeons from around the United States. All of the implants were well fixed by fibrous tissue and a variable amount of bone ingrowth. Forty-four (52%) of the components showed no evidence of bone ingrowth, while 25 (29%) showed bone ingrowth in less than 2% of the available porous surface. Bone ingrowth was seen in only 2% to 10% of the porous surface for the remaining 16 components (19%). There was no difference in the amount of bone ingrowth among tibial, femoral, or patellar components. The authors acknowledged that the majority of specimens were removed at revision surgery, and were frequently associated with poor initial implant position. Considering the large porous surface area of total knee components, the authors concluded that the combination of limited bone ingrowth and extensive fibrous tissue ingrowth is adequate for implant fixation.

Collier et al.[10] recently summarized their analysis of 500 retrieved porous-coated uncemented total knee prostheses. Bone ingrowth of femoral components was frequently seen when compared with other total knee components, and appeared independent of implant design, porous surface structure, and alloy (beaded cobalt-chromium vs. titanium mesh). Distribution of ingrowth by bone was patchy and incomplete. While bone ingrowth into patellar components was similar in extent to femoral components, the authors frequently noted polyethylene wear debris at the periphery of the patellar-component interface. Bone ingrowth of porous tibial components was seen less frequently than with femoral or patellar components. Evidence of bone ingrowth was seen in 75% of titanium tibial implants that provided fixation with four screws. Bone resorption and wear debris within the prosthesis-bone interface were frequently seen in implants that were not bone ingrown. The authors concluded that the femoral component geometry provides sufficient fixation and resistance to micromotion to allow for reliable ingrowth into a large variety of porous surfaces. The frequent presence of polyethylene wear debris at the interface of metal-backed porous-coated patellar components makes long-term fixation of these components uncertain. Although it appears that stable biologic fixation of certain tibial component designs is possible, recognized problems with polyethylene wear debris from the tibial articular surface may also compromise long-term fixation of this component. Tibial component designs that provide for firm initial fixation and implant contact with good-quality bone appear to be prerequisites for bone ingrowth.

Sumner et al.[54] quantified the extent of bone ingrowth and bone apposition in ten uncemented Miller-Galante tibial components retrieved for "reasons unrelated to fixation." The mean extent of bone ingrowth in these implants was 25.1%. Ingrowth was typically observed into the fixation pegs or in the vicinity of the pegs.

Bloebaum et al.[6] reported the results of analysis of two asymptomatic uncemented total knee arthroplasties in a single patient with two different prostheses. Retrieved specimens were taken at the time of postmortem examination. Significant differences in bone apposition and ingrowth were seen between these two prostheses. One titanium tibial implant had appositional bone over 61% to 76% of the sectioned surfaces and bone ingrowth into 22% of the available pore volume. Initial fixation with this implant was provided by four small pegs and two screws. The contralateral asymptomatic cobalt-chromium tibial implant had bone apposition over a mean of only 9% of the sectioned surfaces, but no bone ingrowth into the porous surface. Initial fixation of this component was provided by two short posterior sloping pegs and a single central screw.

In summary, stable biologic fixation appears to occur predictably with uncemented porous ingrowth femoral components. Revision for loosening of uncemented femoral components is extremely rare. Problems related to polyethylene wear and potential degradation of the implant interface, as well as well-documented problems with metal-backed patellar component failure,[2, 3, 33, 41, 44, 45, 53] make uncemented patellar component fixation inadvisable at this time. Although critics of uncemented TKR argue that the limited extent of bone ingrowth into the tibial component makes long-term stable fixation unlikely, this remains conjectural. The extent of bone ingrowth is profoundly influenced by surgical technique and initial fixation inherent in the design of the implant. The extent of actual bone ingrowth fixation necessary for stable biologic fixation is unknown. Despite their methodologic flaws, retrieval studies to date indicate that stable tibial component fixation with fibrous tissue and limited bone ingrowth can be achieved when these prerequisites are met. Satisfactory intermediate clinical follow-up on many patients with uncemented total knee arthroplasties also supports this conclusion.

CLINICAL RESULTS

The development of cementless, porous ingrowth total knee prostheses have recently become a popular alternative to cemented fixation with polymethyl methacrylate. The early clinical results of uncemented total knee arthroplasty have been variable. Dodd et al.[15] reported the clinical and radiographic results in 18 patients with cemented PCA (Porous Coated Anatomic; Howmedica, Rutherford, N.J.) knee arthroplasty of one knee and uncemented PCA arthroplasty of the contralateral knee. At an average follow-up of greater than 5 years, no difference in pain score, function, or patient preference between the cemented and noncemented arthroplasties was apparent. Using fluoroscopic techniques, no femoral lucencies were noted under the uncemented components, and tibial lucencies of less than 1 mm were limited and equally distributed between cemented and uncemented components. Loosening was seen in one cemented tibial tray and in one uncemented patellar component.

Similar results with the uncemented PCA prosthesis have been reported by Hungerford et al.[28] in a group of patients less than 50 years of age. Follow-up of these 48 knees averaged 51 months with a minimum of 28 months. Tibial component revision was performed in one knee for subsidence and patellar revision was performed in three knees for loosening. One other patient had asymptomatic tibial component subsidence which did not warrant revision. No instance of femoral component loosening was noted in these patients.

Rosenberg et al.[44] reported the minimum 3-year follow-up results of their prospective, nonrandomized series of cemented and uncemented total knee arthroplasties with the Miller-Galante prosthesis. Although the clinical results were better with cementless fixation, the indications for the two methods of fixation were significantly different, possibly accounting for these differences. Patients selected for uncemented implant fixation tended to be younger and more active. There was no significant difference in pain score between the two groups. Of note, 2 of 132 tibial components required revision for failure of ingrowth and one patient was revised for pain of undetermined cause. No patients demonstrated evidence of clinical or radiographic femoral component loosening. Three cemented TKRs were revised for pain of undetermined cause. Thirteen uncemented patellar components required revision for patellar component failure. Although clinical results in patients with cemented prostheses deteriorated with time, results in the uncemented TKR group of patients improved over time.

Rorabeck et al.[43] reported the results of their nonrandomized, nonmatched comparison of cemented Kinematic II (Howmedica) and uncemented PCA arthroplasties. Although the results were more favorable with cemented fixation, considerable differences in patient selection regarding age, activity, and bone quality were present for each method of fixation. The authors did not identify any problems with uncemented fixation of the tibial or femoral component, although asymptomatic tibial component subsidence was noted in three patients. Two uncemented patellar components required revision for loosening.

Collins et al.[11] prospectively followed 51 consecutive PCA total knee arthroplasties alternately assigned to either cemented or uncemented fixation groups. The two groups were well matched regarding patient age, weight, diagnosis, and gender. At an average follow-up of 3 years (minimum, 2 years), there was no significant difference in knee score, pain, or range of motion between the two groups. No problems were noted with uncemented femoral component fixation. Tibial component subsidence was noted in 50% of the 26 patients in the uncemented group. Although only one of these patients was revised for tibial component loosening, the authors expressed their concern about nine other uncemented tibial components which have demonstrated subsidence, loose beads, and interface radiolucencies. Based on their results, the authors did not recommend cementless tibial fixation with this prosthesis.

Recently reported results at longer-term follow-up (average, 64 months) with the early PCA design are disappointing.[37] Tibial component revision was necessary in 21 of 108 arthroplasties (19%) by 5 years postoperatively. Subsidence and development of varus deformity occurred in 14 knees. Associated tibial loosening was seen in eight of these cases. Loosening of one other tibial component occurred in the absence of subsidence and five other tibial components required revision for marked polyethylene wear. The cumulative estimate of implant survival at 6 years was 77%. Although no problems with the uncemented femoral component fixation were noted, the authors recommended that uncemented total knee arthroplasty with this prosthesis design be abandoned.

A prospectively studied group of 59 uncemented

PFC (Press Fit Condylar; Johnson & Johnson Orthopaedics, Braintree, Mass.) total knee arthroplasties were compared with a matched, retrospectively studied group of cemented PFC total knee arthroplasties by Rand.[41] The mean ages of the patients in these two groups differed significantly, however. Indications for uncemented fixation were physiologic young age, good bone quality, initial implant stability, bone-prosthesis gaps of less than 1 mm, and ability to cooperate with protected weightbearing for 1 month postoperatively. There were no significant differences in the mean postoperative knee scores, pain scores, or function scores between these two groups at an average follow-up of 2.8 years (minimum, 2 years). Nine patients in the uncemented group required revision for metal-backed patellar failure and one patient in the cemented group developed loosening of all components, requiring revision. Tibial radiolucencies were more frequent in the uncemented group, and were interpreted to be indicative of failure of bone ingrowth into the porous-coated tibial components. Rand concluded that the PFC tibial component appears to function well as a press-fit prosthesis.[41]

Although uncemented total knee arthroplasty has been reserved by most authors for young patients, there is some evidence that this restriction may not be absolutely necessary. Hofmann et al.[24] reported the results of 97 uncemented TKRs in patients greater than 65 years of age. The decision to proceed with uncemented fixation was based on intraoperative assessment of bone quality and the resultant stability of initial implant fixation obtained at the time of surgery. The average age of the patients was 71 years, with a range of 65 to 84 years. Significant improvement in knee score, pain score, and range of motion was noted. Revision was performed in only two patients, both for problems unrelated to loosening. Analysis of these retrieved tibial components showed bone ingrowth into 16% and 22% of the pore volume. The tibial component design incorporated four small fixation pegs and two screws which presumably provided adequate stability for this degree of bone ingrowth and the satisfactory overall results in this older patient population. Whitesides[58] analyzed a series of 1,110 uncemented total knee arthroplasties with respect to postoperative pain relief using two similar tibial component designs that differed primarily by additional fixation with four 6.5-mm cancellous screws. Only one case of loosening involving the tibial and femoral component occurred and results suggested that postoperative pain relief may be related more to quality of fixation than patient age or gender.

Despite concerns about the potential for bone ingrowth in patients with inflammatory arthritis, satisfactory results following uncemented total knee arthroplasty have been reported in this population.[1, 16, 52] Stuchin et al.[52] have suggested that although patients with rheumatoid arthritis may be more prone to osteopenia, the mechanical integrity of bone cannot be inferred by diagnosis alone. As in patients with other diagnoses, biologic fixation of the uncemented femoral component appears to be reliable. Initial implant stability with certain, but perhaps not all, tibial component designs is probably sufficient to provide for stable cementless fixation.

The "hybrid" total knee arthroplasty, with an uncemented femoral and a cemented tibial component, has evolved as a result of the recognized success of uncemented femoral component fixation, and concerns about the long-term fixation of uncemented tibial components. Despite its recent popularity, clinical reports documenting the results with this method of fixation are limited.[30, 59] Wright et al.[59] reported good or excellent results in 94% of 114 hybrid PFC total knee arthroplasties followed for a minimum of 2 years. There were no cases of clinical or radiographic femoral or tibial component loosening. Based on their results, the authors concluded that the hybrid technique provided a predictable result that was comparable to cemented total knee arthroplasty.

COMPLICATIONS

Complications following uncemented total knee arthroplasty are similar to those following cemented knee replacement. Certain problems unique to this mode of implant fixation deserve special mention, however.

Aseptic loosening involving the tibial or rarely the femoral component can occur. The diagnosis can be difficult to confirm in patients with persistent knee pain, as the bone-implant interface is easily obscured by a metal-backed component. Fluoroscopically guided radiographs have been demonstrated to be significantly more sensitive than plain radiographs in the detection of interface lucencies[35] and their use should be considered in the evaluation of the painful uncemented total knee arthroplasty. Assumptions regarding the significance of interface lucencies are extrapolations from previous findings with cemented TKRs and may not be valid for uncemented prostheses.

Although change in implant position has generally been considered to be indicative of loosening, the timing and degree to which this occurs may be significant. Subtle migration of less than 0.5 mm has been demonstrated in clinically well-fixed cemented and uncemented tibial components with RSA.[38] This migration occurs shortly after uncemented total knee arthroplasty and stabilizes within the first 6 to 12 months. An equivalent degree of total migration appears to occur more gradually, during the first 24 months postoperatively, with cemented tibial components. Microscopic trabecular failure and formation of a new "subchondral plate" has been postulated to occur after uncemented TKR[40] and may be related to this early implant settling. Implant migration of this magnitude is likely not detectable with standard radiographic techniques. Migration and change in component position detectable with plain radiography, especially when occurring after the perioperative period, is highly suggestive of loosening.

Because of the well-developed fibrous interface between bone and implant, arthrography may not be helpful in identifying loosening in the patient with a symptomatic prosthesis which may be inadequately fixed by fibrous tissue ingrowth alone. Radionucleotide bone scanning may be useful in cases of suspected loosening, although interpretation of these can be difficult, as local uptake can be increased for a prolonged period of time following uncemented total knee arthroplasty.

When loosening is suspected, frequently only the involved component requires revision. Failure of uncemented fixation usually requires the use of cemented fixation of the revised component. Most current implant systems have cemented revision components that are compatible with the components not requiring revision. Bone deficits due to subsidence or following component removal may require bone grafting or modular prosthetic augmentation. Posterior cruciate ligament competence may be inadequate after component removal and may require substitution with an appropriate prosthesis.

Design problems and failure mechanisms of uncemented metal-backed patellar components have been discussed previously. While patellar component loosening can usually be determined by plain radiography, the diagnosis of polyethylene wear or patellar component failure can be difficult. The clinical presentation of metal-backed patellar component failure is variable.[3, 33, 53] Often the patient will relate an acute onset of audible, grating patellofemoral crepitus after a specific episode involving significant knee flexion and loading of the patellofemoral joint. This is usually associated with either acute or delayed onset of anterior knee pain, and later development of an effusion. This scenario is indicative of catastrophic patellar component failure with resultant metal-on-metal articulation of the failed patellar and femoral components. In other patients, the clinical presentation is more insidious, with gradual development of peripatellar pain and an effusion. We have observed asymptomatic patellar component failure at the fixation peg junction in the presence of a well-developed patellar meniscus.

Regardless of the symptoms, patients with metal-backed patellar components warrant a high index of suspicion in view of the increasing frequency of problems with these designs. Risk factors associated with early component failure have been discussed previously. Prompt diagnosis is essential to prevent the consequences of damage to the underlying femoral component and metallosis. Examination often shows significant patellofemoral crepitus, boggy synovitis, and a massive effusion which makes the diagnosis rather certain. Physical findings in patients presenting early can be subtle and consist only of mild peripatellar pain or a minor effusion. Plain radiography may demonstrate peg failure at the junction with the metal base, or may occasionally demonstrate a lucency in the suprapatellar pouch corresponding with dissociation of the polyethylene from the underlying metal backing. Merchant or other tangential views of the patellofemoral articulation may demonstrate loss of interposed polyethylene between the femoral and patellar component metal backing, or patellar malalignment. Radiographs should be carefully evaluated for limb or component malalignment, which frequently contributes to patellar subluxation and patellar component failure. Joint aspiration may reveal discolored synovial fluid in association with metallosis or even polyethylene wear debris. Frequently, the diagnosis is uncertain and can only be confirmed by arthroscopy or arthrotomy. When metal-backed patellar failure is suspected and arthroscopy or exploration is contemplated, the knee should be immobilized and the diagnosis confirmed without significant delay.

Revision of the failed metal-backed patellar component can be complicated by several factors. Damage to the underlying femoral component frequently makes revision of this component necessary. Uncomplicated removal of the uncemented femoral component often allows for exchange with a new cemented prosthesis. Posterior cruciate ligament competence may be compromised by removal of a well-fixed femoral component or by the extensive synovectomy necessary if associated metallosis is present. Use of a posterior cruciate ligament–substituting prosthesis should be considered in this situation.

Component positioning and axial and rotational alignment should be carefully evaluated intraoperatively because of the frequent association of malalignment with patellar component failure. Component malalignment may warrant tibial or femoral component revision to ensure adequate extensor mechanism alignment. The metal-backed patellar component should be removed carefully to minimize bone stock loss. Usually the failed patellar component can be successfully revised with a cemented all-polyethylene component. Rarely, patellar bone stock will be insufficient to allow for resurfacing, and a patelloplasty will be required.

RESULTS AT UNIVERSITY HOSPITALS OF CLEVELAND

Our current selection criteria for uncemented fixation are slightly more restrictive than previously noted,[30] and as a result our indications for the use of hybrid fixation have expanded. In general, female patients less than 60 years of age and male patients less than 65 years of age are typically candidates for uncemented total knee arthroplasty, provided their medical condition and bone quality are satisfactory. Older patients who are active and in good general health are frequently candidates for the hybrid technique, provided their femoral bone quality is satisfactory. In some patients who might otherwise be candidates for uncemented total knee arthroplasty, intraoperative assessment may reveal inadequate proximal tibial bone quality to allow for insertion of an uncemented tibial component. In this situation, femoral bone stock is frequently adequate and these patients are candidates for hybrid implant fixation. Patients with significant osteopenia or conditions which might adversely affect bone ingrowth, serious medical conditions affecting longevity, or who are relatively inactive are typically candidates for cemented total knee arthroplasty. In addition to intraoperative assessment of bone quality, close apposition of implant to bone and secure press-fit tibial and femoral component stability are necessary for the use of cementless fixation. The presence of significant bone deficits requiring grafting usually warrants cemented implant fixation.

Results of our initial experience with hybrid total knee arthroplasty using the Miller-Galante prosthesis have been reported previously.[30] Twenty-nine consecutive hybrid total knee arthroplasties were followed prospectively according to the guidelines of the Knee Society. Selection of this technique of implant fixation was based primarily on the clinical judgment of the operating surgeon, after consideration of the patients' age, medical condition, activity level, and intraoperative assessment of bone quality. At an average follow-up of 28 months, pain relief and function were good or excellent in 89% of patients in this study. There were no cases of clinical or radiographic femoral component loosening. Evaluation since has shown no evidence of deterioration of these results. Fluoroscopically guided radiographs demonstrated that interface lucencies under the femoral components were limited in distribution and magnitude, with many of these the result of initial incongruities between the cut surface of the anterior femur and the implant. Stable biologic fixation of the uncemented Miller-Galante femoral component appears to occur predictably in all but the most osteopenic patients.

Our initial experience with uncemented fixation of both the tibial and femoral components has also been favorable. We have recently reviewed the results of 124 consecutive uncemented Miller-Galante total knee arthroplasties in 99 patients followed for a minimum of 5 years. Detailed radiographic analysis demonstrated an apparent correlation between outcome and restoration of alignment to within a neutral range defined as: change of the joint line of 4 mm or less, patellar height of 10 to 30 mm, change of the anteroposterior dimension of the medial femoral condyle of 4 mm or less, and deviation of the mechanical axis of the limb of 0 ±2 degrees and the coronal axis of the tibia of 0 ±2 degrees. The average Knee Society Knee Score in 99 TKRs meeting these alignment criteria was 95 ±3.5 points, and the average range of motion was 112 ±15 degrees. None of these knees required revision or demonstrated implant migration or loosening. The average knee score in the remaining 25 TKRs not satisfying these criteria was 86 ±6 points and the average range of motion was 105 ±10 degrees. Tibial component loosening occurred in one of these patients. Seven patients in this group were revised for metal-backed patellar component failure.

Our short-term results with the Miller-Galante II uncemented total knee prosthesis have demonstrated an apparent reduction in complications related to the patellofemoral joint. Design changes include the use of an all-polyethylene modified dome-shaped patellar component that provides for increased patellofemoral congruence and contact without increased constraint (Fig 61-5). More extensive implant size options provide for better tibial coverage, and improved tibial component fixation is provided with the use of larger 6.5-mm cancellous screws. These modifications should further reduce the incidence of patellofemoral complications and rare tibial loosening seen with the early Miller-Galante design.

Uncemented total knee arthroplasty appears to show great promise in providing for long-term biologic implant fixation. Other potential advantages of

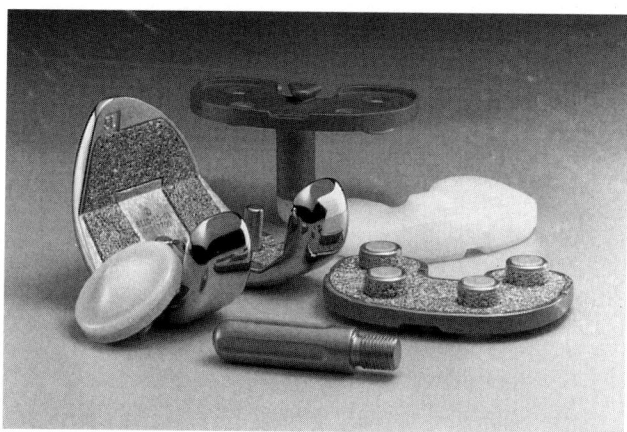

FIG 61–5.
The Miller-Galante II total knee prosthesis. Fixation of the stemmed or four-peg porous-coated tibial component is supplemented with 6.5-mm cancellous screws. The modified dome-shaped patellar component is available as a cemented all-polyethylene component or metal-backed, porous-coated component. (Courtesy of Zimmer, Inc., Warsaw, Ind.)

uncemented component fixation include decreased operative time and reduction of polyethylene wear from polymethyl methacrylate debris. Should revision ever be necessary, more conservative initial bone resection and avoidance of the potential adverse biologic response to polymethyl methacrylate might provide for better bone stock and an improved result following revision. Although these early results are promising, determination of the ultimate durability of this mode of fixation requires long-term follow-up.

REFERENCES

1. Armstrong RA, Whiteside LA: Results of cementless total knee arthroplasty in an older rheumatoid arthritis population, *J Arthroplasty* 6:357–362, 1991.
2. Bayley JC, Scott RD: Further observations on metal-backed patellar component failure, *Clin Orthop* 236:82–87, 1988.
3. Bayley JC, et al: Failure of the metal-backed patellar component after total knee replacement, *J Bone Joint Surg [Am]* 70:668–674, 1988.
4. Bartel DL, Bicknell VL, Wright TM: The effect of conformity, thickness and material on stresses in ultra-high molecular weight components for total joint replacement, *J Bone Joint Surg [Am]* 68:1041–1051, 1986.
5. Bartel DL, et al: Performance of the tibial component in total knee replacement, *J Bone Joint Surg [Am]* 64:1026–1033, 1982.
6. Bloebaum RD, et al: Bilateral tibial components of different cementless designs and materials, *Clin Orthop* 268:179–187, 1991.
7. Bobyn JD, et al: The optimum pore size for the fixation of porous-surfaced metal implants by the ingrowth of bone, *Clin Orthop* 150:263–270, 1980.
8. Bobyn JD, et al: Osteogenic phenomena across endosteal bone-implant spaces with porous surfaced intramedullary implants, *Acta Orthop Scand* 52:145–153, 1981.
9. Collier JP, et al: Macroscopic and microscopic evidence of prosthetic fixation with porous-coated materials, *Clin Orthop* 235:173–180, 1988.
10. Collier JP, et al: Biologic ingrowth of porous-coated knee prostheses, *Instruct Course Lect* 40:91–95, 1991.
11. Collins DN, et al: Porous-coated anatomic total knee arthroplasty, *Clin Orthop* 267:128–136, 1991.
12. Cook SD, et al: Quantitative histologic analysis of tissue growth into porous total knee components, *J Arthroplasty* 4(suppl):33–43, 1989.
13. Dawson JM, Bartel DL: Consequences of an interference fit on the fixation of porous-coated tibial components, *J Bone Joint Surg [Am]* 74:233–238, 1992.
14. Dempsey AJ, et al: Stability and anchorage considerations for cementless tibial components, *J Arthroplasty* 4:223–230, 1989.
15. Dodd CAF, Hungerford DS, Krackow KA: Total knee arthroplasty fixation, *Clin Orthop* 260:66–70, 1990.
16. Ebert FR, et al: Minimum four year follow-up of the PCA total knee arthroplasty in rheumatoid patients, *J Arthroplasty* 7:101–108, 1992.
17. Engh GA, Petersen TL: Comparative experience with intramedullary and extramedullary alignment in total knee arthroplasty, *J Arthroplasty* 5:1–8, 1990.
18. Finley JB, et al: Analysis of the pullout strength of screws and pegs used to secure tibial components following total knee arthroplasty, *Clin Orthop* 247:220–231, 1989.
19. Giori NJ, Beaupré GS, Carter DR: The influence of fixation peg design on the shear stability of prosthetic implants, *J Orthop Res* 8:892–898, 1990.
20. Goldstein SA, et al: Patellar surface strain, *J Orthop Res* 4:372–377, 1986.
21. Goldstein SA, et al: The effect of prosthesis surface geometry on implant stability and tissue ingrowth. In *Proceedings of the 37th Annual Meeting of the Orthopaedic Research Society*, 1991, p 92.
22. Haddad RJ, Cook SD, Thomas KA: Biologic fixation of porous-coated implants, *J Bone Joint Surg [Am]* 69:1459–1466, 1987.
23. Hofmann AA, Bloebaum RD: Bone chip incorporation in porous coated total knee replacement, *Trans Orthop Res Soc* 14:553, 1989.
24. Hofmann AA, et al: Cementless total knee arthroplasty in patients over 65 years old, *Clin Orthop* 271:28–34, 1991.
25. Hollister SJ, Kikuchi N, Goldstein SA: Effects of implant interface design on bone ingrowth predicted using topology optimization. In *Proceedings of the 37th Annual Meeting of the Orthopaedic Research Society*, 1991, p 108.
26. Hsu H, Walker PS: Wear and deformation of patellar

components in total knee arthroplasty, *Clin Orthop* 246:260–265, 1989.
27. Hsu H, et al: Effect of knee component alignment on tibial load distribution with clinical correlation, *Clin Orthop* 248:135–144, 1989.
28. Hungerford DS, Krackow KA, Kenna RV: Cementless total knee replacement in patients 50 years old and under, *Orthop Clin North Am* 20:131–145, 1989.
29. Jasty M, et al: Factors effecting bone ingrowth into porous coated canine acetabular replacements, *Trans Orthop Res Soc* 8:276, 1983.
30. Kraay MJ, et al: "Hybrid" total knee arthroplasty with the Miller-Galante prosthesis, *Clin Orthop* 273:32–41, 1991.
31. Lee RW, Volz RG, Sheridan DC: The role of fixation and bone quality on the mechanical stability of tibial knee components, *Clin Orthop* 273:177–183, 1991.
32. Lewis JL, Askew MJ, Jaycox DP: A comparative evaluation of tibial component designs of total knee prostheses, *J Bone Joint Surg [Am]* 64:129–135, 1982.
33. Lombardi AV, et al: Fracture/dissociation of the polyethylene in metal-backed patellar components in total knee arthroplasty, *J Bone Joint Surg [Am]* 70:675–679, 1988.
34. Matthews LS, Goldstein SA: The prosthesis-bone interface in total knee arthroplasty, *Clin Orthop* 276:50–55, 1992.
35. Mintz AD, Pilkington CAJ, Howie DW: A comparison of plain and fluoroscopically guided radiographs in the assessment of arthroplasty of the knee, *J Bone Joint Surg [Am]* 71:1343–1347, 1989.
36. Miura H, et al: Effects of screws and a sleeve on initial fixation in uncemented total knee tibial components, *Clin Orthop* 259:160, 1990.
37. Moran CG, et al: Survivorship analysis of the uncemented porous-coated anatomic knee replacement, *J Bone Joint Surg [Am]* 73:848–857, 1991.
38. Nilsson KG, et al: Evaluation of micromotion in cemented vs uncemented knee arthroplasty in osteoarthritis and rheumatoid arthritis, *J Arthroplasty* 6:265–278, 1991.
39. Pilliar RM, Lee JM, Maniatopoulos C: Observations on the effect of movement on bone ingrowth into porous-surfaced implants, *Clin Orthop* 208:108–113, 1986.
40. Rackemann S, et al: Uncemented press-fit total knee arthroplasty, *J Arthroplasty* 5:307–314, 1990.
41. Rand JA: Cement or cementless fixation in total knee arthroplasty, *Clin Orthop* 273:52–62, 1991.
42. Reilly DT, Martens M: Experimental analysis of the quadriceps muscle force and patellofemoral joint reaction force for various activities, *Acta Orthop Scand* 43:126–137, 1972.
43. Rorabeck CH, Bourne RB, Nott L: The cemented Kinematic-II and the non-cemented porous coated anatomic prosthesis for total knee replacement, *J Bone Joint Surg [Am]* 70:483–490, 1988.
44. Rosenberg AG, Barden RM, Galante JO: Cemented and ingrowth fixation of the Miller-Galante prosthesis, *Clin Orthop* 260:71–79, 1990.
45. Rosenberg AG, et al: Patellar component failure in cementless total knee arthroplasty, *Clin Orthop* 236:106–114, 1988.
46. Ryd L: Roentgen stereophotogrammetric analysis of prosthetic fixation in the hip and knee joint, *Clin Orthop* 276:56–65, 1992.
47. Shimagaki H, et al: Stability of initial fixation of the tibial component in cementless total knee arthroplasty, *J Orthop Res* 8:64–71, 1990.
48. Soballe K, et al: Tissue ingrowth into titanium and hydroxyapatite-coated implants during stable and unstable mechanical conditions, *J Orthop Res* 10:285–299, 1992.
49. Spector M: Historical review of porous-coated implants, *J Arthroplasty* 2:163–177, 1987.
50. Spector M, et al: Advances in our understanding of the implant-bone interface: Factors affecting formation and degeneration, *Instruct Course Lect* 40:101–113, 1991.
51. Strickland AB: The initial fixation of porous coated tibial components evaluated by the study of rigid body motion under static load. In *Proceedings of the 34th Annual Meeting of the Orthopaedic Research Society,* 1988, p 476.
52. Stuchin SA, Ruoff M, Matarese W: Cementless total knee arthroplasty in patients with inflammatory arthritis and compromised bone, *Clin Orthop* 273:42–51, 1991.
53. Stulberg SD, et al: Failure mechanisms of metal-backed patellar components, *Clin Orthop* 236:88–105, 1988.
54. Sumner DR, et al: The amount and distribution of bone ingrowth in tibial components retrieved from human patients. In *Proceedings of the 35th Annual Meeting of the Orthopaedic Research Society,* 1989, p 375.
55. Volz RG, et al: The mechanical stability of various noncemented tibial components, *Clin Orthop* 226:38–42, 1988.
56. Walker PS, Hsu HP, Zimmerman RA: A comparative study of uncemented tibial components, *J Arthroplasty* 5:245–253, 1990.
57. Walker PS, et al: Fixation of tibial components of knee prostheses, *J Bone Joint Surg [Am]* 63:258–267, 1981.
58. Whitesides LA: The effect of patient age, gender and tibial component fixation on pain relief after cementless total knee arthroplasty, *Clin Orthop* 271:21–27, 1991.
59. Wright RJ, et al: Two to four year results of posterior cruciate sparing condylar total knee arthroplasty with an uncemented femoral component, *Clin Orthop* 260:80–86, 1990.
60. Yoshii I, et al: The effect of central stem and stem length on micromovement of the tibial tray. In *Proceedings of the 37th Annual Meeting of the Orthopaedic Research Society,* 1991, p 555.

62

Posterior Cruciate Ligament–Retaining Total Knee Arthroplasty

KAYVON S. RIGGI, M.D.
JAMES A. RAND, M.D.

Polycentric knee arthroplasty
Geometric total knee arthroplasty
Duocondylar and duopatellar total knee arthroplasties
Cruciate-sparing total condylar knee replacement
Kinematic total knee
Townley and Cloutier resurfacing designs

Miller-Galante prosthesis
Porous coated anatomic total knee arthroplasty
Meniscal bearing prosthesis
Press Fit condylar prosthesis
Summary

The role of the cruciate ligaments is an important feature in the design consideration of total knee arthroplasty. Most authors now favor resection of the anterior cruciate ligament (ACL). The status of the posterior cruciate ligament (PCL), however, remains controversial.[1, 16]

Proponents of PCL retention argue that preservation improves function, range of motion, strength, stability, and reduces interface stresses.[1] Many authors have found that PCL preservation results in a more normal and efficient gait pattern, especially with stair climbing.[2, 13, 29] The PCL induces femoral rollback with knee flexion resulting in posterior translation of the tibiofemoral contact point. This improves potential range of motion by preventing impingement of the posterior tibial plateau on the femur. In addition, this increases the dynamic quadriceps lever arm for improved strength. The PCL is the strongest ligament in the knee joint and stabilizes the knee against a predominantly posteriorly directed shear force during activities of daily living. When the PCL is not present, this shear force must be transmitted to the fixation interfaces where shear stress is not well tolerated. In addition, retention of the PCL helps maintain the joint line and may provide some proprioceptive function.

Proponents of PCL resection argue that removal greatly simplifies correction of deformity, allows for less tibial bone resection for a given thickness of prosthesis, and permits placement of a prosthesis with greater articular conformity and thus improved polyethylene wear characteristics.[16] Ultimately the dilemma is between a PCL-retaining low-conformity prosthesis with reduced interface stresses and a PCL-sacrificing semiconstrained prosthesis with reduced polyethylene stresses. Continued long-term study is necessary to determine where the proper balance lies. This chapter describes the evolution and results of cruciate-retaining total knee arthroplasties. This provides an important baseline for comparison and establishes a minimum standard that future designs must meet.

POLYCENTRIC KNEE ARTHROPLASTY

The Polycentric (Howmedica, Rutherford, N.J.) knee arthroplasty was the first cruciate-sparing, resurfacing total knee arthroplasty[18, 25] (Fig 62–1). Gunston recognized that movement in the normal knee consists of rocking, gliding, and axial rotation and follows a multiple center, or polycentric pathway. The instant center for each increment of flexion moves posteriorly in a spiral pattern. Thus the concept of the Polycentric knee was to simulate normal knee motion by separate prosthetic replacement of each joint surface. The circular configuration of the femoral runners was a compromise between ease of manufacturing and the spiral curve of the femoral condyle in the normal knee. The length of the tibial track allowed both rocking and gliding movements while the articu-

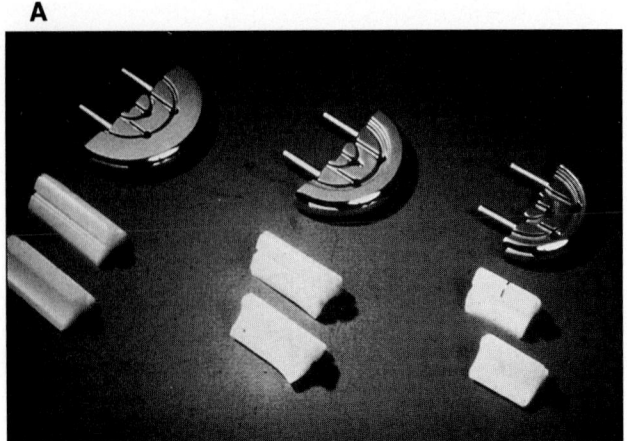
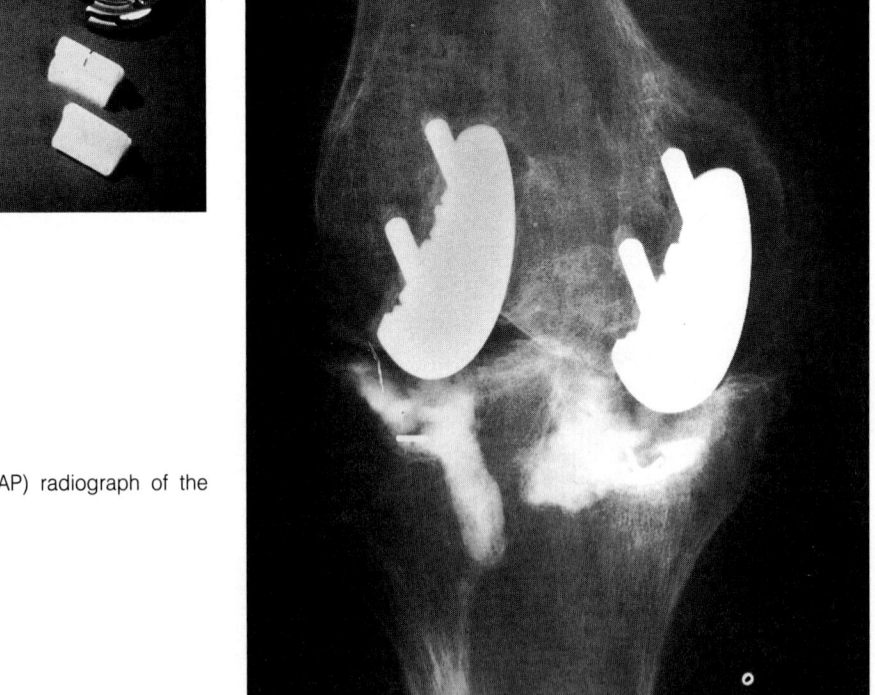

FIG 62-1.
(A) Photograph and **(B)** anteroposterior (AP) radiograph of the Polycentric prosthesis.

lar groove allowed 20 degrees of axial rotation in an effort to reduce rotational stresses on the cement-bone interface.

Gunston in 1971 reported on 22 Polycentric total knee arthroplasties in 20 patients, all with rheumatoid arthritis except for two patients with osteoarthritis and a previous contralateral knee arthrodesis.[18] With 1 to 2½ years follow-up all patients had excellent pain relief. One knee, however, in a patient with a previous patellectomy required reoperation to an arthrodesis for residual lateral instability. Thirteen knees recovered a motion arc of greater than 90 degrees and 19 of 20 patients benefited from an increased overall mobility. Operative complications included delayed wound healing in four knees and peroneal nerve palsy in one.

In 1976 Skolnick[50] reported on 500 Polycentric total knee arthroplasties performed at the Mayo Clinic between July 1970 and October 1971 and followed for 2 years. Patients' ages ranged from 20 to 83 years with a mean of 60 years. Sixty-eight percent were women and 32% men. The diagnosis was rheumatoid arthritis in 60%, osteoarthritis in 34%, and miscellaneous diagnoses in the remaining 6%. Of the 500 knees, 432 (86.4%) obtained excellent pain relief, with similar improvement in function in patients with rheumatoid arthritis and in those with osteoarthritis. The number of patients able to ambulate without aids improved from 23% to 64% and the number of patients unable to walk at all decreased from 8% to 2%. The average postoperative arc of motion was 95 degrees, an average increase of 5 degrees of motion. Overall, 96% of patients expressed satisfaction with their surgical results. Complications included malalignment or imprecise apposition of the components in 19 knees (3.8%), deep infections in 14 (2.8%), 12 instances of loosening (2.4%), and instability in 7 knees (1.4%). A total of 59 reoperations were performed on 51 knees for an overall failure rate of 10.2%.

Gunston[19] in 1980 reported the results of 204 Polycentric knee arthroplasties in 172 patients 2 to 10 years after operation. Patients' ages ranged from 29 to 79 years with a mean of 60 years with the diagnosis of rheumatoid arthritis in 80% and osteoarthritis in 20%. Pain relief was obtained in only 59%; 39% of patients had residual pain from the patellofemoral joint. Loosening occurred in 10.0% and infection in 6.4% of patients. Overall, 24 patients required reoperation (12%) including seven revisions and 13 arthrodeses.

Lewallen et al.[34] in 1984 reported the 10-year results of 209 Polycentric total knee arthroplasties performed in 159 patients at the Mayo Clinic between July 1970 and November 1971. Fifty-two men and 107 women ranged in age from 20 to 82 years with a mean of 56 years. Sixty-seven percent had rheumatoid arthritis, 26% osteoarthritis, and 4% posttraumatic arthritis. Based on the Kaplan-Meier survival curve the probability of still having a successful Polycentric total knee arthroplasty declined to 66% at 10 years. Important determinants of success or failure were the existence of a previous operation and axial alignment. Knees previously operated on had only a 48% probability of success at 10 years compared with a 75% probability of success in the knee not operated on. If components were implanted in any varus angulation or valgus angulation greater than 8 degrees, the failure rate was approximately doubled. Malalignment often leads to ligamentous laxity and instability, which was the most common cause of failure in 27 knees (13%). Loosening, usually of the tibial component, was the cause of failure in 15 knees (7%). Deep infection developed in seven knees (3%). Overall, 71 knees had a failed result (34%), 58 requiring reoperation with most undergoing a revision arthroplasty.

Although the early reports were encouraging, once longer follow-up was obtained it became apparent that instability and loosening would claim many of these prostheses and only slightly more than half of the patients would retain a successfully functioning arthroplasty at 10 years (Table 62–1).

GEOMETRIC TOTAL KNEE ARTHROPLASTY

In the early 1970s, Coventry and colleagues designed the Geometric (Howmedica) total knee arthroplasty[10, 11, 24] (Fig 62–2). The goals of this resurfacing, cruciate-sparing design were to avoid the early recognized pitfalls of the hinge-type prosthesis while at the same time providing enhanced stability compared with its predecessor, the Polycentric total knee. Unfortunately, it was not recognized in that era that a geometrically partially constrained implant with a single axis of rotation that preserves the cruciate ligaments represents a kinematic mismatch and thus is predisposed to loosening.

Skolnick and Coventry[49] reported the 2-year follow-up of 119 knees in 85 patients with Geometric total knee arthroplasties implanted at the Mayo Clinic between April 1971 and June 1972. Thirty-eight percent were men and 62% were women with an age range from 25 to 84 years with a mean of 61 years. Fifty-three percent of patients had rheumatoid arthritis and 41% had osteoarthritis. Satisfactory relief of pain was obtained in 84% of knees with comparable results in those with rheumatoid arthritis and with osteoarthritis. Ninety-three percent of the patients expressed overall satisfaction with their results. Complications included tibial component loosening in 13 knees (11.8%), 8 of which had persistent varus deformity. Deep infection occurred in only 2 knees (1.8%). In contrast to the Polycentric knee, instability was not a significant problem, with only one case of dislocation occurring in a patient with rheumatoid arthritis and absence of both cruciate ligaments. Overall, 17 of 110 knees (15.5%) required a total of 22 reoperations.

In 1981, Lowe and McNeur[35] reported on 150 knee arthroplasties in 106 patients implanted at the Alfred Hospital in Melbourne, Australia between 1973 and 1977. Forty-eight percent of the arthroplasties were performed for rheumatoid arthritis in patients with an average age of 55 years. Fifty-two percent of the arthroplasties were performed for osteoarthritis in patients with an average age of 74 years. Follow-up ranged from 2 to 6 years postoperatively. In the osteoarthritis group 89% of the arthroplasties were considered satisfactory or better while 79% of the knees in the rheumatoid group were satisfactory or better. Complications included loosening in 5 knees (3.3%), deep infection in 7 (4.7%), and patellofemoral pain in 1 knee. Overall, 17 knees (11%) were considered unsatisfactory leading to seven revision arthroplasties (5%).

Riley and Woodyard[44] in 1985 published the results of 71 Geometric knees implanted in 48 patients at the Stafford District Hospital (England) with follow-up of 2 months to 8 years. There were 37 women and 11 men in the study, 68% with rheumatoid arthritis and 32% with osteoarthritis. Ages ranged from 25 to 79 years with a mean of 61 years. Pain relief was considered to be 72% of the maximum possible. Complications included 11 knees (15.5%) with mechanical loosening and 2 knees (2.8%) with deep infection. Overall, 18.3% of knees either had severe pain or underwent revision arthroplasty and were considered failures. By an actuarial technique, a 21% probability of success was predicted at 8 to 9 years.

Rand and Coventry[41] reported the results of 193 Geometric prostheses implanted in 129 patients between February 1972 and March 1975. The study

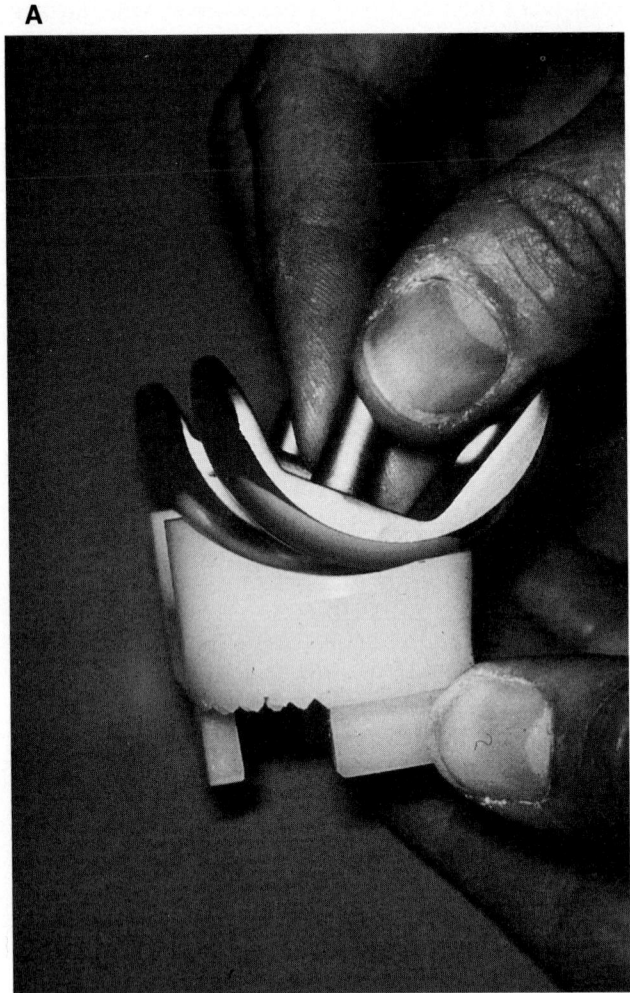 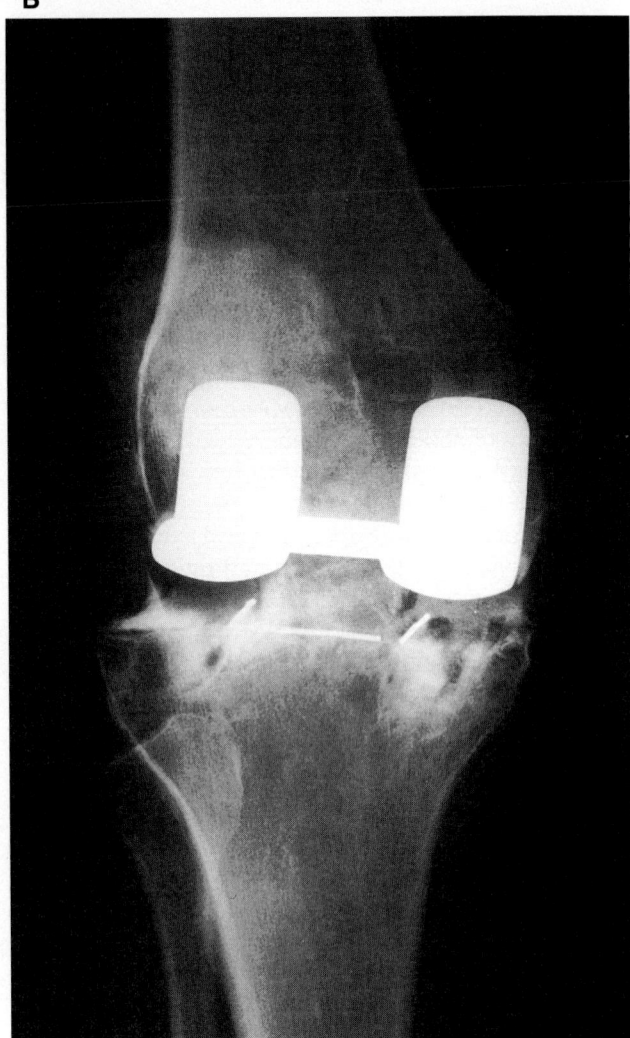

FIG 62–2.
(A) Photograph and **(B)** AP radiograph of the Geometric prosthesis.

comprised 63 men and 66 women, all with osteoarthritis, with a mean age at operation of 69 years. Final follow-up evaluation occurred at an average of 10.8 years with a minimum of 8 years. The actuarial survival of a retained implant was 78% at 10 years. Using implant removal or pain as an end point, the success rate dropped to 69% at 10 years. Loosening occurred in 24 knees (12.5%) necessitating revision. These authors evaluated the development of lucent lines, which almost always occurred at the bone-cement interface of the tibial component. Radiolucent lines wider than 1 mm were present in 38% and progressed in 34%. The initial postoperative axial alignment significantly influenced the development of lucent lines: 9 of 15 knees with greater than 3 degrees of varus alignment compared with 17 of 53 knees with a greater valgus alignment had progressive radiolucent lines. In addition, varus tibial component positioning was associated with the development of lucent lines: 21 of 45 knees with greater than 4 degrees of varus alignment compared with 5 of 23 with a more valgus component orientation. Other complications included infection in 8 (4.1%), and instability in 3 (1.5%). Overall, revision procedures were performed in 38 (20%) of the 193 knees.[41]

Compared with modern standards, the Geometric prosthesis was lacking in design, with an inherent kinematic mismatch, as well as in instrumentation to provide for consistent implant positioning. Even so, the Geometric knee provided approximately 70% successful results at 10 years. These results are important because they serve as a baseline with which the results of more contemporary designs can be compared (Table 62–2).

TABLE 62-1.
Polycentric Total Knee Arthroplasty

Authors	No. of Knees/Patients	Mean Age (yr) (Range)	Rheumatoid Arthritis (%)	Osteoarthritis (%)	Follow-up (yr)	Successful Result (%)	Instability (%)	Loosening (%)	Infection (%)	Reoperations/Failures (%)
Gunston (1971)[18]	22/20	—	91	9	1–2½	95	27	—	—	4.5
Skolnick et al. (1976)[50]	500 knees	X̄ = 60 (20–83)	60	34	2	86	1.4	2.4	2.8	10.2
Gunston (1980)[19]	204/172	X̄ = 60 (29–79)	80	20	2–10	59	—	10	6.4	39
Lewallen et al. (1984)[34]	209/159	X̄ = 56 (20–82)	67	26	10½	66 (actuarial analysis)	13	7	3	34

TABLE 62-2.
Geometric Total Knee Arthroplasty

Authors	No. of Knees/Patients	Mean Age (yr) (Range)	Rheumatoid Arthritis (%)	Osteoarthritis (%)	Follow-up (yr)	Successful Result (%)	Instability (%)	Loosening (%)	Infection (%)	Reoperations or Failures (%)
Skolnick et al. (1976)[49]	119 knees	X̄ = 61 (25–84)	53	41	2	84	0.8	11.8	1.8	15.5
Lowe & McNeur (1981)[35]	150/106	OA 74 RA 55	48	52	2–6	OA 89 RA 79	—	3.3	4.7	11
Riley & Woodyard (1985)[44]	71/48	X̄ = 61 (25–79)	68	32	0–8	72	—	15.5	2.8	18.3
Rand & Coventry (1988)[41]	193/129	X̄ = 69	—	100	10.8	69 (actuarial analysis)	1.5	12.5	4.1	20

OA = osteoarthritis, RA = rheumatoid arthritis.

DUOCONDYLAR AND DUOPATELLAR TOTAL KNEE ARTHROPLASTIES

In the early 1970s Walker, Insall, and Ranawat at The Hospital for Special Surgery in New York City developed the Duocondylar (Johnson & Johnson Orthopaedics, Braintree, Mass.) total knee[38] (Fig 62–3). The metal femoral condylar surfaces closely matched the shape of the normal femoral condyles in an effort to reproduce a normal polycentric motion pattern. The condylar surfaces were connected by an anterior bar providing increased stability and making insertion easier. Two separate polyethylene tibial components each had upward sloping curves toward the intercon-

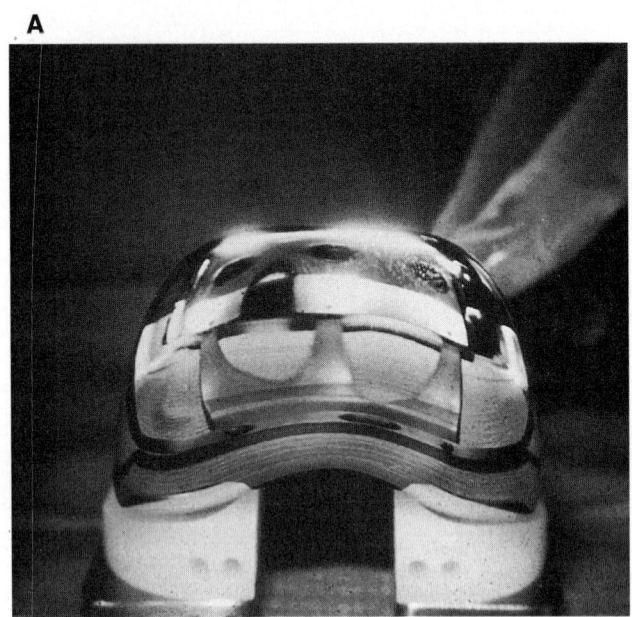

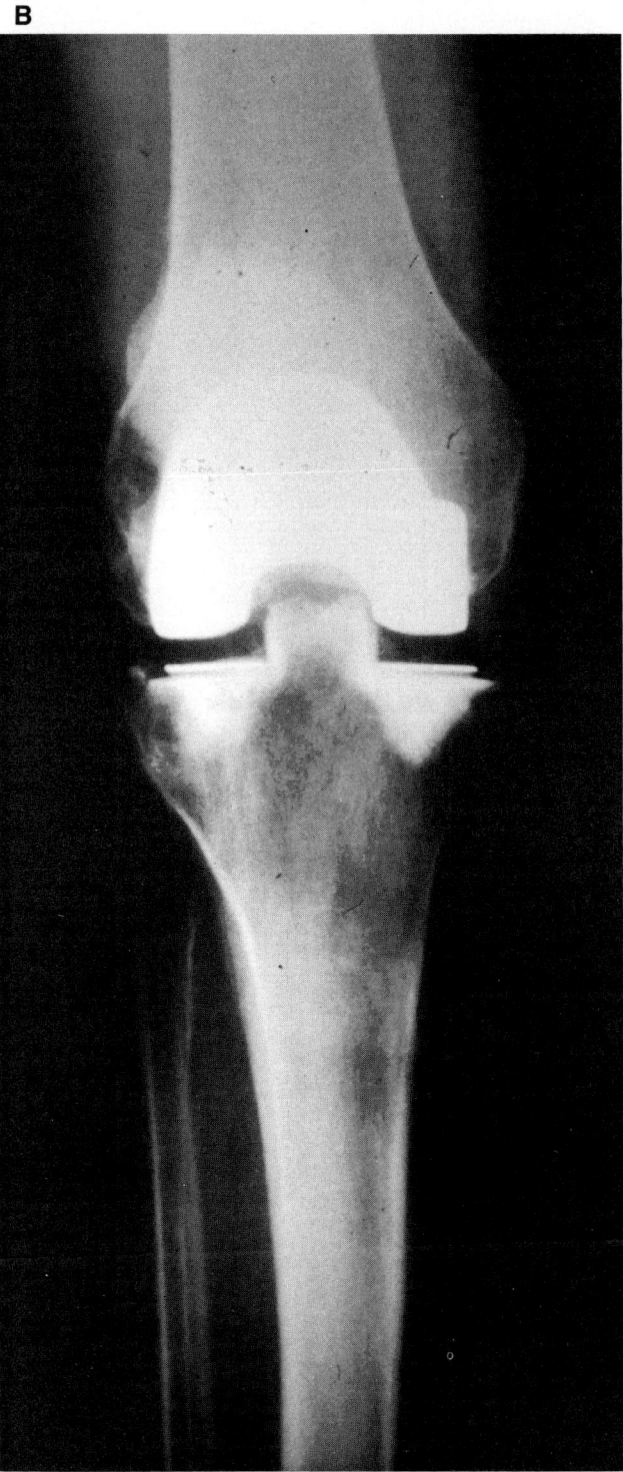

FIG 62–3.
(A) Photograph and **(B)** AP radiograph of the Duocondylar prosthesis.

dylar area in an effort to provide mediolateral stability, but were flat in the sagittal plane to provide no constraint in the anteroposterior direction. The tibial intercondylar eminence and PCL were preserved and there was no replacement of the patellofemoral joint.

In 1976 Ranawat et al.[37] reported the results of 94 Duocondylar knees in 88 patients with an average 3-year follow-up. Seventy-five percent of patients had rheumatoid arthritis and 25% had osteoarthritis. Ages ranged from 25 to 72 years with an average of 65 years. As judged by The Hospital for Special Surgery Knee rating system, good or excellent results were obtained in 75% of the knees. Complications included significant instability in 9.3% and loosening in 5.3%. There were no cases of deep infection. Lucent lines occurred under the tibial component in 76% and were progressive in 26% of knees. Overall, 5.5% required revision arthroplasty. The main causes of failure were under- or overcorrection of deformity leading to instability, loosening of the tibial components, and patellofemoral pain.

Sledge and co-workers[52] in 1978 reported the results of 135 Duocondylar prostheses with an average of 2.7 years' follow-up. The patients ranged in age from 39 to 80 years with a mean of 62 years. Seventy-nine percent of patients had rheumatoid arthritis and 21% had osteoarthritis. Overall, 67% of patients were considered to have good or excellent results. Complications included two knees with component loosening (one tibial and one femoral), instability in one, and residual patellofemoral pain in 20%. Lucent lines occurred at the tibial bone-cement interface in 22%, but in all were less than 1 mm thick, incomplete, and not associated with clinical loosening. Revision operations were required in five knees (3.7%) and patellofemoral pain was noted to be the most common cause of poor results (Table 62-3).

Based on these observations from Harvard Medical School and The Hospital for Special Surgery, the Duocondylar evolved into the Duopatellar (Johnson & Johnson, Braintree, Mass.) total knee with incorporation of an anterior patellar flange on the femur. The tibial component initially remained as two separate components and the surface contour was changed from a flat to a curved surface in the sagittal plane conferring added inherent articular constraint.[14, 48, 51] In 1978, initial 2-year results were reported from both institutions.

Ewald et al.[14] in Boston reviewed 167 knees (70% with rheumatoid arthritis and 30% with osteoarthritis) and found 85% of patients with good or excellent results. The incidence of patellofemoral pain was reduced from 20% with the Duocondylar to only 5% with the Duopatellar prosthesis. Loosening occurred in only 0.9%; however, incomplete lucent lines less than 1 mm in thickness were discovered in 45%. This was a twofold increase in lucent lines at 2 years compared with the Duocondylar knees reviewed at the same institution (45% vs. 22%). Since the patellar flange and the dished tibial articular surface were the only two design changes, the most likely explanation for the increased incidence of lucent lines was that the higher degree of constraint transferred greater stress to the bone-cement interface.[14, 51] Inglis and Lane[26] in New York made similar observations in 53 Duopatellar knees at 2 years with 90% overall good and excellent results, but also with incomplete lucent lines less than 2 mm in thickness in 45%.

In 1980 Thomas et al.[53] evaluated 493 knees with Duopatellar prostheses out of 747 performed with an average 2.7-year follow-up. Overall, 93% of patients experienced marked pain relief. Average preoperative and postoperative scores according to The Hospital for Special Surgery System improved from 39 to 87 in the rheumatoid population and from 39 to 90 in the osteoarthritis population. Clinical loosening occurred in only seven of 747 knees (0.9%). However, in 344 radiographs studied, incomplete lucent lines were present in 50% and lines greater than 1 mm wide or involving greater than 90% of the surface were present in 3% of tibial components. The overall revision rate for the 747 knees was 2.8%.

Extensive bench testing performed in 1979 demonstrated that a one-piece tibia with a central stem enhanced tibial component fixation through increased surface area contact and better distribution of the weightbearing force. As a result, the two-piece Duopatellar tibial components were abandoned in favor of the one-piece design.[51] At the same time the tibial component was made flat in the sagittal plane, imparting less constraint and allowing femoral rollback in flexion.[48]

Scott[48] in 1982 reported the results of the first 100 Duopatellar replacements using the flat one-piece all-plastic tibial components, with a minimum 2-year follow-up. Fifty percent were implanted in patients with rheumatoid arthritis and 45% in patients with osteoarthritis. Ninety-five percent of patients had excellent pain relief with an average of 106 degrees of motion. The incidence of incomplete lucent lines less than 1 mm thick decreased to 24% and only 3% had lucent lines greater than 1 mm in thickness. Two reoperations were necessary for patellar resurfacing, but no revisions were required for tibial loosening (Table 62-4).

Duocondylar and Duopatellar arthroplasties marked a significant era in the evolution of total knee arthroplasties. Important concepts and design con-

TABLE 62–3.
Duocondylar Total Knee Arthroplasty

Authors	No. of Knees/Patients	Mean Age (yr) (Range)	Rheumatoid Arthritis (%)	Osteoarthritis (%)	Follow-up (yr)	Good or Excellent Results (%)	Instability (%)	Loosening (%)	Lucent Lines (%)	Infection (%)	Reoperations or Failures (%)
Ranawat et al. (1976)[37]	94/88	X̄ = 65 (25–72)	75	25	2–4	75	9.3	5.2	76* 26†	—	5.5
Sledge & Ewald (1979)[51]	135 knees	X̄ = 62 (39–80)	79	21	2.7	67	0.75	1.5	22	—	3.7

*Incomplete lucent lines, <1 mm.
†Lucent lines >1 mm and complete, or progressive.

TABLE 62–4.
Duopatellar Total Knee Arthroplasty

Authors	No. of Knees/Patients	Mean Age (yr)	Rheumatoid Arthritis (%)	Osteoarthritis (%)	Follow-up (yr)	Good or Excellent Results (%)	Instability	Loosening (%)	Lucent Lines (%)	Infection (%)	Reoperations or Failures (%)
Ewald et al. (1978)[14]	167 knees	63	70	30	2	85	—	0.9	45*	—	2.7
Inglis & Lane (1978)[26]	53/42	54	85	12	2	90	—	—	45*	—	3.8
Thomas et al. (1980)[53]	493 knees	—	70	30	2.7	93 pain relief	—	0.9	50* 3†	0.4	2.8
Scott (1982)[48]	100 knees (one-piece tibial component)	—	50	45	2	95	—	—	24* 3†	—	2.0

*Incomplete lucent lines, <1 mm.
†Lucent lines >1 mm and complete, or progressive.

siderations that were introduced and confirmed were: (1) the use of an anterior femoral flange to resurface the femoral trochlea; (2) flat tibial surface geometry in the sagittal plane in concert with a retained PCL to preserve motion and reduce interface stresses; and (3) use of a one-piece tibial component with a central stem for improved component stability and fixation.

CRUCIATE-SPARING TOTAL CONDYLAR KNEE REPLACEMENT

The posterior cruciate condylar knee (Howmedica, Rutherford, N.J.) was introduced in 1975. The design was essentially identical to the total condylar knee with the exception of a central posterior cutout section that allows preservation of the PCL (Fig 62–4). The aim of the design change was to improve posterior stability for improved function (e.g., stair climbing) while retaining the wear and motion characteristics of the Total Condylar knee.[45] Potential disadvantages expressed by Insall et al.[28] included the possibility of impingement of the femur on the posterior aspect of the cupped tibial plateau during flexion, which could limit flexion, deform the plastic, and increase interface stresses. In addition, correction of the deformity may be rendered more difficult with retention of the PCL.[28]

Ritter et al.[45] in 1984 reported the 5-year follow-up results of 94 cruciate condylar knee replacements. Sixty-three percent of patients had osteoarthritis and 27% had rheumatoid arthritis. The average age was 67 years (range, 21–85 years). Overall, 96.8% of patients had excellent or good results, which compares well with the 90% rate reported by Insall et al. for the Total Condylar design and 96% for the posterior-stabilized design.[27, 28] The average preoperative flexion was 104 degrees while average post-

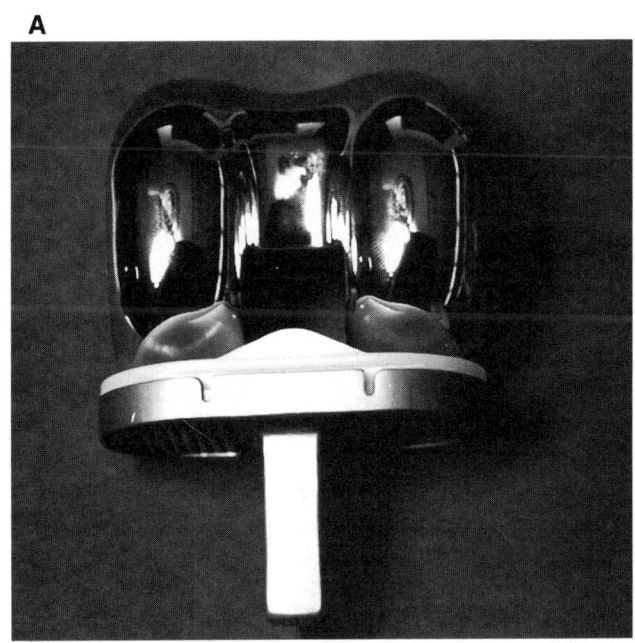

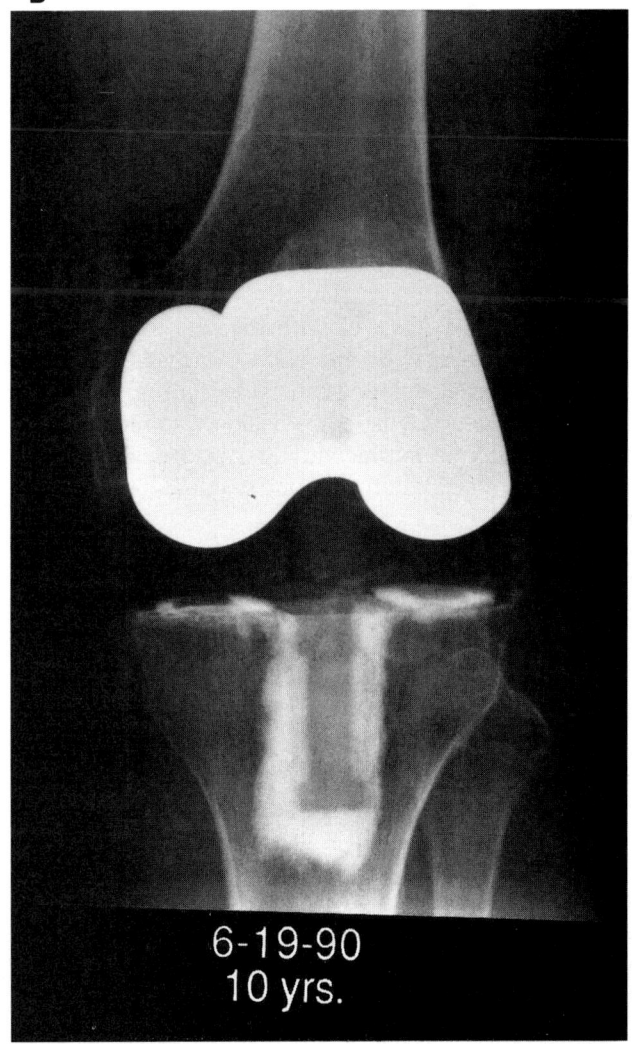

FIG 62–4.
(A) Photograph and **(B)** AP radiograph of the cruciate condylar prosthesis.

operative flexion was 101 degrees. Postoperatively, only one knee showed varus deformity and only one knee had a valgus deformity greater than 10 degrees. Incomplete, nonprogressive tibial radiolucencies less than 1 mm wide occurred in 22% and only one knee demonstrated tibial loosening with a complete radiolucency around the prosthesis. Six percent of knees had a 2+ anterior drawer and 5% had a 2+ posterior drawer. There were no cases of 3+ instability. One knee developed a deep infection requiring revision.

Bourne et al.[4] reported the results of 164 cruciate condylar arthroplasties with an average 5.3-year follow-up. Sixty-one percent of patients had osteoarthritis and 32% had rheumatoid arthritis. The average age was 65 years (range, 26–88 years). Seventy percent of tibial components were solid polyethylene and 30% were metal-backed. Overall, good or excellent results were obtained in 95%, and 97% of knees had no posterior instability. The percentage of patients who could climb stairs without support increased from 37% to 69%. Maximum flexion averaged 107 degrees preoperatively and 101 degrees postoperatively. Ninety-nine knees demonstrated a preoperative deformity of more than 3 degrees of varus or 10 degrees of valgus alignment. Postoperatively, only eight knees had such a deformity. Lucent lines greater than 1 mm in length or width occurred in only 6% and progressed in only 3%. Lucent lines occurred in 5.6% of all-polyethylene tibiae, and in 2.7% of tibiae with metal backing. Of note, no fluoroscopic radiographs were used. Nevertheless, this rate of radiolucency compares well with the 22% incidence of lucent lines seen with the Total Condylar prosthesis.[28] No knees developed clinical loosening, deep infection occurred in one, and revision was required in three knees (one supracondylar fracture, one tibial component malrotation, and one residual varus malalignment).

A survivorship study of 190 cruciate-sparing total condylar knee prostheses was performed.[39] Sixty-one knees with an all-polyethylene tibial component were compared with 129 knees with a metal-backed tibial component at a mean of 10 years. Using an end point of revision, survivorship was 96% for the all-polyethylene compared to 93% for the metal-backed tibial component, which was not statistically significant. Using an end point of moderate or severe pain or revision, survivorship was 83% at 10 years overall (86% in all-polyethylene vs. 79% in metal-backed tibial components). Of 134 knees in 108 patients available for follow-up at 10 years, The Hospital for Special Surgery knee scores were good or excellent in 88%. Radiolucent lines were present adjacent to 59% of the all-polyethylene and 52% of the metal-backed tibial components, which was not statistically significant.

Another study of 144 knees at a mean of 9 years found 94.5% good or excellent results.[32] The mean range of motion was 106 degrees. Radiolucent lines were identified in 41% of which 12% were progressive. There were eight failures leading to three revisions. Elevation of the joint line by greater than 8 mm correlated with aseptic loosening.

The posterior cruciate condylar prosthesis provided good or excellent results in 90% to 95% of knees at 5 or more years' follow-up. Thus the evolution of knee arthroplasty continues to demonstrate benefits. Concerns that cruciate retention would lead to diminished motion, tibial loosening, and persistent deformity were not substantiated by these studies. Despite the excellent results, a subtle kinematic mismatch exists with this prosthesis and a change to a flat tibial plateau in the sagittal plane was recommended[45] (Table 62–5).

KINEMATIC TOTAL KNEE

The Kinematic (Howmedica) total knee is a PCL-sparing prosthesis designed in an attempt to further refine the advancements made in the cruciate-sparing condylar knee (Fig 62–5). The tibial component was flattened in the sagittal plane allowing unconstrained femoral rollback which clears the posterior structures and avoids femoral impingement.[51] A metal-backed short-stemmed tibial component was designed to improve tibial component fixation and load transmission.[55] Finally, the patellar groove in the anterior flange was placed in slight valgus alignment to improve patellar tracking.

In 1984, Ewald et al.[15] from Harvard Medical School reported the results of 124 kinematic knee replacements with an average of 2.25 years' follow-up. Fifty-four percent of patients had rheumatoid arthritis, 5% had juvenile rheumatoid arthritis, and 41% had osteoarthritis. The average age of the patients was 76 years (range, 25–86 years). The patella was resurfaced in all patients with rheumatoid arthritis and in 68% of patients with osteoarthritis. Overall, 90% (111 knees) had excellent or good results. The average postoperative range of motion was 106 degrees of flexion, and extension to 2 degrees short of full extension. Overall, the average postoperative alignment was 5.3 ±2.9 degrees of valgus angulation. Radiolucent lines occurred beneath the tibial component in 22 knees (18%), all of which were less than 1 mm wide, incomplete, and nonprogressive. Lucencies occurred in 19 knees with osteoarthritis and in only 3 with rheumatoid arthritis. A statistically sig-

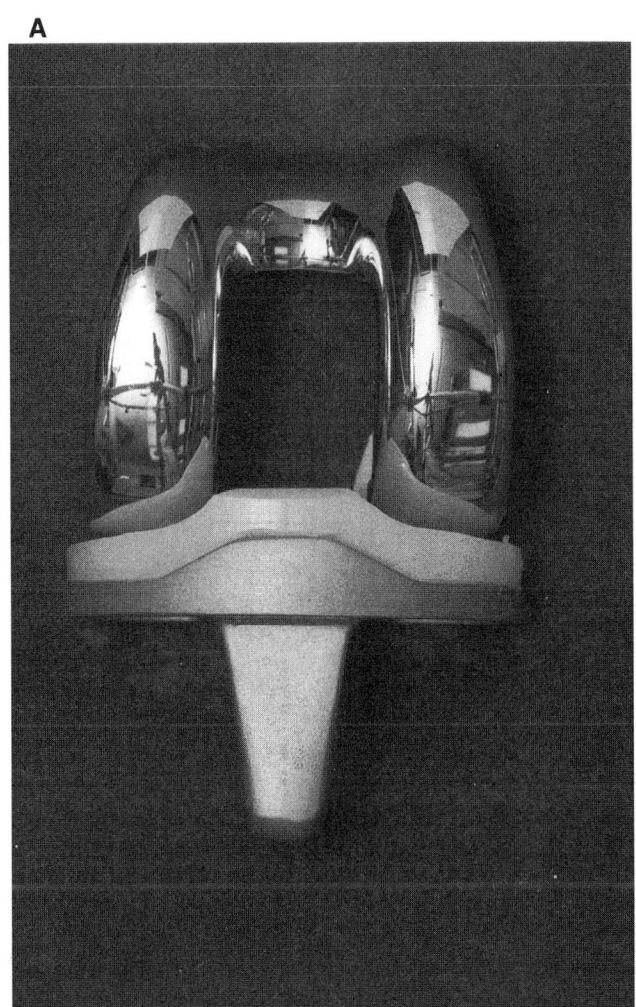 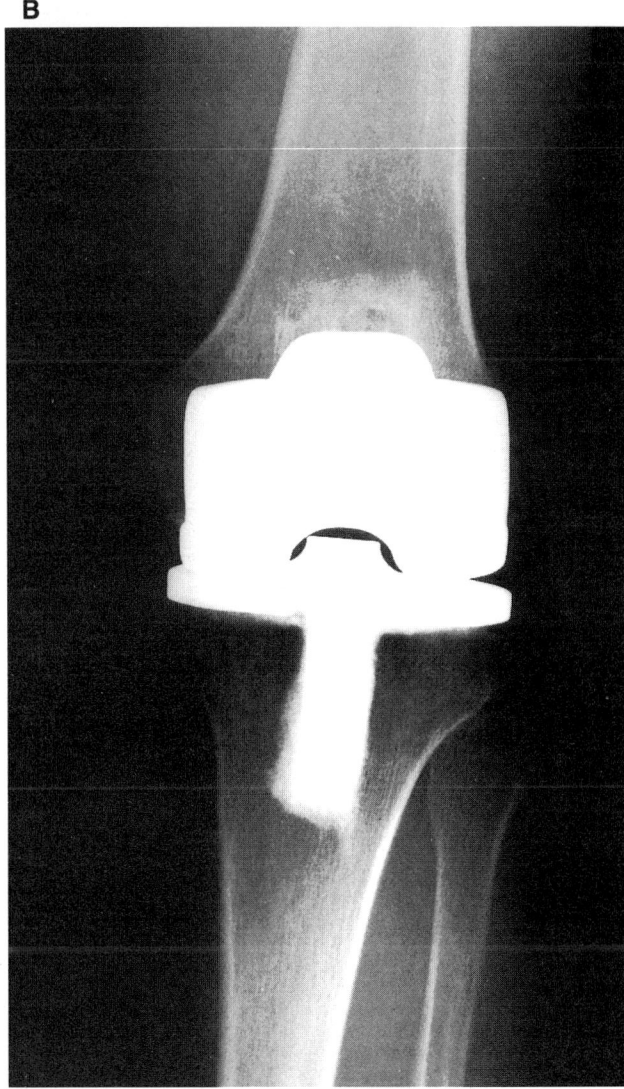

FIG 62-5.
(A) Photograph and **(B)** AP radiograph of the Kinematic condylar prosthesis.

nificant correlation was found between the development of lucent lines and knees with incompletely corrected varus malalignment in which the tibial component was placed in excessive varus angulation. Two knees required reoperation, for an overall rate of 1.6%. One was for a patellar dislocation and 1 was a revision for loosening of the tibial component (0.8%). This occurred in a knee with a 30-degree preoperative varus angulation in which a large medial tibial plateau defect was filled with unreinforced cement, the tibial component was placed in 10 degrees of varus angulation, and the overall postoperative alignment was 0 degrees of valgus angulation. There were no cases of instability or infection.

A subsequent study from the same group reported 192 knees followed for a mean of 6 years.[56]

The mean age of the patients with rheumatoid arthritis was 61 years and 70 years in those with osteoarthritis. Knee motion improved from 104 degrees preoperatively to 109 degrees at last follow-up evaluation. Good or excellent results were achieved in 88% of the knees. The joint line was shifted an average of 1 mm. Radiolucent lesions were present adjacent to 40% of the tibial, 30% of the femoral, and 60% of the patellar components. Complications consisted of four deep and four superficial infections, four patellar implant loosenings, one tibial tray fracture, one patellar fracture, one peroneal nerve palsy, and one patellar subluxation. Reoperations were performed in 11 knees (four patellar loosenings, one tibial tray fracture, one patellar fracture, and four deep infections).

This experience with the Kinematic total knee re-

TABLE 62–5.
Cruciate Condylar Total Knee Arthroplasty

Authors	No. of Knees/Patients	Mean Age (yr)	Rheumatoid Arthritis (%)	Osteoarthritis (%)	Follow-up (yr)	Good or Excellent Results (%)	Instability (%)	Loosening (%)	Lucent Lines (%)	Infection (%)	Reoperations or Failures (%)
Ritter et al. (1984)[45]	94/63	67	27	63	5	96.8	—	1	22*	1	1
Bourne et al. (1988)[4]	164/131	65	32	61	5.3	95	4.2	—	6* 3†	0.6	3.7
Rand (1991)[39]	134/108	63	33	62	10	88	—	1	59	1	1.5
Lee et al. (1990)[32]	144/193	67	21	72	9	94	—	12	42	—	2

*Incomplete lucent lines, <1 mm.
†Lucent lines >1 mm and complete, or progressive.

TABLE 62–6.
Kinematic Condylar Total Knee Arthroplasty

Authors	No. of Knees/Patients	Mean Age (yr)	Rheumatoid Arthritis (%)	Osteoarthritis (%)	Follow-up (yr)	Successful Results (%)	Lucent Lines (%)	Infection (%)	Reoperations/ Failures (%)
Ewald et al. (1984)[15]	121/91	76	59	41	2.2	90	18	—	1.6
Wright et al. (1990)[56]	192/147	70	54	44	6	88	30–40	2.0	5.7

placement not only confirms the excellent results obtained with design changes as total knee prostheses evolve, but also continues to elucidate the important principles of surgical technique, namely component position and axial alignment. Patellar implant fixation remains a problem (Table 62–6).

TOWNLEY AND CLOUTIER RESURFACING DESIGNS

The original Townley (Fig 62–6) and Cloutier (Fig 62–7) prostheses had similar design concepts and hence are discussed together here. The stated goal of both systems was to reproduce as accurately as possible the normal joint anatomy, mechanics, and kinematics of the human knee.[7, 54] Both systems were designed to preserve both cruciate ligaments. Both employed a U-shaped tibial component without a stem that was flat in the sagittal plane so as to provide unconstrained motion to minimize stress transfer to the cement-bone interface. Finally, both designers emphasized the importance of implant position and axial alignment. Each utilized unique instrumentation using an extramedullary alignment system based on intraoperative localization of the femoral head to obtain accurate and reproducible component implantation.

In 1985, Townley[54] reviewed 532 total knees with 1.5 to 11 years' follow-up out of over 700 implants that had been performed since 1972. Seventy-three percent were performed for osteoarthritis, 18% for rheumatoid arthritis, and 9% were revision operations for a previously failed arthroplasty. The tibial component was non-metal-backed and was ideally placed in 2 degrees of varus angulation so that the joint line would remain horizontal during the single-leg stance phase of ambulation to minimize shear stresses.

Overall, excellent or good results were obtained in 89% of knees (i.e., motion beyond 90 degrees, mild or no pain, and no walking aid). Tibial loosening occurred in 10 knees (1.9%) requiring revision; 6 knees (1.1%) had patellofemoral complications necessitating a reoperation. Clinical instability occurred in 3 knees, and deep infection occurred in 9 knees (1.2%). Townley noted that the majority of loosening complications were associated with some degree of technical malalignment of the joint. Overall, 19 knees (3.6%) required reoperation.

A study of 88 Townley knee arthroplasties in 72 patients followed a mean of 2.5 years was performed.[36] The mean relative age of the patients was 68 years. Pain relief was achieved in 94% with "acceptable" results in 86%. Reoperation was performed for tibial loosening in 3, deep infection in 1, and patellar loosening in 1. Incomplete radiolucent lines were identified in 18% (Table 62–7).

The Cloutier prosthesis was developed at the St.

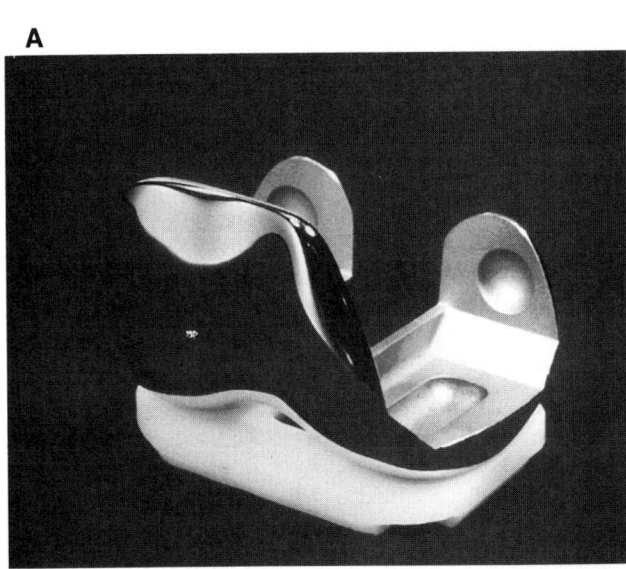
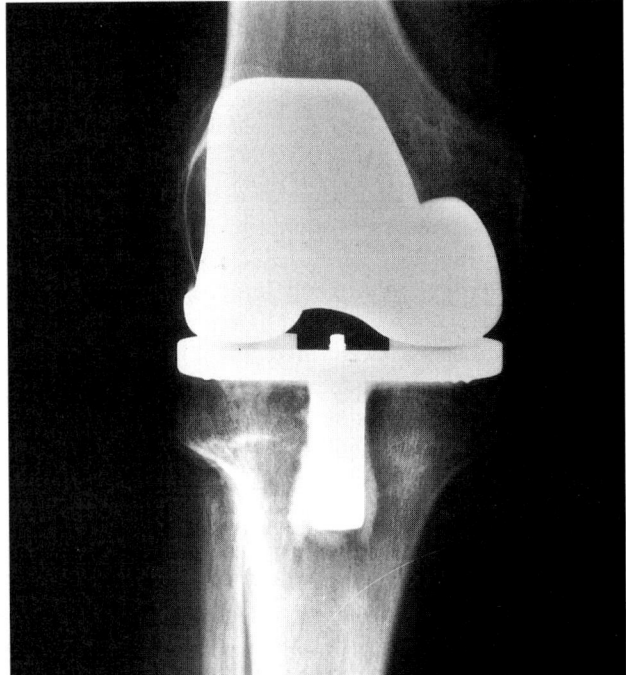

FIG 62–6.
(A) Photograph and **(B)** AP radiograph of the Townley prosthesis.

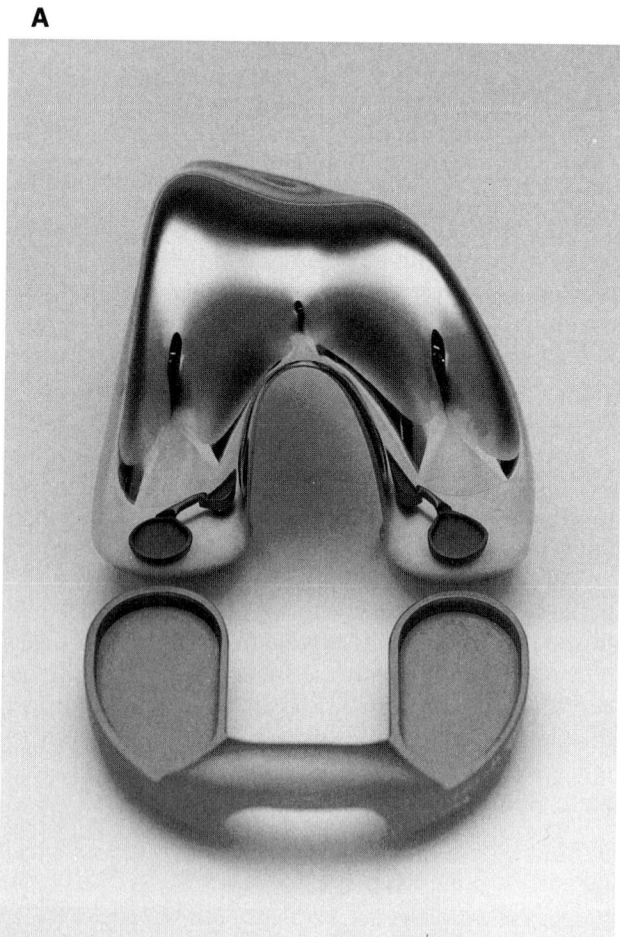
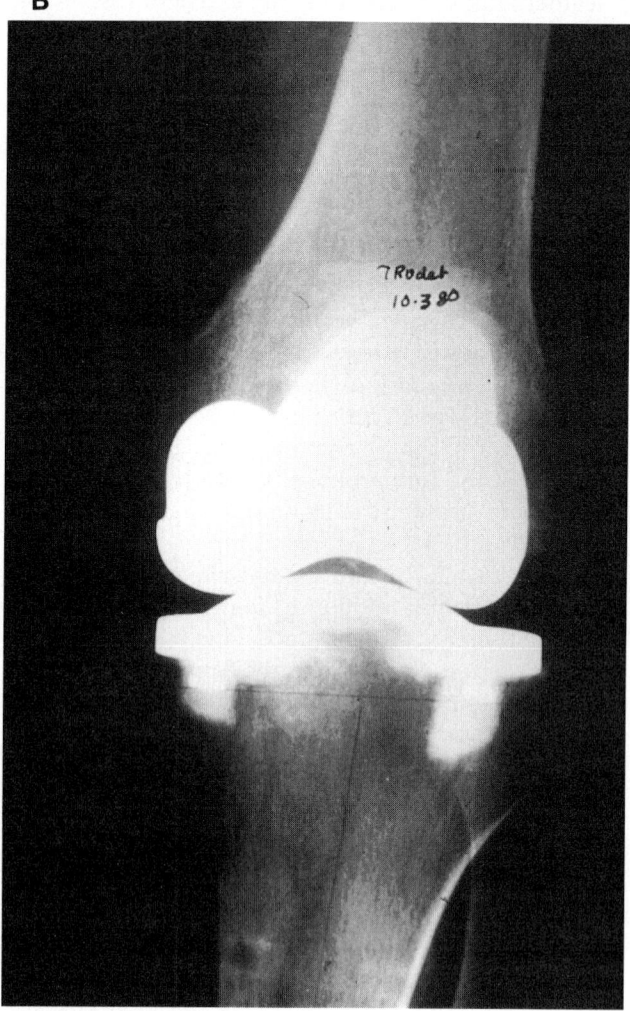

FIG 62-7.
(A) Photograph and **(B)** AP radiograph of the Cloutier prosthesis.

Luc Hospital in Montreal in 1975.[7] Unique features include a metal-backed U-shaped tibial plateau into which two separate polyethylene inserts are press-fitted. In addition, the technique for component implantation relies on a knee joint distractor which maintains axial alignment and ligament tension while the osteotomies are performed.

In 1983, Cloutier published the results of 107 total knee replacements with follow-up of 2 to 4½ years.[7] Sixty-four percent were performed for rheumatoid arthritis and 33% for osteoarthritis in patients with an average age of 58 years (range, 35–81 years). The ACL was found to be attenuated or destroyed in 57% of knees. The PCL was always preserved, and was not found to prevent adequate component positioning or correction of even severe deformities. Using The Hospital for Special Surgery rating system, 91% of knees had good or excellent results at final follow-up. Complications included instability in three knees and deep infection in three knees. Twenty-four percent of knees were found to have lucent lines beneath the tibial component which were less than 1 mm in width and nonprogressive. Only one progressive tibial lucency occurred, which led to the one case of tibial component loosening and required revision. Overall, reoperations were required in eight knees (7.5%). A subsequent study of 85 knees in 61 patients followed for 10 to 12 years was performed.[8] The mean patient age was 59 years. Good or excellent results were achieved in 79%. The results were good or excellent in 93% of the ACL-intact knees and in 62.5% of the ACL-deficient knees. Aseptic loosening occurred in 1.2%. Revision was performed in seven knees (13%): for infection (2), instability (3), aseptic loosening (1), and pain of indeterminant cause (1). Radiolucent lines were identified in 25% of the knees (Table 62–8).

Gait studies were performed on 17 patients with

TABLE 62–7.
Townley Total Knee Arthroplasty

Authors	No. of Knees/Patients	Mean Age (yr)	Rheumatoid Arthritis (%)	Osteoarthritis (%)	Follow-up (yr)	Good or Excellent Results (%)	Instability (%)	Loosening (%)	Lucent Lines (%)	Infection (%)	Reoperations/Failures (%)
Mallory et al. (1982)[36]	88/72	68	12	81	2½	86	—	4.1	18	1.3	6.9
Townley (1985)[54]	532/426	—	18	73	1½–11	89	0.6	1.9	—	1.2	3.6

TABLE 62–8.
Cloutier Total Knee Arthroplasty

Authors	No. of Knees/Patients	Mean Age (yr)	Rheumatoid Arthritis (%)	Osteoarthritis (%)	Follow-up (yr)	Good/Excellent Results (%)	Instability (%)	Loosening (%)	Lucent Lines (%)	Infection (%)	Reoperations/Failures (%)
Cloutier (1983)[7]	107/83	58	64	33	2–4½	91	2.8	1	24* 1†	2.8	7.5
Cloutier (1991)[8]	85/61	59	55	39	10–13	79	3.5	1.2	25	2.3	13

*Incomplete lucent lines, <1 mm.
†Lucent lines >1 mm and complete, or progressive.

Cloutier prostheses that had excellent results and a minimum of 1-year follow-up.[2] Gait was compared with gait of a matched set of 17 patients with a cruciate-sacrificing total condylar knee prosthesis, excellent results, and at least 1-year follow-up. The results demonstrated that both groups walked on level ground with a shorter-than-normal stride length and used a smaller-than-normal flexion during stance phase. However, while ascending and descending stairs, knee flexion was significantly greater in patients with the Cloutier prosthesis and did not differ significantly from normal controls. This suggests that preservation of the PCL may lead to not only improved function in stair climbing but possibly in other activities of daily living as well.

The Townley and Cloutier resurfacing prostheses have been carefully studied by their designers and have demonstrated excellent and good results in approximately 90% of patients at midrange follow-up. Lew and Lewis[33] demonstrated in the laboratory the importance of low-conformity, low-constraint articular surfaces when the cruciate ligaments are preserved. These clinical studies not only document the behavior of a particular prosthesis but also add in vivo confirmation of these important concepts.

MILLER-GALANTE PROSTHESIS

The Miller-Galante total knee (Zimmer, Warsaw, Ind.) (Fig 62–8), one of the first knee replacements designed for use with cement or cementless fixation, was first implanted in 1986.[31] A titanium fiber composite was chosen for the bony ingrowth surface because of its well-recognized biocompatibility in primates, as well as its previous use in limb-salvage tumor surgery. To replicate normal knee kinematics as closely as possible, the designers believed that the slope of the replaced femoral condyles must match that of the native condyles in addition to preservation of the PCL. Seven different femoral component sizes (right and left) were made available. In order to place the tibial component on the cortical rim to avoid subsidence, five sizes of tibial components were designed.[46] Finally, modularity of polyethylene inserts

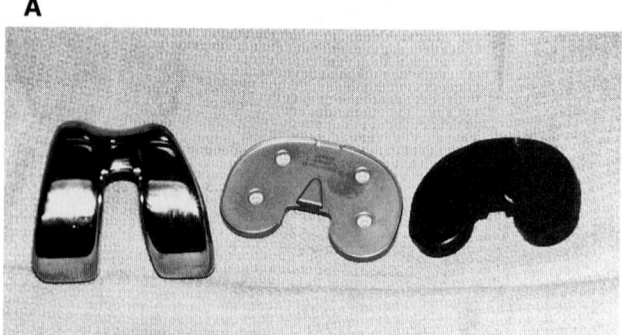

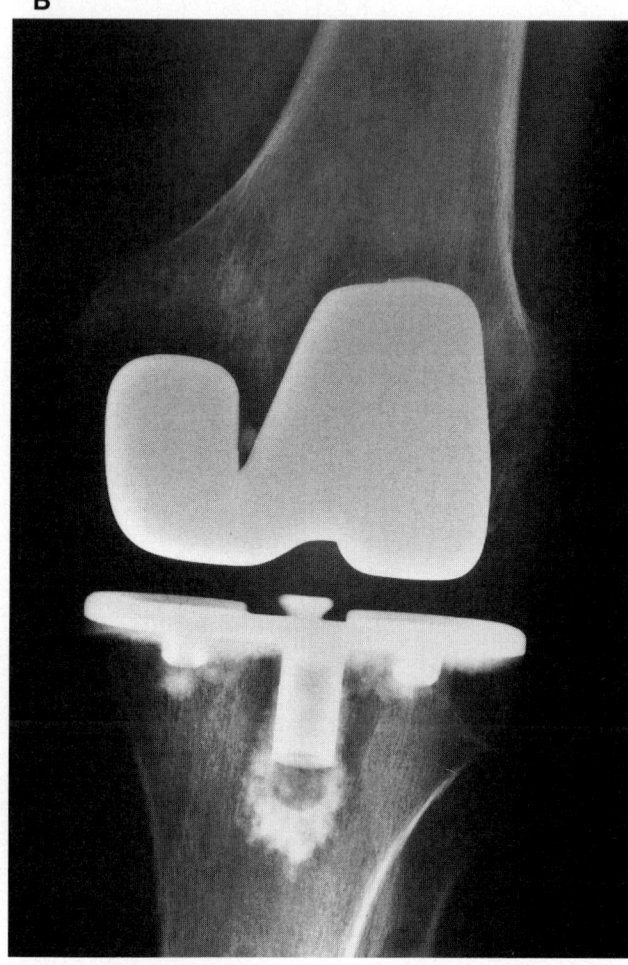

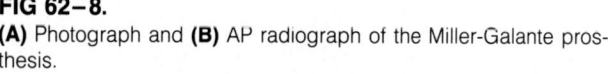

FIG 62–8.
(A) Photograph and **(B)** AP radiograph of the Miller-Galante prosthesis.

was incorporated in order to allow fine-tuning of ligamentous tension, the degree of articular constraint, and the possibility of future isolated polyethylene replacement. Modular polyethylene is an important part of almost all contemporary knee prosthetic designs.

Landon et al.[31] in 1986 reported early 1- to 4-year follow-up on the first 37 cementless knees implanted in 35 patients, 54% of whom had osteoarthritis and 26% rheumatoid arthritis. Using the modified rating of The Hospital for Special Surgery, 32 patients (86%) obtained good or excellent results. Five patients were considered failures: 3 for proven infections and 1 for tibial component loosening. No progressive lucencies were observed in the patients with satisfactory results.

In 1989 Rosenberg et al.[46] reported the results of 133 cemented and 134 cementless total knee arthroplasties. The series was prospective but not randomized. Patients of older age, with poorer bone stock, and with questionable ability to comply with a touch weightbearing-only rehabilitation were selected for a cemented arthroplasty. The average age in the cemented group was 70 years (range, 31–97 years); the average age in the cementless group was 58 years (range, 19–75 years). In both groups, osteoarthritis accounted for 80% and rheumatoid arthritis for 15% of patients. The patients were evaluated at a mean of 22 months for the cemented and 23 months for the cementless arthroplasty group.

Using the modified rating of The Hospital for Special Surgery, 93% of cemented and 95% of cementless knees showed good or excellent results. Postoperative range of motion was similar for both groups, 104 and 107 degrees, respectively. More patients in the cementless group complained of slight pain at final follow-up (34% vs. 19%). Failures requiring revision occurred in 5% (seven knees) of cemented arthroplasties and 3% (four knees) of cementless arthroplasties. Four additional cemented knees required reoperation for extensor mechanism complications (two patellar realignments, one patellar revision, and one quadriceps repair). Eleven cementless knees required reoperation for failure of the cementless patellar component. In all instances there was ingrowth of the patellar pegs, failure of ingrowth of the patellar plate, with subsequent shear failure of the peg-plate junction. There were two cases of infection in each group, one tibial loosening in the cementless group, and two cases of instability in the cemented group.

One hundred twenty-five cementless knees were evaluated for interface radiolucencies. Almost no complete or partial lucencies occurred about the femoral component. Evaluation of the patellar components demonstrated only two complete lucencies. Thirteen percent showed partial lucencies, 55% showed no lucencies, and in 30% the radiographs could not be evaluated. Partial tibial radiolucencies were seen in 36%, complete lucencies in 8%, no lucencies in 47%, and 10% had inadequate radiographs. In ten cementless tibial components removed for reasons other than mechanical loosening, the mean extent of plate bone ingrowth was 25%. In all ten, bony ingrowth was present on at least three of the four pegs.

A subsequent report by Rosenberg et al.[47] compared 116 cemented with 123 cementless knees at 44 months following arthroplasty. Good or excellent results were achieved in 92% of the cementless compared with 88% of the cemented knees. The range of motion was 105 degrees in the cemented and 109 degrees in the cementless knees. Incomplete radiolucent lines were identified in 26% of cementless and in 16% of cemented knees. Three cementless knees had complete radiolucent lines. Reoperation was performed in 11% of cementless and in 9% of cemented knees. Revision occurred in 5% of cementless and in 6% of cemented knees.

Kraay et al.[30] reported on 29 knees in 22 patients with hybrid fixation which were followed for a mean of 28 months. The mean age of the patients was 71 years. The diagnoses were osteoarthritis in 19, traumatic arthritis in 2, and rheumatoid arthritis in 1 patient. The range of motion was 110 degrees. The Knee Society pain score averaged 47 and the function score 79. Radiolucent lines were seen in 39% of knees.

These studies demonstrate equally good short-term results with both the cemented and cementless PCL-sparing Miller-Galante knee with the exception of the cementless metal-backed patellar component. The results closely match those of the previously discussed unconstrained resurfacing designs with at least 90% good and excellent results (Table 62–9).

POROUS COATED ANATOMIC TOTAL KNEE ARTHROPLASTY

The PCA total knee (Porous Coated Anatomic, Howmedica) was designed with the objective of reconstituting normal kinematic function of the knee through minimal articular surface replacement (Fig 62–9).[20] Each of the components simulated the normal anatomy of the surface it replaced. Each of the fixation interfaces was porous-coated with a double layer of sintered cobalt-chromium beads, and could be implanted with or without cement. The femoral condyles were flattened in the mediolateral dimension to improve loading characteristics. There were three separate instant centers of rotation and three differ-

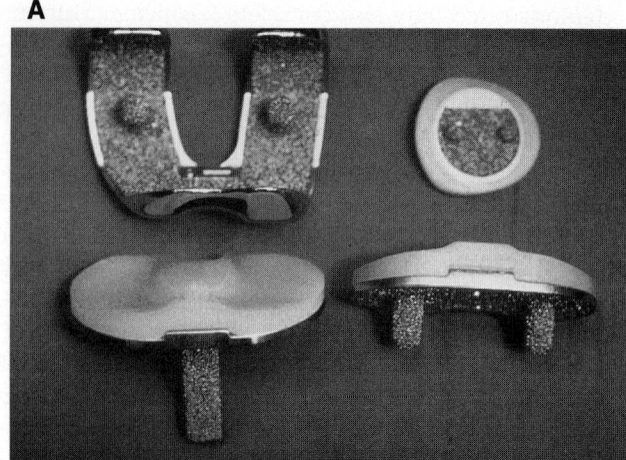

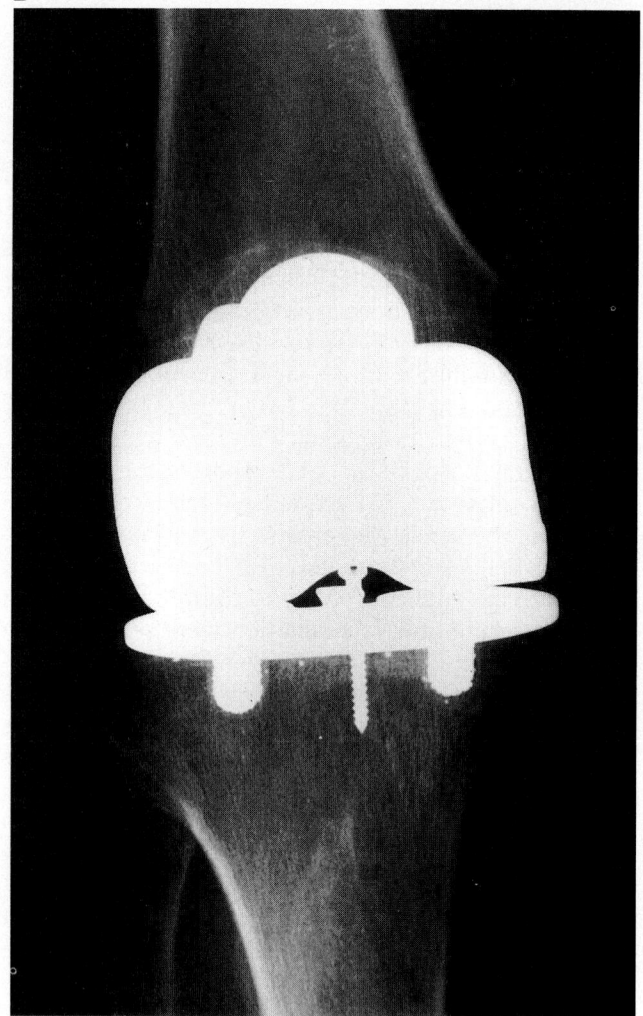

FIG 62-9.
(A) Photograph and (B) AP radiograph of the Porous Coated Anatomic prosthesis.

ent radii of curvature, which were unique for the medial and lateral condyles, thereby mimicking the normal knee. The intercondylar notch was curved to simulate normal anatomy, which contributed to the screw-home mechanism. The tibial component was asymmetric, flat, and sloped posteriorly. The curved posterior slope, which was more anterior on the medial side, also contributed to the automatic rotational or screw-home mechanism. The trochlea was in 3 degrees of valgus angulation and the lateral facet of both the trochlea and patella were more prominent than the medial facet, again simulating the normal knee.

In 1987, Hungerford[22] reported 2- to 5-year follow-up results of 93 cementless PCA knees in 82 patients. Sixty-three percent had osteoarthritis with a mean age of 68 years and 30% had rheumatoid arthritis with a mean age of 56 years. Patients were selected for ingrowth arthroplasties if there was less than 25 degrees of axial malalignment, good bone stock, and satisfactory implant stability intraoperatively. These cementless knees represented less than 50% of all knees performed by the authors, the remainder being cemented knees. However, the authors note that this proportion gradually increased until approximately 90% of femoral components and 80% of tibial and patellar components were being implanted without cement.

Overall, 94.5% of patients obtained excellent or good results using a 100-point evaluation scale that assigns a total of 50 points for pain, 20 points for range of motion, and 10 points each for alignment, stability, and strength. There were no cases of aseptic loosening of femoral or tibial components and no cases of instability. Aseptic loosening of the patellar component requiring revision occurred in six knees and infection occurred in one knee. Using fluoroscopic imaging of the tibial interface, 83% of components showed no radiolucent zones, 17% demonstrated incomplete lucent lines, and no components showed a complete radiolucent line. In addition, the authors noted that interfaces that appeared radio-

TABLE 62-9.
Miller-Galante Total Knee Arthroplasty

Authors	No. of Knees/Patients	Mean Age (yr)	Rheumatoid Arthritis (%)	Osteoarthritis (%)	Follow-up (yr)	Good or Excellent Results (%)	Instability (%)	Loosening (%)	Lucent Lines (%)	Infection (%)	Reoperations/Failures (%)
Landon et al. (1986)[31]	37/35	57	26	54	1–4	86	—	2.7	—	8.1	14
Rosenberg et al. (1989)[46]	Cemented: 133/133	70		80	1–4	93	1.5	—	—	1.5	9
	Uncemented: 134/126	58	15			95	—	0.75	36* 6†	1.5	12

*Incomplete lucent lines, <1 mm.
†Lucent lines >1 mm and complete, or progressive.

TABLE 62-10.
Porous-Coated Anatomic Total Knee Arthroplasty

Authors	No. of Knees/Patients	Mean Age (yr)	Rheumatoid Arthritis (%)	Osteoarthritis (%)	Follow-up (yr)	Good or Excellent Results (%)	Instability (%)	Loosening (%)	Lucent Lines (%)	Infection (%)	Reoperations or Failures
Hungerford et al. (1985)[21]	OA 186/162		—		2–5	Cementless: 96 Cemented: 96	—	—	—	—	7.2
	RA 92/74					Cementless: 92 Cemented: 81	—	—	—	—	7.2
Rand et al. (1987)[43]	50/33 (cemented)	65	32	68	2.2	97	—	—	3*	—	—
	41/33 (cementless)	56	34	61	2.4	83	4.8	2.4	18*	2.4	9.7
Hungerford et al. (1987)[22]	93/82 (cementless)	56	30	63	2–5	94.5	—	—	17†	1.1	8.6

OA = osteoarthritis, RA = rheumatoid arthritis.
*Lucent lines >1 mm and complete, or progressive.
†Incomplete lucent lines, <1 mm.

graphically stable at 6 months postoperatively remained stable throughout the follow-up period.

In another study, Hungerford et al.[21] compared the results of cemented and cementless PCA knees at 2- to 5-year follow-up. In 186 knees implanted for osteoarthritis (54% cementless), 96% showed good or excellent results. In 92 knees implanted for rheumatoid arthritis (59% cementless), 92% of the cementless knees were rated good or excellent, while only 81% of the cemented knees demonstrated good or excellent results. The difference, however, was attributed to the selection criteria, with the more severe bone loss and deformity in the cemented group.

Rand et al.[43] in 1987 also compared the results of cemented vs. cementless PCA total knee arthroplasties. Fifty cemented knees with greater than 2 years' follow-up showed 97% good or excellent results, while only 83% of 41 cementless knees showed good or excellent results. There were no differences in function or range of motion between the two groups. Reoperation was required in 4 cementless knees, including three revision arthroplasties: one each for tibial component breakage, tibial component loosening, and infection. There were no reoperations in the cemented arthroplasty group. Progressive lucent lines occurred in 3% of cemented components and in 18% of cementless components. It is noteworthy, however, that fluoroscopic views were utilized in the cementless group and not in the cemented group; thus the validity of this comparison is questionable. In the cemented group, there were no significant changes in component position; however, in the cementless group, three knees sustained significant shifts in the position of the tibial component. This study demonstrated satisfactory results in both cemented and cementless PCA knees, but raises questions about cementless tibial component fixation.

A study of 48 knees in 39 patients with cementless fixation and an age of less than 50 years was performed.[23] Good or excellent results were achieved in 39 knees (81%) at 4 years after arthroplasty. The mean range of motion was 105 degrees. Radiolucent lines were observed in 35%. Complications consisted of instability (4 knees), patellar loosening (3), subsidence (2), patellar subluxation (2), fibrosis (1) and fat pad impingement (1).

A comparative prospective study of 26 cementless and 25 cemented knees was performed.[9] At 3 years following arthroplasty, good or excellent results were achieved in 18 (69%) of the cementless and in 17 (68%) of the cemented knees. Lucent lines of 2 mm in width were seen adjacent to 44% of the cementless and 12% of the cemented knees ($P = .02$). Tibial component subsidence occurred in 50% of the cementless and 8% of the cemented knees. Reoperation was performed for 1 knee in each group.

A study of 18 patients with a cemented knee on one side and a cementless knee on the other was performed.[12] At 5 years following arthroplasty there were no differences in knee scores of radiolucent lines. There was one reoperation for cemented tibial component loosening and one for cementless patellar component loosening.

The PCA prosthesis demonstrates that with increasing sophistication in the reproduction of normal knee surface anatomy and kinematics, continued improved results can be expected with a resurfacing, PCL-preserving, unconstrained design (Table 62–10).

MENISCAL BEARING PROSTHESIS

The concept of a meniscal bearing prosthesis is to provide congruity of the articulating surfaces and unconstrained tibiofemoral movement[17] (Fig 62–10). The conforming articular surfaces minimize wear, but the bearing motion allows knee motion and ligament function. The original Oxford meniscal bearing prosthesis had a spherical femoral surface of a single size. No soft tissue balancing was performed. Of 125 knees treated with the Oxford prosthesis and reviewed at a mean of 4 years, pain relief was achieved in 89%. Mean motion was 99 degrees. Complications consisted of four loosenings, one deep infection, five dislocated meniscal bearings, one tibial plateau fracture, and two subluxated meniscal bearings. The revision rate was 7%. Radiolucent lines beneath the tibial component were present in 96%.

The low-contact stress (LCS) prosthesis differs from the Oxford prosthesis by having a decreasing posterior femoral condyle radius which results in slight incongruence in the tibial articulation.[5] One hundred seventy knees were treated with cementless fixation in patients with a mean age of 60 years.[5] Ninety-five percent good or excellent results were achieved at 4.5 years. One hundred eight knees were treated with cement fixation in patients with a mean age of 64 years. Eighty-nine percent good or excellent results were obtained at a mean of 7.6 years. Complications were numerous, affecting 32% of the cemented and 27% of the cementless knees. Reoperation was required in 11% of the cemented and 2.9% of the cementless knees. A subsequent study used survivorship analysis with an end point of poor knee score or revision.[6] A 91% survivorship of 46 cemented bicruciate designs at 12 years was predicted.

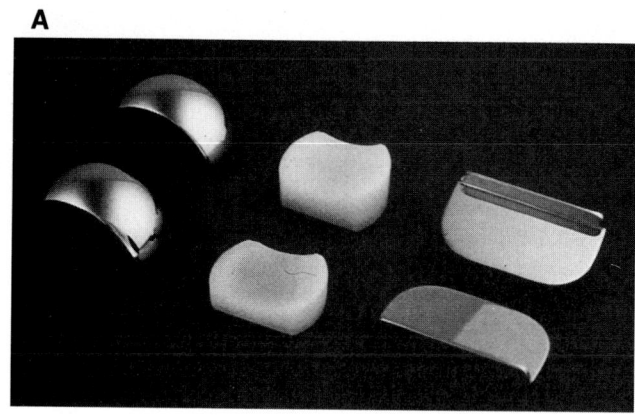
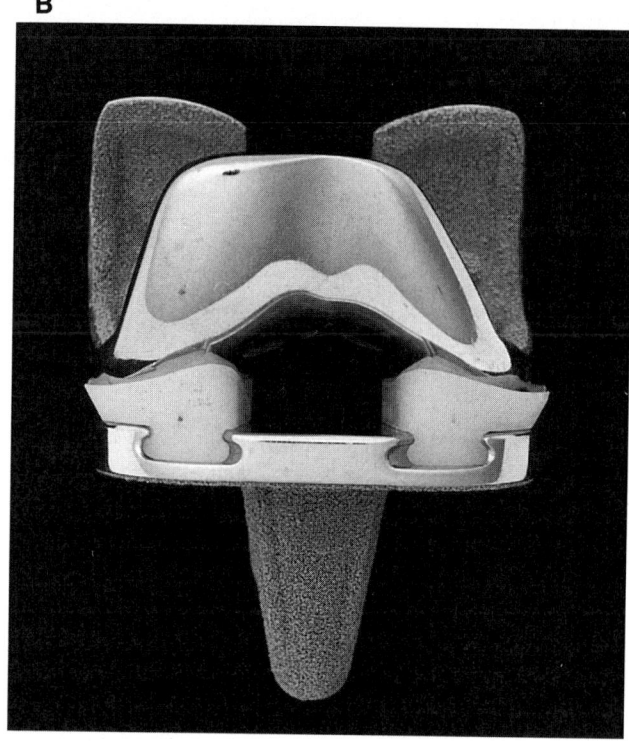

FIG 62-10.
(A) The Oxford meniscal bearing prosthesis; B, low-contact stress (LCS) prosthesis.

A 98% survivorship of 57 PCL-retaining designs at 6 years was predicted. Another 1-year study of 43 LCS knees found 39 knees (91%) good or excellent.[3] However, there was a 9.3% incidence of dislocation of the meniscal bearings. The mean range of motion was 94 degrees. The concept of meniscal bearings is therefore attractive for managing problems of polyethylene wear. The clinical results of 90% to 95% good or excellent appear to be similar to other designs. Whether the long-term results suggest a lower wear rate and greater durability than other condylar prostheses is unknown (Table 62-11).

PRESS FIT CONDYLAR PROSTHESIS

The PFC (Press Fit Condylar, Johnson & Johnson Orthopaedics) prosthesis was designed with a finned keel on the tibial component in an attempt to provide improved resistance to offset loading with minimal removal of tibial bone (Fig 62-11). The implant was designed for cemented or cementless fixation. The results of 114 PFC knees with hybrid fixation (cementless femur, cemented tibia) followed for 2.8 years were reported.[57] The knee society scoring system improved from a preoperative value of 35 to a postoperative value of 92. Ninety-three percent had good or excellent results. The average flexion was 112 degrees. Radiolucent lines were identified adjacent to 30% of the femoral, 30% of the tibial, and 23% of the patellar components. Complications consisted of one wound hematoma, two deep infections, three deep venous thromboses, and two pulmonary emboli. The reoperation rate was 3%.

Another study compared 59 knees with cementless fixation with 59 knees with cemented fixation using the PFC prosthesis.[40] At 2.8 years following arthroplasty, good or excellent results were achieved in 98% of the cemented compared with 90% of the cementless knees. Motion was 101 degrees in the cementless and 103 degrees in the cemented knees. Complications in the cementless group consisted of nine metal-backed patellar failures, and one each of deep infection, fibrous ankylosis, and deep venous thrombosis, for an overall complication rate of 20%. Complications in the cemented knees consisted of two deep venous thromboses, and one each of deep infection, patellar fracture, supracondylar femur fracture, and loosening, for an overall complication rate of 10%. Reoperation was performed in 7% of the cemented and 19% of the cementless knees.

The PFC prosthesis provides satisfactory results in 93% to 94% of knees with or without cement fixation. The complication and reoperation rates are similar to other current condylar prostheses. The use of a metal-backed patella of this design should be avoided (Table 62-12).

TABLE 62–11.
Meniscal Bearing Total Knee Arthroplasty

Authors	No. of Knees/Patients	Mean Age (yr)	Rheumatoid Arthritis (%)	Osteoarthritis (%)	Follow-up (yr)	Successful Results (%)	Lucent Lines (%)	Infection (%)	Reoperations or Failures (%)
Goodfellow & O'Connor (1986)[17]	125/107	65	40	53	4	89	96	1	7
Buechel & Pappas (1989)[5]	170 (cementless)	60	23	69	4½	95	—	—	2.9
	106 (cemented)	64	41	58	7.6	89	—	2.5	11

TABLE 62–12.
Press Fit Condylar Total Knee Arthroplasty

Authors	No. of Knees/Patients	Mean Age (yr)	Rheumatoid Arthritis (%)	Osteoarthritis (%)	Follow-up (yr)	Successful Results (%)	Lucent Lines (%)	Infection (%)	Reoperations or Failures (%)
Wright et al. (1990)[57]	112 knees	65	32	68	2.8	93	30	1.8	3
Rand (1991)[40]	118/102	66	13	62	2.8	94	75	1.8	13

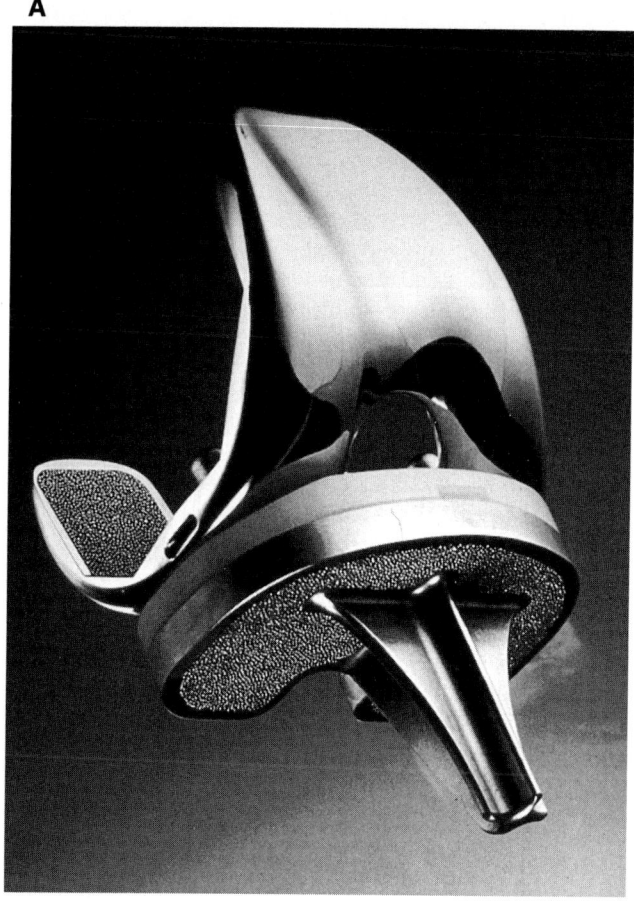
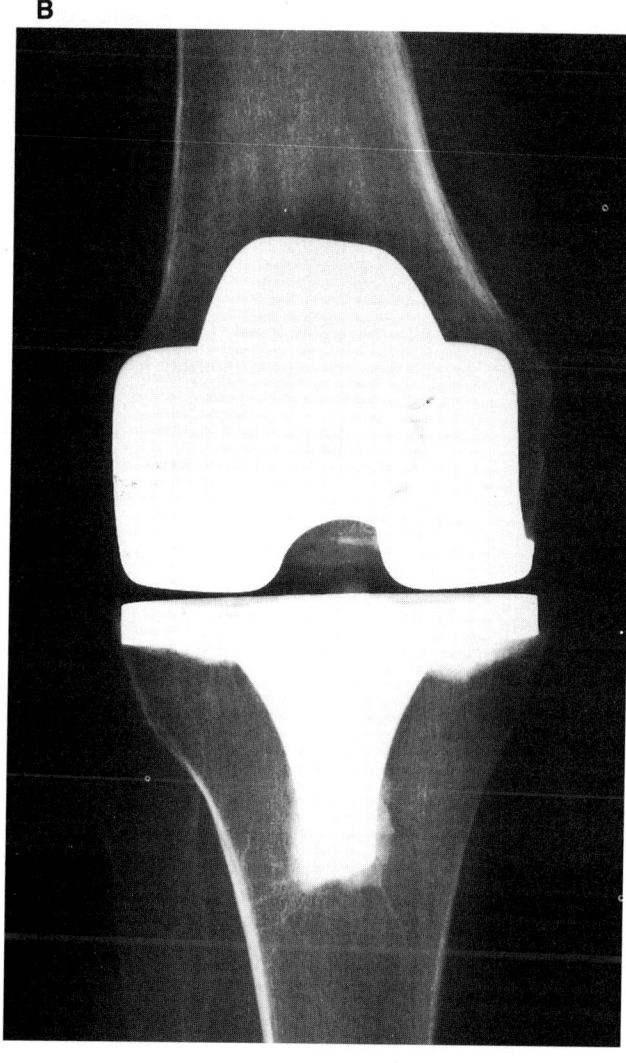

FIG 62–11.
(A) Photograph and (B) AP radiograph of Press Fit condylar prosthesis.

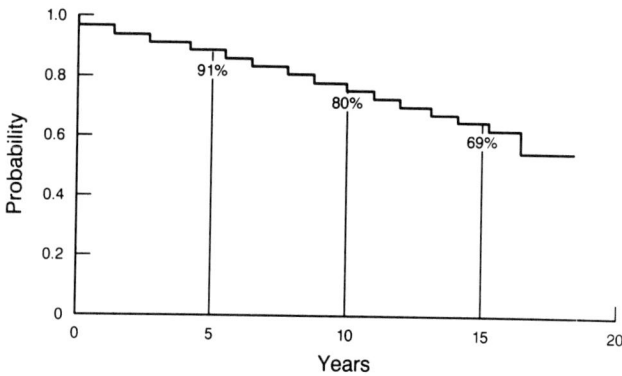

FIG 62–12.
Survivorship of 9,200 total knee arthroplasties was 69% at 15 years. (From Rand JA, Ilstrup DM: *J Bone Joint Surg [Am]* 73:397, 1991. Used by permission.)

SUMMARY

In 1991 Rand and Ilstrup[42] reported the results of 9,200 total knee arthroplasties implanted between 1971 and 1987 using survivorship analysis, with revision of an implant chosen as the end point of survival (Fig 62–12). Of these, 2,947 primary total knee arthroplasties were performed using older resurfacing designs, including the Polycentric and Geometric knees. Cumulative rates of survival were 95% at 2 years, 89% at 5 years, and 78% at 10 years. Primary arthroplasties using condylar resurfacing PCL-retaining designs with metal-backed tibial components, were performed on 3,620 knees. These designs included the cruciate condylar (Howmedica), kinematic condylar, Townley, Cloutier, Miller-Galante, PCA, PFC, and Orthomet (Minneapolis, Minn.) prostheses. Cumulative rates of survival were 99% at 2 years, 98% at 5 years, and 91% at 10 years. Risk of failure was significantly greater for the early resurfacing designs compared with the metal-backed condylar designs. When metal-backed PCL-retaining arthroplasties were compared with PCL-substituting designs (234 posterior-stabilized knees), the results did not differ significantly for primary or revision arthroplasties. However, when primary and revision knees were combined, the PCL-substituting knees had a statistically significant higher cumulative failure rate: 3.8% vs. 1.6% ($P < .03$). Considering all 9,200 knees implanted, use of a proportional-hazard general linear model identified four independent variables associated with a significantly lower risk of failure: (1) primary arthroplasty, (2) diagnosis of rheumatoid arthritis, (3) age of 60 years or more, and (4) use of a condylar PCL-retaining prosthesis with a metal-backed tibial component.

The results of these studies confirm that PCL-retaining total knee arthroplasties have evolved and improved to become one of the most successful orthopaedic operations, with greater than 90% satisfactory results at up to 10 years' follow-up. Continued long-term study is necessary to determine the relative benefits of various design modifications.

REFERENCES

1. Andriacchi TP, Galante JO: Retention of the posterior cruciate in total knee arthroplasty, *J Arthroplasty* 3:S13, 1988.
2. Andriacchi TP, Galante JO, Fermier RW: The influence of total knee replacement design on walking and stair climbing, *J Bone Joint Surg [Am]* 64:1328, 1982.
3. Bert JM: Disclocation/subluxation of meniscal bearing elements after New Jersey low-contact stress total knee arthroplasty, *Clin Orthop* 254:211, 1990.
4. Bourne MH, Rand JA, Ilstrup DM: Posterior cruciate condylar total knee arthroplasty: five year results, *Clin Orthop* 234:129, 1988.
5. Buechel FF, Pappas MJ: New Jersey low contact stress knee replacement system, *Orthop Clin North Am* 20:147, 1989.
6. Buechel FF, Pappas MJ: Long-term survivorship analysis of cruciate sparing versus cruciate-sacrificing knee prostheses using meniscal bearing, *Clin Orthop* 260:162, 1990.
7. Cloutier JM: Results of total knee arthroplasty with a nonconstrained prosthesis, *J Bone Joint Surg [Am]* 65:906, 1983.
8. Cloutier JM: Long-term results after nonconstrained total knee arthroplasty, *Clin Orthop* 273:63, 1991.
9. Collins DN, et al: Porous coated anatomic total knee arthroplasty, *Clin Orthop* 267:128, 1991.
10. Coventry MB, et al: Geometric total knee arthroplasty. I. Conception, design, indications and surgical technique, *Clin Orthop* 94:171, 1973.
11. Coventry MB, et al: Geometric total knee arthroplasty. II. Patient data and complications, *Clin Orthop* 94:177, 1973.
12. Dodd CAF, Hungerford DS, Krackow KA: Total knee arthroplasty fixation, *Clin Orthop* 260:66, 1990.
13. Dorr LD, et al: Functional comparison of posterior-cruciate–retained versus cruciate-sacrificed total knee arthroplasty, *Clin Orthop* 236:36, 1988.
14. Ewald FC, et al: Duo-patella total knee arthroplasty in rheumatoid arthritis, *Orthop Trans* 2:202, 1978.
15. Ewald FC, et al: Kinematic total knee replacement, *J Bone Joint Surg [Am]* 66:1032, 1984.
16. Freeman MAR, Railton GT: Should the posterior cruciate ligament be retained or resected in condylar nomeniscal knee arthroplasty: The case for resection, *J Arthroplasty* 3:S3, 1988.
17. Goodfellow JW, O'Connor J: Clinical results of the Oxford knee, *Clin Orthop* 205:21, 1986.
18. Gunston FH: Polycentric knee arthroplasty. Prosthetic simulation of normal knee movement, *J Bone Joint Surg [Br]* 53:272, 1971.
19. Gunston FH: Ten year results of polycentric knee arthroplasty. In Proceedings of the Canadian Orthopaedic Association, *J Bone Joint Surg [Br]* 62:133, 1980.
20. Hungerford DS, Kenna RV, Krackow KA: The porous-coated anatomic total knee. Symposium on Total Knee Arthroplasty, *Orthop Clin North Am* 13:103, 1982.
21. Hungerford DS, Krackow KA, Kenna RV: Clinical experience with the PCA prosthesis without cement, *Orthop Trans* 9:424, 1985.
22. Hungerford DS, Krackow KA, Kenna RV: Two to five year experience with a cementless porous-coated total knee prosthesis. In Rand JA, Dorr LD, editors: *Total arthroplasty of the knee. Proceedings from the Knee Society, 1985–1986,* Aspen, 1987, Rockville, Md, pp 215–235.
23. Hungerford DS, Krackow KA, Kenna RV: Cementless total knee replacement in patients 50 years old and under, *Orthop Clin North Am* 20:131, 1989.
24. Ilstrup DM, Coventry MB, Skolnick MD: A statistical evaluation of geometric total knee arthroplasties, *Clin Orthop* 120:27, 1976.
25. Ilstrup DM, et al: A statistical evaluation of polycentric total knee arthroplasties, *Clin Orthop* 120:18, 1976.
26. Inglis AE, Lane LB: Total knee replacement using the duo-patella prosthesis, *Orthop Trans* 2:202, 1978.
27. Insall JN, Lachiewicz PF, Burstein AH: The posterior stabilized condylar prosthesis: A modification of the total condylar design. Two to four year clinical experience, *J Bone Joint Surg [Am]* 64:1317, 1982.
28. Insall JN, Scott WN, Ranawat CS: The total condylar knee prosthesis. A report of two hundred twenty cases, *J Bone Joint Surg [Am]* 61:173, 1979.
29. Kelman GJ, et al: Gait laboratory analysis of posterior cruciate-sparing total knee arthroplasty in stair ascent and descent, *Clin Orthop* 248:21, 1989.
30. Kraay MJ, et al: Hybrid total knee arthroplasty with the Miller-Galante prosthesis, *Clin Orthop* 273:32, 1991.
31. Landon GC, Galante JO, Maley MM: Noncemented

total knee arthroplasty, *Clin Orthop North Am* 205:49, 1986.
32. Lee JG, et al: Review of the all polyethylene tibial component in total knee arthroplasty, *Clin Orthop* 260:87, 1990.
33. Lew WD, Lewis JL: The effect of knee-prosthesis geometry on cruciate ligament mechanics during flexion, *J Bone Joint Surg [Am]* 64:734, 1982.
34. Lewallen DG, Bryan RS, Peterson LFA: Polycentric total knee arthroplasty. A ten year follow-up study, *J Bone Joint Surg [Am]* 66:1211, 1984.
35. Lowe GP, McNeur JC: Results of geometric arthroplasty for rheumatoid and osteoarthritis of the knee, *Aust N Z J Surg* 51:528, 1981.
36. Mallory TH, Smalley D, Dray J: Townley anatomic total knee arthroplasty using total tibial component with cruciate release, *Clin Orthop* 169:197–201, 1982.
37. Ranawat CS, Insall J, Shine J: Duo-condylar knee arthroplasty. Hospital for Special Surgery design, *Clin Orthop* 120:76, 1976.
38. Ranawat CS, Shine JJ: Duo-condylar total knee arthroplasty, *Clin Orthop* 94:185, 1973.
39. Rand JA: A comparison of metal backed and all polyethylene tibial components in total knee arthroplasty, Total Knee Replacement 1991, Boston, April 26, 1991.
40. Rand JA: Cement or cementless fixation in total knee arthroplasty? *Clin Orthop* 273:52, 1991.
41. Rand JA, Coventry MB: Ten-year evaluation of geometric total knee arthroplasty, *Clin Orthop* 232:168, 1988.
42. Rand JA, Ilstrup DM: Survivorship analysis of total knee arthroplasty. Cumulative rates of survival of 9.200 total knee arthroplasties, *J Bone Joint Surg [Am]* 73:397, 1991.
43. Rand JA et al: A comparison of cemented versus cementless porous-coated anatomic total knee arthroplasty, In Rand JA, Dorr LD, editors: *Total arthroplasty of the knee. Proceedings of the Knee Society, 1985–1986.* Rockville, 1987, Aspen, p 195.
44. Riley D, Woodyard JE: Long-term results of geometric total knee replacement, *J Bone Joint Surg [Br]* 67:548, 1985.
45. Ritter MA, et al: The posterior cruciate condylar total knee prosthesis. A five year follow-up study, *Clin Orthop* 184:264, 1984.
46. Rosenberg AG, Barden R, Galante JO: A comparison of cemented and cementless fixation with the Miller-Galante total knee arthroplasty, *Orthop Clin North Am* 20:97, 1989.
47. Rosenberg AG, Barden RM, Galante JO: Cemented and ingrowth fixation of the Miller-Galante prosthesis, *Clin Orthop* 260:71, 1990.
48. Scott RD: Duopatellar total knee replacement: The Brigham experience, *Orthop Clin North Am* 13:89, 1982.
49. Skolnick MD, Coventry MB, Ilstrup DM: Geometric total knee arthroplasty. A two-year follow-up study, *J Bone Joint Surg [Am]* 58:749, 1976.
50. Skolnick MD, et al: Polycentric total knee arthroplasty. A two-year follow-up study, *J Bone Joint Surg [Am]* 58:743, 1976.
51. Sledge CB, Ewald FC: Total knee arthroplasty experience at the Robert Breck Brigham Hospital, *Clin Orthop* 145:78, 1979.
52. Sledge CB, et al: Two-year follow-up of the duocondylar total knee replacement, *Orthop Trans* 2:193, 1978.
53. Thomas WH, et al: Duopatella total knee arthroplasty, *Orthop Trans* 4:329, 1980.
54. Townley CO: The anatomic total knee resurfacing arthroplasty, *Clin Orthop* 192:82, 1985.
55. Walker DS, et al: Fixation of tibial components of knee prosthesis, *Trans Orthop Res Soc* 4:95, 1979.
56. Wright J, et al: Total knee arthroplasty with the kinematic prosthesis, *J Bone Joint Surg [Am]* 72:1003, 1990.
57. Wright RJ, et al: Two to four year results of posterior cruciate sparing condylar total knee arthroplasty with an uncemented femoral component, *Clin Orthop* 260:80, 1990.

63

The Role of Congruent Meniscal Bearings in Knee Arthroplasty

JOHN GOODFELLOW, M.S., F.R.C.S.
JOHN O'CONNOR, B.E., M.A., Ph.D.

Articular surface design in the human knee
Articular surface design in the artificial knee
  Congruent joint surfaces
  Incongruent joint surfaces
  Justification for using unconforming designs
    Hinge solution
    Meniscal bearing solution
  Kinematics and mechanics of the knee
    Cruciate ligaments
    Muscles
    Importance of sagittal kinematics of the knee
    Patellofemoral joint
    Summary of kinematics and mechanics of the knee

Principles of design of meniscal bearing arthroplasty
  Femoral condyle
  Tibial plateau
  Meniscal bearing
Oxford knee
  In vitro studies
  Clinical experience
  Unicompartmental arthroplasty for osteoarthritis
  Function of meniscal bearings
Conclusions

In 1978 we published, in the *Journal of Bone and Joint Surgery* (British volume), a paper entitled "The Mechanics of the Knee and Prosthesis Design."[15] In that paper we drew attention to the fact that a prosthesis that aims to restore physiologic movement to the knee must incorporate analogs of the natural menisci. Though the logic of that assertion has not been contradicted, it has been largely ignored during the last decade of prosthesis design. Until recently, few efforts have been made to design prostheses which incorporate the meniscal principle and those that have attempted to do so have failed to realize its full implications.

It would, however, be a mistake to suppose that merely to include meniscal bearings in a prosthesis automatically confers an advantage. It is to be hoped that the too hasty acceptance of the incongruent designs introduced during the last decade will not be repeated in the 1990s in favor of a rash of meniscal bearing implants whose designs are no better founded.

We believe that many of the errors in the design of prostheses for the knee have arisen from an inadequate understanding of that joint's complicated mechanics. In this chapter the design criteria for the articular surfaces are restated and explained in terms, mainly, of the mechanics and kinematics of the joint in the sagittal plane. From these considerations it is possible to deduce the role of meniscal bearings, and not only their use but, equally important, the limitations to their usefulness. The deductions have been validated, at least in part, by our clinical experience with meniscal bearing arthroplasty in more than 600 patients since 1976.

ARTICULAR SURFACE DESIGN IN THE HUMAN KNEE

Lateral radiographs of the knee demonstrate that the articular surfaces of the tibia in the sagittal plane are virtually flat, articulating with the convex femoral condyles only at a point. This appearance is misleading. The dissimilar shapes of the articular surfaces of the two bones are made congruent by the interposed meniscus. The important function of the meniscus in transmitting compressive load from the femur to the tibia was reported from direct measurements in human and porcine joints in the laboratory by Shrive,[30]

Seedhom et al.,[29] Walker and Erkman,[33] and Shrive et al.[31]

The menisci are integral parts of the tibial articular surface, making it conform to the shape of the femoral condyle as the acetabulum conforms to the head of the femur. The details of meniscal movements are complex, but the function of the meniscus is simple in principle. Sliding movements between the femur and the concave upper surface of the meniscus allow flexion and extension; sliding movements between the flattened undersurface of the meniscus and the tibial plateau allow rotation and anteroposterior translation of the tibia. In fact, sliding movements usually occur simultaneously at both the femoromeniscal and the tibiomeniscal joints.

ARTICULAR SURFACE DESIGN IN THE ARTIFICIAL KNEE

The sagittal plane diagrams in Figure 63-1 epitomize three designs of articular surface replacement.

Congruent Joint Surfaces

Figure 63-1,A represents designs in which two spherical condyles articulate in two spherically concave cups. It also represents equally well, in kinematic terms, implants in which a cylindrical femoral component articulates in a cylindrically concave trough.

For the surfaces to conform in all positions, the femoral condyles must have a constant radius. Therefore, only spherical or cylindrical surfaces can be used. Such a prosthesis only allows flexion and extension about a fixed transverse axis, like a simple hinge; neither axial rotation nor anteroposterior translation is possible without dislocation of its surfaces.

In both designs the conforming articular surfaces make contact over large areas and therefore transmit load across the knee at low pressure. Such joints ought to wear out no quicker than do similarly congruent hip prostheses; indeed, since the areas of contact are greater, the rate of wear ought to be less than in hip arthroplasty. Such articulations are therefore mechanically sound in theory and have proved so in practice; failures have not been described from penetration of the femoral component through the polyethylene tibial plateau.

Incongruent Joint Surfaces

The design represented by the diagrams of Figure 63-1,B and C is mechanically unsound and is representative of most of the implants in current use. Such incongruent geometry results in small areas of contact, high loads per unit area, and consequently high rates of polyethylene wear.[27] The least bad of these designs are those that most nearly conform, and the worst are those which provide no more than notional point or line contact between the articular surfaces. In theory all such designs must exhibit more rapid polyethylene wear than do conforming hip replacements, a deduction which has been borne out in prac-

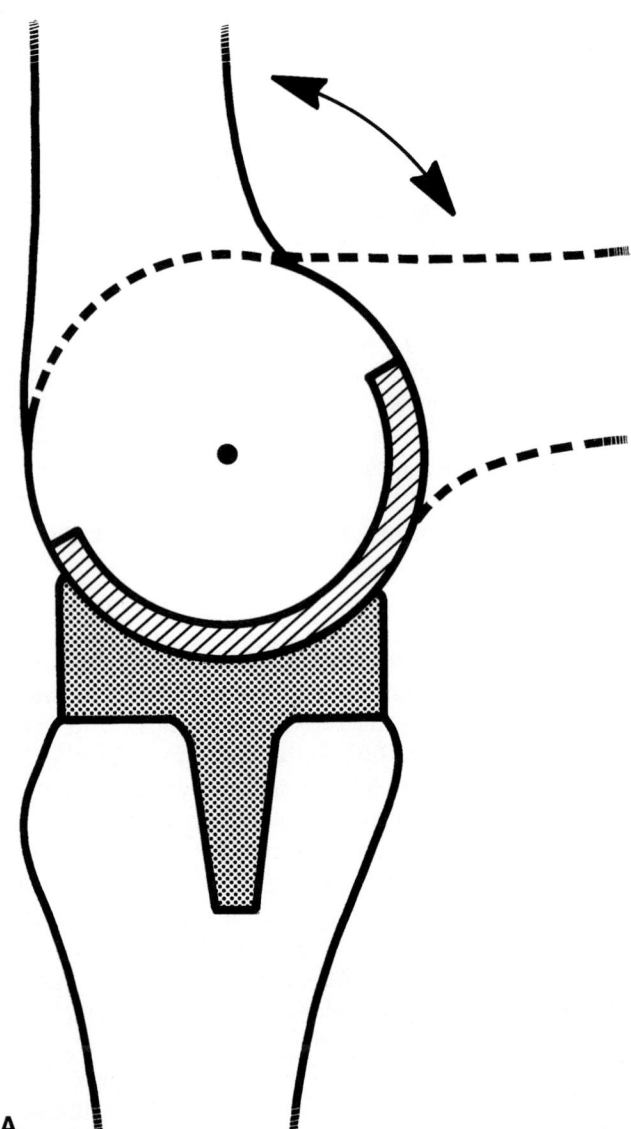

FIG 63-1.
Sagittal plane diagrams of the knee. **A,** fully congruent surfaces give large contact areas and low wear rates, but allow only fixed-axis flexion and extension, like a hinge. **B** and **C,** the surfaces are inevitably incongruent, at least in some positions, if the femoral condyles are polycentric. Such designs provide, at best, line contact and, at worst, point contact. **D,** a fully mobile congruent bearing, between a femoral condyle of constant radius and a flat tibial surface, can maintain full congruence *and* allow flexion and extension about a changing axis as in the natural knee.

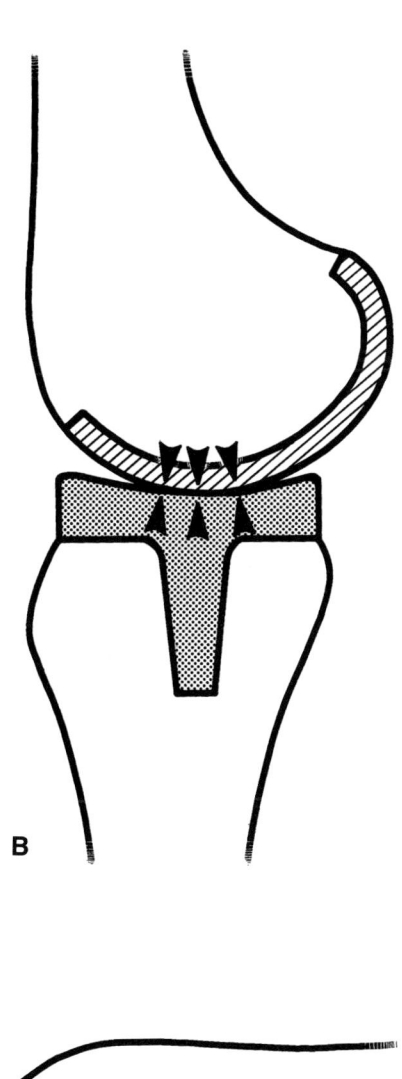

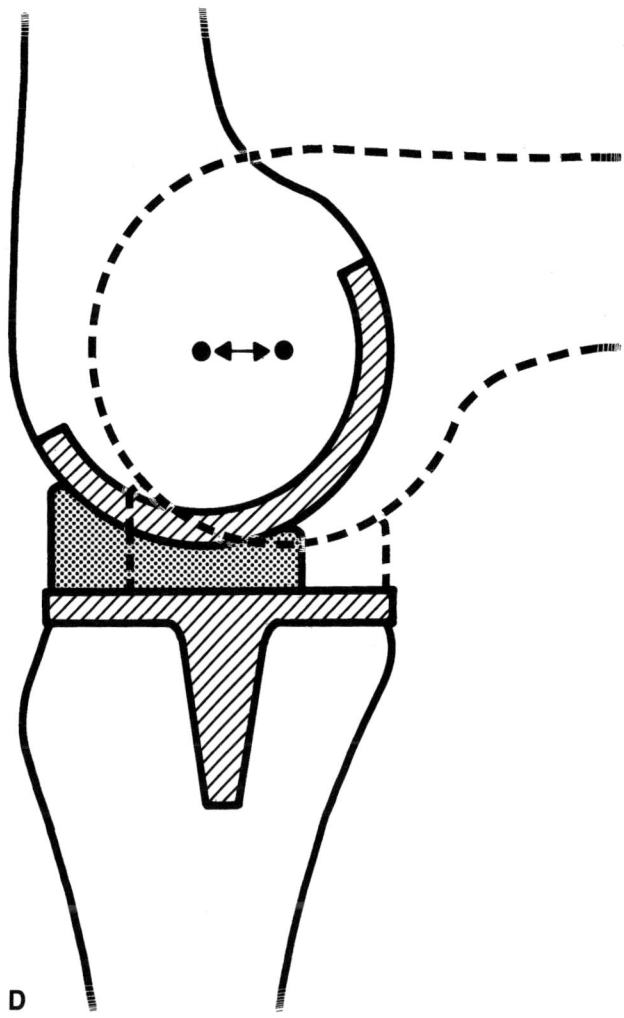

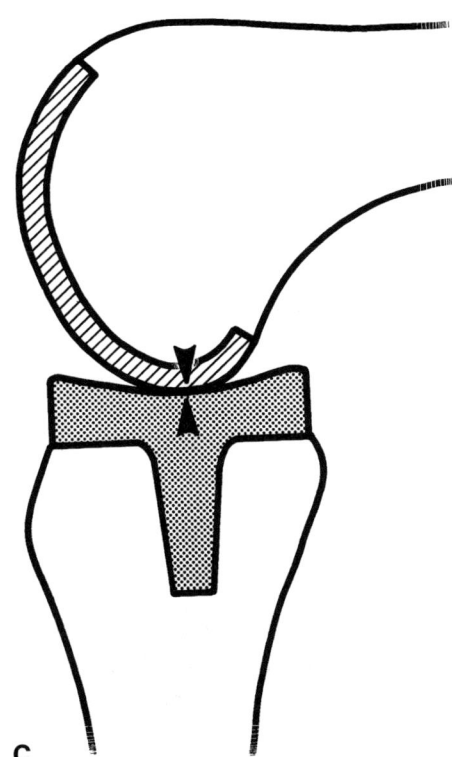

tice. Those that were the least conforming have exhibited the worst features of destructive wear.[11, 32]

Justification for Using Unconforming Designs

It is important to appreciate the arguments which persuaded some designers of knee implants to forsake the mechanically sound principle of congruent articular surfaces.

First, the lateral radiographs of the human knee may have been misinterpreted and the mechanical function of the natural menisci ignored. If nature can manage with unconforming surfaces at the knee, then why cannot an artificial joint do the same? Second, it is still widely believed that physiologic function can only be reproduced by femoral condyles with varying radii of curvature. If the condyles do not have a constant radius, they cannot fit in all positions into *any* socket of fixed dimensions, and therefore incongruence becomes inevitable, at least in some positions (see Fig 63–1,B and C).

However, the designs with extreme forms of incongruence, with completely flat tibial plateaus, were introduced with the intention of reproducing those translational and rotational movements of the femur on the tibia which distinguish the human joint from a simple hinge. Almost any degree of "dishing" of the tibial plateau greatly impedes translational or rotational movements of the femoral condyles upon it.[3] Under load, the condyles locate at the deepest point of any such dish and very large rotational or translational forces are required to persuade them to slide uphill. It follows that if such movements are to be reproduced *under load*, then the tibial plateaus must be relatively flat.

In summary, the designer faces a dilemma to which we first drew attention in 1976.[13] A mechanically satisfactory design, one which will minimize the effects of polyethylene wear, must have conforming articular surfaces, but such surfaces, under load, will allow only uniaxial flexion and extension, as in a simple hinge. Translational and rotational movements require flattened tibial plateaus which are mechanically unacceptable in theory (and have proved so in practice). There are two solutions to this dilemma.

Hinge Solution

In practice, replacement of an arthritic knee with a simplified articulation like that in Figure 63–1,A can successfully relieve the patient's symptoms and restore adequate if not normal function to the limb. The implants which have proved least susceptible to wear over the last decade have been either completely congruent or nearly so. The "nearly congruent" status of the total condylar design, coupled with its use of a thick layer of polyethylene on the tibial plateau, has allowed that prosthesis to function without serious destructive wear for periods up to 15 years.[28]

Meniscal Bearing Solution

The second mechanically sound solution, one which does not require converting the knee into a kinematic hinge, is to employ free meniscal bearings. The diagram in Figure 63–1,D shows how a meniscal bearing, free to slide on a flat tibial plateau, can allow translational movements and yet maintain congruence of all the articular surfaces throughout the range of movements.

Kinematics and Mechanics of the Knee

Cruciate Ligaments

The biomechanics of the human knee in the sagittal plane are largely determined by the anatomy of the cruciate ligaments; they are mainly responsible for locating the femoral condyles on the tibial plateau in the sagittal plane. A simple (indeed oversimplified) explanation of their function is that the posterior cruciate ligament stops the femur sliding forward on the tibia and the anterior cruciate ligament stops the femur sliding backward on the tibia. It is then evident that the position of the femur on the tibia at any time depends upon the integrity of both ligaments.

Because of their crossed form, the geometry of the linkage changes during flexion and extension so that the cruciates hold the femur toward the back of the tibial plateau in flexion and toward the front of the plateau in extension (Fig 63–2).

Muscles

The cruciate ligaments are not the only structures which apply anteroposterior forces at the tibiofemoral articulation.[23] Figure 63–2,A shows that in the extended knee the force exerted through the patellar tendon not only extends the joint but also tends to pull the tibia forward in relation to the femur, a movement which is resisted by the anterior cruciate ligament. Figure 63–2,C shows that in the flexed knee the patellar tendon exerts a backward pull on the tibia which is resisted by the posterior cruciate ligament. The cruciate ligaments act, therefore, in direct opposition to that component of the quadriceps force which is exerted in the plane of the tibial plateau. They cause the femur to roll forward on the tibia in extension when the quadriceps force tends to make it slide backward, and cause it to roll backward in flexion when the muscle force tends to make it slide forward.

Importance of Sagittal Kinematics of the Knee

Why is it important for the proper function of the human knee that the femur should move backward with respect to the tibia during flexion and forward during extension? The answer is that the lever arms of the three great muscle groups which extend and flex the knee are all measured from the instant center of the joint's movement, the axis about which flexion and extension occur. In the knee with intact cruciates, the flexion axis, when viewed from the side, lies at the point at which the cruciate ligaments cross (Fig 63–2,B). In the flexed knee, this point lies toward the back of the joint, maximizing the lever arms available to the quadriceps and the patellar tendon. In the extended knee the instant center moves forward, maximizing the lever arms available to the hamstrings and the gastrocnemius. Though the backward and forward movements of the axis of rotation are small, the lever arms employed by the major muscles are also very short so that the alterations in their lengths occasioned by small movements of the center of rota-

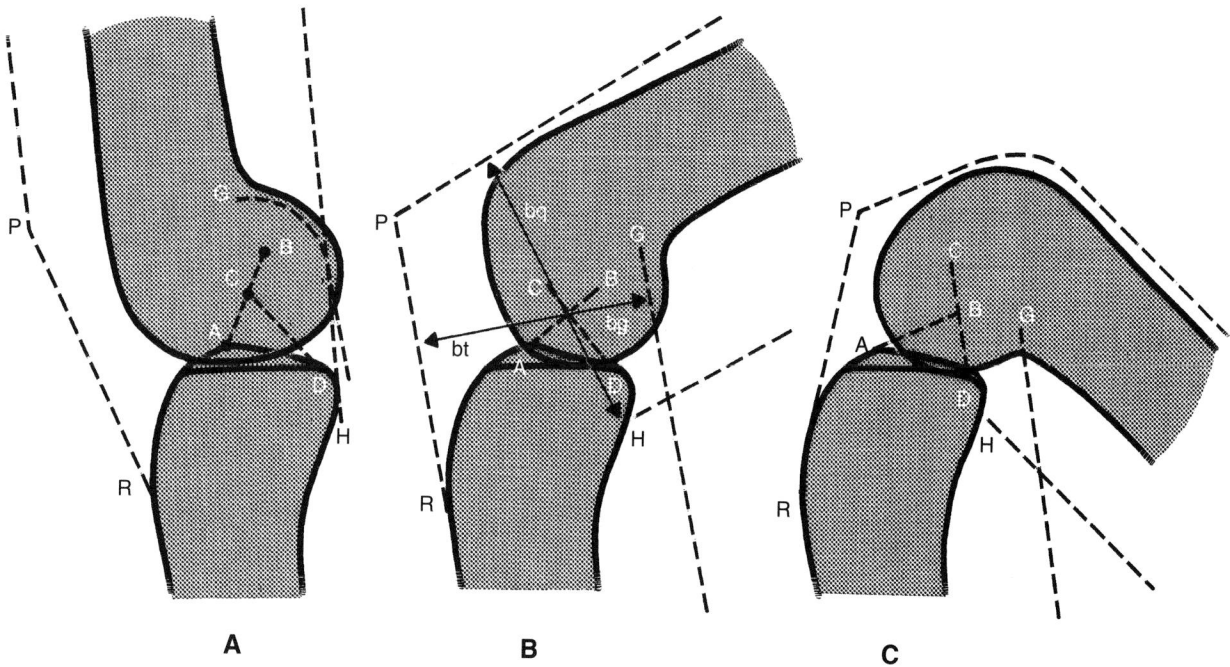

FIG 63-2.
Computer-generated line models of the knee in the sagittal plane. The model bones are joined by a four-bar linkage, AB/CD, to represent the cruciate ligaments. The instant center of the joint, the axis about which flexion-extension movements occur, is at the point at which AB crosses CD. The four-bar linkage constrains the femur to roll backward on the tibia during flexion and forward during extension. The extensor and flexor muscles are represented by *dashed lines*. Their lever arms are measured from the instant center of rotation (*bt*, for the patellar tendon; *bq*, for the quadriceps tendon; *bg* for the gastrocnemius). In **(B)**, at 70 degrees of flexion, the patellar tendon is in line with the tibial axis, but in **(A)**, at full extension, it is inclined forward, and pulls the tibia forward on the femur. In **(C)** the tendon is inclined backward, with the opposite effect.

tion have a relatively large effect on the torques generated.[24]

Patellofemoral Joint

One consequence of a misplaced flexion axis is unphysiologic loading at the patellofemoral joint. Since patellofemoral complications have proved some of the most intractable problems of modern forms of knee arthroplasty, it is worth considering this matter in some detail.

The magnitude of the patellofemoral force, as a proportion of the quadriceps force, varies inversely with the cosine of the angle between the line of action of the quadriceps tendon and the line of action of the patellar tendon. As the knee flexes, that angle diminishes and the patellofemoral force increases. The diagrams in Figure 63-3 show that, for any given angle of knee flexion, the further back the femur is upon the tibial plateau, the greater the angle between the quadriceps and patellar tendon and, therefore, the smaller the patellofemoral force. One effect, then, of the posterior translation of the tibia during flexion is to diminish the patellofemoral force as a proportion of quadriceps force. The analysis would suggest that if femoral rollback did not occur or, worse still, if the femur moved forward on the tibia during flexion, the patellofemoral force would rise above that experienced in the physiologic knee.

This theoretic prediction was tested on cadaver knees by Miller.[22] He simultaneously measured quadriceps force, patellofemoral compression force, tibiofemoral flexion angle, and the angle between the patellar tendon and the long axis of the tibia. When the cruciate ligaments were divided and an unconstrained condylar type of knee replacement was implanted, the patellofemoral forces rose in flexion to 30% above those recorded in the intact knee. This increase in force was related to the reduced angle between the patellar and quadriceps tendons which resulted from subluxation of the femur forward on the tibia during flexion.

Summary of Kinematics and Mechanics of the Knee

From the foregoing overview of the sagittal kinematics and mechanics of the knee, it is possible to draw the following conclusions:

1. The cruciate ligaments are essential for maintenance of the normal mechanics of the knee. They

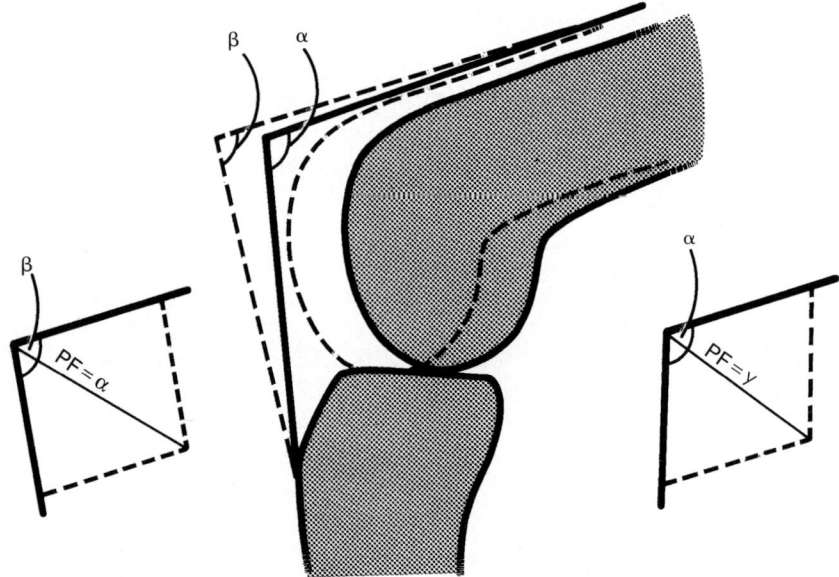

FIG 63–3.
With the knee at 70 degrees of flexion, the angle between the quadriceps and the patellar tendon is α, and the patellofemoral force (PF) is y (see parallelogram on right). If the femur is subluxated forward on the tibia, the angle diminishes to β and the patellofemoral force rises to x (see parallelogram on left).

locate the axis about which flexion and extension occur, maintaining it toward the front of the knee in extension, and toward the back of the knee in flexion.

2. In the absence of a functioning cruciate mechanism the position of the axis of flexion is determined mainly by the balance of muscle forces. When the quadriceps acts it tends to drive the femur to the front of the tibial plateau in flexion and toward the back of the plateau in extension.

3. Such paradoxical movements alter the lever arms of the muscles disadvantageously. In particular, anterior displacement of the femur in flexion increases the patellofemoral force significantly.

Principles of Design of a Meniscal Bearing Arthroplasty

Femoral Condyle

The prosthetic femoral condyles must have a constant radius if they are to be congruent in all positions. Multiradius helical surfaces can fit together exactly in only one position; in all other positions they are incongruent (see Fig 63–1,B and C).

The natural femoral condyles are usually described as having a helical form, with a radius of curvature that is larger anteriorly than posteriorly.[18] In fact, the helical form is more apparent than real. Figure 63–4 demonstrates that when the bone is viewed from the side, the helical appearance arises from the way in which the patellar facets of the femur (in the midline) are flared into its tibial facets (medially and laterally). If sections are cut through the femoral condyles proper, i.e., those parts of the articular surface which make contact with the tibia, they have a nearly spherical form.[21] In considering the complex shape of the end of the femur it is therefore better to regard it not as a continuous articular surface of constantly changing radii and centers of curvature, but instead as a construct of three surfaces, each having contours which are roughly circular when viewed from the side. This interpretation of the anatomy was described by O'Connor et al.[26] and by Elias et al.[8] and is implicit in the engraving in Figure 63–5 which is from William Cheselden's *Osteographia, or the Anatomy of the Bones* (1733).[6]

Tibial Plateau

It has already been remarked that to allow their translational movement the meniscal bearings must seat on a flattened tibial surface.

Such a tibial implant, supporting a mobile meniscal bearing, would (if friction were discounted) experience only compressive force and would therefore transmit only compressive stress to its bone-implant interface; it would be stable, without the need of an intramedullary stem. This is only true if the point of application of the compressive load lies always approximately within the central one third of the plateau. If the load is applied outside this area, then the

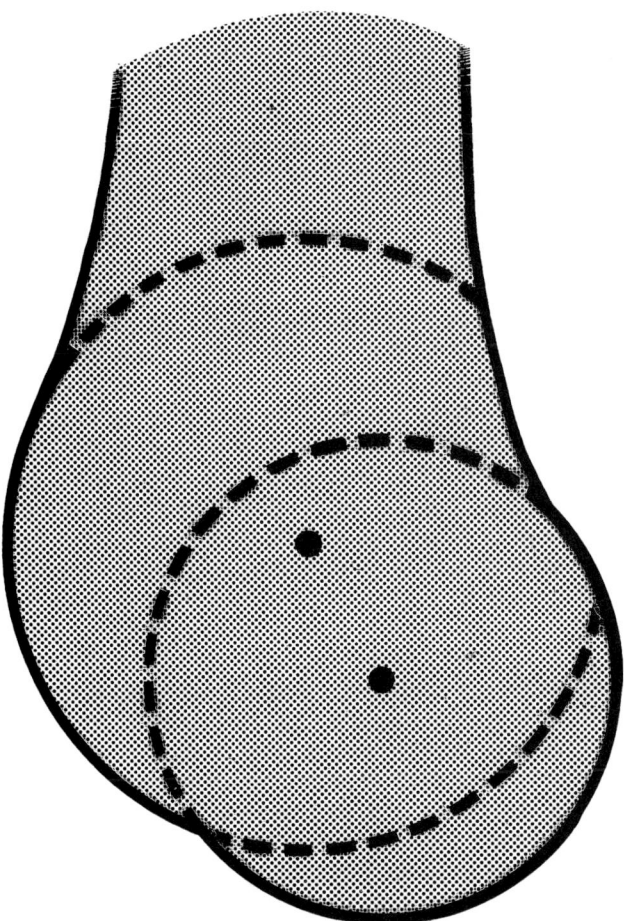

FIG 63–4.
The femoral condyles seen from the side as a construct of two circles, one representing the tibiofemoral and the other the patellofemoral surface.

tilting moment causes tension at the implant interface at the opposite end.[24] As has been described above, an intact cruciate mechanism is required to ensure that the controlled movements of the femur on the tibia do, in fact, lie near the center of the plateau.

Meniscal Bearing

If separate meniscal bearings are used in each compartment, they must be free to translate mediolaterally as well as anteroposteriorly; there are disadvantages to constraining the bearings, to moving in tracks.

Figure 63–6,A demonstrates that if the bearings move along parallel anteroposterior tracks on the tibia, the distance between their centers must increase and decrease during tibial rotation. Since the distance between the centers of the femoral condyles remains constant, congruent bearings would allow rotation only by subluxating with respect to the femur.

Figure 63–6,B shows that if the tracks are curved, in an attempt to keep the bearings equidistant during rotation, anteroposterior translation of the femur on the tibia must result in the bearings approaching or receding from one another; again, congruent bearings would have to dislocate with respect to the femur to allow these movements.

Both the above designs have been employed in practice. The inevitable subluxation of the tibiofemoral articulation in these designs is accommodated by the employment of incongruent meniscofemoral surfaces, a stratagem which diminishes the area of meniscofemoral contact and negates somewhat the advantages of employing meniscal bearings at all. If a pair of congruent bearings is used it is necessary for them to be free to slide in *all* directions on the tibial plateau.

Since the distance between their centers must remain constant, the two bearings can be joined together to function as a rotating and gliding platform. Such a platform, if it is free of constraint, is not kinematically different from two independently unconstrained menisci. However, such a bearing has the practical disadvantage that its shape may preclude the preservation of the tibial eminence and the cruciate ligaments, without which its anteroposterior movements are likely to be paradoxical. A simple rotating platform, able to turn only about a fixed axis and without anteroposterior translational freedoms, is a better compromise if the cruciate mechanism is not functioning. It could not, of course, accommodate intact cruciate ligaments. Such a bearing can allow rotation without loss of congruence, but has no kinematic advantage over rotating-hinge designs.[10]

Oxford Knee

The three components of the Oxford knee replacement are shown articulated in Figure 63–7. The sliding movements of the bearing on the flat tibial plateau are unconstrained. The rail along the straight edge of the tibial component is to protect the polyethylene bearing from abutting directly against the vertical cut surface of the tibial eminence. It limits but does not disallow mediolateral translation (see the top diagram in Fig 63–8).

Dislocation is resisted by the interpenetration of the femoral condyle into the concavity of the meniscal bearing, in which it is held by the tension in the joint's ligaments. The articular surface of the femoral condylar component is spherical and is completely congruent with the meniscal bearing in all positions.

It was remarked above that, in the sagittal plane, a cylindrical femoral condyle would function simi-

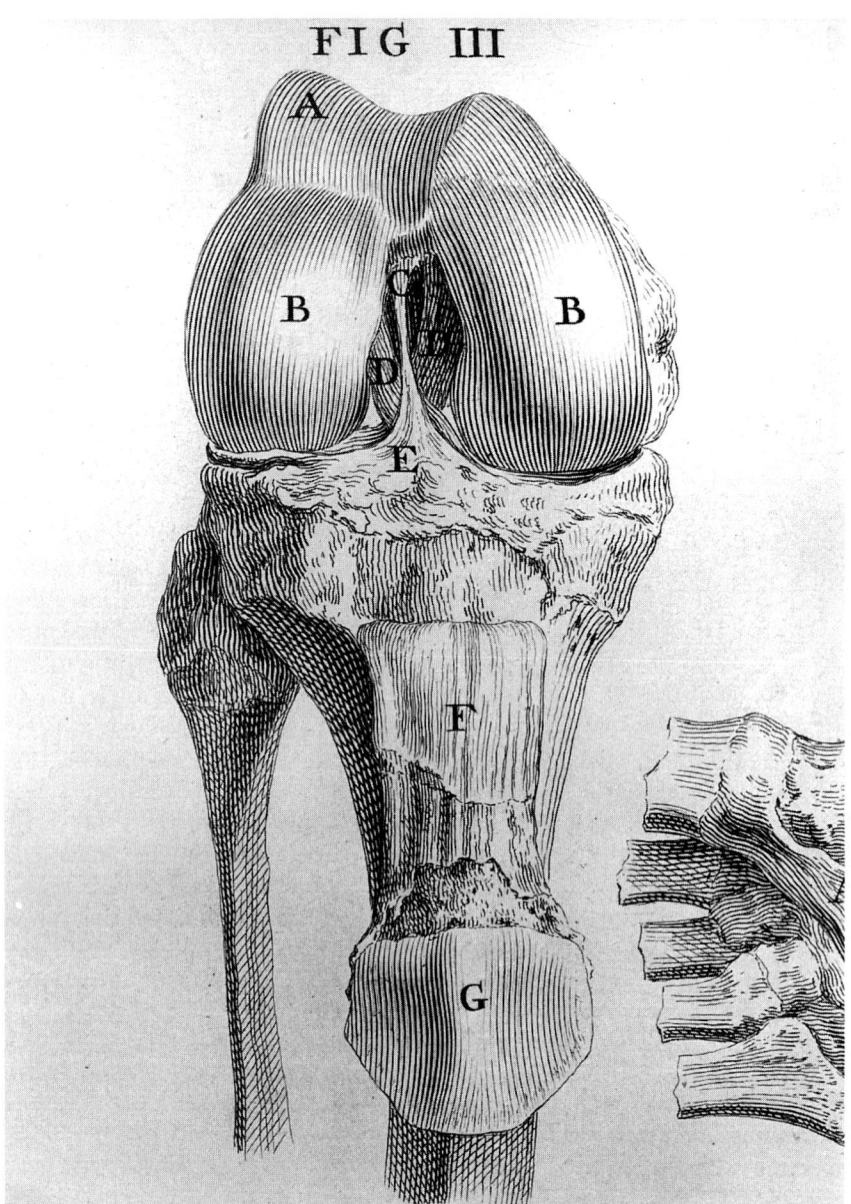

FIG 63–5.
The articular surfaces of the femur are not one continuous polycentric curve, but a construct of two nearly spherical condyles and a nearly cylindrical patellar surface. (From William Cheselden's *Osteographia, or the Anatomy of the Bones*, 1733.)

larly. The advantage of employing spherical surfaces is that they maintain congruence in the coronal plane as well. Figure 63–8 shows that a spherical condyle, unlike a cylinder, can accommodate inaccuracies of implantation and also allow the small varus and valgus angular movements which normally occur at the knee without loss of congruence.

In Vitro Studies

When such components were implanted into both compartments of cadaver knees and the intact ligaments were restored to their normal tension by the choice of an appropriate thickness of bearing, the kinematics of the knee were restored virtually to normal.[14, 15] Experiments in a laboratory rig demonstrated that the natural articular surfaces do not direct the reciprocal movements of the bones but merely allow them, and that the unconstrained components of the meniscal knee perform in the same way when directed by the ligamentous mechanism.

The most striking feature of the function of the implant was the fine control which the choice of bear-

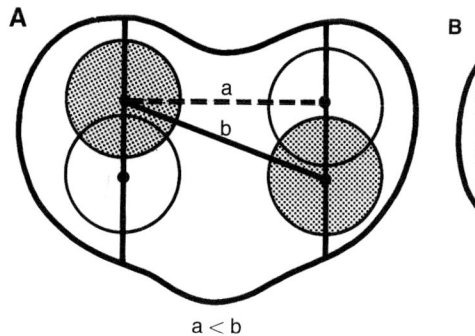

FIG 63–6.
Movements of a pair of tracked bearings during rotation and during anteroposterior translation. **A,** if the tracks are parallel the bearings must approach and recede from one another during tibial rotation ($a < b$). **B,** if the tracks are curved, the bearings must approach and recede from one another during anteroposterior translation ($a > b$).

ing thickness exerted on rotational and translational stability of the knee. An appropriate choice gave complete lateral stability throughout the range of flexion; extension was accurately limited and the joint locked in full extension, allowing no rotation in that position. The drawer test, performed with the knee flexed, demonstrated a normal range of anteroposterior glide, the bearings moving forward and backward near the center of the tibial plateau. If bearings 1 or 2 mm thinner were inserted, instability resulted, *particularly in the anteroposterior directions.*

As was expected, the prosthetic joint also became unstable in the anteroposterior plane if both cruciates were divided. However, it was also found that division of the anterior cruciate alone rendered the joint almost equally unstable. At the same time it made the meniscal bearings, which had previously been of an appropriate thickness to tension the ligaments, appear now to be too thin. If bearings 2 to 3 mm thicker were inserted, some of the original anteroposterior stability was recovered, though the joint could not be restored to normal.

These observations in the cadaver knee throw some light on the interrelation of the cruciate ligaments. When both cruciates are intact, it is they that act with the medial collateral ligament to limit distraction of the joint. Together, they define the size of the gap into which the meniscal bearing is placed. If the anterior cruciate is destroyed the bones come further apart because loss of the anterior ligament allows the tibia to subluxate forward,[7] causing the intact posterior ligament to assume a more vertical alignment (Fig 63–9).

It is, therefore, not possible to retain normal posterior cruciate function if the anterior cruciate—its essential partner—is absent. The more vertical alignment of the posterior cruciate compromises its ability to resist posterior translation of the tibia. The concept of the "posterior cruciate–retaining" prosthesis is therefore fundamentally flawed.

These observations, had they been properly interpreted, should have led us to conclude that the role of unconstrained meniscal arthroplasty would be in joints in which both cruciate ligaments were intact, and that implantation of such a device into a joint in which the anterior cruciate ligament was absent would inevitably lead to anteroposterior instability. The same limitations would apply, of course, to any design of implant which allowed unconstrained anteroposterior translation, whether or not it contained a meniscal bearing. Such instability would have all the ill effects on the biomechanics of the knee referred to above and in addition would result in the applica-

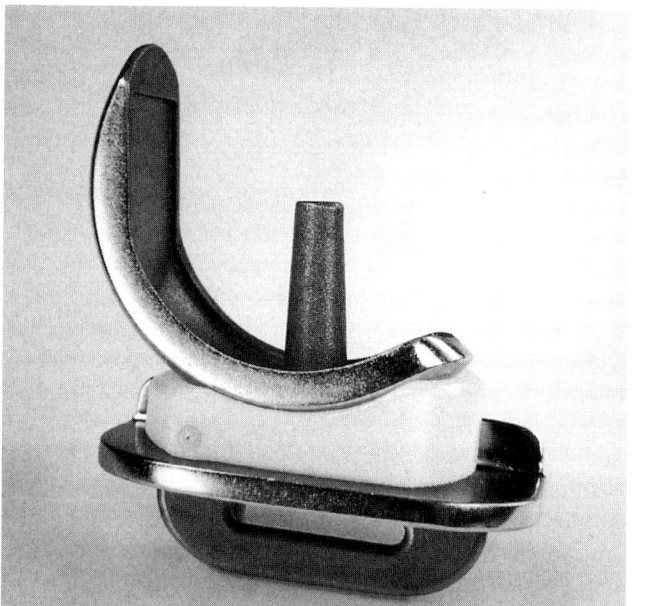

FIG 63–7.
The components of the Oxford knee (phase II) articulated.

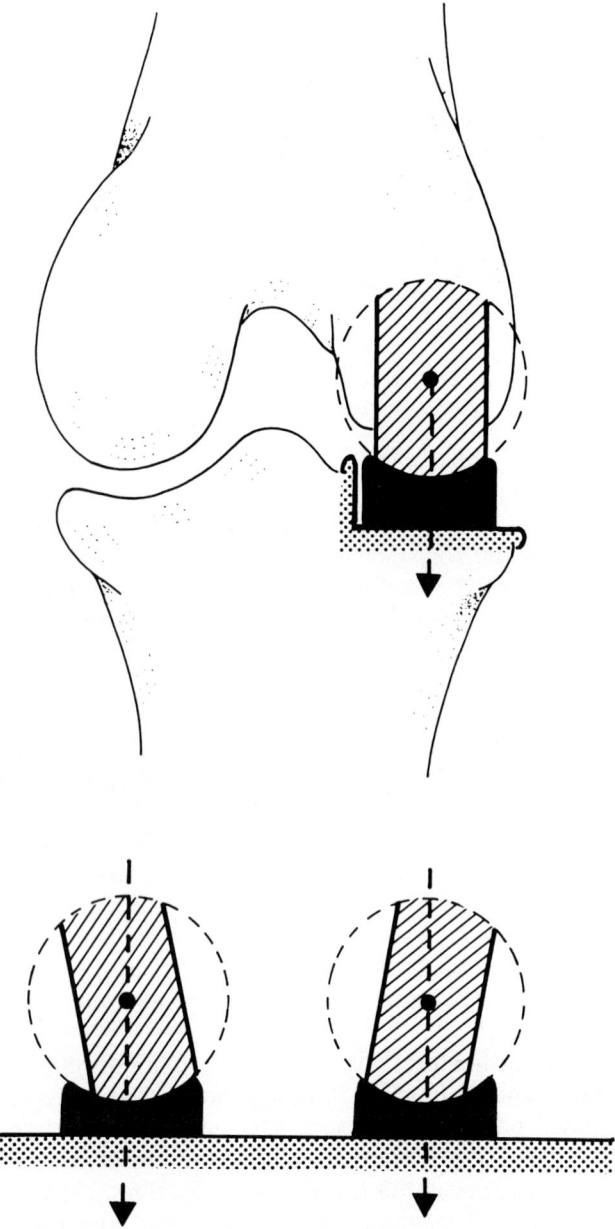

FIG 63-8.
Spherical condyles, unlike cylindrical condyles, maintain congruence in the coronal as well as in the sagittal plane, despite errors of implantation and varus-valgus angular movements of the joint.

tion of tilting loads to the tibial plateau which might cause loosening.

Clinical Experience
Between 1976 and 1985, 321 knees were operated on (by J.G.) in Oxford. For each case a data sheet was prepared that contained preoperative and intraoperative information. The patients have continued to be reviewed at annual intervals ever since at a special monthly clinic where measurements are made and radiographs taken.

In 1986 we published a detailed description of the results of 125 operations for rheumatoid arthritis and osteoarthritis, in all of which the prosthesis had been implanted bicompartmentally and without regard for the state of the anterior cruciate ligament.[14] We reported that the failure rate was 8.8% at 6 years in those with an absent or damaged anterior cruciate ligament and 4.8% in knees with a normal anterior cruciate ($P < .1$). This trend was confirmed by a later review of 301 patients[16] in which the cumulative survival rate at 6 years was 95% in knees in which the anterior cruciate ligament was normal at the time of surgery and 81% in those joints in which the anterior cruciate ligament was absent or severely damaged ($P < .05$).

In both studies the primary disease was also found to be an important determinant of outcome. In the second study, the success rate in rheumatoid arthritis was 95% at 6 years, and there had been too few failures (4.2%, or 4 out of 96 knees) to allow confident distinction between those with or without an intact anterior cruciate ligament. It was among the osteoarthritic knees, with a success rate of only 83%, that the effect of the presence or absence of the anterior cruciate was most marked. In the 102 osteoarthritic knees with an intact ligament at surgery, the success rate at 6 years was 93%; in the 70 knees in which the ligament was absent or damaged the success rate was only 73% ($P < .05$).

Others have found that the success rate of knee replacement is greater in patients with rheumatoid arthritis, perhaps because of the limited mechanical demands which these patients make on their replaced joints. Conclusions about rival designs of implant should only be drawn from the results of their use in patients with one or the other of these diseases.

Unicompartmental Arthroplasty for Osteoarthritis
In about 80% of knees with osteoarthritis the disease begins in the medial compartment of the joint. In the course of our clinical studies it began to appear that there were two stages in the development of medial arthritis of the knee. The first stage was characterized clinically by a mild varus deformity which was passively correctable to neutral, by the pathologic changes on the articular surfaces being mainly limited to the medial compartment, *and by an intact anterior cruciate ligament.* Radiologically, these cases matched those described by Ahlback[1] as grades 2 and 3.

The second phase of the disease was characterized by the development of fixed varus and flexion deformity, involvement of both compartments of the joint, *and an absent or severely disorganized anterior cru-*

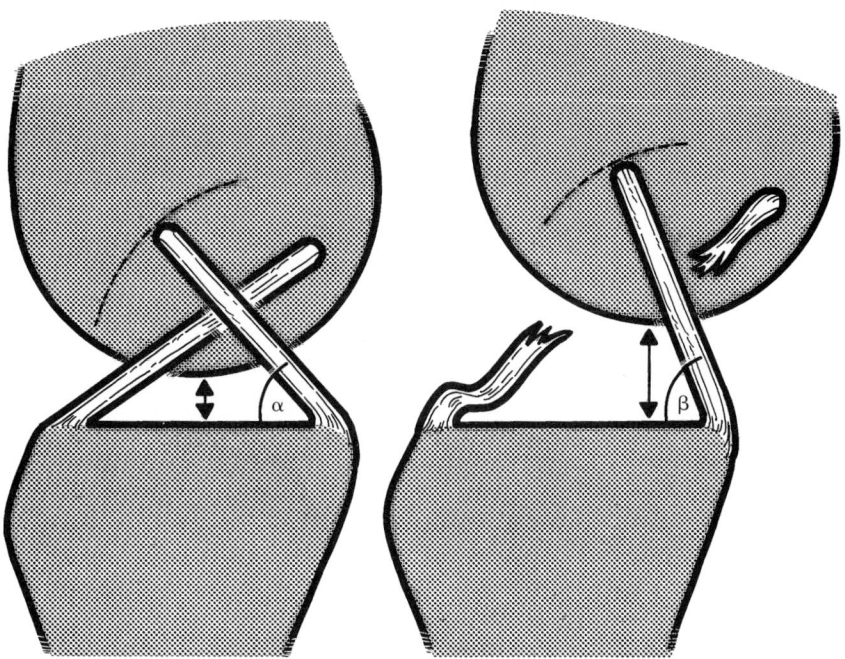

FIG 63-9.
When both cruciate ligaments are intact they limit distraction of the joint and define the size of the gap into which the meniscal bearing is placed. If the anterior cruciate ligament is ruptured the tibia can subluxate forward; the posterior cruciate then becomes more vertical ($\alpha < \beta$) and the bones can be distracted further apart.

ciate ligament. A detailed description of the pathomechanics of the first of these two stages was given by White et al.[34] It was called "anteromedial osteoarthritis" because the surface lesion on the tibia is limited not only to the medial compartment but to the anterior part of that compartment. The close correlation between the anterior site of the cartilage lesion and the presence of an intact anterior cruciate ligament makes it possible to predict the state of that ligament preoperatively from the examination of lateral radiographs, an observation which has led to a suggested modification of Ahlback's radiographic classification.[20]

These considerations combined with our clinical experience suggest, therefore, that it is mainly in the field of unicompartmental osteoarthritis that an unconstrained meniscal bearing implant should be used, since in bicompartmental disease the anterior cruciate ligament is usually damaged. Indeed, if unicompartmental arthroplasty is to be undertaken at all, it would seem essential to employ a meniscal bearing. As has been argued above, the only mechanically sound alternative is a spherical or cylindrical femoral component seated in a matching polyethylene cup or trough, an implant which has the kinematic qualities of a simple hinge. If both compartments of the joint are so replaced, such a simplified articulation has proved to be an acceptable compromise. However, if one compartment with its attendant ligamentous mechanisms is to be preserved, then the artificial components replacing the other *must* be free to follow the complex pattern of motion of its fellow.

Early Clinical Experience. We started to use the components of the Oxford knee for unicompartmental replacement in osteoarthritis in 1982, and the results of the first 103 operations were reported in 1988.[12] The failure rate in 37 knees with absent or damaged cruciate ligaments was 16.2% (6/37) at a mean of 36 months after operation and 4.8% in 63 knees (3/63) in which both cruciates were normal ($P < .02$). The review also revealed a significant difference between the results of medial and lateral unicompartmental replacement. In 63 knees with medial replacement only one bearing dislocated; laterally there were five dislocations in 27 knees. From the experience of this series we deduced strict criteria for the future selection of patients and recognized the need to improve the precision and reproducibility of the operation.

Instrumentation. Initially the method of implantation of the components had been relatively unsophisticated, as were most of the techniques for unicompartmental replacement at that time. In 1986 we redesigned the nonarticular surfaces of the femoral component to enable it to be placed with greater precision on the femur. Instruments were devised which allowed the surgeon to ensure that the flexion and extension gaps were exactly similar. This had long been recognized as a necessary requirement for maintaining ligamentous tension and alignment in total condylar replacements, but the same rigor had not been applied, before, to the location of unicompartmental components. The phase II Oxford instrumentation allows the flexion and extension gaps to be accurately matched.

The instruments also ensure that the prosthetic joint line, the level of articulation between the femur and the upper surface of the meniscal bearing, lies at the same level as it did before the arthritic process developed. This is a particularly important point in any reconstruction in which both cruciate ligaments are retained. The components of a unicompartmental prosthesis require that they be implanted with even greater accuracy than is required for tricompartmental arthroplasty because the cruciate ligaments can only function normally if the joint cleft is appropriately related to their geometry. The importance of ensuring that the gap between the bones is similar in flexion and extension is, of course, to ensure that the tension in the cruciate and medial collateral ligaments is constant throughout the range of movement.

The principles of the method of implanting the Oxford knee have been described elsewhere.[25]

Recent Results. In 1991, we reviewed 121 knees which had been treated for anteromedial osteoarthritis by medial unicompartmental replacement with the Oxford Knee.[5, 19] All the patients had fulfilled the following strict criteria: (1) the anterior cruciate ligament was intact; (2) the surfaces of the lateral compartment of the knee were covered by articular cartilage of normal thickness; (3) the varus deformity was passively correctable to neutral. The patients were followed by annual visits to a special clinic *and no patient was lost to follow-up.* One patient, with bilateral operations, died at 10 days from a pulmonary embolus. Five other patients died during the period of follow-up from causes unrelated to the operation.

During a mean period of follow-up of 44.4 months (SD 21.9; range, 12–108 months) only one patient required revision. In this case, the tibial plateau loosened 3 months after the original operation and the meniscal bearing became secondarily subluxated. The knee was successfully revised with a posterior-stabilized total condylar implant.

The cumulative success rate was 99.1% at 7 years.

Function of Meniscal Bearings

The question arises whether the meniscal bearings do perform, in fact, those functions which we have attributed to them in theory. Do they move backward and forward on the tibial plateau during rotation and during flexion and extension of the knee? Does the employment of fully congruent surfaces minimize the problem of polyethylene wear? Can the leg be realigned with reproducible precision?

Bearing Movements. Theoretic analysis of the cruciate ligament geometry suggests that the meniscal bearings ought to translate backward in flexion and forward in extension over a distance of about 12 mm.[26] We have measured the bearing movements in cadaver knees mounted in a rig to simulate weight-bearing stance and have confirmed that the movements are of a similar order.[26] Cadaver specimens also demonstrated reciprocal movements of the meniscal bearings, one forward and one backward during internal and external rotation.[15]

When the movements were measured in living patients who had undergone medial or lateral unicompartmental meniscal arthroplasty, it was found that the bearings did slide on the tibial plateau in the same directions as had been seen in the laboratory.[4] In 20 knees, radiographed in full extension and then in full flexion, all the bearings moved backward in flexion, an average distance of 4.4 mm in the medial compartment and 6.0 mm in the lateral compartment. When the tibia was internally rotated, all the medial bearings moved forward and the lateral bearings moved backward; the opposite happened during external rotation. The average bearing movement between these extremes was 6.6 mm in the medial compartment and 5.1 mm in the lateral.

As has already been remarked in the discussion of knee mechanics, the effect of the quadriceps muscles is generally opposite to that of the cruciate ligaments, tending to pull the tibia forward in extension and backward in flexion. This contrary effect, produced by muscle tone, may explain why the bearings moved during flexion and extension through a smaller range in vivo than in vitro.

In a study of another design of meniscal bearing prosthesis, the posterior cruciate–saving Low-Contact-Stress (LCS) knee system (DePuy, Warsaw, Ind.), the bearings were observed in four joints to translate, paradoxically, forward in flexion and backward in extension,[17] movements which suggest that the femur was moving under the control of the muscles rather than under the direction of an intact cruciate mechanism.

Polyethylene Wear. Wear rates for the Oxford Knee have been computed from thickness measurements of 18 bearings retrieved after periods of use in vivo which ranged from 1 to 9 years.[2] Depending on the statistical method used, the rate of penetration of the metal components into the bearings was reported as either 0.043 mm or 0.026 mm per year. These rates are much lower than the 0.19 mm/yr reported for the Charnley hip.[35] This result might be expected from the fact that the area available for the transmission of load through the unicompartmental Oxford knee (5.7 cm) is larger than that available in the Charnley hip (3.8 cm). Of importance, the rate of penetration in the Oxford Knee was not related to the thickness of the meniscal bearings. These low wear rates were achieved despite the presence of sliding movements at both the femoromeniscal and tibiomeniscal interfaces.

The measurements confirm the theoretic prediction that high-density polyethylene can be expected to function well if it is employed in a congruent articulation and that a properly designed knee replacement should last as long or longer than a hip replacement. The study showed, too, that a thin layer of polyethylene can be used if it is congruent. The thinnest bearing employed in the Oxford knee is only 3.5 mm thick at its center allowing minimal resection of the tibial bone.

Alignment of Leg. The bearings of the Oxford Knee are retained in place by the elastic recoil of the ligaments. The thickness of the bearing has therefore to be that which restores ligamentous tension approximately to normal. But the thickness of the bearing also determines the alignment of the leg. Are these two requirements incompatible? In theory they are not. If preoperative selection ensures that the operation is only performed on knees which are passively correctable to neutral, then the size of bearing needed to restore normal ligamentous tension will be the same as that required to restore normal alignment. Emerson et al.[9] have reported that in 27 consecutive Oxford unicompartmental arthroplasties performed on varus knees, the average postoperative alignment was 6 degrees of valgus (range, 0–12 degrees), with no knee left in varus. This was in contrast to the authors' experience with a nonmeniscal implant which had given a 15% incidence of undercorrection in 42 knees.

CONCLUSIONS

We have reached the following conclusions about the role of meniscal bearings in knee arthroplasty from theoretic analysis and from practical experience.

1. The implantation of freely mobile bearings into knees which lack an intact and functioning anterior cruciate ligament is theoretically mistaken, and has proved in our hands to be unsatisfactory in practice. It is irrational to build into a prosthesis the freedom to translate anteroposteriorly in the absence of a mechanism to control that freedom. The paradoxical translational movements of the femur on the tibia which would result are biomechanically even less desirable than those which result from the fixed axis of a simple hinge, and may result, among other disadvantages, in high loads at the patellofemoral joint.

2. The meniscal bearing prosthesis is the only mechanically sound design that allows physiologic movement at the knee. If the cruciates are intact, such a prosthesis is theoretically appropriate, and our experience has shown that it is effective in practice.

3. In most cases of osteoarthritis the disease remains limited to the medial compartment until the anterior cruciate ligament fails. It follows that, in osteoarthritis, the commonest indication for meniscal bearing arthroplasty is in unicompartmental replacement.

4. Medial unicompartmental replacement with a meniscal bearing prosthesis has proved more reliable than high tibial osteotomy and at least as reliable, in the medium term, as the more invasive, more expensive, and less physiologic tricompartmental type of replacement.

5. The very low wear rates reported for the Oxford knee are probably the result of the congruence of its surfaces as well as the mobility of its bearings.

REFERENCES

1. Ahlback S: Osteoarthrosis of the knee. A radiographic investigation, *Acta Radiol Suppl* (Stockh) 277:7–72, 1968.
2. Argenson J-N, O'Connor JJ: Polyethylene wear in meniscal knee replacement: A 1-9 year retrieval analysis of the Oxford Knee, *J Bone Joint Surg [Br]* 74B:228–232, 1992.
3. Bourne RB, Goodfellow JW, O'Connor JJ: A functional analysis of various knee arthroplasties, Transactions of the 27th Annual Meeting of the Orthopaedic Research Society, Las Vegas, 1981.
4. Bradley J, Goodfellow JW, O'Connor JJ: A radiographic study of bearing movement in unicompartmental Oxford knee replacements, *J Bone Joint Surg [Br]* 69B:598–601, 1987.
5. Carr A, et al: Medial unicompartmental arthroplasty with the Oxford knee, *Clin Orthop* 1993 295:205-213, 1993.
6. Cheselden W: *Osteographia, or the Anatomy of the Bones.* London, 1733.
7. Deschamps G, Lapeyre B: Rupture of the anterior cruciate ligament: A frequently unrecognised cause of failure of unicompartmental knee prostheses, *Fr J Orthop Surg* 4:323–330, 1987.

8. Elias SG, Freeman MAR, Goksan EI: A correlative study of the geometry and anatomy of the distal femur, *Clin Orthop* 260:98–103, 1990.
9. Emerson RH, Head WH, Peters PC: Soft tissue balance and alignment in medial unicompartmental knee arthroplasty, *J Bone Joint Surg [Br]* 74B:807–810, 1992.
10. Engelbrecht E, Heinert K: Experience with a surface and total knee replacement: Further development of the model St George. In Niwa S, et al, editors: *Total knee replacement,* Tokyo, 1988, Springer-Verlag, pp 257–275.
11. Engh GA, Dwyer KA, Hanes CK: Polyethylene wear of metal-backed tibial components in total and unicompartmental knee prostheses, *J Bone Joint Surg [Br]* 74:9–17, 1992.
12. Goodfellow JW, et al: The Oxford Knee for unicompartmental osteoarthritis, *J Bone Joint Surg [Br]* 70:692–701, 1988.
13. Goodfellow JW, O'Connor JJ: The mechanics of the knee and prosthesis design, *J Bone Joint Surg [Br]* 59:358-369, 1977.
14. Goodfellow JW, O'Connor J: Clinical results of the Oxford Knee, *Clin Orthop* 205:21–42, 1986
15. Goodfellow J, O'Connor J: The mechanics of the knee and prosthesis design, *J Bone Joint Surg [Br]* 60:720–726, 1978.
16. Goodfellow J, O'Connor JJ: The anterior cruciate ligament in knee arthroplasty: A risk factor with unconstrained meniscal prostheses. *Clin Orthop* 276:245–252, 1992.
17. Hodge WA, Banks SA, Riley PO: In vivo meniscal bearing motion after mobile bearing total knee replacement. *Orthop Trans* 16:367, 1992.
18. Kapandji IA: *The physiology of the joints,* vol 2, Edinburgh, 1970, Churchill Livingstone.
19. Keyes GW, et al: Oxford meniscal prosthesis for anteromedial osteoarthritis of the knee and intact ACL, *J Bone Joint Surg [Br]* 73(Suppl 2):140, 1991.
20. Keyes GW, et al: The radiographic classification of medial gonarthrosis: Correlation with operation methods in 200 knees, *Acta Orthop Scand* 63:497, 1992.
21. Kurosawa H, et al: Geometry and motion of the knee for implant and orthotic design, *J Biomech* 18:487–499, 1985.
22. Miller RK: Biomechanics of the patellofemoral joint (thesis). Oxford, University of Oxford, 1991.
23. O'Connor JJ: Can muscle co-contraction protect knee ligaments after injury or repair? *J Bone Joint Surg [Br]* 75:41–48, 1993.
24. O'Connor JJ, Goodfellow JW, Perry N: Fixation of the components of the Oxford Knee, *Orthop Clin North Am* 13:65–87, 1982.
25. O'Connor J, Goodfellow J: The role of meniscal bearing vs. fixed interface in unicondylar and bicondylar arthroplasty. In Goldberg VM, editor: *Controversies of total knee arthroplasty,* New York, 1991, Raven Press, pp 27–49.
26. O'Connor JJ, et al: The geometry of the knee in the sagittal plane. *Proc Inst Mech Eng [H]* 203:223–233, 1989.
27. Rostoker W, Galante JO: Contact pressure dependence of wear in ultra high-molecular weigh polyethylene, *J Biomed Mater Res* 13:957–964, 1979.
28. Scuderi GR, et al: Survivorship of cemented total knee replacements, *J Bone Joint Surg [Br]* 71:798–803, 1989.
29. Seedhom BB, Dowson D, Wright V: Functions of the menisci, a preliminary study. In *International Congress series, no. 324,* Amsterdam, 1974, Excerpta Medica.
30. Shrive NG: The transmission of load through animal joints (thesis), Oxford, University of Oxford, 1974.
31. Shrive NG, O'Connor JJ, Goodfellow JW: Load-bearing in the knee joint, *Clin Orthop* 131:279–287, 1978.
32. Tsao A, et al: Failure of the porous coated anatomic prosthesis in total knee arthroplasty due to severe polyethylene wear, *J Bone Joint Surg [Am]* 75:19–26, 1993.
33. Walker PS, Erkman MJ: The role of the menisci in full transmission across the knee, *Clin Orthop* 109:184–192, 1975.
34. White S, Ludkowski PF, Goodfellow JW: Anteromedial osteoarthritis of the knee, *J Bone Joint Surg [Br]* 73:582–586, 1991.
35. Wroblewski BM: Direction and rate of socket wear in Charnley low friction arthroplasty, *J Bone Joint Surg [Br]* 67:757–761, 1985.

64

Meniscal Bearing Knee Replacement: Development, Long-Term Results, and Future Technology

FREDERICK F. BUECHEL, M.D.

History and development of mobile bearings
Surface geometry
Contact stress analysis of mobile bearings and fixed bearings
Wear properties of mobile bearings and fixed bearings
Failure modes of rotating bearing patella replacements
Fixation of mobile meniscal bearings
Clinical application of mobile meniscal bearings
   Unicompartmental knee replacement
   Bicompartmental knee replacement
   Tricompartmental knee replacement

Bicruciate-retaining meniscal bearing total knee replacement
Posterior cruciate ligament–retaining meniscal bearing
Cruciate-sacrificing rotating platform
Isolated patellofemoral replacement
Revision total knee replacement
   Septic revision using mobile bearings
Survivorship analysis of cemented and cementless meniscal bearing knee replacements
Future directions

HISTORY AND DEVELOPMENT OF MOBILE BEARINGS

Artificial human joint replacements have been developed with specific bioengineering requirements to provide normal kinematics, maintain fixation, and minimize wear. A mechanical solution to the bearing overload problem which causes wear has been to use more congruent meniscal bearing surfaces[19, 38, 43, 63] to lower the contact stresses below 10 MPa,[41] which is reported as the maximum permissible compressive stress limit of ultrahigh-molecular-weight (UHMW) polyethylene. Lowering contact stresses to within the reported medical load limit of 5 MPa[27] while allowing kinematically acceptable motion provides a meniscal bearing surface that is resistant to fatigue wear and demonstrates normal abrasive wear behavior over a 10-year period as seen in both simulator and retrieval studies[20, 21, 33, 38, 53] (Figs 64–1 and 64–2).

The first mobile bearing application was seen in shoulder replacement in which two eccentrically placed spherical elements improved the range of motion over simple ball-and-socket systems. These "floating-socket"[25] bearings were developed in 1974 and used clinically from 1975 to 1979, when less constrained shoulder implants were developed.[24] Later, knee[21] and ankle[12] bearings were developed using similar concepts.

The first complete systems approach to total knee replacement using meniscal bearings was developed in 1977 and reported in 1986.[19] Unicompartmental, bicompartmental, and tricompartmental disease were managed with a variety of primary and revision components that allowed retention of both cruciates, the posterior cruciate ligament (PCL) only, or no cruciate ligaments. Additionally, the first metal-backed, rotating-bearing patella replacement was developed in 1977 to provide mobility with congruence in patellofemoral articulation. This New Jersey Low-Contact-Stress (LCS) total knee system (DePuy, Warsaw, Ind.), initially used with cement in 1977, was expanded to noncemented use in 1981 with the availability of sintered-bead porous coating[59] and remains the only knee system in the United States to have undergone formal Food and Drug Administration (FDA)–Investigational Device Exemption (IDE) clinical trials in both cemented and cementless applications before being released for general clinical use[18, 28, 29, 31] (Fig 64–3).

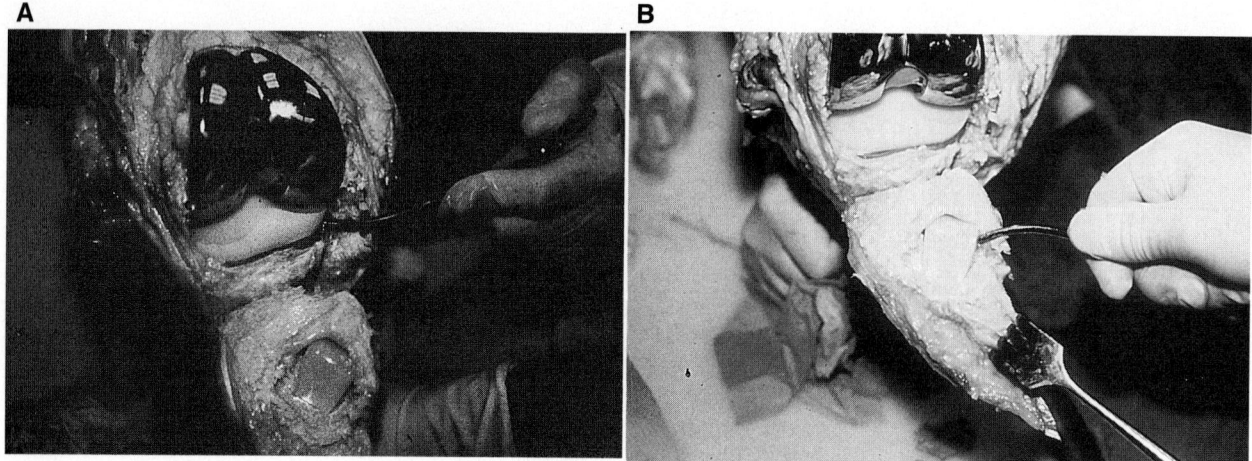

FIG 64–1.
A, Ten-year postmortem retrieval of an asymptomatic rotating platform prosthesis demonstrating continued rotation of the tibial bearing. **B,** the same retrieval specimen demonstrating continued axial rotation of the rotating patella bearing.

SURFACE GEOMETRY

Surface congruence is essential to improve wear life in UHMW polyethylene bearings, especially in major repetitive load-bearing activities, such as walking, which generates loads of 2.5 times body weight, and stair-climbing, which can generate loads of 8 times body weight. Aside from direct compressive loading, however, the tibiofemoral bearings must be able to accommodate flexion of 155 degrees, varus-valgus movements of 10 degrees, axial rotation of 30 degrees, and anteroposterior (AP) translation of 15 mm when the cruciate ligaments are retained. The patellofemoral articulation is also loaded mainly in compression and needs to accommodate similar flexion to 155 degrees, axial rotation of 6 degrees, and the ability to tilt laterally and medially in the femoral groove without dislocating or rubbing on an edge.

These kinematic tibiofemoral motion requirements dictate the use of spherical upper tibial bearing surfaces and a flat undersurface to accommodate the variety of movements in the most congruent way. The Oxford meniscal knee[38] uses matching spherical surfaces for the femoral component and the upper meniscal bearing surface and a flat surface to match a flat tibial component. This preferred geometry appears to work well as a medial unicompartmental replacement,[32] but has evinced dislocation problems in other applications.[39] These were most likely caused by a larger-than-normal single radius of curvature of the femoral component, which under the pull of the PCL in flexion moves the bearing too far posteriorly (Fig 64–4).

A design solution to the Oxford problem in the presence of cruciate ligaments is seen in the LCS[21] femoral component which uses the same spherical surface of revolution in the mediolateral plane, but decreases the radius of curvature from extension to flexion, thus maintaining full area contact on the upper meniscal bearing surface from 0 to 45 degrees at which walking loads are encountered, and maintaining at least spherical line contact at deeper flexion angles (Fig 64–5). This surface geometry allows a more central femoral component position in flexion by reducing the PCL tension, which tends to pull the femur posteriorly when overstretched (Fig 64–6). Another design solution to prevent meniscal bearing dislocation is the use of radial tracks on the LCS tibial components. These tracks allow axial rotation and controlled AP translation, which impedes direct dislocation by means of the cruciate bone bridge poste-

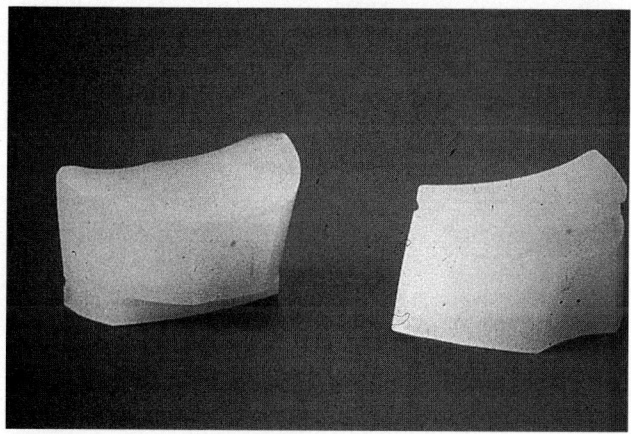

FIG 64–2.
Meniscal bearing simulator specimen after 10 million cycles under loads of 2,200 Ns.

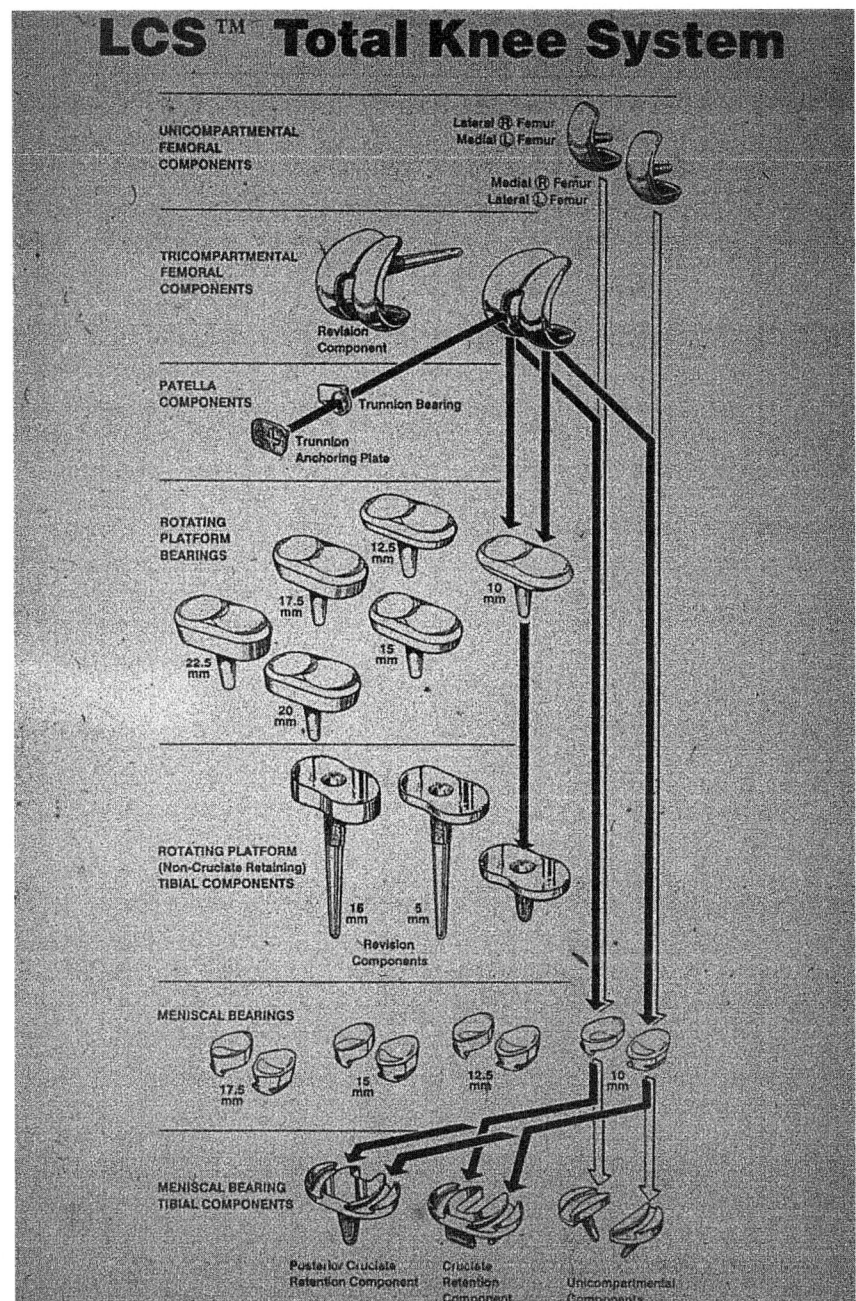

FIG 64–3.
New Jersey LCS knee replacement system components.

riorly and the patellar tendon anteriorly (Fig 64–7). When combined with stable flexion and extension gaps at surgery, the LCS meniscal bearings can be used safely when both cruciate ligaments are intact or if only the PCL is intact.

In the event of a nonfunctional or absent PCL, central stability with the ability to axially rotate is essential. The long-term survivorship studies of Scuderi et al.[64] and Ranawat et al.[60] have demonstrated that a centrally stabilized total condylar knee replacement can last for 15 years in over 90% of cases when used in elderly patients with low loading demands. These important studies prove that cruciate function is not essential for successful long-term fixation and function in low-demand situations.

Since wear increases as loads and demands increase, it seems most appropriate to utilize the proven fixation and central stabilizing concepts of the

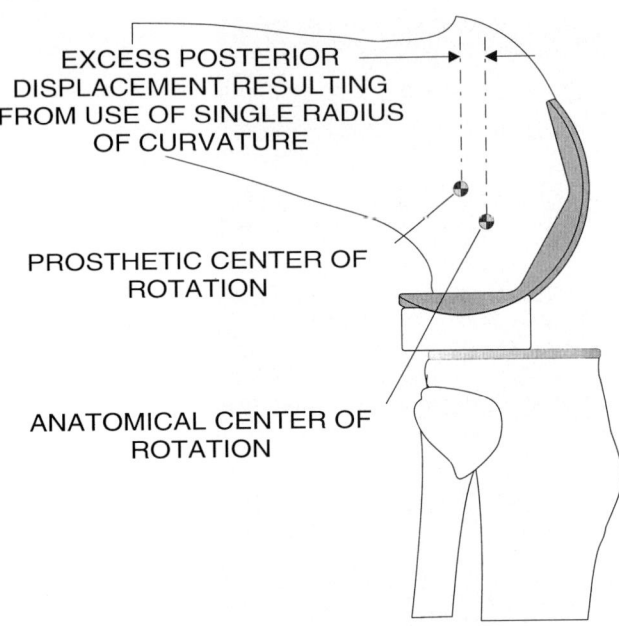

FIG 64–4.
Excessive posterior bearing displacement due to use of a single radius of curvature of the femoral component.

total condylar device and provide a more wear-resistant and dislocation-resistant bearing surface to achieve better long-term survivorship and reduce wear-related failures. This concept led to the development of a rotating platform total knee device which employs the same spherical surface geometry as the meniscal bearings, centrally stabilized by a UHMW polyethylene trunnion cone (Fig 64–8).

The patellofemoral design process, like the tibiofemoral design process, seeks to provide proper motion and maintain contact stresses below 5 MPa during walking, stair-climbing, and deep-knee-bending. Button or nonrotating anatomic-type patellar replacements suffer from either high point or line contact stresses or from overconstraint. High contact stress will cause early wear failure,[61] while overconstraint will cause early loosening failure.[4] For these reasons a rotating-bearing patellar replacement was developed to maintain spherical area contact on the medial and lateral facets while congruent with the surface of revolution of the deep-sulcus femoral groove (Fig 64–9). The rotating-bearing patella replacement of the LCS design improves greatly upon the contact stress seen in other configurations (Fig 64–10,A and B).

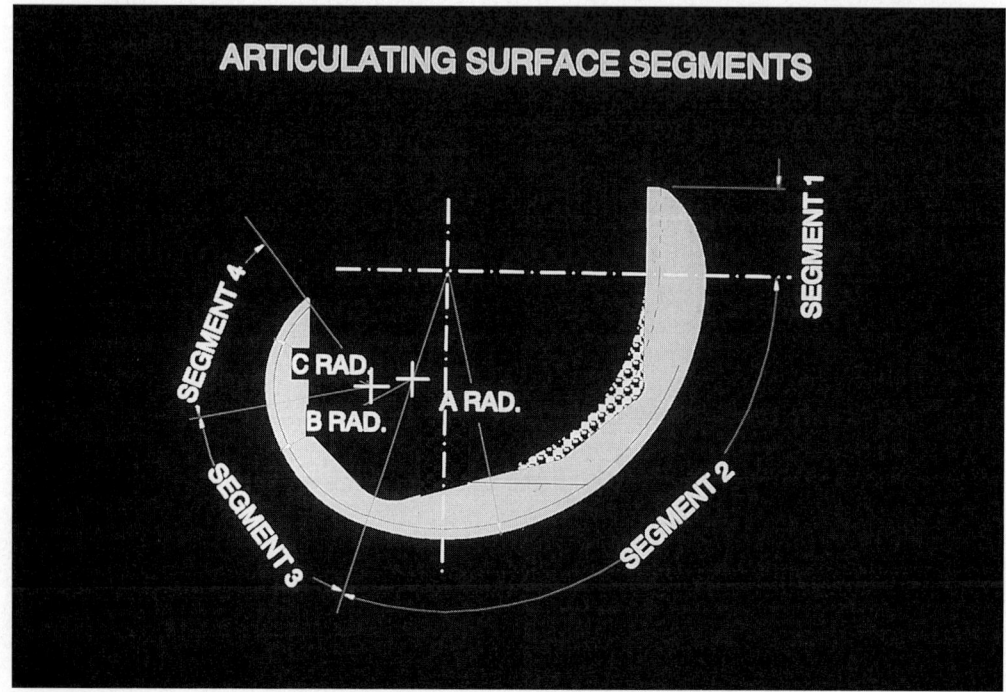

FIG 64–5.
Lateral surface geometry of the New Jersey femoral component: *S1* represents the patellofemoral bearing surface in full extension; *S2* is the primary load-bearing surface of the femoral component for both patellar and tibial articulation; *S3* and *S4* are the posterior bearing surfaces used during full flexion.

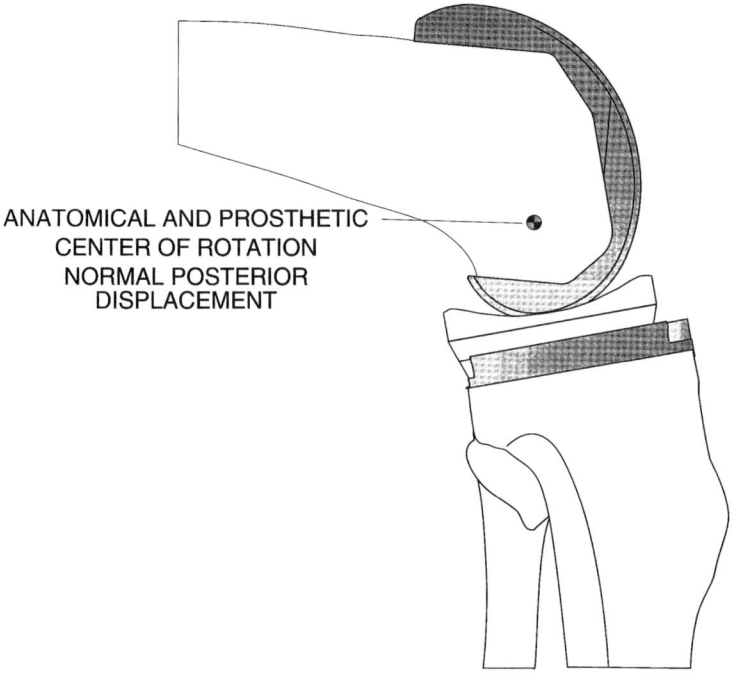

FIG 64–6.
Decreasing radius of curvature of the femoral component maintains central positioning of meniscal bearings.

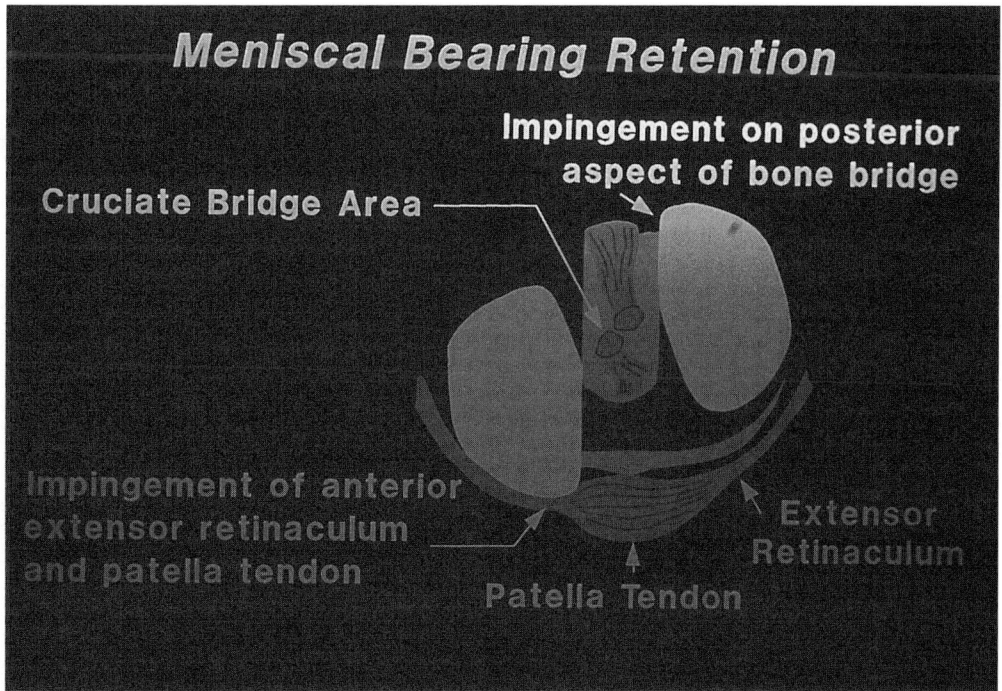

FIG 64–7.
Effective use of radial tracks to allow controlled axial rotation, controlled AP translation, and impede direct dislocation of meniscal bearings.

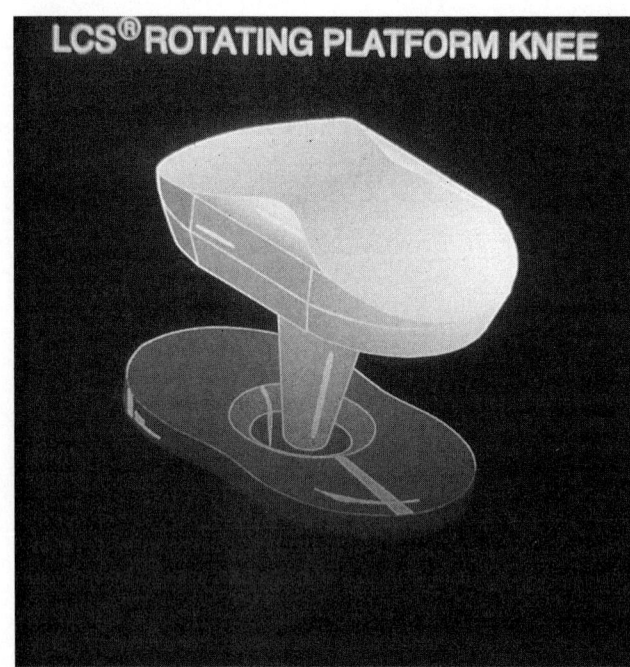

FIG 64–8.
New Jersey LCS Rotating Platform Tibial Component.

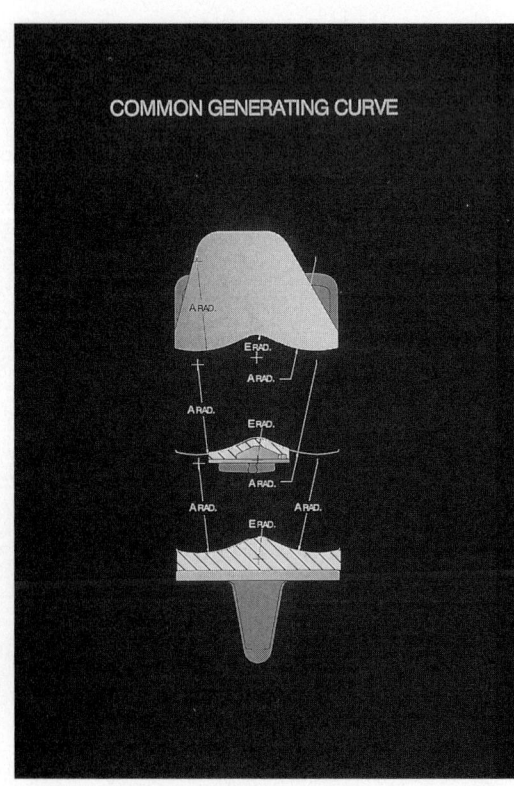

FIG 64–9.
Common generating curve. The same curve is used to form the tibial and patellar articulating surfaces ensuring that at least line contact will be maintained for all motion phases.

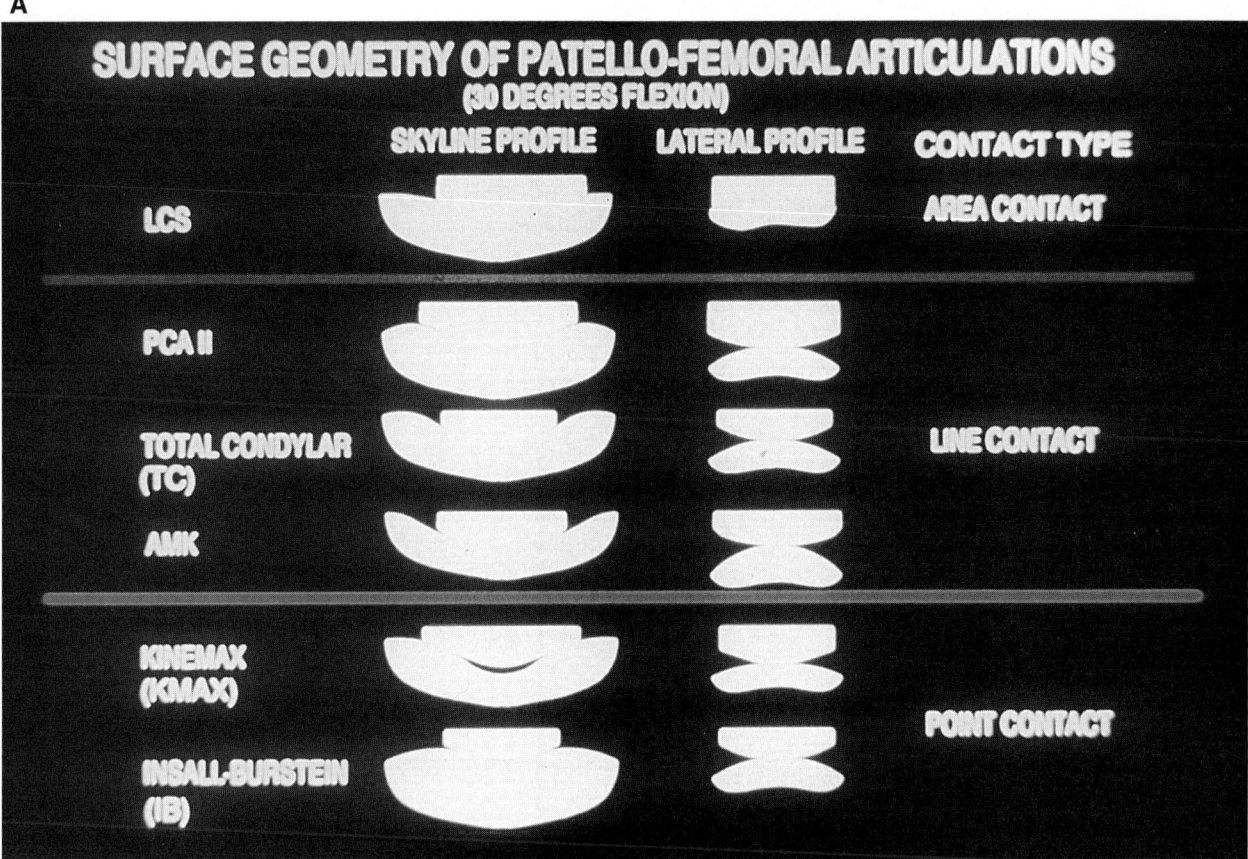

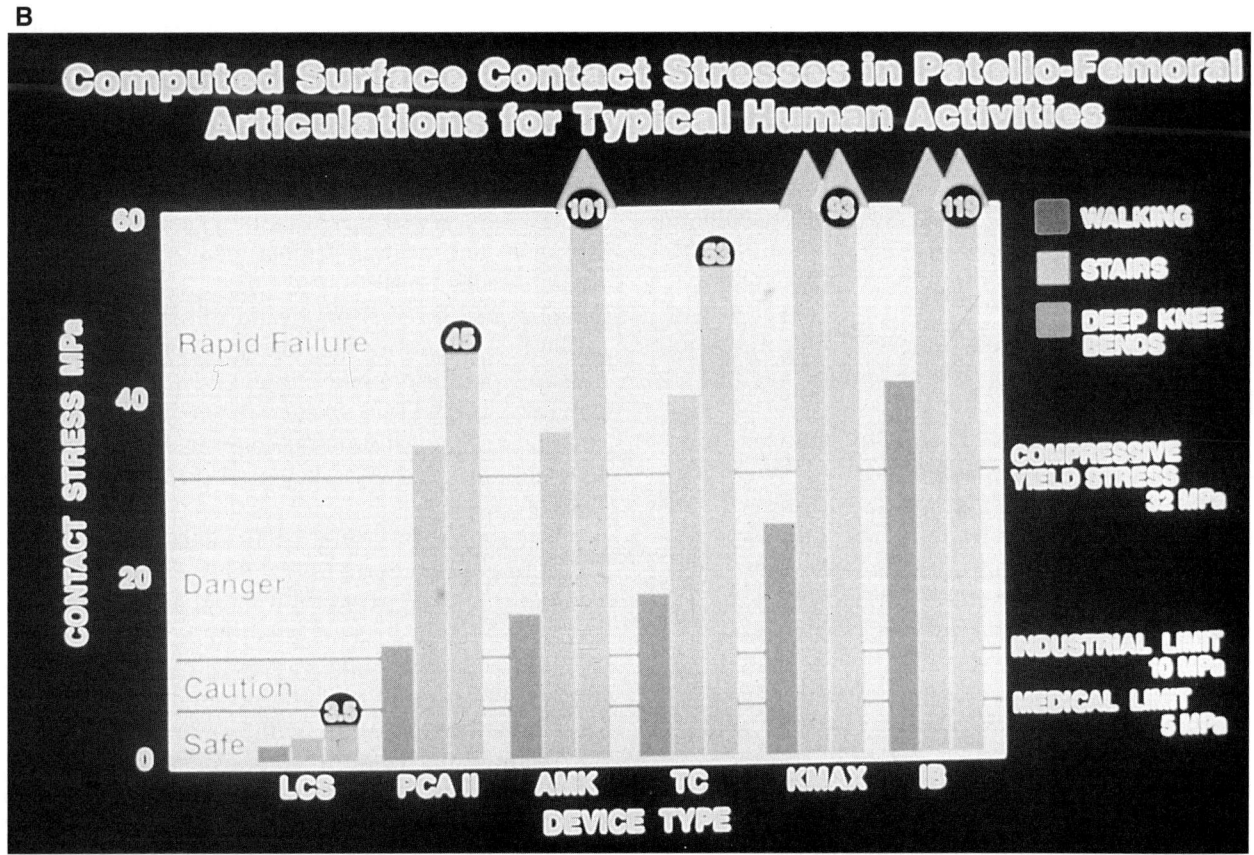

FIG 64–10.
A, surface geometry of various patellofemoral articulation types. **B,** computed contact stresses in patellofemoral articulations for typical human activities.

CONTACT STRESS ANALYSIS OF MOBILE BEARINGS AND FIXED BEARINGS

The industrial contact stress limit for UHMW polyethylene is given as 10 MPa by Hoechst,[41] a major manufacturer of this material. This load limit defines the maximum stress that gear teeth made of UHMW polyethylene can endure under cyclic loading in a machine. Pappas and colleagues[27, 55] defined 5 MPa as the medical load limit for UHMW polyethylene for use in repetitively loaded bearings for human joint replacements. Pappas and co-workers believed that a safety factor of 50% for human use was a prudent value to assure increased longevity of such bearings. The repetitive walking loads on these bearings should be under 5 MPa, while less repetitive activities such as stair-climbing or deep-knee-bending may allow increased loads for shorter durations without major concerns for wear failure. In no case, however, should peak bearing loads exceed 32 MPa, as this represents the compressive yield stress of UHMW polyethylene, above which rapid wear can be expected. It can been seen from contact stress analysis that certain tibiofemoral and patellofemoral geometries greatly exceed these load limits,[2, 26, 27, 34, 67] and as such are destined for earlier wear-related failure than more congruent meniscal bearing designs (see Figs 64–10 and 64–11, A and B).

WEAR PROPERTIES OF MOBILE BEARINGS AND FIXED BEARINGS

Retrieval analysis of the tibiofemoral and patellofemoral bearing surfaces have demonstrated a high clinical wear rate of nonconforming fixed-bearing knee replacements.[34, 35, 37, 48, 58] Similar retrieval analysis of meniscal bearings, rotating platform bearings, and rotating patellar bearings demonstrated significantly less wear than fixed bearings.[18]

Although, mobile bearings allow reduced contact stress, they can be overloaded to failure by excessive weight, activity, malalignment, or a combination of these factors. The overall failure rate of the bicruciate-retaining meniscal bearing total knee replacement (TKR) as a result of fracture, dislocation, or bearing wear-through has been 2 out of 95 TKRs, or 2.1%, in my series of primary and multiply-operated (mo) TKRs followed for 2 to 15 years (mean, 8.5 years).

The overall failure rate of the PCL-retaining meniscal bearing TKR as a result of fracture, dislocation, or bearing wear-through has been 2 out of 178 TKRs, or 1.1%, in my series of primary and mo TKRs followed for 2 to 8 years (mean, 5 years).

The overall failure rate of rotating platform TKRs due to bearing dislocation has been 1 out of 294 TKRs, or 0.3%, in my series of primary and mo TKRs followed for 2 to 14 years (mean, 8 years). No rotating platform bearing wore through or fractured in this series.

FAILURE MODES OF ROTATING BEARING PATELLA REPLACEMENTS

Failures of the rotating-bearing patella have been rare[30, 47] and usually associated with displaced patellar fractures, malposition, subluxation, or excessive, repetitive hyperflexion loads.

The overall complications of rotating bearing patellar replacements that required revision surgery in 515 knees originally followed for 6 months to 11 years[30] and now followed for 4 to 15 years (mean, 8 years) was 3 in 515 (0.6%). Long-term rotating patella replacement retrievals have demonstrated continued mobility and minimal wear (Fig 64–12.)

FIXATION OF MOBILE MENISCAL BEARINGS

Methyl methacrylate bone cement was the initial adjunctive method of bony attachment in the first unicompartmental meniscal bearing used in 1977,[13] and in subsequent bicompartmental and tricompartmental devices.

The tibial fixation surface of the LCS unicompartmental knee replacement employs a flat, tibial loading plate and a short-angled stem to resist tipping and shear loads. Bicruciate-retaining LCS tibial components use three short fixation fins for anchorage, while PCL-retaining LCS meniscal bearing and LCS rotating platform tibial components utilize a short, conical metaphyseal fixation stem centered in the proximal tibia. All femoral components utilize shallow cement locking pockets and centralized femoral fixation pegs.

The rotating-bearing patella replacement (Fig 64–13) utilizes a cruciform fin geometry for fixation. This geometry reinforces the thin metal plate against torsional failure and reinforces the patellar remnant against fractures while engaging the patellar bone stock sufficiently to prevent loosening.

Cementless fixation with sintered-bead cobalt-chromium-molybdenum porous coating on the Co-Cr-Mo substrate (Porocoat, DePuy, Warsaw, Ind.) using the same articulating and fixation geometries of the LCS knee system was first used clinically in 1981.

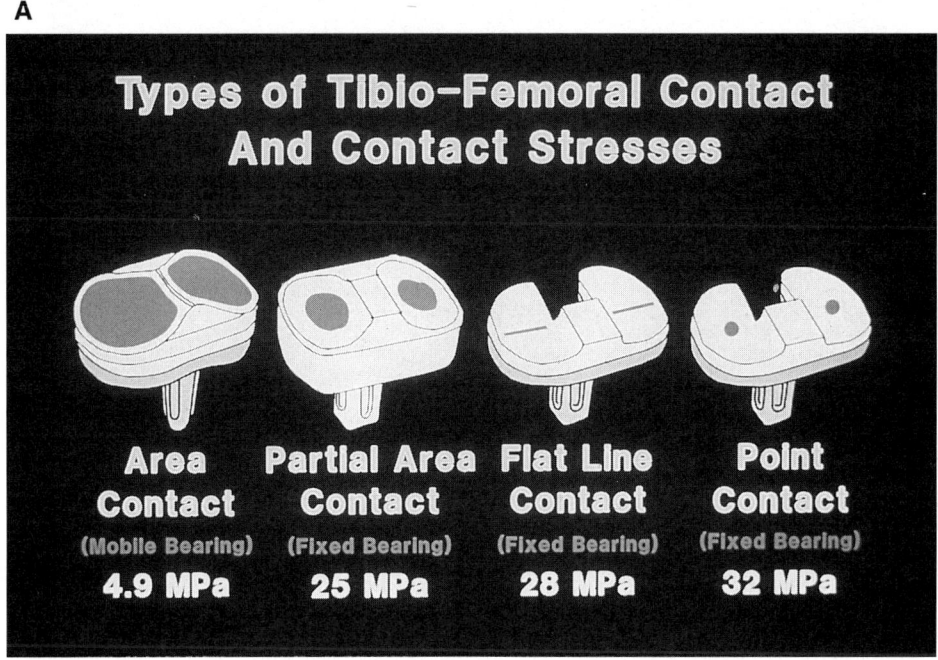

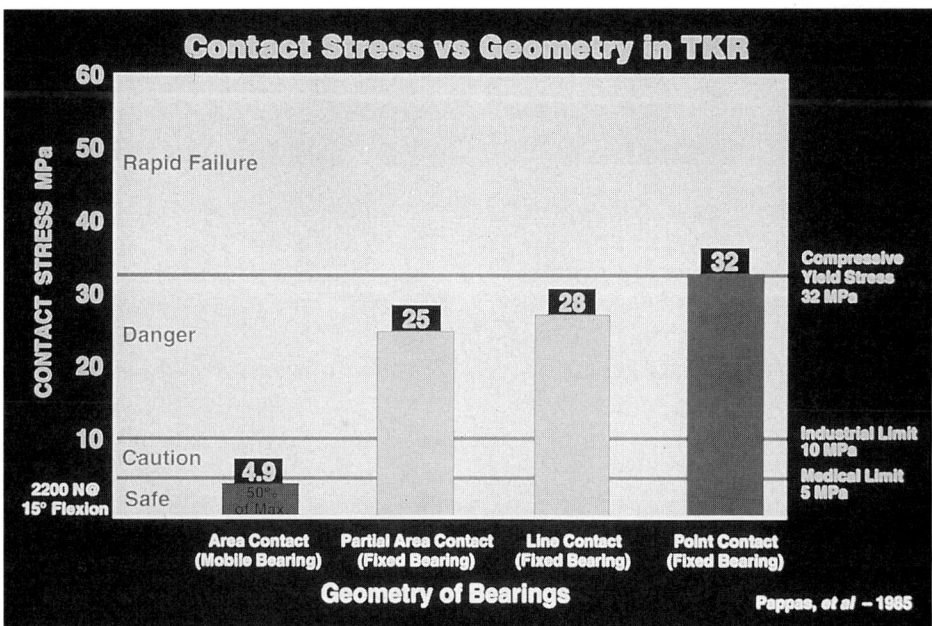

FIG 64-11.
A, surface geometry and contact stress of various tibiofemoral articulation types during walking. **B,** computed contact stress in tibiofemoral articulations during walking.

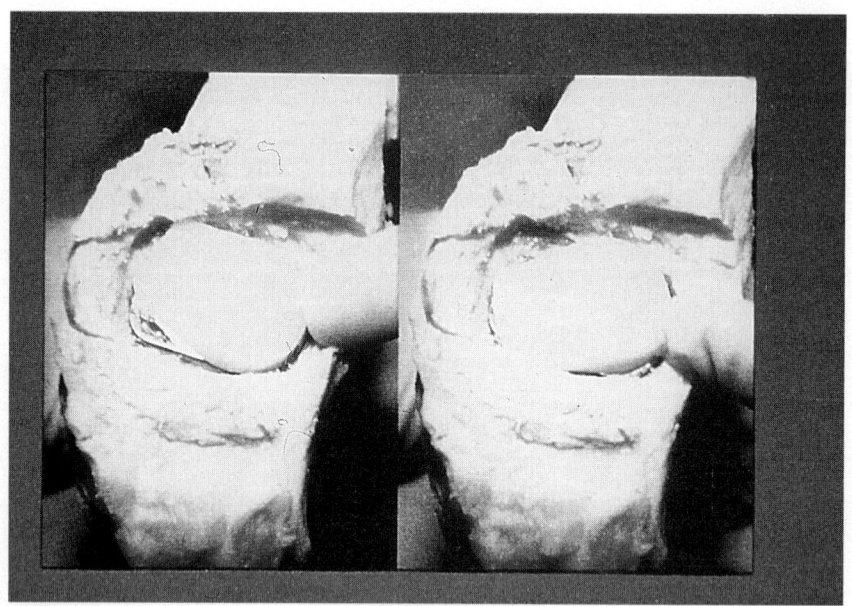

FIG 64–12.
Ten-year postmortem retrieval of an asymptomatic rotating-bearing patella replacement demonstrating continued rotational ability and minimal abrasive wear.

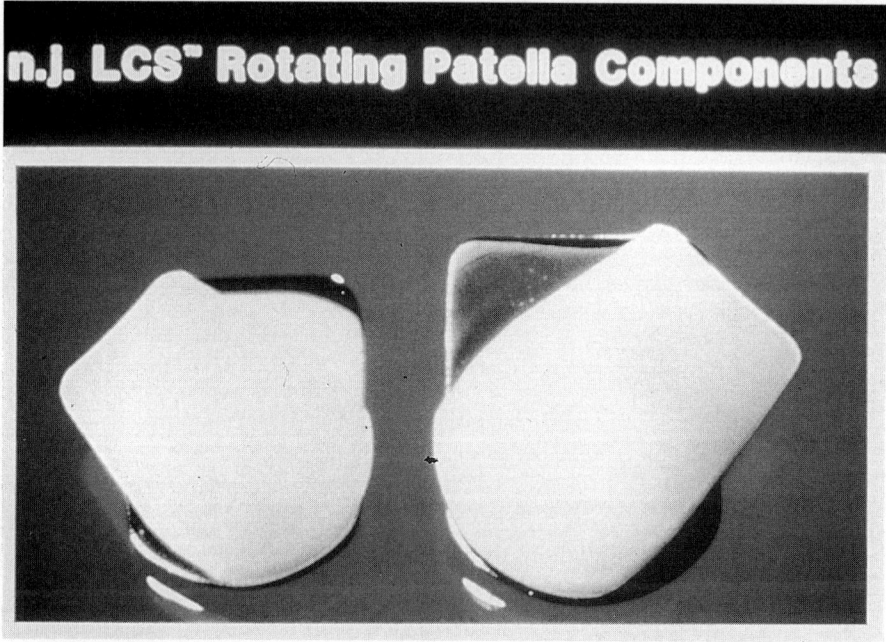

FIG 64–13.
Rotating-bearing patella components demonstrating limits of axial rotation.

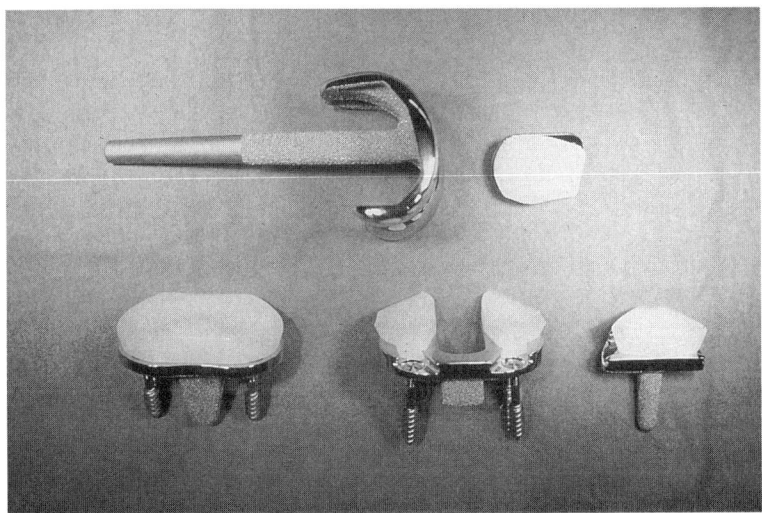

FIG 64–14.
Porous-coated LCS tibial components with fixation screws—1981.

Bicruciate-retaining and rotating platform tibial components were developed with four screw holes and spherical seats. These implants used 6.5-mm cancellous bone screws to augment fixation (Fig 64–14).

Our concerns over fretting, screw breakage, osteolysis, and potential neurovascular injuries from screw penetration led us away from screw fixation later in the same year. These early concerns have since been documented by several authors.[34, 58, 62]

Press-fit, non-screw-fixed LCS knee replacements with porous coating have been in clinical use since late 1981 (Fig 64–15).

Ten-year survivorship studies have demonstrated a 96.5% overall survivorship using non-screw-fixed, press-fit, porous-coated, cementless fixation, justifying its continued use.[13–16] The cementless fixation success of the LCS mobile bearing knee replacement has improved upon a similar group of ce-

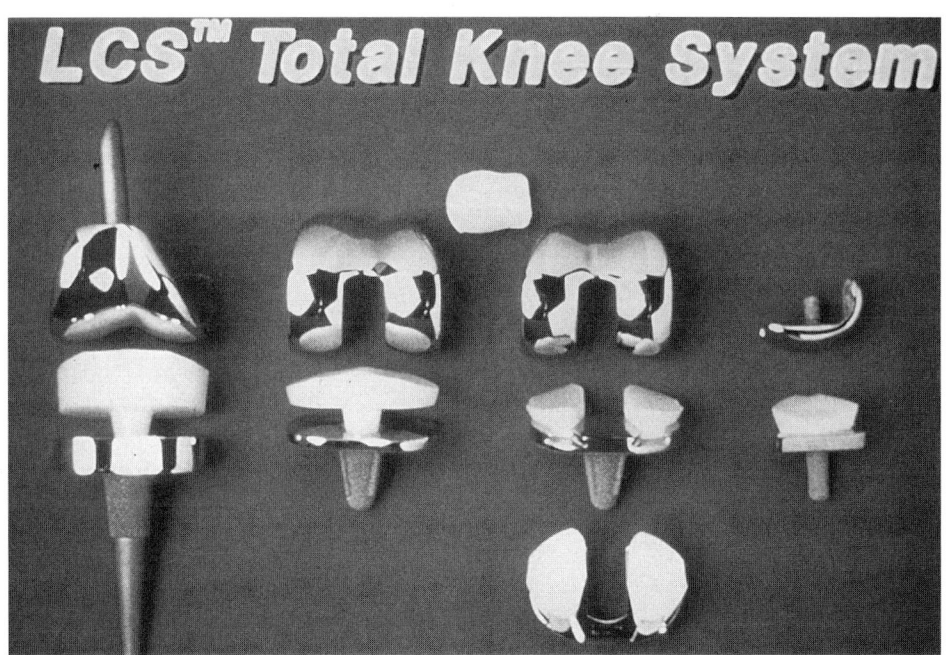

FIG 64–15.
Porous-coated LCS total knee fixation elements in use since 1981—without screws.

mented implants which demonstrated a 10-year overall survivorship of 90%. The specifics of individual component survivorship are presented later in this chapter.

CLINICAL APPLICATION OF MOBILE MENISCAL BEARINGS

Unicompartmental Knee Replacement

The first meniscal bearing knee replacement used clinically was a cemented Oxford meniscal knee, implanted as a medial, unicompartmental device in June 1976.[39]

The first LCS meniscal bearing knee replacement used clinically, was also a cemented medial, unicompartmental device, implanted in September 1977, into a 64-year-old, 82-kg postmenisectomy osteoarthritic man (Fig 64–16,A–C) who maintained an excellent clinical result until his death from cardiac failure 10 years after surgery.

Unicompartmental meniscal bearings are well adapted for knee replacement. They allow retention of both cruciate ligaments, normal forward and backward translational movement of the femur on the tibia, as well as axial rotation and varus-valgus movement, with excellent congruence of the bearing surfaces. The Oxford meniscal bearing unicompartmental device has had excellent success when used as a medial unicompartmental replacement,[32] but has functioned less consistently as a lateral compartment replacement because of significant dislocation problems[39] resulting from the use of a femoral component with single radius of curvature.

The cementless LCS unicompartmental knee was approved by the FDA orthopaedic advisory panel in August 1991 and released for general use by the FDA in November 1992 after successful completion of an FDA-IDE clinical trial. Good or excellent results us-

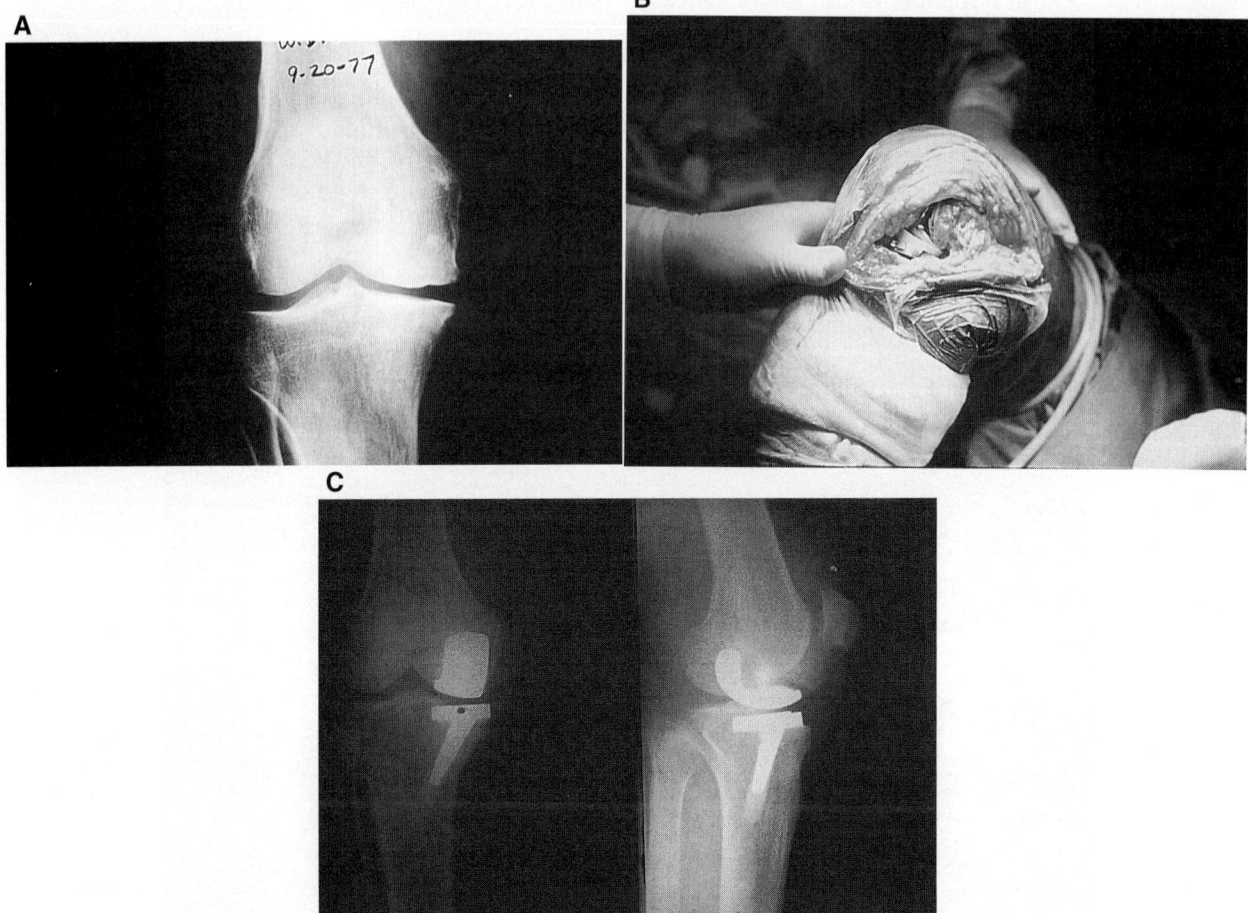

FIG 64–16.
A, preoperative AP radiograph of a 64-year-old, 82-kg osteoarthritic male knee showing medial compartment joint disease. **B,** intraoperative photograph of unicompartmental meniscal bearing replacement of the same knee. **C,** postoperative radiographs.

ing a strict knee scoring scale[5] were seen in 98.4% of 122 patients followed for 2 to 6 years (mean, 3.3 years). One bearing fractured, and one tibial component loosened in a patient with posttraumatic, osteoporotic bone deficiency. Progressive disease in the opposite knee compartment was an additional cause for revision. Such disorders represent the current failure mechanisms for this device.

Bicompartmental Knee Replacement

The articulating geometry of the femoral component is critical to the success or failure of the patellar component. A bispherical femoral groove with a continuous surface of revolution matching a bispherical congruently tracking patellar component provides a long life for the patellar bearing. This same femoral groove can match the anatomic patellar geometry and allow retention of the natural patella, with highly predictable results[46] (Fig 64–17). Keblish,[45] in a 10-year series comparing biocompartmental (retention of the natural patella) vs. tricompartmental (replaced patella) knee replacements using the femoral groove of the LCS design,[17] found no differences between the groups.[44] Such predictability can allow patella retention in patients such as farmers or laborers who require repetitive squatting loads that may increase patellar component wear. Additionally, patella retention in conditions such as patella infera or alta, or hypoplasia, can facilitate central tracking without fear of early knee replacement failure.[8] Lastly, those patients with previous patellectomies can undergo a patellar tendon bone grafting[11] (Fig 64–18) and enjoy a well-functioning bicompartmental replacement with improvement in both quadriceps leverage and tibiofemoral dislocation resistance.

Tricompartmental Knee Replacement

Bicruciate-Retaining Meniscal Bearing Total Knee Replacement

The concept of retaining both viable cruciate ligaments is appealing, since normal knee kinematics depends on the AP translation of the femur on the tibia which is under the direct control of these intact structures.[65] Ligament loads greater than body weight have been recorded for all knee ligaments. Thus, in theory at least, in the absence of each ligament, these loads would need to be carried by the remaining ligaments and perhaps transferred to the prosthesis itself. As such, retention of all load-bearing ligaments would be ideal if normal kinematic knee motion were allowed. Based on these concepts, the bicruciate-

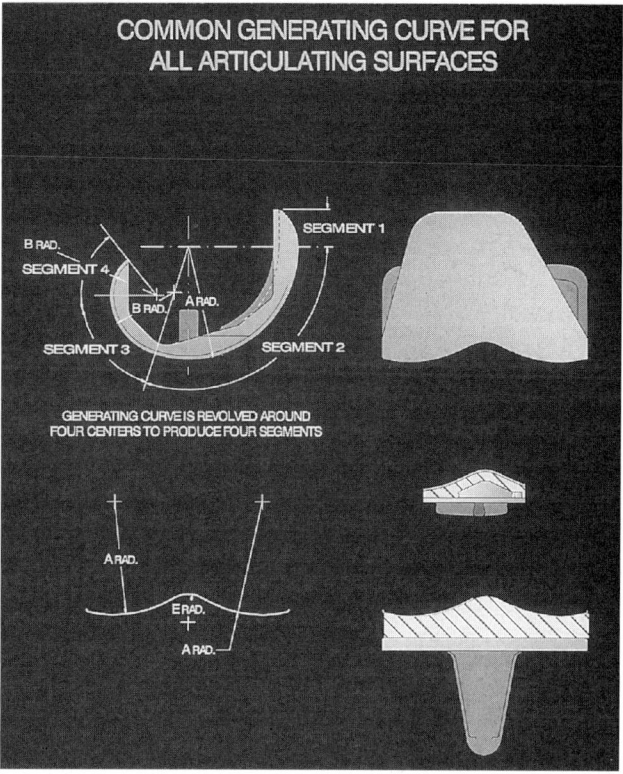

FIG 64–17.
Bispherical continuous surface-of-revolution femoral groove is used to match either a bispherical congruently tracking patellar component or the natural patella.

retaining, LCS meniscal bearing knee replacement was developed and successfully tested in FDA-IDE clinical trials.[18]

The use of three fixation fins, rather than a central conical peg, has led to a greater incidence of tibial component loosening with this device than with central conical peg devices.[22] Also, Hamelynck[40] in the Netherlands has reported that loosening of these trifinned components is increased in patients with previous high tibial osteotomies or proximal tibial fractures. Such conditions appear to alter blood flow and impede osseointegration in cementless bicruciate-retaining knees and as such remain contraindications to their cementless use. Additionally, early or late rupture of the anterior cruciate ligament (ACL) degrades the arthroplasty to the level of an ACL-deficient knee in many cases and raises doubts as to whether ACL retention should be attempted except in circumstances of youth, good bone stock, and a perfect ACL, which is a rare situation at best. Still, those knees with intact ACLs, excellent bone stock, and solid fixation of components represent the best possible TKRs because they function and act as normal knees.[14]

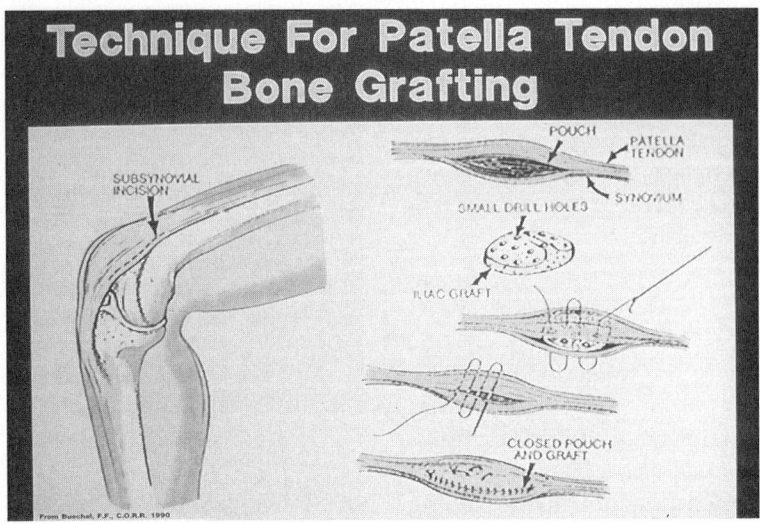

FIG 64–18.
Technique of patellar tendon bone grafting: (1) subsynovial incision along the border of the patellar tendon–synovial junction at the level of the original patella; (2) development of a subsynovial pouch of 3 × 3 cm between the synovial layer and the patellar tendon; (3) bone graft with 2.5-mm holes spaced 5 mm apart; (4) suturing the predrilled bone graft into the subsynovial pouch; (5) the subsynovial pouch is closed with a running suture; (6) the bone graft is stabilized completely in the closed subsynovial pouch.

Posterior Cruciate Ligament–Retaining Meniscal Bearing

Retention of the PCL has been reported to improve quadriceps leverage, increase extension torque, and improve flexion over cruciate-sacrificing designs.[54] In fixed bearings, this increased motion and function is related to increased posterior rollback on the incongruent tibial bearing surface, which increases wear over cruciate-sacrificing, fixed-bearing designs.[36] A meniscal bearing device allows more congruent rollback in flexion to improve wear resistance over fixed-bearing designs.

The Oxford meniscal knee, however, functioned poorly with only an intact PCL. As such, the Oxford knee developers did not recommend using the Oxford device in any ACL-deficient knee and cautioned against the use of any meniscal bearing device in the absence of the ACL. With this in mind, the significant dislocation rate of 9.3% reported by Bert in 1990[3] using rotating platform and PCL-retaining LCS knee replacements would tend to support this caveat. However, as was pointed out in rebuttal to the Bert article,[10] meniscal or rotating bearings require adequate control of the flexion and extension gaps during surgery to maintain contact stability of the prosthesis. As such, failure to maintain flexion and extension gap stability will compromise the results of any mobile bearing knee replacement, whether both, one, or no cruciate ligaments are preserved.

The successful FDA-IDE cementless clinical trial of the PCL-retaining, meniscal bearing LCS knee replacement documented the ability to retain only the PCL and maintain long-term stability and function with a meniscal bearing device.[28, 51]

Tibial component loosening and dislocations were seen in knees with poor flexion stability and were noted to be related to technique rather than to the implant, as was noted in the Bert study.[10] Early or late PCL instability remains a concern for this arthroplasty. Intraoperative diligence to avoid any release of this ligament attachment is desirable and if PCL compromise is noted, then replacement with a centrally stabilized, rotating platform device is advisable for long-term stability and function.

Cruciate-Sacrificing Rotating Platform

Cruciate sacrifice is often desirable in conditions such as fixed flexion, fixed valgus, and in some severe fixed varus deformities. It is often unavoidable in conditions where significant trauma, rheumatoid arthritis, or inflammatory osteoarthritis has destroyed these structures. In such cases, a centrally stabilized device with long-term fixation and excellent wear properties would be most desirable. The cemented total condylar knee replacement has been used in elderly patients over a 10- to 15-year period with exceptionally good results with a reported 90% survivorship using revision as an end point.[64] Considering these results to represent the standard for future design comparisons, any cemented or cementless cruciate-sacrificing design should demonstrate at least a 90% 10-year survivorship and have contact stresses less than the total condylar device.[26] Additionally, since total condylar range of motion was only considered to be fair and reported dislocations were fairly frequent, any new design should improve upon motion and dislocation resistance.

The LCS rotating platform knee replacement represents an improvement over the total condylar device in concept and in clinical performance. Conceptually, the deeper engagement of the rotatable, spherically congruent surfaces allow lower contact stresses during normal walking, namely, 25 MPa for the total condylar and 4.9 MPa for the LCS device.[55] This deeper engagement also improves dislocation resistance over the total condylar device (Fig 64–19). The LCS device utilizes a conical central tibial component stem which approximates the successful total condylar stem. Thus, similar fixation is achieved with rotational relief of shear stresses to tibial fixation with the rotating platform design.

The FDA-IDE clinical trials demonstrated long-term safety and efficacy of the rotating platform in a wide variety of primary and MO knees in both cemented and cementless applications. The FDA orthopaedic advisory panel recommended approval of the cemented LCS rotating platform device in 1984[18] and of the cementless device in 1991,[31] making the rotating platform the first, and currently the only total knee device to be approved for both cemented and cementless application in the United States after an FDA-IDE clinical trial.

Isolated Patellofemoral Replacement

The complex shape of the femoral groove impedes the design of a patellofemoral flange that will congruently accept a patellar bearing and yet avoid invading the tibiofemoral and meniscal articulations. In my experience, this situation requires a custom femoral flange to match each particular femoral groove and avoid the tibiofemoral and meniscal attachments. Such a device can be constructed by taking a dental-like impression of the femoral groove and then, using a positive plaster model, constructing a wax model and mold for the final flange dimension, followed by using the lost wax technique to fabricate the correct implant dimension.

A rotating-patellar bearing can then be constructed to match the primary surface curvature of the femoral flange, providing a custom patellofemo-

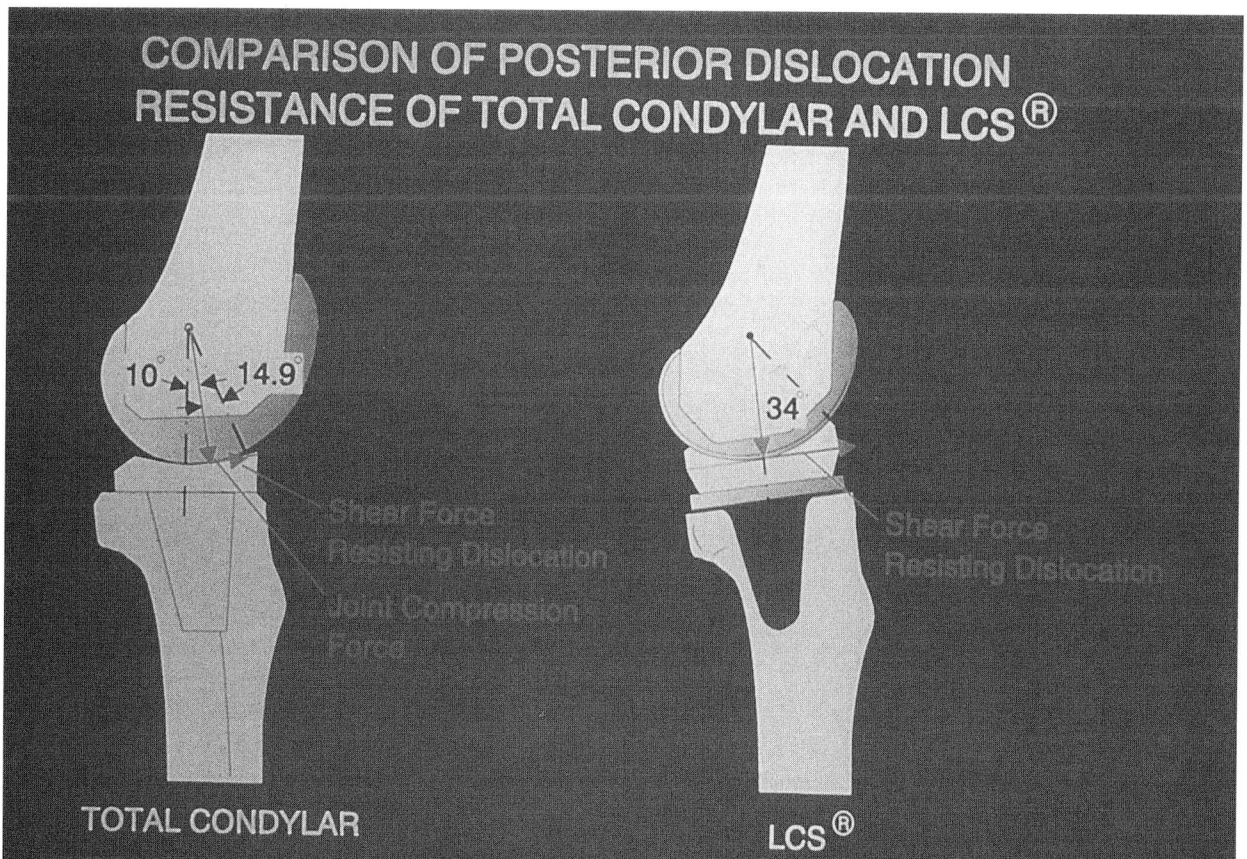

FIG 64–19.
Comparison of Total Condylar and LCS rotating platform articulating geometries in the lateral plane.

ral component with maximum congruence of the bearing surfaces.

Isolated patellofemoral replacement is complex and I believe it requires a custom approach to design. Current use of computed tomography (CT) scanning may obviate the need for two operations, and may make this procedure more practical. Use of a rotating-bearing patellar replacement allows for long-term fixation and function with few short-term problems. One out of six knees required revision over a 13-year period using this technique.

REVISION TOTAL KNEE REPLACEMENT

Aseptic failed knee replacement surgery is usually accompanied by a loss of bone stock and loss of the cruciate ligaments. In such cases, a centrally stabilized, rotating platform device with intramedullary stems can be used to salvage a wide variety of complex pathologic conditions.[7] These stems can be fixed to the femoral or tibial components (Fig 64–20) or be modular constructs with the ability to increase or decrease diameter as well as length similar to that found in current revision hip replacements.[23]

Attention to surgical technique, in regard to flexion-extension stability as well as varus-valgus ligamentous balancing, remains crucial to revision success. In those few cases in which AP stability continued to be a problem, the use of a high central post, posterior-stabilized prosthesis of the Total Condylar III design[49] was preferred while awaiting the final development of a suitable rotating platform with high central post stabilization.

Septic Revision Using Mobile Bearings

An infected TKR is a devastating complication which requires expert surgical judgment and the advice of infectious disease consultants to achieve a satisfactory outcome. The surgical principles of thorough debridement of infected and nonviable tissues as well as the mechanical principles of maintaining satisfactory flexion and extension stability with mechanical axis alignment remain paramount for success. Delayed exchange revision arthroplasty has been the standard of care[66] for the infected TKR, but it should be augmented by the concept of primary exchange revision replacement,[1, 9] which, when successful, limits surgery to one rather than multiple attempts. Perhaps 10% of patients will require at least a second operation after a primary exchange replacement, but 90% of patients will not require a second procedure as long as the implants used do not have a problem with stability, wear, or fixation.

Choice of revision implant from the patients' point of view is even more critical in this situation than the choice of primary implant, since they must now undergo a revision of their original surgery. These patients, whether infected or aseptic, want to know how long their revision will last. Having undergone total knee surgery, their question is important, since the severe pain associated with either the primary or the revision procedure is focused in the mind of the patient, and must not be underestimated by the surgeon. Thus, it is important to consider using the most wear-resistant implants with proven fixation for revision in either

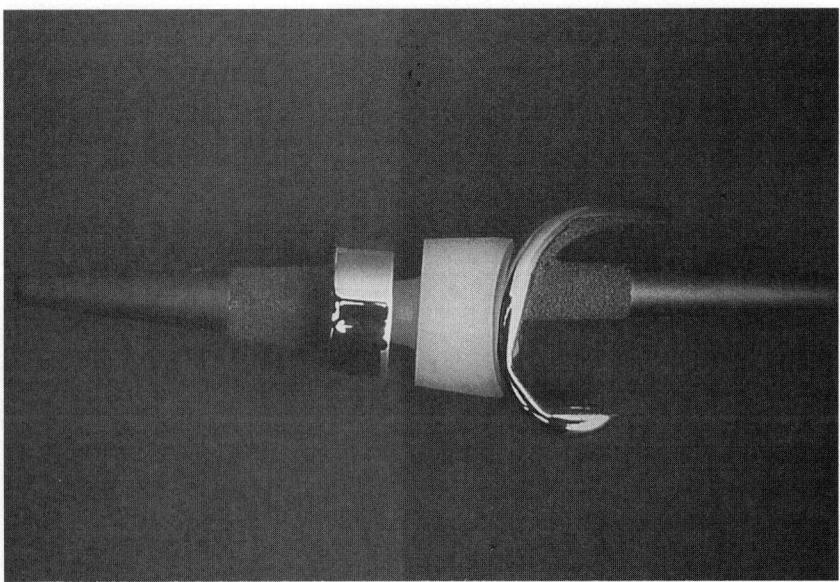

FIG 64–20.
LCS rotating platform fixed stem revision components.

septic or nonseptic situations. The LCS rotating platform revision implant offers long-term fixation and wear resistance for these applications and remains a superior implant choice, although expected revision results remain at about 80% good or excellent on the first revision attempt.[7]

SURVIVORSHIP ANALYSIS OF CEMENTED AND CEMENTLESS MENISCAL BEARING KNEE REPLACEMENTS

Survivorship of a least 90% at the 10-year interval, using as an end point revision of any component for any reason, has been recommended as the standard for primary TKR.[26] Any knee replacement that does not achieve this level of success should not be routinely used until design improvements can clearly demonstrate advantages over other standard designs to warrant further clinical use.

Meniscal bearing knee replacements have demonstrated this high level of survivorship in several designs. The Oxford meniscal knee has been specifically indicated for medial, unicompartmental, noninflammatory arthritis, and in such conditions, when both cruciate ligaments are intact, has a reported 99.1% survivorship at 10 years when used with methyl methacrylate bone cement.[32] Cementless long-term use of the Oxford device has not been reported and its use in bicompartmental and lateral unicompartmental applications is not recommended because of loosening and dislocation problems.[39]

The cemented LCS unicompartmental meniscal knee replacement has a reported 91% survivorship at 10 years when used for either the medial or lateral compartments in conjunction with intact cruciate ligaments in noninflammatory degenerative arthritis. The cementless LCS unicompartmental replacement has a reported 98% survivorship at 10 years when indicated for the same conditions as the cemented device. Inflammatory conditions such as rheumatoid arthritis, severe osteoporosis, and ACL deficiency are contraindications for LCS meniscal bearing unicompartmental replacement and are a documented source of failure in such cases.[29]

The cemented LCS bicruciate-retaining meniscal bearing TKR has a reported 90% survivorship at 10 years and the cementless device has a 95% survivorship at the same follow-up. Undersizing the tibial component in the cemented group and previous high tibial osteotomy or tibial plateau fracture in the cementless group are causes for failure and are now contraindicated for these devices. Additionally, it is not recommended to use the bicruciate device when the ACL has been disrupted or is deficient, but rather the centrally stabilized, PCL-retaining meniscal bearing tibial component is preferred.

The cementless LCS PCL-retaining meniscal bearing TKR has a 97% survivorship over the initial 8 years. It was released for clinical use in 1984 and remains the most popular meniscal bearing knee replacement worldwide at the present time. Flexion instability[3, 10] and late rupture of the PCL can compromise the long-term results with this device. It is important to be sure of PCL integrity and balanced flexion-extension gaps at surgery[6] for reproducible long-term results with this implant.

The cemented LCS rotating platform TKR used for cruciate ligament deficiency has a reported 97% survivorship at 10 years and the cementless device has a 98% survivorship at the same follow-up. Flexion instability has been identified as an unusual but the main problem with this device. The successful cemented and cementless survivorship of this implant represents a new standard for successful TKR to which future designs should be compared.

Cementless total knee fixation represents an advance over cemented fixation in that a temporary bone-cement interface is eliminated in favor of a permanent bone-prosthesis interface. Thus, it is reasonable to assume that a 10-year survivorship of a cementless device that improves upon a cemented device of the same design would be preferred as a means of long-term fixation. As such, the improved contact stresses of mobile bearings over fixed bearings would also be preferred, especially if long-term survivorship studies demonstrate such improvement. Such is the case, when one reviews the reported survivorship of a wide variety of fixed-bearing knee replacements used in cementless applications compared to the long-term survivorship of LCS cementless knee replacements (Fig 64–21).

The fact that wear resistance is also superior to fixed-bearing designs makes cementless mobile bearings the current implant choice for joint replacement of the knee in patients with active loading demands.

FUTURE DIRECTIONS

Meniscal bearings represent the logical approach to the future development of human knee joint replacement. This fact is supported by long-term survivorship and contact stress studies that favor mobile bearings over fixed bearings in a wide variety of clinical applications varying from unicompartmental to tricompartmental arthroplasty (references 2, 21, 22, 27, 32, 35, 42, 43, 50, 52, 63). It is important to explore alternative bearing geometries and biomaterials to optimize future designs.

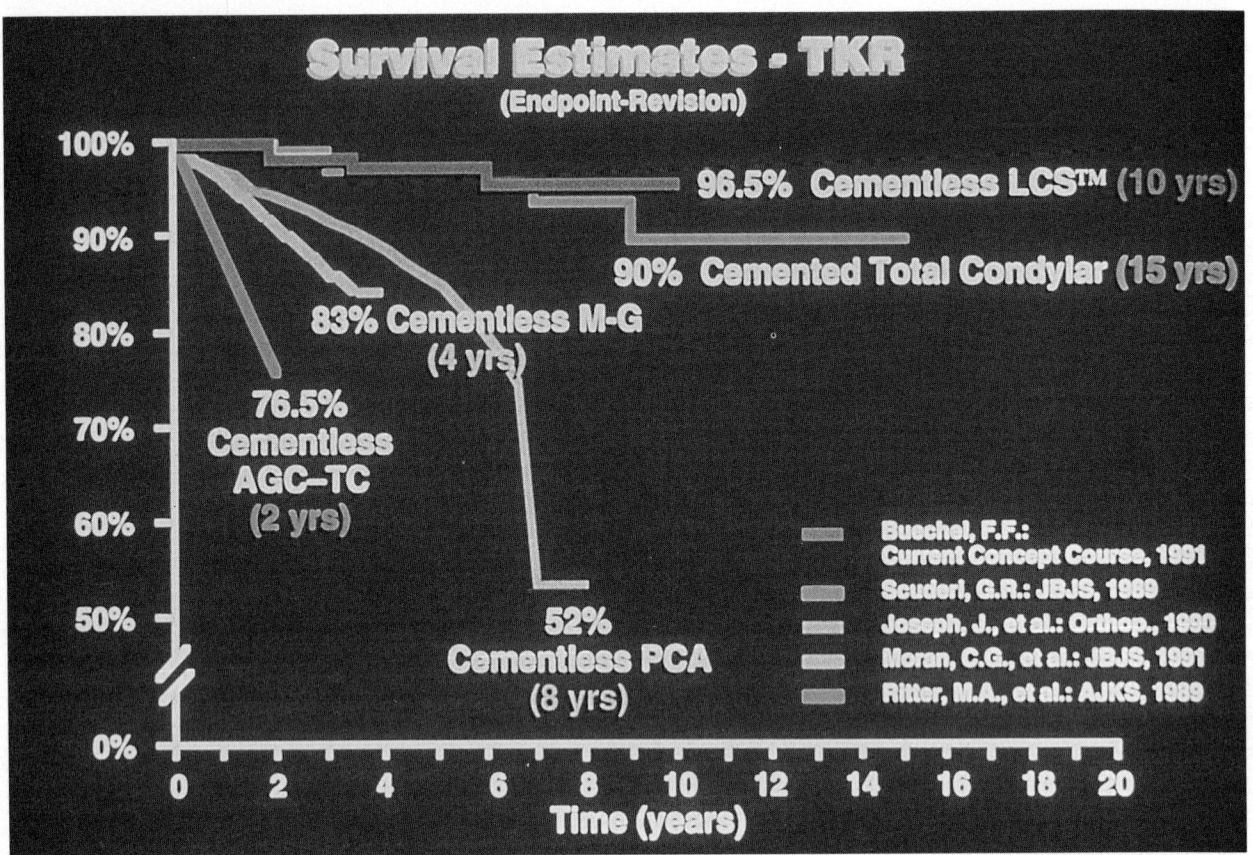

FIG 64-21.
Survival estimates of cementless TKRs compared with the cemented total condylar knee.i

Improved ceramic biomaterials such as aluminum oxide, zirconium oxide, and titanium nitride appear to offer improved wear resistance over polished metal surfaces. Bulk ceramics such as alumina and zirconia, however, have mechanical limitations, in that they are sensitive to notching and impact, which precludes their use in thin-shell applications. Polished titanium nitride ceramic, on the other hand, can be applied by a physical vapor deposition process[33] as a thin film on a metallic substrate to offer both impact and wear resistance.

Thin-film, polished, titanium nitride ceramic surfaces against UHMW polyethylene offer wear resistance greater than three times that of similar polished Co-Cr-Mo surfaces,[56] thus offering a strong potential as a bearing material for more active patient use.

This material has been developed and used clinically in active patients undergoing cementless meniscal bearing knee joint replacement with no clinical difference in performance outcome over a 2-year interval compared with similar cementless Co-Cr-Mo meniscal bearing knee replacements.

This observation leads one to accept that the performance of titanium nitride ceramic-coated devices is similar to the time-tested Co-Cr-Mo counterpart. Thus, the titanium nitride–coated devices are clinically acceptable in the short term. The important point is the fact that simulator studies[56, 57] demonstrate a significant improvement in wear resistance of polished titanium nitride ceramic over polished Co-Cr-Mo when used with the same UHMW polyethylene bearings. This leads one to anticipate improved longevity of ceramic bearings over their metallic counterparts.

With documented improvement of wear resistance of such ceramics on polyethylene meniscal bearings, it is reasonable to assume that athletic performance, e.g., running and jumping, may be possible and predictable with these improved bearing materials. Limited clinical trials in patients involved in such activities have been initiated and are being closely monitored for performance.

Future meniscal bearing knee joint development will undoubtedly rely on some of the basic principles presented in this chapter. It is of utmost importance for orthopaedic surgeons and mechanical engineers to work together in this area of implant design, to ensure that our future joint replacements are practical improvements over past misadventures.

REFERENCES

1. Barrett J: Primary exchange of the infected knee replacement, Fifth Annual Boston Knee Replacement Symposium, Boston, 1990.
2. Bartel DL, Bicknell VL, Wright TM: The effect of conformity, thickness, and material on stress in ultra-high molecular weight polyethylene components for total joint replacement, *J Bone Joint Surg [Am]* 68:1041–1051, 1986.
3. Bert JM: Dislocation/subluxation of meniscal bearing elements after New Jersey Low-Contact Stress total knee arthroplasty, *Clin Orthop* 254:211, 1990.
4. Bourne RB, Goodfellow JW, O'Connor JJ: A functional analysis of various knee arthroplasties. Transactions of the 24th Annual Meeting of the Orthopaedic Research Society, Dallas, Texas, Feb 21–23, 1978, p 156.
5. Buechel FF: A simplified evaluation system for the rating of knee function, *Orthop Rev* 97–101, 1982.
6. Buechel FF: *New Jersey LCS API surgical procedure.* Warsaw, Ind, 1989, DePuy Division of Boehringer Mannheim Corp.
7. Buechel FF: Cemented and cementless revision arthroplasty using rotating-platform total knee implants: A 12-year experience, *Orthop Rev* (suppl)71–75, 1990.
8. Buechel FF: Treatment of the patella in revision total knee surgery using a rotating-bearing patellar replacement, *Orthop Rev Suppl* 76–82, 1990.
9. Buechel FF: Primary exchange revision arthroplasty using antibiotic-impregnated cement for infected total knee replacement: An alternative to delayed exchange techniques, *Orthop Rev Suppl* 83–87, 1990.
10. Buechel FF: Dislocation/subluxation of the LCS knee replacement [letter]. *Clin Orthop* 264:309, 1991.
11. Buechel FF: Patella tendon bone grafting for patellectomized patients undergoing knee replacement, *Clin Orthop* 271:72–78, 1991.
12. Buechel FF: Total ankle replacement—State of the art. In Jahss MH, editor: *Disorders of the foot and ankle: Surgical and medical management,* Philadelphia, 1991, WB Saunders, pp 2671–2687.
13. Buechel FF: Cementless LCS endoprostheses: Concepts and 10 year evaluation, Presented at the Fourth World Biomaterials Congress, Berlin, April 27, 1992.
14. Buechel FF: Cementless mobile bearing TKR: 10 year results, Presented at the Seventh Annual Joint Replacement Symposium, Palm Beach, Fla, Oct 23, 1992.
15. Buechel FF: Fourteen year survivorship analysis of mobile bearing total knee arthroplasties. Presented at the State of the Art in Total Joint Replacement Symposium, Phoenix, Ariz, Nov 24, 1992.
16. Buechel FF: Cementless meniscal bearing TKA, Presented at the Eighth Annual Current Concepts in Joint Replacement Symposium, Orlando, Fla, Dec 18, 1992.
17. Buechel FF, Pappas MJ: New Jersey Meniscal Bearing Knee [July 27, 1982], Patent No. 4,340,978.
18. Buechel FF, Pappas MJ: New Jersey integrated total knee replacement system: Biomechanical analysis and clinical evaluation of 918 Cases. FDA Panel Presentation, Silver Spring, Md, July 11, 1984.
19. Buechel FF, Pappas MJ: The New Jersey Low Contact Stress knee replacement system: Biomechanical rationale and review of the first 123 cemented cases, *Arch Orthop Trauma Surg* 105:197–204, 1986.
20. Buechel FF, Pappas MJ: New Jersey LCS Knee replacement system: Biomechanical rationale and comparison of cemented and noncemented results (a two to five year follow-up), *Contemp Orthop* 14:52–60, 1987.
21. Buechel FF, Pappas MJ: New Jersey LCS Knee replacement system: 10 year evaluation of meniscal bearings, *Orthop Clin North Am* 20:147–177, 1989.
22. Buechel FF, Pappas MJ: Long-term survivorship analysis of cruciate sparing versus cruciate sacrificing knee prostheses using meniscal bearings, *Clin Orthop* 260:162–169, 1990.
23. Buechel FF, Pappas MJ: Efficacy and application of modular stems in THR, Presented at the Combined Meeting of the Orthopaedic Associations of the English-Speaking World. (poster exhibit), Toronto, June 21–26, 1992.
24. *Buechel-Pappas total shoulder system implants and instruments,* South Orange, NJ, Endotec, Inc., 1992.
25. Buechel FF, Pappas MJ, DePalma AF: Floating-socket total shoulder replacement: Anatomical, biomechanical and surgical rationale, *J Biomed Mater Res* 12:89–114, 1978.
26. Buechel FF, Pappas MJ, Greenwald AS: Use of survivorship and contact stress analyses to predict the long term efficacy of new generation joint replacement designs: A model for FDA device evaluation, *Orthop Rev* 20:50–55, 1991.
27. Buechel FF, Pappas MJ, Makris G: Evaluation of contact stress in metal-backed patellar replacements: A predictor of survivorship, *Clin Orthop* 273:190–197, 1991.
28. Buechel FF, et al: New Jersey LCS posterior cruciate retaining total knee replacement: Clinical, radiographic, statistical, and survivorship analyses of 395 cementless cases performed by 13 surgeons, Food and Drug Administration Panel Presentation. Rockville, Md, June 1, 1990.
29. Buechel FF, et al: New Jersey LCS unicompartmental knee replacement: Clinical, radiographic, statistical and survivorship analyses of 106 cementless cases performed by 7 surgeons. Food and Drug Administra-

---

*The author would like to acknowledge Linda A. Carter for her excellent technical assistance in the research and preparation of this manuscript.

tion Panel Presentation. Rockville, Md, August 16, 1991.
30. Buechel FF, Rosa RA, Pappas MJ: A metal backed, rotating-bearing patellar prosthesis to lower contact stress: An 11-year clinical study, *Clin Orthop* 248:34–49, 1989.
31. Buechel FF, Sorrels B, Pappas MJ: New Jersey Rotating Platform total knee replacement: Clinical, radiographic, statistical, and survivorship analyses of 346 cases performed by 16 surgeons, Food and Drug Administration Panel Presentation, Gaithersburg, Md, Nov 22, 1991.
32. Carr AJ, Keyes G, Miller RK: Medial unicompartmental arthroplasty: A survival study of the Oxford Meniscal Knee. Presented at the Ninth Combined Meeting of the Orthopaedic Association of the English-Speaking World (poster exhibit), Toronto, June 21–26, 1992.
33. Coll BF, Jacquot P: Surface modification of medical implants and surgical devices using TiN layers, *Surface Coating Technol* 36:867–878, 1988.
34. Collier JP, et al: The biomechanical problems of polyethylene as a bearing surface, *Clin Orthop* 261:107–113, 1990.
35. Engh GA, Dwyer DA, Hanes CK: Polyethylene wear of metal-backed tibial components in total and unicompartmental knee prosthesis, *J Bone Joint Surg [Br]* 74:9–17, 1992.
36. Ewald FC, et al: Kinematic total knee replacement, *J Bone Joint Surg [Am]* 66:1032, 1984.
37. Freeman MAR, Railton GT: Should the posterior cruciate ligament be retained or resected in condylar non-meniscal knee arthroplasty: The case for resection, *J Arthroplast Suppl* S3–S12, 1988.
38. Goodfellow J, O'Connor J: The mechanics of the knee and prosthesis design, *J Bone Joint Surg [Br]* 60:358, 1978.
39. Goodfellow JW, O'Connor J: Clinical results of the Oxford Knee surface arthroplasty of the tibio-femoral joint with a meniscal bearing prosthesis, *Clin Orthop* 205:21–42, 1986.
40. Hamelynck K: Results of 106 cementless bi-cruciate retaining meniscal bearing knee replacements in osteoarthritis, Personal communication, 1991.
41. Hostalen GUR: Hoechst aktiengellschaft, Frankfurt, Germany, 1982, p 22.
42. Huang CH, et al: Clinical results of the New Jersey Low Contact Stress knee arthroplasty with two to five years follow-up, *J Orthop Surg* 8:295–303, 1991.
43. Huson A, Spoor CW, Verbout AJ: A model of the human knee derived from kinematic principles and its relevance for endoprosthesis design, *Acta Morphol Ned Scand* 270:45, 1989.
44. Keblish PA: Patella retention vs. patella resurfacing, Presented at the 18th Annual Orthopaedic Surgery and Trauma Society Scientific Meeting, Peter Island, British Virgin Islands, June 13–20, 1992.
45. Keblish PA: Patella retention vs. re-surfacing, Presented at the Issues in Orthopaedic Implant Technology Symposium, Rancho Mirage, Calif, Nov 10–15, 1992.
46. Keblish PA, Greenwald SA: Patella retention versus patella resurfacing in total knee arthroplasty (scientific exhibit), Presented at the 58th Annual Meeting of the American Academy of Orthopaedic Surgeons, March 7–12, 1991.
47. Keblish PA, Pappas MJ: Rationale and selection of prosthetic types in mobile bearing total knee arthroplasty (scientific exhibit), Presented at the 59th Annual American Academy of Orthopaedic Surgeons. Washington, DC, Feb 20–25, 1992.
48. Landy M, Walker PA: Wear in condylar replacement knees. A 10 year follow-up, *Trans Orthop Res Soc* 10:96, 1985.
49. Lombardi AV, et al: The Total Condylar III prosthesis in complex primary total knee arthroplasty: A three to ten year clinical and radiograph evaluation (poster exhibit), Presented at The Combined Meeting of the Orthopaedic Associations of the English-Speaking World, Toronto, June 21–26, 1992.
50. Moran CG, et al: Survivorship analysis of the uncemented porous coated anatomic knee replacement, *J Bone Joint Surg [Am]* 73:848–857, 1991.
51. New Jersey Low Contact Stress Posterior Cruciate Retaining Cementless Total Knee Replacement Approval for United States Distribution, Letter to DePuy, Warsaw, Ind, from Food and Drug Administration, Rockville, Md, October 2, 1990.
52. Nielsen PT, Hansen EB, Rechnagel K: Cementless total knee arthroplasty in unselected cases of osteoarthritis and rheumatoid arthritis: A 3 year follow-up study of 103 cases, *J Arthroplasty* 7:137–143, 1992.
53. O'Connor J, Goodfellow J, Biden E: Designing the human knee. In Stokes IAF, (editor): *Mechanical factors and the skeleton,* London, John Libbey, 1981.
54. Oshsner JL, et al: Prospective comparison of posterior cruciate–retaining versus cruciate sacrificed total knee arthroplasty, Presented at the 55th Annual Meeting of the American Academy of Orthopaedic Surgeons, Atlanta, Feb 4–9, 1988.
55. Pappas MJ, Makris G, Buechel FF: Biomaterials for hard tissue applications. In Pizzoferrato PG, et al, editors: *Biomaterials and clinical applications: Evaluation of contact stresses in metal-plastic knee replacements,* Amsterdam, 1987, Elsevier, pp 259–264.
56. Pappas MJ, Makris G, Buechel FF: Comparison of wear of UHMWPe cups articulating with Co-Cr and Ti-Ni coated titanium femoral heads, *Transactions of the 16th Annual Meeting of the Society for Biomaterials,* Charleston, SC, May 20–23, 1990, p 36.
57. Pappas MJ, Makris G, Buechel FF: High cycle wear simulation of TiN coating on UHMWPe, a thirty-five million cycle test, Presented at the 19th Annual Meeting of the Society for Biomaterials, Birmingham, Ala, April 28–May 2, 1993.
58. Peter PC, Engh GA, Dwyer KA: Osteolysis after total knee arthroplasty without cement, *J Bone Joint Surg [Am]* 74:864–876, 1992.

59. Pilliar RM, et al: Radiographic and morphologic studies of load-bearing porous-surfaced structured implants, *Clin Orthop* 156:249–257, 1981.
60. Ranawat CS, et al: Long-term results of the Total Condylar knee arthroplasty. A 15 year survivorship study, Presented at the Ninth Combined Meeting of the Orthopaedic Association of the English-Speaking World, Toronto, June 21–26, 1992.
61. Rose RM, et al: Wear of the tibial component of the knee prosthesis, *Transactions of the 28th Annual Orthopaedic Research Society,* New Orleans, Jan 19–21, 1982, vol 7, p 252.
62. Schatzker J, Horne JG, Sumner-Smith G: The effect of movement on the holding power of screws in bone, *Clin Orthop* 111:257–262, 1975.
63. Schlepckow P: Three dimensional kinematics of total knee replacement systems, *Arch Orthop Trauma Surg* 3:204–209, 1992.
64. Scuderi GR, et al: Survivorship of cemented knee replacements, *J Bone Joint Surg [Br]* 71:798–803, 1989.
65. Tria AJ, Klein KS: *An illustrated guide to the knee,* New York, Churchill Livingstone, pp 31–38, 1992.
66. Windsor RE, Insall JN, Urs WK: Two-stage reimplantation for the salvage of total knee arthroplasty complicated by infection, *J Bone Joint Surg [Am]* 72:272–278, 1990.
67. Wright TM, Bartel DL: The problem of surface damage in polyethylene total knee components, *Clin Orthop* 205:67–74, 1986.

65

Cruciate-Substituting Knee Arthroplasty

STEVEN STERN, M.D.
JOHN N. INSALL, M.D.

History of knee arthroplasty at the hospital for special surgery
Advantages of posterior cruciate ligament sacrifice or substitution
Total condylar prosthesis
   Design
   Long-term results
     The Hospital for Special Surgery
     Other institutions
Posterior stabilized prosthesis
   Design rationale

Insall-Burstein posterior stabilized prosthesis
   Clinical results
     The Hospital for Special Surgery
     Other Institutions
Posterior cruciate ligament sacrifice or substitution
   Clinical function
   Clinical results of posterior substitution at Mayo Clinic
   Survivorship analysis
   Complications of posterior cruciate substitution
Conclusion

Total knee arthroplasty has become one of the most common procedures performed in the United States. Excellent results have been reported by many authors working at different institutions (references 1, 2, 7, 9, 12, 14, 16, 18, 20, 22, 24, 25, 26, 30, 31, 36, 37, 38, 40, 42, 43, 45, 46, 50, 51, 59, 61). These results have been achieved with assorted component types utilizing various modes of fixation. However, there is no unanimity regarding which total knee construct will maximize clinical function.

Thus, while great progress has been made in knee arthroplasty, questions and issues still remain. Should none, one, or both of the cruciate ligaments be sacrificed at the time of surgery? What is the optimal shape for the tibial polyethylene? Should knee components be fixed to the host bone with bone cement, or does porous technology result in a more stable interface? Is better function achieved with patellar resurfacing, or do the complications attendant to this additional step outweigh the benefits? Fully answering these questions is impossible at this time, but examination of prior results can serve as a useful frame of reference. It is in this context that "newer" ideas can be assessed, and older techniques preserved, modified, or discarded.

This chapter examines the modern concept of cruciate sacrifice, with special emphasis on the work from The Hospital for Special Surgery in New York City. Since the surgeons at The Hospital for Special Surgery have been relatively staunch advocates of bone cement, the results in this discussion are restricted to this mode of fixation. While it is possible to combine posterior cruciate ligament sacrifice and noncemented fixation, we know of no studies in which these two concepts have been coordinated. Therefore, the results and outcomes in this chapter are restricted to the use of polymethyl methacralate.

HISTORY OF KNEE ARTHROPLASTY AT THE HOSPITAL FOR SPECIAL SURGERY

The modern age of total knee arthroplasty was ushered in during the early 1970s with the advent of the total condylar prothesis. The original Total Condylar prothesis was a semiconstrained, nonlinked condylar replacement (Fig 65–1). The femoral component was designed so that its geometry roughly approximated that of the average knee. An anterior phalange was incorporated into the femoral design to allow for replacement of the patellofemoral articulation. The patella was resurfaced with an all-polyethylene patellar dome. The tibial component had conforming concave surfaces that contributed some inherent stability to the device.[22, 25] The Total Condylar device was

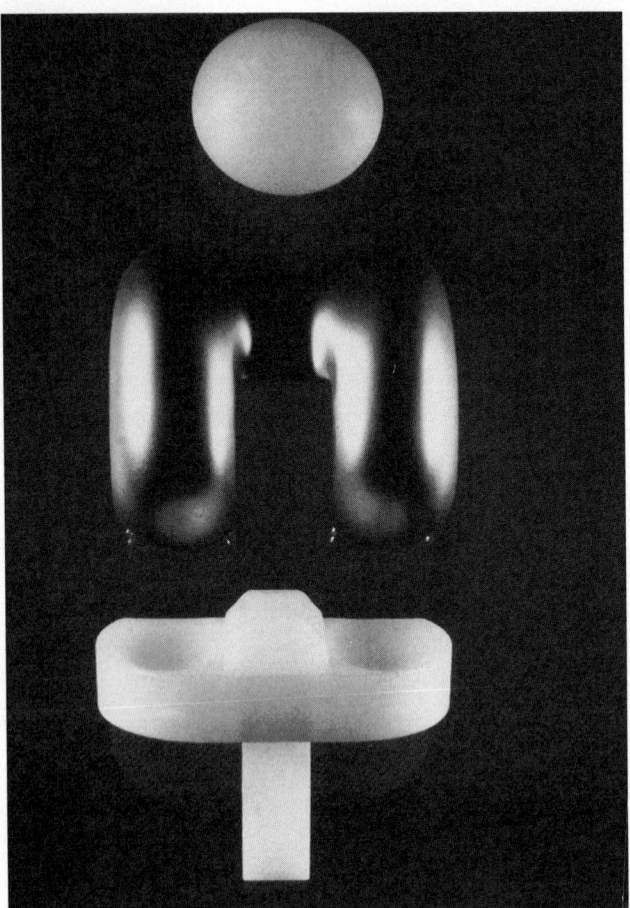

FIG 65-1.
The Total Condylar prosthesis. This was a semiconstrained device which required sacrifice of both cruciate ligaments for implantation. The femoral component consisted of symmetric condyles connected by an anterior flange. The tibial component had conforming concave surfaces.

one of the first designs to yield predictable and durable total knee arthroplasty results.[22, 26] The long-term clinical results with this prosthesis still offer a standard of comparison for other knee designs.[37, 38, 59]

However, certain weaknesses became apparent with the Total Condylar prosthesis as clinicians accumulated experience with its use. Specifically, some early studies revealed limited knee motion with this design.[22] In cases where the flexion gap was inadequately balanced, the tibial component had a propensity to subluxate posteriorly. It was believed that sacrifice of the posterior cruciate ligament played an intrinsic role in these problems. Theoretically, an intact ligament would cause the femur to roll back on the tibia during knee flexion, and hence promote a greater arc of motion. In addition, an intact posterior cruciate ligament would resist posterior tibial subluxation. In an attempt to address these concerns, designers envisioned a prosthesis in which a posterior cruciate ligament–substituting mechanism was built directly into the prosthesis.

The initial attempt at a posterior-stabilized knee prosthesis was the Total Condylar type II. This prosthesis, introduced in 1976, featured a central tibial post to deter posterior tibial subluxation. However, the tibial post was not designed to effect femoral rollback, nor to substitute for the collateral ligaments. Early results with the Total Condylar II were poor, with a relatively high rate of tibial loosening.[23] These failures were believed to be caused by problems inherent in the design of this particular device.

The original posterior stabilized prosthesis was introduced at The Hospital for Special Surgery in 1978 as a further modification of the Total Condylar design[21] (Fig 65–2). The prosthesis was intended to improve stair climbing, increase range of motion, and prevent posterior tibial subluxation. The femoral component, composed of cobalt-chromium, had a

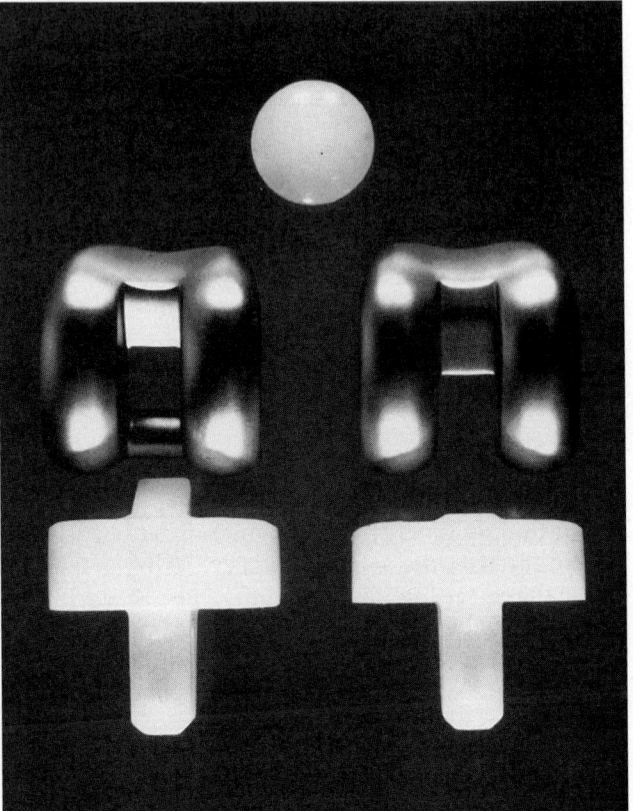

FIG 65-2.
The original Insall-Burstein Posterior Stabilized prosthesis. This design introduced the concept of ligament substitution as compared to the Total Condylar. The original tibial component was composed entirely of polyethylene.

transverse cam that contacted with a central tibial polyethylene spine in knee flexion. The cam and spine mechanism was designed to substitute for the posterior cruciate ligament. The tibial component was fabricated entirely of ultrahigh-molecular-weight polyethylene (UHMWPE). The patellar bone was resurfaced with a domed component composed of polyethylene with a central round peg. All components in this arthroplasty were implanted with the use of polymethyl methacralate.

Several design modifications of the Insall-Burstein Posterior Stabilized (Zimmer, Warsaw, Ind.) prosthesis have been introduced over the years. The tibial component was the first area in which these alterations were done. Initially, the tibial tray was composed entirely of polyethylene. However, finite element analysis demonstrated enhanced load transmission to the underlying bone with the addition of metal backing to the tibial component.[3] Therefore, in the latter portion of 1980, metal backing was added to the tibial tray. By 1981 the all-polyethylene tibial component had been totally replaced at The Hospital for Special Surgery by its metal-backed counterpart.

A brief use of carbon-reinforced polyethylene occurred in the early 1980s. Carbon-reinforced polyethylene was used because of its theoretic increased strength. However, the clinical results with carbon-reinforced polyethylene proved disappointing, with several reports of failures with this biomaterial.[63, 64] Therefore, the Posterior Stabilized arthroplasty resumed use of standard (nonreinforced) polyethylene (Fig 65–3).

The next major prosthetic change occurred in 1983 with the introduction of modified Posterior Stabilized components. Modifications occurred, in part, because of concern regarding the patellofemoral joint. The femoral component was altered in order to allow for a smoother patellofemoral transition. This transition occurs as the patellofemoral contact point moves along the femoral component's anterior flange to its distal runners as the knee goes from extension to flexion. Modifications included rounding of the anterior portion of the femoral component, as well as a deepening of the femoral groove. Both of these changes represented an attempt to enhance patellar tracking. In addition, the implant was manufactured in various sizes, since the original version had only been available in one intermediate size. This sizing limitation had occasionally resulted in mismatches between component and host bone, which was minimized with the introduction of these multiple sizes.

The prosthesis then continued in use without

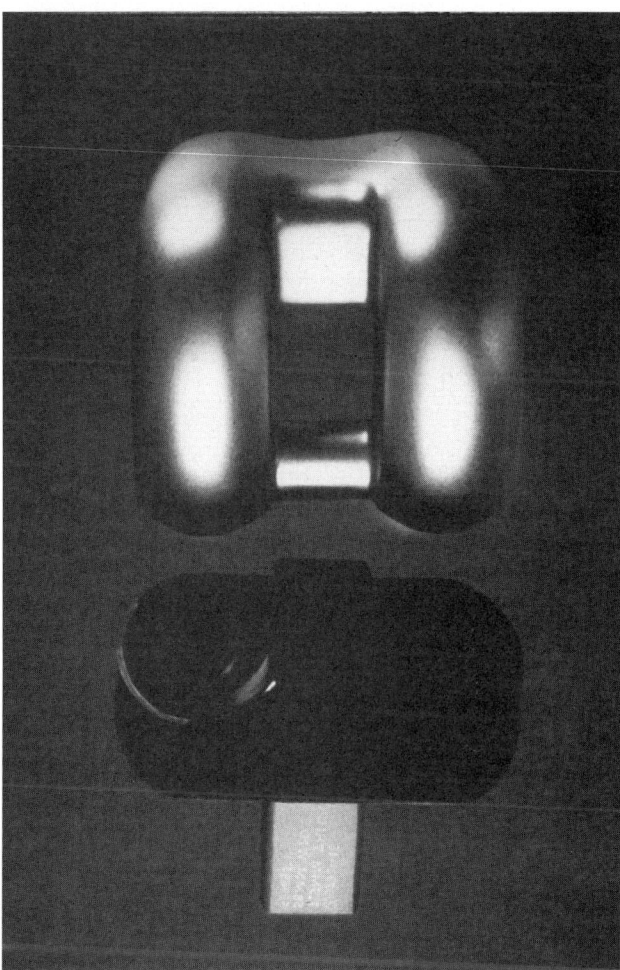

FIG 65–3.
An early modification of the Insall-Burstein Posterior Stabilized design included a carbon-reinforced tibial component.

major change until the late 1980s. At that time, the Insall-Burstein II Posterior-Stabilized prosthesis was introduced (Fig 65–4). This newer prosthesis incorporated several major design and instrument changes. Intramedullary instruments were utilized for prosthetic implantation, and the "tenser" (used in the original design to balance the flexion and extension gaps) was abandoned. However, the concept of ligamentous balance was not discarded, remaining an essential factor for successful arthroplasty. The Insall-Burstein II prosthesis also inaugurated the concept of component modularity to the posterior-stabilized design. It was thus possible to assemble various metallic tibial tray base plates, polyethylene inserts, intramedullary rods, and wedges at the time of surgery.

In addition, the inauguration of the Insall-Burstein II prosthesis heralded a slight modification

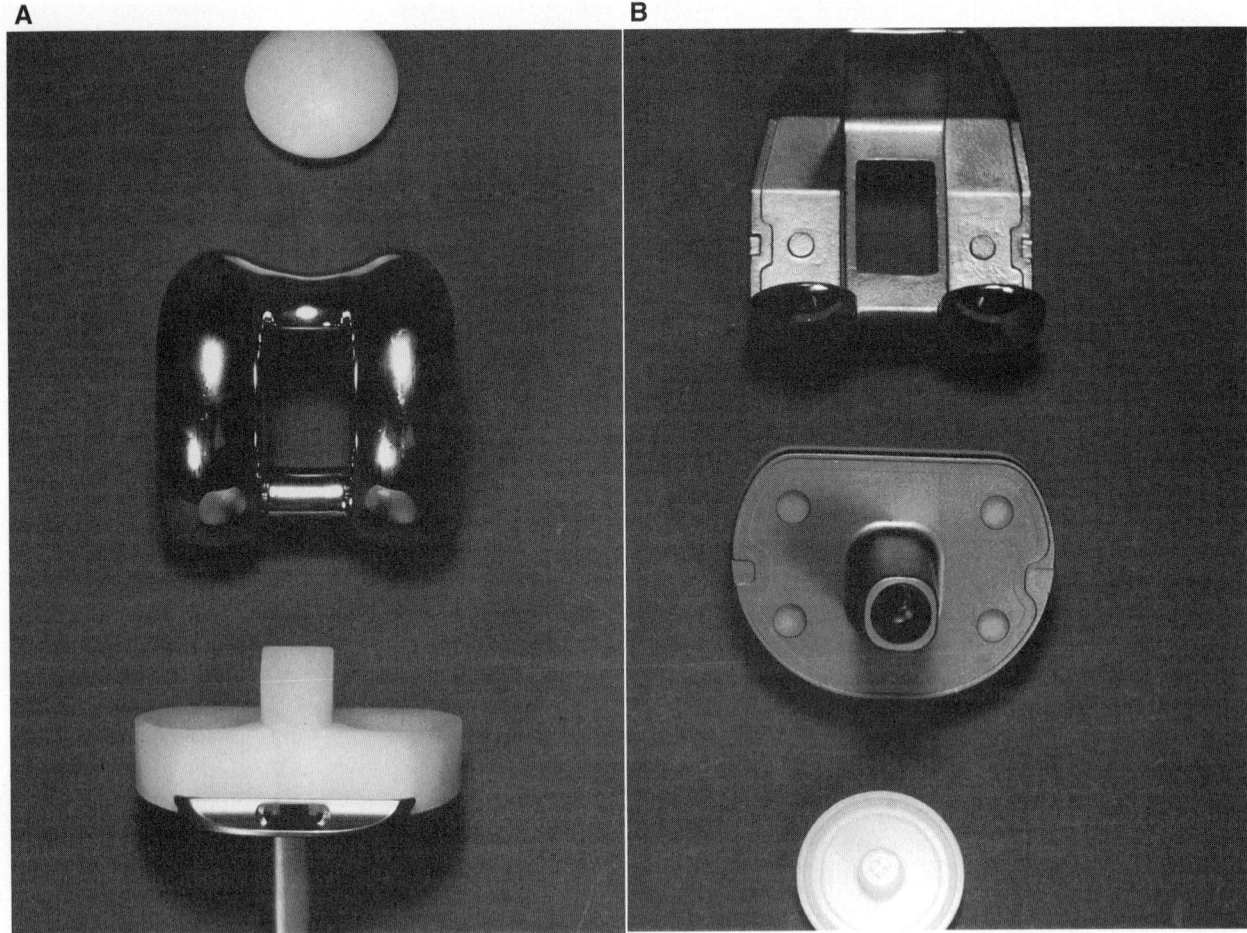

FIG 65–4.
The Insall-Burstein II prosthesis. **A,** front view; **B,** posterior view.

in the mechanism of ligament substitution. This was done in an attempt to further enhance femoral rollback and increase knee flexion. Unfortunately, there were reports of component dislocations with the new prosthesis.[36] These dislocations, while rare, were especially worrisome in knees with a preoperative valgus deformity or those that attained large flexion angles.[10] Because of concern regarding this problem, a modification of the tibial insert was carried out. These changes were restricted to the tibial insert, and included both elevation and a relative anterior translation of the tibial spine. These revisions served to increase the inherent stability of the device.

Thus, the current Insall-Burstein II prosthesis offers the advantages of modularity, while maintaining the basic aspects of ligament substitution. It employs essentially the same arthroplasty philosophy that has been used successfully for the past 15 years, thereby remaining one of the few prostheses fundamentally unchanged in concept after more than a decade of use.

ADVANTAGES OF POSTERIOR CRUCIATE LIGAMENT SACRIFICE OR SUBSTITUTION

1. Minimal tibial resection possible. Sacrifice of the posterior cruciate ligament removes some restrictions inherent in attempting to perform a knee arthroplasty with posterior cruciate ligament retention. Specifically, the surgeon does not have to "balance" the posterior cruciate ligament, and thus is not restricted to a particular depth of tibial bone resection. This allows for a minimal tibial bone resection with implantation of the tibial tray in the strong subchondral bone. The tibial component is then placed in a sturdy bone bed, as opposed to the weaker metaphyseal cancellous bone encountered with larger tibial resections.

2. Easier surgery technique. Sacrifice of the posterior cruciate ligament is a straightforward and reproducible surgical technique. A posterior bone island is not needed for preservation of the posterior cruciate ligament and the tibial bone cut can be made

with impunity. The ligament can be sharply excised from its femoral attachment. Thus, ligamentous balancing is not complicated by the possible tethering effect of this posterior structure.

3. Polyethylene wear. The long-term durability of polyethylene is an increasing concern as implant survival lengthens. There is expanding evidence that polyethylene may prove to be the weak link in modern knee arthroplasty.[17, 29, 39, 57, 62] Posterior cruciate ligament substitution or sacrifice allows for a tibial component designed in a more protective fashion for the polyethylene. This is achieved by the increased conformity of the articular polyethylene surface. The conforming surfaces increase the contact area at the femorotibial articulation, thus decreasing the stress to which the plastic is subjected. Evidence of significant polyethylene wear with less conforming posterior cruciate ligament–retaining tibial articular surfaces has already been reported.[52]

4. Correction of deformity. Posterior cruciate ligament excision allows easier deformity correction in severely deformed knees.[32]

TOTAL CONDYLAR PROSTHESIS

The name total condylar denoted a specific prosthesis developed at The Hospital for Special Surgery by Insall, Ranawat, and Walker.[60] However, the term eventually became generic for a class of prostheses. These prostheses were generally semiconstrained designs, necessitating sacrifice of both cruciate ligaments. They were anatomic in shape, with a conforming geometry. Implantation of these devices usually required the use of bone cement.

The Total Condylar prosthesis was introduced at The Hospital for Special Surgery in 1974. This specific prosthesis was an outgrowth of earlier work with the Duocondylar and Duopatellar prostheses. Knee arthroplasty using the Total Condylar required sacrifice of both cruciate ligaments. Cruciate excision was originally undertaken to allow an extensive exposure and afford easier correction of angular deformities. Special attention was paid to the patellofemoral articulation. The Total Condylar's femoral component included an anterior phalange which mated with the polyethylene dome used to resurface the patella. This had not been routinely done prior to the introduction of this prosthesis.

The prosthetic design integrated several other concepts that had evolved to that point.[60] These included straight bone cuts to maximize the accuracy of the component fit. The prosthesis was designed to be "semiconstrained." Thus, the components were constructed so that their shape would provide some inherent stability. However, there was a small amount of laxity built into the design so that the ligaments would also take up stress. Contact area between the femoral and tibial surfaces was maximized in order to decrease stress at the polyethylene surface.

There have been multiple reports in the literature on results with the Total Condylar arthroplasty.[18–20, 22, 24, 25, 27, 30, 41, 49, 56] The first report on the Total Condylar prosthesis appeared in 1976.[25] This preliminary report dealt mainly with surgical technique and a method for accurate placement of the components. Later reports detailed the long-term results achieved with this prosthesis, which proved to be both predictable and durable.[12, 26, 31, 37, 38, 42] The efficacy of this prosthesis, as well as its versatility in various situations, was demonstrated in these reports. Because of the excellent results, some centers continued its use with only relatively minor changes through the 1980s.

Design

The Total Condylar prosthesis designed at The Hospital for Special Surgery consisted of a cobalt-chromium femoral component. This was anatomically shaped with a symmetric anterior phalange for articulation with the patellar dome. The femoral component's anterior phalange interconnected two symmetric condyles. Each of these condyles had a decreasing radius of curvature posteriorly. This resulted in femoral condyles that were more steeply curved posteriorly than distally. As the knee went into flexion, the decreased radius of the femoral component allowed some rotation. The prosthesis, therefore, had a greater area of contact in extension when the distal femoral condyles articulated with the tibial tray. This was done to promote stability and decrease polyethylene wear.

The tibial component was composed of high-density polyethylene incorporating two separate concave conforming wells. These were machined to conform exactly with the femoral component in extension, thereby minimizing rotation in this position. The symmetric tibial wells were interconnected by an intercondylar eminence, designed to prevent translocation. The anterior and posterior peripheral margins of the tibial component were of equal height. Thus, the tibial component was specifically designed to offer inherent stability to the knee. Finally, the tibial component had a central fixation peg to enhance fixation. All components were fixed with a bone cement.

The patellar component was composed of high-density polyethylene. Its articulating surface was dome-shaped, designed to conform closely to the anterior femoral flange. An advantage of the dome geometry was that it did not require rotatory alignment, which would be necessary with an anatomic patellar replacement. The patellar dome had a central rectangular fixation peg to augment cement fixation.

The original Total Condylar prosthesis was available in only one femoral size, designed to mate with one of three different tibial thicknesses. However, the prosthesis was eventually manufactured in an increased range of sizes. In addition, other changes were made in the prosthetic design during its time in use. The original Total Condylar prosthesis did not have a posteriorly sloped tibial tray. This was later modified with the Insall-Burstein Total Condylar prosthesis, in which a posterior slope was incorporated in the tibial tray.[58] This was done to improve knee flexion by avoiding posterior impingement of the femur against the tibial polyethylene. In addition, metal backing was added to the tibial component in order to enhance load distribution.[3]

Long-Term Results

The Hospital for Special Surgery

The majority of the Total Condylar results from The Hospital for Special Surgery have been in surgical cases performed under the direction of either Insall or Ranawat. An early report in 1979 gave their combined experience,[22] but in subsequent longer-term follow-ups, results have been reported separately (Table 65–1).

The first report on the long-term results for the Total Condylar prosthesis was published in 1983.[26] This paper analyzed the first 100 consecutive patients that underwent Total Condylar knee arthroplasty at The Hospital for Special Surgery. The patient population was limited to knees with gonarthrosis (degenerative joint disease). Patients were reviewed 5 to 9 years after index arthroplasty. The average age was 68 years. There were 69 women and 10 men. Patellar replacements were done in all cases, except for ten knees operated on early in the series. At follow-up, 64% were rated excellent, 27% were rated as good, 2% were rated fair, and 7% were rated poor. Range of motion averaged 98 degrees. There was no survivorship analysis done with this initial long-term report.

There were seven failures in this group. One was secondary to a deep infection that developed after a wound problem. One knee underwent revision to a constrained prosthesis secondary to posterior subluxation. One knee was in varus malignment at the time of initial arthroplasty and eventually required revision secondary to medial knee pain. One knee had inadequate soft tissue balancing and a recurrent varus instability which eventually deteriorated requiring a revision. One knee had been performed in a patient status post patellectomy. Post arthroplasty, this patient continued to have extensor weakness and complaints of pain. Because of this continued pain, 7 years post surgery, an arthrodesis was done at another institution. Two knees had loosening of the tibial component requiring revision. One knee had medial pain in the proximal tibia after the arthroplasty was in varus malalignment at the time of initial arthroplasty. The other tibial component loosening occurred in a knee that was initially correctly aligned. However, a progressive radiolucency associated with escalating knee pain necessitated revision.

Vince et al.[59] reported the 10- to 12-year results of the Total Condylar prosthesis in 1989. This report represented the results of patients implanted between 1974 and 1975. The average age of patients at the time of surgery was 67 years. Women made up 79%. Seventy-four of the original 130 Total Condylar prostheses were evaluated 10 to 12 years post sur-

TABLE 65–1.
Total Condylar Prosthesis: Comparison of Knee Scores*

Institution†	Follow-up (yr)	No. of Knees	Mean Flexion (degrees)	Excellent	Good	Fair	Poor	Survivorship Analysis (%)
HSS (1979)[22]	3–5	220	90	62	28	4.5	5.5	
HSS (1983)[26]	5–9	100	98	64	27	2.0%	7.0	
HSS (1989)[59]	10–12	74	90	51	37	4.0	8.0	93
HSS (1988)[37]	8–11	90	95	53	39	4.0	4.0	94
HSS (1989)[38]	2–9	100	109	64	35	0	1.01	99
Cleveland Clinic (1987)[42]	8–11	64	101	41	36	16	7.0	
Case Western Reserve[12]	7.0–11.5	109	95	34	30	9.0	27	

*As judged by The Hospital for Special Surgery rating system, except for the Case Western Reserve study, which used the University Hospitals of Cleveland rating system.
†HSS = The Hospital for Special Surgery.

gery. Of these, 51% (38 knees) were rated excellent, 37% (27 knees) good, 4% (3 knees) fair, and 8% (6 knees) poor. The average flexion arc achieved was 91 degrees. Of the 6 knees with poor results, 5 required revision. Four of these were secondary to tibial loosening (these cases had been reported in detail earlier[26]) related to technical errors. One femoral component insidiously loosened over time in a knee with a preoperative valgus deformity. One knee was categorized as poor after a cerebrovascular accident dropped the rating, though the knee had scored excellent prior to the infirmity. The authors concluded that preservation of the posterior cruciate ligament, in order to spare the interface between component and bone, was not necessary to achieve satisfactory long-term arthroplasty results. This was an argument that had been advanced in the past by others.[43, 48] In addition, the authors believed that there was no need to develop cementless fixation for knee arthroplasties in patient populations similar to the one reported on in their study.

Ranawat and Boachie-Adjei[37] reported on their results with the Total Condylar replacement. Their 9- to 11-year analysis revealed 53% excellent, 39% good, 4% fair, and 4% poor results. At 11 years survivorship was 94.1% using revision or recommended revision as the end-point criterion. Average range of motion was 95 degrees. There were four poor results in this series. One was secondary to a deep infection, one knee required revision for a loose tibial component, and one knee had loosening of the patellar component. The final poor result was in an overweight patient with multiple joint arthritis and mild knee pain.

In a follow-up report, Ranawat and Hansraj[38] published the results of the second 100 Total Condylar replacements. This represented results after Ranawat and colleagues had theoretically progressed along the learning curve for implantation of this device. In this group, there were 64% excellent, 34% good, and 1% poor results. The one poor result was in a knee infected with *Escherichia coli*. Survival tables generated a cumulative survivorship rate of 98.9% at 9 years' follow-up. Average range of motion was 109 degrees, a significant improvement over results from prior reports with the total condylar.[22] Thus, this report attested that knee flexion greater than 90 degrees could be achieved with the total condylar prosthesis.

Other Institutions

In 1990 Laskin[31] reported his results with the Total Condylar prosthesis in a cohort of patients with rheumatoid arthritis. There were 80 knees available for analysis at follow-up of 10 years. Nineteen of these failed and required a revision procedure. The major mode of failure in this study was loosening of the tibial component (12 knees) and late bacteremic seeding (5 knees). Average range of motion was 96 degrees. Cumulative survival was 81% at 10 years. Laskin did note a decline in knees scores with age. He attributed this to the overall debilitation that occurs with the aging process, rather than a problem inherent to knee arthroplasty. While there was a relatively high incidence of tibial loosening, the patient population differed significantly from that seen in The Hospital for Special Surgery studies. This is because Laskin's report was restricted to patients with rheumatoid arthritis. Additionally, 89% of his patients needed chronic steroid treatment, which may have resulted in poor bone quality and contributed to component loosening.

Shurman et al.[42] reported on the 8- to 11-year follow-up of the first 129 Total Condylar prostheses performed at the Cleveland Clinic. In this study, there were nine knees that had been revised for infection, instability, or loosening. Average flexion in this group was 101 degrees. Of the original 129 knees, the authors were able to assess 64 of the original joints. They found 41% excellent, 36% good, 16% fair, and 7% poor results.

In 1988 researchers at Case Western Reserve also reported on a long-term study of Total Condylar prostheses.[12] Their paper dealt with arthroplasties performed between 1975 and 1979. They had 109 knees in 82 patients available for analysis. This initial cohort had been performed with an all-polyethylene tibial component. The knees were evaluated at an average of 9 years after arthroplasty. The authors used the rating system of the University Hospitals of Cleveland. This is somewhat different from The Hospital for Special Surgery scoring system. Overall results with this system were 34% excellent, 30% good, 9% fair, 11% poor, and 16% failed. Range of motion averaged 95 degrees. The authors noted a decline in scores at long-term follow-up from values found at an interim 4-year study. They also believed that this decline represented a general debilitation associated with the aging process, rather than a problem related to the knee arthroplasty. The report concluded that the Total Condylar implant was an excellent prosthesis, achieving consistent pain relief with predictable and durable results.

POSTERIOR STABILIZED PROSTHESIS

The Posterior Stabilized prosthesis was designed in the late 1970s in an effort to overcome some of the limitations of the Total Condylar design. The basic concept of substitution for the posterior cruciate ligament has proved extremely reliable over the ensuing years. While the specifics of the original design have undergone slight modifications over time, the basic philosophy behind this design remains unchanged.

Because of its extended history of use, there is abundant clinical evidence attesting to the results achieved with the posterior cruciate substitution design. These results, available from a multitude of centers, have been uniformly excellent,[1, 2, 9, 14, 16, 21, 35, 36, 44, 46, 50, 51] They refute the concern of many surgeons, who at the time of the implant's introduction, thought that the increased constraint of the device might result in an increased incidence of aseptic component loosening.[43]

The concept of posterior ligament substitution is now widely accepted, with many prosthesis manufacturers currently producing some version of a posterior-stabilized implant. The contemporary Posterior Stabilized implant is available in a modular format with metal backing of the tibial base plate. Modularity allows for the interchangeability of parts, and the addition of wedges, blocks, and rods to the basic implant construct. The implant persists as one of the few prosthesis with excellent long-term clinical results, and continues to offer a standard of comparison for the multitude of other designs.

Design Rationale

The rationale for substitution of the posterior cruciate ligament evolved over time as an outgrowth of results achieved with the original Total Condylar prosthesis. As already detailed, results with the Total Condylar were quite encouraging, but some functional shortcomings remained. Specifically, posterior subluxation in flexion occurred in some cases in which adequate ligamentous balance was not obtained. In addition, early reports demonstrated an average of "only" 90 degrees of knee flexion with the Total Condylar design.[22, 26]

The Posterior Stabilized prosthesis was developed in order to deal with these potential limitations. The designers of this new knee built a ligament-substituting mechanism directly into the construct of the prosthesis, while adhering to the basic principles that had made the Total Condylar prosthesis so successful. Thus, implantation of the Posterior Stabilized knee required sacrifice of both cruciate ligaments, and the use of bone cement to secure the components to the host bone. In addition, the Posterior Stabilized knee substituted for the posterior cruciate ligament by the interaction of a transverse femoral cam, and a polyethylene tibial spine. Ligament substitution was intended to improve stair-climbing ability, prevent posterior tibial subluxation, and enhance range of motion.

The Posterior Stabilized arthroplasty components encompassed a tibial articulating surface composed of conforming bicondylar wells. The shape of the tibial wells roughly corresponded to that of the femoral component. The tibial tray was posteriorly sloped, so that the component would more closely resemble the posterior angulation of the proximal portion of the tibia. This tilt was designed to improve flexion by helping to clear the posterior tibial condyles at maximum flexion angles and avoid edge-loading (Fig 65–5). The posterior slope also augmented knee stability, especially in resisting posterior subluxation, throughout the knee's arc of motion.

The actual ligament substitution mechanism of the Insall-Burstein prosthesis is unique to this particular prosthesis. The components are designed so that the cam will contact the tibial spine at about 70 degrees of flexion. At this point the cam and spine mechanism cause rollback of the femur and a posterior femoral tibial contact point. The mechanism also prevents subluxation of the components throughout the arc of motion. Of note is the fact that the cam has no effect on knee stability in extension, since it does not articulate at these lesser flexion angles. At these angles knee stability is dependent solely on soft tissue balance, the inherent conformity of the components, and the posterior slope. The ligament substitution mechanism does not prevent anterior tibial subluxation, nor does it substitute in any way for the collateral ligaments (Fig 65–6). Consequently, mediolateral stability of the arthroplasty is entirely dependent on intact collateral ligaments. In those cases in which the collateral ligaments are insufficient, and the knee is unstable to varus or valgus stress, the prosthesis will not provide sufficient support. These cases must be addressed with a constrained implant,

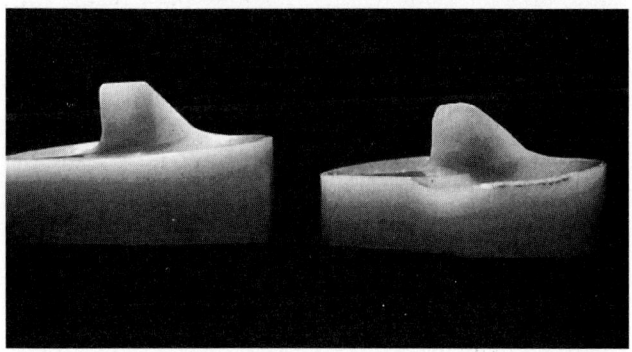

FIG 65–5.
An example of edge-loading wear.

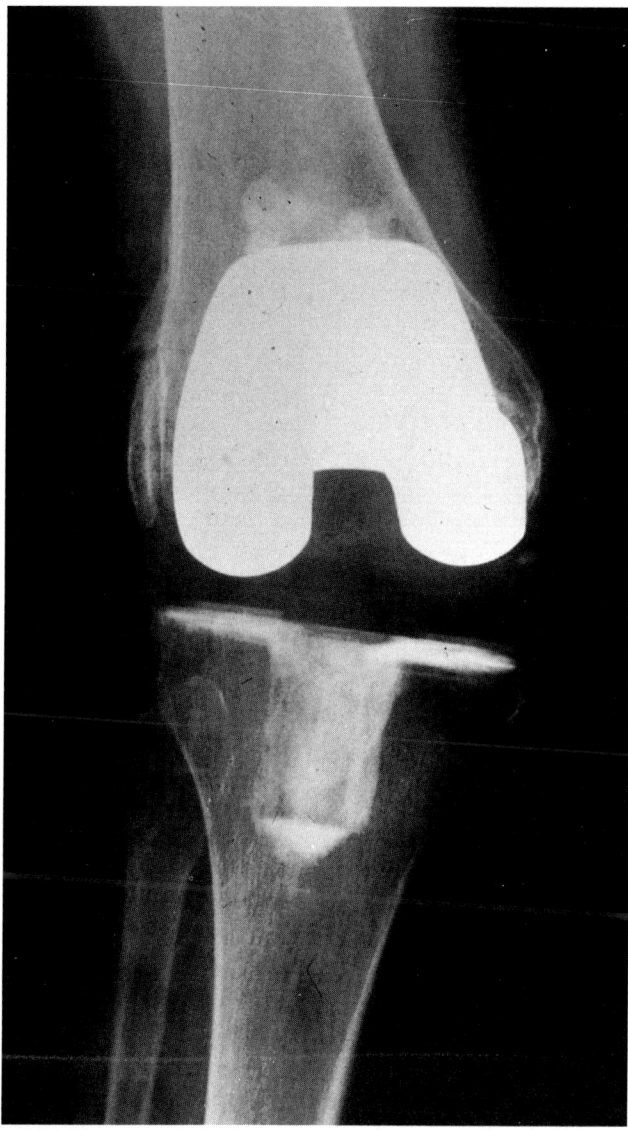

FIG 65–6.
The Posterior Stabilized prosthesis does not substitute for the collateral ligaments. Therefore, mediolateral stability must be achieved with adequate balance of these ligaments. Note the results of a Posterior Stabilized prosthesis implanted in a patient with medial collateral ligament insufficiency.

such as the Total Condylar type III or Constrained Condylar knee (CCK).

Since the particular ligament substitution mechanism for the Insall-Burstein prosthesis is patented,[4] other posterior-stabilized implants utilize slightly different mechanisms for posterior cruciate ligament substitution. Differences include variations in shape, placement, and height of the tibial spine. By changing these design parameters, other prostheses may have inherent anterior or mediolateral stability, as well as cam and spine contact throughout the entire range of knee motion.

The current Insall-Burstein II prosthesis retains the essential design features of the original Posterior Stabilized knee. It has undergone updating and modifications over the years. However, the basic mechanism for ligament substitution has remained essentially unchanged, and the current design adheres to the basic principles of ligament substitution.

INSALL-BURSTEIN POSTERIOR STABILIZED PROSTHESIS

Clinical Results

The Hospital for Special Surgery

Multiple reports on the clinical results achieved with the Posterior Stabilized prosthesis at The Hospital for Special Surgery have been published. Initial reports contributed preliminary results for the concept of cruciate substitution. Longer follow-up with this design philosophy is now available, as it has been in continuous use since the late 1970s (Table 65–2).

The earliest report on posterior cruciate ligament substitution appeared in 1981. Of note, the paper was misleadingly titled "The Correction of Knee Alignment in 225 Consecutive Total Condylar Knee Replacements."[16] In fact, the paper represents the initial report on posterior-stabilized arthroplasty. At that time the Posterior Stabilized prosthesis was referred to generically as a type of "total condylar" replacement. This problem was corrected and in future reports the prosthesis is properly designated as Posterior Stabilized. This initial article was a preliminary report on 225 knees. Its focus was the importance of soft tissue releases in knee arthroplasty. The thrust of the paper was that excellent correction of knees with severe malalignment could be achieved with this prosthesis. The authors dealt with clinical results in a cursory manner, mentioning three clinical failures. One failure was due to sepsis, while the other two were secondary to tibial component loosening in obese patients who had undergone revision-type procedures.

The first extensive report on the Posterior Stabilized knee was published in 1982.[21] This paper dealt with 118 Posterior Stabilized arthroplasties at 2- to 4-year follow-up. The Hospital for Special Surgery knee scoring system was used to evaluate the results: 88% were rated excellent, 9% were good or fair, and 3% were poor. Range of motion was 115 degrees, an average increase of 20 degrees from the preoperative value of 95 degrees. The authors believed that the Posterior Stabilized prosthesis achieved better function than the total Condylar had in previous reports. Seventy-six percent of patients with a Posterior Sta-

TABLE 65–2.
Posterior Stabilized (PS) Prosthesis: Comparison of Knee Scores*†

Institution‡	Prosthesis	Follow-up (yr)	No. of Knees	Rating (%)			
				Excellent	Good	Fair	Poor
HSS (1982)[21]	Original PS	2–4	118	88	8	1.0	3.0
HSS (1991)[51]	Original PS	9–12	194	61	26	6.0	7.0
HSS (1990)[50]	Modified PS	2–6	257	87.5	11	1.0	0.5
Lenox Hill (1986)[44]	Original PS	3–6	56	87	7	2.0	4.0
Lenox Hill (1988)[45]	Mixed group	2–8	119	83	15	0	2.0
University of Florence, Italy (1988)[1]	Mixed group	3–8	85	57	33	5.0	5.0
Case Western Reserve (1986)[1]	Original PS	2.5–5.0	116	65	23	3.0	9.0
Veterans Administration Hospital, Columbia, Mo.[14]	Mixed group	1–6	137	91	7	0.5	1.5

*Adapted from In Insall JN, editor: *Surgery of the knee*, ed 2, New York, 1993, Churchill Livingstone, pp Used by permission.
†Knees were judged by the The Hospital for Special Surgery rating system, except for the Case Western Reserve study, which uses the University Hospital of Cleveland rating system.
‡HSS = The Hospital for Special Surgery.

bilized arthroplasty attained what the authors called "normal function," as compared to 22% at that level of function after Total Condylar replacement.

Of concern was the surprisingly high incidence of patellar complications (11%) in this original report. There were stress fractures of ten (8.4%) patellae. While this was reason for concern, the vast majority of these (eight of ten) were asymptomatic and not associated with any quadriceps weakness or extensor lag. The fracture incidence appeared to be related to the size of the patellar button. The fracture rate was 13% with the use of a 38-mm prosthesis, and 7.7% with a 35-mm prosthesis. No fractures were noted in knees with a 32-mm component. As has been pointed out by others,[44] it is not clear if this difference is related to the size of the prosthesis or to the size and weight of the patient. Symptomatic patellar subluxation was reported in two knees (1.7%) that required reoperation. One knee with a peripatellar nodule required surgical excision to relieve anterior impingement against the femoral component's intercondylar box. Two other cases of presumed patellar impingement, both of which were asymptomatic at that time, were also mentioned.

Concern over the patellofemoral articulation was partially responsible for modification of the prosthesis in 1981. Changes included deepening the femoral component's patellar groove, and an alteration in the shape of the patellar flange. This resulted in the modified component having a more rounded anterior contour. The prosthesis was also made available in multiple sizes, in order to achieve better match between prosthesis and host bone. Finally, metal backing was added to the tibial base plate to enhance load transfer.

Stern and Insall[50] in 1990 reported on the results attained with the modified Posterior Stabilized prosthesis. Follow-up was available on 257 knees at 2 to 6 years postsurgery. Of these, 225 knees (87.5%) were rated as excellent, 28 were good (11%), 3 were fair (1.0%), and 1 was poor (0.5%). The poor result was in a knee that required revision after becoming secondarily infected from a urinary tract infection. Prior to the infection the knee had been rated excellent at follow-up of 5 years.

In this report, special attention was paid to the function of the patellofemoral joint, which was analyzed separately for each knee. Flexed knee symptoms that were believed referable to the patellofemoral joint were given a patellar score.[50] Grade 0 meant no symptoms; grade 1, a mild ache anteriorly, perceived only with stair climbing; and grade 2, moderate or severe pain with rising from a chair or pain that limits stair climbing to a nonreciprocal gait. Knees with patellar fractures were graded with the same criteria, but the fracture was also noted. The 213 knees (83%) that had no anterior knee complaints attributable to the patellofemoral joint were classified as grade 0. Forty-one knees (16%) were grade 1, and 3 (1%) knees were grade 2. There were four patellar fractures, and one loose patellar component without evidence of fracture. Interestingly, patellofemoral symptoms were found to be statistically higher in moderately and severely obese patients. Overall these results were considered to be encouraging, as the prosthesis continued to function well, while the incidence of severe patellofemoral problems was reduced. The decreased frequency of patellar problems served as confirmation that the prosthetic modifications had functioned as theorized.

The above papers detailed intermediate-term results for both the original and modified Posterior Stabilized arthroplasty. Long-term results are now available on the initial cohort of knee replacements with the original components.[51] Follow-up was attained on the 289 Posterior Stabilized knees (218 patients) implanted with an all-polyethylene tibial tray at The Hospital for Special Surgery. The average age of this group of patients was 66 years, ranging from 17 to 87 years. The patient population, as in other studies from The Hospital for Special Surgery, was predominately osteoarthritic (73%) and female (73%).

Each patient was assessed between 9 and 12 years post arthroplasty. There were 180 intact knee prostheses in 139 patients available for analysis. Fourteen knees (14 patients) had undergone revisions (Five patients with bilateral arthroplasties had one knee which required revision and an intact implant on the contralateral side.) Forty-eight patients (66 knees) had died prior to their 9-year follow-up. Twenty-nine knees (22 patients) were lost to follow-up prior to the 9-year evaluation.

The average age at arthroplasty was 63 years of the 194 knees studied, 117 knees (61%) were rated excellent, 51 (26%) good, 12 (6%) fair, and 14 (7%) poor. The average range of motion postoperatively was 110 degrees (range, 40–135 degrees) (Fig 65–7).

Fourteen Posterior Stabilized knees were revised because of failure of their index arthroplasty. Five of these required revision because of sepsis. These were treated by removal of the components, an extended course of intravenous antibiotics, and eventual reimplantation. This protocol was effective in four cases. The fifth knee became reinfected 26 months after reimplantation. This reinfection was treated with a successful knee arthrodesis after removal of the revision prosthesis. Two of the patients with septic loosening had acquired immunodeficiency syndrome. Six of the 14 revised knees had aseptic loosening of their tibial components, while the other three had femoral loosening. All of these aseptic loosenings were success-

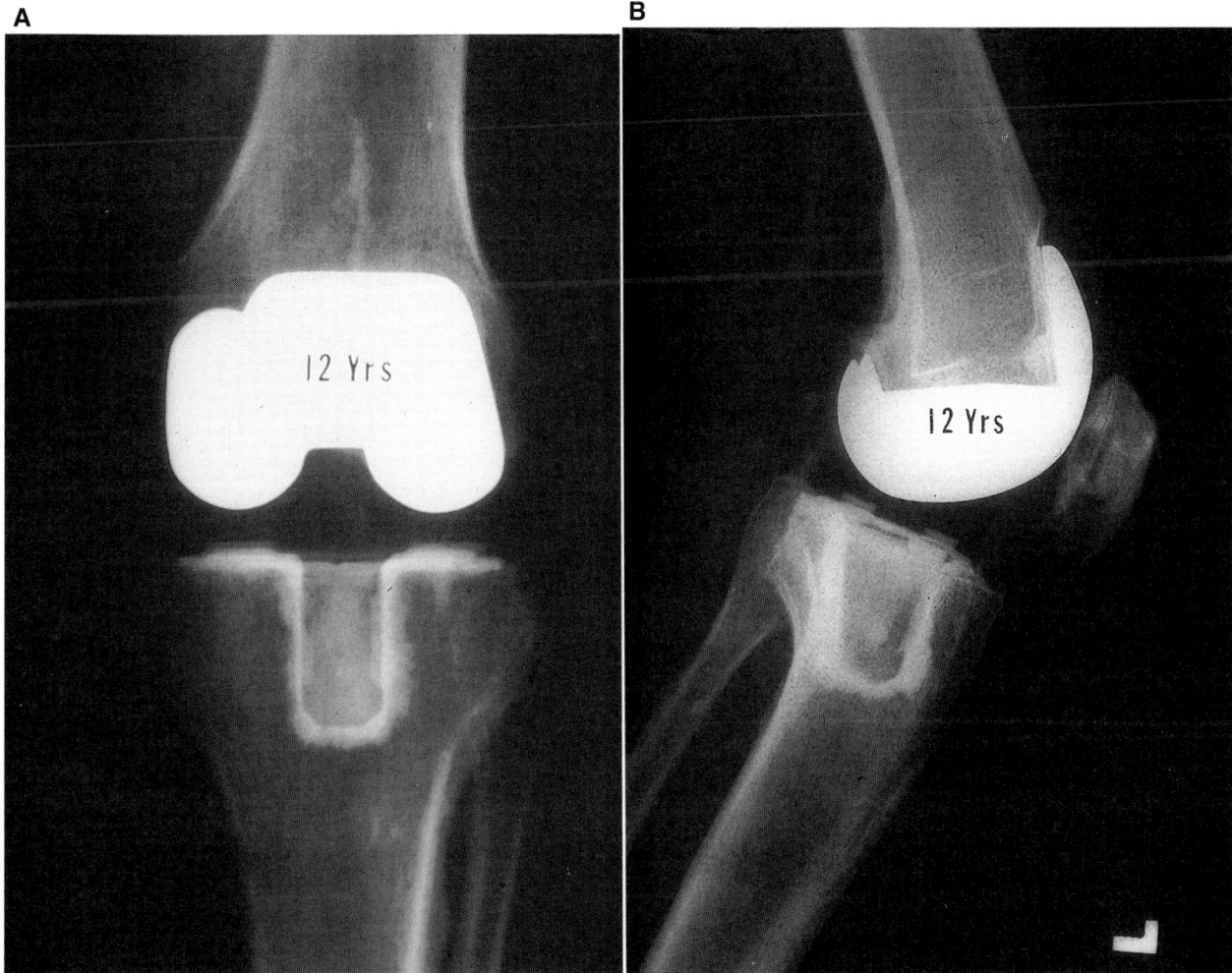

FIG 65–7.
A and **B,** Insall-Burstein Posterior Stabilized prosthesis at 12-year follow-up.

fully revised in one-stage procedures using components with intramedullary stems (Fig 65–8).

This study on long-term component function had fewer knees graded excellent (61%) than those in the original report[21] (88%) on Posterior Stabilized arthroplasty. In comparison, the original report dealt with a smaller group of patients with shorter (2–4 years) follow-up than seen in this long-term study. A possible explanation for this decline in percentage of excellent results is the increased age of patients at final follow-up (average, 73 years) in the long-term study. It would be expected that knee scores would decrease with advancing age as patient frailty increased. This phenomenon has been reported by other authors.[5, 12]

The intact prosthesis (180) was also rated with the new Knee Society scoring system.[28] This method classifies patients into one of three categories depending on their overall musculoskeletal status. In addition, each knee receives both a knee score, based on prosthetic knee function, and a function score, based on the patient's overall functional status. The average postoperative knee score was 92 (range, 35–100). The average function score was 66 (range, 0–100). Figure 65–9 demonstrates both knee and function scores stratified by patient musculoskeletal status. Utilizing this method, knee scores were similar among the three different patient categories. However, function scores declined for each subgroup as medical infirmity increased. This was an expected finding, in that the Posterior Stabilized prosthesis yielded relatively uniform results with respect to motion and pain relief, but functional results declined in patients with greater medical disabilities.

As in the study on the modified Posterior Stabilized prosthesis, special analysis of the patellofemo-

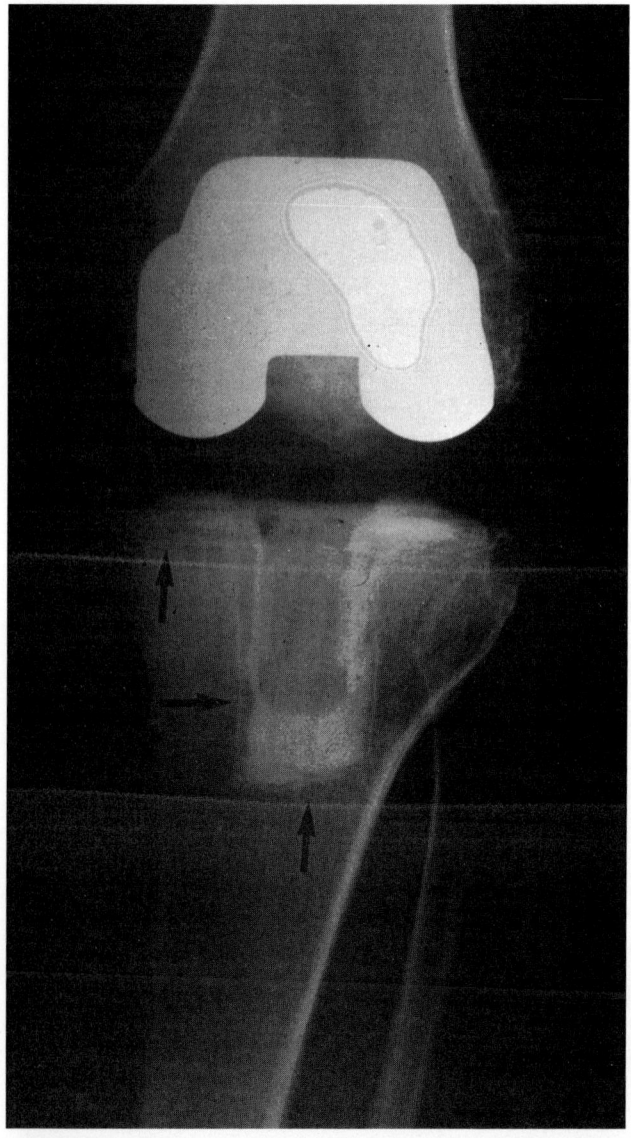

FIG 65–8.
Radiolucent zones *(arrows)* around an all-polyethelene tibial component.

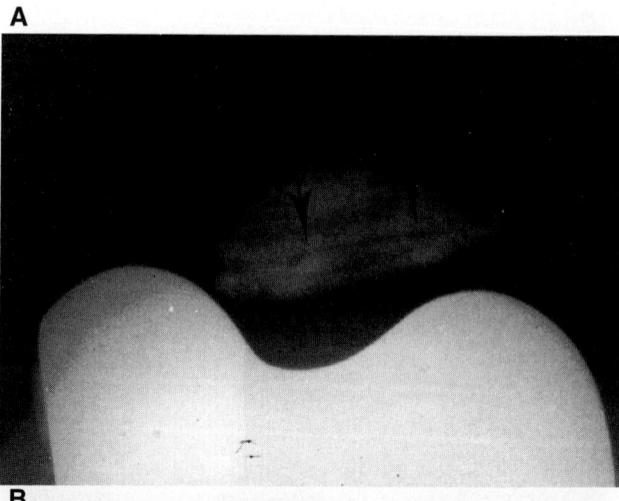

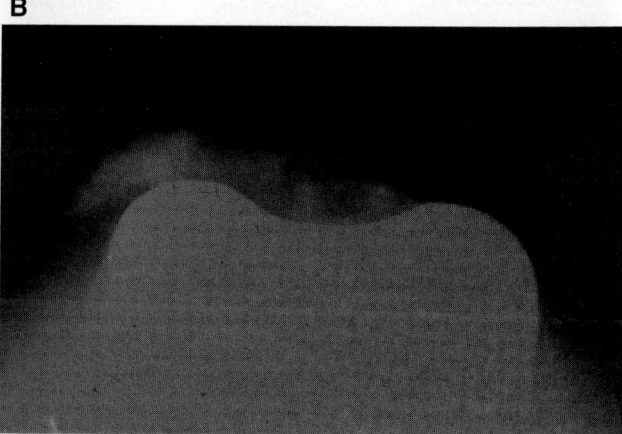

FIG 65–9.
Merchant view showing **(A)** patellar radiolucencies *(arrows)* and **(B)** a fractured patella.

ral articulation was carried out. The same scoring system used in the prior report for symptoms believed referable to the patellofemoral joint was employed[50] (Table 65-3). The clinical function of the patellofemoral articulation was grade 0 in 88%, grade 1 in 11%, and grade 2 in 1%. Consequently, 12% of knees had some degree of anterior knee complaints believed referable to the patellofemoral joint. Seven patellar fractures (4%) were noted in these 180 knees. All of these knees were asymptomatic at long-term follow-up and received a patellar grade of 0.

Other Institutions

Other institutions that have reported an extensive experience with the Posterior Stabilized prosthesis include Lenox Hill Hospital in New York City. A preliminary report was published in 1982,[46] and a more extensive analysis in 1986.[44] The latter evaluates results of 56 original Posterior Stabilized implants followed for 3 to 6 years. The average age (68 years) and predominantly osteoarthritic (79%) patient population are similar to those seen in other reports. Nevertheless, there was a relatively small percentage of women (53%) in this study. Analysis with The Hospital for Special Surgery score demonstrated 87% excellent, 7% good, 2% fair, and 4% poor results. A major area of concern remained the patellar component, with bony fractures in three cases (5%). As in the report from The Hospital for Special Surgery,[21] fractures were associated with larger patellar buttons, with all fractures occurring in knees with a 41-mm patellar dome.

Scott et al.[45] in 1988, reported results of a series of knees which included both the original and the modified version of the Posterior Stabilized prosthesis. Their series comprised 119 knees with follow-up ranging from 2 to 8 years (average, 5 years). The mean patient age was 67 years and once again the principal diagnosis was osteoarthritis (74%). Postoperative range of motion averaged 107 degrees. Eighty-three percent of the knees were rated as excellent, 15% as good, none were fair, and 2% were poor. Stratifying results by preoperative diagnosis showed that the patients with osteoarthritis attained statistically better outcomes than patients that had rheumatoid arthritis. In addition, a preoperative varus alignment was a statistical predictor of improved results, compared with knees with a preoperative valgus malalignment. There was 93% survival using survivorship analysis at 8 years. The authors also reported on a smaller subgroup of 41 knees followed to 6 years. In this subgroup, results were still satisfactory with 96% achieving a good or excellent result.

Aglietti and co-workers[1,2] reported on the University of Florence (Italy) experience with the Posterior Stabilized prosthesis in two similar studies published in 1988. The larger series[1] reviewed 85 knees, in which either the original or the modified implant was used. The average age in this population was 66.5 years. The patient population, as in other reports, was predominantly osteoarthritic (72%). Mean follow-up was 5 years (range, 3-8 years). Forty-nine knees (57%) had excellent, 28 had good (33%), 4 had fair (5%), and 4 (5%) had poor results.

TABLE 65-3.
Posterior Stabilized (PS) Prosthesis: Patellofemoral Problems*

Institution†	Prosthesis	Follow-up (yr)	Fracture(%)	Impingement(%) Mild	Impingement(%) Severe	Miscellaneous(%)
HSS (1982)[21]	Original PS	2-4	8.0		1	1.7‡
HSS (1992)[51]	Original PS	9-12	4.0	11	1	
HSS (1990)[50]	Modified PS	2-6	2.0	16	1	0.5§
Lenox Hill (1986)[44]	Original PS	3-6	5.0			
Lenox Hill (1988)[45]	Mixed group	2-8	5.0			
University of Florence, Italy (1988)[2]	Entire group	3.5-8.0	2.7	10	15	1.4‖
	Original PS			12	3	
	Modified PS					
Case Western Reserve[9]	Original Ps	2.5-8.0	2.5-5.0	5	7	
Veterans Administration Hospital Columbia, MO.[14]	Mixed group	1-6	0.7	21¶	0	0.7**

*Adapted from In Ingalls JN, editor: *Surgery of the knee*, ed 2, New York, 1993, Churchill Livingstone. Used by permission.
†HIS = The Hospital for Special Surgery.
‡Two knees with subluxation.
§One knee with a loose patelar component.
‖One knee with subluxation.
¶Includes all knees with mild postoperative pain (26 knees), as the authors stated that most patients with mild pain had anterior knee pain.
**One knee with patellar dislocation.

In the second report,[2] 73 knees were evaluated with specific attention to patellofemoral complaints. *Impingement,* which was defined as catching and locking occurring at 30 to 40 degrees of knee flexion, was found in 15 (21%) of knees. One knee was found to have a peripatellar synovial frond which was catching on the anterior edge of the femoral component's intercondylar box. This was the only case in which the symptoms were severe enough to require surgical intervention. The overall incidence of impingement symptoms decreased from 25% with the original design to 15% in knees implanted with the modified prosthesis. The authors believed that locking, which they classified as the most severe problem, also decreased, from 15% to 3%, after the change to the modified component. Only two patellar fractures were noted (one after a motor vehicle accident), and both were asymptomatic at the time of last follow-up.

The study by Figgie et al.[9] on the original Posterior Stabilized prosthesis correlated knee function with tibial and patellofemoral component location. In this report 116 implants were evaluated $2\frac{1}{2}$ to 5 years post surgery. Average age at arthroplasty was 65 years. Once again females (70%) and those with osteoarthritis (70%) predominated. A modified Mayo Clinic knee score was used to assess the knees. Evaluation with this rating system yielded 65% excellent, 23% good, 3% fair, and 9% poor results. Range of motion averaged 101 degrees. Patellofemoral symptoms were found in 12% of knees, with a subgroup making up 7% who had severe persistent symptoms requiring revision procedures. Radiographic and statistical analysis was used to define a *neutral range* for component implantation that would maximize clinical and functional results. The neutral range included posterior position of the prosthesis in the anteroposterior plane, a joint line change of less than 8 mm, and a patellar height of 10 to 30 mm. Of 41 knees that fell within this neutral range, 95% were rated excellent, and 5% were good. No knee within this region had patellofemoral symptoms. While these results are compelling, the concept of a neutral range has not been confirmed in other reports.[8]

Lombardi et al.[35] reported on the Columbus, Ohio experience of Thomas Mallory with the Posterior Stabilized arthroplasty. This study on 47 knees had 85% component survival at 6 years. The patient population was unremarkable with an average age of 67 years, with females (71%), and osteoarthritis (83%) predominant. The Hospital for Special Surgery mean knee score was 85, but results were not stratified into the four categories (excellent, good, fair, poor). The average arc of flexion was 97 degrees. There were four failures in this study: one deep infection, two aseptic component loosenings, and one stiff, chronically painful knee. No mention was made of patellar fractures.

Groh et al.[14] reported on their results in 137 Insall-Burstein Posterior Stabilized knee arthroplasties. This study was performed in patients at a Veterans Administration (VA) Hospital in Columbia, Missouri. The average age at arthroplasty was 61 years. Follow-up was from 1 to 6 years, with an average of 29 months. The authors reported 124 excellent results (91%), 11 good results (7%), 1 fair, and 3 poor results. There were three knees that underwent revision procedures. There were two aseptic tibial loosenings, and one had a deep infection. The authors reported that both of the aseptic loosenings were in obese patients. Mild pain complaints were found in 19% of knees, which was most often patellar in origin. Two percent of knees had moderate pain symptoms and no knee had severe pain. One patellar fracture (1%) and one asymptomatic lateral patellar dislocation was noted. Of particular note is that the overall excellent results seen in this report were achieved in a VA Hospital setting.

POSTERIOR CRUCIATE LIGAMENT SACRIFICE OR SUBSTITUTION

Clinical Function

Long-term results are now available for implants in which either posterior cruciate sacrifice (Total Condylar) or posterior cruciate substitution (Posterior Stabilized) concepts were employed. It is also possible to compare the results obtained with these methods with the results with implants in which efforts were made to retain the ligament. However, the difficulty in directly comparing results with different prostheses—the large number of confounding variables—must always be borne in mind. Confounding variables include possible differences in preoperative populations (diagnosis, age, extent of preoperative disease, etc.), institutional protocols, surgical skill and experience, and the knee evaluation methods employed. Nevertheless, comparisons are useful in critically examining implant function over time.

Long-term evaluation of both Total Condylar[59] and Posterior Stabilized[51] arthroplasties from the knee service at The Hospital for Special Surgery have been completed. Since both of these studies were done under the direction of the same senior author, are from the same institution, have similar patient populations, and employ similar evaluation methods, confounding variables are lessened. However, they still represent knee replacements performed over different time periods. The Total Condylar group of patients were implanted several years prior to the Posterior Stabilized cohort. Over this time span changes occurred outside of those related to the change in prosthetic design. Surgical instruments and technique continued to evolve. As the senior surgeon gained increased confidence and experience with successful knee arthroplasty, the indications for the procedure may have been modified, resulting in an increase in the different types of deformities undergoing reconstruction.[57]

The Total Condylar report[59] reviews the 10- to 12-year follow-up of 130 prostheses implanted from 1974 to 1975. The Posterior Stabilized study examines 289 knees operated on from 1978 to 1981. In the latter study, only the original prosthesis with an all-polyethylene tibial component is analyzed. The patient populations examined in the two reports are otherwise comparable, with similar ages, weights, diagnoses, and female predominance.

Results for 74 of the original 130 Total Condylar prostheses at 10 to 12 years postarthroplasty have been described. In 51% results were rated excellent, in 37% good, in 4% fair, and in 8% poor. The average flexion arc achieved was 91 degrees. This is in contrast to the results seen in the 194 Insall-Burstein Posterior Stabilized implants, evaluated at 9 to 12 years post surgery.[51] The results with this prosthesis were rated excellent in 61%, good in 26%, fair in 6% percent, and poor in 7%. The average range of motion for the Posterior Stabilized knees was 110 degrees.

Thus, 87% of the Posterior Stabilized implants achieved an excellent or good rating at long-term follow-up. This is the same rate of excellent and good results (88%) seen in the long-term Total Condylar study. There was a slight difference, in that 61% of Posterior Stabilized arthroplasties were in the excellent category, as contrasted with 51% of the Total Condylar replacements. The average flexion of the knees with the Total Condylar implant was 91 degrees, compared to 110 degrees in knees with the Posterior Stabilized design. Consequently, while both prostheses have yielded excellent results at extended follow-up, there is a slight trend to better motion and functional outcomes in knees utilizing a Posterior Stabilized device.

There are relatively few long-term results of cruciate-retaining knees to compare with the above results. Wright et al.[61] reviewed the Brigham and Women's Hospital (Boston) experience with the Kinematic I prosthesis (Howmedica, Rutherford, N.J.). In this report, 192 knees were followed for 5 to 9 years (average, 6 years). The cohort of patients in this study had a high percentage of rheumatoid arthritis (104/192, or 54%) compared with populations from The Hospital for Special Surgery. The Brigham knee scoring system was used to evaluate these arthroplasties. There were 59% excellent, 29% good, 6% fair, and 6% poor results. A more appropriate comparison may be gotten by examining only the subset of 85 patients with osteoarthritis. In this group, as might be expected, the results were significantly better: 71% excellent, 24% good, 4% fair, and 1% poor.

Ritter et al.[40] reported on survival results with posterior cruciate condylar knee arthroplasty. They found 94.6% survival at 10 years with this device in which the posterior cruciate ligament was retained. While this report is encouraging, it must still be viewed as preliminary. The paper is subtitled "A 10-year Evaluation," but the average follow-up period for the 394 knees examined was only 4.75 years. Ten-year data were available for only 31 knees, representing 8% of the total cohort. In addition, the authors mention four infections noticed less than 1 year after surgery, and these appear to have been deleted from the study. Inclusion of these knees would decrease the survival rates reported for all follow-up intervals. In contrast, septic knees are routinely counted as failures in survival studies on the Insall-Burstein Posterior Stabilized arthroplasty,[47, 51] and are not excluded from analysis.

Clinical Results of Posterior Substitution at Mayo Clinic

There have been only a few reports on the results with posterior-stabilized designs other than the Insall-Burstein prosthesis. In 1988, Hanssen and Rand[15] reported the Mayo Clinic experience with the Kinematic Stabilizer prosthesis (Howmedica, Rutherford, N.J.). The Kinematic Stabilizer prosthesis, like the Insall-Burstein, accomplishes cruciate substitution by the action of a central tibial post articulating with a femoral housing mechanism. The two prostheses differ otherwise in several ways. The Insall-Burstein prosthesis substitution mechanism engages only in knee flexion with the femoral cam impacting on the tibial spine causing femoral rollback. This design allows for an increased range of motion, an improved lever arm for the quadriceps, and prevention of posterior tibial subluxation. In contrast, the Kinematic Stabilizer has a central tibial post residing within the femoral housing which restrains anterior, as well as posterior, motion of the tibia between 0 and 30 degrees of flexion. At flexion angles greater than 30 degrees, as in the Insall-Burstein prosthesis, the substituting mechanism replicates only the function of the posterior cruciate ligament in enhancing femoral rollback. Neither design substitutes for the collateral ligament.

The report by Hanssen and Rand[15] involved 79 arthroplasties (66 patients) with an average follow-up of 37 months. There were 53 revisions and 26 primary arthroplasties in their series. Postoperatively, of the entire group, 34 knees (43%) were rated excellent, 33 (42%) good, 7 (9%) fair, and 5 (6%) poor. However, in this group of knees a majority were undergoing revision procedures. Separate analysis of the results of the 26 knees undergoing index procedures revealed 54% with excellent results, 38% good, 4% fair, and 4% poor. Postoperative range of motion averaged 101 degrees.

Of note, despite the good results reported in this series, the patient population differed from the population implanted with Insall-Burstein Posterior Stabilized knees at The Hospital for Special Surgery. Since the Mayo Clinic surgeons are advocates of posterior cruciate ligament retention, cases in which a substituting mechanism is employed at their institution are either revisions or index arthroplasties performed in knees with instability or malalignment. Preoperatively, moderate or severe instability was present in 42% of their knees, while 12 of the 26 primary knees had preoperative flexion contractures greater than 10 degrees. In addition, the diagnoses were osteoarthritis in 37 knees, rheumatoid arthritis in 36 knees, and posttraumatic arthritis in 6 knees. They had a relatively high percentage of patients with rheumatoid or traumatic arthritis in their series, because they reserved the use of this prosthesis for their most difficult cases.

The results must therefore be viewed with the knowledge that knees with inflammatory arthropathy,[22, 31, 53] posttraumatic arthritis,[65] or with a preoperative valgus alignment[52] tend not to achieve as satisfactory results as knees with minimal deformity and osteoarthritis. Therefore, although the 92% excellent and good results seen with the Kinematic Stabilizer in knees undergoing index arthroplasty is encouraging, one would expect even superior outcomes if this prosthesis had been used routinely, as is done in other institutions.

Survivorship Analysis

Survivorship analysis has been advocated by many as a way to evaluate the results of joint arthroplasties.[6, 13, 33, 34, 47, 54, 55] Long-term survival curves have been generated for both the Total Condylar and Posterior Stabilized prostheses in the standard fashion of Armitage. *Success* is defined as a prosthesis still in place at the end of any interval. *Failure* is defined as a prosthetic revision for any reason, or an implant in which revision has been recommended for any reason.

The survival table for the Total Condylar prosthesis at long-term follow-up has been generated by Vince.[57] This prosthesis yielded a survival rate of 93% at 11 years, with an average annual failure rate of 0.6%[57] (Table 65–4). The survival table for the original Posterior Stabilized prosthesis with an all-polyethylene tibial component was generated in the comprehensive long-term study[51] (Table 65–5). This prosthesis had an average annual failure rate of 0.4% and a 12-year overall success rate of 94%.

In a separate report, Scuderi et al.[47] generated survival curves for all knees (Total Condylar, Posterior Stabilized with an all-polyethylene tibial component, Posterior Stabilized with a metal-backed tibial component) implanted on the knee service at The Hospital for Special Surgery. In this study, 224 Total Condylar arthroplasties were entered into the table and yielded a success rate of 91% at 15 years. Preliminary survival curves for 917 Posterior Stabilized prostheses with a metal-backed tibial tray were also constructed. The survival percentage for this prosthesis was 99% at 7 years with an annual failure rate of 0.2%.

Analysis of the long-term survival curves reveals that they are essentially identical for the all-polyethylene Posterior Stabilized prosthesis and for the Total Condylar design. However, the Posterior Stabilized design achieved improved functional outcomes as discussed above. Despite the concern expressed by some regarding the inherent constraint with the Posterior Stabilized prosthesis,[43] there is no evidence from the survival data that long-term substitution for the posterior cruciate ligament causes failure at the bone-cement interface.

Complications of Posterior Cruciate Substitution

Complications are inherent with total knee arthroplasty, as they are with other surgical procedures. However, there are certain problems which are relatively peculiar to substitution for the posterior cruciate ligament. Posterior cruciate substitution prevents subluxation of the knee, which can occur with retention of an incompetent posterior cruciate ligament. This is precluded by the stability provided by the design's interaction between the femoral cam and the tibial spine. However, while the problem of subluxation of the components is essentially eliminated (Fig 65–10), there does exist the possibility of anterior dislocation of the femoral cam over the tibial spine.

TABLE 65-4.
Survivorship Analysis of the Posterior Stabilized Prosthesis*

Follow-up Interval X to X + 1 (yr)	No. of Knees at Start of Each Interval	No. of Failures During Interval	No. of Knees Withdrawn†	No. of Knees at Risk‡	Predicted Annual Percentage		Cumulative Survival Percent at X Years
					Failure	Survival	
0-1	289	1	6	286.0	0.3	99.7	100.0
1-2	282	3	9	277.5	1.1	98.9	99.7
2-3	270	2	11	264.5	0.8	99.2	98.6
3-4	257	1	9	252.5	0.4	99.6	97.8
4-5	247	1	5	244.5	0.4	99.6	97.4
5-6	241	0	10	236.0	0.0	100.0	97.0
6-7	231	0	14	224.0	0.0	100.0	97.0
7-8	217	1	14	210.0	0.5	99.5	97.0
8-9	202	2	12	196.0	1.0	99.0	96.6
9-10	188	2	32	172.0	1.2	98.8	95.6
10-11	154	1	90	109.0	0.9	99.1	94.5
11-12	63	0	54	36.0	0.0	100.0	93.6
12-13	9	0	9	4.5	0.0	100.0	93.6

*Adapted from In Insall JN, editor: *Surgery of the knee,* ed 2, New York, 1993, Churchill Livingstone. Used by permission.
†Lost to follow-up.
‡These are the average number at risk during each time interval calculated as follows: Number of knees at start of interval minus the number withdrawn divided by half.

TABLE 65-5.
Survivorship Analysis of Total Condylar Prosthesis*

Follow-up Interval X to X + 1 (yr)	No. of Knees at Start of Each Interval	No. of Failures During Interval	No. of Knees Withdrawn†	No. at Risk‡	Predicted Annual Percentage		Cumulative Survival Percent at X Years
					Failure	Survival	
0-1	130	0	5	127.5	0.0	100.0	100.0
1-2	125	1	14	118.0	0.8	99.2	100.0
2-3	110	0	5	107.5	0.0	100.0	99.2
3-4	105	0	0	105.0	0.0	100.0	99.2
4-5	105	1	19	95.5	1.0	99.0	99.2
5-6	85	1	4	83.0	1.2	98.8	98.2
6-7	80	1	0	80.0	1.3	98.7	97.0
7-8	79	0	2	78.0	0.0	100.0	95.7
8-9	77	2	2	76.0	2.6	97.4	95.7
9-10	73	0	31	57.5	0.0	100.0	93.2
10-11	42	0	36	24.0	0.0	100.0	93.2
11-12	6	0	6	3.0	0.0	100.0	93.2

*Adapted from In Insall JN, editor: Surgery of the knee, ed 2, New York, 1993, Churchill Livingstone. Used by permission.
†Lost to follow-up.
‡These are the average number at risk during each time interval calculated as follows: Number of knees at start of interval minus the number withdrawn divided by half.

Dislocations have been reported with both the Insall-Burstein Posterior Stabilized arthroplasty[10, 36] and the Kinematic II Stabilizer prosthesis.[11] It is not surprising that this problem has been seen with these two designs, because they are the oldest and most widely used of the currently available posterior-substituting designs.

The exact mechanism of dislocation is somewhat controversial in that it is unclear if this phenomenon occurs with the knee in mild flexion with a straight posterior mechanism, or occurs at high flexion angles with a combination of posterior and rotatory stress.[35] Dislocations have happened in knees with a preoperative valgus alignment[10, 11] and in knees status post patellectomy.[11] While preoperative valgus alignment apparently does increase the possibility of this problem, dislocations have also been reported in varus alignment.

A dislocated implant normally presents with the acute inability to extend the knee. Dislocations can occur during sleep, causing the patient to awaken with a sudden limitation to knee extension. In many instances, the patient is unable to explain the exact mechanism, nor the position of the knee, when the actual dislocation occurred. There is usually an obvious knee deformity that can be found on inspection of the knee. Radiographs reveal the femoral cam translated anteriorly to the polyethylene tibial spine.

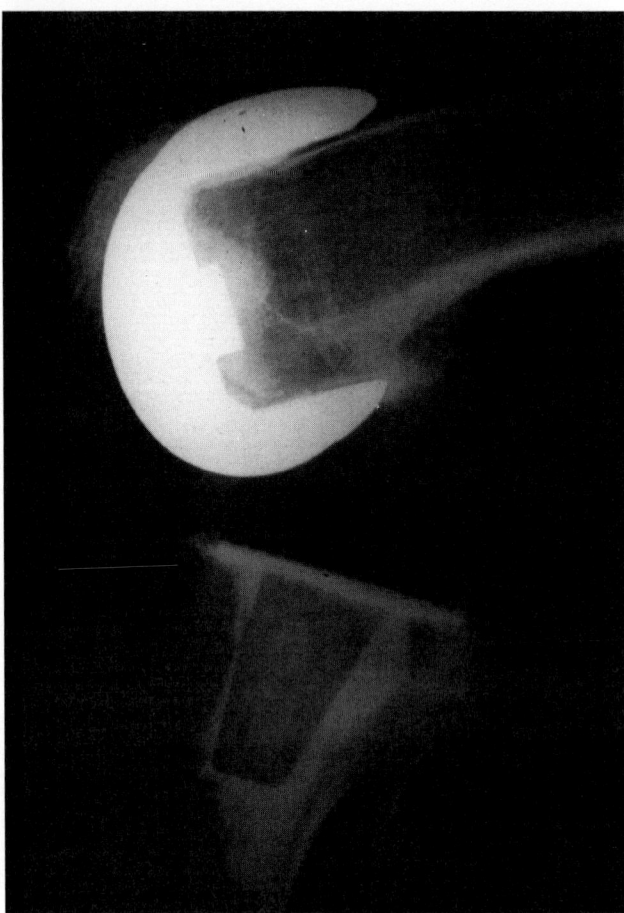

FIG 65–10.
Dislocation of early posterior cruciate–sacrificing designs is virtually eliminated with the posterior-stabilized design.

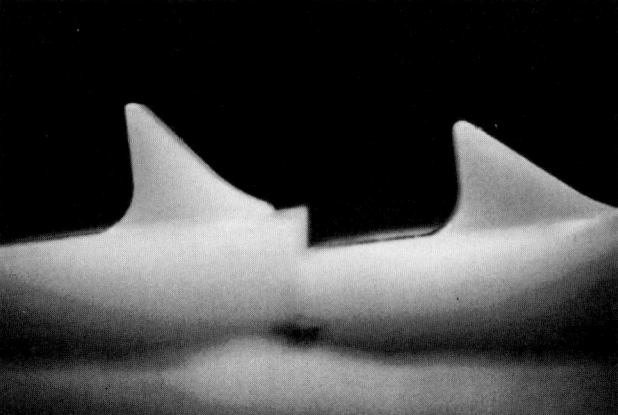

FIG 65–11.
Modification of the Insall-Burstein II arthroplasty. The height of the tibial spine was increased and its location of tibial plastic was moved further anterior. The original Insall-Burstein plastic is on the *left;* the modified plastic is on the *right.*

Dislocations were rare with the original Insall-Burstein prosthesis. The introduction of the Insall-Burstein II prosthesis, however, coincided with an increased incidence of this problem. Six dislocations occurred in the first 600 implants done at The Hospital for Special Surgery with the Insall-Burstein II prosthesis. The patients in whom dislocations occurred tended to be those who had achieved excellent postoperative results with flexion angles greater than 120 degrees. These dislocations were treated with closed reduction and bracing, in order to prevent flexion greater than 90 degrees for several weeks. This conservative regimen was successful in a majority of cases, but two patients required revision of the tibial polyethylene to a thicker size.

Because of this issue, the tibial polyethylene was modified. This was accomplished by increasing the height of the tibial spine and moving it anteriorly (Fig 65–11). These alterations were undertaken to increase the inherent stability of the Posterior Stabilized prosthesis. Subsequent to this modification, there has not been a dislocation in the next 400 knees implanted at The Hospital for Special Surgery.

In order to minimize the problem of knee dislocations, it is important that the surgeon strive to balance the knee in both flexion and extension. While this should be done in all cases, knees with a preoperative valgus deformity may require special attention. In addition, therapists should be instructed that it may be undesirable to achieve large flexion angles (greater than 100 degrees) in the immediate postoperative period.

CONCLUSION

The concept of cruciate sacrifice has proved to be a versatile and durable concept in the success of knee arthroplasty. This was first seen with the Total Condylar prosthesis, which encompassed sacrifice of both cruciate ligaments. The Posterior Stabilized prosthesis eventually supplanted the Total Condylar, incorporating the concept of posterior substitution. Both designs have stood the test of time and achieved excellent long-term clinical results. Concern that the inherent increased constraint of these designs would lead to an increased incidence of component loosening has proved unfounded.

Posterior cruciate ligament substitution has yielded increased range of motion of the knee, prevention of posterior tibial subluxation, and improved clinical function without sacrifice of long-term component survival. With the advent of modular components (see Fig 65–11) the surgeon can customize the arthroplasty at the time of surgery. This allows the surgeon to obtain the benefits of posterior cruciate substitution, while meeting the needs of the individual patient.

REFERENCES

1. Aglietti P, Buzzi R: Posterior stabilized total condylar knee replacement. Three to eight years' follow-up of 85 knees, *J Bone Joint Surg [Br]* 70:211, 1988.
2. Aglietti P, Buzzi R, Gaudeni A: Patellofemoral functional results and complications with the posterior stabilized total condylar knee prosthesis, *J Arthroplasty* 3:17–25, 1988.
3. Bartel DL, et al: Performance of the tibial component in total knee replacement. Conventional and revision designs, *J Bone Joint Surg [Am]* 64A:1026–1033, 1982.
4. Burstein AH, Insall JN: Posteriorly stabilized total knee joint prosthesis, US Patent 4,298,992.
5. Cohn BT, et al: Results of total knee arthroplasty in patients 80 years and older, *Orthop Rev* 19:451–460, 1990.
6. Dobbs HS: Survivorship of total hip replacements, *J Bone Joint Surg [Br]* 62:168–173, 1980.
7. Ecker ML, et al: Long term results after total condylar knee arthroplasty, *Clin Orthop* 216:151–158, 1987.
8. Faris PM, Insall JN, Stern SH: Patellar symptoms in the posterior stabilized knee: A critical analysis. 57th Annual Meeting of the Academy of Orthopaedic Surgeons. New Orleans, 1990.
9. Figgie HE, et al: The influence of tibiopatellofemoral location on function of the knee in patients with the posterior stabilized condylar knee prosthesis, *J Bone Joint Surg [Am]* 68:1035–1040, 1986.
10. Galinat BJ, et al: Dislocation of the posterior stabilized total knee arthroplasty. A report of two cases, *J Arthroplasty* 3:363–367, 1988.
11. Gebhard JS, Kilgus DJ: Dislocation of a posterior stabilized total knee prosthesis. A report of two cases, *Clin Orthop* 254:225–229, 1990.
12. Goldberg VM, et al: Use of a total condylar knee prosthesis for treatment of osteoarthritis and rheumatoid arthritis. Long-term results, *J Bone Joint Surg [Am]* 70:802–811, 1988.
13. Grimer RJ, Karpinski MRK, Edwards AN: The long-term results of Stanmore total knee replacements, *J Bone Joint Surg [Br]* 66:55–62, 1984.
14. Groh GI, et al: Results of total knee arthroplasty using the posterior stabilized condylar prosthesis. A report of 137 consecutive cases, *Clin Orthop* 269:58–62, 1991.
15. Hanssen AD, Rand JA: A comparison of primary and revision total knee arthroplasty using the Kinematic stabilizer prosthesis, *J Bone Joint Surg [Am]* 70:491–499, 1988.
16. Hood RW, Vanni M, Insall JN: The correction of knee alignment in 225 consecutive total condylar knee replacements, *Clin Orthop* 160:94, 1981.
17. Howie DW, et al: A rat model of resorption of bone at the cement-bone interface in the presence of polyethylene wear particles, *J Bone Joint Surg [Am]* 70:257, 1988.
18. Hvid I, Nielson S: Total condylar knee arthroplasty: Prosthetic component positioning and radiolucent lines, *Acta Orthop Scand* 55:160–165, 1984.
19. Hvid I, et al: Knee arthroplasty in rheumatoid arthritis: Four to six year follow-up study, *J Arthroplasty* 2:233–239, 1987.
20. Insall JN, Kelly M: The total condylar prosthesis, *Clin Orthop* 205:43–48, 1985.
21. Insall JN, Lachiewicz PF, Burstein AH: The posterior stabilized condylar prosthesis: A modification of the total condylar design, *J Bone Joint Surg [Am]* 64:1317–1323, 1982.
22. Insall JN, Scott WN, Ranawat CS: The total condylar knee prosthesis. A report of two hundred and twenty cases, *J Bone Joint Surg [Am]* 61:173–180, 1979.
23. Insall JN, Tria AJ: The total condylar knee prosthesis type II, Annual Meeting of the American Academy of Orthopaedic Surgeons, San Francisco, 1979.
24. Insall JN, Tria AJ, Scott WN: The total condylar knee prosthesis: The first 5 years, *Clin Orthop* 145:68–77, 1979.
25. Insall JN, et al: Total condylar knee replacement. Preliminary report, *Clin Orthop* 120:149–154, 1976.
26. Insall JN, et al: The total condylar knee prosthesis in gonarthrosis. A five to nine-year follow-up of the first one hundred consecutive replacements, *J Bone Joint Surg [Am]* 65:619–628, 1983.
27. Insall JN, et al: Total knee arthroplasty, *Clin Orthop* 192:13, 1985.
28. Insall JN, et al: Rationale of the Knee Society clinical rating system, *Clin Orthop* 248:13, 1989.
29. Landy MD, Walker PS: Wear of ultra-high molecular weight polyethylene components of ninety retrieved knee prostheses, *J Arthroplasty* 3(suppl 1):S73, 1988.
30. Laskin RS: Total condylar knee replacement in rheumatoid arthritis, *J Bone Joint Surg [Am]* 63:29–35, 1981.
31. Laskin RS: Total condylar knee replacement in patients who have rheumatoid arthritis. A ten-year follow-up study, *J Bone Joint Surg [Am]* 72:529–535, 1990.
32. Laskin RS, et al: The posterior stabilized total knee prosthesis in the knee with a severe fixed deformity, *Am J Knee Surg* 1:199, 1988.
33. Lettin AWF, et al: Assessment of the survival and the clinical results of Stanmore total knee replacements, *J Bone Joint Surg [Br]* 66:355–361, 1984.
34. Lewallen DG, Bryan RS, Peterson LFA: Polycentric total knee arthroplasty. A ten-year follow-up study, *J Bone Joint Surg [Am]* 66:1211–1218, 1984.
35. Lombardi AV, et al: Six year survivorship analysis of the Insall-Burstein posterior stabilized knee: A clinical and radiographic evaluation, *Orthop Trans* 12:711, 1988.

36. Lombardi AV, et al: Dislocation following primary posterior stabilized total knee arthroplasty, 58th Annual Meeting of the American Academy of Orthopaedic Surgeons, Anaheim, Calif, 1991.
37. Ranawat CS, Boachie-Adjei O: Survivorship analysis and results of total condylar knee arthroplasty. Eight- to eleven-year follow-up period, *Clin Orthop* 226:6–13, 1988.
38. Ranawat CS, Hansraj KK: Effect of posterior cruciate sacrifice on durability of the cement-bone interface, *Orthop Clin North Am* 20:63–69, 1989.
39. Revell PA, et al: The production and biology of polyethylene wear debris, *Arch Orthop Trauma Surg* 91:167, 1978.
40. Ritter MA, et al: Long-term survival analysis of the posterior cruciate condylar total knee arthroplasty, *J Arthroplasty* 4:293–296, 1989.
41. Schurman DJ, Parker JN, Ornstein D: Total condylar knee replacement: A study of factors influencing range of motion as late as two years after arthroplasty, *J Bone Joint Surg [Am]* 67:1006–1014, 1985.
42. Schurman JR, Borden LS, Wilde AH: Long term results of total condylar knee prosthesis, *Orthop Trans* 11:443, 1987.
43. Scott RD, Volatile TB: Twelve years' experience with posterior cruciate retaining total knee arthroplasty, *Clin Orthop* 205:100–107, 1986.
44. Scott WN, Rubinstein M: Posterior stabilized knee arthroplasty: Six year experience, *Clin Orthop* 205:138–145, 1986.
45. Scott WN, Rubinstein M, Scuderi G: Results after knee replacement with a posterior cruciate-substituting prosthesis, *J Bone Joint Surg [Am]* 70:1163–1173, 1988.
46. Scott WN, Schosheim P: Posterior stabilized knee arthroplasty, *Orthop Clin North Am* 20:71, 1982.
47. Scuderi GR, et al: Survivorship of cemented knee replacement, *J Bone Joint Surg [Br]* 71:798–803, 1989.
48. Sledge CB, Walker PS: Total knee replacement in rheumatoid arthritis. Insall JN, editor: *Surgery of the knee.* New York, 1984, Churchill Livingstone, pp 697–715.
49. Sneppen O, Gudmundsson GH, Bunger C: Patellofemoral function in total condylar arthroplasty, *Int Orthop* 9:65–68, 1985.
50. Stern SH, Insall JN: Total knee arthroplasty in obese patients, *J Bone Joint Surg [Am]* 72:1400–1404, 1990.
51. Stern SH, Insall JN: Posterior stabilized prosthesis: Results after 9–12 years follow-up, *J Bone Joint Surg [Am]* 74:980–986, 1992.
52. Stern SH, Moeckel BH, Insall JN: Total knee arthroplasty in valgus knees, *Clin Orthop* 273:5–8, 1991.
53. Stern SH, et al: Total knee arthroplasty in patients with psoriasis, *Clin Orthop* 248:108–111, 1989.
54. Tew M, Waugh W: Estimating the survival time of knee replacements, *J Bone Joint Surg [Br]* 64:579–582, 1982.
55. Tew M, Waugh W, Forster IW: Comparing the results of different types of knee replacement. A method proposed and applied, *J Bone Joint Surg [Br]* 67:775–779, 1985.
56. Tauber C, et al: The total condylar knee prosthesis: A review of 71 operations, *Arch Orthop Trauma Surg* 104:352–356, 1986.
57. Vince KG: The posterior stabilized knee prosthesis. *In* Laskin RS, editor: *Total knee replacement,* New York, 1991, Springer-Verlag, pp 113–149.
58. Vince KG, Insall JN: The total condylar knee prosthesis. *In* Laskin RS, editor: *Total knee replacement,* New York, 1991, Springer-Verlag, pp 85–111.
59. Vince KG, et al: The total condylar prosthesis: 10 to 12 year results of a cemented knee replacement, *J Bone Joint Surg [Br]* 71:793–797, 1989.
60. Walker PS: The total condylar knee and its evolution. *In* Ranawat CS, editor: *Total condylar knee arthroplasty, technique, results and complications,* New York, 1985, Springer-Verlag, pp 7–16.
61. Wright J, et al: Total knee arthroplasty with the Kinematic prosthesis, *J Bone Joint Surg [Am]* 72:1003–1009, 1990.
62. Wright TM, Bartel DL: The problem of surface damage in polyethylene total knee components, *Clin Orthop* 205:67, 1986.
63. Wright TM, et al: Failure of carbon fiber–reinforced polyethylene total knee replacement components. A report of two cases, *J Bone Joint Surg [Am]* 70:926–932, 1988.
64. Wright TM, et al: Analysis of surface damage in retrieved carbon fiber–reinforced and plain polyethylene tibial components from posterior stabilized total knee replacements, *J Bone Joint Surg [Am]* 70:1312–1319, 1988.
65. Zelicof SB, et al: Total knee arthroplasty in post-traumatic arthritis, *Orthop Trans* 12:547–548, 1988.

66

Ligament Releases in the Arthritic Knee

FRANCIS D'AMBROSIO, M.D.
W. NORMAN SCOTT, M.D.

Anatomy
Balancing
  Varus deformity

Valgus deformity
Flexion contracture
Conclusion

Soft tissue contractures around the knee joint are adaptive ligamentous changes which invariably occur in advanced arthritic disease.[6, 9] Bone and cartilage deficiency initiates a shortening of the capsule and periarticular soft tissue. Akeson et al.[1] studied the etiology of joint contractures and found that the fibrous capsular structures of the knee contain collagen fibers oriented in a crisscross weave. By immobilizing the knee joint (stress deprivation), the capsular and ligamentous supporting structures had an increased collagen turnover and degradation, decreased collagen mass, increased reducible collagen cross-links, and reduced glycosaminoglycans and water. The collagen disorientation led to decreased motion and shortening of the tissue.[2]

Blinkley and Peat[3] studied the effects of immobilization on the ultrastructural and mechanical properties of rat medial collateral ligaments. They concluded that the capsule contributes to contracture while ligaments decrease in stiffness. It appears that bone and cartilage loss initiate a pain- or instability-induced lack of motion which causes a shortening of the adjacent soft tissues.

A contracture can occur singly or in combination on the medial, lateral, or posterior aspects of the knee, depending on the location of the bone and cartilage loss.[6, 9] In the case of osteoarthritis, the loss is usually asymmetric and medial. In an attempt to redistribute forces across a larger surface area, osteophytes (reparative bone and cartilage) are formed. Although osteophytes increase the absolute surface area of the joint, they add further to the adjacent capsular shortening, thereby creating a vicious circle.

The medial bone loss and osteophyte formation seen in osteoarthritis alter the physiologic balance of the knee joint and lead to a shortening of the medial collateral ligament (Fig 66–1). Consequently, the lateral collateral ligament and capsule are elongated by the stresses of ambulation on a contracted medial compartment. The end result of these adaptive changes is a varus contracture, the most common angular contracture seen in patients undergoing total knee arthroplasty.[12, 13]

Similar physiologic events occur in the lateral compartment of the knee although with far less frequency. Bone and cartilage loss, osteophyte formation, lateral capsular shortening, and medial collateral ligament stretching does occur in some cases of osteoarthritis. Valgus contracture, however, is more often seen in the symmetric, synovitis-induced joint destruction of rheumatoid arthritis. Characteristically, in rheumatoid arthritis, lateral capsular contracture proceeds to include the iliotibial band (ITB), thereby adding an external rotational component to the valgus deformity[6] (Fig 66–2).

Flexion contractures occur in a fashion similar to a varus or valgus deformity. Bone and cartilage loss, osteophytes, and immobilization lead to a posterior capsular shortening and extension loss. Flexion contractures occur in both osteoarthritis and rheumatoid arthritis with the more extreme cases found in the latter condition.[22]

ANATOMY

In order to fully understand the rationale for soft tissue release and balancing about the knee joint, it is necessary to familiarize oneself with the anatomy of

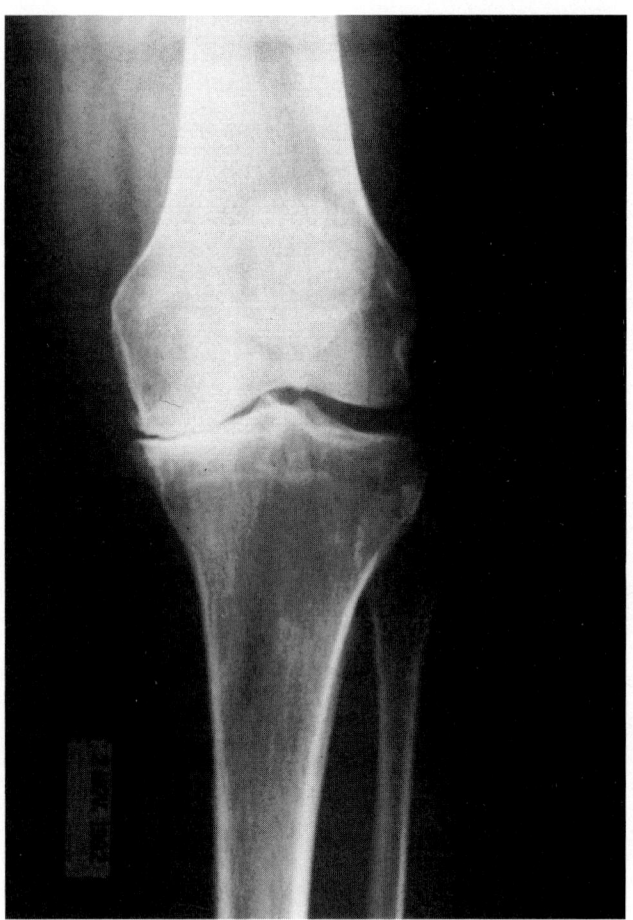

FIG 66–1.
Roentgenogram of a varus knee. In addition to the medial compartment narrowing, flattening, and osteophyte formation, the medial soft tissue structures will often develop a compensating contracture.

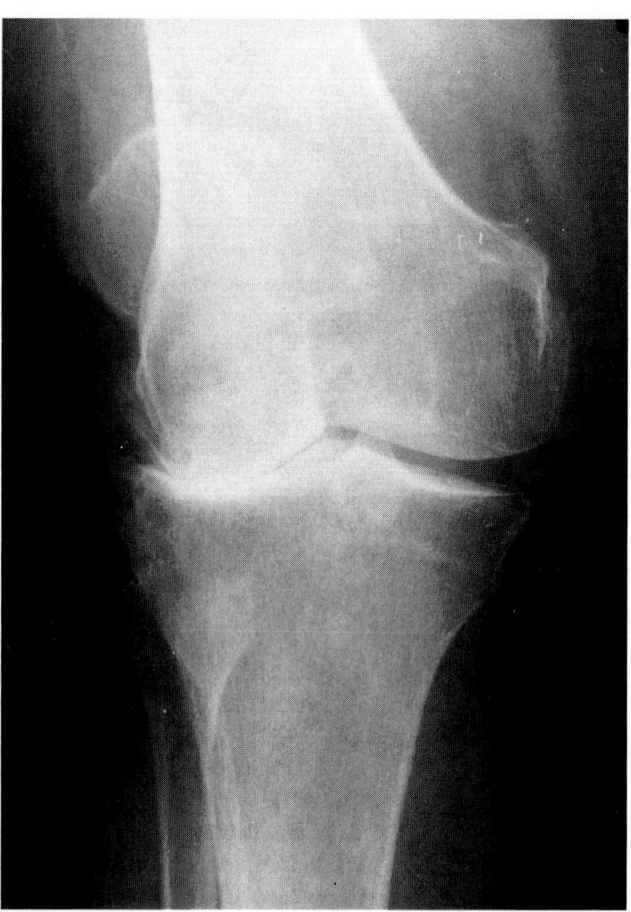

FIG 66–2.
In the valgus knee, the lateral compartment arthritic changes are often accompanied by lateral soft tissue contractures and medial lengthening.

the area. The soft tissue envelope which surrounds the knee consists of a joint capsule, ligaments, fascia, and musculotendinous units.[7, 10, 19, 25]

The anatomy of the medial aspect of the knee was described by Warren and Marshall as having three layers.[24] Layer 1 consists of the deep or crural fascia. Layer 2 contains the superficial medial collateral ligament and layer 3, the deep medial collateral ligament and knee joint capsule. The sartorius insertion, which defines the first layer, lies anterior to the tibial attachments of the deep and superficial medial collateral ligaments. Lying between layers 1 and 2 are the tendons of the gracilis and semitendinosus at the posteromedial corner. Slightly more posteromedially, the semimembranosus tendon, with its five different insertions, fuses with layers 2 and 3 (Figs 66–3 to 66–5).

The anatomy of the lateral aspect of the knee was described by Seebacher[21] as having a similarly layered organization. The superficial portion of the biceps femoris and the iliotibial tract compose layer 1. Layer 2, in an anteroposterior direction, is comprised of the quadriceps retinaculum, lateral collateral ligament, the two patellofemoral ligaments, and the patellomeniscal ligament. Layer 3 consists of the lateral part of the knee joint capsule and the fabellofibular and arcuate ligaments. These latter two ligaments may act to fortify the area of junction of the popliteus muscle with the capsule of the knee joint[16] (Figs 66–6 to 66–8).

The posterior portion of the knee joint contains the posterior cruciate ligament, the capsule with its reinforcing structures, and the musculature that plantarflexes the ankle. The posteromedial corner is supported by the medial collateral ligament, the pes anserinus tendon, semimembranosus insertions, and the oblique popliteal ligament. Posterolaterally, the capsule is fortified by the ITB, popliteus, biceps femoris, and the lateral collateral, arcuate, and fabellofemoral ligaments.[21] The posterior cruciate ligament and medial and lateral menisci are found in a

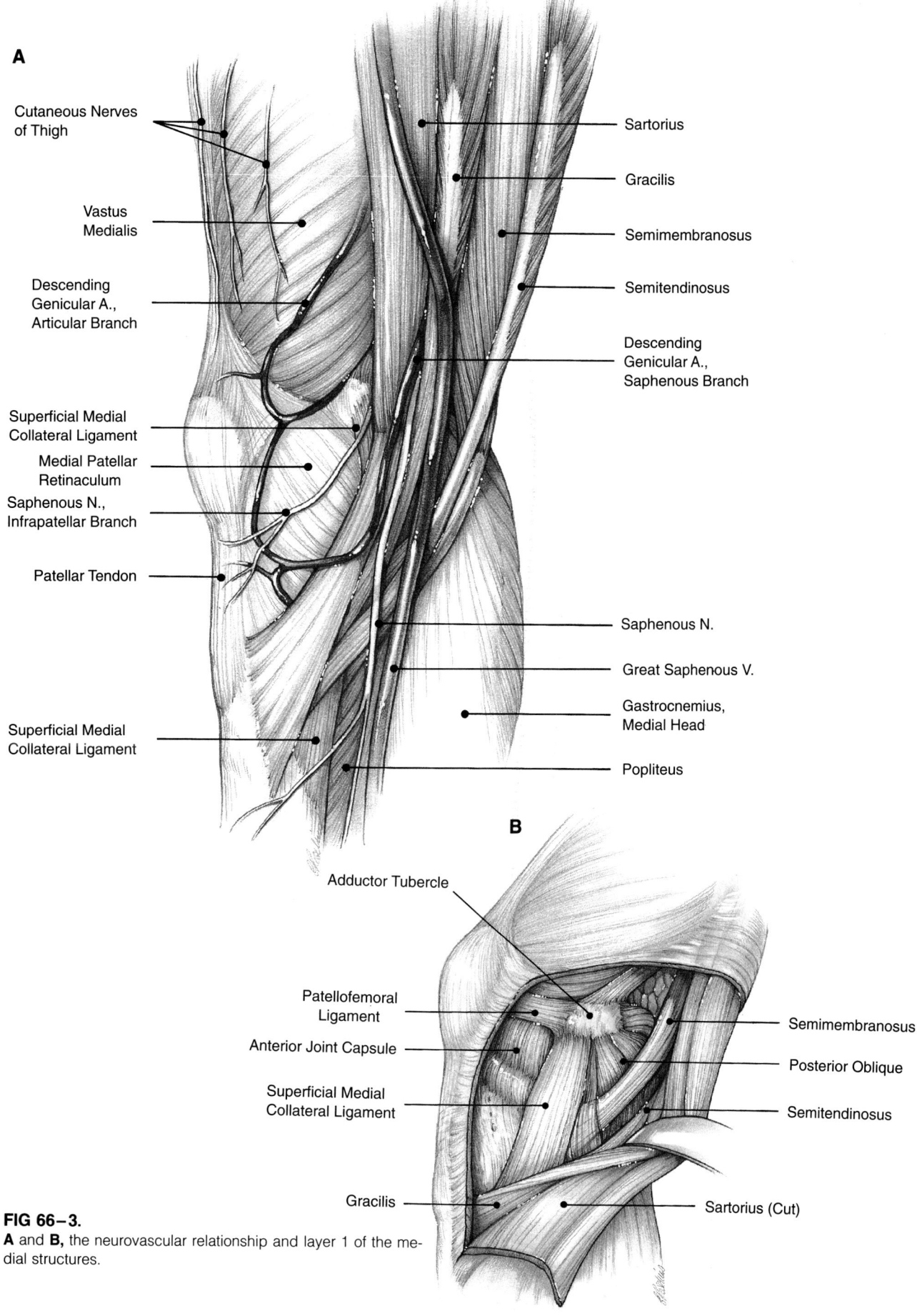

FIG 66-3.
A and **B,** the neurovascular relationship and layer 1 of the medial structures.

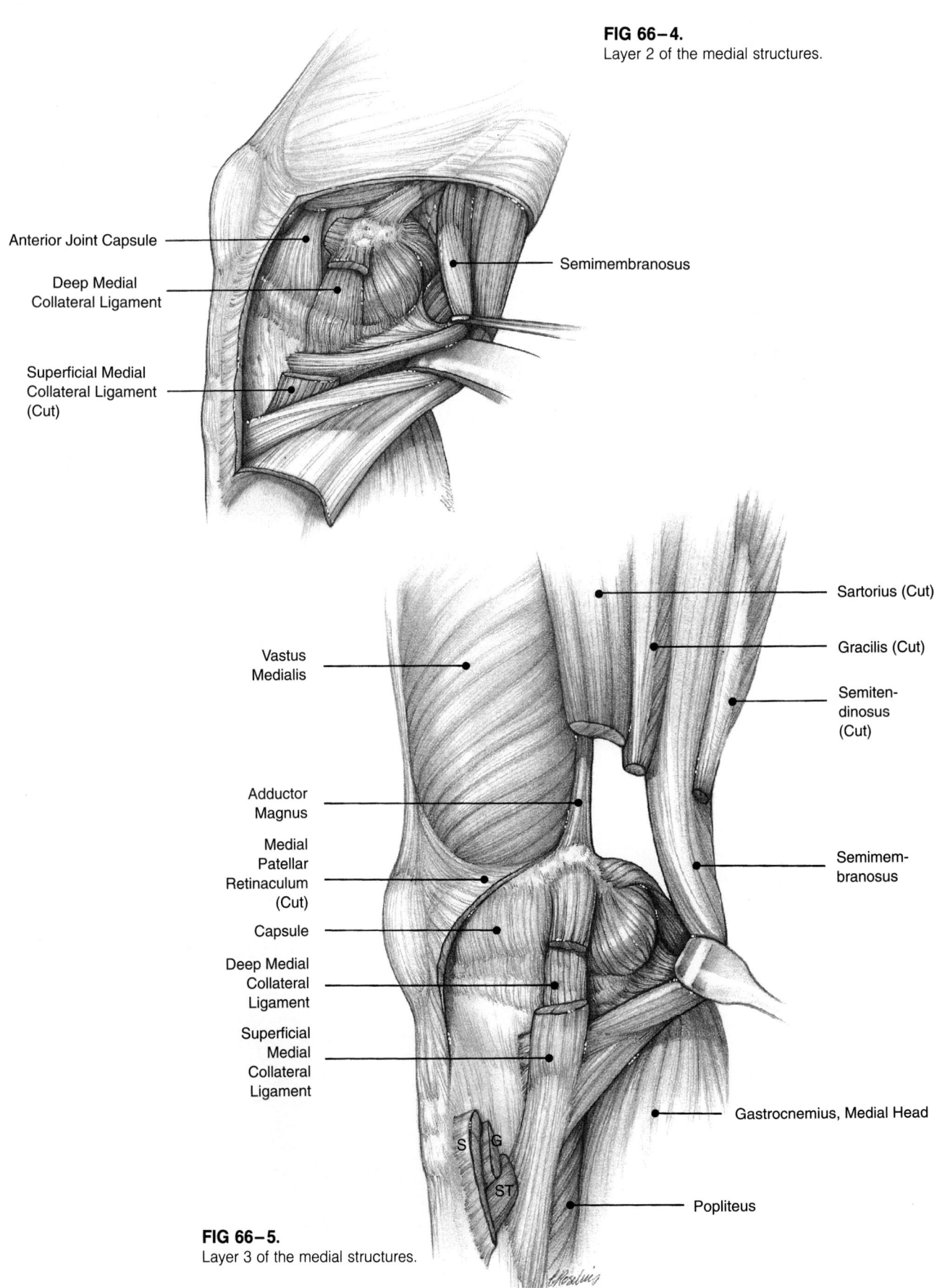

FIG 66-4.
Layer 2 of the medial structures.

FIG 66-5.
Layer 3 of the medial structures.

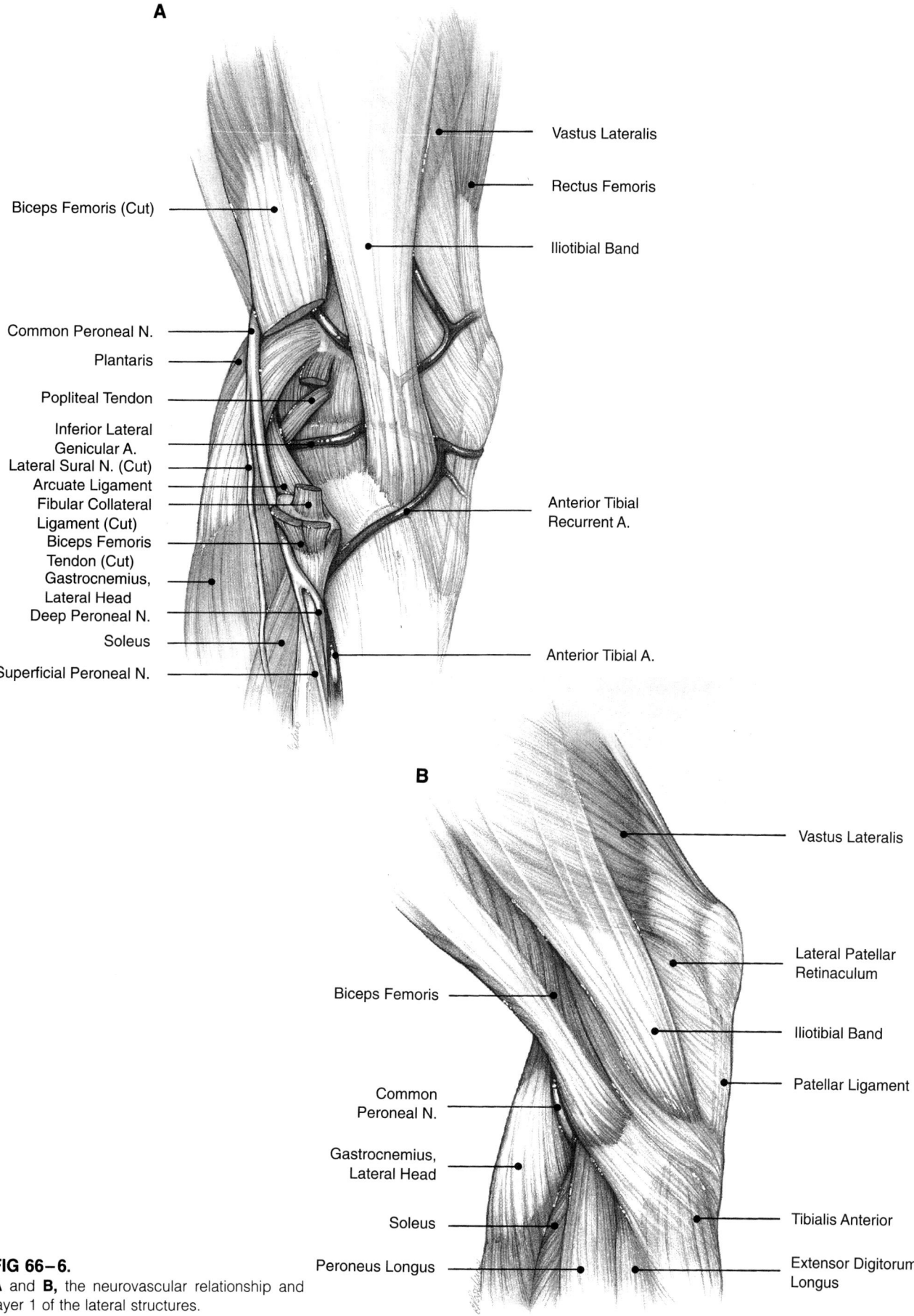

FIG 66-6.
A and **B,** the neurovascular relationship and layer 1 of the lateral structures.

1204 OSTEOTOMY AND PRIMARY TOTAL KNEE REPLACEMENT

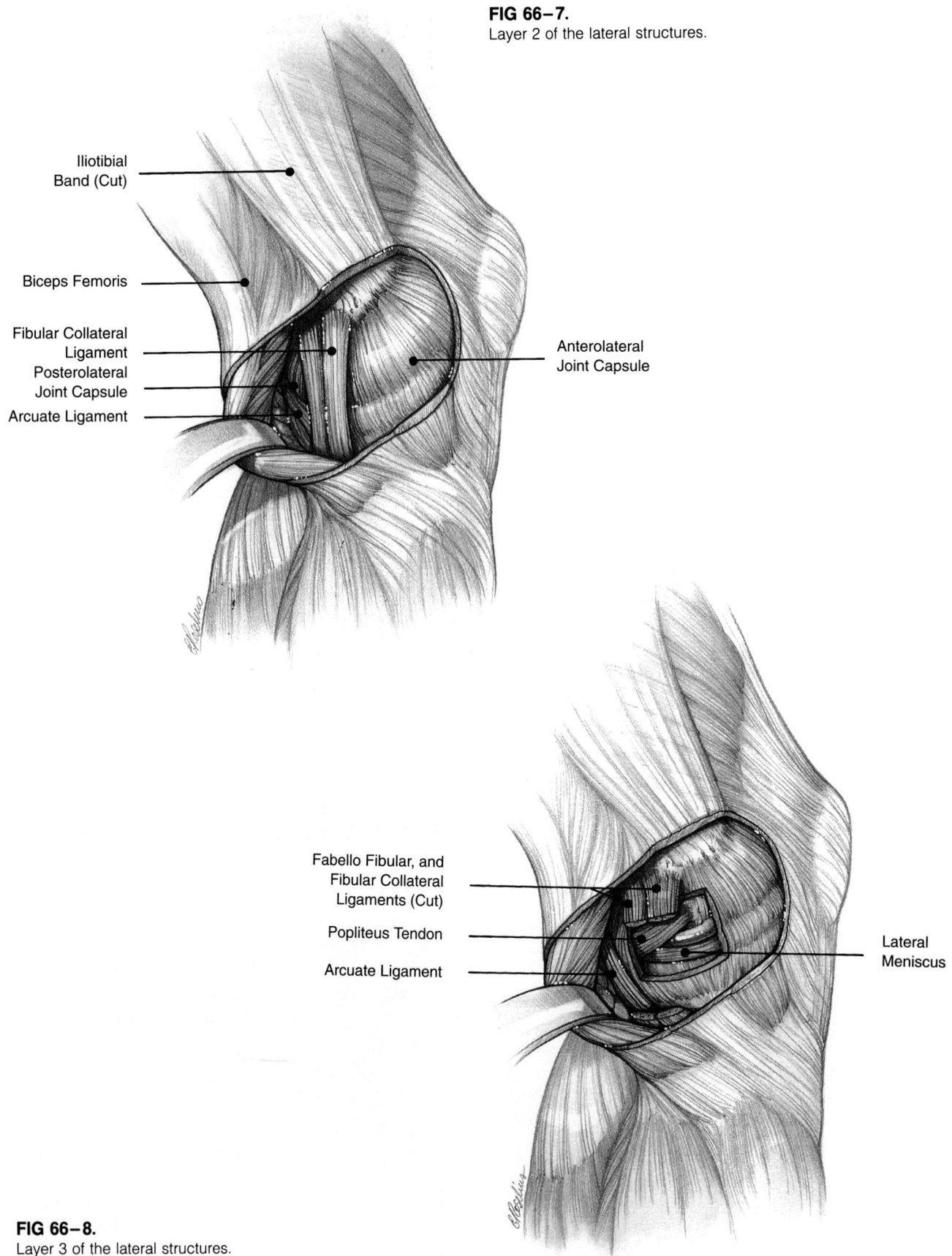

FIG 66–7.
Layer 2 of the lateral structures.

FIG 66–8.
Layer 3 of the lateral structures.

more central location.[23] Finally, on the posterior aspect of the femur, extending distally, are the origins of the plantaris and both heads of the gastrocnemius muscles.

BALANCING

In order to properly balance the knee ligaments, the surgeon performs a surgical release for contracture, and in extremely rare circumstances, for excessive laxity. With the completion of the arthroplasty, the ligaments will reattach at a new resting level predicated on the spacing effect of the prosthesis.

Varus Deformity

In a fixed varus deformity, a contracture of the medial soft tissue structures, including the deep and superficial medial collateral ligaments, capsule, pes anserinus tendons, and posterior cruciate ligament, occurs with a concomitant laxity in the lateral joint soft tissue. Ligament balancing initially should address the removal of all medial osteophytes from the tibia and femur. If osteophyte removal does not fully correct the soft tissue inequality, as can be seen in relatively small contractures, the medial soft tissue sleeve must be progressively released until the medial structures become the same length as the lateral structures.[12, 14] A complete release of the contracture will allow the surgeon to return the joint to a neutral alignment.

Routine exposure in knee arthroplasty often requires a posteromedial elevation of the semimembranosus insertion into the tibia (Fig 66–9,A and B). The medial varus release includes a tibial subperiosteal elevation of the superficial medial collateral ligament and pes anserinus tendon (Fig 66–10). Distally, the periosteum can be elevated on the anteromedial surface for 8 to 10 cm.

For a more severe contracture, Laskin et al.[17] have found it necessary to elevate the insertion of the superficial collateral ligament distally. Insall[13] has found that this is rarely needed and suggests further posterior periosteal stripping, which can include the fascia of the soleus and popliteus.

Insall and others believe that the cruciate ligaments should be completely resected prior to any ligamentous balancing because they prevent full correction when left intact.[8, 11, 12, 15, 18, 23] The cruciate ligaments, with their central location, are affected by either medial or lateral compartment contractures. Recent histologic evidence illustrates the involvement of the posterior cruciate ligament in the arthritic process. Failure to remove these ligaments will not al-

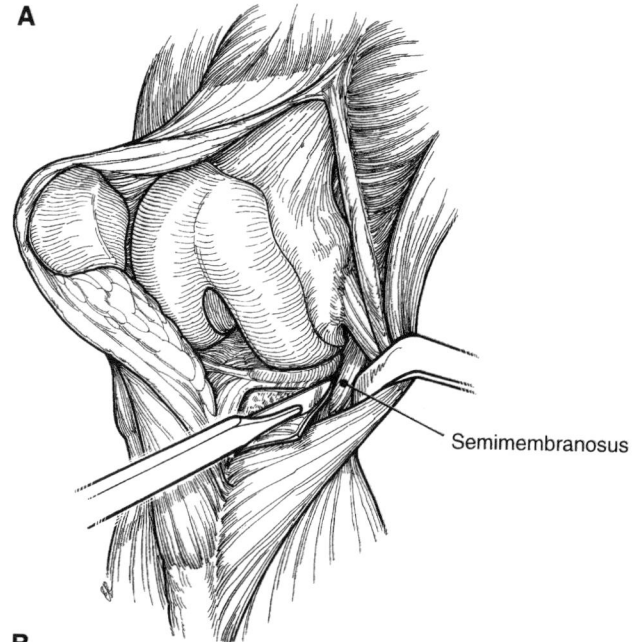

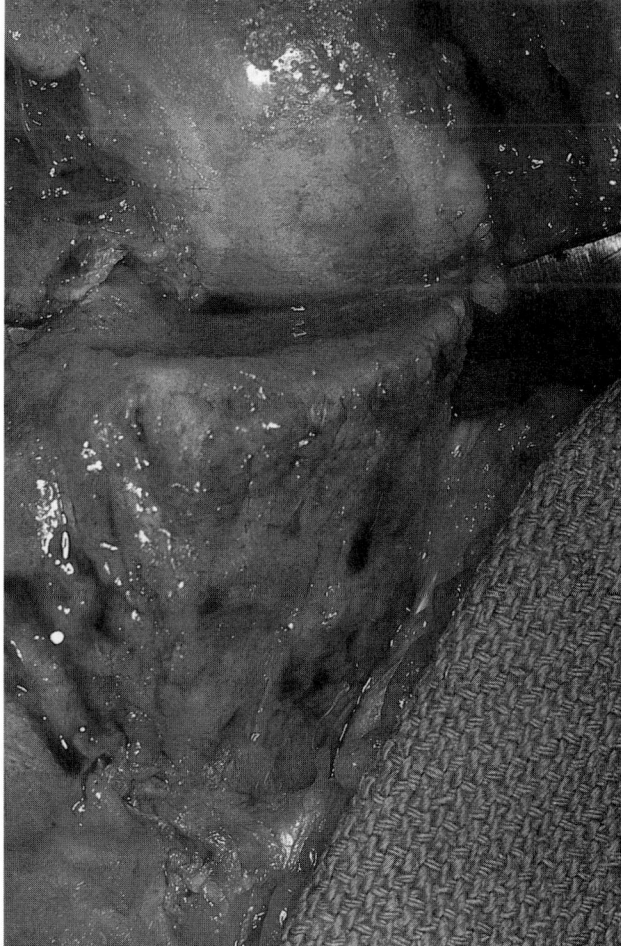

FIG 66–9.
Diagrammatic **(A)** and operative **(B)** demonstration of release of the semimembranosus insertion on the posteromedial aspect of the tibia.

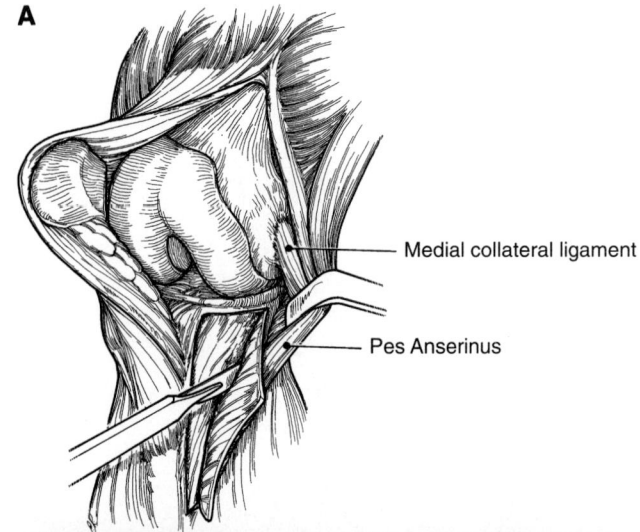

low proper balancing of the contracted soft tissue sleeve (Fig 66–11).

The majority of varus deformities can be managed with medial soft tissue elevation and resection of the cruciates. For the severe deformity, Hungerford et al.[12] have advocated a lateral soft tissue advancement to be used when ligamentous balancing is unrealistic, cannot be achieved, or when medial bone loss cannot be successfully augmented with a bone graft. In our own experience, we have not appreciated the necessity for this approach. In this technique, a proximal fibular osteotomy is made 1 in. from the tip and perpendicular to the long axis. The fibular head is then advanced with the knee in mild flexion and reattached with a lag screw. Preservation of the peroneal nerve as it wraps around the fibular neck is of paramount importance while performing this procedure.

Valgus Deformity

Valgus deformities can be corrected using the same basic principles employed for the varus deformity with two noticeable differences. First, the presence of the peroneal nerve on the contracted lateral aspect of the knee necessitates caution when performing the dissection and elevation. Extensive soft tissue release may stretch the nerve with a resultant neuropraxia.

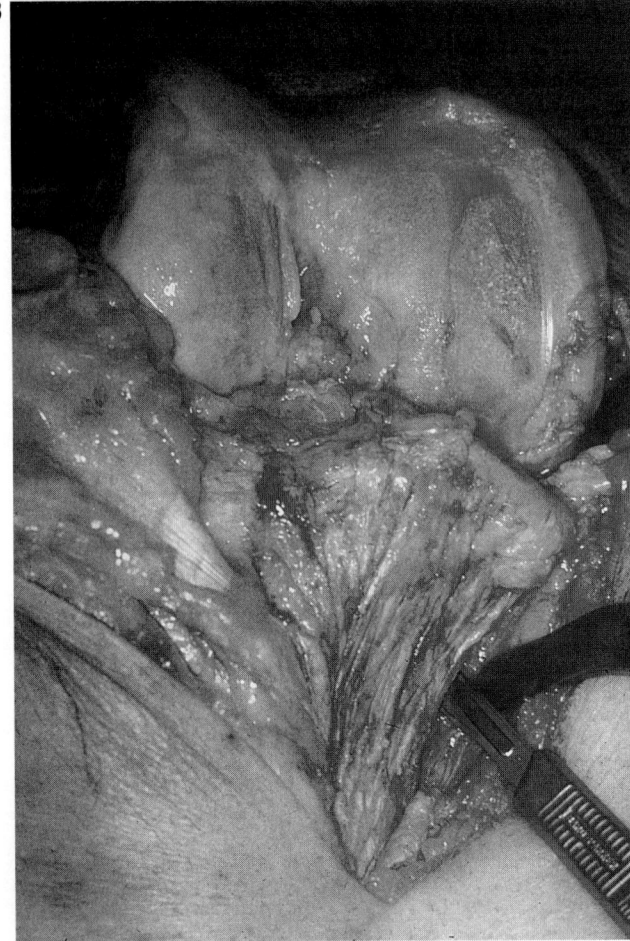

FIG 66–10.
A and **B**, a complete medial varus release includes elevating the medial capsule, deep and superficial medial collateral ligament, and pes anserinus conjoint tendon.

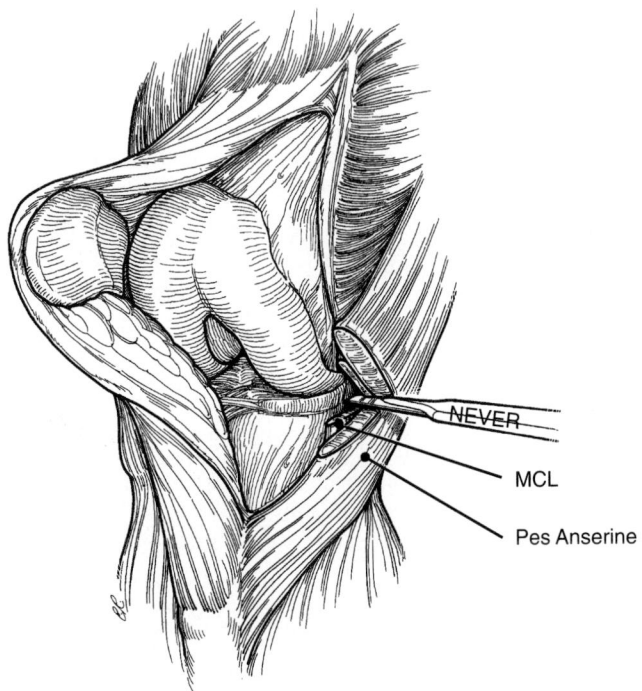

FIG 66–11.
Transecting the medial structures should NEVER be considered a part of the medial release.

Owing to the proximity of the peroneal nerve on the tibia, the valgus soft tissue release is done proximally. For a complete release, the procedure addresses both the extraarticular (ITB) and intraarticular contractures (popliteus and lateral collateral ligament).

As in correction of the varus deformity, peripheral osteophytes on the femoral condyle and tibial plateau are removed first. If osteophyte removal results in an incomplete correction, the contracted soft tissues can be released sequentially. There is some debate as to whether the extraarticular or intraarticular structures should be released first. Our own preference is to release the ITB first as it most often appears to be the major deforming force (Fig 66–12,A and B). Experience has shown that it is somewhat irrelevant whether the release is performed proximal to the patella, at the joint line, or at Gerdy's tubercle. The ITB is transected rather than lengthened. The intraarticular release of the lateral collateral ligament and popliteus can be done by either a sharp dissection off the lateral condyle or an osteotomy (approximately 2–3 mm) of the lateral femoral condyle (Fig 66–13,A and B).

Several authors previously suggested surgical dissection of the peroneal nerve prior to correction of severe valgus deformity. This exploration, if done at all, is now reserved for the combined flexion and valgus deformity.

Hungerford et al.[12] divide fixed valgus deformities into two types based on medial stability. Type I valgus deformity includes contracted lateral soft tissues, lateral bone and cartilage loss, and intact medial stabilizers. The type II deformity differs from type I by having attenuated medial stabilizers. Type I is the more common valgus deformity and can usually be corrected with soft tissue from the distal femur and lateral tendinous resection. For severe type II deformity, the authors include a medial soft tissue advancement in combination with the lateral release, although results with this technique have met with mixed results.

Flexion Contracture

As with the varus and valgus contractures, the first step in treating a fixed flexion contracture is removal of osteophytes.[4, 13] A large anterior tibial osteophyte may contribute significantly to a small fixed flexion contracture and can be removed with the proximal tibial cut during arthroplasty. If this does not correct the deformity fully, one can increase the depths of the femoral and tibial cuts. Although this technique can correct any degree of flexion contracture, a short leg and quadriceps lag may ensue.

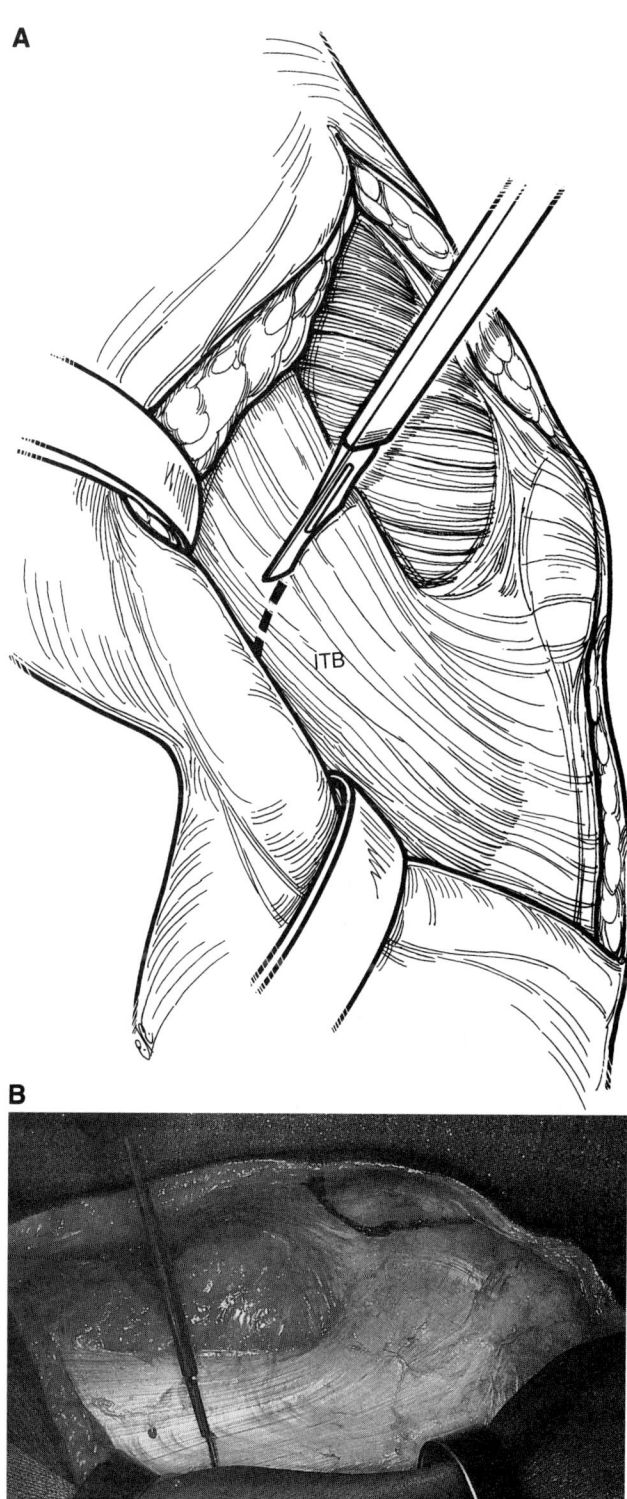

FIG 66–12.
A and **B,** transecting the iliotibial band *(ITB)* as part of the lateral valgus release can be done at the level of the joint line or proximal to the patella, as seen here.

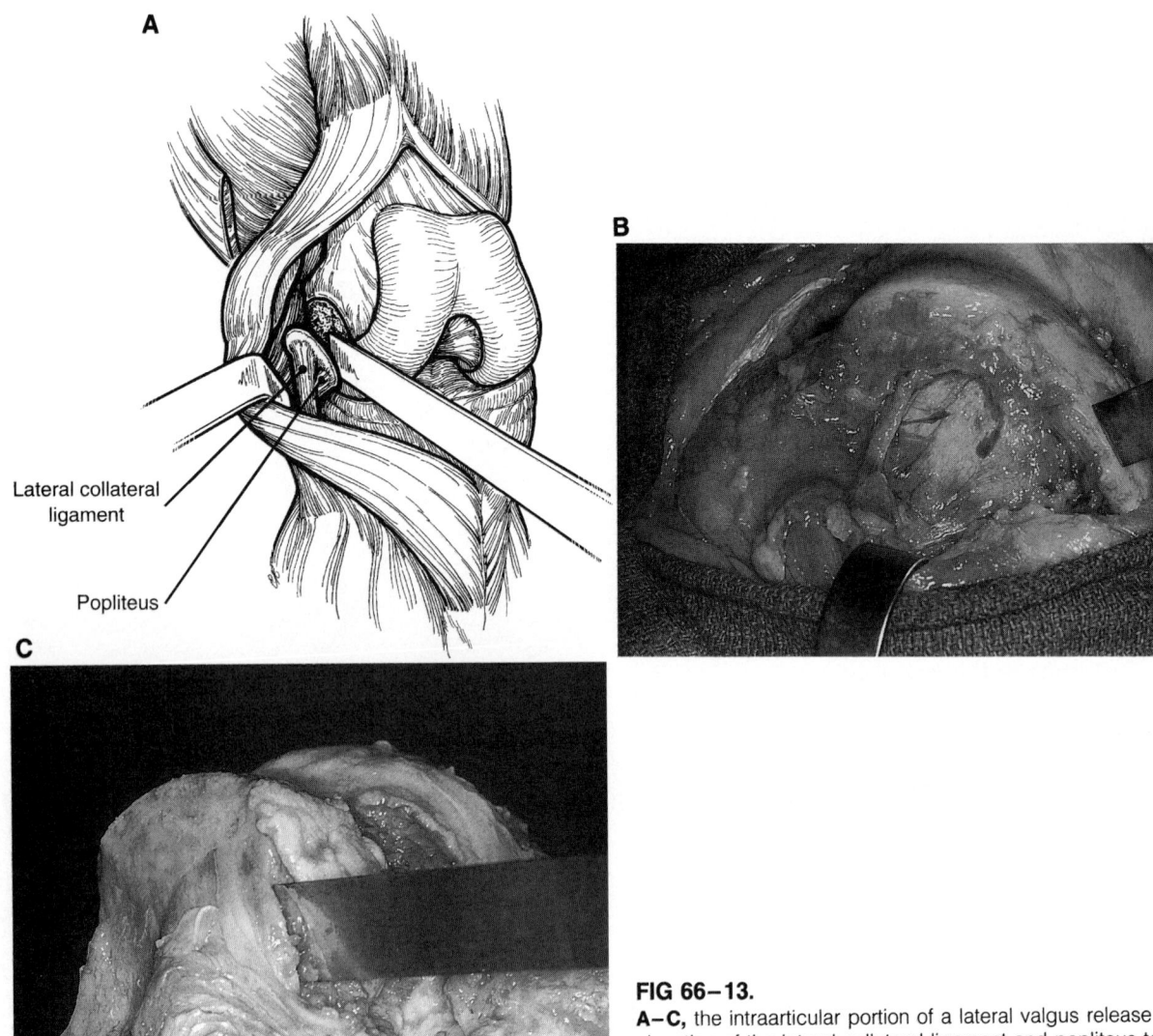

FIG 66–13.
A–C, the intraarticular portion of a lateral valgus release includes elevation of the lateral collateral ligament and popliteus tendon either sharply or via an osteotomy.

For these reasons, most surgeons perform extensive posterior soft tissue releases rather than bone resections (Fig 66–14). Elevation of the posterior capsule does not usually provide enough length to overcome the contracture; hence, posterior capsulotomy should be performed. The posterior cruciate ligament should be sacrificed in all cases of flexion contractures as this structure contributes significantly to the deformity.[13] If further soft tissue release is necessary, the gastrocnemius tendons can be elevated subperiostially from the distal femur. One must be aware continuously of the inherent dangers of a posterior knee dissection and exercise extreme caution when performing the release.

Long-term follow-up studies on the effect of knee replacement on flexion deformities have been done. Tew and Forster[22] reviewed 697 primary and revision replacements and found that 61% of knees had a flexion deformity before the primary operation. Total knee arthroplasty reduced this to 17% and the improvement was maintained. They found that flexion contractures affected rheumatoid knees more often and more seriously than osteoarthritic knees, but arthroplasty was more successful in correcting the deformity in the former.

The indications for ligament releases are in anesthetized patients whose knee cannot be corrected to neutral alignment. Sequential releases are sufficient if, indeed, neutral alignment is achieved. One must, however, make sure that the balance is sufficient; otherwise, the arthroplasty will be adversely affected. Albeit somewhat controversial, it appears that the ligament releases should be performed prior to bone resection.

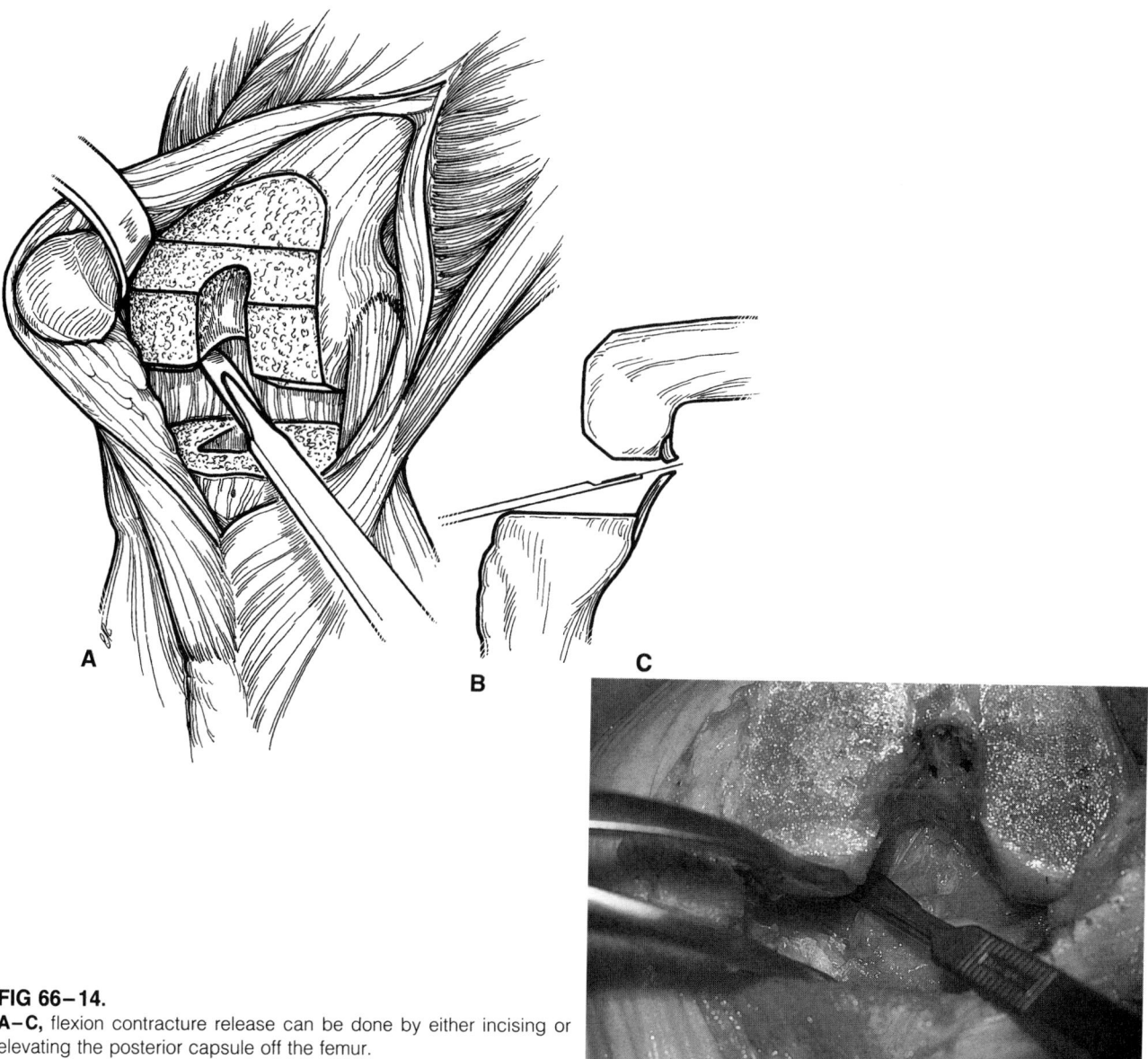

FIG 66–14.
A–C, flexion contracture release can be done by either incising or elevating the posterior capsule off the femur.

CONCLUSION

Contractures can occur at any location in the soft tissue envelope which surrounds the knee. Bone and cartilage loss, osteophytes, and stress deprivation can lead to a shortening of the ligamentous structures on one side of the knee with a concomitant laxity on the opposite side. Except in cases of a severe fixed flexion deformity, ligamentous balancing can be adequately achieved with periosteal elevation of the contracted soft tissues, thereby obviating excessive bone resection. Careful preoperative evaluation and intraoperative balancing with mandatory resection of the posterior cruciate ligament will increase the likelihood of a successful knee replacement.

REFERENCES

1. Akeson W, et al: Effects of immobilization on joints, *Clin Orthop* 219:28–37, 1987.
2. Amiel D, et al.: Stress deprivation effect on metabolic turnover of the medial collateral ligament collagen: A comparison between 9 and 12 week immobilization, *Clin Orthop* 172:265–270, 1983.
3. Blinkley JM, Peat M: The effects of immobilization on the ultrastructure and the mechanical properties of the medial collateral ligaments of rats, *Clin Orthop* 203:301–308, 1986.
4. Don, LD, Boirdo, RA: Technical consideration in total knee arthroplasty, *Clin Orthop* 205:5–11, 1986.
5. Dorr, LD: Technique of correction of varus deformity. In Ranowat CS, editor: *Total condylar knee arthro-*

plasty: Technique, results and complications. New York, 1985, Springer-Verlag.
6. Freeman MAR: *Arthritis of the knee,* New York, 1980, Springer-Verlag.
7. Fulkerson JP, Gossling HR: Anatomy of the knee joint lateral retinaculum, *Clin Orthop* 153:188–196, 1981.
8. Girgis FG, et al: The cruciate ligaments of the knee joint, *Clin Orthop* 106:216–231, 1975.
9. Helfet AJ: *Disorders of the knee,* Philadelphia, 1974, JB Lippincott, p 10.
10. Hollinshead WH: *Textbook of anatomy,* New York, 1974, Harper & Row.
11. Hood RW, Vanni M, Insall JN: The correction of knee alignment in 225 consecutive total condylar knee replacements, *Clin Orthop* 160:94, 1981.
12. Hungerford D, Krackow K, Kenna R: Management of fixed deformity at total knee arthroplasty. In *Total knee arthroplasty, a comprehensive approach,* Baltimore, 1984, Williams & Wilkins pp 163–192,
13. Insall JN: Total knee replacement. Insall JN, editor: *Surgery of the knee,* New York, 1984, Churchill Livingston, pp 587–695.
14. Insall, JN: Surgical approaches to the knee joint. *In* Insall JN, editor: *Surgery of the knee,* New York, 1988, Churchill-Livingstone, pp 41–54.
15. Insall JN, Scott WN, Ranawat CS: The total condylar knee prosthesis. A report of two hundred and twenty cases, *J Bone Joint Surg* 61:173, 1979.
16. Kaplan, EB: the fabellofibular and short lateral ligaments of the knee joint, *J Bone Joint Surg* 43:169–179, 1961.
17. Laskin, RS, Schob CJ: Medial capsular recession for severe varus deformities and arthroplasty, 2:313–316, 1989.
18. Laskin, RS, et al: The effect of posterior cruciate resection during total knee replacement in the deformed knee, 55th Annual Meeting of the American Academy of Orthopaedic Surgeons, Atlanta, Feb 15, 1988.
19. Pansky B: *Review of gross anatomy,* New York 1979, Macmillan.
20. Sculco TP: Techniques of correction of contracture during total knee arthroplasty. *In* Ranawatt CS editor: *Total condylar knee arthroplasty: Techniques, results and complications.* New York, 1985, Springer-Verlag.
21. Seebacher JR, et al: The structure of the posterolateral aspect of the knee. *J Bone Joint Surg* 64:536–541, 1982.
22. Tew M, Forster IW: Effect of knee replacement on flexion deformity, *J Bone Joint Surg* 69:395–399, 1987.
23. Van Dommelen BA, Fowler PJ: Anatomy of the posterior cruciate ligament, *Am J Sports Med* 17:24–29, 1989.
24. Warren LF, Marshall JL. The supporting structures and layers on the medial side of the knee, *J Bone Joint Surg* 61:56–62, 1979.
25. Williams PL, Warwick R: *Gray's anatomy,* ed 36, Philadelphia, WB Saunders, 1980.

67

Transfusion Considerations in Total Knee Arthroplasty

PHILIP M. FARIS, M.D.

Preoperative period
Intraoperative period

Postoperative period
Summary

Total knee arthroplasty has enjoyed a relatively long and successful reign as a beneficial adjunct in the treatment of various maladies of the painful knee. Complication rates have been relatively low, consisting predominantly of mechanical, infectious, and thromboembolic phenomena. However, as concerns over viral disease transmission through blood and blood product transfusion mount, more clinical and basic science research is being directed toward controlling and preventing disease transfer. Not only has extensive investigation begun into the identification and treatment of these viruses, which is beyond the scope of this chapter, but more practically, into methods of preventing their transmission. Three perioperative time periods should be considered, as the need for the use of blood products may be determined preoperatively, intraoperatively, and postoperatively. This chapter considers each of these perioperative periods and attempts to elucidate hematologic changes that occur and how these can affect blood usage during total knee arthroplasty.

PREOPERATIVE PERIOD

Patient factors are important in determining the necessity for postoperative blood usage. Primarily the patient's coagulation status should be assessed. Bleeding time is the best general test for coagulation status but probably is not a necessary study in the mature patient with no medical history of a bleeding diathesis. Any patient or family history of coagulation defect should be evaluated. Anticoagulants such as warfarin (Coumadin) should be discontinued, if possible, prior to surgery. Since the half-life of warfarin is $2\frac{1}{2}$ days, the drug should be discontinued at least 3 days prior to surgery. Some residual effect may be seen for 4 to 5 days; however, this effect is negligible and the drug can usually be resumed the evening before surgery for thromboembolic prophylaxis. Serum prothrombin time should be determined prior to surgery to verify adequate coagulability and vitamin K may aid in reversing the warfarin effect.

Nonsteroidal anti-inflammatory drugs inhibit platelet aggregation and may prolong bleeding times.[1] The effect of these agents is dependent on their half-lives. Drugs with longer half-lives, e.g., piroxicam with a mean half-life of 50 hours, should be discontinued at least 5 days prior to surgery. Drugs with shorter half-lives, such as indomethacin, may be continued until 2 days prior to surgery. Because aspirin has a more direct and profound effect on platelet function, it should be discontinued 10 days prior to surgery, if possible.

The remainder of the preoperative patient preparation is devoted to preparing the patient for the expected blood loss of surgery. This is achieved currently by autologous self-donation.[4, 8, 12, 41, 42, 52, 54, 58] The future may hold the ability to chemically "jump-start" the hematopoietic system and this is discussed later. Discussion of these techniques should, however, be preceded by a review of the reasons for their use, primarily to prevent the transmission of viral diseases. The most common transfusion-transmitted viral disease is cytomegalovirus (CMV), which occurs in approximately 20% of donors who are 20 years of age or less and 70% of donors of 70 years of age.[5, 10, 18, 24, 41, 42] CMV is harbored in leukocytes and may be transmitted years after donor exposure. In the immunocompetent patient, CMV infection is clinically insignificant; however, in the immunocompromised patient such as the patient with acquired immunodeficiency syndrome

(AIDS) or the transplant patient, CMV infection may create significant clinical sequelae including fever, jaundice, and hepatosplenomegaly.

The incidence of transfusion-transmitted hepatitis, particularly non-A, non-B hepatitis, was estimated in the late 1970s to be between 6% and 11% of recipients. With the advent of donor testing for aminolevulinic transferase and hepatitis B core antigen, the incidence of homologous transfusion transmission of this disease is estimated to be between 1% and 4%. This translates to between 40,000 and 160,000 people yearly. Considering that 40% of these patients will develop chronic liver transaminase elevation, 16% will develop chronic active hepatitis, and 8% will develop cirrhosis, the devastating magnitude of this disease far exceeds that of the AIDS virus. Of great importance was the discovery that hepatitis C was the main cause of posttransfusion chronic liver disease. Approval of the test for hepatitis C should further purify the blood donor pool.[5, 10, 18, 21, 50]

Despite the economic and medical implications of these viral diseases, it was not until the appearance of the AIDS virus and its devastating consequences that public attention became focused on blood and blood product transfusion. As of January 1990, 3,027 (2.5%) of the 121,711 reported cases of human immunodeficiency virus (HIV) infections were transfusion-related. Of these 3,027 transfusion-related infections, 6.8% occurred in the pediatric population. It is estimated that as many as 12,000 additional transfusion-related AIDS cases may occur as a result of blood or blood product transfusions that were performed prior to the implementation of a screening test in 1985.[18]

Currently, two mechanisms for screening prospective donors are used. These are donor deferral for high-risk donors and enzyme-linked immunoabsorbent assay (ELISA) for antibody to HIV. These techniques have reduced the risk of transfusion-associated HIV transmission to from 1 in 20,000 to 1 in 1 million (average estimate, 1 in 156,000). These odds are comparable to the odds of dying from a fatal hemolytic transfusion reaction and an estimated 60 to 230 patients die each year from each of these causes.[18, 49]

Postoperative transfusion after unilateral total knee arthroplasty is unusual in our experience. However, it is much more common after bilateral procedures. In the name of defensive medicine, it has been our practice to have all unilateral total knee replacement (TKR) patients predeposit 1 unit of autologous blood. This practice must now be questioned because of the economic implications of discarding greater than 50% of these donations. We are currently evaluating our patient population to determine which patients in this group will benefit from predonation. Our experience suggests that predonation for those undergoing bilateral, simultaneous procedures is indicated, and rarely is this blood discarded.

Patients should be offered the opportunity to predonate. Some patients, however, will be at high risk for phlebotomy. As predonation has become more prominent, blood bank personnel acceptance of higher-risk and more elderly patients has increased. Spiess et al.[49] categorize high-risk patients as having one or more of the following: a history of angina, myocardial infarction, cardiac dysrhythmia, hypertension requiring two or more medications for control, congestive heart failure, valvular heart disease, congenital heart disease, seizure disorder, previous cerebrovascular accident, or cerebrovascular insufficiency. They exclude from predonation those patients with unstable angina, aortic stenosis, and those who have suffered a myocardial infarction in the last 6 months. Using hemodynamic monitoring, they noted systolic blood pressure drops of 20% or more in 49 of 123 high-risk patients. Although this does not preclude predonation by this group of patients, it does point out the importance of monitoring these patients during phlebotomy.[41]

Spacing of preoperative donations in the normal knee replacement patient population is generally 10 to 14 days. This conservatively spaced period is allowable because of the elective nature of the procedure and the normal physiology of the hematopoietic response. Without the use of oral iron replacement, reticulcytosis peaks at approximately 9 days post phlebotomy and 1 unit of red blood cells can be replaced in 3 to 4 weeks. Red blood cell synthesis can be maximized with routine oral doses (i.e., 300 mg three times a day) of iron, which can result in the replacement of 1 unit of red cells in 3 to 5 days. With oral iron replacement, significant responses can be attained even in iron-deficient patients. Oral iron supplementation should be initiated 2 to 3 days prior to phlebotomy. Through maximization techniques, autologous donations may be procured every fourth day and surgery should be delayed until the fourth day after the last donation.[17-19, 41, 48]

A promising technique for maximizing the availability of autologous units for preoperative donation is recombinant human erythropoietin.[17, 20, 28] Long used for the chronic anemia of renal failure, rheumatoid arthritis, and AIDS patients, it has recently been evaluated in our institution and others for use in the preoperative preparation of elective surgical patients. In a prospective blinded study at our institution using a placebo group, a 100-mg/day group, and a 300-mg/day group, we found a significant increase in the reticulocyte counts of both experimental groups. We also found that transfusions of homologous blood were eliminated in both experimental groups, even when bilateral total hip arthroplasties were performed. In this study, all doses were given intramuscularly beginning 10 days prior to surgery and ending 5 days after surgery. There were no differences in any hematologic parameter between the experimental groups. The dosage schedule and economics of this protocol prohibit the current use of this therapy. Other protocols are currently being evaluated and hold promise for making the use of human recombinant erythropoietin economically feasible in the future.[20]

THE INTRAOPERATIVE PERIOD

Unlike orthopaedic procedures performed above the thigh, total knee arthroplasty is amenable to the use of a tourniquet. Tourniquet use allows a clean, dry surgical field and prevents significant blood loss during the procedure. Intraoperative techniques for blood loss prevention, then, are mainly to prevent postoperative drainage losses. Careful hemostasis during the procedure should be obtained, but it is not necessary to release the tourniquet prior to wound closure. In separate articles by Lotke et al.,[29] Newman et al.,[37] Erskine et al.,[13] and Gannon et al.,[15] tourniquet release prior to wound closure had no effect on total blood loss. Other techniques, such as the smearing of fibrin on the bone and soft tissue surfaces, have likewise had no effect on measurable postoperative blood loss; however, inapparent patient blood loss, which may amount to 31% of the postoperative loss, may be reduced by this method.[32, 38] The superior lateral genicular artery should be sought during lateral retinacular release and either preserved or coagulated because substantial blood loss and tense hematomas may result from its laceration.

The only significant factor in intraoperative blood loss appears to be the use of polymethyl methacrylate for prosthetic fixation. Whether polymethyl methacrylate decreases blood loss via simple tamponade, as suggested by Charnley, an increase in venous pressure which blocks sinusoids, as suggested by Tronzo, protein coagulation by monomer, as described by Jeffries, or heat cauterization of vessels caused by the exothermic curing reaction, cement decreases significantly the blood loss associated with TKR.[9, 13, 34]

The postoperative dressing should be a soft compressive dressing made of burn gauze and elastic bandages. The dressing is designed to improve patient comfort and to allow some knee motion. Various forms of ice application have been designed which may improve patient comfort; however, good prospective, randomized studies are lacking relating to blood loss prevention, pain control, and economic justification that would allow us to recommend them for routine use.

POSTOPERATIVE PERIOD

The postoperative period in TKR seems to hold the greatest promise for salvage and preservation of blood and blood products. Prior to discussing these techniques, note should be made of the effects of tourniquet use and surgery in general on the coagulation system. During surgical procedures, activation of both the fibrinolytic and coagulation systems occurs. This appears to be a general response and is noted after all surgical cases. An in-depth discussion of the multitude of factors involved in these cascades is beyond the scope of this chapter. In general, elevation of fibrinogen and fibrin degradation products occurs along with a decrease in platelet count. Stimulation of the system begins with tissue trauma, whether it be soft tissue or bone, and is mediated by a variety of kinins.[3, 7, 11, 26, 51, 56] Of interest in total knee surgery is the enhanced effect on this system by the hypoxia of tourniquet use.[11, 23, 26, 39] A study on dogs using tourniquet application for 4 hours in three separate groups demonstrated increased bleeding from the anterior tibial muscle, and prolongation of the bleeding time just prior to tourniquet release, maximizing at 5 minutes after release, and normalizing at 15 minutes after release. Blood platelet counts increased slightly throughout the study and capillary permeability increased in the ischemic muscle. Venous occlusion without arterial occlusion can, of itself, increase fibrinolytic activity in the occluded extremity. These concepts, when combined with the tissue trauma occurring during knee arthroplasty, would seem to portend significant hematologic postoperative changes.[35]

Stern et al.[51] studied platelet counts, fibrinogen, and fibrin degradation products in unilateral and bilateral total knee arthroplasties. Overall blood platelets decreased from a mean of 314/nL to a postoperative mean of 173/nL, fibrinogen increased from 304 mg/dL to 647 mg/dL, and variable elevations of fibrin degradation products occurred. All of these changes were enhanced by the performance of bilateral procedures; however, only platelet counts were statistically lower. They suggest that evaluation of preoperative platelet counts are important, especially in patients undergoing bilateral procedures in whom platelet counts decreased by an average of 60%.[51] Stern et al. did not give guidelines for maintenance of platelet counts; we prefer to maintain counts of above 25/nL and will transfuse platelets preoperatively to ensure that these levels are maintained in the postoperative period.

Since most blood loss in TKR occurs in the postoperative period, techniques for postoperative salvage of shed blood have been developed. These techniques derive from techniques previously used for intraoperative blood salvage and include both washed and unwashed blood salvage. Washed and centrifuged red blood cells for reinfusion have been used successfully and safely since the introduction of the Cell Saver (Haemonetics, Braintree, Mass.) in the mid-1970s. This device has been safely and efficaciously adapted to postoperative red blood cell salvage after TKR. However, unless the device is used intraoperatively, the expense of using it in the postoperative period is prohibitive since it requires a technician for operation and the machine is extremely expensive (references 2, 6, 20, 24, 27, 30, 31, 32, 40, 45, 46, 52, 54, 56).

A second method of postoperative shed blood salvage is through the use of unwashed shed red blood cells. This is accomplished via collection through a sterile drainage and filtration system,[14, 15, 43] e.g., Solcotrans (Solco Basle Illingham, Mass.). Ansell et al.[2] demonstrated comparable survival rates of red blood cells between these two different techniques of shed blood collection and preparation. Direct reinfusion of the shed, unwashed, filtered red blood cells and blood products can be accomplished. We have demonstrated in detail the hematologic properties of the shed blood and also the safety of the product when it is used properly.[14] The only major side effect was febrile reactions occurring in 2% of patients in whom shed blood collection lasted less than 6 hours at the time of reinfusion. Our study, however, failed to document efficacy. Reduction of postoperative transfusions using this system were documented by Groh et al.[22] in 1990 and Majkowski et al.[31] in 1991. These studies, however, were retrospective and the factors that led to transfusion are not documented. In a recent prospective study using a triggering hematocrit of 27%, we found no significant difference in transfusion requirements, postoperative drainage, wound problems, or retardation of physical therapy progress regardless of whether a drainage system was used.[44] Consequently, we currently do not use any form of postoperative wound evacuation system after unilateral or bilateral TKR.

Continuous passive motion machines have not been associated with increased blood loss or wound problems in the postoperative period; however, controversy exists as to their benefits in improving postoperative range of motion in knee replacement patients.[16, 29, 36, 45, 52] At this time, based on the current literature, we do not think the expense justifies their use.

SUMMARY

Total knee replacement surgery has proved to be a highly successful form of management of the painful, arthritic knee. Methods of preoperative, intraoperative, and postoperative management of blood loss, blood preservation, and hematopoietic stimulation can reduce the amount of homologous blood usage. However, sorting out of these techniques as to their efficacy and economic feasibility requires closely controlled prospective studies. These studies are not currently available and predonation of autologous blood remains the mainstay of blood loss management in TKR patients.

REFERENCES

1. Anderson SK, Shaikh A: Dicolofenac in combination with opiate infusion after joint replacement surgery, *Anaesth Intensive Care* 19:535, 1991.
2. Ansell J, et al: Survival of autotransfused red blood cells recovered from the surgical field during cardiovascular operations, *J Thorac Cardiovasc Surg* 84:387, 1982.
3. Aranda A, Paramo JA, Rocha E: Fibrinolytic activity in plasma after gynecological and urological surgery, *Haemostasis* 18:129, 1988.
4. Blaise G, Jackmusth R: Preoperative autotransfusion for total hip prosthesis, *Acta Anaesthesiol Belg* 3:175, 1979.
5. Bove J: Transfusion transmitted diseases: Current problems and challenges. *Prog Hematol* 14:123, 1986.
6. Bovill DF, et al: The efficacy of intraoperative autologous transfusion in major orthopedic surgery: A regression analysis, *Orthopedics* 9:1403, 1986.
7. Bredbacka S, et al: Activation of cascade systems in hip arthroplasty, *Acta Anaesthesiol Scand* 58:231, 1987.
8. Chambers LA, et al: Directed donor programs may adversely affect autologous donor participation, *Transfusion* 30:246, 1990.
9. Cushner FD, Friedman RJ: Blood loss in total knee arthroplasty, *Clin Orthop* 269:98, 1991.
10. Dodd RY: Transfusion and AIDS, *Int Ophthalmol Clin* 29:83, 1989.

11. Donadoni R, et al: Coagulation and fibrinolytic parameters in patients undergoing total hip replacement: Influence of the anaesthesia technique, *Acta Anaesthesiol Scand* 33:588, 1989.
12. Editorial. *Am J Clin Pathol* 2978, 1992.
13. Erskine JG, et al: Blood loss with knee joint replacement. *J R Coll Surg Edin* 26:295, 1981.
14. Faris PM, et al: Unwashed filtered shed blood collected after knee and hip arthroplasties, *J Bone Joint Surg [Am]* 73:1169, 1991.
15. Gannon DM, et al: An evaluation of the efficacy of postoperative blood salvage after total joint arthroplasty, *J Arthroplasty* 1:109, 1991.
16. Goletz TH, Henry JH: Continuous passive motion after total knee arthroplasty, *South Med J* 79:1116, 1986.
17. Goodnough LT, Brittenham GM: Limitations of the erythropoietic response to serial phlebotomy: Implications for autologous blood donor programs, *J Lab Clin Med* 115:28, 1990.
18. Goodnough LT, Shuck JM: Risk, options, and informed consent for blood transfusion in elective surgery, *Am J Surg* 159:602, 1990.
19. Goodnough LT, et al: Limitations to donating adequate autologous blood prior to elective orthopedic surgery, *Arch Surg* 124:494, 1989.
20. Goodnough LT, et al: Increased preoperative collection of autologous blood with recombinant human erythropoietin therapy, *N Engl J Med* 321:1163, 1989.
21. Goulet JA, et al: Intraoperative autologous transfusion in orthopaedic patients, *J Bone Joint Surg [Am]* 71:3, 1989.
22. Groh, GI, Buchert PK, Allen WC: A comparison of transfusion requirements after total knee arthroplasty using the Solcotrans autotransfusion system, *J Arthroplasty* 3:281, 1990.
23. Holemans R: Increase in fibrinolytic activity by venous occlusion, *J Appl Physiol* 18:1123.
24. Isbister JP: Autotransfusion: an impossible dream?, *Anaesth Intensive Care* 12:236, 1984.
25. Isbister JP: Strategies for avoiding or minimizing homologous blood transfusion: A sequel to the AIDS scare, *Med J Aust* 142:596, 1985.
26. Kambayashi J, et al: Activation of coagulation and fibrinolysis during surgery, analysed by molecular markers, *Thromb Res* 60:157, 1990.
27. Keeling MM, et al: Intraoperative autotransfusion experience in 725 consecutive cases, *Ann Surg* 197:536, 1982.
28. Levine EA: Increasing autologous blood donation with recombinant human erythropoietin, *Surgery* 88:327, 1991.
29. Lotke PA, et al: Blood loss after total knee replacement. Effects of tourniquet release and continuous passive motion, *J Bone Joint Surg [A]* 73:1037, 1991.
30. Mayer ED, et al: Reduction of postoperative donor blood requirement by use of the cell separator, *Scand J Thorac Cardiovasc Surg* 19:165, 1985.
31. Majkowski RS, Currie IC, Newman JH: Postoperative collection and reinfusion of autologous blood in total knee arthroplasty, *Ann R Coll Surg Engl* 73:381, 1991.
32. Marmor L, Avoy DR, McCabe A: Effect of fibrinogen concentrates on blood loss in total knee arthroplasty, *Clin Orthop* 273:136, 1991.
33. McCarthy PM, et al: Effect of blood conservation efforts in cardiac operations at the Mayo Clin, *Mayo Clin Proc* 63:225, 1988.
34. Mylod AG, et al: Perioperative blood loss associated with total knee arthroplasty, *J Bone Joint Surg [Am]* 72:1010, 1990.
35. Nakahara M, Sakahashi H: Effect of application of a tourniquet on bleeding factors in dogs, *J Bone Joint Surg [Am]* 49:1345, 1967.
36. Nielsen PT, Rechnagel K, Nielsen SE: No effect of continuous passive motion after arthroplasty of the knee, *Acta Orthop Scand* 59:580, 1988.
37. Newman JH, Jackson JP, Waugh W: Timing of tourniquet removal after knee replacement, *J R Soc Med* 72:492, 1979.
38. Page HP, Shepherd BD, Harrison JM: Reduction of blood loss in knee arthroplasty. *Aust N Z J Surg* 54:141, 1984.
39. Petaja J, et al: Fibrinolysis after application of a pneumatic tourniquet, *Acta Chir Scand* 153:647, 1987.
40. Popovsky MA, Devine PA: Intraoperative autologous transfusion, *Mayo Clin Proc* 60:125, 1985.
41. Preoperative autologous blood donations by high-risk patients (editorial). *Transfusion* 32:1, 1992.
42. Rebulla P, et al: Autologous blood predeposit for elective surgery: A program for better use and conservation of blood, *Surgery* 97:463, 1984.
43. Reilly TJ, et al: The use of postoperative suction drainage in total knee arthroplasty, *Clin Orthop* 208:238, 1986.
44. Ritter, MA, Keating, EM, Faris, PM: Closed wound drainage: A prospective randomized study, Unpublished manuscript.
45. Romness DW, Rand JA: The role of continuous passive motion following total knee arthroplasty, *Clin Orthop* 226:34, 1988.
46. Ronai AK, Glass JJ, Shapiro AS: Improving autologous blood harvest: Recovery of red cells from sponges and suction, *Anaesth Intensive Care* 15:421, 1987.
47. Semkiw LE, et al: Postoperative blood salvage using the cell saver after total joint arthroplasty, *J Bone Joint Surg [Am]* 71:823, 1989.
48. Special communication. The use of autologous blood. The national blood resource education program expert panel, *JAMA,* 263:414, 1990.
49. Spiess BD, et al: Autologous blood donation: Hemodynamics in a high-risk patient population, *Transfusion* 32(1):17–22, 1992.
50. Starkey JM, et al: Markers for transfusion-transmitted disease in different groups of blood donors, *JAMA* 262:3452, 1989.
51. Stern SH, Insall JN: Hematological effects of total knee arthroplasty: A prospective evaluation. Annual Meeting

of the American Academy of Orthopaedic Surgery, 1992.
52. Thomson JD, et al: Prior deposition of autologous blood in elective orthopaedic surgery, *J Bone Joint Surg [Am]* 69:325, 1987.
53. Vince KG, et al: Continuous passive motion after total knee arthroplasty, *J Arthroplasty* 2:281, 1987.
54. Wasman J, Goodnough LT: Autologous blood donation for elective surgery, *JAMA* 258:3135, 1987.
55. Williamson KR, Taswell HF: Intraoperative blood salvage: A review, *Transfusion* 31:1991.
56. Wilson J, et al: Coagulation and fibronolysis during hip surgery, *Hip Surg* 51:439, 1988.
57. Wilson WJ: Intraoperative autologous transfusion in revision total hip arthroplasty, *J Bone Joint Surg [Am]* 71:8, 1989.
58. Woolson ST, Marsh JS, Tanner JB: Transfusion of previously deposited autologous blood for patients undergoing hip-replacement surgery, *J Bone Joint Surg* 69:320, 1987.
59. Young JN, et al: Autologous blood retrieval in thoracic, cardiovascular, and orthopedic surgery, *Am J Surg* 144:48, 1982.

68

Thrombophlebitis in Knee Arthroplasty

PAUL A. LOTKE, M.D.

Pathophysiology
Deep venous thrombosis
    Methods of detection
    Incidence
Pulmonary embolism
Prophylaxis for thromboembolic disease
    Warfarin

Aspirin
Heparin
Intermittent compression boots
Vena cava filters
Recommendations
Treatment for thromboembolic disease
Summary

Pulmonary embolism (PE) presents a life-threatening risk to patients after total knee arthroplasty (TKA). This chapter discusses thromboembolic disease (TED) and the controversies that surround the problem. TED includes both deep venous thrombosis (DVT) and PE. First, the pathogenesis is discussed, then DVT, including methods of detection, incidence, and clinical significance. We then review PE and its methods of detection, incidence, and clinical significance. Prophylaxis and therapy for TED are reviewed last. This chapter describes not only what is known but reviews ongoing controversies and how they are being resolved.

PATHOPHYSIOLOGY

For many years, investigators thought they understood the fundamental factors promoting venous thromboembolic disease.[23] Virchow's triad of stasis, vessel injury, and alteration in blood coagulation still seems to apply. However, it has been difficult to determine precisely the specifics of these factors, that is, to define a potential hypercoagulable state. Acute DVT appears to start with eddy currents about a valve cusp that can activate platelets, leading to aggregation and attachment of a red fibrin thrombus. Similarly, injury to a venous wall, as during surgery, can release thrombogenic tissue agents initiating thrombogenesis. These events must be coupled with stasis, which allows thrombus attachment and growth to proceed to a clinically significant size. The thrombus can grow quickly in situ. This growth occurs through progressive layering of fibrin and platelets, forming the lines of Zahn. At any time during the process of growth a fragment on the entire length of the thrombus can break loose and embolize through the right ventricle to the lung. The risk of embolism is highest soon after formation, for two reasons: the thrombus is poorly attached to the venous wall early on, and the thrombus structure is then most fragile and subject to fragmentation. Over a period of days, the thrombus becomes more firmly attached and the endogenous lytic system tends to dissolve it. Then, embolization becomes less likely.

The acute PE event is associated with a number of hemodynamic and pulmonary events. The severity of these events is determined by the magnitude of embolic occlusion, the status of the patient before the embolic event, and the operation of incompletely defined humeral and reflex mechanisms. The outcome depends on the previous cardiopulmonary status of the patient.

A clot will eventually be resolved by the fibrinolytic system and the process of organization. Tissue plasminogen from endothelial cells may completely resorb a clot. However, some clot may remain and become an organized scar and an irregularity of the venous wall, or render a valve incompetent. Large residual scarring may permanently narrow the vein and induce chronic venous stasis. The extent of the thrombotic residual can lead to recurrent thromboembolism.

The overall pathophysiologic sequences involved in DVT and PE are generally established and can provide a structure for decisions regarding diagnosis and management. However, considerable controversy still exists in regard to the definition, diagnosis, management, and significance of thromboembolic phenomena in the postoperative arthroplasty patient.

DEEP VENOUS THROMBOSIS

A primary source of controversy arises from the very definition of this problem.[20] DVT appears to have a very simple definition: any thrombi existing in the deep venous system in the lower extremity. However, a full spectrum of thrombi exists, from very small to extensive thrombi in the distal (Fig 68–1) or proximal (Fig 68–2) venous systems. Recognizing that risk from thrombi in different locations may be different, investigators have only recently begun to segregate DVT into calf (distal) or thigh (proximal) DVT.[22] In addition, appreciating that small thrombi around the valve cusp in the proximal system may not be as threatening to the patient as an extensive thrombus in the same location, authors have begun to quantitate the size of thrombi in each of these locations.[11, 27] We now expect the literature discussing DVT to clearly define both location and size of DVTs in the lower extremity in order to better define what a DVT is.

Methods of Detections

Past and present methods of detection of DVT allow unclear definitions and their clinical significance to persist. Today B-mode duplex ultrasonography challenges the gold standard of detection, which is the venogram. Older tests, such as plethysmography, fi-

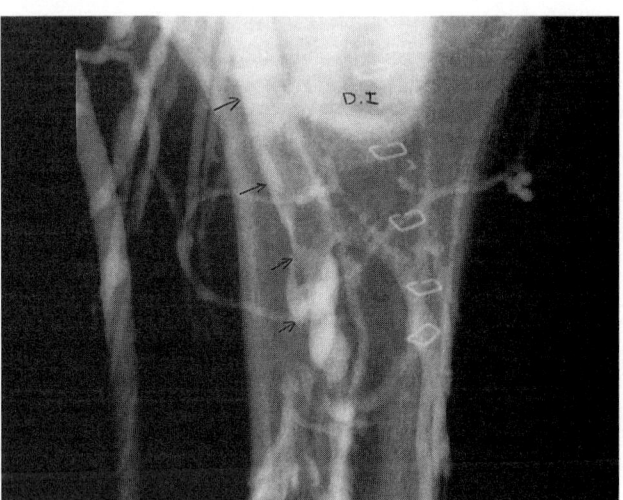

FIG 68–1.
Venogram illustrating a medium-sized clot in the popliteal vein below the knee after total knee arthroplasty. Does this thrombus require treatment?

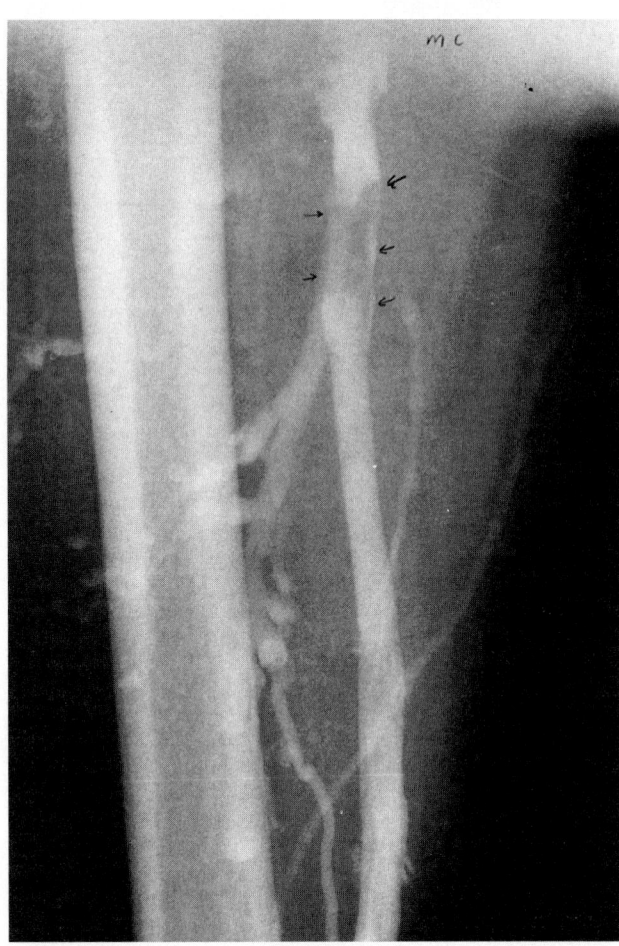

FIG 68–2.
Venogram illustrating a medium-sized clot in the proximal thigh 7 days after total knee arthroplasty. Does this thrombus require treatment?

brinogen scanning, and clinical evaluation, continue to lose popularity. These older imprecise tests are part of the reason why definitions of DVT remain inaccurate and inconsistent. A brief review of each of these studies will make this more apparent.

Ascending venography is a contrast study which has the potential to clearly define, localize, and quantitate thrombi in the lower extremity (see Figs 68–1 and 68–2).[26] It has good accuracy throughout the entire lower extremity, even above the inguinal ligament into the iliofemoral systems. Nonfilling veins or obstruction by prosthetic implants diminishes some of the accuracy, but, in general, clots can be localized and quantitated. Disadvantages include the invasive nature of the test and a chemical phlebitis associated with the use of the contrast dye. In addition, the study is contraindicated in patients who are allergic to intravenous iodine dyes or have poor renal function. However, because of its accuracy and ability to visualize clot, it still remains the gold standard.

B-mode duplex compression ultrasonography (Fig 68–3) is becoming a very popular and widespread technology used to detect DVT.[4, 34] It also has the potential to localize and quantitate clot. The terminology which has been used for this technology has been confusing and we will review it briefly here.

B-mode duplex compression ultrasonography refers to a type of ultrasonography that is related to the evolution and development of the technical aspects of ultrasound. "Duplex" refers to its ability to visualize clots as well assess the functional flow within the veins by Doppler analysis (Fig 68–4). The compression aspect of ultrasound appears to be the most accurate method of detecting DVT (Fig 68–5). This component of the test requires visualization of the vein by ultrasound and then compression with a probe. If the vein compresses, it indicates that no thrombus is present within the vessel and it there-

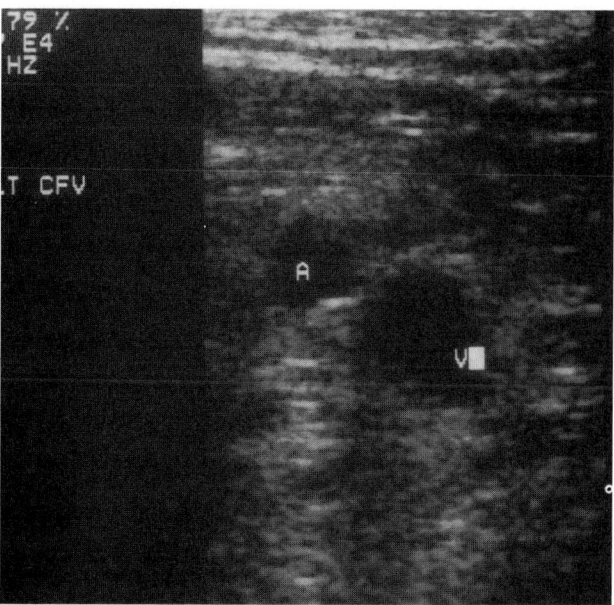

FIG 68–4.
Ultrasound images of superficial femoral artery *(A)* and vein *(V)* which demonstrate normal size lumina and patent vasculature.

fore is patent. On the other hand, if there is a thrombus within the vein, it will not compress. Compression is the most valuable component of this diagnostic study because some thrombi, especially those formed early, are not echogenic and therefore cannot be visualized. If a clot is mature and echogenic, its visualization by ultrasound can be quite dramatic and diagnostic. If the clot is visualized, its length and location can be quantitated. Compression ultrasonography is particularly effective in the proximal deep venous system, from the popliteal vein to the inguinal ligament. Gas in the bowel precludes its use above the inguinal ligament and its accuracy falls off dramatically in the calf. The primary advantage of this study is that it is noninvasive, which allows for repeated evaluations. The secondary advantage is its potential to both localize and quantitate a clot. Disadvantages include variable sensitivity with difficulty in picking up small clots in the proximal system and at the adductor hiatus and the apparent technician-dependency accompanied by a significant learning curve. The importance of experience in performing this study cannot be overemphasized. The variability with the use of technetium may account for the wide variability in the reported accuracy of this study.

Adjuncts have been used to augment the sensitivity of ultrasonography. The principal adjunct is Doppler augmentation of venous flow with calf compression. A flow recording is obtained before and after the calf is compressed. If the proximal veins are

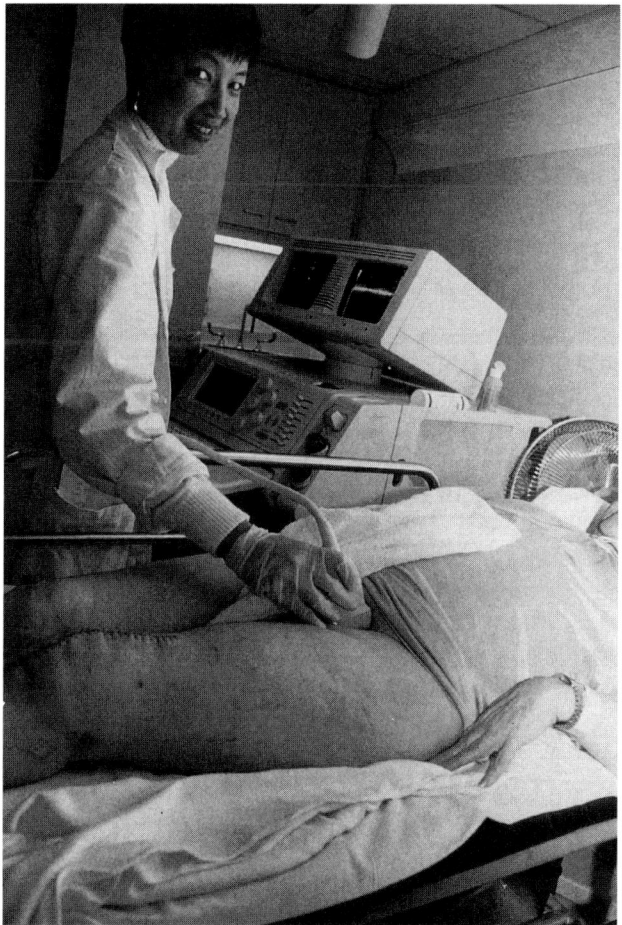

FIG 68–3.
Technician places an ultrasound probe on the proximal femur over the femoral vein in a patient after total knee arthroplasty. The probe is used to isolate the vein and then compression determines if a clot is present. Many clots are not echogenic and therefore cannot be directly visualized.

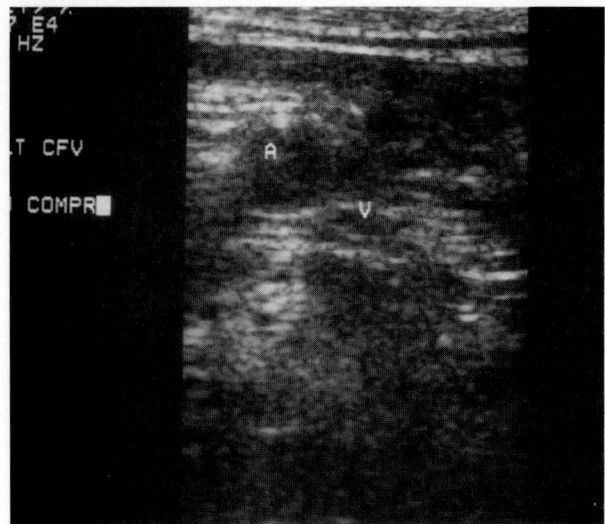

FIG 68–5.
Ultrasound images of the same patient in Figure 67–4 with compression applied to the vein by the ultrasound probe. This has completely occluded the vein and therefore no thrombus is present.

patent, calf compression significantly increases the flow, which is determined by either audio or graphic signals. This augmentation allows the examiner to more carefully evaluate veins which do not show normal flow dynamics. Despite its limitations the potential of this study is great, and in the next decade we may expect to find numerous studies utilizing compression ultrasonography as the principal method for diagnosis of DVT.

The three principal methods of detection of DVT that have been used in the past and that may have contributed to some of the controversy because of their reduced accuracy include fibrinogen scan, plethysmography, and clinical evaluation. It has been shown that the clinical evaluation of DVT in the postoperative patient after total knee surgery is almost a random event.[20, 29] The classic clinical findings of tenderness or Homan's sign being diagnostic of the presence of a DVT are not reliable in the postoperative patient. The sudden onset of thigh swelling 5 to 7 days after surgery may indicate that a proximal thrombus exists and should be followed with appropriate studies. However, calf swelling is so common there is no reliable association with thrombosis.

The iodine 131–labeled fibrinogen scan has been equally inaccurate. In this study, patients are given labeled fibrinogen and then scanned serially over the next 3 to 5 days. If a clot has formed in the lower extremity, a concentration of increased radionuclide will be noted and therefore define the presence of a DVT. This test has limited accuracy, is reduced by postsurgical trauma around the knee, and is technician-dependent. This study will probably be unavailable in the future.

Plethysmography has been particularly popular in the diagnosis of proximal thrombi.[15] This study places a venous tourniquet in the upper thigh and then measures the rate of blood flow out of, or volume decreases in, the calf as the tourniquet is released. Depending on the slope of the curve, the presence or absence of a proximal thrombus is postulated. Obviously, the rate is significantly diminished with large occluding proximal thrombi and although the diagnosis can be established, the clot cannot be quantified. On the other hand, partially occluding smaller thigh thrombi may neither be detected nor quantitated. This study will probably also have diminished use in the future.

In summary, part of the controversy existing in this area of TED results from the diagnostic modalities utilized to study DVT. Many of the tests have been inaccurate or insensitive and yet conclusions have been drawn from these studies. With the recognition of the accuracy of venography and the increasing clinical experience with ultrasonography, we expect that some of the diagnostic problems associated with TED will be diminished.

Incidence

The incidence of DVT in the postoperative patient after total knee surgery is relatively high. Using venographic data, the incidence is between 50% and 70%.[20, 29, 30] Most of these are in the calf and two thirds of them may be defined as small, or less than 3 cm in length. Approximately one third of them will be longer than 3 cm and involve an area up to the popliteal vein. Thigh thrombi will be present in 5% to 7% of the postoperative total knee patients. Most of these will be relatively small, less than 3 cm, or associated with proximal valve cusps, or both. However, there are a few which will be rather extensive, involving the iliofemoral vein of the venous system. Contralateral DVT will develop in 3% to 5% of patients.

The clinical significance of DVT in the distal venous system is still controversial. Some authors believe that the presence of a calf thrombus in the postoperative total knee patient is a normal pathophysiologic event after surgery and does not identify the patient at risk for developing PE. Other authors feel that any clot in the lower extremity is a risk to the patient. At this time there is general agreement that DVTs are common after surgery and that the greater the clot burden, the greater the risk to the patient.

The critical size and location of this clot burden remain controversial.

PULMONARY EMBOLISM

The three main methods to detect PE include (1) clinical evaluation, (2) ventilation perfusion (V/Q) scans, and (3) pulmonary angiography. The accuracy of clinical evaluation in detecting PE varies from 5% to 20%. Only 15% of those patients who are suspected of having a PE on clinical evaluation are subsequently shown to have a PE with further laboratory studies.[28] The classic findings of lethargy and reduced arterial blood oxygen are so common in the postoperative total knee patient with analgesia that PE is frequently overdiagnosed. After the clinical assessment for possible PE is completed, the next step, in most diagnostic studies, has been the V/Q scan (Fig 68–6). A recent multicenter study[25] evaluating the effectiveness of the V/Q scan in the diagnosis of PE has shown that it is not entirely reliable. If clinical suspicion is very high, that is, chest pain, shortness of breath, sudden onset of symptoms, and low arterial blood gas values, a positive V/Q scan may indicate a PE in approximately 95% of patients. On the other hand, if the clinical presentation is relatively indeterminate, the accuracy of a high-probability V/Q scan is less than 70%. It has also been shown that the accuracy of the V/Q scan depends on the size of the clot.[14] Those clots that occlude large segmental systems have a much higher incidence of being identified on the V/Q scan than those with subsegmental defects. We believe that the dependence on the V/Q scan for clinical decisions should be carefully reevaluated in the next decade.

The most accurate way of diagnosing PE continues to be the pulmonary arteriogram. This is considered to be between 90% and 100% accurate and remains the gold standard for detection of PE. However, it has the obvious disadvantage of being invasive and expensive.

Fat embolism syndrome (FES) is a significant problem just recently recognized to mimic a PE in the very early postoperative period. In this syndrome, the patient becomes short of breath, lethargic, and has diminished blood oxygenation. The most severe episode may occur suddenly in the recovery room and be associated with mental obtundation. Less severe episodes demonstrate a narrower spectrum of symptoms. FES should not be confused with PE and should be considered as the primary diagnosis within the first 24 hours after surgery.

If the result of a diagnostic study initiates a therapeutic regimen, then the accuracy of the study should be as high as possible because of the great risk of therapy and the inherent risks of bleeding complications. This is discussed later.

PEs have also been subject to considerable variation in classification. They can be classified as asymptomatic, symptomatic, and fatal. Fatal PE appears to be the simplest to define. However, many patients do not have postmortem examinations and in fact only approximately half of the deaths attributed to PE are clearly caused by a PE. Many may be cardiogenic, FES, or septic in origin, and the differentiation between the direct or indirect cause of death is frequently unclear. Symptomatic PE would also appear to be easy to define. However, as noted above, of the patients who are assumed to have PE serious enough to warrant a pulmonary angiogram, only 20% will indeed have a confirmed diagnosis after all tests are completed.[28] Therefore, although PE is frequently suspected by its symptoms, a definitive diagnosis is more difficult to establish.

Asymptomatic PE has recently been recognized to occur in the postoperative period.[10, 19] These have been found by V/Q scans performed in association with prospective studies on total knee and hip patients. Since these patients are totally asymptomatic and the PE is discovered only in the course of a prospective study, they have not been included in most reports on the incidence of TED. The clinical significance of asymptomatic PE is still undetermined. Its presence also complicates the determination of the cause of death in patients undergoing postmortem examinations.

The incidence of PE after total knee surgery has

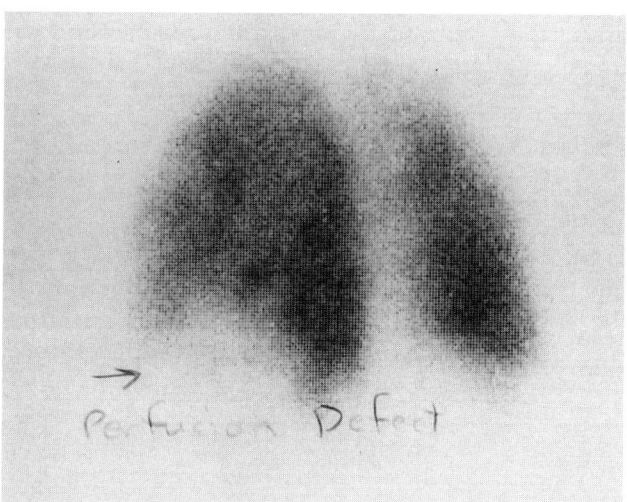

FIG 68–6.
A perfusion defect in the right lower lobe in a patient with a normal ventilation scan. This ventilation-perfusion mismatch was interpreted as high probability for pulmonary embolism.

been variably reported in the literature, which is partly due to the lack of accuracy of diagnostic studies. However, in general, the incidence of fatal PE is believed to be between 0.2% and 0.7%. Symptomatic PE occurs in from 1.0% to 1.9% of patients.

Asymptomatic PE, the new category of PE, has been variably reported at between 10% and 18%.[10, 19] The recognition that many patients have PE after total knee surgery has been a surprise to the medical community. Additional information is being gathered. It is noted that there is an increasing incidence of asymptomatic PE associated with a large DVT. Patients with large calf and thigh thrombi have a higher incidence of asymptomatic PE than those with smaller calf thrombi or those who have no thrombi. However, asymptomatic PE also occurs in a significant number of patients who have no thrombi and therefore the relationship is not clearly defined.

The recognition that asymptomatic PE exists after total knee surgery is important clinically. This is particularly true in patients who become ill and need full medical evaluations. It must be appreciated that the presence of a positive V/Q scan may only indicate an asymptomatic PE and may not be related to the patient's present acute symptoms. This may affect the differential diagnosis and treatment recommendation in the ill postoperative patient.

An unanswered treatment dilemma exists in patients with asymptomatic PE. If prospective studies identify a patient with a PE within the pulmonary vasculature, should this asymptomatic PE be treated? This remains an unanswered question, but at present I have not found these asymptomatic thrombi to be an increased risk to patients and have elected not to initiate treatment but to continue a prophylactic regimen.

PROPHYLAXIS FOR THROMBOEMBOLIC DISEASE

The definition of prophylaxis, as opposed to a therapeutic regimen, has varied over the years and the terms have been frequently interchanged in the literature. Prophylaxis should always be considered as an agent which is given pre- and postoperatively in order to prevent TED. Theoretically, any regimen should have low morbidity and prevent sequelae of emboli. A therapeutic regimen may be defined as any treatment program that is initiated after the discovery of a thromboembolic event. In general, these have been aggressive anticoagulation methods and as such have greater risks from bleeding.

It is generally agreed that some form of prophylaxis should be utilized in the postoperative patient after total knee surgery. However, there are a large number of treatment alternatives and the regimen that is most effective remains to be determined.

Currently, the most popular prophylactic regimens include the use of warfarin, aspirin, low-molecular-weight heparin, intermittent compression boots, and vena cava filters. Each is discussed briefly here. Other, less frequently used modalities include continuous passive motion (CPM), dextran, elastic stockings, antithrombin III, and combinations of these.

Warfarin

Warfarin has become one of the more popular prophylactic agents in the management of the postoperative total knee replacement patient.[6, 7, 16] Amstutz et al.[1] found no in-hospital fatalities secondary to PE in over 3,000 total hip arthroplasty patients treated with warfarin. The effectiveness of this agent appears to be high and has subsequently gained support. The regimen that has been utilized is 10 mg of warfarin given either the night of or the night before surgery and then dose-adjusted throughout the postoperative period to a level of 1.2 to 1.5 times control values. The advantages of warfarin are that it is an oral drug which may be continued in the postdischarge period and it appears to have relatively low potential for excessive bleeding if good control is maintained. The principal disadvantage of warfarin is that the dose response may be variable and therefore careful monitoring is required to achieve appropriate levels. In addition, patients who are on anti-inflammatory medications for other reasons, such as rheumatoid arthritis, are generally excluded from warfarin regimens unless they discontinue their aspirin or other nonsteroidal medications.

Aspirin

Aspirin is a popular method of prophylaxis and recently has been shown to be as effective as warfarin in the prevention of DVT or asymptomatic PE.[9, 18] If one believes that these are appropriate indicators of the effectiveness of an agent, then aspirin may be considered to be equivalent to warfarin in the prevention of TED after total knee surgery. The required dose of aspirin is low, 320 mg/day. The principal advantages of aspirin are its ease of use, high patient tolerance at low dosage, and its oral form, which may be continued after discharge from the hospital. Its disadvantages include some gastrointestinal intolerance and a reluctance to accept the fact that such a common medication may be effective.

Heparin

Heparin has also gained significant popularity as prophylaxis after total knee surgery.[2, 13, 31] There are two forms of heparin which are or will become available. The traditional heparin, an extract from pig intestines, is being challenged by a low molecular weight heparin developed from a subfraction of traditional heparin. The advantages of low molecular weight heparin are believed to be fewer side effects, such as thrombocytopenia, and a prolongation of the half-life, which reduces its dosage requirements. At present, current recommendations for either heparin or low molecular weight heparin are subcutaneous administration twice daily. With this regimen, a significant reduction in the incidence of thrombosis and PE has been demonstrated.[5] The principal disadvantage to the use of heparin is related to its subcutaneous administration and the difficulty of using it in the postdischarge patient.

Intermittent Compression Boots

Intermittent compression boots have recently been shown to reduce the incidence of DVT in the postoperative period.[8, 12, 33] Compression boots may be applied intraoperatively or shortly thereafter and are placed over one or both legs. While the patient is in bed, the boots are intermittently inflated and deflated to assist venous outflow. They have also been used in combination with other antithrombotic agents. The long-term effectiveness of compression boots and their relationship to the prevention of PE are still to be determined.

Vena Cava Filters

Vena cava filters, such as the Greenfield filter, have been used to prevent PE in high-risk patients, especially if there are contraindications to other antithrombotic agents.[30, 32] Such situations may occur in the postoperative total knee patient who has had gastrointestinal bleed. Vena cava filters are small wire cages which are inserted through the femoral vein and left in the vena cava. They have been shown to prevent major PE. They do have complications, such as chronic lower extremity edema and some inhibition to normal venous circulation, which at times can create major circulatory compromise. Despite the occasional downside risks from vena cava filters, there are some authors who advocate using them in the postoperative total arthroplasty patient.

A variety of other modalities and drug therapies have been used over the decades to prevent PE. They include CPM,[21] dextran, and elastic stockings. In addition, antithrombin III, a potentiator of heparin, has also been advocated for use in preventing PE.[28] Most of the above agents have been used in combination or sequentially in the posthospitalization patient.

Recommendations

We must ask why the best regimen to prevent PE is still undecided after more than five decades of investigation. Warfarin and heparin have been used since the early 1940s when warfarin was isolated as the hemorrhagic agent in spoiled sweet clover.[3] There are many possible reasons for the diverse results and conclusions. The first is that a variety of inaccurate diagnostic techniques have been employed. Most of these noninvasive studies, e.g., fibrinogen scans and plethysomography, have only modest accuracy and have not been able to quantitate clot. In addition, venographic data have been inconsistently reported. Early studies did not routinely record the location or size of the thrombus. Furthermore, the inclusion of a variety of patients with varying diagnoses within the same study has contributed to inconsistent results. The risk of PE from calf DVT in a carcinoma patient or congestive heart failure (CHF) patient may be entirely different from that in the postoperative total knee patient. The importance of stratifying patient populations has only recently become apparent. Indeed, some of the most frequently cited articles on this subject have pooled patient populations with varying diagnoses and risk factors and have drawn conclusions from this diverse group which may not apply to specific patients.

PE is a problem with a relatively low incidence. This makes well-controlled studies with clear statistical significance a critical factor in determining the efficacy of prophylactic regimens. However, because of nonstratification of patients and poorly defined diagnostic end points, obtaining true statistically significant data has been difficult.

In addition, there has been a significant change in the care of orthopedic patients over the years. The data accumulated from the era of cup arthroplasty and tibial osteotomies in which patients were placed in casts or immobilized for long periods of time may not apply to the postoperative total knee patient who is mobilized 1 to 3 days after surgery. The historic risks of TED may not apply to current practice. Recommendations for specific anticoagulation regimens for current orthopedic practice continue to be difficult to formulate.

TREATMENT FOR THROMBOEMBOLIC DISEASE

The standard treatment regimen for a life-threatening thromboembolic event is immediate heparinization to 1.5 to 2.0 times control value followed 5 to 10 days later by oral anticoagulation with warfarin.[16] This may be continued for 6 to 24 weeks. This regimen is associated with a significant risk and therefore has been modified in the past few years to allow lower doses of heparin for shorter periods of time.

There is a significant risk in initiating heparin and warfarin therapy in the postoperative total joint patient.[24] One study demonstrated a 30% chance of a bleeding complication with the use of heparin. If the heparin was administered within the first week, there was a 45% chance of a significant bleed. A major prospective study incorporating both total hip and total knee patients showed that there was a 10% risk of major bleeding with the use of heparin given at therapeutic doses, and a 1% death rate from a bleeding complication.[16] With this risk, the indications to initiate therapeutic intervention must be carefully assessed.

The indications to obtain diagnostic studies for TED vary among institutions and clinical settings. We do not yet recommend routine venographic screening for DVT or asymptomatic PE for every patient undergoing TKA. This is partly due to the fact that we do not have valid recommendations as to how to respond to the data obtained on routine screening, and second, the value of a reliable noninvasive test such as ultrasound is still under investigation. However, clinical situations will arise in which it seems appropriate to consider TED and obtain diagnostic tests. The responses to the results of these tests should be individualized to the patient and the risk-benefit ratio carefully assessed.

It is my recommendation that heparin-warfarin therapy be instituted very carefully.[17] Our current regimen for therapy for TED is the following:

Thrombi	Treatment
Calf thrombi	Continue prophylaxis
Popliteal thrombi	Continue prophylaxis
Small thigh thrombi	Continue prophylaxis
Asymptomatic PE	Continue prophylaxis
Large thigh thrombi	Initiate therapy
Symptomatic PE	Initiate therapy

SUMMARY

Thromboembolic disease in the form of thrombi in the lower extremity or PE presents a worrisome risk to patients after total knee surgery. The best method to prevent and treat this problem is yet to be determined. Part of the problem in reaching a consensus is by nature inherent to problems of low incidence. In addition, the problems have been poorly defined and imprecise diagnostic modalities have been used in the past. With newer methods of detection, such as ultrasound, and the wider acceptance of venography, more accurate definitions of patients at risk will be established. Fatal, symptomatic, and asymptomatic PE occur in postoperative total knee patients. Fortunately, symptomatic and fatal PE occur infrequently. The clinical significance of asymptomatic PE is undetermined, but its recognition is important in understanding the pathophysiology of this problem.

There have been numerous investigations into appropriate prophylactic agents to prevent PE and the single consensus is that prophylaxis is important and that orthopedic surgeons should choose one that they feel is best for their patients. The goal of any prophylactic regimen is to reduce the incidence of symptomatic or fatal PE without causing adverse reactions. A change in the incidence of DVT is only important if one believes that it is a significant precursor of PE. This is probably true only for large thrombi in the thigh or more proximally, not for those in the calf. Current choices include warfarin, aspirin, and heparin, but intermittent compression boots, vena cava filters, elastic stockings, antithrombin III, and combinations of the above may be useful in preventing PE. The treatment of thromboembolic phenomena should be carefully weighed because there are significant risks with heparin therapy. The indications are not clearly defined at this time, but it appears that distal and small thrombi may not require therapeutic intervention other than continued prophylactic regimens. With continued investigation, and recognition of the deficiencies in past studies, forthcoming studies should help elucidate the best methods to prevent TED in the total knee patient.

REFERENCES

1. Amstutz, HC, et al: Warfarin prophylaxis to prevent mortality from pulmonary embolism after total hip replacement, J Bone Joint Surg [Am] 71:321–326, 1989.
2. Beisaw NE, et al: Dihydroergotamine/heparin in the prevention of deep-vein thrombosis after total hip replacement, J Bone Joint Surg [Am] 70:2–10, 1988.
3. Bingham JB, Meyer OO, Pohle FJ,: Studies on the hemorrhagic agent 3,3'-methylene-bis-(4-hydroxycoumarin): Its effect on the prothrombin and coagulation time of the blood of dogs and humans, Am J Med Sci 202:563–578, 1941.

4. Camerota, A, et al: Venous duplex imaging: Should it replace hemodynamic tests for deep venous thrombosis?, *J Vasc Surg* 4:53–61, 1990.
5. Collins R, et al: Reduction in fatal pulmonary embolism and venous thrombosis by perioperative administration of subcutaneous heparin, *N Engl J Med* 318:1162–1173, 1988.
6. Francis CW, et al: Two-step warfarin therapy, *JAMA* 249:374–378, 1983.
7. Francis CS, et al: Prevention of venous thrombosis after total knee arthroplasty, *J Bone Joint Surg [Am]* 72:976–982, 1990.
8. Haas B, et al: Pneumatic sequential-compression boots compared with aspirin prophylaxis of deep-vein thrombosis after total knee arthroplasty, *J Bone Joint Surg [Am]* 72:27–31, 1990.
9. Harris WH, et al: High and low-dose aspirin prophylaxis against venous thromboembolic disease in total hip replacement, *J Bone Joint Surg [Am]* 64:63–66, 1982.
10. Harris WH, et al: Detection of pulmonary emboli after total hip replacement using serial $C^{15}O_2$ pulmonary scans, *J Bone Joint Surg [Am]* 66:1388–1393, 1984.
11. Harris WH, et al: Prophylaxis of deep-vein thrombosis after total hip replacement, *J Bone Joint Surg [Am]* 67:57–62, 1985.
12. Hartman JT, et al: Cyclic sequential compression of the lower limb in prevention of deep venous thrombosis, *J Bone Joint Surg [Am]* 64:1059–1062, 1982.
13. Hull RH et al: Adjusted subcutaneous heparin versus warfarin sodium in the long-term treatment of venous thrombosis, *N Engl J Med* 306:189–194, 1982.
14. Hull RD, et al: Diagnostic value of ventilation perfusion lung scanning in patients with suspected pulmonary embolism, *Chest* 88:819–829, 1984.
15. Hull RD, et al: A new noninvasive management strategy for patients with suspected pulmonary embolism, *Arch Intern Med* 149:2549–2555, 1989.
16. Hull RD, et al: Heparin for 5 days with 10 days in the initial treatment of proximal venous thrombosis, *N Engl J Med* 322:1260–1264, 1990.
17. Lotke PA,: Thromboembolic disease: Summary and conclusions *Semin Arthroplasty* 3:137–140, 1992.
18. Lotke PA, Palevsky HI, Steinberg MD.: Warfarin compared to aspirin in the prevention of thromboembolic disease after total hip and total knee surgery. Annual Meeting of the American Academy of Orthopaedic Surgeons, Anaheim, Calif, March 12, 1991.
19. Lotke PA, Wong RY, Ecker ML.: Asymptomatic pulmonary embolism after total knee replacement, *Orthop Trans* 10:490, 1986.
20. Lotke PA et al: Indications from the treatment of deep venous thrombosis following total knee replacement, *J Bone Joint Surg [Am]* 66:202–208, 1984
21. Lynch AF, et al: Deep-vein thrombosis and continuous passive motion after total knee arthroplasty, *J Bone Joint Surg [Am]* 70:11–14, 1988.
22. Moser KM, LeMoine JR: Is embolic risk conditioned by location of deep venous thrombosis? *Ann Intern Med* 94:439–444, 1981.
23. Moser KM: Pathophysiology of venous thromboembolism. *Semin Arthroplasty* 3:64–71, 1992.
24. Patterson BM, Marchard R, Ranawat CS: Complications of heparin therapy after total joint arthroplasty, *J Bone Joint Surg [Am]* 71:1130–1134, 1989.
25. PIOPED: Value of the ventilation perfusion scan in acute pulmonary embolism: Results of the prospective investigation of pulmonary embolism diagnosis, *JAMA* 263:2753–2759, 1990.
26. Ravinov K, Paulin S.: Roentgen diagnosis of venous thrombosis in the leg, *Arch Surg* 104:134–144, 1972.
27. Sharrock NE et al: The effect of intravenous fixed-dose heparin during total hip arthroplasty on the incidence of deep-vein thrombosis, *J Bone Joint Surg [Am]* 72:1456–1461, 1990.
28. Stevens PM: Spurious pulmonary embolism: A non-disease, *Heart Lung* 8:141–147, 1979.
29. Stulberg BN, et al: Deep-vein thrombosis following total knee replacement, *J Bone Joint Surg [Am]* 66:194–201, 1984.
30. Sutherland CJ, Schurman JR,: Complications associated with warfarin prophylaxis in total knee arthroplasty, *Clin Orthop* 219:158–162, 1987.
31. Trupie AGG, et al: A randomized controlled trial of low molecular weight heparin (Eroxaparin) to prevent deep venous thrombosis in patients undergoing elective hip surgery, *N Engl J Med* 315:925–929, 1986.
32. Vaughn BK, et al: Use of the Greenfield filter to prevent fatal pulmonary embolism associated with total hip and knee arthroplasty, *J Bone Joint Surg [Am]* 71:1542–1547, 1989.
33. Woolson ST, Watl MJ: Intermittent pneumatic compression to prevent proximal deep venous thrombosis during and after total hip replacement, *J Bone Joint Surg [Am]* 73:507–512, 1991.
34. Woolson S, et al: B-mode ultrasound scanning in the detection of proximal venous thrombosis after total hip replacement, *J Bone Joint Surg [Am]* 72:983–987, 1990.

Part XV

Revision Total Knee Replacement

69

Nursing Care of a Patient Having a Total Knee Arthroplasty

MARY ANN UNDERHILL, M.S., R.N., O.N.C.

Preoperative program
   Patient education
   Pain management
   Mobility
Preparation for surgery
Postoperative care

Continuous passive motion
   Pain management
   Clinical monitoring
   Occupational therapy
Discharge planning

Total joint replacement has revolutionized orthopaedic medicine. These procedures, coupled with changes in the health care reimbursement system and the subsequent effect on length of stay, have had a profound effect on how orthopaedic nurses care for patients. Historically, nurses have set goals for patients, planned interventions to meet those goals, and then evaluated the effectiveness of their interventions. The patient was a passive recipient of nursing care. Prior to diagnosis-related groups (DRGs), the patient anticipating a total knee arthroplasty was admitted to the hospital 1 or 2 days prior to surgery for a thorough medical workup, ambulation training, and preoperative teaching. Postoperatively, the patient was immobilized for 3 or 4 days before physical therapy was initiated. The patient remained hospitalized for 19 to 21 days, leaving the 6-week follow-up appointment only 2 weeks away. Today, that same patient is admitted to the hospital hours, not days, prior to surgery, is mobilized within 24 hours postoperatively, and is discharged 4 to 6 days following a total knee replacement. This patient is more than a month away from the 6-week follow-up appointment. The orthopaedic nurse today has less than 1 week to prepare this patient to become autonomous in his or her care.

With such a short hospital stay, it is critical that the patient be involved in setting goals for recovery. These goals represent measurable behaviors that reflect the patient's ability to be safe in a home environment. The evaluation process focuses on the patient's progress toward meeting these goals. The patient having a total knee arthroplasty thus becomes a partner, an active participant if you will, in his or her care. The role of the orthopaedic nurse in this partnership is one of expert clinician, patient and family educator, and advocate/facilitator in helping the patient define and meet his or her goals. The purpose of this chapter is to describe the interactive role of the orthopaedic nurse in coordinating this partnership of care with the patient, physician, physical therapist, and other members of the health care team. Inherent in this description is the patient's reaction or response to being an active participant in this experience.

PREOPERATIVE PROGRAM

In response to changes in reimbursement that preclude admitting the patient to the hospital the day before surgery, some hospitals have implemented preadmission planning or testing programs that are provided 5 to 7 days prior to the scheduled surgery. While these programs may take various formats depending upon the availability of resources within a given institution, all have components of preoperative teaching, preoperative testing, physical therapy evaluation and instruction, and discharge planning. The programs may be offered on a one-to-one basis or the teaching phase may be offered as a class for groups of patients anticipating total knee replacement. Some programs are offered on site where the surgery is scheduled, whereas other institutions take the service into the patient's home or into the physician's office. When possible, the program may be scheduled to coincide with an autologous blood draw. The key element, regardless of location or format, remains that the patient, prior to the day of surgery, have access to information and instructions that facilitate active participation in care, and a knowledge base that will allow the patient to be safe at home after surgery. In all situations, it is the registered nurse who assesses the needs of the patient and coordinates the involvement of other disciplines. In this chapter one model is used to describe the assessments and activities that occur 5 to 7 days prior to the patient being admitted to the hospital. During this outpatient visit, which takes approximately $2\frac{1}{2}$ hours, the patient is interviewed by a registered nurse, and based upon the information gathered, a plan of care for the hospital stay is developed and shared with the patient. The patient's learning needs related to surgery and the postoperative period, as well as the patient's plans for post-hospital care, are addressed during this initial nursing assessment using a multidisciplinary approach. A physical therapy evaluation that includes gait training and instruction in postoperative exercises is provided. An electrocardiogram (ECG) and any laboratory tests, radiographs, or other tests ordered prior to surgery are also done during this visit.

The orthopaedic nurse uses this pre-admission planning session to assess the patient's perception and understanding of total knee replacement. The nurse encourages the patient to tell his or her own story. The total knee replacement candidate is frequently a person, who because of severe knee pain, has had to give up or decrease participation in leisure activities and forego hobbies in an attempt to simply remain employed. Degenerative joint disease threatens the person's ability to earn a living. Many candidates for a total knee replacement are within a few years of retirement, not at a point in life to be forced into a job change. Merely being able to remain employed is a goal for many patients. For other patients, being ambulatory without pain is most important. Independence in self-care is a key factor for all patients in their decision to proceed with surgery.

The patient who has decided to proceed with a total knee arthroplasty has had a detailed discussion with the orthopaedic surgeon regarding the procedure, the components of the new joint, and the expected outcome. Potential complications and individual risk factors have also been addressed. Typically, a recovery and rehabilitation program has been discussed. Patients vary in their ability to comprehend the magnitude of this information. Many times a patient hears little of what the surgeon is saying after hearing that a total knee replacement offers pain relief, improved stability, and increased mobility in the affected knee.

It is important to note what the patient expects to have happen or change as a result of this surgery in terms of pain or discomfort, mobility, and return to activities of daily living (ADL). Questioning the patient about previous treatment regimens and his or her perception of success or failure can be a good indicator of the patient's compliance with a prescribed regimen. A detailed discussion and review of the information and instructions received from the orthopaedic surgeon allows the registered nurse to determine what the patient has been told and how that information was interpreted. This is the time when a reality check is carried out to determine what the patient knows about the anticipated length of stay, postoperative pain management, and limitations to mobility, including weightbearing status after surgery, restrictions on activity, and any equipment needed for post-discharge care. In addition to the orthopaedic surgeon, the patient anticipating a total knee replacement has received information about the procedure from friends and relatives, as well as the media. The challenge for the orthopaedic nurse lies in being able to help the patient sort out the meaning of the information received to determine what is valid and what is not. For example, the patient after being told about a weightbearing restriction or the need to use a walker or crutches to ambulate does not automatically translate this information into not being able to drive a car or climb stairs. Following a total knee arthroplasty, taking a shower may be acceptable with a step-in shower, but, climbing over the side of a bathtub without an appropriate handrail or tub seat could be dangerous. The registered nurse helps the patient to understand and incorporate these instructions into his or her lifestyle.

In a pre-admission program, admission assessment and discharge planning go hand in hand. Following the nurse's assessment, a social worker or discharge planner meets with the patient and family to discuss the patient's post-discharge plans and provide assistance in identifying sources of services or equipment. By initiating discharge planning at this time, the patient begins to comprehend that the hospital stay will be relatively short and assistance with ambulation and activities of daily living may be needed beyond the hospital stay. To many people, the length of the hospital stay is related to the seriousness of the surgery and a 1-week hospitalization may imply a simple, short recovery. The perception is that if the new joint eliminates knee pain and it was the pain that hampered their independence, then pain-free independence should be attainable by discharge. Discharge planning dispels this myth. Initiating discharge planning at this time is advantageous because the patient is still very much in control. The patient can return home and make any necessary modifications with regard to bathroom safety, obtaining a rocking chair or straight chair with arms, and so on, prior to being admitted to the hospital the day of surgery. The patient is now actively involved in planning for the recovery period. Timely discharge planning that takes into consideration the patient's support system at home, the early identification of postdischarge options, and goals related to activity that are both realistic and attainable within the time of the hospital stay eliminates unnecessary and costly delays in discharging the patient while last-minute arrangements are made.

Patient Education

It is during this preadmission visit that the registered nurse assesses the patient's learning needs. The learning needs of each person are different, being affected by factors such as level of knowledge, past experience, values and beliefs, and most important, the person's willingness to change or modify behavior and lifestyle to accommodate the new joint. Adults need and want information that will help them live their lives; they are performance-centered, and interested in information they can use immediately. Teaching efforts must also be individualized to meet each patient's needs and learning style. Throughout the teaching process, the nurse must determine what it is this patient wants to know about the procedure and the postoperative course. The issue is not what the nurse thinks the patient wants to know, and therefore the process must be interactive based on the needs of each individual patient. A multimedia approach that combines printed and audiovisual materials helps to clarify and reinforce the information being given (Fig 69–1). While the education component must be tailored to meet individual needs, it is important that there be consistency in the information provided so that reinforcement of the teaching effort can occur at different phases of the postoperative and recovery periods. The National Association of Orthopaedic Nurses (NAON) has a patient education video on total knee replacement that guides a patient through all phases of the surgery and recovery periods. A brochure that gives the patient material to refer to at home is also available for use with the NAON video. As a part of the preoperative planning process, the nurse takes the patient through the schedule of events for the day of surgery to decrease anxiety and encourage questions.

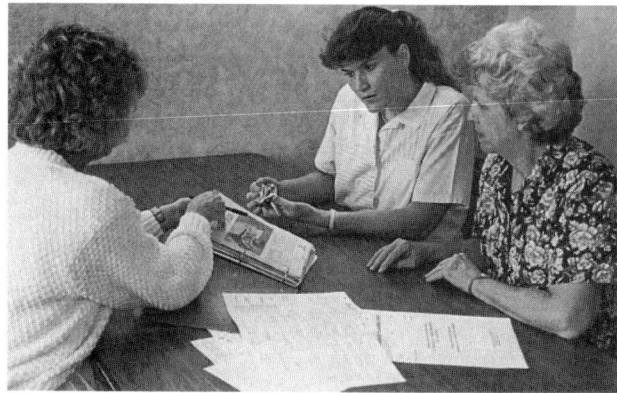

FIG 69–1.
Use of visual aids, including the actual total knee components, enhances preoperative teaching for both the patient and family members.

For adults who are visual learners, it is very helpful if they can see and practice with the actual equipment. Ideally, the patient should experience the slow, steady motion of a continuous passive motion (CPM) unit and either a sequential or intermittent compression device if these pieces of equipment are to be a part of the postoperative treatment.

Pain Management

Pain management is a major concern of the patient anticipating a total knee replacement. As a part of the preadmission assessment, the patient is asked to describe past pain experience and the techniques that were used to achieve pain control. Printed material describing techniques for pain management that the patient may take home and review prior to surgery has proved beneficial. The concept of self-reporting of pain intensity must be thoroughly explained to the patient. The patient needs reassurance that after surgery pain assessments will be done frequently and the information used to guide both pharmacologic as well as nonpharmacologic interventions. The patient may be asked to choose a pain assessment tool that would be useful to him. Examples of three pain assessment tools are shown in Figure 69–2.

These scales help the patient describe the intensity and personal distress caused by pain. Nurses primarily use one of these three types of pain rating scales. A visual analog scale (VAS) should always be represented graphically with a 10-cm baseline and end-point descriptive adjective. Patients are asked to place a mark on the line at a point that best describes their pain. The VAS is scored by measuring the dis-

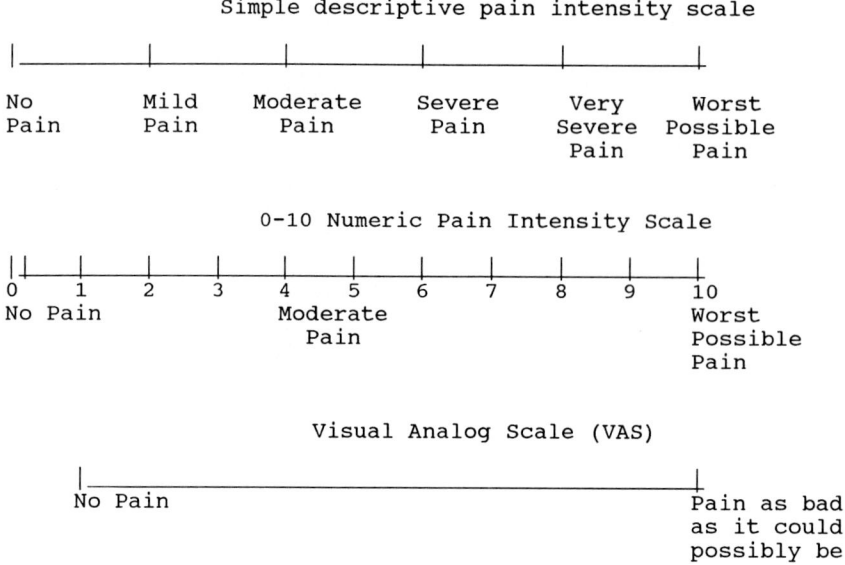

FIG 69-2.
Examples of pain intensity assessment scales. (From Acute Pain Management Guideline Panel: *Acute pain management: Operative or medical procedures and trauma. Clinical practice guideline,* Rockville, Md, Agency for Health Care Policy and Research, Public Health Service, US Dept of Health and Human Services, AHCPR Publication No. 92-0032, 1992.)

tance of the patient's mark from point 0 or no pain. An adjective rating scale may be presented as a list of pain descriptors from which the patient makes a choice (see Fig 69-2). In some situations a numeric scale in which the patient is asked to rate his or her pain on a scale of 0 to 10 with 0 being no pain and 10 being the worst pain possible (see Fig 69-2) will be sufficient to guide the nurse to appropriate interventions. It should be clear to the patient that a nurse will help to identify acceptable levels of pain and implement specific interventions to keep the level of pain within those limits. As a part of this education phase, the nurse describes for the patient the difference between pain intensity and the emotional distress or anxiety produced by the surgical experience. Similar scales can be used to identify the degree of distress the patient is experiencing (Fig 69-3).

If patient-controlled analgesia (PCA) is to be used for postoperative pain management, it should be demonstrated and the concept of PCA thoroughly explained to the patient and family members at this time. Any fears or concerns the patient may have about self-administering an intravenous (IV) narcotic needs to be addressed at this time. The patient needs to know that:

1. PCA allows the self-administration of pain medication through an IV line.
2. By the simple push of a button a predetermined amount of medication is released directly into the bloodstream.
3. Pain control is seconds away rather than 10 to 15 minutes as estimated following an intramuscular injection, or 20 to 25 minutes if an oral agent is used.
4. If the prescribed medication is not effective in achieving pain control, the nurse will consult with the orthopaedic surgeon to adjust the regimen.

The response of patients to PCA has been positive in that it allows them to remain in control, thereby reducing the anxiety experienced when pain intervention was based on a strict time schedule. With PCA, the administration of pain medication is no longer tied to a clock with set intervals of administration that may exceed the peak efficiency of the drug itself. Putting the patient in control of pain medication administration also serves as a distractor to pain. Knowing that relief is seconds away reduces the anxiety of hurting and not being able to intervene on one's own behalf. The administration of narcotics IV has proved to be more effective by reducing or eliminating the peaks and valleys that the patient receiving IM or oral pain medication frequently experiences.

Instead of PCA, some patients may have continuous epidural analgesia during the first 48 hours postoperatively. If this technique has been discussed with the patient by the orthopaedic surgeon, the nurse assesses the patient's understanding of the information he or she received and reinforces the following points:

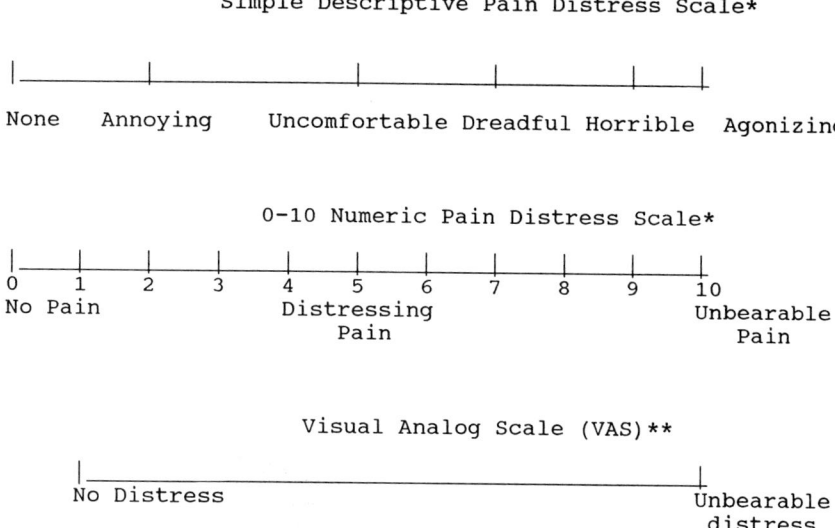

FIG 69-3.
Pain distress scales. (From Acute Pain Management Guideline Panel: *Acute pain management: Operative or medical procedures and trauma. Clinical practice guideline*, Rockville, Md, Agency for Health Care Policy and Research, Public Health Service, US Dept of Health and Human Services, AHCPR Publication No. 92-0032, 1992.)

1. The catheter will be placed by an anesthesiologist.
2. A clear dressing will secure the catheter in place.
3. Frequent assessments will be done by the nurse to monitor for potential side effects and to be certain that the medication is providing adequate pain control.
4. Possible side effects of the medication may cause changes in respiratory status (i.e. respiratory depression), itching, nausea and vomiting, and urinary retention.

It is important for patients to understand that pain control is an important aspect of their postoperative recovery and that they share in the responsibility of accurately reporting the status of their pain so that appropriate and timely interventions can occur. Patients should be aware of other strategies to manage postoperative pain that are nonpharmacologic. Unless identified as pain-relieving techniques, the patient may not perceive them as such. Nonpharmacologic techniques commonly employed following total knee arthroplasty include repositioning, the application of ice packs or cryotherapy, protective immobilization of the knee with a knee immobilizer, gentle exercise, and structured relaxation exercises.

Mobility

Another aspect of the patient's recovery following a total knee arthroplasty is related to mobility and the new joint. During the preadmission planning program, the registered nurse and the physical therapist collaborate in collecting baseline data related to the patient's history of knee problems and mobility status. The stability and range of motion of both knees are assessed and the involved knee is inspected for symmetry, swelling, and deformity as compared with the uninvolved knee. The physical therapist measures both legs to identify any discrepancies in length or muscle mass. Using a goniometer, the range of knee flexion and extension is measured and the findings recorded. The patient's gait is observed, noting dependence and the use of any assistive device. Other joints are also assessed at this time to determine the patient's ability to use a walker or crutches. The physical therapist evaluates the patient and makes recommendations related to the need for a walking aid for postoperative use. Gait training based on the anticipated postoperative weightbearing status is provided. Special attention is given to activities such as getting in and out of bed, rising to a standing position from a chair, and getting on and off the commode. An elevated commode seat is not required for the total knee patient in terms of safe positioning and joint protection, but for many patients the added seat height makes it easier for them to get up. This is especially true for the patient whose uninvolved knee is unstable or for the patient having bilateral total knee arthroplasty. Providing the patient with an opportunity to see and try this equipment prior to surgery helps to reinforce the patient's plans for postdischarge care.

The physical therapist also discusses and demonstrates exercises designed to strengthen and increase the mobility of the affected knee. These exercises, which include quadriceps setting, gluteal setting, and straight leg raises, are initiated postoperatively and continued by the patient at home after discharge. The patient is encouraged to practice these exercises at home once or twice a day as comfort permits until surgery. Written instructions that include pictures provide a quick reference for the patient to use at home.

A nutritional assessment is completed and the patient receives instructions describing the role diet plays in wound healing. Diet counseling is provided for the patient who is obese or who has a nutritional deficit. The importance of weight control to prevent the premature failure of the new joint is addressed. Some patients, because of knee problems, have sedentary lifestyles that make exercise and weight loss difficult. The perception of the obese patient anticipating a total knee is that, once he or she becomes more active, weight reduction and subsequent weight control will be easier. In reality, this has not proved to be true in the majority of cases.

It is very important to continuously solicit feedback as to how the patient is processing the information being shared. Research has demonstrated that patients who have been taught prior to surgery require less pain medication, experience fewer postoperative complications, have a shorter hospital stay, and resume normal activities sooner than patients who received no information. At the conclusion of the preadmission planning session, the patient knows what to expect on the day of surgery, and in the weeks to follow. Using the data obtained during the interview and assessment, the registered nurse, together with the patient, outlines a plan of care that reflects what the patient can expect each hospital day.

PREPARATION FOR SURGERY

Preadmission planning creates a win-win situation for the patient, the orthopaedic surgeon, the nursing staff, and the hospital. Since the results of laboratory tests drawn during the preadmission visit have already been received by the physician, there are no surprise laboratory results the morning of surgery that necessitate the surgery being postponed or cancelled. The patient is truly prepared for surgery. The patient's anxiety level is low because the patient knows what to expect and can anticipate maintaining some sense of control and involvement in his or her care. This patient did his or her own bowel preparation, monitored medications, and fasted.

The time between admission to the hospital and surgery is spent in review and reinforcement of instructions already received. No new information is presented. The assessment data collected during the preadmission visit is updated to include when the patient took the last dose of any routine medications, and the results of the laxative or enema if the patient was to administer one or the other the evening before surgery. The nurse verifies that the patient has taken nothing by mouth for the specified time period. A baseline assessment of the neurovascular status of both lower extremities is documented. If ordered, the patient will have antiembolism stockings and a sequential or intermittent compression device applied. Measuring and fitting the patient with a CPM device may occur at this time. Antibiotic prophylaxis is initiated with the first dose being administered IV prior to surgery. Routine preoperative measures that include removal of jewelry, glasses, hearing aids, and dentures as well as verification of the operative permit and the administration of a preoperative medication all serve to keep the patient busy right up to the time of surgery. For the patient who did not participate in a preadmission program, a thorough nursing assessment and health history must be completed. The nurse must be skilled in being able to query the patient regarding the presence of other health problems or symptoms. This patient may have a high anxiety level and forget significant health information. Situations have been reported where the patient has been so focused on the knee pain and limited mobility, especially when both knees were involved, that warning signs of other health problems went unnoticed and unreported. These physiologic warnings go on to manifest themselves as serious postoperative complications, e.g., myocardial infarction, or gastrointestinal bleed secondary to stress ulcer.

Regardless of their participation in a preadmission program, patients who are admitted just hours before major joint replacement surgery have endured some of the hardships imposed by the current health care system. These patients have had to awaken very early, dress, and travel to the hospital. For the patient with degenerative joint disease severe enough to warrant a total knee replacement, this much activity in a relatively short period of time is exhausting. The patient does not enter the operative arena well rested. The orthopaedic nurse must attempt to create a therapeutic environment for this patient prior to surgery.

During the intraoperative phase, the nurse assists with positioning the patient on the operating table, protecting bony prominences by means of an air or foam pad, and placement of the tourniquet and ground plate for cautery. If an autotransfusion system is used, the nurse is responsible for labeling the collection chamber with the patient's name, room number, and the time the collection was started. In some hospitals, the patient is taken from the operating table and placed directly onto a hospital bed to eliminate the need for a painful move from cart to bed once the patient returns to the nursing unit.

POSTOPERATIVE CARE

Postoperatively, the patient's vital signs are monitored closely, along with Hemovac drainage, the neurovascular status of the affected extremity, intake and output, and pain level. The leg may be elevated and ice packs or some form of cryotherapy may be ordered.

Continuous Passive Motion

There are variations on the use of CPM therapy. These variations range from if it should be used, to when to begin its use in order to achieve the greatest therapeutic effect. Nursing assessments during the time the patient is using a CPM machine include the range of flexion and extension, and the patient's ability to tolerate this range of motion. Key nursing activities associated with positioning the patient following a total knee arthroplasty focus on the prevention of complications and the restoration of maximal knee function. This involves not allowing the patient to flex the operative knee over a pillow when supine, and not resting in the CPM with the unit turned off and the knee flexed. All caregivers must recognize that inability to extend the knee is just as serious a complication in terms of mobility and knee stability as is inability to achieve flexion greater than 90 degrees.

Physician preference as well as standards of care guide the use of CPM with total knee patients. The patient needs to have a clear understanding of the purpose and goal of CPM. The patient's active participation in achieving a goal of 90 degrees of flexion by a specified day is desirable. To ensure consistency in the use of CPM some institutions implement standards of care to address such concerns as when CPM will be initiated; methods to increase flexion; directions for time in use, or some combination of a use-rest cycle; and guidelines for use at night.

Some patients feel that the constant motion interferes with their ability to rest at night and this affects their performance in physical therapy the next day. For the patient who prefers not to use the CPM unit during the night, initiating CPM before breakfast allows the patient to exercise the knee before physical therapy and the day's activities begin. The patient's ability to tolerate CPM or other attempts at mobilizing the new knee is dependent on how well the postoperative knee pain is being managed.

Pain Management

Assessments of pain after surgery should be frequent and simple. In the immediate postoperative period, physiologic responses such as heart rate, blood pressure, and respiratory rate provide critical information about pain. Once the patient has recovered from anesthesia, the patient's self-report is the most reliable indicator of the existence and intensity of postoperative pain (Fig 69–4). Effective pain management requires that the nurse be familiar with the various methods of pain control. The challenge for clinicians is to create a balance that allows the patient to be comfortable without jeopardizing the patient's safety or exposing him or her to negative side effects from the medication itself. To further compound this challenge, not only must the nurse be aware of potential

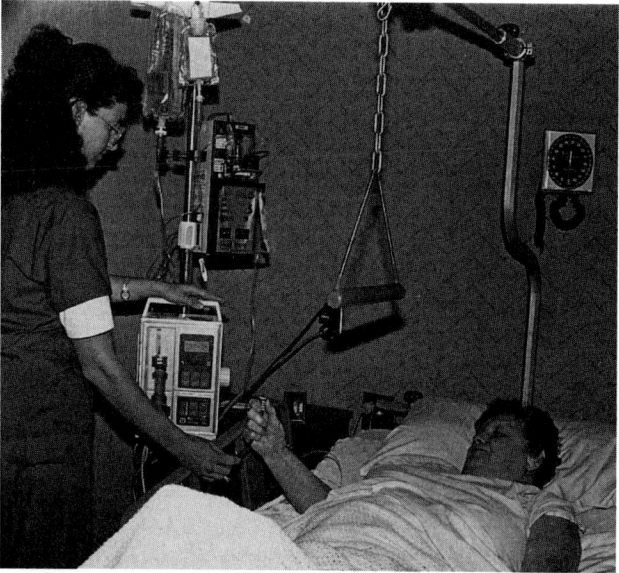

FIG 69–4.
Following a pain assessment, the patient may need to be reminded to self-administer pain medication.

variations in how this patient responded to surgery and the medications used but must also be cognizant of how this individual responds to pain and of any personal preference for treatment. For example, some patients have difficulty swallowing oral medications, whereas others do not want an injection, no matter how severe the pain.

A number of techniques have been identified to increase the degree of pain relief obtained with opioid use. These techniques include such things as giving medications on a regularly scheduled basis rather than as needed. This technique has proved especially beneficial with elderly patients who may be reluctant to request pain medications. Frequently, this is the patient who refuses physical therapy or who does poorly with ambulation and exercise because of inadequate pain control. This technique has proved effective with total knee replacement patients if implemented when the patient first comes off the PCA or following the removal of an epidural catheter. Changing from morphine sulfate IV to oral acetaminophen as needed may not be an effective transition for pain control. A second technique involves combining a tranquilizer with a narcotic to reduce the anxiety associated with the actual or anticipated pain created by increased postoperative mobility. This technique requires frequent assessments and close monitoring, especially if used in an older adult who may become confused and fall while attempting to get out of bed unassisted.

Clinical Monitoring

The selection of a pain management regimen for the total knee replacement patient must take into account the increased risk of thromboembolic complications. The patient's pain must be kept manageable without compromising early ambulation and exercise. Whichever method of opioid administration is prescribed, the nurse must be vigilant in monitoring for signs and symptoms of pulmonary embolism and deep vein thrombosis.

The registered nurse maintains an ongoing assessment of respiratory function by encouraging the patient to take deep breaths, and if secretions are present, to cough gently. An incentive spirometer may be ordered every 2 hours while the patient is awake. Once the registered nurse validates the patient's ability to perform these treatments independently, the patient can be in charge of doing his or her own incentive spirometry treatments. This allows the patient to assume some control over recovery and rehabilitation activities.

The neurovascular status of the operative or affected leg is assessed frequently by the nurse, noting the presence of the dorsalis pedis and posterior tibialis pulses, capillary refill, temperature, motion, and sensation. The nurse assesses for a positive Homan's sign realizing that both false-positive and false-negative results occur in approximately 50% of all patients with a total knee arthroplasty. The registered nurse monitors those interventions designed to reduce the patient's risk of pulmonary embolism or deep vein thrombosis. From early postoperatively until discharge, the patient is encouraged to do ankle pumps and circumduction exercises of both feet and ankles. These in-bed exercises and early ambulation lessen the patient's risk of deep vein thrombosis secondary to inadequate venous return.

The registered nurse coordinates measures to prevent infection such as care of the drains, sterile dressing changes, daily wound assessment, and monitoring the patient's temperature. Parenteral antibiotics are administered prophylactically as ordered. From the first dressing change, the incision is inspected daily, noting the integrity of the skin, erythema, amount and character of drainage, and the status of wound sutures or staples. Once the patient's oral intake is adequate, the IV line is discontinued, and the patient's nutritional status is monitored daily until discharge. At specified intervals, the patient's hemoglobin is checked to identify the need for blood replacement. Today it is common practice for the patient anticipating a total knee arthroplasty to donate 1 or 2 units of blood. Standards of practice vary as to whether the patient receives this blood as a replacement transfusion regardless of the volume of blood lost postoperatively.

Some patients may require an indwelling catheter for a short time postoperatively. Research has demonstrated that in-and-out catheterization for the purpose of emptying the bladder creates less risk of urinary tract infection than an indwelling catheter. As soon as the patient is allowed out of bed, a bedside commode is preferable to catheterization.

As the patient's activity tolerance increases, nursing staff support and encourage the patient's progress toward independence and self-care. As the length of stay following a total knee arthroplasty becomes shorter, orthopaedic nurses must think in terms of a rehabilitation model within an acute care setting. Once the total knee arthroplasty patient is able to be up in a chair, no meals should be taken in bed; once bathroom privileges are accomplished, then daytime bedpan use should cease. The activity of using a walker to get to the bathroom not only provides exercise and builds endurance, it demonstrates progress toward self-care and increased self-confidence (Fig 69–5). As soon as the orthopaedic surgeon allows, the patient should be encouraged to flex the affected knee to tolerance when sitting in a chair. The more comfortable and confident the patient is with ambulation, exercises, and ADL while in the hospital, the more likely he or she is to transfer those behaviors into the postdischarge routine at home.

Occupational Therapy

As the registered nurse monitors the patient's progress toward meeting the discharge goals, a consultation with an occupational therapist (OT) may be indicated. The OT is expert in advising and assisting the patient with special equipment to facilitate independence in self-care. It is the OT who makes suggestions for ways to modify daily activities to protect the new joint. At this point in the postoperative course, the patient has gained a more realistic appreciation of what he or she will need to be independent at home. Some examples of assistive devices commonly selected by total knee arthroplasty patients include reachers, a long-handled shoehorn, a sock aid to assist with putting stockings on without bending, and a long-handled sponge to assist in bathing independently. The OT helps the patient to plan a daily routine that combines activity with periods of rest.

DISCHARGE PLANNING

While actual length of stay varies depending upon the patient's prior physical condition and postoperative course, many total knee patients today are being discharged 4 to 6 days following surgery. The key to timely discharge is a plan or pathway that defines specific patient outcomes and offers specific measurements of the patient's progress toward defined discharge goals. Having behavior-based criteria rather than calendar-based discharge assures that the patient is moving toward desired outcomes that take into account the patient's recovery and level of motivation. Some examples of behavior-based discharge criteria are ability to get in and out of bed with standby assistance; to rise from a chair or commode; to walk a specified distance using a walking aid, according to weightbearing instructions; to actively flex the affected knee 70 to 90 degrees; and to perform prescribed exercises to promote knee flexion. When the patient has been made aware of these criteria from the outset, discharge will not be a surprise. The patient knows day by day where he or she is in relation to where he or she needs to be.

Prior to discharge the patient should receive written instructions explaining exercises and any activity restrictions. Having a list of "Do nots" serves as a reminder about crossing the legs, stooping, and avoiding activities that force the new knee into hyperextension or greater than 90 degrees of flexion. The patient's questions about resuming sexual activity should be addressed, recognizing that the main concern in any physical activity after a total knee arthroplasty is how much stress or potential for injury is placed on the knee during the activity. The nurse discusses with the patient the signs or symptoms that should be brought to the attention of the orthopaedic surgeon, for example, the knee becomes more swollen or red; drainage occurs from a previously dry wound; fever develops (temperature above 101° F); or there is calf tenderness or pain, redness of the calf, or pain in the calf with passive stretch of the foot.

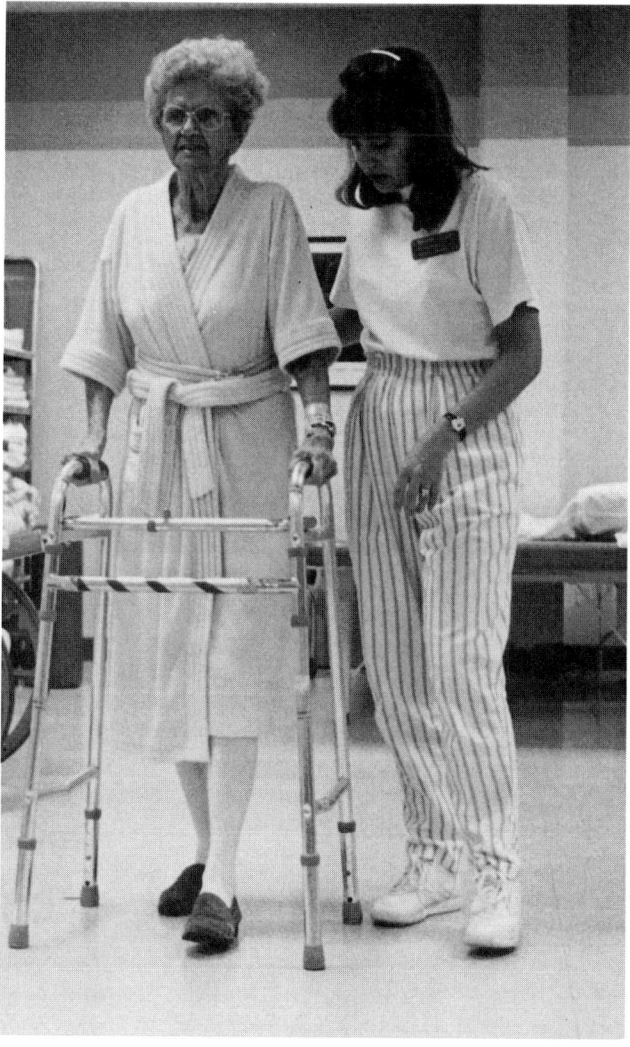

FIG 69–5.
Under the direction of a physical therapist, the patient gains confidence and endurance using a walker.

Instructions to call for a follow-up appointment should also be provided before the patient leaves the hospital.

Patients with prosthetic joints must be informed of the need for continued protection against infection. The patient should be advised to inform his or her dentist and any other health care providers of the total knee prosthesis. Prior to dental work, including routine cleaning, or any invasive diagnostic procedure, a round of prophylactic antibiotics is recommended. Since the components of the knee joint are made of metal, the patient should also be aware that he or she may activate certain types of security systems, such as those at the airport.

The registered nurse as the manager of patient care frequently maintains contact with the patient after discharge. Phone calls to the patient provide the nurse with an opportunity to reinforce instructions for exercise and activity, but most important, an opportunity is provided for the patient to ask questions that may have come up since discharge. The questions most frequently asked are related to intolerance of activity owing to fatigue, and the patient's unrealistic expectation of what he or she should be able to do by that time postoperatively. Even though this discussion was a part of the preadmission planning session, it is only now very real to this patient. The transition from hospital to home can be difficult, especially for the older patient. The patient who is recovering at home 1 week after a total knee replacement needs reassurance and encouragement. The registered nurse counsels this patient in restructuring the daily routine and modifying the home environment to accommodate the rehabilitation phase. Some hospitals provide a post–acute care service in the form of a skilled care facility or a rehabilitation unit that extends the continuum of care for those patients who would benefit from additional days of physical therapy and simulated home living activities.

The orthopaedic nurse working in collaboration with the orthopaedic surgeon maintains an emphasis on patient needs and patient outcomes. A total knee replacement program that focuses on the patient and promotes the outcomes of a return to pain-free ambulation, joint stability, and independence in ADL, drives the use of technology toward more effective care delivery and a use of available resources that is compatible with reimbursement allowances.

SUGGESTED READING

Acute Pain Management Guideline Panel. *Acute pain management: Operative or medical procedures and trauma. Clinical practice guideline,* Rockville, Md, Agency for Health Care Policy and Research, Public Health Service, US Dept of Health and Human Services, AHCPR Publication No 92-0032, 1992.

American Nurses Association and National Association of Orthopaedic Nurses: Orthopaedic nursing practice process and outcome criteria for selected diagnoses, *Orthop Nurs* 6:11–16, 1987.

Core curriculum for orthopaedic nurses, ed 2, National Association of Orthopaedic Nurses, Anthony J. Jannetti, Inc., Pitman, New Jersey, 1991.

Ecker M, Lotke P: Postoperative care of the total knee patient, *Orthop Clin North Am* 20:55–62, 1989.

Genge M: Epidural analgesia in the orthopaedic patient, *Orthop Nurs* 7:11–19, 1988.

Hackett C: Neurovascular assessment technique, *Nursing 83:* 40–43, 1983.

Kelley H: Patient perceptions of pain and disability after joint arthroplasty, *Orthop Nurs* 10:43–50, 1991.

Kyle B, Pitzer S: A self care approach to today's challenges, *Nurs Manage* 21:37–39, 1990.

Mengel A: Getting the most from patient interviews, *Nursing* 82:46–49, 1982.

Miller A: When is the time ripe for teaching, *Am J Nurs* 7:801–804, 1985.

Olson B, et al: Variables associated with hypotension in post operative total knee arthroplasty patients receiving epidural analgesia, *Orthop Nurs* 11:31–37, 1992.

Orr P: An educational program for total hip and knee replacement patients as part of a total arthritis center program, *Orthop Nurs* 9:61–69, 1990.

Strange E, Johns J: Nursing care of the patient treated with continuous passive motion following total knee arthroplasty, *Orthop Nurs* 3:27–32, 1984.

Walsh C, Wirth C: Total knee arthroplasty: Biomechanical and nursing considerations, *Orthop Nurs* 4:29–34, 1985.

70

Mechanisms of Failure of Total Knee Arthroplasty

LAWRENCE D. DORR, M.D.
JOHN H. SEROCKI, M.D.

Mechanical failure of the interface
   Failure of initial fixation
   Cementless knee
Instability

Stiff total knee replacement
Wear
Conclusions

The mechanisms of failure of total knee arthroplasty (TKA) have changed dramatically in the course of the last decade. In the 1970s the predominance of hinged knee replacements and constrained replacements, such as the Geometric (Howmedica, Rutherford N.J.), failed by loosening. Loosening occurred because the highly constrained articulation caused high stress transfer to the fixation interface. Loosening also occurred in the UCI (Dow Corning Wright), which failed because of the thin polyethylene and rapid deformation and sinking of the tibial component. The design of the Total Condylar device (Howmedica) changed the failure mechanism of total knee replacement. The Total Condylar was designed to prevent rotation in extension, but allow rotation in flexion to minimize the constraint between the femoral and tibial surfaces. This reduced the adverse forces on the cement-bone interface. Furthermore, the emphasis on valgus limb alignment was the most significant factor in permitting correct transfer of load from the femur to the tibia. High stresses in the bone and at the cement-bone interface caused by varus or severe valgus alignment were evaluated as well. The instrumentation of the PCA knee (Porous Coated Anatomic; Howmedica) was the second most significant factor to reduce failure by loosening. These sophisticated instruments allowed surgeons to have a simple set of tools to facilitate correct component positioning.

Thus the incidence of loosening with cemented implants was significantly reduced in the 1980s. However, with the advent of cementless fixation of the femur and tibia, loosening remained a common cause of failure in cementless knees. Throughout the 1980s fixation with cementless components was improved, primarily by the use of screws for initial fixation. With the improvement in initial fixation in cementless tibiae, and the decrease in enthusiasm for cementless fixation, failure of cementless knees by failure of fixation has also been reduced. In the 1980s instability became a more common mechanism of failure than did loosening. The number of instability failures increased primarily because of the vast increase in the number of total knee replacements being performed. In addition, the popularity of flat tibial and femoral articulation surfaces increased the incidence of instability because less inherent constraint was present within the design of the knee.

Finally, in the 1990s, the failure of total knee replacement by wear products and the consequences of these wear products has emerged. The surface finish of polyethylene has also been implicated in more rapid wear, particularly a heat-pressed surface finish.[8, 33] The wear products have been significantly greater in knees with flat femoral and tibial articulation surfaces. The use of thin polyethylene in metal-backed tibial trays has increased the amount of polyethylene debris which can cause osteolysis. Engh et al.[16] have shown cyst formation in the tibia, particularly around screws. Cysts have begun to be observed behind the noncemented femur which has resulted in pain necessitating revision.[25]

The common thread throughout all of these failure mechanisms is the failure of bone and bone support for total knee replacement.[4, 10] The early failures in knees which had too much constraint were caused by failure of bone support at the interface because of overload of the interface by forces transmitted to it. The failure of the tibia in cementless knees has primarily been by subsidence, again an overload phenomenon of the bone caused by the position or motion of the component.[34] The cementless tibia and femur must be placed against cancellous bone because this bone structure is all that is available in the knee. The necessity for fixation and load transfer into cancellous bone in cementless components places this form of fixation in severe jeopardy. Not only is the initial fixation compromised by the failure of cortical bone support for the implant but late failure will be much more common because debris products can much more easily infiltrate cancellous bone than cortical bone. Therefore, wear debris cysts and failure of fixation from wear debris will be much more common in cementless knees than in cemented knees.[9] The cemented knee has a seal which protects cancellous bone from easy infiltration of wear debris products. Furthermore, cement fixation in cancellous bone provides a large area of fixation rather than the spot-weld type of fixation that occurs with cementless components against cancellous bone.

The influence of bone is also easily seen in failures that occur because of poor alignment of components or of the knee. Poor alignment causes increased load of the medial or lateral tibia and this can cause overload of the underlying bone.[29, 34, 41] Overload causes bone necrosis, reducing support for the component. Subsidence and a loose component are the result. Therefore, if improper cuts are done, the knee is left unstable, which results in eccentric loading. Alternatively, inadequate fixation leads to component motion, excessive loading of the underlying bone, and failure by overload. The most predictable method by which to avoid failure of a total knee replacement is therefore to avoid overload. If overload of the bone and ligaments is avoided by correct bone cuts and proper soft tissue balance, the fixation surface encounters minimal adverse forces. If overload of the polyethylene is avoided by the use of proper thickness of plastic and avoiding the motion of plastic in a metal reinforcement tray, polyethylene debris is minimized and failure from wear is reduced. In this chapter we discuss mechanical failure of TKA, which can be caused by interface failure, instability, stiffness, or wear. Each of these factors can occur alone or in combination, as in the case of instability leading to off-center loading, increased wear, and eventual interface failure. In the discussion of these mechanisms, we provide factors of design and technique which will prevent failure.

MECHANICAL FAILURE OF THE INTERFACE

Historically, failure of the cement-bone interface has been the most common reason for failure of TKA. Early prosthetic designs were highly constrained, causing increased shear stresses at the bone-cement interface, resulting in loosening rates of 10% to 20%.[17, 39] Two important reasons for these early failures were given as causative factors: prosthetic obliquity[2, 21] and constraint of design.[23] Prosthetic obliquity refers to the varus-valgus position of the components in the mediolateral plane or to the anteroposterior position of the components in the anteroposterior plane. Examples of prosthetic obliquity are severe varus position of the tibial component, which leads to rapid subsidence or loosening, and anterior tilt of the tibial component, which can lead to stiffness of the knee (Fig 70–1). Ducheyne et al.[15] emphasized the eccentric loading of the prosthesis with prosthetic obliquity adversely affecting the fixation interface. Laboratory studies of a Total Condylar knee have shown that a uniform load distribution occurs when the femoral component is in 7 degrees of valgus alignment and the tibial component is neutral. In contrast, malalignment of 5 degrees leads to a 40% change in load distribution.[18] Clinically, the adverse consequences of prosthetic obliquity have been confirmed. Windsor et al.[46] reported that varus tibiofemoral alignment or a varus tibial cut of more than 5 degrees was related to five of nine tibial components that failed due to mechanical loosening. Dorr et al.[12] found that 93% of knees in less than 3 degrees of valgus alignment had radiolucent lines compared with 35% of knees in 3 to 9 degrees of valgus alignment. The consequence of this varus malalignment most likely is an overload of the underlying cancellous bone and subsequent necrosis of the bone. Dorr et al. also studied the effect on bone of malalignment, using radiographic densitometry.[12] The normal ratio of lateral to medial bone was 0.89. In knees in less than 3 degrees of valgus alignment (i.e., in varus alignment), the mean ratio was 1.06. These data indicate that malalignment creates an adverse bone environment which will lead to abnormal bone remodeling. With an adverse bone environment, bone can become overloaded, which leads to necrosis and fibrous interface tissue. Fibrous tissue at the interface creates an interface demarcation with inferior fixation, which can lead to subsidence or sinking of the component into the bone.

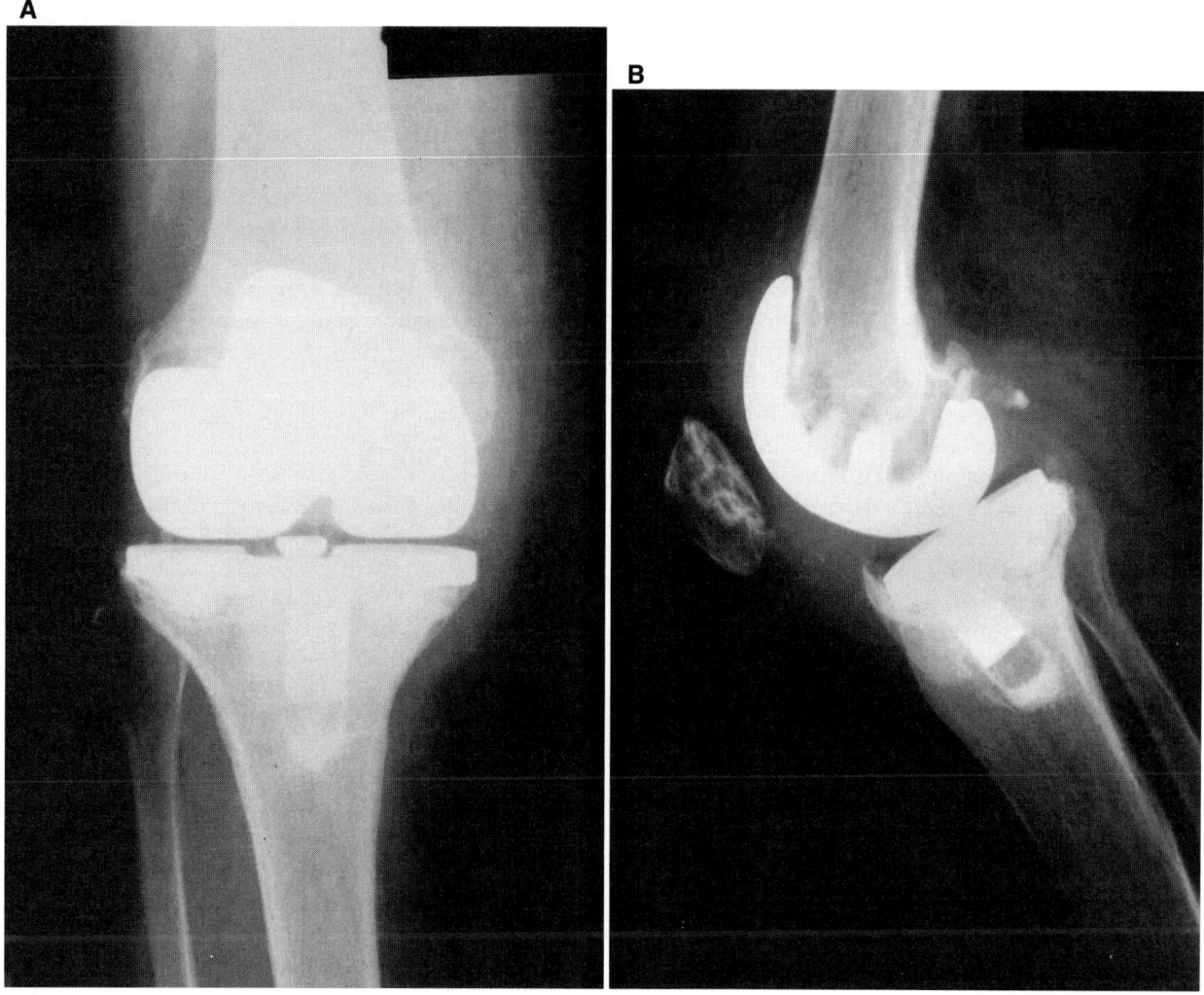

FIG 70-1.
A, anteroposterior (AP) and **B,** lateral radiographs of a loose total knee replacement. A radiolucent line around the tibial component is seen on the AP view and subsidence is demonstrated on the lateral film. Note that the tibia is cut in the varus position.

Bone biopsies support the probable failure of bone as the primary cause of sinking of tibial components. In knees with a total knee replacement and good alignment, which were reoperated on for patella problems 6 months after the index procedure, a bone biopsy of the medial condyle with the cancellous and subchondral bone was done. This bone was studied by histomorphometry. The bone demonstrated a high metabolic state at the cement-bone junction, where a new cortical subchondral layer of bone had formed. The bone was in a high turnover state, which most likely reflects the regional accelerating phenomenon (RAP) of Frost, which is common in injured bone.[19] In this high metabolic state, RAP can easily tilt the bone into a rapid resorption phase in varus total knees. This can be seen in biopsies with an increased osteoclastic index compared to the osteoblastic index. With resorption of the bone at the cement-bone interface, a radiolucent line is seen and the possibility of subsidence of the tibial component secondary to inadequate bony support is present. If subsidence occurs, particularly subsidence of more than 5 degrees, then the tibial component will be loose.

The femoral component can also be a source of component malalignment leading to aseptic loosening. This most commonly occurs when the femoral component is left in internal rotation.[24] Flexion or extension of the femoral component of no more than 10 degrees has not been shown to be destructive. Internal rotation of the femoral component can lead to asymmetric loading in flexion. This asymmetric loading will result again in overload on the compression side and tensile failure on the unloaded side. Once again, as described for the tibial component, this overload of the tibia on the compression side secondary to asymmetric loading can lead to collapse of the bone. As collapse of the bone and sinking of the tibial plastic occurs, the opposite condyle is placed under severe tensile stress and failure of that cement-bone bond can occur.

Failure of Initial Fixation

Loosening can also be caused by inadequate initial fixation, which results in rocking of a component. In cemented total knee replacement this is most commonly caused by poor initial fixation from poor cement technique. In the early days of total knee replacement, when sizes of components were limited, this initial failure could also be caused by inadequate sizing of the implants on the bone. Today this should not be a cause of failure. Multiple sizes are available with all total knee replacement designs. The initial reaction to small tibial size failures was to design a tibial component that was asymmetric and that would therefore cover all of the tibial surface. This entire coverage is not necessary, as Walker[43] has shown that only 85% of the tibia need be covered to give optimal tibial coverage. Furthermore, the use of an asymmetric component results in medial overhang of the tibial component in many knees.

Walker et al.[44] suggested that the ideal depth of cement penetration is 3 to 4 mm. A depth of at least 2 to 3 mm is required to engage at least one level of transverse trabeculae, which is adequate for excellent fixation. A depth of 5 mm or more may lead to heat necrosis of bone as well as increased bone loss if revision is required.[44] Ewald has popularized the use of holding the leg in extension so that compression is provided across the joint during cement fixation. Using this technique, Walker and Ewald found that the depth of cement penetration of 3 to 4 mm can be achieved with the cement placed 4 minutes after initial mixing.[44] Dorr et al.[13] found that intrusion was superior in bone repaired using pulsatile lavage and manual pressurization after mixing the cement for no longer than 3 minutes. This study was done in cadaver tibiae and was controlled by measuring the bone density and correlating the density with the level of intrusion of the cement.

Cement technique is critical to the durability of fixation (discussed in detail in Chapter 74). Bindelglass et al.[5] have outlined our recommended technique of simultaneous cementing of all components. All bone surfaces are cleaned with pulsatile lavage and dried with a sponge. The patella is cemented at 2 minutes and held by an assistant. The tibia is cemented at 3 to 4 minutes. The tibial cement column is then pressurized by extending the leg with the femoral trial prosthesis in place. At 6 to 7 minutes the cement is applied to the cut femoral surface, and the femoral component, with cement on the posterior condyles, is malleted into position. Again, the knee is extended to compress the cement. Finally, the knee is flexed and all excess cement surrounding the femoral and tibial components is removed. The leg is again held in extension during completion of cement polymerization.

Cementless Knees

Achieving good initial fixation of the cementless knee has proved to be a problem. Kavolus et al.[26] have presented data on the high level of subsidence of tibial components that have only a central peg for fixation. Samuelson and Nelson[37] have reported data on the failure of fixation by subsidence of "magic pegs." The difficulty in achieving good initial fixation in uncemented tibiae is that distractive motion in excess of 150 μm will prevent bone ingrowth into a porous-coated implant.[38] With a solid metal tray without good initial mechanical fixation, teeter-totter motion can result in failure of fixation. In addition, radial spread of the flat tibial surface also occurs under an applied load. This spread can be as high as 150 μm.[47] This is an additional source of motion that can prevent bone ingrowth. Volz et al.[42] and Whiteside[45] have both shown the positive influence of screw fixation on initial mechanical stability of the metal tray on the flat tibial surface. Volz et al. demonstrated that a tibial base plate design with four 6.5-mm cancellous screws limited motion to 100 μm. In a design using a porous-coated implant, pegs exhibited subsidence and liftoff displacements of 500 μm.

Clinical studies have been reported by Whiteside,[45] Rosenberg et al.[36], and Hofmann et al.[20] which indicate the advantage of initial screw fixation for the tibia. Our own data comparing tibial component fixation with and without screws confirm that better results are obtained with initial screw fixation. In our series, 7 of 17 cementless tibial components fixed without screws showed some subsidence. Two of the tibial components required revision because they were loose; one exhibited gross subsidence and sinking (Fig 70–2). Use of screws can be a source of metal debris and can act as a track for debris to reach the tibial condylar cancellous bone. This is discussed later under Wear.

Achieving good cementless fixation requires a

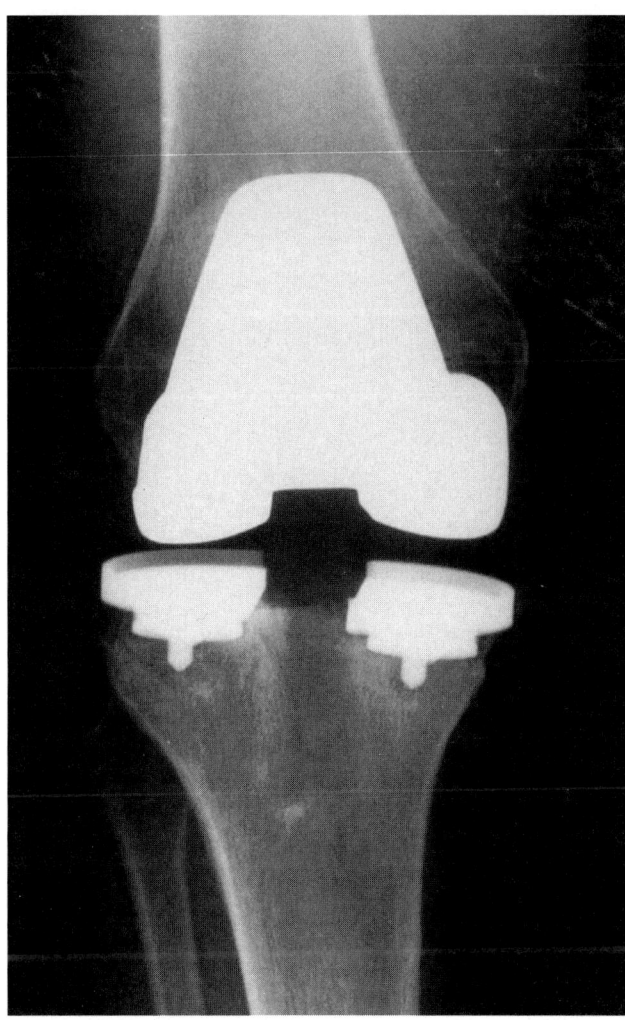

FIG 70–2.
AP radiograph of a total knee with a cementless bicondylar tibial component fixed without screws. The medial tibial component demonstrates subsidence and sinkage.

sidence is much more frequently encountered in cementless knees and almost always occurs with varus alignment of 5 degrees or more.

Initial failure of fixation with cementless knees can also be associated with bone grafting of tibial defects. If an entire condyle is bone-grafted, then bone ingrowth fixation may occur only in the condyle that is host bone. The grafted condyle may have fibrous fixation. This creates a differential deflection between the fixed and unfixed condyle which has resulted in broken metal trays and subsidence. This possibility must be kept in mind when bone grafting is used for a cementless tibial or femoral component.

Failure of cementless femoral components has recently been reported by Jones et al.[25] Initial fixation has been uniformly successful and the "hybrid total knee" is a common procedure. However, these authors have shown the occurrence of cysts in the femoral bone from debris (Fig 70–3). This is ominous in

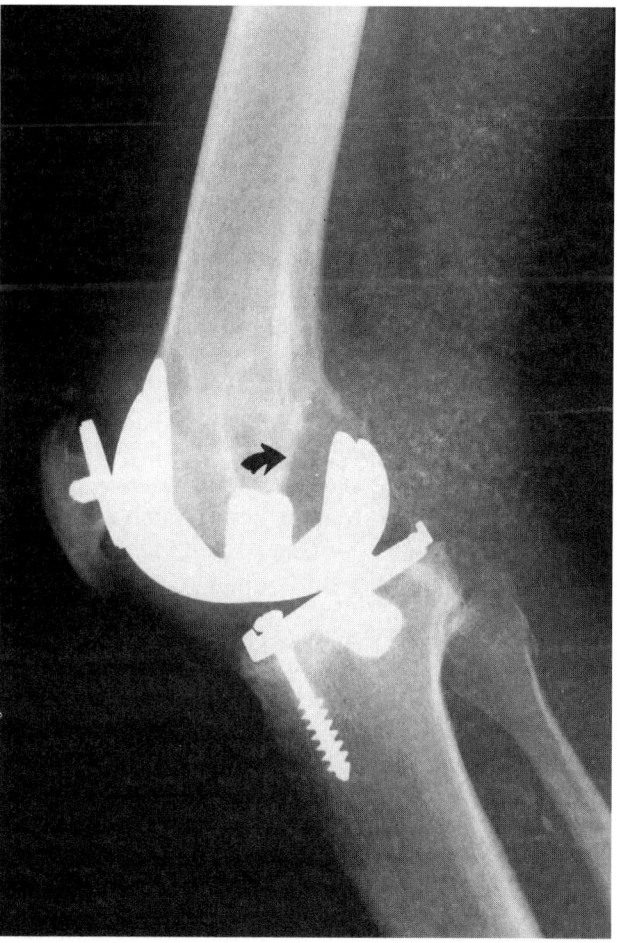

FIG 70–3.
Lateral radiograph of a cementless total knee with flat articulating surfaces demonstrating severe osteolysis *(arrow)* secondary to wear debris.

flat, uniform tibial cut. A cadaver study has demonstrated that creating such a cut is difficult.[40] When a flat metal component is placed on the uneven cut surface of the tibia, rocking may occur which will result in failure of bone fixation. Alignment is even more critical in cementless knees because cement fixation is not present to help protect against excessive point loading which can occur with malalignment. With cement fixation load is more evenly distributed across the tibia even when malalignment is present. Without cement fixation this even distribution of load is not present and a point-load situation is created which will certainly cause necrosis of bone under the overloaded tibial component. Furthermore, without the protective effect of cement fixation, failure of fixation at the opposite condyle occurs from excessive tension at the interface. This is the reason that sub-

regard to the durability of cementless components. The problem is failure of a seal which protects the cancellous bone from having plastic debris pumped through the bone. Cement provides such a seal. This problem is discussed further under Wear.

INSTABILITY

Instability of the femoral and tibial articulation surfaces can be a primary cause of failure. Instability can also be a source of intolerable pain. Instability can also cause eccentric loading, bone overload, and aseptic loosening of the tibia, as described above (Fig 70–4).

With the sophisticated instrumentation that is available today for making bone cuts for total knee replacement, the critical job of the total knee surgeon is to ensure that component position and ligament balance are such that the knee is stable. For us, stability means that there is no rocking motion between the femur and tibial components in full extension or at 30 degrees of flexion. For others, a rocking motion of 5 to 10 mm is acceptable in full extension and at 30 degrees of flexion. Those who advocate 5 to 10 mm of motion are the same surgeons who prefer flat femoral and tibial surfaces. The recent increased failure rates by wear in knee designs with flat articulation surfaces is both a reflection of the flat surfaces and the laxity of ligaments provided by the surgical technique. What is sometimes forgotten by some surgeons and designing engineers is that a knee with a total knee replacement is not a normal knee. Our gait studies have certainly demonstrated this.[14] Because the articulation surface of a total knee replacement is metal on plastic, certain compromises are necessary to enhance the durability of these surfaces. One of these compromises is that the knee be stable and that rocking between the two components be held to an absolute minimum within the constraints of design and technique.[7]

This means that the articulating surface of the femoral component should be round in both the mediolateral and anteroposterior planes and that the tibial surface have some congruence with the femur. The congruent surfaces can be such that there is 10 degrees of rotation present in flexion and extension. No more rotational freedom is necessary to protect the fixation interface and this degree of congruence provides improved protection for the ligament. With these principles in mind, one of the biggest problems that occurs with stability is the presence of a large angular deformity. With a large angular deformity the ligaments on the convex side of the deformity will be stretched. This means that release of the ligament on

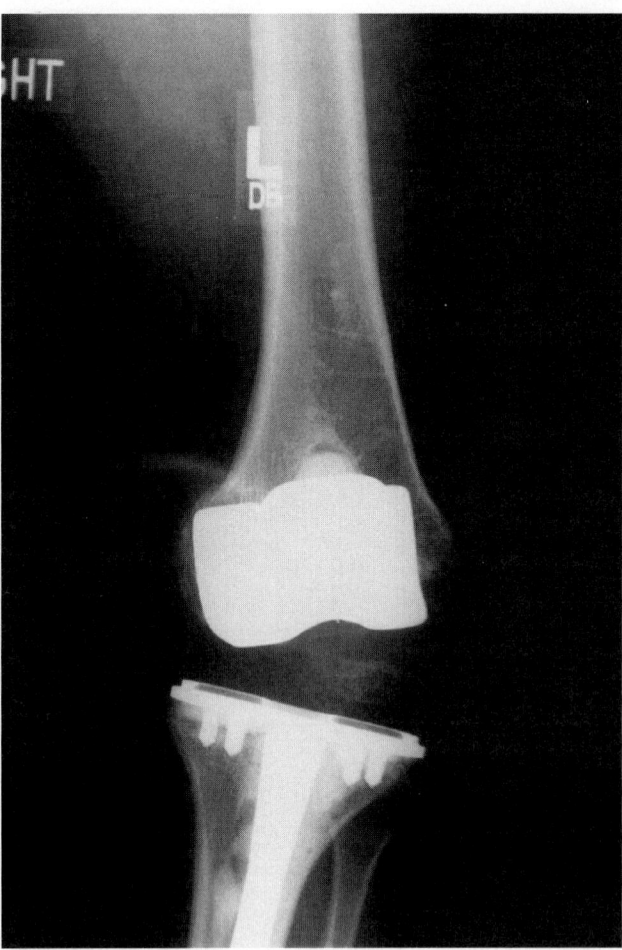

FIG 70–4.
AP radiograph of an unstable total knee arthroplasty causing pain and disability in a postpoliomyelitis patient.

the concave side of the deformity will produce a gap between the tibia and the femur that is larger than expected. Furthermore, with release of a large deformity, the flexion space is usually larger than the extension space. In this situation the thickness of the tibial insert required for stability in flexion is too great to allow full extension. Here one of two choices is present. First, more distal femur can be resected to allow stability in both flexion and extension. This is the better choice when a primary arthroplasty is being performed and when there is no more than a 4-mm difference between the flexion and extension spaces. The second choice is to use a constrained knee design such as the Total Condylar III (Johnson & Johnson Orthopaedics, Brockton, Mass.). With this knee design, the high tibial eminence provides mediolateral and anteroposterior stability in flexion when the flexion gap is greater than the extension gap. This knee has shown an excellent record over a 10-year time period in our experience. There has been no loosening during this period in our series. This knee is almost exclusively a revision knee for us.

The most important ligament for stability of a total knee replacement is the medial collateral ligament (MCL). If the MCL is present, then a total knee replacement can be stabilized almost always without the necessity of using designs with increased constraint. Flexion instability will occur if the length of the MCL relative to the joint line is not preserved. This occurs if the posterior femoral condyles are removed and not replaced with bone graft or metal wedges. The MCL then becomes lax in flexion, and mediolateral and anteroposterior stability are compromised. In this situation, whether a primary or revision arthroplasty is being performed, a posterior-stabilized design of knee replacement should be used to provide improved stability in flexion. In a revision knee in which the posterior condyles are absent and an increased flexion gap is present, the Total Condylar III should be used.

Posterior instability may occur if the posterior cruciate ligament (PCL) is sacrificed. Again, for many surgeons, the use of a posterior-stabilized design will substitute for the absent PCL and provide improved anteroposterior stability.

Salvage of the PCL can also result in instability and asymmetric loading. If the PCL is saved the knee may "hang" on the PCL if balance between flexion and extension is not present. This cause of instability is more likely to occur with the measured resection technique of bone cuts, which in combination with a medial release can create unequal flexion and extension gaps. If this unequal gap situation occurs, correction is done by either again removing more distal femoral bone or by recession of the PCL, which may require the use of a thicker plastic insert.

The most common type of poorly balanced knee replacement is with the measured resection type of bone cut and salvage of the PCL. Often this results in the tibia failing to seat under the femur in flexion. If the PCL is tight, the femur will slide to the posterior half of the plastic tibial component and the entire anterior one half to two thirds of the plastic will sit anterior to the distal femoral condyles. In this situation, there is always asymmetric loading of the tibia with an anterior tilt force present. This asymmetric loading situation can result in more rapid loosening of the tibial component; subsidence, if the posterior sliding is also tilted medially or laterally; posterior pain in the knee from a tight PCL; and increased wear of the plastic from sliding of the femur on the tibia. If the PCL is retained and after the trial prostheses are in place the tibia sits anterior to the femur (Fig 70–5), then recession of the PCL should be done.[30]

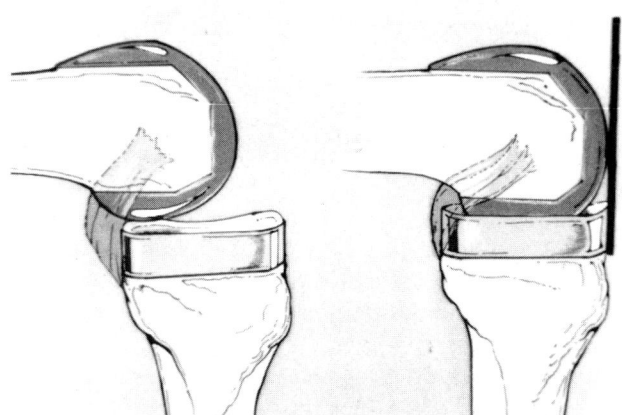

FIG 70–5.
Recession of the posterior cruciate ligament allows the tibia to be reduced under the femur.

Recession of the PCL is done by incising fibers from the femoral attachment in the intercondylar notch and manually putting posterior directional pressure on the proximal tibia. When enough recession has been done, the tibia will slide posteriorly to fit correctly under the femur. This removes the potential of eccentric loading from the femorotibial articulation in flexion.

STIFF TOTAL KNEE REPLACEMENT

A stiff TKA can lead to pain, disability, and the need for further surgery. In our review[11] of 13 stiff knee replacements which required reoperation, the results were dependent upon the cause of the stiffness. If the stiffness is caused by malposition of the components, correction can be successful. If stiffness is caused by excessive scarring or by patella baja, then reoperation is limited in its results. In our series, revision succeeded in relieving pain in 12 of the 13 knees.[11] There was no significant improvement in range of motion except in knees which had incorrect component position. Anterior tibial tilt was present in 5 knees, medial tibial tilt in 2, and an oblique femoral component in 1 knee. Range of motion was not improved in knees which had stiffness from scarring, such as the "stiffening" type of rheumatoid arthritis, or in knees which had patella baja. Patella baja is particularly common in posttraumatic arthritis. When patella baja is present and a primary arthroplasty is being performed, attention should be directed toward increasing the tibial resection and minimizing the femoral resection to avoid raising the joint line. A second option in this situation is to cut the patella but not to resurface it, thereby decreasing the height of the patella without disrupting the mechanical advantage of the quadriceps mechanism. This results in increased anterior knee pain for 3 to 4 months until the usual fibrous meniscus forms around the cut patelllar bone. However, knee range of motion is superior with this technique. The performance of primary TKA in knees which are stiff has been reported to be successful by Aglietti et al.[1]

The technical aspects of operating on a stiff TKA include management of the patellofemoral extensor mechanism and release of the MCL from the tibia. The MCL should be elevated subperiosteally from the tibia during the approach for every stiff knee, either primary or revision. This prevents tearing of the MCL as the knee is taken into flexion. Secondly, the patella may require either a V-Y quadricepsplasty[5] or elevation of the tibial tubercle. Proximal or distal release of the extensor mechanism prevents tearing of the patellar ligament. Lastly, all of the stiff, thickened capsule must be excised from the knee. The excision should be done medially until the MCL is visualized and laterally until the popliteus and lateral collateral ligament (LCL) can be visualized and palpated. Posteriorly, the capsule should be excised until the medial and lateral quadriceps muscle fibers can be seen. The PCL should be excised. This will often give an increased flexion gap as compared to an extension gap, and this should be treated as described above under Instability.

WEAR

We have mentioned that mechanical failure by loosening was the most frequent cause of failed TKA until the latter 1980s when instability and failure of the extensor mechanism became more common. The reason for the decline in loosening was the advent of precision instrumentation and less constrained designs. Windsor et al.[46] reported a loosening rate of 0.86% with the Insall-Burstein knee in a review of 1,430 TKAs. In this and all early studies on failures of TKA, there were no reports of failure due to wear.

The changes of the 1980s were made in an effort to decrease the shear stress at the fixation interface.[22] These changes were made in an attempt to make the TKA as close as possible to the normal knee in regard to rotational freedom. The articular surfaces of the femur and tibia were flattened. This provided more rotational freedom of the femur on the tibia which, it was hoped, would reduce shear stress at the interface. Additionally, metal-backed tibial components became popular because finite element analysis suggested that metal backing would improve stress transfer to bone.[3] The use of metal-backed tibial components mandated the use of thinner polyethylene inserts to avoid excessive tibial resection. Furthermore, the inserts were modular so that an exchange of worn inserts could be made. The modular insert allowed access to the base plate and to screw holes in the base plate to permit screw fixation in cementless fixation. Lastly, the PCA knee used a heat-pressed treatment of the polyethylene to enhance the surface finish of the plastic.

Recent reviews of the performance of total knees incorporating these design changes are notable for the high rates of failure due to wear of the tibial polyethylene component. Kilgus et al.[27] reported eight revisions in a series of 176 PCA knees for tibial polyethylene wear at an average of 60 months. Five of these had severe periprosthetic osteolysis as a response to polyethylene wear debris. Nine additional knees had thinning to less than 30% of the initial component thickness. Jones et al.[25] reported five revisions for severe tibial polyethylene wear in a series of 108 PCA knees at an average of 56 months. Patients were noted to have pain, effusion, and progressive varus instability. Gross wear was present on the medial sides of the insert in five cases; in two cases disintegration of the plastic resulted in metal-on-metal articulation. Mintz et al.[31] found that 43 of 487 PCA knees developed symptoms related to polyethylene particulate synovitis at an average of 54 months; 32 of these eventually required revision. In this study the increased polyethylene wear was found in heavier, younger, and more active patients. Wear was associated with flat articular surfaces, thin polyethylene, heat-pressed fabrication, and nonrigid mechanical attachment of polyethylene to the metal base plate.

Engh et al.[16] examined 86 polyethylene inserts retrieved from a variety of total and unicondylar knee prostheses after an average time in situ of 39.5 months. The authors found severe wear with delamination and deformation of the polyethylene in 44 (51%) of the implants. The degree of wear was associated with time in situ, lack of congruence (flat surfaces), thin inserts, third-body wear debris, and heat-pressed polyethylene. Undersurface cold flow of the plastic was identified in some areas of unsupported polyethylene (over screw holes) and was associated with delamination in load-bearing areas in thin inserts above screw holes in the metal tray. Seven of these 86 cases were revised specifically because of wear.

Wear is now recognized as a significant cause of failure or impending failure in TKA.[28] In order to avoid failure due to wear, the surgeon must understand the factors that affect wear resistance in polyethylene. These include appropriate polyethylene thickness (at least 8 mm), congruent articular geometry but which still affords 10 to 12 degrees of rotational freedom, and limb alignment. Modular tibial inserts should be avoided, if possible. This means that for cemented tibiae, an all-plastic component should be used when possible. In those situations in which the tibial component height is 13 mm or more, metal backing is preferred. If a metal tibial stem is required, metal backing is preferred. For cementless fixation, metal backing at this time is necessary. The presence of screw holes in trays has been associated with underlying cold flow and surface delamination.[16] Last, with modular tibial trays, particulate polyethylene debris can accumulate at the interface between the insert and the tray as a result of micromotion and accelerated wear. In uncemented implants this debris may track down through screw holes and cause osteolysis of the proximal tibia[27, 32] (Fig 70–6).

Polyethylene quality can be affected by the manufacturing process. Heat pressing used in the fabrication of the plastic in the PCA knee has been shown to predispose the polyethylene to delamination. A demarcation line in the plastic has been found to occur 1 mm below the surface, which coincidentally is at the highest level of shear stress within the component.[8] Nelson and Lyman[33] have reported a 52% incidence of delamination in a series of heat-pressed tibial polyethylene components at 2 to 4 years. Bloebaum et al.[6] found that 54% of 33 heat-pressed PCA inserts showed severe delamination within 4 years of implantation. Analysis demonstrated increased crystallinity in the surface and middle regions of the insert. This increase is associated with higher stress magnitudes, which increase the risk of surface delamination.

In summary, wear and the consequences of wear, such as osteolysis, are becoming the leading cause of revision of TKA. To reduce this complication polyethylene that is at least 8 mm thick and has congruent articular surfaces to maximize contact areas should be used. This means that in most cemented TKAs an all-polyethylene tibial component should be used. Flat tibiofemoral articulations should be avoided. The tibial component should have dishing that is consistent with 10 to 12 degrees of rotational freedom between the femur and tibia. The femoral component should have round surfaces in both the mediolateral and anteroposterior planes to optimize contact areas. The most critical round surface is the mediolateral radius of the femoral condyles. Polyethylene should not be heat-pressed.

CONCLUSIONS

Mechanical failure of TKA continues to evolve in its etiology. The initial failures of TKA were caused by loosening. It is of interest that failures in the last 10 years have not been by mechanical loosening. This is a testament to the initial design of the Total Condylar knee. Much like the initial Charnley hip, the mechanisms of failure have changed over time. Once surgeons improved their technique, the loosening rate diminished. With TKA in the last 10 years, failures have been primarily extensor mechanism failures such as patellofemoral loosening, patellofemoral dislocation, or failure of metal-backed patellae. Second, in the last 10 years, instability of the tibiofemoral joint has been a cause of failure, as described above. Today, failures are primarily caused by wear and the consequences of wear such as osteolysis. For longevity of total knee replacement, we recommend cementing all three components. Surgery time is not increased.[5] A knee design should be used that fulfills the requirement of a round condylar surface on

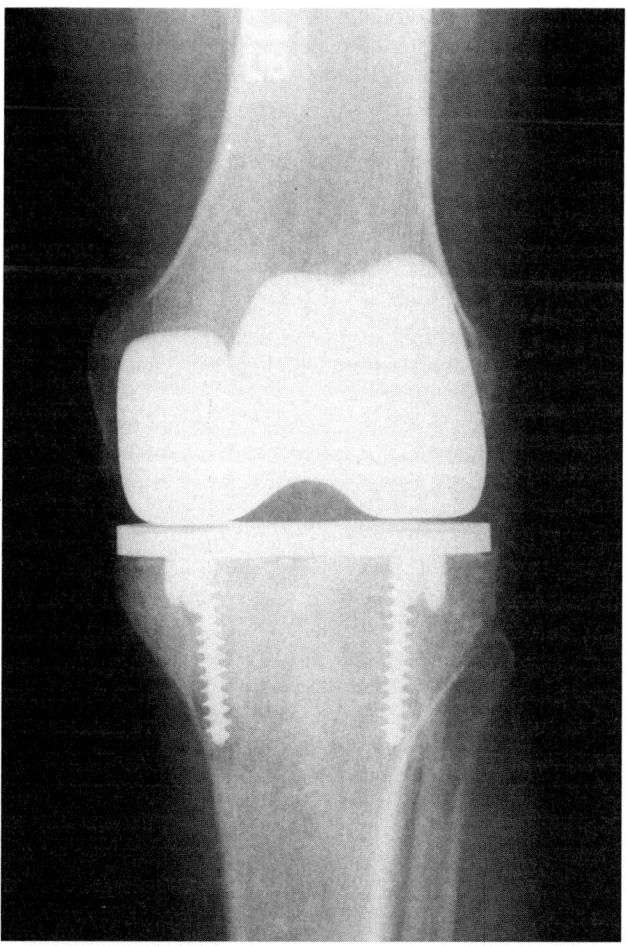

FIG 70–6.
AP radiograph of cementless total knee arthroplasty 4.5 years postsurgery demonstrating osteolysis about the tip of the medial screw.

the femur, both mediolaterally and anteroposteriorly, and provides a congruent surface on the tibia that optimizes the contact areas.

The longevity of a total knee replacement appears to be easily 15 to 20 years.[46] We believe that this does not require a PCL-substituting mechanism. The same result can be obtained if the knee is balanced in regard to the tibia seating under the femur. This can be done by recession of the PCL. Our opinion is that mechanical failure of total knee replacements will be minimized if the knee is correctly aligned, soft tissue balance is correct, and a correct design, as described above, is used. We believe that cementless knees in their present form do not match cemented knees. Because cementless knees are necessarily implanted into cancellous bone, conceptual changes are needed for their durability to match that of cemented knees. Cancellous bone is susceptible to debris migration and osteolysis. The difference between cementless fixation in the hip and in the knee is that in the hip the acetabulum and femur can achieve a seal into cortical bone at the periphery of the acetabulum and the proximal femur that protects against debris infiltration. This is also what cement fixation provides. At the present time, to minimize mechanical failure of the total knee, we recommend that all components be cemented.

REFERENCES

1. Aglietti P, et al: Arthroplasty for the stiff or ankylosed knee, *J Arthroplasty* 4:1, 1989.
2. Bargren J, et al: Alignment in total knee arthroplasty, *Clin Orthop* 173:68–79, 1983.
3. Bartel DL, Bicknell VL, Wright TM: The effect of conformity, thickness, and material on stress in ultrahigh molecular weight components for total joint replacement, *J Bone Joint Surg [Am]* 68:1041–1051, 1986.
4. Behrens JC, Walker PS, Shoji H: Variation in strength and structure of cancellous bone of the knee, *J Biomech* 7:201, 1974.
5. Bindleglass DF, Cohen JL, Dorr LD: Technique for TKA using simultaneous cementing of components, *Tech Orthop* 6:47–56, 1991.
6. Bloebaum RD, et al: Investigation of early surface delamination observed in retrieved heat-pressed tibial inserts, *Clin Orthop* 269:120–127, 1991.
7. Burstein AH: Design principles of total knee arthroplasty. Knee Society State of the Art Total Knee Review Course, Laguna Nigel, Calif, Oct 5, 1990.
8. Collier JP, Mayer MD, McNamara JL: Analysis of failure of 122 polyethylene inserts from uncemented tibial knee components, *Clin Orthop* 273:232–242, 1991.
9. Cooke TDV, Collins A, Wevers HW: Failure of a knee prosthesis accelerated by shedding of beads from the porous metal surface, *Clin Orthop* 258:204–207, 1990.
10. Dorr LD, Boiardo RA: Mechanisms of failure of TKA. In Scott WN, editor: *Total knee revision arthroplasty*, Orlando, Fla, 1987, Grune & Stratton.
11. Dorr LD, Nicholls DW: Revision surgery for stiff total knee arthroplasty, *J Arthroplasty* 5 (suppl): S73–77, 1990.
12. Dorr LD, et al: Technical factors that affect mechanical loosening of total knee arthroplasty. In Dorr LD, editor: *The knee: Papers of the First Scientific Meeting of the Knee Society*, Baltimore, Md, 1985, University Park Press, pp 121–135.
13. Dorr LD, et al: Factors influencing the intrusion of methylmethacralate into human tibiae, *Clin Orthop* 196:12–20, 1985.
14. Dorr LD, et al: Functional comparison of posterior cruciate retained vs. cruciate-sacrificed total knee arthroplasty, *Clin Orthop* 236:36–43, 1988.
15. Ducheyne P, Kagan A, Lacey JA: Failure of TKA due to loosening and deformation of the tibial component, *J Bone Joint Surg [Am]* 60:384–391, 1978.
16. Engh GA, Dwyer KA, Hanes CK: Polyethylene wear of metal-backed tibial components in total and unicompartmental knee prostheses, *J Bone Joint Surg [Br]* 74:9–17, 1992.
17. Evanski PM, et al: UCI knee replacement, *Clin Orthop* 120:33, 1976.
18. Ewald F, et al: Kinematic total knee replacement, *J Bone Joint Surg [Am]* 66:1039, 1984.
19. Frost HM: *Bone remodelling and its relationship to metabolic bone diseases. Orthopaedics lecture series*, vol 3, Springfield, Ill, 1973, Charles C Thomas.
20. Hofmann AA, et al: Total knee arthroplasty—Two to four year experience using an asymmetric tibial tray and a deep trochlear-grooved femoral component. Meeting of the Western Orthopaedic Association, San Antonio, October 1990.
21. Hsu H-P, et al: Effect of knee component alignment on tibial load distribution with clinical correlation, *Clin Orthop* 248:135, 1989.
22. Hungerford DS: Technique of total knee replacement, *Tech Orthop* 6:1–7, 1991.
23. Insall JN: Total knee arthroplasty. In Insall JN, editor: *Surgery of the knee*, New York, 1984, Churchill-Livingston, pp 587–598.
24. Insall JN, Burstein AH, Freeman MAR: *Principles and techniques of knee replacement*, New York, 1983, Zimmer.
25. Jones SMG, et al: Polyethylene wear in uncemented knee replacements, *J Bone Joint Surg [Br]* 74:18–22, 1992.
26. Kavolus CH, et al: Survivorship of cementless total knee arthroplasty without tibial plateau screw fixation, *Clin Orthop* 273:170–176, 1991.
27. Kilgus DJ, et al: Catastrophic wear of tibial polyethylene inserts, *Clin Orthop* 273:223, 1991.
28. Landy MM, Walker PS: Wear of UHMWPE components of 90 retrieved knee prostheses, *J Arthroplasty* 3 (suppl):73, 1988.

29. Laskin RS, Riager MA, Mark A: Surgical technique for performing a total knee replacement, *Orthop Clin North Am* 20:31–48, 1989.
30. Mallory TH, Smalley D, Danyi J: Townley anatomic TKA using total tibial component with cruciate release, *Clin Orthop* 169:197, 1982.
31. Mintz L, et al: Arthroscopic evaluation and characteristics of severe polyethylene wear in total knee arthroplasty, *Clin Orthop* 273:215–222, 1991.
32. Miura H, et al: Effects of screws and sleeves on initial fixation of uncemented total knee tibial components, *Trans Orthop Res Soc* 13:474, 1988.
33. Nelson KJ, Lyman DJ: Origins of delamination in heat-pressed polyethylene tibial components, *Trans Orthop Res Soc* 15:30, 1990.
34. Passick JM, Dorr LD: Primary total knee arthroplasty for the 1990's *Tech Orthop* 5:57–66, 1990.
35. Ranawat CS, Rose HA: Clinical and radiographic results of total-condylar knee arthroplasty: A 3–8 year followup. In Ranawat CS, editor: *Total-condylar knee arthroplasty,* New York, 1985, Springer-Verlag, pp 140–148.
36. Rosenberg AG, Burden RM, Galante JO: Cemented and ingrowth fixation of the Miller-Galante prosthesis: Clinical and roentgenographic comparison after three to six year followup studies, *Clin Orthop* 260:71–79, 1990.
37. Samuelson K, Nelson L: An all-polyethylene cementless tibial component, *Clin Orthop* 260:93–97, 1990.
38. Shimagaki H, et al: Stability of initial fixation of the tibial component in cementless total knee arthroplasty, *J Orthop Res* 8:64–71, 1990.
39. Skolnick MD, Coventry MB, Ilstrup DM: Geometric TKA: A two-year follow-up study, *J Bone Joint Surg [Am]* 58:749–753, 1976.
40. Toksvig-Larsen S, Ryd L: Surface flatness after bone cutting, a cadaver study, *Arch Orthop Scand* 62:15–18, 1991.
41. Townley CO: The anatomic total knee: Instrumentation and alignment technique. In Dorr LD, editor: *The Knee. Papers of The First Scientific Meeting of the Knee Society.* Baltimore, 1985, University Park Press, pp 39–52.
42. Volz RG, et al: The mechanical stability of various noncemented tibial components, *Clin Orthop* 226:38–42, 1988.
43. Walker PS: Technique and results in cemented total knee arthroplasty, Summer Meeting of the Knee Society, Scottsdale, Ariz, November 1989.
44. Walker PS, et al: Control of cement penetration in TKA, *Clin Orthop* 185:155–169, 1984.
45. Whiteside LA: Clinical results of the Whitesides Ortholoc total knee replacement, *Orthop Clin North Am* 20:113–124, 1987.
46. Windsor RE, et al: Mechanisms of failure of the femoral and tibial components in total knee arthroplasty, *Clin Orthop* 248:15–20, 1989.
47. Yang A, et al: Direct measurement of micromotion at the bone-implant interface of the tibial component in a canine model, *Trans Orthop Res Soc* 15:233, 1990.

71

Retrieval Analysis of Knee Replacements

CLARE M. RIMNAC, PH.D.
TIMOTHY M. WRIGHT, PH.D.

Methods for retrieval analysis
Factors affecting performance
  Articulating surfaces
Metal backing
Fixation
Summary

Observations made from examining total knee components retrieved from revision or removal surgery and at autopsy provide valuable information on the performance of total knee arthroplasty. Specifically, these observations can be used to identify problems and to correlate these problems with clinical, design, material, and manufacturing variables. Because of the importance of retrieval analysis in identifying problems, observations of retrieved components are an integral part of outcome measures. This has been recognized by Congress and the Food and Drug Administration (FDA), first through medical device reporting legislation, in which problems identified on retrieved components are to be reported to the FDA by the implant manufacturer, and, more recently, by the Safe Medical Devices Act of 1990, in which the reporting burden falls on user facilities, such as hospitals. In these instances, retrieval analysis is used in efforts to assure safety and efficacy of total joint replacements.

More important, however, retrieval analysis closes the design loop (Fig 71–1). Retrieval analysis provides evidence of design and material problems. These problems can be studied both analytically and experimentally to establish potential design solutions that can be incorporated into new joint replacement systems. The success of the new design must then be verified through further retrieval analysis.

Problem identification is the key to successful retrieval analysis. Many retrieval programs emphasize undirected, large-scale data gathering. This approach is time-consuming and expensive and often does not provide sufficient specific information to justify the required resources. Successful programs rely on the scientific approach of testing well-constructed hypotheses.

In this chapter, emphasis is placed on factors influencing the performance of total knee replacements as identified from observations on retrieved components. Consideration is given to the articulating surface, the use of metal backing, and the problem of fixation in contemporary total knee designs.

METHODS FOR RETRIEVAL ANALYSIS

At The Hospital for Special Surgery in New York City, all implants retrieved at revision or removal surgery are sent to the pathology department and then forwarded to the Department of Biomechanics. To ensure patient anonymity, each implant is assigned a unique identification number. Implants are soaked in a dilute solution of chlorine bleach in water (1:5) for 20 minutes to kill any potential human immunodeficiency virus (HIV) or hepatitis virus. The implants are then cleaned with warm water and a mild detergent, followed by a final rinse with acetone. Throughout the cleaning process, care is taken not to introduce additional damage to the implants beyond that which occurred in vivo and during surgical removal.

Ultrahigh-molecular-weight polyethylene components are examined visually and with light microscopy (at ten times magnification). In particular, the articulating surfaces are subjectively graded for surface damage modes (burnishing, abrasion, delamination, pitting, surface deformation, scratching, and embedded cement and metallic debris).[40, 41] To correlate surface damage with the location on the com-

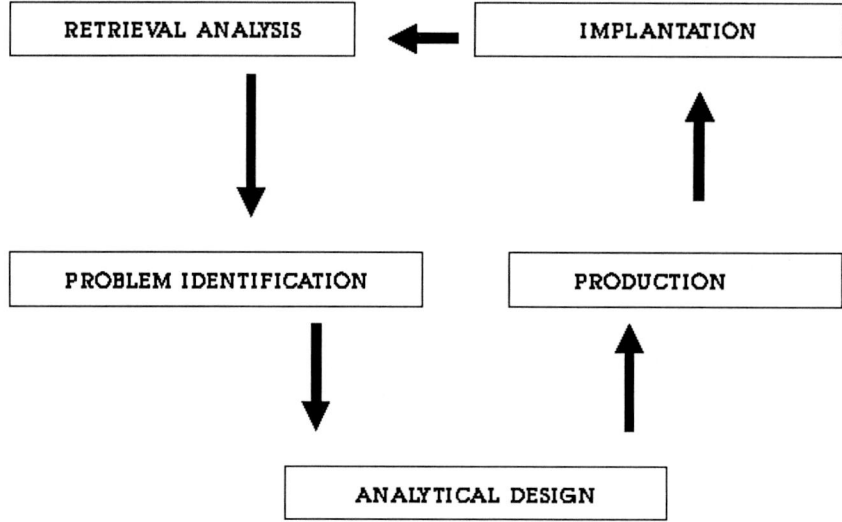

FIG 71-1.
Retrieval analysis closes the design loop.

ponent where the damage occurred, the articulating surface is divided into sections. Each condyle of a tibial component is divided into four quadrants (anterior, posterior, medial, and lateral), and the intercondylar area is divided into anterior and posterior halves. A patellar component is divided into four quadrants (superior, inferior, medial, and lateral). The grading system uses a scale of 0 to 3 to determine the presence of each damage mode. A grade of 0 means the damage mode is absent from the section. A grade of 1, 2, or 3 means that the damage mode is evident on less than 10%, on 10% to 50%, or on more than 50% of the surface, respectively. The resulting damage scores can be compared with respect to clinical, design, and material factors. For metal-backed components, the back face of the polyethylene can also be examined.

In addition to analysis of surface damage to polyethylene components, the polyethylene can be characterized with respect to changes in density and infrared spectra, using standard methods.[18, 32] Cylindrical cores, taken perpendicular to the surface, are cut using a microtome into sequential slices (about 150 μm thick). Profiles of density and infrared spectra can then be obtained as a function of depth below the articulating surface. These measurements reflect changes in the chemical, physical, and mechanical properties of the polyethylene due to gamma radiation sterilization and oxidative degradation.

Metallic components are also examined visually and with light microscopy. The articulating surfaces of femoral components are examined for evidence of wear damage. Similarly, the mating surfaces of metallic tibial trays and patellar metal backings are also examined for wear damage. Porous coatings (sintered beads, wire mesh, and plasma spray) are examined to determine the presence and type of tissue ingrowth, and the integrity of the coating. In the rare case of a fractured component, the fracture surfaces are examined using electron microscopic and metallographic techniques.[30, 31]

For components intended to be fixed by biologic ingrowth, retrieval analysis can be used to determine the extent and type of tissue ingrowth. One typical technique involves embedding the component in acrylic. Sections are then cut, ground, and polished for histologic examination.[12] The presence of calcified tissue within the porous coating can be identified using methods such as backscattered scanning electron microscopy[6] or energy dispersive x-ray analysis.[30]

Demographic and clinical information for each retrieved implant can be obtained from the patient's medical record. Observations made at the time of revision or removal surgery are important in documenting the condition of the implant prior to efforts to remove it. These observations can be obtained from the operative record. Radiographs provide additional information concerning the location and alignment of the joint components. Serial radiographs can provide historical information of time-dependent problems, such as wear and gross deformation of components.

FACTORS AFFECTING PERFORMANCE

Articulating Surfaces

Wear damage has been observed on the polyethylene articulating surfaces of tibial and patellar knee components, as well as on metallic femoral component surfaces. Wear of the polyethylene articulating surface is a significant long-term problem in total knee replacement. Cystic bony changes associated with abundant polyethylene debris have been reported.[15] In addition, certain total knee replacement designs have been shown to fail in less than 7 years due to excessive wear and fracture of the tibial component.[37] Finally, failure and dissociation of metal-backed patellar components have been attributed to excessive and permanent deformation of the polyethylene.[26, 35]

Wear damage to polyethylene is influenced by both clinical and design factors. Observations performed on tibial components of a single design showed statistically significant positive correlations between the amount of polyethylene damage to the articulating surface and both patient weight and the length of time the components had been implanted.[40] Other observations on retrieved tibial components of a number of different designs also found a significant positive correlation between the amount of damage and the length of time of implantation.[24] Wear damage was also found to be greater in patients who achieved a better ambulatory status postoperatively. Similarly, observations of dome-type, all-polyethylene patellar components revealed a significant positive correlation between the amount of polyethylene damage and the range of motion achieved postoperatively.[19]

Analytic studies predicted that thickness is an important design variable affecting the stresses occurring on and within polyethylene joint components.[3] For condylar total knee replacements, a polyethylene thickness below approximately 8 mm was associated with large stresses. These stresses have been particularly linked with the damage modes of delamination and pitting, caused by fatigue fracture of the polyethylene. Retrieval studies of thin tibial components (typically less than 6 mm thick) confirmed that excessive delamination, pitting, and catastrophic failure occur in these implants,[23, 43] though there may have been mitigating factors, such as the way in which the polyethylene was attached to the tibial tray.[4] The catastrophic failures of metal-backed patellar components have also been partly attributed to the lack of sufficient polyethylene thickness.[35]

Both analytic and experimental studies predicted that conformity is also an important design variable affecting the stresses on and within polyethylene joint components.[3, 8] As the difference in radii of curvature increases between the polyethylene tibial component and the metallic femoral component, the stresses associated with pitting and delamination increase. An in vitro experiment,[8] using repeated (cyclic) loading of flat, nonconforming polyethylene specimens, produced subsurface cracks similar to those observed in delaminated regions of retrieved tibial knee components with nonconforming articulating surfaces. In a recent retrieval study,[41] the prevalence of damage modes between a cruciate-sparing, relatively nonconforming knee design and a cruciate-substituting, more conforming knee design were compared. Delamination was commonly observed in the tibial components of the relatively nonconforming design. In contrast, delamination was absent from all of the components of the more conforming cruciate-substituting design (Table 71-1).

The effects of conformity on wear of polyethylene components must be considered in both the anteroposterior and mediolateral directions. Implant designs for total knee replacement in which the posterior cruciate ligament is to be spared often employ polyethylene tibial articulating surfaces that are nonconforming in the anteroposterior direction. The flat tibial surface is believed to be necessary to allow sufficient posterior translation of the tibia relative to the femur to ensure adequate constraint by the ligament.[21] Though it is possible to design the femoral component to be relatively conforming (i.e., flat) with the tibial component near full extension, the more curved posterior condyles of the femoral component articulate against the flat tibial surface when the knee moves into flexion. The resulting nonconformity increases the contact stresses and the stresses associated with pitting and delamination. This increase is exacerbated by the high functional loads that can occur across the knee in flexion, as in stair climbing and rising from a chair.

In the mediolateral direction, more conforming articulating surfaces tend to resist rotation in the presence of compressive joint loads. Flatter, nonconforming surfaces have the least resistance to rotation.

TABLE 71-1.

Subjective Point Scores for Damage of Posterior Stabilized Total Condylar and PCA (Porous Coated Anatomic) Tibial Components*

Mode of Damage	PCA (n = 12)	Posterior Stabilized (n = 20)†
Cement debris	0.0 ± 0.0	1.2 ± 2.3
Pitting	13.7 ± 3.4	10.5 ± 6.7
Scratching	14.4 ± 4.9	12.5 ± 6.5
Burnishing	16.2 ± 4.8	14.0 ± 6.8
Delamination	12.7 ± 6.8	0.0 ± 0.0
Surface deformation	7.9 ± 4.1	1.4 ± 1.8
Abrasion	1.8 ± 1.5	0.4 ± 1.3

*Data from Wright TM, et al: Clin Orthop 276:126–134, 1992.
†Values are means plus or minus standard deviation.

Many posterior cruciate ligament–sparing designs that have flat tibial surfaces in the anteroposterior direction also have flat tibial surfaces in the mediolateral direction. By designing the femoral component to likewise be flat in the mediolateral direction, the implant designer achieves rotational laxity. Having flat tibial and femoral surfaces in the mediolateral direction also maximizes contact area in such a design, but only when the load is equally distributed on both plateaus. When varus or valgus moments are applied across the knee, the load may shift totally to one plateau. With flat contacting surfaces, this shift results in all of the load being distributed over a small contact area near the extreme outer edge of the tibial component. The resulting excessive stresses are associated with large amounts of delamination and even with gross component fracture (Fig 71–2, A and B).

Other confounding, though poorly understood, variables affecting the performance of articulating surfaces of polyethylene components are the types of resin used to manufacture the polyethylene material and the manner in which these resins are fabricated into bulk shapes. Several types of resins have been commonly used to manufacture polyethylene joint components. These include : RCH 1000 (Ruhrchemie, Oberhausen, Germany); GUR 412 and GUR 415 (Hoechst Celanese, Houston); and Hifax 1900cm (Himont USA, Wilmington, Del.). The differences in physical properties (molecular weight, density, crystallinity) and mechanical properties (elastic modulus, strength, creep resistance) between these resins are significant[25] and probably affect the performance of polyethylene implants. A controlled retrieval study comparing the performance of implants made from the different resins has been difficult to perform, so that no data demonstrating differences in performance exist. Implant manufacturers are aware of the potential problem, however, and most have recently chosen to manufacture implants from a single resin source.

The manner in which the resin is fabricated into a bulk shape may also be important to the wear resistance of the resulting component. Implant components have been machined from both extruded rods and compression-molded sheets of polyethylene. In addition, implant components have also been molded directly into final form. These fabrication techniques are known to influence the properties of the polyethylene.[25] In our experience, however, there was no significant difference in the amount of surface damage to machined and molded tibial components of a single design.[41]

Methods have been employed to modify polyethylene components in hopes of improving performance. In the late 1970s, carbon fiber reinforcement was advocated as a means for improving the mechanical and wear properties of polyethylene.[2] Some mechanical tests and in vitro wear tests showed improved properties when carbon fibers were added. However, the amounts and types of surface damage observed on tibial components made from plain and carbon fiber–reinforced polyethylene did not differ.[41] In this comparison, as many factors as possible were matched (implant design, patient weight, the length of time the component had been implanted, the ra-

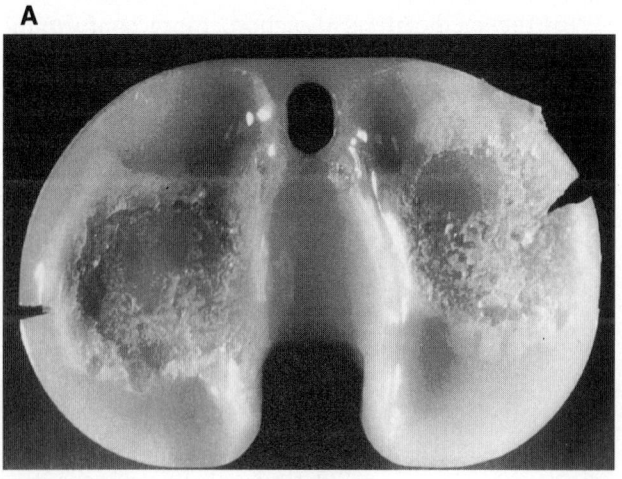
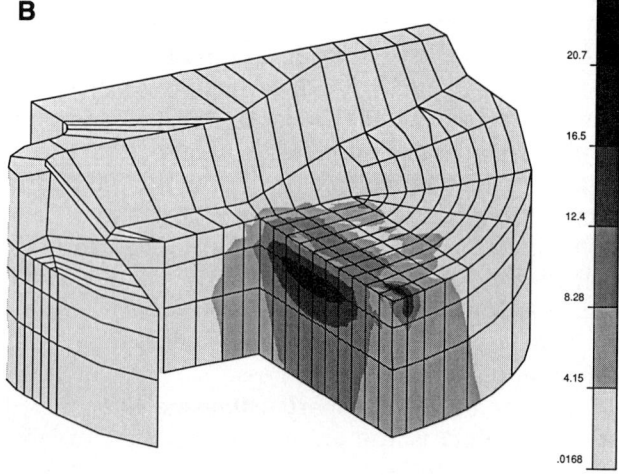

FIG 71–2.
A, retrieved tibial component showing severe delamination of the articulating surface and gross fracture initiating from the periphery. **B,** analytic contour plot showing significant shear stresses below the articulating surface, consistent with the modes of damage observed on the retrieved component. The scale is in megapascals. (Courtesy of D. Bartel.)

diographic position and angular alignment of the components, the original diagnosis, and the reason for removal), so that any difference in performance should have been due to material. Furthermore, components molded from carbon fiber–reinforced polyethylene have been shown to experience gross failure because of poor consolidation of the polyethylene powder particles around the carbon fibers during fabrication.[42]

Another method used to modify polyethylene components was heat polishing. Heat polishing involved localized heating, resulting in a smooth, close-tolerance articulating surface. At the same time, however, the heat-polishing process resulted in a thin surface layer (approximately 1 mm thick) of polyethylene with altered physical properties from those of the underlying polyethylene substrate[7] (Fig 71–3). It has been suggested that the interface between the heat-polished polyethylene and the substrate is partly responsible for the significant delamination observed in retrieved heat-polished components.[7, 43]

The physical and mechanical properties of polyethylene are also altered in an uncontrolled manner by oxidative degradation, arising from the process of gamma radiation sterilization,[33] as well as from exposure to the body environment.[18] The changes to the polyethylene are nonuniform and are greatest near the surface. The variation in properties caused by degradation as a function of depth from the articulating surface was found to be similar between components in a series of retrieved tibial implants of a single design[43] (Fig 71–4). In most retrieval studies, the state of the polyethylene prior to implantation is unknown. Therefore, it is difficult to assess reliably the extent of oxidative degradation that has oc-

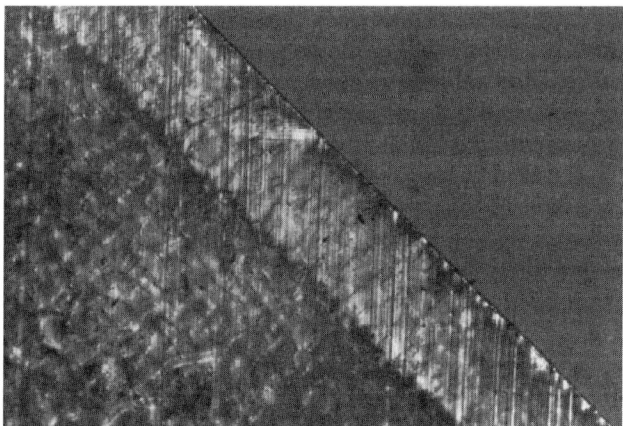

FIG 71–3.
Light photomicrograph of the cross section of a polyethylene component that had been heat-polished during manufacture. Note the alteration in the appearance of the material within 1 mm of the component surface. (Courtesy of S. Li.)

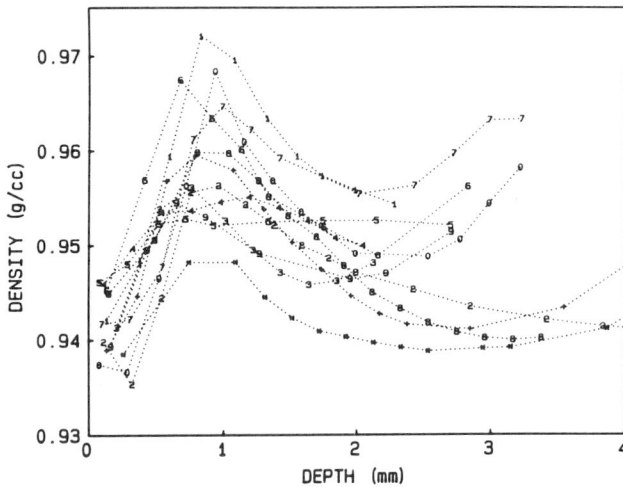

FIG 71–4.
Polyethylene density as a function of depth below the articulating surface for a series of 12 retrieved PCA tibial components.[43] The components were retrieved after 4 to 7 years of implantation.

curred in the component. However, comparison of the properties measured from retrieved tibial knee components with typical properties for bulk polyethylene have revealed differences significant enough to predict an increase in the stresses associated with wear damage.[17]

To rigorously establish the effects of degradation requires comparison of retrieved components with the original stock material from which they were fabricated. In an effort to collect such data, a unique study has been initiated in which the material properties of retrieved polyethylene tibial inserts are being measured and compared with the initial stock properties in the as-received and as-sterilized conditions.[32] Preliminary results demonstrate that significant changes occur to the polyethylene properties beyond those caused by the sterilization process (Fig 71–5). The associated mechanical property changes are being incorporated into stress analyses in an effort to understand the role of degradation in the creation of wear damage.

Wear damage to the articulating surfaces of metallic femoral components is not generally considered a severe problem. Severe metallic wear has only been observed in cases in which cement or metallic debris became entrapped between the articulating surfaces or metal-backed polyethylene components fractured or dissociated, leading to direct articulation between the femoral component and the metal backing (Fig 71–6). As with polyethylene wear, the concern with metallic wear is not simply damage to the articulating surface, but the release of metallic debris into the surrounding tissues and fluids. In total hip replacements, for example, large amounts of metallic debris

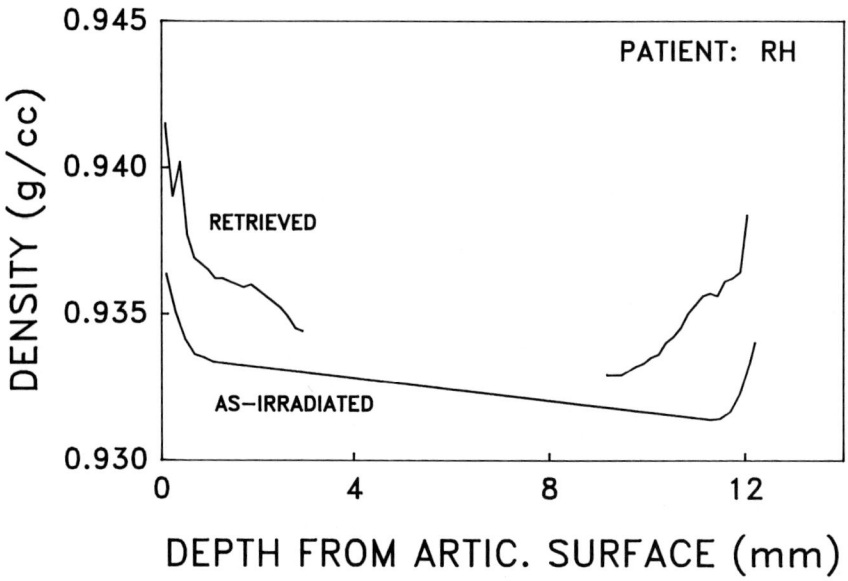

FIG 71–5.
Polyethylene density as a function of depth below the articulating surface and above the bottom surface of a bulk specimen (as-irradiated) and of a retrieved Insall-Burstein Posterior Stabilized tibial component. The component was retrieved after 11 months of implantation.

have been measured, particularly around components employing titanium alloy articulating surfaces.[1, 38] On the other hand, serum concentrations of titanium, aluminum, and vanadium were not found to be elevated after about 2 years around successful porous-coated total knee replacements using a titanium alloy femoral component.[22] The clinical significance of elevated metal levels is unknown. Indications are that much of the debris probably results from the failure process, though this conclusion is based on measurements from around the total hip (rather than total knee) replacements.[9]

Metal Backing

Polyethylene total knee components act as surface replacements and, as such, transfer load directly to the underlying trabecular bone. Failure of the underlying bone as a reason for removal of these components led implant designers to examine methods for reducing the stresses in the bone by more evenly distributing the loads transferred from the component. The theoretic basis for achieving this goal through the use of metal backing has been well established through stress analysis.[5] Added advantages of a metal backing include the ability to attach metallic porous structures for fixation by tissue ingrowth, and the ability to design modular systems with stem, wedge, and polyethylene insert options.

A number of design factors influence the performance of metal-backed total knee components. The importance of these factors has been demonstrated from observations of retrieved components. For example, it is usually necessary to decrease the thickness of the polyethylene when adding a metal backing to maintain the overall thickness of the implant within anatomic constraints. As was noted earlier, with a decrease in polyethylene thickness, the stresses associated with damage to the articulating surface increase. In fact, the severe wear observed on metal-backed tibial components has been attributed, in part, to the thickness (less than 6 mm) of the polyethylene inserts.[23, 43]

Another factor influencing the performance of metal-backed components is the design of the metal backing itself. Fatigue failures have been reported in metallic tibial trays due to stress concentrations around screw holes, at the posterior cutout necessary for retention of the posterior cruciate ligament (Fig 71–7), and at the junction between the metallic tray and the metallic peg.[11, 14, 20, 28–30, 34] Trays with porous metallic coatings for tissue ingrowth are more susceptible to fatigue failures because of the introduction of numerous sites for a crack to initiate and because of the alteration in microstructure caused by the sintering treatment used to attach the porous coating to the tray.

The method of fixation between the polyethylene insert and the metallic tray can also influence the performance of metal-backed knee components. Analytic studies have shown that when the polyethylene is not rigidly fixed to the metal backing, the stresses

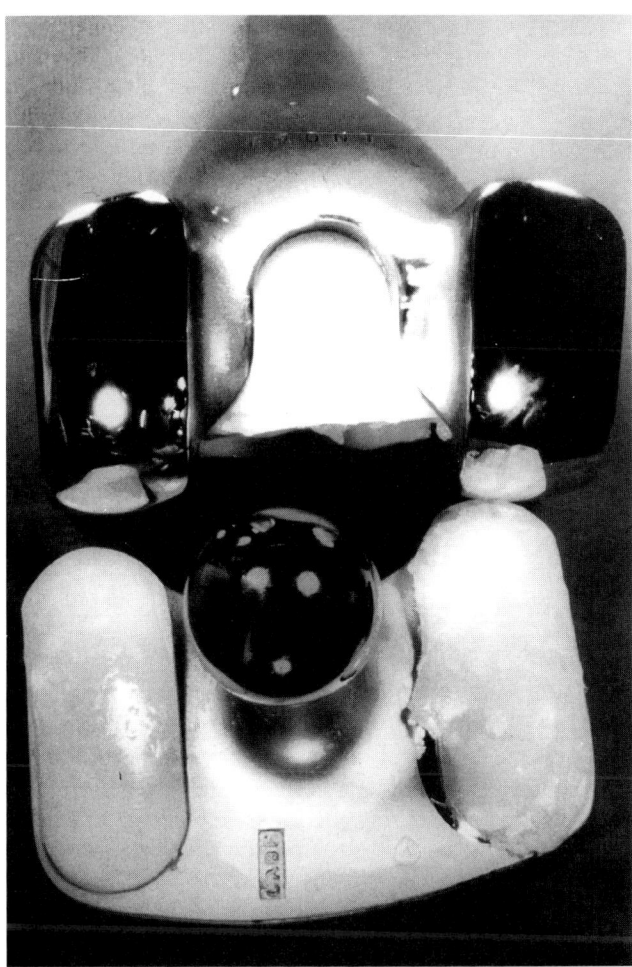

FIG 71–6.
Retrieved Spherocentric knee replacement showing wear of the tibial metal backing at the periphery of the severely worn polyethylene insert *(lower right)*.

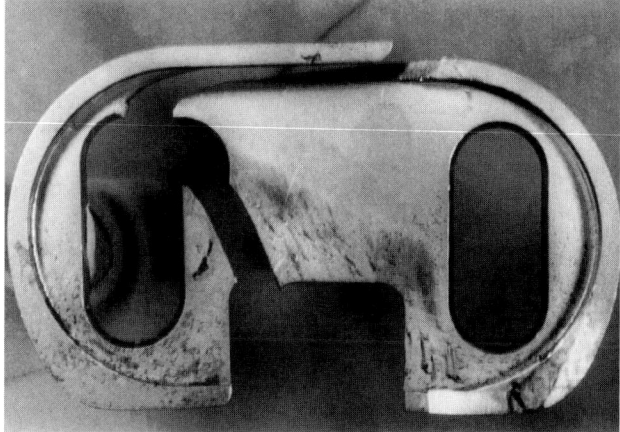

FIG 71–7.
Tibial metallic tray from a retrieved posterior cruciate ligament–retaining knee replacement showing fatigue fracture initiating at the posterior cutout.

associated with surface damage increase.[4] In addition, the lack of rigid fixation can allow significant motion at the interface and the metal backing, creating another wear surface from which debris can be released (Fig 71–8).

Metal-backed patellar components suffer from many of the same design problems as metal-backed tibial components. The addition of a metal backing reduces even further an already thin polyethylene component, leading to increased wear, deformation, and fracture. The gross deformation that occurs in the polyethylene portion of the component makes fixation to the metal backing difficult to design. A solution involving any form of interference fit must rely on the polyethylene maintaining its shape throughout the life of the component. Similarly, plastic tabs extending through the metal backing must resist cyclic loading and gross deformation. Consequently, dissociation of the polyethylene from the metal backing is a common failure mode[26, 35, 36] (Fig 71–9). Dissociation is a serious complication requiring revision and resulting in the generation of considerable metallic debris in addition to polyethylene debris.

Fixation

Historically, total knee components have been fixed to the surrounding bone using acrylic bone cement. Even with the introduction of porous-coated metal-backed components for fixation by tissue ingrowth, cemented components remain the gold standard for long-term success. Certainly, observations from retrieved knee components demonstrate that excellent fixation between metal and cement, and plastic and cement can be achieved by the use of simple under-

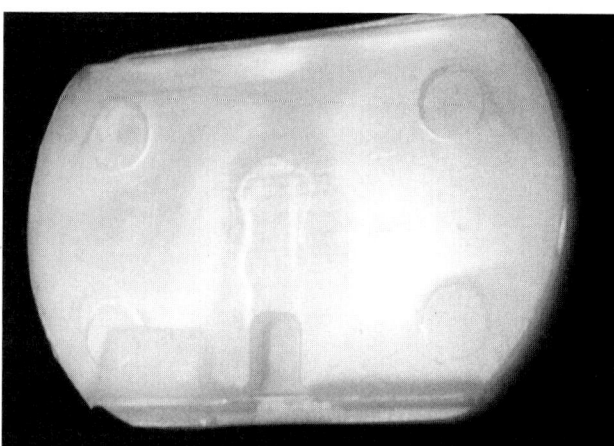

FIG 71–8.
Bottom surface of a polyethylene tibial insert showing burnishing and scratching consistent with articulation against the metallic tibial tray.

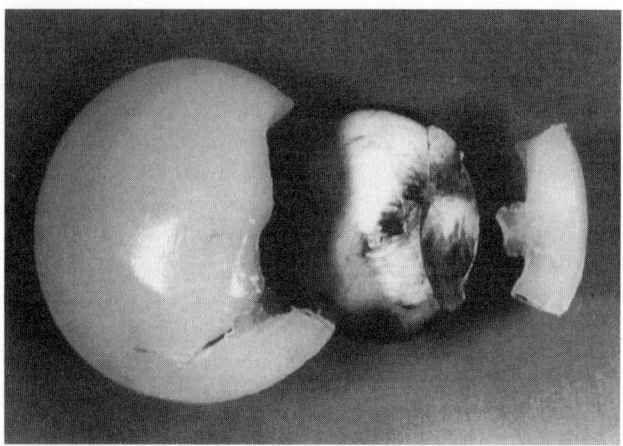

FIG 71-9.
Failed metal-backed patellar implant showing severe wear and fracture of the polyethylene component and subsequent severe wear of the metal backing, consistent with articulation against the femoral component.

cuts and macrotexturing. Failure at the cement-bone interface is more difficult to assess from retrieved components as this interface has usually already failed in vivo or is disrupted during the removal process. Failures due to loosening are often associated with crushing of the underlying cancellous bone. Loss of bony support can result in gross deformation of all-polyethylene tibial components[39] (Fig 71-10) and can contribute to fatigue failures of metallic trays.

Several contemporary designs for total knee replacement employ metallic porous-coated surfaces with the hope of achieving permanent fixation through bone ingrowth. The extent of bone ingrowth is difficult to assess radiographically and clinical symptoms do not always reflect stable long-term fixation. Observations from retrieved porous-coated knee components can be used to accurately assess the type and amount of tissue ingrowth remaining on the component at the time of removal. However, implants are usually recovered at failure so that their condition does not reflect successful in vivo performance. In this regard, the information that can be obtained about the performance of porous-coated implants from retrieval analysis is limited.

Retrieval analysis of porous-coated knee components has shown restricted bony ingrowth, usually confined to regions around porous-coated pegs used to enhance initial fixation of femoral, tibial, and patellar components[13, 30] (Fig 71-11, A and B). Ingrowth has also been noted in peripheral regions of tibial components where contact with the cortical shell had occurred.[13] The predominance of bone ingrowth into fixation pegs is supported by analytic results. An interference fit between fixation pegs and the surrounding cancellous bone leads to residual stresses in the bone that inhibit interface motion and enhance ingrowth into the pegs.[16] The interference fit and subsequent bone ingrowth serve to unload the bone under the remainder of the component, making bone ingrowth in regions away from the pegs less probable.

In a recent study of components retrieved from 58 total knee replacements, 46% of the components showed no evidence of bone ingrowth and only 11% showed evidence of bone ingrowth extending over more than 5% of the porous-coated area.[13] No differences were found in the amount of bone ingrowth between tibial, femoral, and patellar components. Similarly, no difference was found between components with a beaded cobalt alloy porous coating and components with a titanium fiber mesh coating. It must be remembered, however, that 60% (35 of 58) of the implants were removed for reasons that could be expected to compromise the quality of bone ingrowth (e.g., persistent subluxation and infection).

An unanticipated problem with porous-coated devices is failure of the porous coating itself. Fracture of the porous coating can lead to loss of fixation and to the release of beads or mesh fragments to the surrounding tissues.[10, 27, 30] Beads and mesh fragments can migrate considerable distances. In fact, beads have become entrapped in the polyethylene articulating surfaces, leading to increased polyethylene and metallic wear (Fig 71-12).

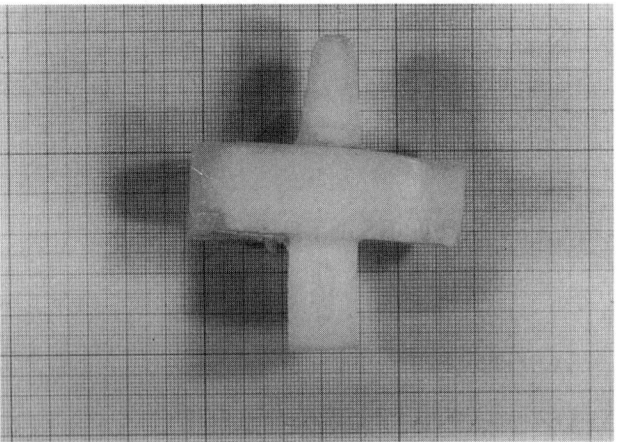

FIG 71-10.
Excessive deformation noted in a retrieved Total Condylar II tibial component.[39] The time implanted was 25 months. Loosening was due to failure of the underlying cancellous bone, leading to permanent deformation of the polyethylene plateau.

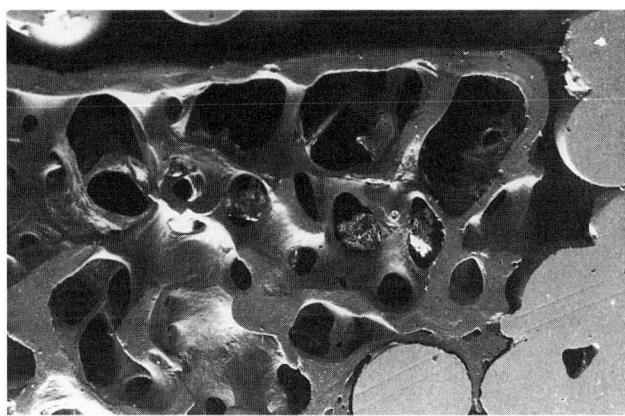 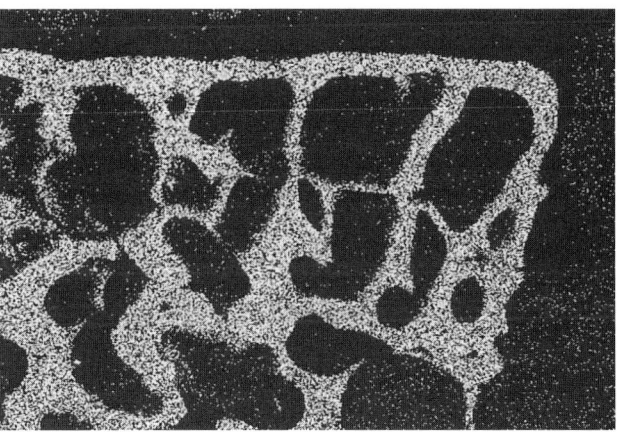

FIG 71-11.
A, scanning electron photomicrograph of a cross section through a retrieved PCA tibial component.[30] Bone tissue is seen in close apposition to the porous-coated peg *(lower right)*, but no bone ingrowth is noted at the bottom surface of the porous-coated tibial tray *(top)*. **B,** the presence of bone tissue is confirmed by a calcium dot map *(white regions)* obtained from energy dispersive spectroscopy of the surface of the section.

SUMMARY

Retrieved total knee components are a valuable resource from which mechanical performance can be evaluated on the basis of design and material factors. Observations from retrieved implants have been used to support analytic predictions about the designs of articulating surfaces and of metal backings and about the patterns of bone ingrowth into porous-coated knee prostheses. Measurements performed on retrieved polyethylene components have been used to establish the extent of oxidative degradation and to identify design and manufacturing parameters affecting both mechanical and chemical degradation. Despite the importance of these findings, the usefulness of retrieval analysis is limited in that components are usually retrieved from implants that have already failed clinically. Until similarly large numbers of specimens can be obtained from well-functioning knee replacements at autopsy and at amputation, the clinician and implant designer must rely on retrieved components from revision and removal surgery.

REFERENCES

1. Agins HJ, et al: Metallic wear in failed titanium-alloy total hip replacements, *J Bone Joint Surg [Am]* 70:347–356, 1988.
2. Ainsworth R, Farling G, Bardos D: An improved bearing material for joint replacement prostheses: Carbon fiber reinforced UHMW polyethylene, *Trans Orthop Res Soc* 2:120, 1977.
3. Bartel DL, Bicknell VL, Wright TM: The effect of conformity, thickness, and material on stresses in UHMWPE components for total joint replacement, *J Bone Joint Surg [Am]* 68:1041–1051, 1986.
4. Bartel DL, Wright TM, Edwards D: The effect of metal-backing on stresses in polyethylene acetabular components. In Hungerford DS, editor: *The hip, Proceedings of the Eleventh Meeting of the Hip Society,* St Louis, Mo, 1983, Mosby–Year Book, pp 229–239.
5. Bartel DL, et al: Performance of the tibial component in total knee replacement, *J Bone Joint Surg [Am]* 64:1026–1033, 1982.
6. Bloebaum RD, Bachus KN, Boyce TM: Backscattered electron imaging: The role in calcified tissue and implant analysis, *J Biomater Appl* 5:56–85, 1990.
7. Bloebaum RD, et al: Investigation of early surface delamination observed in retrieved heat-pressed tibial inserts, *Clin Orthop* 269:120–127, 1991.

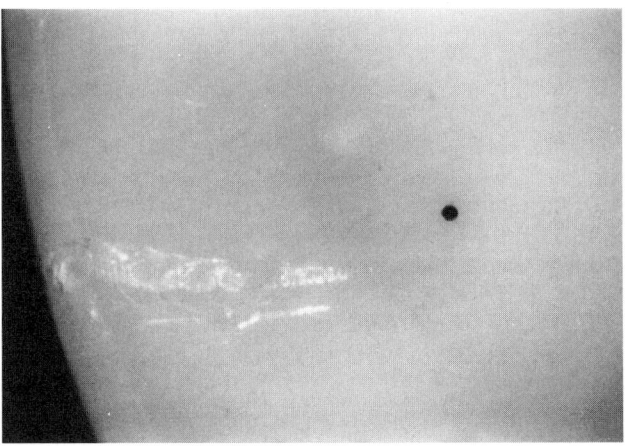

FIG 71-12.
Light photomicrograph of the articulating surface of a polyethylene tibial component showing an embedded cobalt alloy bead.

8. Blunn GW, et al: The dominance of cyclic sliding in producing wear in total knee replacements, *Clin Orthop* 273:253–260, 1991.
9. Brien WW, et al: Metal levels in cemented total hip arthroplasty: A comparison of well-fixed and loose implants, *Clin Orthop* 276:66–74, 1992.
10. Buchert PK, et al: Excessive metal release due to loosening and fretting of sintered particles on porous-coated hip prostheses, *J Bone Joint Surg [Am]* 68:606–609, 1986.
11. Cheal EJ, Gerhart TN, Hayes WC: Failure analysis of a porous coated patellar component. In Lewis, JL, editor: *Computational methods in bioengineering,* New York, 1989, American Society of Mechanical Engineers, pp 211–221.
12. Collier JP, et al: Results of implant retrieval from postmortem specimens in patients with well-functioning, long-term total hip replacement, *Clin Orthop* 274:97–112, 1992.
13. Cook SD: Clinical, radiographic, and histologic evaluation of retrieved human noncement porous coated implants, *J Long-Term Effects Med Implants* 1:11–51, 1991.
14. Cook SD, Thomas KA: Fatigue failure of noncemented porous coated implants, *J Bone Joint Surg [Br]* 73:20–24, 1991.
15. Dannenmaier WC, Haynes DW, Nelson CL: Granulomatous reaction and cystic bony destruction associated with high wear rate in a total knee prosthesis, *Clin Orthop* 198:224–230, 1985.
16. Dawson JM, Bartel DL: Consequences of an interference fit on the fixation of porous coated tibial components in total knee replacement, *J Bone Joint Surg [Am]* 74:233–238, 1992.
17. Elbert KE, et al: In vivo changes in material properties of polyethylene and their effects on stresses associated with surface damage of polyethylene components, *Trans Orthop Res Soc* 13:53, 1988.
18. Eyerer P, Ke Y-C: Property changes of UHMW polyethylene hip cup endoprostheses during implantation, *J Biomed Mater Res* 18:1137–1151, 1984.
19. Figgie MP, et al: Performance of dome-shaped patellar components in total knee arthroplasty, *Trans Orthop Res Soc* 14:531, 1989.
20. Gradisar IA, Hoffman ML, Askew MJ: Fracture of a fenestrated metal-backing of a tibial knee component, *J Arthroplasty* 4:27–30, 1989.
21. Hungerford DS, Kenna RV: Preliminary experience with a total knee prosthesis with porous coating used without cement, *Clin Orthop* 176:95–107, 1983.
22. Jacobs JJ, et al: Metal release and excretion from cementless titanium total knee replacements, *Trans Orthop Res Soc* 16:558, 1991.
23. Kilgus DJ, et al: Catastrophic wear of tibial polyethylene inserts, *Clin Orthop* 273:223–231, 1991.
24. Landy MM, Walker PS: Wear of ultra-high-molecular-weight polyethylene components of 90 retrieved knee prostheses, *J Arthroplasty* 3(suppl):S73–S85, 1988.
25. Li S, Nagy EV, Wood BA: Chemical degradation in hip and knee replacements, *Trans Orthop Res Soc* 17:41, 1992.
26. Lombardi AV, et al: Fracture/dissociation of the polyethylene in metal-backed patellar components in total knee arthroplasty, *J Bone Joint Surg [Am]* 70:675–679, 1988.
27. Manley MT, et al: Effects of repetitive loading on the integrity of porous coatings, *Clin Orthop* 217:293–302, 1987.
28. Mendes DG, et al: Breakage of the metal tray in total knee replacement, *Orthopedics* 7:860–862, 1984.
29. Morrey BF, Chao EYS: Fracture of the porous coated metal tray of a biologically fixed knee prosthesis, *Clin Orthop* 228:182–189, 1986.
30. Ranawat CS, et al: Retrieval analysis of porous coated components for total knee arthroplasty: A report of two cases, *Clin Orthop* 209:244–248, 1986.
31. Rimnac CM, et al: Failure of orthopaedic implants: Three case histories, *Mater Characterization* 26:201–209, 1991.
32. Rimnac CM, et al: Characterization of material properties of ultra high molecular weight polyethylene before and after implantation, *Society for Biomaterials Implant Retrieval Symposium,* 15:16, 1992.
33. Roe RJ, et al: Effect of radiation sterilization and aging on ultra high molecular weight polyethylene, *J Biomed Mater Res* 15:209–230, 1981.
34. Scott RD, Ewald FC, Walker PS: Fracture of the metallic tibial tray following total knee replacement, *J Bone Joint Surg [Am]* 66:780–782, 1984.
35. Stulberg SD, et al: Failure mechanisms of metal-backed patellar components, *Clin Orthop* 236:88–104, November 1988.
36. Sutherland CJ: Patellar component dissociation in total knee arthroplasty, *Clin Orthop* 228:178–181, 1988.
37. Tsao A, et al: Severe polyethylene failure in PCA total knee arthroplasties, *J Bone Joint Surg [Am]* 75:19–26, 1993.
38. Wright TM: Implant debris from total joint arthroplasties. In Hirohata K, Mizumo K, and Matsubara T, editors: *Trends in research and treatment of joint diseases,* Tokyo, 1992, Springer-Verlag, pp 116–121.
39. Wright TM, Burstein AH: The method of implant retrieval analysis at The Hospital for Special Surgery. In *Proceedings of the Conference on Implant Retrieval Analysis,* Gaithersburg, Md, 1981, National Bureau of Standards, pp 559–570.
40. Wright TM, Hood RW, Burstein AH: Analysis of material failures, *Symposium on Total Knee Arthroplasty, Orthop Clin North Am* 13:33–44, 1982.
41. Wright TM, et al: Analysis of surface damage in retrieved carbon fiber–reinforced and plain polyethylene tibial components from posterior stabilized total knee replacements, *J Bone Joint Surg [Am]* 70:1312–1319, 1988.
42. Wright TM, et al: Failure of carbon fiber–reinforced polyethylene total knee components. A report of two cases, *J Bone Joint Surg [Am]* 70:926–932, 1988.
43. Wright TM, et al: Wear of polyethylene in total joint replacements: Observations from retrieved PCA knee implants, *Clin Orthop* 276:126–134, 1992.

72

Infected Total Knee Arthroplasty

MICHAEL A. MASINI, M.D.
JAMES H. MAGUIRE, M.D.
THOMAS S. THORNHILL, M.D.

Defining infection in total knee arthroplasty
Factors associated with increased infection rate
   Choice of prosthesis
   Wound problems
Prevention of infection in total knee arthroplasty
   Preoperative planning
   Perioperative antibiotics
   Controlled surgical environment
   Postoperative management
   Long-term prevention of infection
Diagnosis of infection
   Clinical findings
   Laboratory findings
   Causative organisms

Treatment and results
   Antibiotic therapy
   Specific regimens
   Long-term suppression with oral antibiotics
   Antibiotic-loaded cement in prevention and treatment of infected total knee replacements
   Surgical options
   Aspiration and antibiotics
   Open debridement
   Immediate exchange
   Early exchange
   Delayed exchange
   Arthrodesis
   Resection arthroplasty
   Amputation
Summary

Infection is the most dreaded complication of total knee arthroplasty (TKA). The psychological and monetary costs of multiple surgical procedures, prolonged courses of intravenous (IV) antibiotics, and rehabilitation are staggering. Revision arthroplasty following infection may fail and result in a markedly decreased functional status.

Most recent series report a deep infection rate of 1% to 2%. In a recent article analyzing infection in TKA at the Brigham and Women's Hospital (BWH) in Boston, a 1.6% rate of infection occurred in 1,693 knees during the interval from 1973 to 1980 and a 1.5% rate was found in 2,478 knees operated on between 1980 and 1987.[1] These rates remain similar to those of reports published earlier in the 1980s and may represent the lowest achievable rates using available preventive techniques.

Intraoperative contamination has been decreased by shorter operative times, total body exhaust systems, ultraviolet light, laminar flow systems, and even isolation facilities, but to date a true "sterile" field has not been achieved. In addition, it is currently impossible to completely prevent hematogenous infection in either the perioperative or late postoperative periods.

Treatment of the infected TKA requires a cooperative approach between the orthopedic surgeon and an infectious disease consultant familiar with infection of prosthetic devices. Successful management requires an awareness of changing resistance patterns among pathogenic organisms and an ability to analyze serum concentrations of antibiotics in relation to the susceptibility of the infecting organism.

In this chapter, we discuss the variable manifestations of deep infection, factors associated with an increased risk of infection, surgical options available for treatment, and a rational approach to the use of prophylactic and therapeutic antibiotics.

DEFINING INFECTION IN TOTAL KNEE ARTHROPLASTY

It is important to identify noninfectious wound problems that may lead to wound infection. It is also essential to distinguish between wound contamination and wound infection and between superficial infection and deep infection. When the number of bacteria contaminating a wound following secondary closure exceed 10,000 organisms per gram of tissue, abscess formation and wound breakdown are likely to ensue.[2] Wound problems that predispose to infection include dehiscence, persistent drainage, skin slough, and hematoma. Superficial infection is confined to the skin and subcutaneous tissues and does not penetrate the fascia. Deep infection implies involvement of the prosthesis and is inferred when evidence of infection is found deep to the fascia. Wound problems and superficial infection may lead to deep infection and should be treated promptly and aggressively.

The time of onset of infection and the duration of deep infection have important pathophysiologic implications for prognosis and treatment. In the past, early infection was defined as that occurring within 3 months of the index arthroplasty, and late infection as that appearing 3 months or more after surgery. Late infections were then subdivided into acute, subacute, and chronic.[3] Because persistence of infection seems to be common in treatment protocols which preserve the prosthesis when the infection is present 2 weeks or more after index arthroplasty,[4] a more practical classification would be to designate early infections as those that occur within 2 or 3 weeks of the index arthroplasty and late infections as those that occur after 3 weeks.

Late infections may result from hematogenous seeding of the prosthesis or direct penetration of the joint space. Acute late infections would be those that had a documented bacteremic event within 3 weeks of presentation and chronic late infections would be those in which the bacteremic event occurred greater than 3 weeks prior to presentation or in which no bacteremic event or penetrating injury could be documented.

FACTORS ASSOCIATED WITH AN INCREASED INFECTION RATE

Patients with rheumatoid arthritis (RA) have a rate of infection following TKA greater than two times that of patients with osteoarthritis.[1] This is because rheumatoid patients often have deficient wound healing, impaired immune responses, and breaks in the integrity of the skin due to ulcers, nodules, and bed sores.[5] Rheumatoid males appear to have a higher incidence of infection than rheumatoid females.[1] This may be due to the fact that most rheumatoid males are seropositive, have an acquired hypogammaglobulinemia, and tend to suffer from immune system compromise.

The use of steroids does not appear to be an independent risk factor for infection, but may reflect disease severity.[1] Rheumatoid patients are hospitalized more frequently than their osteoarthritic counterparts and thus are more predisposed to nosocomial infections.

Although similar pathogenic mechanisms would seem to apply to other inflammatory arthropathies such as systemic lupus erythematosus, psoriatic arthritis, arthritis of inflammatory bowel disease, and ankylosing spondylitis, an increased incidence of infection in TKA has not been documented in these conditions. Other disease states which result in altered immunity and an increased incidence of infection in TKA include diabetes mellitus,[6] chronic renal failure with subsequent renal transplantation, malignancy, chronic alcoholism, and the use of immunosuppressive agents.[1,7] Table 72–1 provides a list of factors predisposing to infection in TKA.

Choice of Prosthesis

The increased rate of both early and late infection of hinged prostheses is well documented. In the BWH series, 17 of 156 (10.9%) hinged arthroplasties became infected compared with 0.57% of the unconstrained metal-on-polyethylene prostheses during a comparable time period.[8] Constraining forces across hinged devices are transmitted to the bone-cement interface and often lead to tibial and femoral loosening. A poorly vascularized macrophage-lined membrane

TABLE 72–1.
Factors Associated With Increased Rate of Infection in Total Knee Arthroplasty

Underlying disease
   Rheumatoid arthritis
   Systemic lupus erythematosus
   Diabetes mellitus
   Chronic renal failure
   Chronic alcoholism
Host factors
   Chronic immunosuppression
   Distant focus of infection
   Previous infection in the knee
   Previous surgery in the knee
Type of prosthesis
   Hinge knee arthroplasty
Wound problems
   Skin slough
   Dehiscence
   Hematoma

then forms at the bone-cement interface, providing an environment conducive to bacterial growth isolated from host defense mechanisms. These macrophages engulf wear debris that impairs phagocytosis, a critical factor in bacterial surveillance. Different rates of infection have not been identified for posterior cruciate ligament–retaining and posterior cruciate ligament–sacrificing prostheses despite their differences in constraint. Host factors are also responsible for higher rates of infection as hinged prostheses are used primarily in patients with severe RA, severe deformity, or complex revision procedures.

Wound Problems

Wound complications are the leading cause of perioperative infection after TKA. Poss et al.[8] reported that 25 of 26 patients with perioperative (within 15 days) joint infections had wounds that did not heal primarily. Wound problems in this series included persistent drainage, hematomas, skin slough, stitch abscesses, superficial cellulitis, and persistent effusions or synovitis. More recently, Teeny et al.[4] found wound complications in 10 of 24 patients who had developed deep infection after TKA. Seven patients had wound slough or dehiscence and 3 patients had persistent drainage.

Some degree of hemarthrosis follows every total knee replacement. A tense, painful hemarthrosis may require arthrocentesis, both for control of pain and to allow proper rehabilitation. Hemarthrosis may lead to a capsular dehiscence and subsequent wound drainage. Persistent drainage in the immediate postoperative period usually indicates infection, active bleeding, or capsular dehiscence. When drainage occurs, physical therapy should be discontinued for 24 hours, and if the drainage continues, surgical exploration or at least arthrocentesis and culture should be considered.

The later onset of wound drainage (after institution of physical therapy) usually indicates capsular dehiscence or acute infection. Capsular dehiscence exposes the prosthesis to the external environment and interferes with patellar tracking. Dehiscence is best prevented by closing the capsule with interrupted sutures and testing the repair by flexing the knee before closing the subcutaneous tissues. If capsular dehiscence is suspected postoperatively, early surgical exploration and closure should be performed.

Skin slough is a major cause of perioperative sepsis that can be avoided by careful preoperative planning. The blood supply to the skin on the extensor surface of the knee is derived directly from cutaneous arteries rather than from segmental perforating arteries that course through muscle, such as those that supply the skin overlying the hip. The cutaneous arteries are branches of the lateral and medial genicular system and run superficial to the deep investing fascia.[9] The supramedial genicular artery is a major source of blood for the skin overlying the knee. Interruption of this artery is tolerated as long as the lateral genicular system remains intact. If, however, a previous lateral incision has interrupted the lateral supply, a long medial incision that interrupts the superomedial genicular artery may cause acute ischemia of the lateral flap. A single long medial incision will heal, as collaterals from the lateral genicular vessels will restore the vascularity of the lateral flap.

Skin necrosis is observed most commonly when a medial incision is placed near a previous lateral scar (Fig 72–1). When possible, the previous lateral scar should be incorporated in the new incision and a flap

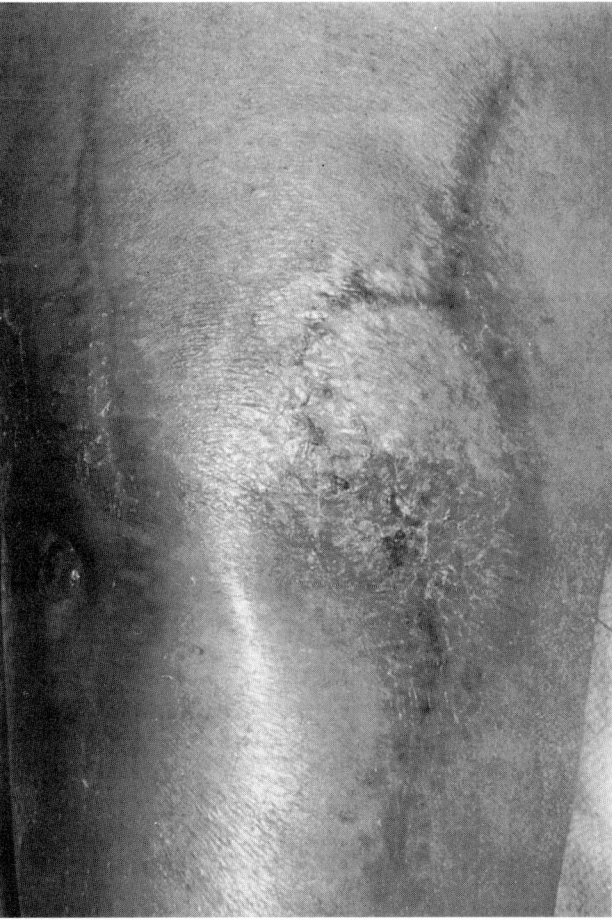

FIG 72–1.
Skin necrosis from a medial incision placed near the old lateral incision.

developed deep to the deep investing fascia until a medial capsular parapatellar incision can be performed. This is particularly important in the reconstruction of anterior cruciate ligament-deficient knees, which are prone to osteoarthritis and the need for eventual TKA because of meniscal damage and ligamentous laxity.

PREVENTION OF INFECTION IN TOTAL KNEE ARTHROPLASTY

Careful preoperative planning, meticulous intraoperative soft tissue management, and attention to detail in the early and late postoperative period are critical to prevention of infection following TKA.

Preoperative Planning

Patients with RA, diabetes, malignant disease, and malnutrition are all at increased risk of infection following major surgery. Patients with diabetes should not have uncontrolled hyperglycemia or metabolic acidosis at the time of surgery. Patients with malignant disease should undergo surgery only during periods in which they do not require chemotherapy. Malnourished patients should receive oral or parenteral hyperalimentation prior to an elective TKA. Patients with gingival or dental disease, established urinary tract infections, or other types of infection must be treated preoperatively.

Perioperative Antibiotics

Controlled clinical trials have demonstrated the efficacy of prophylactic antibiotics in reducing the incidence of deep wound infection after total hip arthroplasty and open reduction and internal fixation of hip fractures.[10, 11] Standard practice now mandates the use of perioperative antibiotics for any orthopaedic procedure that involves implantation of foreign materials, including knee prostheses. Parenterally administered semisynthetic penicillins and first-generation cephalosporins are usually chosen because of their activity against staphylococci and streptococci, the most common pathogens in joint replacement surgery. No study to date has shown superiority of any one agent and standard doses of all yield inhibitory levels in bone and joint fluid. Cefazolin, a first-generation cephalosporin, is the preferred antibiotic for perioperative prophylaxis in many institutions, including our own. Its long plasma half-life of 1½ hours leads to high sustained levels of the drug in bone and allows dosing at 8-hour intervals. The shorter half-life of the semisynthetic penicillins (nafcillin, oxacillin) and the other first-generation cephalosporins (cephalothin, cephapirin) requires 4-hour dosing with higher costs for drug acquisition and administration. Several second-and third-generation cephalosporins such as ceforanide, cefonicid, and ceftriaxone have extremely long half-lives and are administered every 12 to 24 hours. Despite the obvious advantages, studies to compare the efficacy of these agents with that of older agents are needed before their widespread use for the prevention of gram-positive infections can be recommended.

In recent years, there has been an increased incidence of infection due to methicillin-resistant strains of coagulase-negative staphylococci and *Staphylococcus aureus*. Vancomycin alone or in combination with gentamicin has been proposed for use in institutions particularly troubled with methicillin-resistant staphylococci or gram-negative organisms. However, the efficacy of vancomycin for prophylaxis is not well studied and its widespread use may promote the emergence of resistant organisms. Increasing numbers of organisms have been detected since the mid-1980s which exhibit vancomycin resistance, including several species of enterococci and staphylococci.[12] Cefuroxime, a second-generation cephalosporin, appears to have superior in vitro activity against methicillin-resistant staphylococci, but there are no comparative studies that document its superiority over the first-generation cephalosporins in either the treatment or prevention of orthopaedic infections with this pathogen.

Vancomycin is an acceptable alternative for patients with a history of allergy to cephalosporins or with a history of immediate-type hypersensitivity reaction to a penicillin. Disadvantages of vancomycin include its high cost and the common occurrence of rashes and hypotension with rapid administration (red syndrome). Clindamycin is a less satisfactory alternative because 5% or more of isolates of *S. aureus* are resistant and because the drug is bacteriostatic rather than bactericidal.

The optimal timing of prophylaxis has recently been confirmed. Effective prophylaxis requires inhibitory concentrations of the antibiotic against the likely pathogens in the operative site during the surgical procedure. Classen et al.[13] published the results of a prospective study of 2,847 surgical patients and found a statistically significant increased rate of infection if antibiotics were administered earlier than 2 hours before incision or at any period after incision. In addition, it appears that antibiotics should be administered at least 5 minutes before inflation of the tourniquet.[14, 15] Because antibiotic probably needs to be present only during the procedure itself, it is likely that a single dose of cefazolin 30 to 45 minutes prior to the incision would be sufficient. It has been shown that antibiotics administered for 24 hours are as effective as antibiotics administered for 7 days.[16] For this reason, courses longer than 24 hours are not recommended. All patients should receive perioperative antibiotics according to regimens such as those shown in Table 72-2.

Controlled Surgical Environment

Wound infection occurs when host defenses are unable to contain the bacterial contamination that probably occurs in all surgical wounds. Host resistance depends on systemic factors (listed in the previous section) and local factors, including tissue necrosis, presence of dead space, extent of hemostasis, and duration of surgery. The use of ultraviolet light, body exhaust facilities, and vertical laminar airflow systems reduces the amount of bacterial contamination that occurs in conventional operating room suites.[17, 18] For years it has been accepted that prophylactic antibiotics significantly reduce the incidence of infection in total joint arthroplasty. The further diminution of infection by altering the surgical environment is more controversial.

J.P. Nelson and co-workers[19] demonstrated that prophylactic antibiotics significantly reduced the incidence of postoperative infection when compared with cases in which antibiotics were not used. Moreover, the use of vertical laminar flow significantly improved the infection rate when large numbers of patients were examined. In the study of Nelson et al., the use of ultraviolet light decreased the incidence of infection but fell short of significance owing to the relatively low numbers of patients studied.[19] Lidwell et al.[20] showed a decrease in infection when unidirectional airflow was used and a further decrease with exhaust systems. Salvati et al.[21] surprisingly reported an increased incidence of infection in TKA but not in total hip arthroplasties when using a horizontal airflow system. They concluded that the position of the surgeon at the foot of the table blocked airflow and created eddys over the wound, thus increasing local contamination. Current data suggest that, when properly employed, secondary measures to control the surgical environment will reduce contamination of the surgical field.

Postoperative Management

Prophylactic antibiotics should not be continued for greater than 24 to 48 hours. Specific postoperative infections involving the urinary tract, the skin, the lungs, or an IV line should be treated aggressively to avoid bacteremic seeding of the wound. A short course of postoperative antibiotics may decrease the incidence of urinary tract infection in patients requiring an indwelling Foley catheter, but prolonged courses increase the risk of infection with highly resistant organisms. Persistent drainage, increasing pain, erythema, or rise in temperature are not indications for blind antibiotic therapy but necessitate an aggressive attempt to culture an organism from the wound. The temptation to place a patient on oral antibiotics for swelling and erythema around the wound must be avoided. If infection is documented or the suspicion of infection is high, a broad-spectrum IV antibiotic regimen should be instituted once adequate wound and blood cultures have been obtained.

Long-Term Prevention of Infection

The majority of late infections in TKA occur by hematogenous spread of organisms from elsewhere in the body. Infections of the skin, genitourinary tract, gastrointestinal tract, and respiratory tract should be treated promptly before there is spread to the prosthetic joint.[22] Surgical procedures involving the mucosal surfaces of the mouth, genitourinary tract, and lower gastrointestinal tract frequently produce a transient bacteremia, but documented cases of total joint infection resulting from such procedures are rare. The results can be catastrophic, however, as noted by a case report by Wilde et al.,[23] who documented a hematogenously acquired case of *Clostridium perfringens* infection after cholecystitis in a patient with a recently implanted TKA. The patient failed an attempt at debridement and delayed exchange of the prosthesis and ultimately required arthrodesis.[23]

TABLE 72-2.
Perioperative Antibiotic Prophylaxis for Total Knee Arthroplasty*

Preferred regimen
　Cefazolin, 1 g IV q8h × 3 doses
Alternative regimen (for cephalosporin-allergic patient or patient with immediate-type hypersensitivity to penicillin)
　Vancomycin, 1 g IV infused over 1 hr
Other regimens
　Nafcillin
　Oxacillin
　Cephalothin
　Cephapirin　　　　1-2 g IV q4h × 6 doses
　Clindamycin, 600 mg IV q8h × 3 doses

*The first dose in all instances is administered approximately 30 minutes before the joint space is entered.

TABLE 72-3.
Antibiotic Prophylaxis for Patients With Total Knee Arthroplasty Undergoing Procedures Likely to Result in Transient Bacteremia*

Dental, upper respiratory tract, gastrointestinal, and genitourinary procedures
  Amoxicillin 3 g PO 1 hr before procedure and 1.5 g 6 hr after initial dose
Amoxicillin, penicillin allergy:
  Erythromycin ethylsuccinate 800 mg, or erythromycin stearate, 1 g, PO 2 hr before procedure and one-half dose 6 hr after initial dose
  Clindamycin 300 mg PO 1 hr before procedure and 150 mg 6 hr after initial dose

*Data from JAMA 264:2920, 1990.

The efficacy of prophylactic antibiotics in preventing infection of any prosthetic device (including heart valves as well as orthopaedic appliances) following such procedures has not been studied. Despite the absence of data to support the practice, prophylaxis is advocated by many surgeons because of the catastrophic consequences of total joint infection and the possible legal ramifications. In our institution, prophylaxis is recommended especially for patients with RA in whom the risk of late hematogenous infection is high.[1] In each case, the risk of serious allergic reactions to the antibiotics should be weighed against the unknown but extremely low risk of hematogenous seeding of a joint replacement. The oral antibiotic regimens (Table 72-3) are the same as those currently recommended for the prevention of bacterial endocarditis in patients with valvular heart disease.[24]

DIAGNOSIS OF INFECTION

Clinical Findings

The diagnosis of an acute infection is easily made when a febrile patient presents with a painful, erythematous, swollen knee, as seen in Figure 72-2. In many cases, however, such cardinal features of acute infection are not present. There may be minimal swelling and no erythema or drainage. It is frequently difficult to differentiate normal postoperative pain with the pain of an acute infectious process and it is a change in findings rather than the findings themselves that indicates a problem. The persistence of pain, an increase in pain or swelling, or the failure to reach standard rehabilitation goals should raise the suspicion of an infectious process. Figure 72-3 illustrates a case initially presumed to be a stitch granuloma which was, in fact, a deep periprosthetic infection.

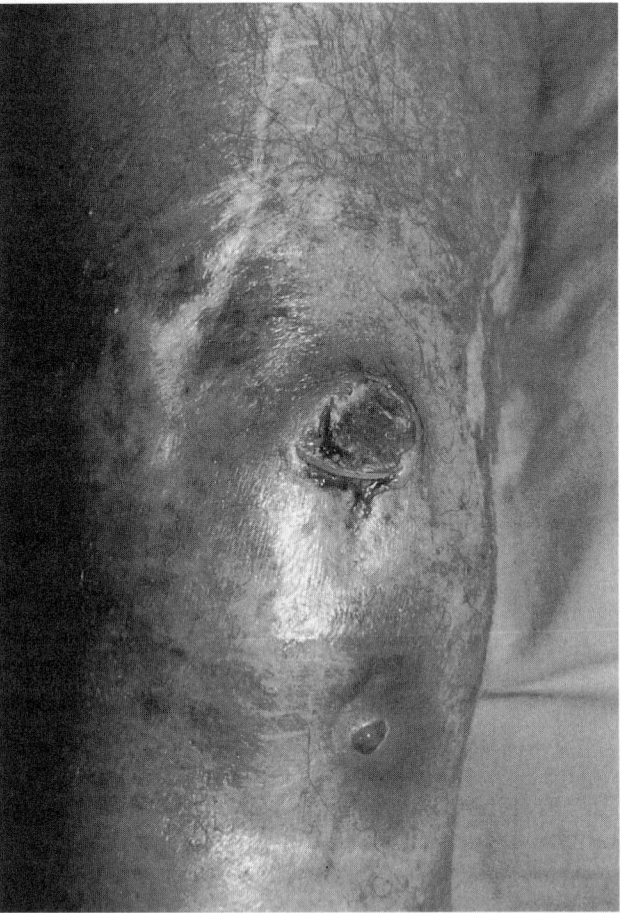

FIG 72-2.
Staphylococcal infection with sinus formation, cellulitis, and skin necrosis.

Laboratory Findings

Acute phase reactants such as sedimentation rate and C-reactive protein are usually elevated while the white blood cell (WBC) count may be elevated or normal. The acute phase reactants, however, may be elevated normally in the postoperative period. The most helpful laboratory test is analysis of synovial fluid including aerobic and anaerobic cultures, a cell count, differential, and Gram stain. Additional tests such as determination of synovial fluid sugar and protein values are useful in monitoring the response to treatment. Plain radiographs that include anteroposterior (AP), lateral, and skyline views may show periprosthetic osteolysis, periosteal elevation, or bony erosion. A positive technetium bone scan does not distinguish between aseptic loosening and infection, and the bone scan remains positive for months after surgery. The combination of technetium and gallium scans is more specific for diagnosing infection.[25] Infection results in increased uptake of gallium relative to that seen with loosening.[26] Indium scan

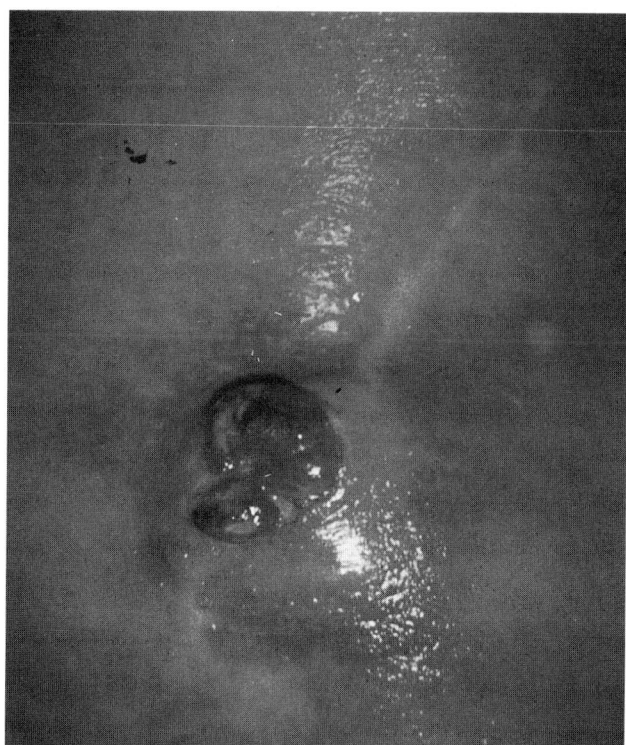

FIG 72–3.
Apparent granuloma actually represented a deep wound infection.

imaging used after a positive technetium scan may also increase the sensitivity of detecting infection about a prosthesis.[27] Arthrograms or sinograms or both may demonstrate a communication between a sinus tract and the prosthesis.

Causative Organisms

A broad spectrum of bacteria and, less frequently, mycobacteria or fungi have been implicated in infections of total joint prostheses. The species of offending organism reflects the route of acquisition of infection and susceptibility factors of the host (Table 72–4). Different pathogens occur with varying frequency among institutions as a result of different patient populations and infection rates in different series. Staphylococci account for the majority of TKA infections in reported series. Table 72–5 includes the organisms isolated from culture of all the infected TKAs at BWH. The incidence of early infection due to intraoperative contamination with *S. aureus* (coagulase-positive staphylococcus) has declined because of the routine use of perioperative antibiotics. However, *S. aureus* is responsible for many early infections and also remains the leading cause of late infections acquired by the hematogenous route in our hospital because of our large population of patients with RA. Rheumatoid patients seem to be at particular risk for hematogenous infection with *S. aureus*. The source of infection is often a lesion in the skin,[1, 28] but in many cases there is no apparent portal of entry. Defects in neutrophil function have been demonstrated in RA and staphylococcal infections of rheumatoid nodules, ulcers, and bursae are common. Many rheumatoid patients require corticosteroids for control of their arthritis, which further impairs their host defenses against this organism.

In some institutions, coagulase-negative staphylococci (usually *Staphylococcus epidermidis*) are the most common pathogen associated with total joint infections.[29] Nearly all cases of prosthetic joint infection caused by this organism occur as a result of intraoperative contamination with the normal bacterial flora of the patient's or operating team's skin. Infections due to coagulase-negative staphylococci typically run an indolent course, and hence months or even several years may elapse after surgery before the infection is detected. Despite their relative "avirulence" when compared to organisms such as *S. aureus*, coagulase-negative staphylococci are rarely eradicated without removal of the prosthesis because of the ability of pathogenic strains to adhere to inert surfaces and to secrete a protective glycocalyx.[30]

The streptococci, as a group, are responsible for a large proportion of total knee infections. Group A streptococcal infections are seen most commonly in patients with cellulitis or erysipelas, and group B streptococci seem to have a predilection for diabetic patients. Viridans streptococci usually originate in the oropharynx and lead to total joint infections in patients with dental or periodontal infections and in patients with subacute bacterial endocarditis. Enterococci are common in patients whose infections occur as a result of breakdown of the wound. In these cases, the wound becomes colonized with enterococci (and other organisms) because of their resistance to semisynthetic penicillins or cephalosporins. Enterococci also occur by bacteremic spread from infections of the genitourinary or gastrointestinal tract.

Gram-negative enteric bacilli such as *Escherichia coli*, *Proteus*, and *Klebsiella* usually originate in the genitourinary and gastrointestinal tracts. *Pseudomonas aeruginosa*, *Enterobacter*, and *Serratia* occur most frequently in patients with open wounds who have received various courses of antibiotics.

Anaerobic bacteria are increasingly recognized as pathogens in total knee infections. In some cases, organisms such as peptostreptococci (including organisms formerly known as peptococci) or *Propionibacterium acnes*, which are part of the normal flora of the skin, are introduced at the time of surgery. In other

TABLE 72-4.

Bacteriology of Total Joint Infection According to Route of Infection and Predisposing Conditions

Infection acquired by intraoperative contamination
    Coagulase-negative staphylococci (usually *Staphylococcus epidermidis*) *Staphylococcus aureus*
    Propionibacterium acnes and other diphtheroids
    Microaerophilic and anaerobic streptococci

Infection acquired hematogenously

Underlying condition or risk factor	Common organisms
Rheumatoid arthritis	*S. aureus*
Corticosteroid therapy	*S. aureus*
Bacteremic pneumonia	*Streptococcus pneumoniae* (pneumococcus)
Skin infections	*S. aureus*, group α-hemolytic streptococcus, other streptococci
Diabetes mellitus	*S. aureus*, group B streptococci
Hemodialysis	*S. aureus*
IV catheter infections	*S. aureus*, gram-negative bacilli
Urinary tract infection	*Escherichia coli, Klebsiella, Proteus, Pseudomonas*, other gram-negative bacilli, enterococcus
Gastrointestinal infections (e.g., diverticulitis, intraabdominal abscesses, cholangitis)	Gram-negative enteric bacilli, *Bacteroides fragilis*, enterococcus
Intraoral infections	Viridans streptococci

Infections caused by direct extension
    Early wound breakdown
        S. epidermidis
        S. aureus
        Enterococci
        Streptococci
    Longstanding wound breakdown
    Often a mixture of bacteria, including staphylococci; streptococci; enterococci; anaerobes; gram-negative bacilli, including *Pseudomonas*
    Intraarticular injection
    Coagulase-negative staphylococci (usually *S. epidermidis*), *S. aureus*
    Peptococcus
    P. acnes and other diphtheroids
    Microaerophilic and anaerobic streptococci

TABLE 72-5.

Organisms Isolated From III Infected Total Knee Arthroplasties (Brigham and Women's Hospital)

Organism	Number	Percent
Staphylococcus aureus	55	50
Gram-negative rods	11	10
Streptococcus	9	8
Staphylococcus epidermidis	7	6.5
Enterococcus	4	3.8
Peptostreptococcus	4	3.8
Pseudomonas	4	3.8
Others	8	7.3
Mixed infections	9	8

cases, the source of an anaerobic infection lies elsewhere in the body. *Bacteroides fragilis* has been isolated from patients with diverticulitis and other intraabdominal infections, and peptostreptococcal infections have originated from upper respiratory sources. Patients whose infections are due to an open wound often have several pathogens occurring simultaneously, and frequently anaerobes are present along with aerobes.

Fungal infections are decidedly rare in TKA. Levine et. al.[31] reported the first case of *Candida albicans* infection in TKA, although other species of *Candida* had been isolated previously. Fungal infections generally occur after prolonged antibiotic treatment for bacterial sepsis or in immunocompromised patients and should be considered in symptomatic patients whose bacterial cultures are sterile. Review of the literature has indicated that successful eradication of infection requires debridement, removal of the prosthesis, and prolonged IV antifungal therapy with agents such as amphotericin B, 5-fluorocytosine, and ketoconazole.[21, 32] Successful prosthetic reimplantation after fungal infection has been reported only rarely and arthrodesis is usually required for eradication of infection.

TREATMENT AND RESULTS

The selection of antibiotics and determination of the duration of treatment should be made in conjunction with an infectious disease consultant.

Antibiotic Therapy

Antibiotics should not be administered before appropriate samples of synovial fluid and tissue are obtained for culture. Empiric therapy should be based on the findings of the Gram-stained smear of synovial fluid and definitive therapy should be based on the culture results. Antibiotics selected should be bactericidal against the responsible agent and should be administered parenterally in doses that will yield adequate concentrations in the serum and tissues (Table 72–6).

TABLE 72–6.

Doses of Antibiotics Commonly Used for Treatment of Infected Total Knee Replacements

Antibiotic	Dose*
Penicillin G	3×10^6 U IV q4h
Ampicillin	
Nafcillin	
Oxacillin	2 g IV q4h
Cephalothin	
Cephapirin	
Cefazolin	1 g IV q8h
Vancomycin†	500 mg IV q6h
	or
	1 g IV q12h
Clindamycin	600 mg IV q8h
Gentamicin‡	2.0 mg/kg loading dose, then 1.7 mg/kg IV q8h
Tobramycin	2.0 mg/kg loading dose, then 1.7 mg/kg IV q8h
Metronidazole	15 mg/kg IV, then 7.5 mg/kg IV q8h
Ciprofloxacin	400 mg IV q12h
	or
	750 mg PO q12h

*Doses are for adults with normal renal and hepatic functions.
†Initial doses and dosing intervals are estimates that should be based on body weight, body composition, and renal function. Subsequent doses are determined following measurement of serum levels.
‡Dose for treating most gram-negative bacillary infections; 1 mg/kg IV q.8h. is recommended for treating enterococcal infection (in addition to penicillin, ampicillin, or vancomycin).

The optimal duration of antibiotic therapy has not been established. Because the relapse rate in cases of acute hematogenous osteomyelitis is unacceptably high when antibiotics are given for less than 3 weeks, we routinely treat all patients with an infected TKA for a minimum of 4 weeks and some authors suggest that 6 weeks of antibiotic therapy may be most prudent.[33, 34] There are no controlled studies, however, to suggest that treatment for 6 weeks is superior to treatment for 4 weeks, and the duration of treatment should be determined after discussion with the infectious disease consultant.

After removing an infected prosthesis, we administer 4 weeks of antibiotics, even if additional therapy had been given preoperatively. Some authorities recommend the routine use of serum and synovial fluid bactericidal levels to monitor antibiotic therapy.[22, 35] We have not seen a good correlation between these levels and the outcome of treatment and do not request them as routine. Parenthetically, there has been little correlation between serum bactericidal levels and the outcome of treatment of bacterial endocarditis, an infection in which there has been widespread use of such levels.

Standard doses and common adverse effects of commonly used antibiotics are listed in Tables 72–6 and 72–7.

Specific Regimens

Empiric therapy should he based on the Gram-stained smear of synovial fluid and a consideration of predisposing conditions in each patient. If the smear shows gram-positive cocci, vancomycin should be given because of the high incidence of methicillin-resistant coagulase-negative staphylococci in total joint infections. Vancomycin is active against most gram-positive organisms. If gram-negative rods are present on the smear, an aminoglycoside or a third-generation cephalosporin should be given, unless an intraabdominal source of infection is suspected, in which case an agent active against *Bacteroides fragilis* such as metronidazole should also be added. Gentamicin is the aminoglycoside of choice for empiric therapy in our hospital, but in centers with a high prevalence of gentamicin resistance, amikacin is preferable. If no organisms are present on the smear, we begin therapy with vancomycin and gentamicin in the acutely ill patient until culture results become available. Definitive therapy is based on the results of the culture and sensitivity testing.

Staphylococci and streptococci sensitive to penicillin should be treated with penicillin G. Penicillin-resistant staphylococci that are sensitive to methicil-

TABLE 72-7.
Selected Adverse Effects Associated With Antibiotic Therapy

Antimicrobial Agent	Common Adverse Effects	Comments
Penicillins and cephalosporins	Allergic reactions (rash, drug fever, interstitial nephritis, hepatitis, neutropenia, anaphylaxis	Requires discontinuation of drug; occasionally topical or systemic steroids are indicated
		Elevated eosinophil count supports the diagnosis of hypersensitivity; 5%–15% cross-reactivity between penicillins and cephalosporins
Aminoglycoside	Eighth cranial nerve toxicity	Serum levels and renal function should be monitored closely to avoid toxic concentrations of drugs in serum and tissues
		Patients with renal impairment should have dosages reduced or intervals between doses prolonged depending on peak and trough serum levels
Vancomycin	Phlebitis of veins used for infusion	Central line desirable for long courses of therapy
	Red syndrome (erythematous rash, hypotension)	Infuse slowly (over at least 1 hr)
	Nephrotoxicity	Monitor serum levels and renal function closely, especially if an aminoglycoside is used at the same time
	Allergic reactions (fever, rash, neutropenia, eosinophilia)	May require discontinuation of drug
All antibiotics except vancomycin Increased incidence with clindamycin	Pseudomembranous colitis (due to toxin of *Clostridium difficile*)	Toxin-induced illness ranges from mild diarrhea to fulminant course with hemorrhage or perforation
		Diagnosis made by detecting toxin in stool
		Treatment includes stopping the drug when possible; in some cases oral metronidazole or vancomycin is required

lin, oxacillin, or nafcillin should be treated with oxacillin or nafcillin. For patients allergic to penicillin, a first-generation cephalosporin may be substituted unless there is a history of immediate-type hypersensitivity. Vancomycin is indicated for patients who are allergic to cephalosporins or who have immediate-type hypersensitivity to penicillin. Cephalosporins should never be used to treat infections due to methicillin-resistant staphylococci even if in vitro sensitivity testing indicates susceptibility to cephalosporins. Such organisms are best treated with vancomycin, and clinical studies are underway to examine the possible benefit of adding gentamicin or rifampin to the regimen.[36] The new quinolone antibiotics such as ciprofloxacin or ofloxacin should not be used to treat total knee infections due to staphylococci because of the well-documented risk of emerging resistance. Enterococcal infections should be treated with two drugs: an aminoglycoside (usually gentamicin) and either penicillin or ampicillin (or vancomycin in the case of penicillin allergy or resistance to penicillins).

The treatment of gram-negative infections varies according to the organism and the sensitivity pattern. Antibiotic resistance may develop if *Pseudomonas, Enterobacter,* or *Serratia* spp. are treated with a penicillin or cephalosporin alone. These bacteria are usually treated initially with an aminoglycoside and either an antipseudomonal penicillin or cephalosporin. Gram-negative infections may be treated with quinolone antibiotics (ciprofloxacin or ofloxacin), but caution should be used in *Pseudomonas* infections because resistance to quinolones can develop during therapy.

The prolonged courses of therapy required for treatment of infected TKAs are associated with a high incidence of adverse effects and allergic reactions. Careful monitoring of serum levels of antibiotics such as vancomycin and the aminoglycosides will help prevent toxicity. Close observation of patients will allow the early detection of allergic reactions or side effects that necessitate discontinuation or substitution of an antibiotic. Table 72-7 lists some of the most common problems associated with long-term antibiotic therapy and appropriate preventive and therapeutic measures. Outpatient administration of IV antibiotics has become a common practice and has helped reduce length of stay in hospitals and hospital costs. In selected cases, an oral quinolone antibiotic can be used to complete therapy after initial IV treatment. Serum bactericidal levels should be measured to ensure compliance and adequate serum levels.

Long-Term Suppression With Oral Antibiotics

There is rarely any indication for the prolonged use of oral antibiotics in the management of the infected

TKA. Chronic suppression of an infected implant may be considered for the unusual case in which surgery is contraindicated for medical reasons or in which removal of the prosthesis would result in an outcome such as amputation that would be unacceptable to the patient. However, occasionally suppression may be indicated to suppress a distant focus such as a chronic urinary tract infection.

Suppression of a TKA infection should never be viewed as a permanent solution, but rather as a possible means of delaying removal of the prosthesis. The hazards and disadvantages of prolonged suppressive oral antibiotics are multiple. Suppression frequently fails and places the patient at risk for serious systemic infection or for further loss of bone stock or soft tissue structures. Suppression may lead to the emergence of antibiotic-resistant organisms and thus compromise definitive treatment at a later date. Finally, chronic antibiotic therapy exposes the patient to side effects and allergic reactions and the cost of the drugs may be substantial.

In the event that suppression is to be attempted, several criteria should be fulfilled. All clinical signs of infection must be resolved and synovial fluid cultures must be negative before switching from parenteral to oral antibiotics. The responsible organism must be susceptible to an antibiotic that can be taken orally and that can achieve serum and tissue levels sufficient for inhibition of the organism.

Despite following the above indications, suppression must still be considered only temporary and is frequently unsuccessful. Tsukayama et al.[37] recently reported the outcome of 13 patients treated with surgical debridement, retention of the components, and suppressive antibiotics. At a mean follow-up of 37.6 months, only 3 patients (23%) had retained their prosthesis. In addition, 5 patients (38%) had experienced adverse effects which led to changes in antibiotic therapy.[37]

Antibiotic-Loaded Cement in Prevention and Treatment of Infected Total Knee Replacements

Powdered antibiotics mixed in polymethyl methacrylate before polymerization are released in high concentrations from the surface of the hardened polymer into the adjacent bone and soft tissue. The concentrations obtained are many times higher than the minimal level that inhibit growth of most bacteria. Several authorities therefore have advocated the routine use of antibiotic-loaded cement for prophylaxis in joint replacement and for therapy of deep infection.[38] Currently available clinical data, however, are insufficient to demonstrate the superiority of this means of antibiotic delivery over standard parenteral administration. The theoretic advantages of antibiotic-loaded cement are several. The concentrations of antibiotics in bone and soft tissues following release from cement are many times greater than concentrations obtained by IV administration of the same antibiotic. The serum concentrations of antibiotics released from cement at the same time are low, thus offering little risk of toxicity. Released antibiotics may diffuse into poorly vascularized tissues that are not reached by parenterally administered antibiotics. The sustained release of antibiotics may offer prolonged protection or therapy in the adjacent tissue.

Potential disadvantages of antibiotic-loaded cement include allergic reactions and mechanical weakening of the polymer. The occurrence of an allergic reaction to the antibiotic in cement could necessitate removal of the prosthesis and cement. Fortunately, the incidence of allergy to gentamicin or tobramycin, the antibiotics most commonly added to cement, is low, and there are no reports of allergic reactions among persons who received cement containing these compounds. However, hypersensitivity to other antibiotics, especially the penicillins and cephalosporins, is common.

In vitro studies have documented mechanical weakening of cement following the addition of antibiotics. Increased rates of mechanical failure of prostheses in patients have not been reported, but long-term follow-up is lacking. In the absence of comparative data to substantiate the efficacy of antibiotic-loaded cement and long-term studies of its safety, its use should be considered experimental in prophylaxis. It should not be used as the sole form of perioperative antibiotic for either initial or repeat joint replacement because the antibiotic is unlikely to reach all parts of the wound in therapeutic concentrations. In one prospective study, the rate of superficial wound infections was significantly higher among persons receiving antibiotic-loaded cement when compared with persons receiving parenteral antibiotic prophylaxis for total hip replacement.[39] Moreover, streptococci and some strains of staphylococci are not inhibited by gentamicin or tobramycin alone. Whether the combined use of systemic antibiotics and antibiotic-loaded cement offers advantages over the use of systemic prophylaxis alone is not known.

Antibiotic-containing cement beads and spacers are employed with increasing frequency for the treatment of infected joint prostheses and chronic osteomyelitis. After removal of the infected implant and cement, dead space in the bone and soft tissues is filled with the beads or spacers which release high concentrations of the antibiotic into adjacent bone and soft tissue. The beads or spacers are later removed at the time of further debridement or reimplantation of a prosthesis. Systemic antibiotics should be administered concomitantly to assure penetration of drug to all parts of the wound. Superinfection with a resistant organism or later difficulty in removing the beads or spacer is a potential complication of this practice. The major advantage of the spacer over the beads is improved control of soft tissue tension. The potential disadvantage of both spacers and beads is that they are foreign bodies which remain in the wound and may paradoxically protect organisms which have the capacity to form a glycocalyx.

Use of antibiotic-loaded cement is best restricted to gentamicin or tobramycin because of their low risk for causing hypersensitivity. Treatment with cement containing these antibiotics should be restricted to infections due to susceptible organisms. Lack of efficacy against streptococci and some staphylococci requires that another antibiotic be administered for routine prophylaxis, preferably by the parenteral route. For both gentamicin and tobramycin, the powder form only is mixed in a dose of 500 to 600 mg in 40 g of cement powder. The dose may be doubled for use in beads or spacers. Although our experience is limited, we believe that the spacer has advantages over beads. The spacer block helps prevent soft tissue contracture, provides increased knee stability, and facilities ambulation in addition to providing local delivery of antibiotic.

Surgical Options

Surgical options for treatment of an infected total TKA include:

1. Retention of prosthesis
   a. Aspiration
   b. Open debridement
2. Removal of prosthesis
   a. Immediate exchange
   b. Early exchange
   c. Delayed exchange
   d. Arthrodesis
   e. Resection arthroplasty
   f. Amputation

Factors that influence choice of surgical option for an infected TKA include:

1. Early detection
2. Host resistance
3. Species of organism
4. Radiographic findings
5. Skin and soft tissue coverage
6. Response to treatment
7. Type of prosthesis

Treatment of infection without removing the prosthesis should be attempted only in an otherwise healthy patient infected with an organism that is easily eradicated, such as a streptococcus. Treatment must be instituted as soon as possible, and ideally within 24 to 48 hours of onset of symptoms to prevent invasion of the bony interface and subsequent loosening or osteomyelitis. The prosthesis must be in good position with no radiographic evidence suggestive of loosening. Retention of the prosthesis or performance of direct exchange requires adequate soft tissue coverage, sufficient bone stock, and a functioning quadriceps mechanism. Our experience with infected hinge knees suggests that component removal is always necessary.

Aspiration and Antibiotics

Under rare circumstances, an acutely infected TKA can be cured by aspiration and treatment with parenteral antibiotics. The knee is amenable to this form of therapy because it is easily drained and examined for reaccumulation of fluids. This form of therapy is only indicated in an immunocompetent patient with an infection of short duration (less than 24–48 hours) caused by a streptococcus which can be easily eradicated. The prosthesis must be firmly fixed and well aligned. The overlying skin and soft tissues must be viable and functional. The presence of a draining sinus tract indicates a chronic infection and precludes this form of therapy. The joint is aspirated repeatedly over the first 72 hours, during which time the effusion must disappear, the cultures turn negative, and the cell counts decrease. If these goals are not achieved or if the knee remains swollen immediately after arthrocentesis (indicating loculated fluid or a boggy synovitis), an open debridement at least is indicated. In the BWH experience, 12 acutely infected TKAs have been treated by aspiration and antibiotics alone. At follow-up of at least 2 years, only five patients were successfully treated and three of these continued to take oral antibiotics.

Open Debridement

Surgical debridement with synovectomy and component retention may cure an infected TKA in an otherwise healthy patient with an infection of short duration in a firmly fixed metal-to-plastic TKA. Limited open drainage or arthroscopic debridement and joint lavage of the infected TKA offer few advantages over simple joint aspiration and irrigation. Surgical debridement is best achieved by opening the entire wound and performing a formal synovectomy. The wound is closed primarily over surgical drains attached to simple suction. A closed irrigation system is not necessary to deliver antibiotics and may introduce additional pathogens. Range-of-motion exercises are begun on the second or third postoperative day to prevent soft tissue contractures and loculation of fluid. Drains are removed at approximately 48 to 72 hours. Persistent purulent drainage beyond 72 hours usually indicates failure of this form of therapy and the need for removal of the prosthesis. As noted earlier in this chapter, this type of therapy is most efficacious when the index arthroplasty was performed within 2 weeks of identification of infection and when infection is due to a "favorable" organism such as a streptococcus.[3]

Immediate Exchange

Immediate exchange is defined as placement of a new prosthesis at the time of removal of the infected prosthesis. The advantages of an immediate exchange over a delayed exchange include fewer operations, shorter hospitalization, and a decrease in soft tissue contractures. Immediate exchange is rarely practiced in the United States, but has been successful, especially in an acute infection due to susceptible organisms.[40] It is an unsuitable alternative when there is component loosening or malalignment.

Early Exchange

Rand et al.[41] reported the results of early exchange in 14 acutely infected TKAs. The protocol involved removal of the component with extensive debridement repeated every 2 to 3 days until the wound was judged suitable for reimplantation. After reimplantation, the patient received IV antibiotics for 4 to 6 weeks. Infection was eradicated in six of the seven knees infected with "low virulence" organisms in contrast to only two of seven knees that were infected with "high virulence" organisms. Of the eight knees cured bacteriologically, two were stiff and one was painful, so that only 5 patients (36%) had a good result. The authors concluded that early exchange offered little advantage over delayed exchange. Recent interest in antibiotic-impregnated cement and the use of antibiotic-impregnated acrylic beads may improve the results of early and immediate exchange. Several prospective trials are underway to assess the efficacy of antibiotic-impregnated cement and acrylic beads in conjunction with early exchange.

Delayed Exchange

A delayed exchange protocol was reported from The Hospital for Special Surgery in New York City.[21] The protocol included component removal, thorough debridement, primary closure, and 6 weeks of IV antibiotics with doses adjusted to achieve serum bactericidal activity at a dilution of 1:8 or greater. After 6 weeks of antibiotic therapy, the joint was inspected in the operating room and Gram staining and frozen section microscopy were performed. If the wound was clean and the Gram stain and the frozen section failed to show acute inflammation or microorganisms, a prosthesis was reimplanted. Prophylactic antibiotics were continued for 48 hours after surgery. Of the 44 knees treated in this manner, there were no recurrences with the same organism after 2 years follow-up. One patient with a *Pseudomonas* infection developed a new infection with *S. aureus*.

Rosenberg et al.[34], using a protocol of delayed exchange after debridement and parenteral antibiotics, found no recurrences of infection in a population of 25 patients with 26 infected knee arthroplasties. Nineteen (76%) patients had a good or excellent functional rating using The Hospital for Special Surgery Rating Scale. Five of the six patients with poor ratings had joint problems unrelated to the infected TKA. Table 72–8 shows the results of several series utilizing a delayed exchange protocol. In all of these, improved results were obtained with the delayed exchange protocol compared with treatment modalities that attempted to salvage the index prosthesis. The worst results in these reports occurred in the Mayo Clinic series, in which reimplantation was performed at 2 weeks. It thus appears that immediate exchange would result in a higher failure rate than delayed exchange; the duration of interim antibiotic therapy seems to be important in controlling infection.

Appropriate technique is vital to eradication of infection and to the ultimate outcome of the reimplanted arthroplasty. Figure 72–4 illustrates the membrane which remains after removal of an infected total knee. Meticulous debridement must be performed in all cases of sepsis. Time, patience, and pulsatile lavage are necessary to provide a clean bed for later reimplantation.

The surgeon must be prepared to address bone loss and deformity when performing reimplantation. Figure 72–5 illustrates the usual amount of bone loss one can expect after removal of components and thorough debridement. Stems, wedges, and spacers should be available at the time of reimplantation. Reimplantation can be one of the most challenging revision procedures. The posterior cruciate ligament can rarely be preserved and semiconstrained implants that provide anteroposterior and varus-valgus stability are often required (Fig 72–6).

Our current protocol for delayed exchange involves component removal, extensive debridement,

TABLE 72-8.
Results of Delayed Exchange Protocols

Series	Time to Reimplant (wk)	Antibiotic-Impregnated Cement	Postoperative Regimen	Infection Eradicated No.	%
Rand[41]	2	NA	NA	8/14	57
Insall et al.[33]	6–14	NA	Dressing Antibiotic Monitoring	44/44	100
Borden[47]	3	Yes	Beads Cast Dressing	18/21	92
Rosenberg et al.[34]	6–8	Yes	Skeletal traction	26/26	100
Teeny et al.[4]	0–12	NA	NA	10/10	100
Wilson et al.[1]	6–24	Yes, 40%	Variable	16/20	80

NA = not available.

and primary closure with suction drainage. After 48 to 72 hours, the knee is flexed from 0 to 30 degrees in a continuous passive motion (CPM) machine to prevent loculation of fluid and to maintain the soft tissues for subsequent reimplantation. Antibiotics are administered for 4 to 6 weeks and then discontinued unless there is evidence of continued infection. The patient is observed off antibiotics for a period of 2 weeks or more, and if there is no clinical evidence of active infection and the sedimentation rate has declined, reimplantation is scheduled. If there is clinical suspicion of ongoing infection (fever, local signs, leukocytosis, persistently elevated sedimentation rate), the knee is aspirated for culture and cell counts and repeat debridement is performed. At the time of reimplantation, the wound is examined visually and by Gram stain and frozen section microscopy. If there is suspicion of continued infection, further debridement without reimplantation or arthrodesis is performed. It is generally technically easier to perform reimplantation shortly after debridement, but delays of several months may be necessary to ensure against possible relapse of infection. The technique of delayed exchange is similar to that described for revision of noninfected TKAs except for the correction of bony defects and the use of antibiotic-impregnated cement rather than allograft. Bony defects are filled with autologous cancellous bone when possible, but a custom implant may be required. Antibiotic-impregnated cement may be used if the causative microorganism is susceptible to an antibiotic appropriate for addition to acrylic cement. After reimplantation, perioperative antibiotics are continued until intraoperative cultures are proved negative. Prolonged antibiotic therapy following reimplantation is not recommended.

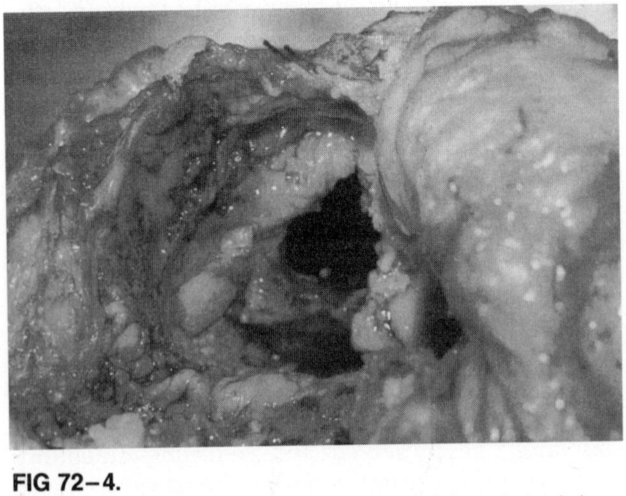

Arthrodesis

Arthrodesis for the infected TKA is indicated for patients who have failed attempts at revision or in cases in which skin coverage and soft tissue are insufficient to allow a functional arthroplasty. Broderson et al.[42] reviewed 45 arthrodeses for failed TKA and reported an 81% fusion rate following failure of metal-to-plastic implants, but only a 56% fusion rate following failure of hinged implants. Stulberg[43] similarly reported a higher fusion rate following removal of unconstrained prostheses than after removal of hinged implants. In a small series from the BWH, similar rates of fusion were reported. Following resection of a failed hinged TKA, prolonged periods of immobili-

FIG 72-4.
Fibrous membrane surrounding removed infected total knee implant.

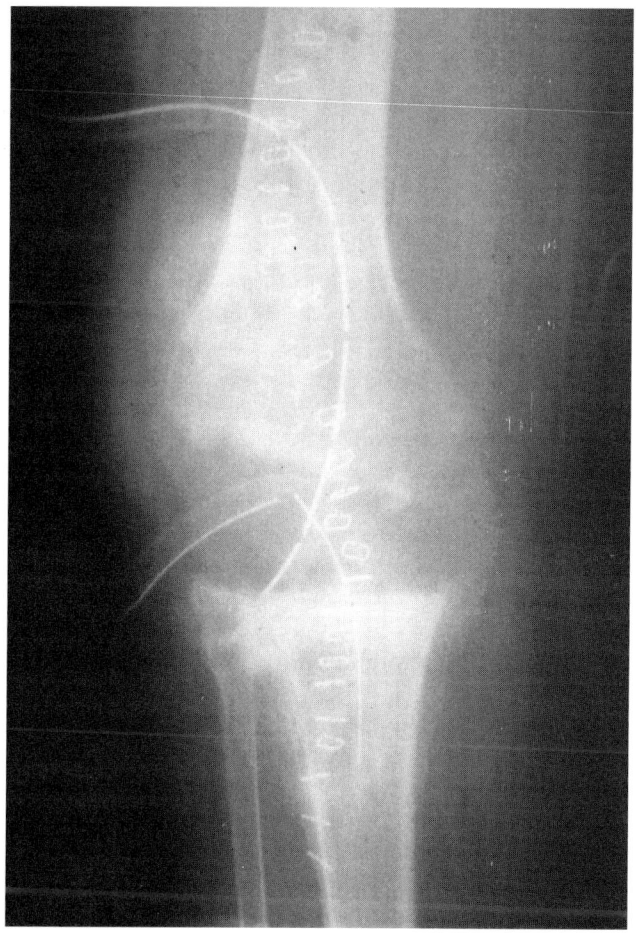

FIG 72–5.
Radiograph exhibiting bone loss after component removal for infection.

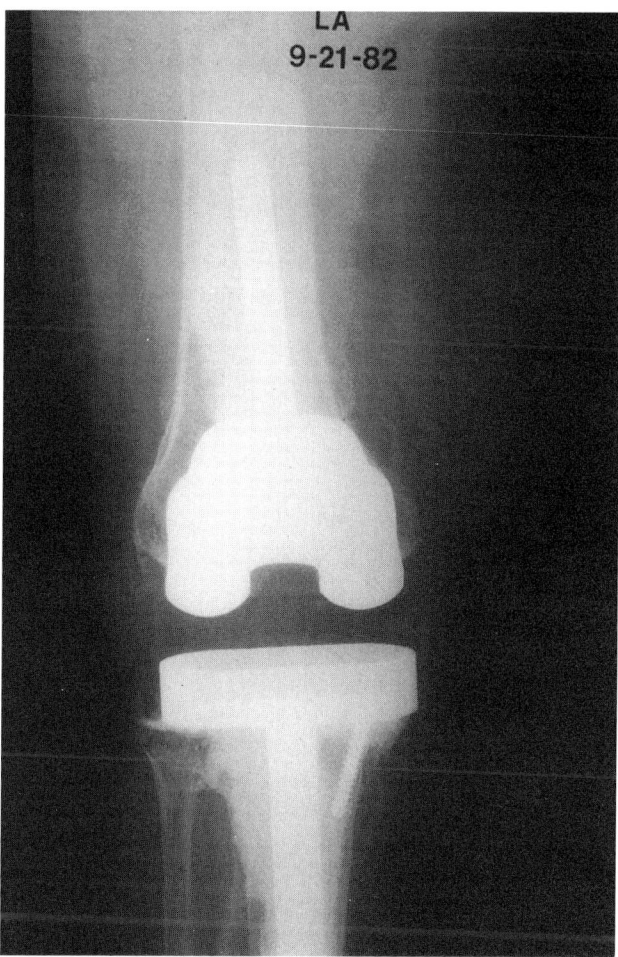

FIG 72–6.
Reimplanted total knee arthroplasty.

zation and multiple operations were often required to achieve fusion, and significant shortening (average 6.24 cm) resulted.[44]

There are essentially three techniques for arthrodesis: external fixation, internal fixation, and intramedullary fixation. The selection of mode of fixation should be individualized.[33] A period of 4 to 6 months is usually required before successful fusion. Repeat autogenous bone grafting may be required if union is delayed. While successful fusion is generally considered the desired end point, a recent case report has documented persistent infection despite arthrodesis.[45]

Resection Arthroplasty

Removal of the components without reimplantation or attempted arthrodesis has been reported by Falahee et al.[46] for treatment of failed TKA. They emphasized the importance of prolonged immobilization following resection arthroplasty to allow sufficient scarring for joint stability. They believe resection arthroplasty is most suitable for patients who have had severe disability before the TKA owing to systemic or multiarticular disease.[46] The senior author's (TST) current indications for resection arthroplasty include life-threatening infections or failures of revision in nonambulators or infections in patients with contralateral arthrodesis. Multiple failed attempts at reimplantation or significant bone loss may also necessitate resection arthroplasty.

Falahee et al. described the surgical technique and postoperative management of patients undergoing resection arthroplasty. The operation consists of thorough debridement with removal of all infected tissue, the component, and cement. The wound is closed loosely or left open depending on the character of the tissue. A cast or splint is applied postoperatively. Patients are allowed to bear weight as soon as they are physically capable. A removal universal splint is provided for use as desired after the cast or splint is removed.[46]

Amputation

Above-knee amputation is reserved for those patients in whom multiple attempts at fusion have failed or in whom infection cannot be eradicated by more conservative means. Amputation is rarely indicated in cases of life-threatening sepsis that cannot be managed by radical debridement and open packing. In such cases, a guillotine-type above-knee amputation is performed and the stump revised once the infection is controlled.

SUMMARY

An understanding of the factors associated with an increased incidence of infected TKA will identify the patient at risk but will not necessarily prevent infection. Careful preoperative evaluation to eliminate possible sources of infection, meticulous operative technique for handling skin and soft tissues, use of perioperative antibiotics, limiting bacterial contamination by controlling the surgical environment during operation, and long-term surveillance will not only lower the incidence of infection but will facilitate its early detection. A high index of suspicion and early detection of an infected TKA will affect treatment outcome. A promptly recognized infection in an immunocompetent host may, in rare instances, respond to treatment by aspiration and IV antibiotics. This form of treatment is limited to patients with an intact bony interface, no bony reaction, and organisms such as viridans streptococci, which are easily eradicated. The patient must respond promptly to antibiotics with a decrease in fluid accumulation, a decrease in cell count, cultures turning negative, increasing joint sugar, and an improved clinical appearance.

Treatment of an infected TKA by open debridement, synovectomy, and retention of the prosthesis is indicated in patients who have failed attempted aspiration and antibiotics alone, but who are otherwise healthy and infected with a "favorable" organism. The prosthesis must be removed when there is a significant delay in establishing a diagnosis of infection (possibly as short as 2 weeks) or when there is any evidence of component loosening. Periosteal elevation, bone resorption, or the presence of a sinus tract also mandates removal of the prosthesis. Immunocompromised patients and patients who have failed an attempted debridement with component retention should undergo removal of the prosthesis.

We have little data to support an immediate or early exchange protocol but recognize that the expanded use of antibiotic-impregnated cement and antibiotic-impregnated acrylic beads might enhance the success of such an option.

At present, the preferred method of treating an infected TKA when there is delay in diagnosis, loose components, immunoincompetence, or failure of open debridement is a delayed exchange protocol. The components are removed and a formal synovectomy is performed. When possible, the wound is closed primarily over a suction drain. Gentle motion is begun on approximately the third day to maintain the joint space and prevent loculation of fluid. Alternatively, an antibiotic-impregnated spacer block or beads may be utilized. An IV antibiotic is used for 4 to 6 weeks as determined by the infecting microorganism, the host defense status, and the patient's response. The patient is observed for persistent infection for approximately 2 weeks after the antibiotics are stopped. At the time of revision, the wound is inspected, and a Gram stain, cultures, and frozen section microscopy are performed, and a decision made to proceed with further debridement, reimplantation, or arthrodesis.

Arthrodesis is limited to those patients who have failed an attempted revision; patients with skin, muscle, and soft tissue defects that would render a second implant nonfunctional; and immunocompromised patients with virulent microorganisms. Resection arthroplasty is limited to nonambulatory patients, patients with contralateral arthrodesis who have failed a revision attempt, or patients who are too ill for subsequent surgery. Amputation is indicated in life-threatening situations where a radical debridement and open packing will not suffice or in patients who have failed multiple attempts at revision, arthrodesis, or resection arthroplasty.

REFERENCES

1. Wilson MG, Kelley K, Thornhill TS: Infection as a complication of total knee-replacement arthroplasty, J Bone Joint Surg [Am] 72:878–883, 1990.
2. Schwartz SJ, Shires TG, Spencer FC, editors. Principles of surgery, ed 5, New York, 1989, McGraw-Hill, p 320.
3. Eftekhar NS: The natural history of infection in joint replacement surgery. In Infection in joint replacement surgery, St Louis, 1984, Mosby–Year Book, p 26.
4. Teeny SM, et al: Treatment of infected total knee arthroplasty: Irrigation and debridement versus two-stage reimplantation, J Arthroplasty 5:35–39, 1990.
5. Garner RW, Mowat AG, Hazelman BL: Wound healing after operations on patients with rheumatoid arthritis, J Bone Joint Surg [Br] 55:134–144, 1973.
6. Hood RW, Insall JN: Infected total knee joint replace-

ment arthroplasties. In Evarts CMcC, editor: *Surgery of the musculoskeletal system,* vol 4, New York, 1983, Churchill Livingstone, pp 173–195.
7. Schwartz SJ, Shires TG, Spencer FC, editors: *Principles of surgery,* ed 5, New York, 1989, McGraw-Hill, p 184.
8. Poss R, et al: Factors Influencing the incidence and outcome of infection following total joint arthroplasty, *Clin Orthop* 182:117–126, 1985.
9. Manchot C: Die Hautarterien des menschlichen Körpers, Leipzig, 1889, Vogel.
10. Norden CW: Prevention of bone and joint infections, *Am J Med* 78(suppl 6B):229–232, 1985.
11. Boyd RJ, Burke JF, Colton T: A double-blind clinical trial of prophylactic antibiotics in hip fractures, *J Bone Joint Surg [Am]* 55:1251–1258, 1973.
12. Ruoff KL: New and emerging Gram-positive pathogens, *Mediguide Infect Dis* 11:1–4, 1991.
13. Classen C, et al: Timing of prophylactic administration of antibiotics and the risk of surgical-wound infection, *N Engl J Med* 326:281–286, 1992.
14. Bannister GC, et al: The timing of tourniquet application in relation to prophylactic antibiotic administration, *J Bone Joint Surg [Br]* 70:322–324, 1988.
15. Friedman RJ, et al: Antibiotic prophylaxis and tourniquet inflation in total knee arthroplasty, *Clin Orthop* 260:17–23, 1990.
16. Nelson CL, et al: One day versus seven days of preventive antibiotic therapy in orthopedic surgery, *Clin Orthop* 176:258–263, 1983.
17. Ritter MA, Stringer EA: Laminar air-flow versus conventional air operating systems: A seven-year patient follow-up, *Clin Orthop* 150:177–180, 1980.
18. Ad Hoc Committee of the Committee on Trauma, Division of Medical Science, National Research Council: Postoperative wound infections: The influence of ultraviolet irradiation of the operating room and of various other factors. *Ann Surg* 160(supplement):1964.
19. Nelson JP, et al: The effect of previous surgery, operating room environment, and preventive antibiotics on postoperative infection following total hip arthroplasty, *Clin Orthop* 147:167–169, 1980.
20. Lidwell OM, et al: Ultraclean air and antibiotics for prevention of postoperative infection. A multicenter study of 8,052 joint replacement operations, *Acta Orthop Scand* 58:4–13, 1987.
21. Salvati EA, et al: Infection rates after 3175 total hip and total knee replacements performed with and without a horizontal unidirectional filtered air-flow system, *J Bone Joint Surg [Am]* 64:525–535, 1982.
22. Stinchfield FE, et al: Late hematogenous infection of total joint replacement, *J Bone Joint Surg [Am]* 62:1345–1350, 1980.
23. Wilde AH, Sweeney RS, Borden LS: Hematogenously acquired infection of a total knee arthroplasty by *Clostridium perfringens,* *Clin Orthop* 229:228–231, 1988.
24. Nelson PJ, et al: Prophylactic antimicrobial coverage in arthroplasty patients (editorial), *J Bone Joint Surg [Am]* 72:1, 1990.
25. Kirchner PT, Simon MA: Current concepts review. Radioisotopic evaluation of skeletal disease, *J Bone Joint Surg [Am]* 63:15–23, 1981.
26. Merkel KD, Fitzgerald RH Jr, Brown ML: Scintigraphic evaluation in musculoskeletal sepsis, *Orthop Clin North Am* 15:401–415, 1984.
27. Wukich DK, et al: Diagnosis of infection by preoperative scintigraphy with indium-labeled white blood cells, *J Bone Joint Surg [Am]* 69:1353–1359, 1987.
28. Thomas BJ, Moreland JR, Amstutz HC: Infection after total joint arthroplasty from distal extremity sepsis, *Clin Orthop* 181:121–125, 1983.
29. Inman RD, et al: Clinical and microbial features of prosthetic joint infection, *Am J Med* 77:47–53, 1984.
30. Gristina AG, Costerton JW: Bacterial adherence to biomaterials and tissue. The significance of its role in clinical sepsis, *J Bone Joint Surg [Am]* 67:264–273, 1985.
31. Levine M, Rehm SJ, Wilde AH: Infection with *Candida albicans* of a total knee arthroplasty, *Clin Orthop* 226:235–239, 1988.
32. Koch AE: *Candida albicans* infection of a prosthetic knee replacement: A report and review of the literature, *J Rheumatol* 15:362–365, 1988.
33. Insall JN, Thompson FM, Brause BD: Two-stage reimplantation for the salvage of infected total knee arthroplasty, *J Bone Joint Surg [Am]* 65:1087–1098, 1983.
34. Rosenberg AG, et al: Salvage of infected total knee arthroplasty, *Clin Orthop* 226:29–33, 1988.
35. Brause BD: Infected total knee replacement. Diagnostic, therapeutic, and prophylactic considerations, *Orthop Clin North Am* 13:245–249, 1982.
36. Karchmer AW: Staphylococcal endocarditis. Laboratory and clinical basis for antibiotic therapy, *Am J Med* 78(suppl 6B):116–127, 1985.
37. Tsukayama DT, Wicklund B, Gustilo RB: Suppressive antibiotic therapy in chronic prosthetic joint infections, *Orthopedics* 14:841–844, 1991.
38. Josefsson G, Lindberg L, Wiklander B: Systemic antibiotics and gentamicin-containing bone cement in the prophylaxis of post-operative infections in total hip arthroplasty, *Clin Orthop* 159:194–200, 1981.
39. Elson RA: Antibiotic-loaded acrylic cement (ALAC). In Uhthoff HK, editor: *Current concepts of infections in orthopedic surgery,* Berlin, 1985, Springer-Verlag, pp 247–250.
40. Freeman MAR, et al: The management of infected total knee replacements, *J Bone Joint Surg [Br]* 67:764–768, 1985.
41. Rand JA, Bryan RS: Reimplantation for the salvage of an infected total knee arthroplasty, *J Bone Joint Surg [Am]* 65:1081–1086, 1983.
42. Broderson MP, Fitzgerald RH, Peterson LF: Arthrodesis of the knee following total knee arthroplasty, *J Bone Joint Surg [Am]* 61:181, 1979.
43. Stulberg SD: Arthrodesis in failed total knee replacements, *Orthop Clin North Am* 13:213–224, 1982.
44. Thornhill TS, Dalziel R, Sledge CB: Alternatives to ar-

throdesis for the failed total knee arthroplasty, *Clin Orthop* 170:131, 1982.
45. Schoifet S, Morrey BF: Persistent infection after successful arthrodesis for infected total knee arthroplasty. A report of two cases, *J Arthroplasty* 5:277–279, 1990.
46. Falahee MH, Matthews LS, Kaufer H: Resection arthroplasty as a salvage procedure for a knee with infection after a total arthroplasty, *J Bone Joint Surg [Am]* 69:1013–1021, 1987.
47. Borden LS, Gearen PF: Infected total knee arthroplasty. A protocol for management, *J Arthroplasty* 2:27–36, 1987.

73

Soft Tissue Considerations in the Failed Total Knee Arthroplasty

SUSAN M. CRAIG, M.D.

Anatomy
Wound healing
Postoperative monitoring

Coverage options
Summary

Wound healing per primam is the goal in total knee arthroplasty; failure to achieve this goal gives added complexity to an already major undertaking. The opportunity for rapid patient mobilization and rehabilitation is lost when skin slough requires debridement and grafting; if the prosthesis becomes exposed, joint infection requiring prosthesis removal, extended hospitalization, and even fusion may result. Anticipation and prevention of soft tissue problems are the key to primary healing; once present, such problems must be dealt with aggressively to preclude further deterioration and compromise of the outcome.

ANATOMY

The skin and soft tissue envelope, which encloses the knee, covers the patella and the patellar tendon as well as the tendinous muscle origins and insertions. There is no underlying muscle layer to provide a pathway for direct arterial perforators, nor, at least anteriorly, are there intermuscular septa through which arteries might also course. The blood supply of the anterior surface of the knee between the quadriceps tendon and tibial tubercle is completely random. The multiple contributions to this random blood supply overlap extensively, and are well outlined in several detailed anatomic studies.[1, 12, 114, 144] They provide an extensive and plentiful source of skin and soft tissue nutrition, but their random nature provides clues to the source of trouble in certain postoperative situations.

The distal femur, proximal tibia and fibula, and patella receive their arterial inflow directly from bony perforators derived from the superior and inferior medial and lateral genicular arteries; in fact, these arteries reach the bone by coursing through and first supplying the ligamentous and tendinous supporting structures of the joint.[55, 70, 72]

The blood supply to the soft tissue which stabilizes and supports the knee is from the genicular branches of the popliteal artery (Fig 73–1). In the upper portion of the popliteal space just above the level of the intercondylar notch, the medial and lateral superior genicular arteries take their origin: the medial artery passes beneath the tendons of the semimembranosus, semitendinosus, sartorius, and gracilis directly on the femur. In a similar fashion, the lateral superior genicular artery passes on the femur beneath the biceps femoris tendon. These arteries then perforate the intermuscular septum and anastomose in the muscle fibers of the vastus lateralis and vastus medialis, respectively; their terminal branches reach the skin anteriorly traveling subcutaneously in the fat and subdermal plexus. While these branches are small, there does exist the potential for direct communication between these medial and lateral vessels within the skin if local demand so dictates. Such "intrinsic" vessel sources form the uppermost of the arches supplying the patella and skin on the anterior aspect of the knee.

The lower arch, which provides blood supply to the anterior knee, is formed from the inferior medial and lateral genicular arteries, which leave the lower segment of the popliteal artery in the popliteal space just above its bifurcation. These medial and lateral arteries pass along the posterior surface of the tibia; the medial vessel travels beneath the medial collateral ligament and then more superficially reaches the an-

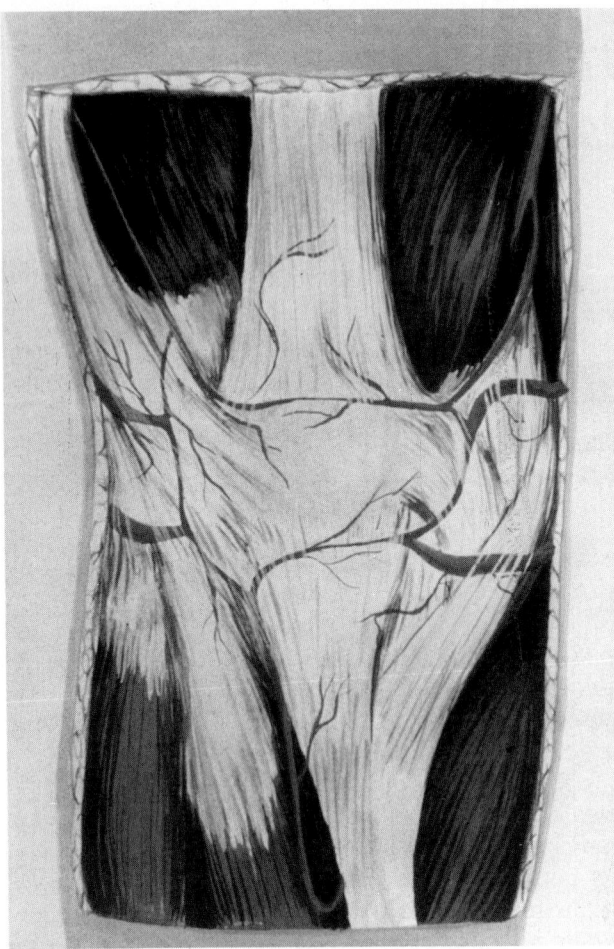

FIG 73–1.
Medial and lateral genicular arteries contribute to the cutaneous circulation by way of multiple small perforating vessels supplying the skin on the anterior surface of the knee.

teroinferior skin of the knee, where its terminal branches have the potential to meet with the lateral branch that has come along the upper border of the fibular head at the level of the soleus muscle origin, around the head of the fibula itself, and under the lateral collateral ligament.

It must be emphasized that this intrinsic blood supply to the joint primarily maintains the soft tissue in immediate proximity to the joint, as well as supplying the distal femur and proximal tibia. The superior and inferior genicular arteries contribute to the blood supply of the overlying skin only through their terminal branches; such contribution can be increased if local demand warrants. The anterior aspect of the knee, with its overlap of random blood supply, provides an excellent example of Taylor and Palmer's[130] concept of "choke-vessels"; local soft tissue ischemia or interruption of primary vessel sources will cause potential anastamotic communicating channels to open and provide new sources of nutritional inflow. The genicular contribution to the blood supply of the skin exists in conjunction with, and augments the primary soft tissue blood supply provided by three additional, separate, and extrinsic sources.

The first of these extrinsic sources originates as a branch of the profunda femoris artery. Approximately two fingerbreadths below the inguinal ligament, the profunda femoris gives off the lateral circumflex femoral artery; this vessel then subdivides, sending its branches coursing deep to and directly supplying the rectus femoris, vastus intermedius, and vastus lateralis muscles. In the distal one third of the thigh, small perforators leave these muscles and pass into the overlying skin in an inferior direction where they meet in the skin with small end-arteries of the lateral genicular system.

The second extrinsic source of blood supply originates superomedially as the supreme or descending genicular artery, the arteria genus suprema. This vessel leaves the superficial femoral artery in the lower part of the adductor canal. It has two branches: the musculoarticular branch, and the saphenous artery. The musculoarticular branch runs medially in the vastus medialis and inferiorly meets the superior medial genicular artery within the muscular and musculotendinous portion of the vastus medialis, sending vessels to the medial joint. The saphenous artery heads inferiorly, perforates through or inferior to the sartorius tendon at about the level of the joint line, ending in a well-defined vessel which supplies the skin overlying and below the medial tibial plateau.[3]

The third extrinsic source is the recurrent branch of the anterior tibial artery, which arises from the anterior tibial vessel just beyond its origin in the lower leg. As the anterior tibial artery leaves the popliteal artery, it runs directly forward and penetrates the interosseous membrane at about the level of the tibial tubercle. At this point the recurrent branch leaves the main artery and heads superiorly and laterally where it meets with branches of the lateral inferior genicular artery as that vessel emerges from beneath the fibular collateral ligament; at the same time, the recurrent anterior tibial artery sends branches upward and medially to the areolar tissue and skin overlying and lateral to the patellar ligament.[87, 103, 137, 143]

The plentiful random vessels which supply the skin overlying the knee, in the absence of systemic vascular disease, infection, hematoma, or other untoward condition, richly nourish this thin, distensible skin envelope. It is clear that any single incision which gives access to the knee joint cannot interrupt this prodigeous blood supply and this is certainly true in the patient who presents for primary total knee arthroplasty. However, patients requiring revision arthroplasty always have one and not infrequently two or more incisions present, in a variety of locations and orientations (Fig 73–2). It is the revision patient whose preexisting incision must be considered in the preoperative planning phase, for dire consequences can result when the incision is ignored. There is no evidence to support the commonly held concept that an older scar can virtually be ignored because it is sufficiently vascular. While a healed scar does contain within it some blood vessels which cross the scar, such vessels are neither predictable nor reliable in the long run. In planning the surgical approach to revision, first consideration should always be given to using the existing incision. If the existing incision does not allow adequate access for joint replacement, several questions need to be answered. First, is a completely new incision needed or is it possible to use a portion of the preexisting incision to minimize skin flap compromise?[119] Second, in using a new incision, can it be designed with as wide a base as possible, and as distant from the existing incision as possible? Third, how can the incision be oriented so that the most predictable and reliable skin circulation is over the patella tendon? Fourth, will preoperative skin expansion be of benefit? (Fig 73–3).

WOUND HEALING

Tissue survival depends on the delivery of adequate oxygen to support metabolism; wound healing also depends on oxygen supply, as well as the unfolding of the orderly series of events leading to collagen synthesis, cross-linkage, and wound strength. Both tis-

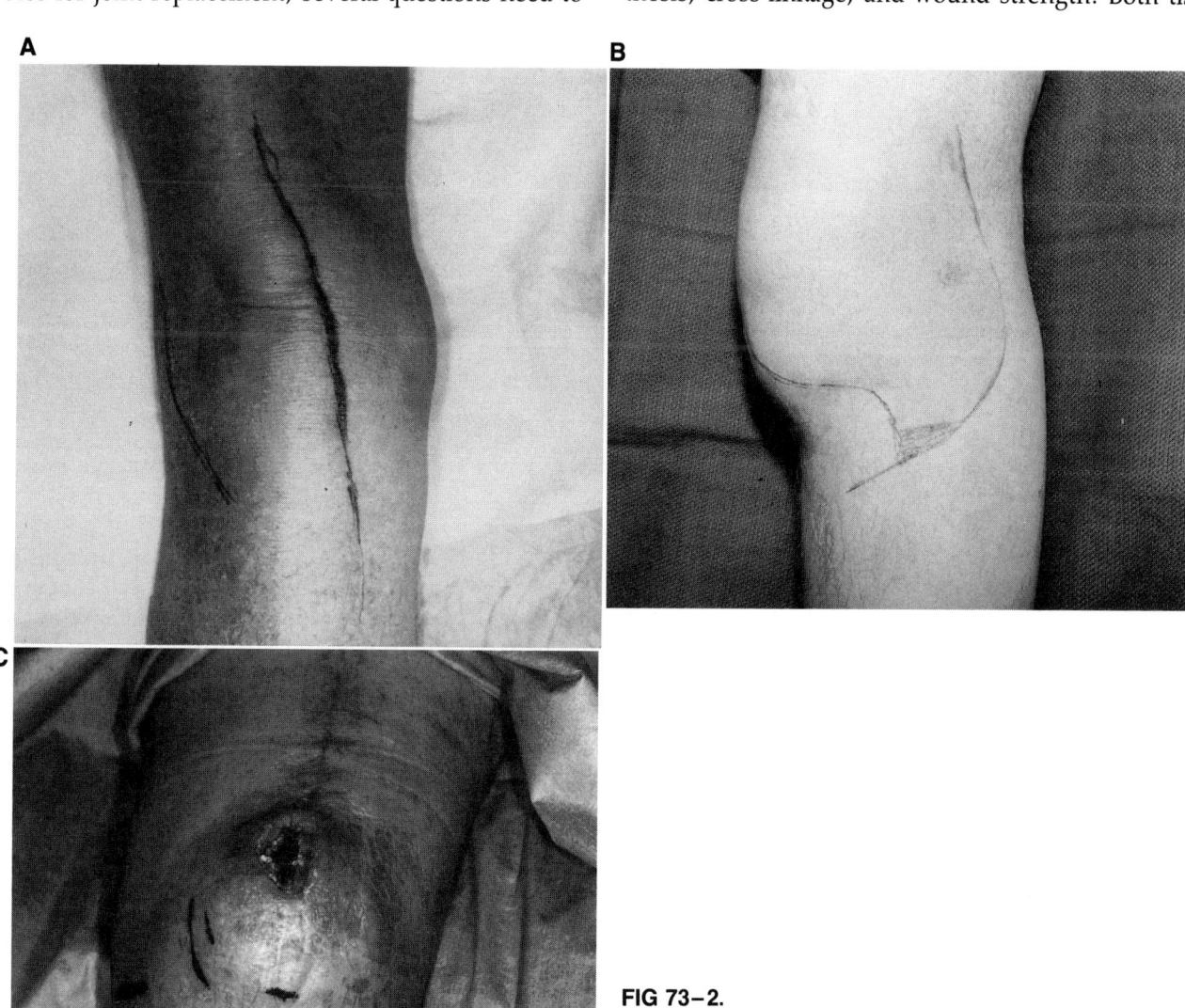

FIG 73–2.
Presence of preexisting skin incisions as seen in **A** and **B,** can lead to necrosis of soft tissue covering **(C),** even with the most meticulous preoperative planning.

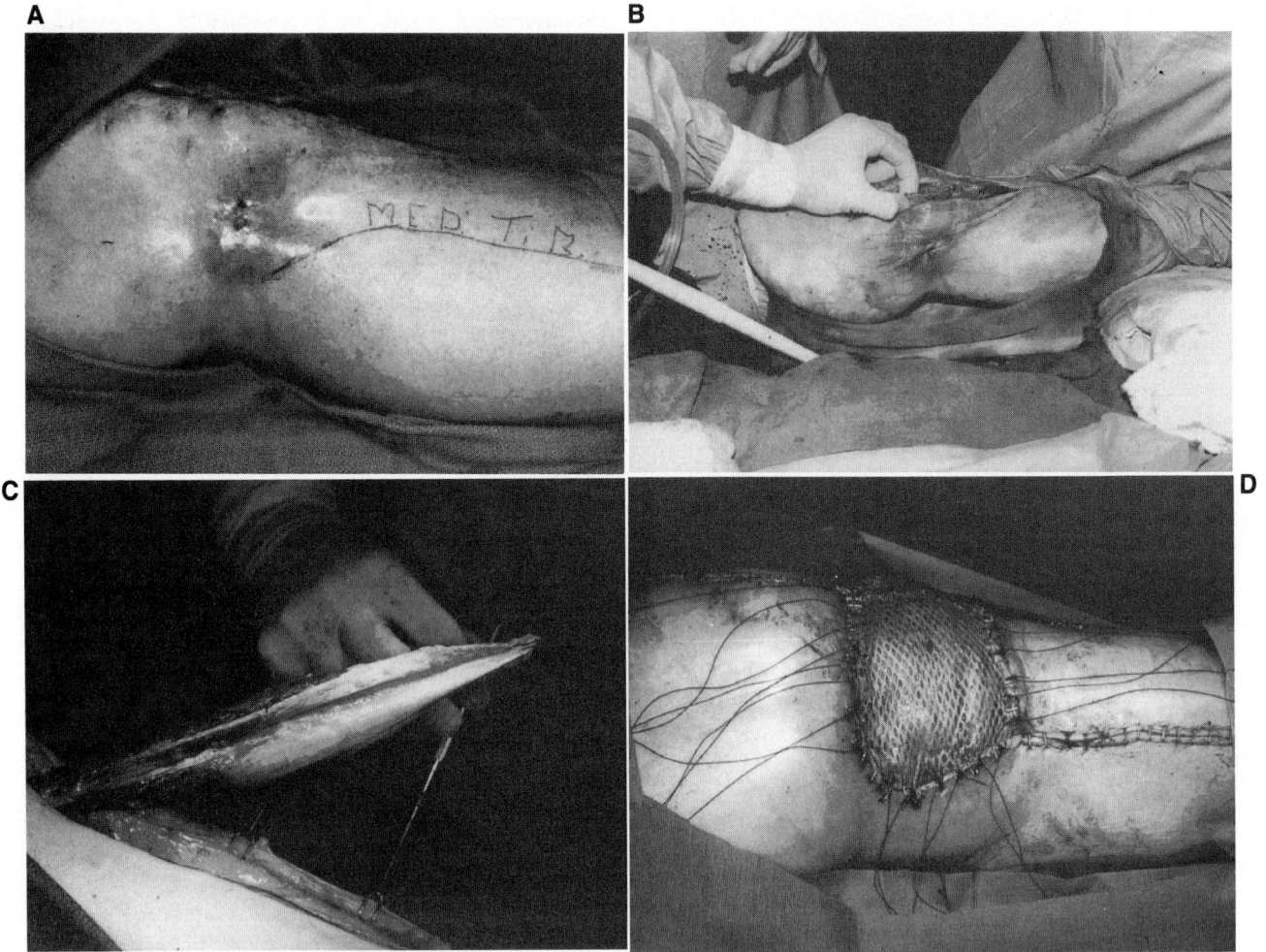

FIG 73-3.
Preoperative skin assessment is essential for a successful outcome. **A** and **B,** this patient's infected prosthesis was removed; skin overlying drain exit sites was densely fibrotic and avascular. **C** and **D,** at the time of prosthesis reinsertion, all compromised skin was excised and a healthy muscle flap was rotated into position. Healing ensued.

sue survival and wound healing can be influenced by local and systemic factors. An understanding of how these factors influence healing enables the surgeon to take steps pre- and postoperatively to control them.

The dermal plexus, the layer of vessels that bleeds so profusely when a skin incision is made, and which supplies the dermis and epidermis with nutrients, is the end-organ of the arterial tree. The dermal vessels have ultimate responsibility for the circulatory integrity of the skin and the healing wound (Fig 73-4).

Blood vessels reach the dermal plexus in one of three ways. These three pathways—direct subcutaneous perforators, musculocutaneous perforators, and septocutaneous perforators—represent the only existing communications between segmental divisions from the aorta and the blood supply to the skin.

When intact skin is wounded, the ability of the wound to heal depends on the immediate inflammatory response and the subsequent phases of wound healing, whose goal is the synthesis of collagen of adequate tensile strength to again function as a mechanical barrier to the outside world. Wound healing problems and skin loss in the patient undergoing total knee revision arthroplasty depend in part on the surgeon's awareness of local and systemic factors which influence wound healing.

With a few specific exceptions, the patient's nutritional state influences wound healing only in the most severe deficiency states. A wound cannot heal when the building blocks for protein synthesis are unavailable; however, the body will use protein preferentially to heal a wound even in situations where protein is in short supply.[58, 74, 75, 96, 98, 110, 118]

In considering the effect of anti-inflammatory medications on wound healing, two categories of

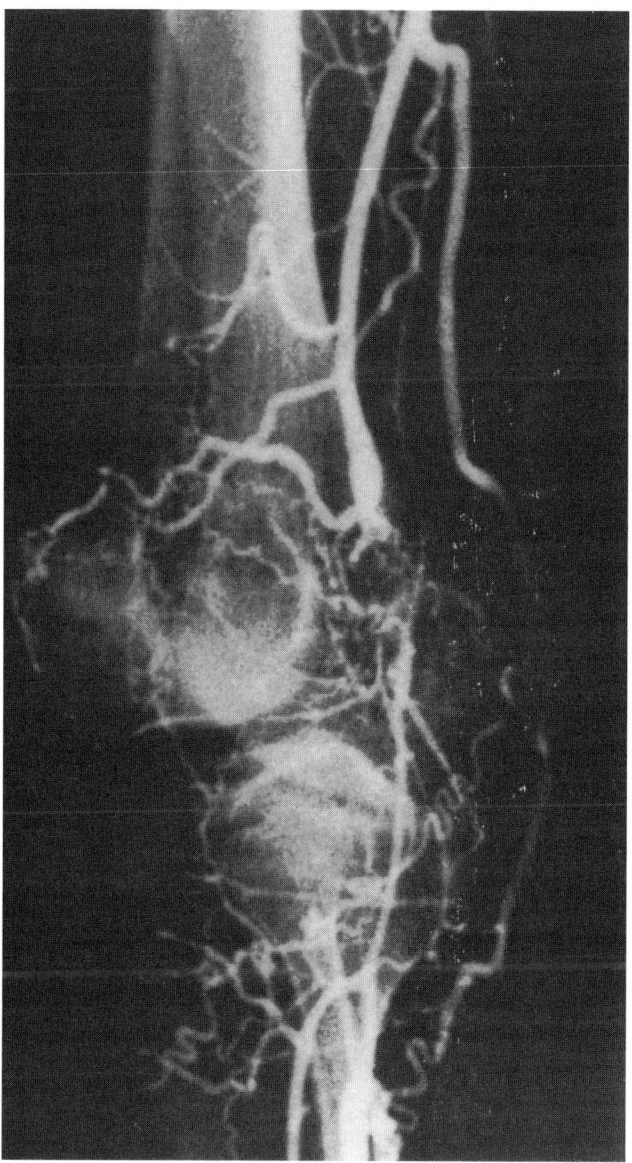

FIG 73-4.
Patients with occlusive peripheral vascular disease develop an extensive cutaneous collateral circulation. This patient, whose anteriogram shows a complete popliteal artery occlusion, has extensive collateralization; the superior genicular vessels, rarely seen on a normal arteriogram, are clearly visualized.

anti-inflammatory medication must be considered separately. The nonsteroidal anti-inflammatory medications have the potential to alter, prolong, or prevent wound healing only to the extent that they inhibit the acute inflammatory response, the earliest phase of wound healing. Indomethacin and aspirin, for example, act by inhibiting the synthesis of prostaglandin E_1 and E_2, two terminal mediators of the acute inflammatory response; this action is dose-related and requires much larger dosages than those usually encountered clinically.[84]

Corticosteroids have a much more profound effect on wound healing because they interfere at several different points in the healing sequence of events and because this interference occurs at clinically relevant dosages. This effect of corticosteroids is quite apart from the known effects on the incidence of wound infection.

While experimental models of the effect of cortisone on wound healing vary somewhat in exact dosage, duration, and preparation used, as well as the exact criteria used to assess healing, some cortisone effects on tissue and its repair are proven.

First, cortisone inhibits fibroblast proliferation; this has the effect of slowing the accumulation of wound collagen and delaying gain in tensile strength. This effect on wound healing is enhanced by even mild starvation, a condition common to all patients in the early postoperative phase.[17, 18, 27, 35, 48, 73]

In addition, cortisone increases collagenase activity; this enzyme, always present in the healing wound, gradually decreases in activity as the time from surgery lengthens in the normally healing wound. Administration of cortisone slows the decrease in activity of this enzyme, causing increased collagen destruction.[60, 141, 145]

The effect of glucocorticoids on fibroblast proliferation and collagen breakdown is reversed by the systemic administration of vitamin A; increased numbers of fibroblasts and increased collagen synthesis result in gains in wound strength equivalent to those in patients not receiving corticosteroids.[33, 34, 53, 59, 112, 113]

The quality of the skin in patients with rheumatoid arthritis is often cited as a cause of poor tissue healing; indeed, the thin atrophic skin of such patients will at times tear with even an adherent surgical drape, or abrasive clothing contact. There is no good evidence that the disease process itself results in structural weakening of skin, and these effects are most probably due to long-term, high-dose systemic corticosteroid administration which these patients require.

Cigarette smoking has a direct inhibitory effect on the dermal microcirculation. Excellent experimental evidence exists that inhaled cigarette smoke is highly toxic; recent reports, in addition, place the blame for delayed healing of primary wounds on two circulating substances resulting from smoke inhalation.[9] Nicotinic acid and its more potent longer-lived breakdown product, cotinine, both appear in the circulatory system during cigarette smoke inhalation. Both are potent vasoconstrictors. Nicotinic acid also increases plasma catecholamine levels, further increasing peripheral vasoconstriction. Nicotinic acid is rapidly broken down and its direct metabolic effect is short-lived; cotinine, however, is stored in body fat and released to the peripheral circulation in the weeks following exposure. Release can be stimulated by stress; it is cotinine which is believed to be responsible for defects in primary healing noted in patients who smoke, and for the continued effect even after cigarette smoking has been stopped.[9, 10, 11, 26, 29, 88, 89, 100, 104, 142, 146]

The *diabetic* patient presents special problems of wound healing. While it is difficult to separate the effect of age and obesity from the effect of glucose control in these difficult patients, adequate treatment with insulin will ensure optimal conditions for wound repair. Simple epithelialization is not hindered in diabetes mellitus; collagen synthesis and gain in tensile strength of the deep wound, however, are delayed. The risk of wound infection and peripheral microangiopathy contribute to healing problems. Meticulous control of blood sugar with insulin is the most satisfactory treatment.[45, 85, 105, 107]

Any discussion of factors that negatively affect wound healing is not complete without mentioning conditions commonly seen in the revision population whose effect on tissue healing is marginal. The presence of occlusive peripheral vascular disease jeopardizes wound healing only to the extent that it lowers oxygen tension in the healing wound. The slow progression of vessel occlusion in most patients with peripheral vascular disease allows for the development of collateral circulation around the knee, which is usually adequate to prevent necrosis of skin and in fact has a protective effect.[57, 64, 93, 128] (see Fig 73–4). There is no evidence to implicate *anemia* as a factor in poor wound healing. Hypovolemia can affect oxygen delivery to the wound and cause skin necrosis; correction to normovolemia, even in the presence of a hematocrit in the 18% to 20% range, reverses the deleterious effect of inadequate volume and perfusion. Similarly, patients whose general nutritional status is poor or patients receiving chemotherapy have no significant difference in ability to heal a cutaneous wound in the absence of infection.[117] Such patients preferentially allocate the building blocks for protein synthesis to the macrophages and fibroblasts present and necessary for wound healing.[37, 117]

Local factors also contribute to prompt wound healing and influence adequate skin circulation. Gentle handling of tissue during revision surgery is essential, particularly in the diabetic patient, the cigarette smoker with high circulating catecholamines, or the patient with an old incision nearby. Overzealous retraction, crushing clamps, and heavy, toothed forceps place an added burden on tissue which is already compromised, and may push marginal but viable skin toward wound compromise.

Hemostasis must be meticulous at the time of wound closure. Careful ligature of obvious bleeding vessels, the use of evacuating drains, and a brief postoperative period of immobilization to allow blood clotting to occur are sensible steps which help avoid postoperative hematoma formation. Hematomas must be evacuated; they can, by mechanical pressure, induce necrosis of overlying skin. In addition, they are an excellent culture medium, and as such represent an unacceptable risk for wound infection. The use of anticoagulants in the total knee revision patient for prophylaxis against a postoperative thromboembolic complication is undertaken with full understanding of associated risks, but there is no evidence that the use of anticoagulants has any adverse effect on soft tissue healing.[61, 95]

Perioperative broad-spectrum antibiotics are always used in joint replacement surgery and a full 10-day course is given if there is any sign of wound compromise; if operative cultures are positive, a longer period may be necessary. Revision arthroplasty is at times a lengthy procedure; certainly, in the general surgical literature, the incidence of wound infection correlates directly with the length of surgery. Even adjusted for patient age and other associated risk factors, this increased rate of infection with prolonged surgery is real, ranging from 3.6% for operations lasting less than 30 minutes to 16.4% for operations lasting over 5 hours.[4] Certain suture materials are known to be minimally reactive during the weeks required for skin healing. Provided skin edge-to-skin edge coaptation is attended to, closure of a skin wound with a synthetic, monofilament permanent suture such as nylon or polypropylene (Prolene) is ideal. The fine stainless steel clips which significantly shorten the time required for closure also have the advantage of being nonreactive; certainly stainless steel has an admirable track record as a fine, permanent suture material. The everting nature of stainless steel clips requires a very precise subcutaneous supporting layer to avoid delay in primary wound healing which can result from inaccurate edge-to-edge approximation.

When drains are used it is advisable not to bring them out through the incision, and to remove them as soon as possible. Drains are a potential path for bacterial wound contamination and this potential is more likely to be realized the longer the drain is in place.[76, 123, 147]

POSTOPERATIVE MONITORING

Wound healing postoperatively proceeds in an orderly and predictable sequence. The wound in which there is circulatory compromise, however, or in which infection or hematoma intervene to prevent healing and cause loss of tissue, must be recognized early and treated aggressively so that tissue damage is kept to a minimum and simple problems that are easily solved do not become complex tissue coverage problems.

Certainly, the earlier circulatory compromise is recognized, the earlier it can be treated. Recent advances in microsurgical tissue transfer have necessitated lengthy operating times for the transfer of composite tissue with its own vascular supply. These complex surgical procedures have broadened our capability for monitoring and evaluating the adequacy of circulation in transferred tissue. Parallel with the development of microsurgical techniques has been a proliferation in sophisticated tools for monitoring tissue viability. Certain of these techniques are applicable to the cutaneous circulation in the postoperative total knee, or revision total knee patient.

The direct visual assessment of a surgical wound for circulatory embarrassment by the same reliable experienced observer under reproducible conditions has been the standard against which current advances in assessment of dermal circulation are measured. Just after World War II, fluorescein, a water-soluble dye, was investigated as an aid to visual inspection which might give some quantifiable and reproducible support for the admittedly subjective eye of a human observer.[28, 67, 68] Despite this early start, however, technology has only recently been devised which enables the observer to precisely evaluate and predict physiologic changes in the microcirculation; in the intervening years, multiple methods of evaluating circulatory integrity have been tried and discarded.

Direct penetration of the tissue in question and observation of the rate and color of the resultant bleeding, a popular early technique for the evaluation of reattached parts, is subject to the same errors as is direct visualization; its reliability is only as good as the observer. In addition, the technique introduces a disturbing element of contamination which makes it particularly inappropriate for monitoring the skin wound of a postoperative total knee replacement patient.

Clearance studies with washout techniques using radioactive isotopes such as xenon 133, technetium 99m, and sodium 22 are precise and reproducible, but they are unsatisfactory for continuous monitoring because they may be used only once in a 24-hour period. The substance being monitored is injected directly into the skin and its rate of decrease from the infection site is monitored. The method has obvious limitations: first, it reflects only the circulation of the 1- to 2-mm site injected; second, the radioactivity of the substance in multiple doses is worrisome; and last and most important, the test can only be repeated every 24 hours.[7, 51, 115, 129, 139, 140]

Cutaneous temperature monitoring as an indicator of intact circulation is imprecise because of transmitted heat from underlying tissue, variations in room temperature and room air circulation, and the insulating effect of overlying dressings.[52] The elimination of these temperature-influencing conditions with the use of implantable thermocouple probes is quite reliable when placed beside a patent artery; unfortunately this monitoring method is not applicable to cutaneous circulation.[21, 79] The current techniques for evaluating cutaneous circulation most applicable to knee surgery are laser Doppler flow metering, transcutaneous oxygen monitoring, and fluorescein injection.

Doppler flow metering uses the Doppler principle to evaluate circulation; a beam of light of a certain wave length is deflected when it collides with a moving object (red blood cells) in a quantifiable way, which alters when red cell flow is decreased, reflecting tissue ischemia. This technique is a surface-applicable one; it is noninvasive, uses nonsurgical skin areas for comparison, and is available for continuous clinical dermal blood flow monitoring.[41]

Transcutaneous oxygen monitoring accurately assesses tissue viability by creating a maximally dilated vascular bed with local temperature elevation; the surface probe then measures oxygen diffusion through the skin from the capillary bed. Originally used only to monitor high-risk neonates, the technique is reproducible and the instrumentation simple. It can provoke a continuous readout, and for that reason has predictive value as well.[2, 56, 116]

Fluorescein injection resulting in tissue fluorescence is perhaps the most extensively used perfusion monitor today. The dye diffuse from the intravascular to the extravascular extracellular space; tissue fluorescence is then observed using a Wood's lamp that emits ultraviolet light with a wavelength of 450 to 500 nm. The electrons within the fluorescein molecule achieve an excitation state and give off a greenish-gold glow as they return to their original energy level. The single drawback to the use of fluorescein is its long half-life; in currently used doses, 10 to 15 mg/

kg, the dye is excreted over several days following injection and persists in the tissue so long that the injection test cannot be repeated more often than once every 24 to 48 hours.[66, 82, 90, 99, 102, 124, 134]

Continuous monitoring of skin flap circulation based on tissue fluorescence with low doses of flourescein is now available. Using fibroptic cables to both transmit blue light and act as afferent pathways for emitted fluorescence, an instrument known as a dermoflourimeter employs a filter to increase its ability to detect small amounts of flourescein.[69] The flourescein dose required is significantly less than the dose needed for visual perception: 4 to 8 mg/kg need be injected intravenously for fluorescein to be detected. This greatly decreases the incidence of complications related to intravenous fluorescein injection[16, 20, 36, 71, 77, 127] and more important, allows repetition of the test every 2 to 3 hours, as the low dose of fluorescein is rapidly excreted in the urine. This simple, effective continuous monitoring device is not affected by variations in temperature, hematocrit, or in the patient's natural skin pigmentation, and does not rely on the subjective visual evaluation of an observer.[46, 47, 54, 120, 121, 133]

Finally, a word must be said about what to do when the postoperative viability monitoring shows compromised skin circulation (Fig 73–5). First, of course, any constricting dressings should be loosened. Elevation of the affected limb and the addition of intravenous antibiotics to the postoperative regimen should be initiated if this has not been done. Skin sutures should be released; if hematoma is suspected, exploration and evacuation are mandatory. Continuous passive motion, which is usually begun immediately postoperatively, must cease. While there are no medications available which reliably reverse compromised cutaneous circulation, certain drugs with an indirect effect on circulation are usually added when the above steps are not successful. Low molecular weight dextran is used for its ability to decrease platelet aggregation and intravascular sludging; while these conditions are results, not causes, of circulatory compromise, dextran 40 can be useful in some circumstances.[101] Less helpful is heparin, which in low doses inhibits platelet aggregation and in high doses completely prevents clot formation.[63] While there is some experimental evidence that certain pharmacologic agents that have as their primary effect sustained vascular smooth muscle relaxation and vasodilation, which may improve skin blood supply, the clinical applicability of this evidence remains to be determined.[31, 40]

More recently intravenous nitroglycerin,[43] topical nitroglycerin,[108] phenoxybenzamine,[91] and prostaglandin E_2[122] analog have all shown promise in improving circulation to tissue compromised by ischemia. Finally, hyperbaric oxygen is helpful in increasing oxygen availability to the tissue by a local increase in oxygen saturation. Whether this actually reverses impending necrosis or simply delays the inevitable is not known; unfortunately hyperbaric oxygen requires specially designed equipment not widely available or frequently needed and extensive clinical series are lacking.

The wound with compromised circulation must be dressed with care; excellent evidence exists that a local environment designed to prevent dessication and evaporative loss by exposure minimizes ultimate tissue loss.[83, 109]

COVERAGE OPTIONS

When wound healing per primam does not occur and tissue is lost, the reconstructive solution must proceed from the simplest to the most complex. It is always appropriate to allow skin whose survival is questionable to declare itself. In the absence of infection, debridement of tissue can safely wait until an eschar forms and begins to separate. Wound contracture also works very much in the surgeon's favor and often the final deficit is considerably smaller than predicted.

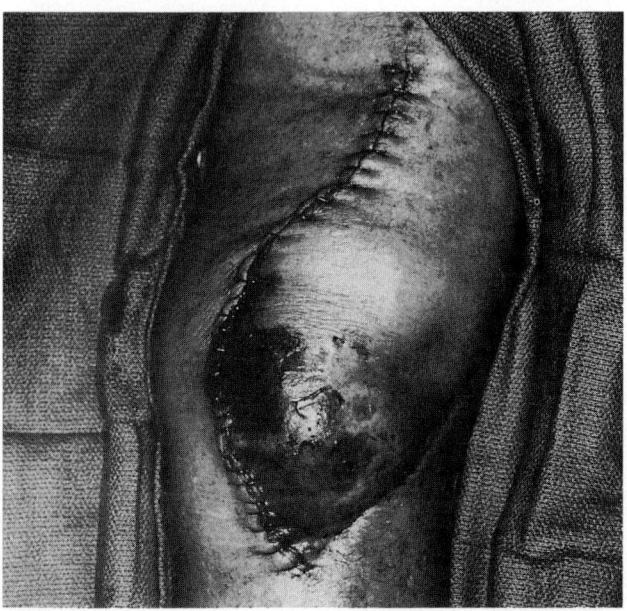

FIG 73–5.
By postoperative day 3 to 4, frank compromise of cutaneous circulation is in evidence. In this patient, constricting stockings were removed and continuous passive motion was discontinued. The ultimate area of skin necrosis was considerably smaller than that involved on initial examination.

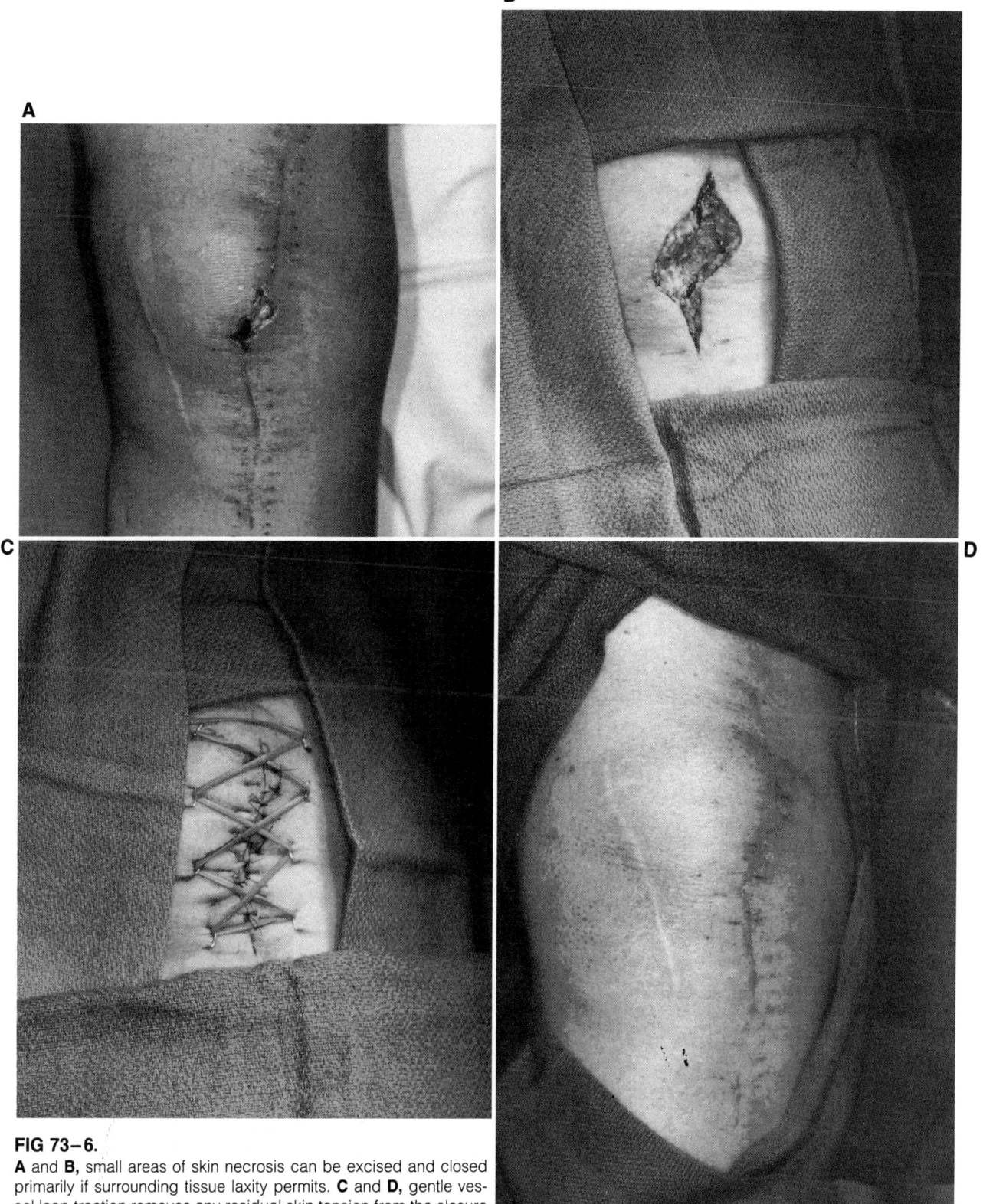

FIG 73-6.
A and **B**, small areas of skin necrosis can be excised and closed primarily if surrounding tissue laxity permits. **C** and **D**, gentle vessel loop traction removes any residual skin tension from the closure and allows unimpeded healing.

Small areas of superficial, partial, or even full-thickness loss may be allowed to contract and granulate on their own or may be excised and closed primarily (Fig 73-6). Small areas of crusting with no surrounding erythema can safely be observed as the eschar separates on its own. Such wounds are allowed to heal by secondary intention; such healing is permissible when the time to closure is brief and when the prosthesis is not at risk of exposure. Two processes occur simultaneously resulting in a closed wound. The first, wound contracture, gently pulls the periphery of the wound toward the center. As this occurs, eschar, which is inelastic, separates gradually allowing wound size to progressively decrease.

In addition, secondary intention involves the advancement of epithelial cells from the wound margin and from any dermal elements within the wound itself. Both processes will often surprise us with their remarkable ability to salvage that which appears unsalvageable.

Skin grafting is indicated when the time to healing by secondary intention would be considerably longer than the 5 to 7 days of protected immobilization required for skin graft healing. An area of a few square centimeters will heal almost as rapidly by a combination of wound contracture and epithelialization as by skin grafting, without the added burden of donor site morbidity, provided there is no exposure of the prosthesis or of bone without periosteal cover. Even exposed tendon, provided it is sufficiently small and protected from dessication, will heal in this way. Active and passive motion can continue while this is allowed to occur, a major advantage in the reconstructed joint.

The last decade has seen remarkable advances in topical dressings for open wounds to enhance healing. Debridement of any necrotic tissue is essential if topical agents are to be used, even if there is no local inflammation. I use a topical regimen of acetic acid 0.25%, followed by Neosporin solution (bacitracin zinc–neomycin sulfate–polymyxia B sulfate), followed by amphotericin B in a concentration of 50 g/L. These three topical agents are alternated in a thrice-daily regimen. As healing progresses platelet-derived growth factor is added in an alternating regimen administered three time a day.[15, 32, 42, 65, 92] This course is ideal in the patient who is not a candidate for more complex surgical attempts at coverage, or whose wound bed is not adequate for grafting (Fig 73-7).

Skin grafting is the simplest method of closure in the wound deemed unsuitable for healing by secondary intention. If certain technical points are adhered to, the graft take is quite predictable. To heal, a skin graft must be penetrated by the outgrowth of vascular buds from the underlying wound bed. As vessels penetrate the graft, usually within about 48 hours of placement, oxygen delivery is provided, as are vascular channels to carry away metabolic wastes. If the graft is not adequately immobilized, vascular ingrowth cannot occur, and the graft will become ischemic.[22, 23, 111, 125]

A skin graft will not adhere to an infected bed. Krizek and Robson[66, 106] have cited a bacterial count of 10^5 organisms per gram of tissue as sufficiently high to require further debridement for healing to progress. This number is considerably lower for more virulent organisms such as streptococci and other enzyme-producing bacteria that loosen the fibrin layer upon which early skin graft adherence depends and which provides a structural framework for vascular penetration.[131] All open wounds are necessarily contaminated; the significance of the contamination can best be determined by culture, biopsy, and precise bacterial count. Finally, the bed on which the graft is placed must have absolute hemostasis; a collection of blood or seroma beneath a graft will prevent vascular penetration. A hematoma can be evacuated up to 48 hours with graft survival; a longer period jeopardizes not only the graft but the underlying bed as well.

When bone without periosteum or a significant amount of quadriceps tendon without paratenon is exposed or when infection or tissue loss has caused exposure of the knee joint and of the prosthesis, the coverage requirements are more complex. Such developments require tissue that brings its own blood supply. Two options are available: local tissue can be rotated or advanced in to cover the defect or, if this is not possible, free transfer of distant tissue is available (Fig 73-8).

The most commonly used local rotation flap for coverage of the anterior aspect of the knee is the gastrocnemius muscle, with or without its overlying skin.[49, 50] This muscle occupies the most superficial segment of the posterior compartment of the lower leg. The medial and lateral heads arise from the medial and lateral femoral condyles respectively; they coalesce as they receive their blood supply at about the level of the tibial plateau. For most of their length, they remain identifiable as medial and lateral bellies; as they approach their insertion into the Achilles tendon, their anatomically separate identities are lost and form one muscle coalescing with one tendon.

The two heads of the gastrocnemius muscle are supplied by medial and lateral divisions of the sural artery; these enter the muscle on its deep surface and run longitudinally through the fibers, sending perfo-

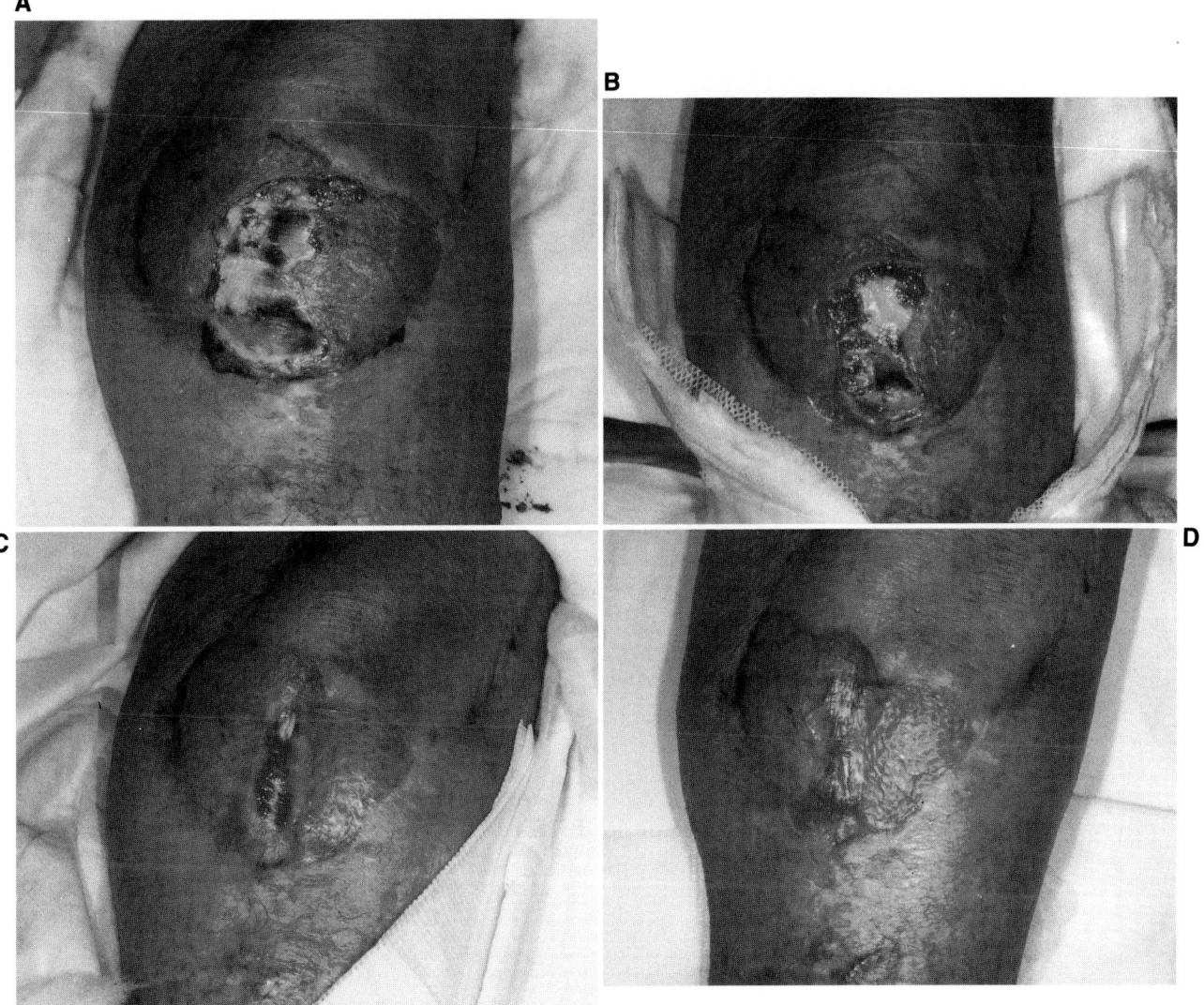

FIG 73–7.
Care with topical wound management can salvage a situation in which coverage is needed in patients who represent a significant risk for further reconstructiion. This patient had had both medial and lateral gastrocnemius flaps placed following a revision total knee replacement complicated by extensive skin necrosis. **A,** after flap placement, further debridement was necessary directly over the patellar tendon. **B,** following debridement, the wound was treated with dressing changes four times a day, and antibacterial and antifungal agents followed by platelet-derived growth factor, topically applied. **C,** this treatment, aided by wound contracture and epithelialization, resulted in complete closure and preservation of tendon function. The wound was completely epithelialized at discharge.

rators which supply the overlying fascia and skin. The remarkably robust blood supply to skin and fascia allows the skin to be transposed with muscle. Provided the perforating vessels are not disturbed, a 5- to 7-cm skin extension beyond the lowermost limit of the muscle fiber may be included with the flap. The arc of rotation, determined by its proximal attachment to the femoral condyle and by the point where its arterial supply enters, allows the muscle to be transposed to cover the entire anterior surface of the knee; the muscle can be split and used as a single belly if only a small area of coverage is needed.

Recently our understanding of the anatomy of this area has allowed modifications of this flap to eliminate its two main drawbacks: bulk and an unsightly donor defect. First, extensive experience with the flap has taught that muscle alone can be rotated on its vascular pedicle; the muscle is then skin grafted in place providing cover and contour. The donor defect is minimal since skin and subcutaneous tissue are left behind. Alternatively, when a relatively thin flap is required, the skin overlying the muscle may be transposed provided that on its deep surface it includes the fascia on the muscle surface; the donor site

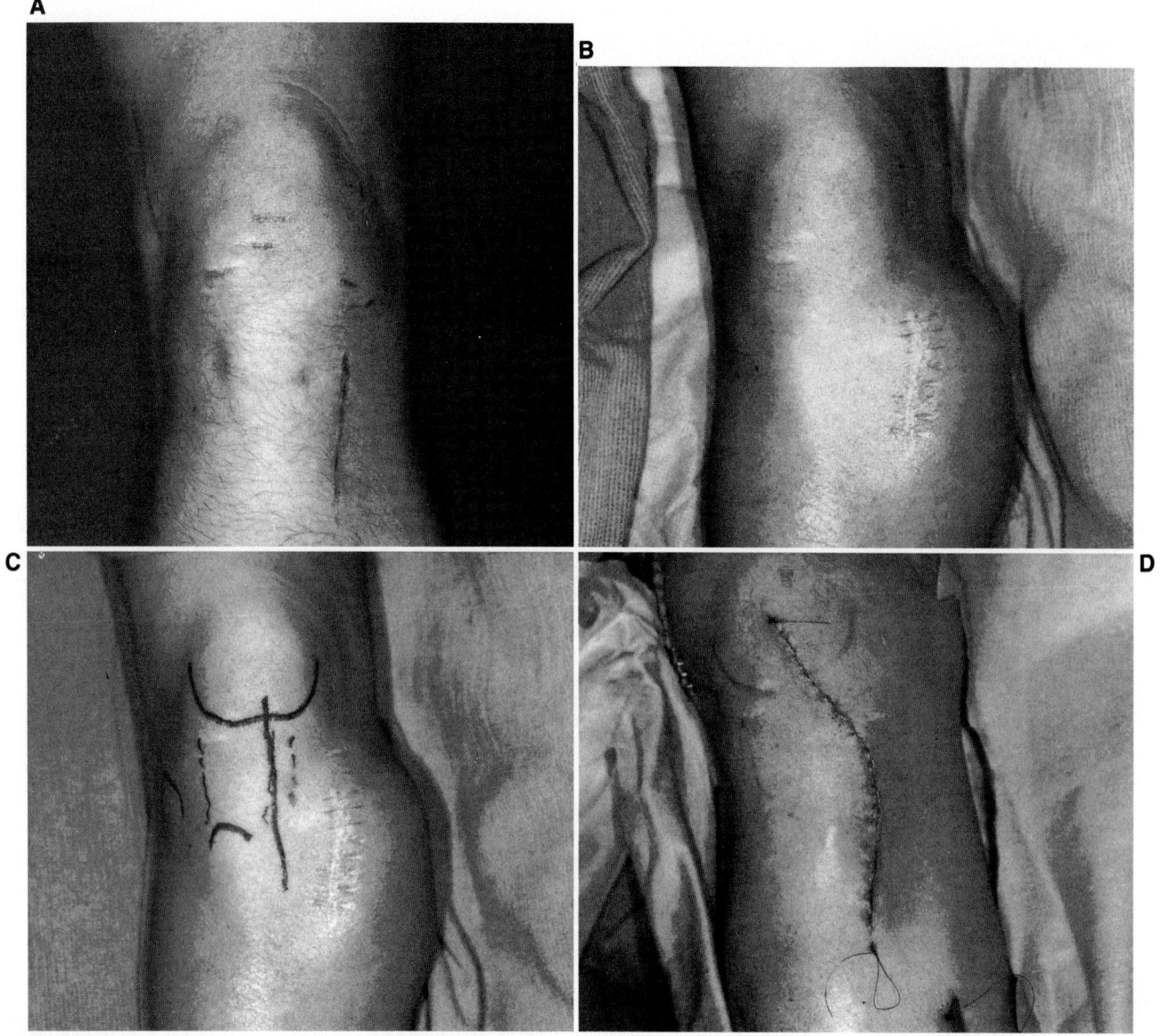

FIG 73–8.
A, preoperative planning for the wound in which compromised healing is likely can include insertion of a tissue expander. This patient had three previous reconstructive procedures on her knee. **B,** 6 weeks prior to surgery, a tissue expander was inserted and inflated weekly to a total volume of 200 cc. **C,** at surgery, the planned incision was made; the skin between the new and the old incision was at risk. **D,** the intervening skin at risk was excised and the expanded tissue advanced to cover the defect. Healing progressed uneventfully.

is then skin-grafted. The rich vascular network both above and below the fascia is the reason for skin survival.[6, 8, 19, 24, 25, 97, 132, 136]

The soleus muscle, the second muscle belly just beneath the gastrocnemius in the posterior calf, can be rotated to cover the tibial tubercle area; in rotating this flap it is important to remember that its muscle belly extends much further down the calf than the gastrocnemius muscle, and in dissecting and raising this flap one must begin distally to adequately isolate and ligate small distal arterial perforations from the peroneal artery. The blood supply to this muscle has two dominant vascular pedicles, and this limits its arc of rotation and consequently its usefulness for all but the smallest, most inferior defects about the knee.[138]

A third flap is adequate for coverage of small superior defects in the anterior knee. The vastus medialis muscle lying deep to the sartorius is a type IV muscle. It can be raised with care on its vascular pedicle and transposed distally; the muscle is then skin-grafted as it has no skin territory of its own. The muscle can be completely detached proximally from its origin for additional length.[5, 135]

Before leaving the subject of local rotation flaps for coverage of the knee, the skin and subcutaneous tissue of the medial aspect of the knee supplied by the saphenous artery must be described.[3] This artery arises as a terminal branch of the supreme genicular artery. It penetrates the tendinous insertion of the sartorius muscle and heads inferiorly. When it is present, it can reliably supply a skin and subcutaneous tissue flap to cover limited defects in the area of the patella and patellar tendon.

Finally, free tissue transfer can be accomplished if no local rotation flap is available, if lower leg deformity will not be tolerated, or if the loss of muscle function in the lower leg cannot be accepted. Experience with free tissue transfer has served to demonstrate that excellent coverage can be provided in this way; shortened operating time, hidden donor defects, and a good cosmetic result make this solution, in experienced hands, at least equal to and in some instances better than local rotation flaps for the patient who requires it.

Free tissue for transfer may be harvested as a cutaneous, fasciocutaneous, or musculocutaneous flap. While the choice of ideal donor for coverage of the anterior knee is not agreed upon, several excellent flaps exist with well-defined anatomy, a single dominant vascular pedicle, and minimal patient-to-patient variation, and some experience has been gained in their application.

Large defects with an exposed prosthesis require well-padded, protective coverage consisting usually of both skin and muscle. The latissimus dorsi muscle, the rectus abdominis muscle, and the scapular free flaps, the first with or without overlying skin, have all proved to be reliable, reproducible, and satisfactory for this purpose.[13, 30, 38, 44, 80, 81, 86, 94, 138]

The recently described temporalis fascia flap can be taken with no donor deformity and immediately skin-grafted in situ. This supple flap may in fact be the best replacement for the anterior surface of the knee where thin, stretchable skin provides the best functional and cosmetic results.[14, 62, 126]

Muscle flaps are divided into five types according to the pattern and distribution of major and minor vascular pedicles on which they are dependent for their nutrition[78]:

Type I: single dominant vascular pedicle
Type II: dominant pedicle on which the entire muscle can survive, and a minor pedicle
Type III: paired, equally dominant vascular pedicles; the muscle can survive on either one
Type IV: multiple segmental vascular pedicles, none dominant; muscle cannot survive without one or more delays
Type V: one dominant pedicle and several small minor pedicles

Clearly, the muscle that can survive on a single dominant pedicle is technically the most satisfactory muscle for transfer. In addition, the muscle that is thin, flat, or can be segmentally divided is ideally suited to this recipient bed. Donor selection rests on these factors and on the experience of the operating surgeon.

SUMMARY

The great increase in procedures done to reconstruct and resurface the deteriorating knee joint, the longevity of an active aging population, and the need for revision in reconstruction have provided a wealth of experience in wound healing and coverage in the area of the knee. The particular demands of this joint and the unique anatomy of the blood supply of its skin envelope make these efforts challenging and rewarding.

REFERENCES

1. Abbott LC, Carpenter WF: Surgical approaches to the knee joint, *J Bone Joint Surg* 27:277, 1945.
2. Achauer BM, Black KS, Litke DK: Transcutaneous PO$_2$ in flaps: A new method of survival prediction, *Plast Reconstr Surg* 65:738, 1980.
3. Ackland RD, et al: The saphenous neurovascular free flap, *Plast Reconstr Surg* 67:763, 1981.
4. Ad Hoc Committee of the Committee on Trauma, Division of Medical Sciences, National Research Council: Postoperative wound infections: The influence of ultraviolet irradiation of the operating room and of various other factors. *Ann Surg* 160(suppl 1):1, 1964.
5. Arnold PG, Prunes-Carrillo F: Vastus medialis muscle flap for functional closure of the exposed knee joint, *Plast Reconstr Surg* 68:69, 1981.
6. Barclay TL, et al: Repair of lower leg injuries with fascio-cutaneous flaps, *Br J Plast Surg* 35:127, 1982.
7. Barron JN, et al: Observations on circulation of tubed skin pedicles using local clearance of radioactive sodium, *Br J Plast Surg* 5:171, 1952.
8. Bashir AH: A gastrocnemius tenocutaneous island flap, *Br J Plast Surg* 35:436, 1982.
9. Benowitz NL, Jacob P III: Daily intake of nicotine during cigarette smoking, *Clin Pharmacol Ther* 35:499, 1984.
10. Benowitz NL, Kuyt F, Jacob P III: Influence of nicotine on cardiovascular and hormonal effects of cigarette smoking, *Clin Pharmacol Ther* 36:74, 1984.
11. Benowitz NL, et al: Cotinine disposition and effects. *Clin Pharmacol Ther* 34:604, 1983.

12. Bjorkstrom S, Goldie IF: A study of the arterial supply of the patella in the normal state, in chondromalacia patellae and in osteoarthrosis. *Acta Orthop Scand* 51:63, 1980.
13. Boyd JB, Taylor GI, Corlett R: The vascular territories of the superior epigastric and the deep inferior epigastric systems, *Plast Reconstr Surg* 73:1, 1984.
14. Brent B, et al: Experience with the temporoparietal fascial free flap, *Plast Reconstr Surg* 76:177, 1985.
15. Brown GL, et al: Enhancement of wound healing by topical treatment with epidermal growth factor, *N Engl J Med* 321:76, 1989.
16. Buchanan RT, Levine NS: Blood pressure drop as a result of fluorescein injection, *Plast Reconstr Surg* 70:363, 1982.
17. Cahill GF, et al: Hormone-fuel interrelationships during fasting, *J Clin Invest* 45:1751, 1966.
18. Carpenter NH, Gates DJ, Williams HT: Normal processes and restraints in wound healing—review article, *Can J Surg* 20:314, 1977.
19. Carriquiry C, Aparecida Costa MM, Vasconez LO: An anatomic study of the septocutaneous vessels of the leg, *Plast Reconstr Surg* 76:354, 1985.
20. Chazan BI, Balodimos MC, Konez L: Untoward effects of flourescein angiography, *Ann Ophthalmol* 3:42, 1971.
21. Cohn KH, May JW Jr: Thermal-energy dissipation: A laboratory study to assess patency in blood vessels, *Plast Reconstr Surg* 70:475, 1982.
22. Converse JM, Rapaport FT: The vascularization of skin autografts and homografts, *Ann Surg* 153:306, 1956.
23. Converse JM, Uhlschmid GK, Ballantyne DL Jr: "Plasmatic circulation" in skin grafts. The phase of serum imbibition, *Plast Reconstr Surg* 43:495, 1969.
24. Cormack GC, Lamberty BGH: A classification of fasciocutaneous flaps according to their pattern of vascularization, *Br J Plast Surg* 37:80, 1984.
25. Cormack GC, Lamberty BGH: Fasciocutaneous vessels in the upper arm: Application to the design of new fasciocutaneous flaps, *Plast Reconstr Surg* 74:244, 1984.
26. Craig SM, Rees TD: The effects of smoking on experimental skin flaps in hamsters, *Plast Reconstr Surg* 75:842, 1985.
27. Creditor MC, et al: Effect of ACTH on wound healing in humans, *Proc Soc Exp Biol Med* 74:245, 1950.
28. Crismon JM, Fuhrman FT: Studies on gangrene following cold injury: Use of fluorescein as an indicator of local blood flow; distribution of fluorescein in body fluids after intravenous administration, *J Clin Invest* 26:259, 1947.
29. Cryer PE, et al: Norepinephrine and epinephrine release and adrenergic mediation of smoking-associated hemodynamic and metabolic events, *N Engl J Med* 295:573, 1976.
30. dos Santos LF: The vascular anatomy and dissection of the free scapular flap, *Plast Reconstr Surg* 73:599, 1984.
31. Douglas B, et al: Improved flap tolerance to warm ischemia after ibuprofen, *Plas Reconstr Surg* (in press).
32. Eaglstein WH, Mertz PM: Effect of topical medicaments on the rate of repair of superficial wounds. In Dineen P, Hildick-Smith G, editors: *The surgical wound,* Philadelphia, 1981, Lea & Febiger, pp 55–70.
33. Ehrlich HP, Hunt TK: Effects of cortisone and vitamin A on wound healing, *Ann Surg* 167:324, 1968.
34. Ehrlich HP, Tarver H: Effects of beta-carotene, vitamin A, and glucocorticoids on collagen synthesis in wounds, *Proc Soc Exp Biol Med* 137:936, 1971.
35. Eilon A, Rousso M, Wexler MR: The effect of systemic corticosteroid therapy on the breaking strength of skin, *Chir Plast* 4:207, 1978.
36. Ellis PP, Schoenberger M, Rendi MA: Antihistamines as prophylaxis against side reactions to intravenous flourescein, *Trans Am Ophthalmol Soc* 78:190, 1980.
37. Falcone RE, Nappi JF: Chemotherapy and wound healing. *Surg Clin North Am* 64:779, 1984.
38. Feldman JJ, Cohen BE, May JW: The medial gastrocnemius myocutaneous flap, *Plast Reconstr Surg* 61:531, 1978.
39. Ferner H, Staubesand J, editors: *Sobotta's atlas of human anatomy,* ed 10, Baltimore, 1983, Urban & Schwarzenberg, pp 310–312.
40. Finseth F, Adelberg MG: Prevention of skin flap necrosis by a course of treatment with vasodilator drugs, *Plast Reconstr Surg* 61:738, 1978.
41. Fischer JC, Parker PM, Shaw WW: Comparison of two laser Doppler flowmeters for the monitoring of dermal blood flow, *Microsurgery* 4:164, 1983.
42. Fox CL Jr: Silver sulfadiazine—A new topical therapy for *Pseudomonas* in burns, *Arch Surg* 96:184, 1968.
43. Galli, et al: Intravenous NTG as a means of improving ischemic tissue hemodynamics and survival, *Ann Plast Surg* 16:521, 1986.
44. Gilbert A, Teot L: The free scapular flap, *Plast Reconstr Surg* 69:601, 1982.
45. Goodson WH III, Hunt TK: Wound healing and the diabetic patient, *Surg Gynecol Obstet* 149:600, 1979.
46. Graham BH, et al: Surface quantification of injected fluorescein as a predictor of flap viability, *Plast Reconstr Surg* 71:826, 1983.
47. Graham BH, et al: Serial quantitative skin surface fluorescence: A new method for postoperative monitoring of vascular perfusion in revascularized digits (abstract). *J Hand Surg* 10A:226, 1985.
48. Green JP: Steroid therapy and wound healing in surgical patients, *Br J Surg* 52:523, 1965.
49. Haertsch P: The surgical plane of the leg, *Br J Plast Surg* 34:464, 1981.
50. Haertsch PA: The blood supply to the skin of the leg: A post-mortem investigation, *Br J Plast Surg* 34:470, 1981.
51. Handel N, Zarem HA, Graham LS: Computerized determination of blood flow in pedicle flaps by the clearance of epicutaneously applied ^{133}xenon, *J Surg Res* 20:579, 1976.

52. Harrison DH, Girling M, Mott GT: Discussion of Ackland RD: Experience in monitoring the circulation in free-flap transfers, *Plast Reconstr Surg* 68:554, 1981.
53. Hatz RA, Kelley S, Ehrlich HP: The ICDO complex reverses the effect of cortisone on wound healing,
54. Hidalgo DA: Lower extremity avulsion injuries, *Clin Plast Surg* 13:701, 1986.
55. Hollinshead WH, Rosse C: *Textbook of anatomy*, ed 4. Philadelphia, 1985, Harper & Row, pp 432–433.
56. Huch A, et al: Continuous transcutaneous oxygen tension measured with a heated electrode, *Scand J Clin Lab Invest* 31:269, 1973.
57. Hunt TK, Pai P: The effect of varying ambient oxygen tensions on wound metabolism and collagen synthesis, *Surg Gynecol Obstet* 135:561, 1972.
58. Hunt TK, Zederfelt B: Nutritional and environmental aspects in wound healing. In Dunphy JE, Van Winkle J Jr, editors: *Repair and regeneration. The scientific basis for surgical practice,* New York, 1969, McGraw-Hill, p 217.
59. Hunt TK, et al: Effect of vitamin A on reversing the inhibitory effect of cortisone on healing of open wounds in animals and man, *Ann Surg* 170:633, 1969.
60. Jeffrey JJ, Coffey RJ, Eisen AZ: Studies on uterine collagenase in tissue culture: II. Effect of steroid hormones on enzyme production, *Biochim Biophys Acta* 252:143, 1971.
61. Kakkar VV, Stringer MD: Prophylaxis of venous thromboembolism, *World J Surg* 14:670, 1990.
62. Kaplan IB, Gilbert DA, Terzis JK: The vascularized fascia of the scalp, *J Reconstr Microsurg* 5:7, 1989.
63. Kashtan J, Conti S, Blaisdell FW: Heparin therapy for deep venous thrombosis, *Am J Surg* 140:836, 1980.
64. Knighton DR, Silver IA, Hunt TK: Regulation of wound-healing angiogenesis—effect of oxygen gradients and inspired oxygen concentration, *Surgery* 90:262, 1981.
65. Knighton DR, et al: Classification and treatment of chronic nonhealing wounds: Successful treatment with autologous platelet-derived wound healing factors (PDWHF), *Ann Surg* 204:322, 1986.
66. Krizek TJ, Robson MC, Kho E: Bacterial growth and skin graft survival, *Surg Forum* 18:518, 1967.
67. Lange K, Boyd LJ: Use of fluorescein to determine adequacy of circulation, *Med Clin North Am* 26:943, 1942.
68. Lange K, Boyd LJ: Use of fluorescein method in establishment of diagnosis and prognosis of peripheral vascular disease, *Arch Intern Med* 74:175, 1944.
69. Lange K, Krewer SE: The dermofluorimeter. Instrument for objective measurement of fluorescence of skin and organs and objective determination of circulation time and capillary permeability, *J Lab Clin Med* 28:1746, 1943.
70. Langman J, Woerdeman MW: *Atlas of medical anatomy,* Philadelphia, 1982, WB Saunders, p 311.
71. LaPiana F, Penner R: Anaphylactoid Reaction to intravenously administered flourescein, *Arch Ophthalmol* 79:161, 1968.
72. Last RJ: *Anatomy: Regional and applied,* ed 7. Edinburgh, 1984, Churchill Livingstone.
73. Leibovich SJ, Ross R: The role of the macrophage in wound repair: A study with hydrocortisone and anti-macrophage serum, *Am J Pathol* 78:71, 1975.
74. Levenson SM, Birkhill FR, Waterman DF: The healing of soft tissue wounds: The effects of nutrition, anemia and age, *Surgery* 28:905, 1950.
75. Levenson S, Seifter E: Dysnutrition, wound healing and resistance to infection, *Clin Plast Surg* 4:375, 1977.
76. Magee C, Rodeheaver GT, Golden GT: Potentiation of wound infection by surgical drains, *Am J Surg* 131:547, 1976.
77. Marfuggi RA, Greenspan M: Reliable intraoperative prediction of intestinal viability using a fluorescein indicator, *Surg Gynecol Obstet* 152:33, 1981.
78. Mathes SJ, Nahai F: Classification of the vascular anatomy of muscles: Experimental and clinical correlation, *Plast Reconstr Surg* 67:177, 1981.
79. May JW Jr, et al: Removable thermocouple probe microvascular patency monitor: An experimental and clinical study, *Plast Reconstr Surg* 72:366, 1983.
80. McCraw JB, Fishman JM, Sharzer LA: The versatile gastrocnemius myocutaneous flap, *Plast Reconstr Surg* 62:15, 1978.
81. McCraw JB, Penix JO, Baker JW: Repair of major defects of the chest wall and spine with latissimus dorsi myocutaneous flap, *Plast Reconstr Surg* 62:197, 1978.
82. McCraw JB, et al: The value of fluorescein in predicting the viability of arterialized flaps, *Plast Reconstr Surg* 60:710, 1977.
83. McGrath M: How topical dressings salvage "questionable" flaps: Experimental study, *Plast Reconstr Surg* 67:653, 1981.
84. McGrath MH: The effect of prostoglandin inhibitors on wound contraction and the myofibroblast, *Plast Reconstr Surg* 69:74, 1982.
85. McMurry JR Jr: Wound healing with diabetes mellitus, *Surg Clin North Am* 64:769, 1984.
86. Milloy FG, Anson BJ, McAfee DK: The rectus abdominis muscle and the epigastric arteries, *Surg Gynecol Obstet* 122:293, 1960.
87. Morrison WA, Shen TY: Anterior tibial artery flap: Anatomy and case report, *Br J Plast Surg* 40:230, 1987.
88. Mosely LH, Finseth F: Cigarette smoking: Impairment of digital blood flow and wound healing in the hand, *Hand* 9:97, 1977.
89. Mosely LH, Finseth F, Goody M: Nicotine and its effect on wound healing, *Plast Reconstr Surg* 61:570, 1977.
90. Myers MB: Prediction of skin sloughs at the time of aspiration with the use of fluorescein dye, *Surgery* 51:158, 1962.
91. Myers MB, Cherry G: Enhancement of survival in

devascularized pedicles by the use of phenoxybenzamine, *Plast Reconstr Surg* 41:254, 1968.
92. Nanney LB: Epidermal growth factor–induced effects on wound healing (abstract). *Clin Res* 35:706A, 1987.
93. Niinikoski J, Hunt TK, Dunphy JE: Oxygen supply in healing tissue, *Am J Surg* 123:247, 1972.
94. Olivari N: The latissimus flap, *Br J Plast Surg* 29:126, 1976.
95. Pachter HL, Riles TS: Low dose heparin: Bleeding and wound complications in the surgical patient: A prospective randomized study, *Ann Surg* 186:669, 1977.
96. Peacock E: *Wound repair,* ed 3, Philadelphia, 1984, WB Saunders, pp 124–125.
97. Ponten B: The fasciocutaneous flap: Its use in soft tissue defects of the lower leg, *Br J Plast Surg* 34:215, 1981.
98. Powanda MC, Moyer ED: Plasma proteins and wound healing, *Surg Gynecol Obstet* 153:749, 1981.
99. Prather A, et al: Evaluation of tests for predicting the viability of axial pattern skin flaps in the pig, *Plast Reconstr Surg* 63:250, 1979.
100. Rees TD, Liverett DM, Guy CL: The effect of cigarette smoking on skin-flap survival in the face-lift patient, *Plast Reconstr Surg* 73:911, 1984.
101. Reilly DT: Prophylactic methods against thromboembolism. *Act Chir Scand Suppl* 550 (suppl):115, 1989.
102. Reinisch JF: The pathophysiology of skin circulation, *Plast Reconstr Surg* 54:585, 1974.
103. Rich NM, Spencer FC: *Vascular trauma,* Philadelphia, 1978, WB Saunders.
104. Riefkohl R, et al: Association between cutaneous occlusive vascular disease, cigarette smoking and skin slough after rhytidectomy, *Plast Reconstr Surg* 77:592, 1986.
105. Robson MC, Heggers JP: Effect of hyperglycemia on survival bacteria, *Surg Forum* 20:56, 1969.
106. Robson MC, Krizek TJ: Predicting skin graft survival, *J Trauma* 13:213, 1973.
107. Robson MC, Krizek TJ, Heggers JP: Biology of surgical infection, *Curr Probl Surg* 1–62, 1973.
108. Rohrich, et al: Enhancement of skin survival utilizing 2% NTG ointment, *Surg Forum* 33:592, 1982.
109. Rovee DT, Kurowsky CA, Labun J: Local wound environment and epidermal healing: Mitotic response, *Arch Dermatol* 106:330, 1972.
110. Ruberg RL: Role of nutrition in wound healing, *Surg Clin North Am* 64:705, 1984.
111. Rudolph R, Klein L: Healing processes in skin grafts, *Surg Gynecol Obstet* 136:641, 1973.
112. Salmela K: The effect of methylprednisolone and vitamin A on wound healing, *Acta Chir Scand* 147:313, 1981.
113. Salmela K, Ahonev J: The effect of methylprednisolone and vitamin A on wound healing, *Acta Chir Scand* 147:307, 1981.
114. Scapinelli R: Studies on the vasculature of the human knee joint, *Acta Anat* 70:305, 1968.
115. Sejrsen P: Measurement of cutaneous blood flow by freely diffusable radioactive isotopes, *Dan Med Bull* 18 (suppl 3):1–40, 1971.
116. Serafin D, et al: Transcutaneous PO_2 monitoring for assessing viability and predicting survival of skin flaps: Experimental and clinical correlations, *J Microsurg* 2:165, 1981.
117. Shamberger R: Effect of chemotherapy and radiotherapy on wound healing: Experimental studies, *Recent Results Cancer Res* 98:17, 1985.
118. Shizgal HM, Forse RA: Protein and caloric requirements with total parenteral nutrition, *Ann Surg* 192:562, 1980.
119. Silver L: Personal communication, July 1992.
120. Silverman DG, et al: Quantification of tissue fluorescein delivery and prediction of flap viability with the fiberoptic dermofluorimeter, *Plast Reconstr Surg* 66:545, 1980.
121. Silverman DG, et al: Monitoring tissue elimination of fluorescein with the perfusion fluorimeter: A new method to assess capillary blood flow, *Surgery* 90:409, 1981.
122. Silverman DG, et al: The effects of topical PGE_2 analogue on global flap ischemia in rats, *Plast Reconstr Surg* 84:794, 1989.
123. Simchen E, Rozin R, Wax Y: The Israeli study of surgical infection of drains and the risk of wound infection in operations for hernia, *Surg Gynecol Obstet* 170:331, 1990.
124. Singer ER, et al: Fluorescein test for prediction of flap viability during breast reconstructions, *Plast Reconstr Surg* 61:371, 1978.
125. Smahel J: The healing of skin grafts, *Clin Plast Surg* 4:409, 1977.
126. Smith RA: The free fascial scalp flap, *Plast Reconstr Surg* 66:204, 1980.
127. Stein MR, Parker CW: Reactions following intravenous fluorescein, *Am J Ophthalmol* 72:861, 1971.
128. Stephens FO, Hunt TK: Effect of changes in inspired oxygen and carbon dioxide tensions on wound tensile strength, *Ann Surg* 173:515, 1971.
129. Tauxe WN, et al: Determination of vascular status of pedicle skin flaps by use of radioactive pertechnetate (^{99m}Tc), *Surg Gynecol Obstet* 130:87, 1970.
130. Taylor GI, Palmer JH: The vascular territories (angiosomes) of the body: Experimental study and clinical applications, *Br J Plast Surg* 40:113, 1987.
131. Teh BT: Why do skin grafts fail?, *Plast Reconstr Surg* 63:323, 1979.
132. Thatte RL, Laud N: The use of the fascia of the lower leg as a roll-over flap: Its possible clinical applications in reconstructive surgery, *Br J Plast Surg* 37:88, 1984.
133. Thomson JG, Kerrigan CL: Dermoflourimetry: Thresholds for predicting flap survival, *Plas Reconstr Surg* 83:859, 1984.
134. Thorvaldsson SE, Grabb WC: The intravenous fluorescein test as a measure of skin flap viability, *Plast Reconstr Surg* 53:576, 1974.
135. Tobin GR: Vastus medialis myocutaneous and

musculocutaneous-tendinous composite flaps, *Plast Reconstr Surg* 75:677, 1985.
136. Tolhurst DE, Haeseker B, Zeeman RJ: The development of the fasciocutaneous flap and its clinical applications, *Plast Reconstr Surg* 71:597, 1983.
137. Torii S, Namiki Y, Hayashi Y: Anterolateral leg island flap, *Br J Plast Surg* 40:236, 1987.
138. Townsend PLG: An inferiorly based soleus muscle flap, *Br J Plast Surg* 31:210, 1978.
139. Tsuchida Y, Tsuya A: Measurement of skin blood flow in delayed deltapectoral flaps, using local clearance of ^{133}xenon, *Plast Reconstr Surg* 62:763, 1978.
140. Wagner HN: *Regional blood flow measurements with krypton 856 and xenon 133 in dynamic clinical studies with radioisotopes. No 3 Report T.I.D. 7678, AFC Symposium,* Oak Ridge, Tenn, US Atomic Energy Commission.
141. Wahl LM: Hormonal regulation of macrophage collagenase activity, *Biochem Biophys Res Commun* 74:838, 1977.
142. Webster RC, et al: Cigarette smoking with facelift: Conservative versus wide undermining, *Plast Reconstr Surg* 77:596, 1986.
143. Wee JTK: Reconstruction of the lower leg and foot with the reverse pedicled anterior tibial flap: Preliminary report of a new fasciocutaneous flap, *Br J Plast Surg* 39:327, 1986.
144. Weisbrod H, Treiman N: Intraosseous venography in patellofemoral disorders, *J Bone Joint Surg [Br]* 62:454, 1980.
145. Werb Z: Biochemical actions of glucocorticoids on macrophages in culture, *J Exp Med* 147:1695, 1978.
146. Westfall TC, Watts DT: Catecholamine excretion in smokers and non-smokers, *J Appl Physiol* 19:40, 1964.
147. Willett KM, Simmons CD, Bentley G: The effect of suction drains after total hip replacement, *J Bone Joint Surg [Br]* 70:607, 1988.

74

Principles of Planning and Prosthetic Selection for Revision Total Knee Replacement

CHITRANJAN S. RANAWAT, M.D.
WILLIAM F. FLYNN, JR., M.D.

Indications for revision
General considerations
Preoperative surgical assessment and planning
Surgical considerations

Prosthesis selection
Approach
Implant removal
Final implant selection and fixation

INDICATIONS FOR REVISION

Preoperative planning is essential in revision total knee replacement (TKR) surgery if intra- and postoperative problems are to be avoided. First, the general health of the patient ought to be good enough that the patient will benefit from and be able to use a revised TKR. The next decision is whether or not to revise the existing prosthesis. Revisions are performed for many reasons, such as infection, loosening, patellar complications, instability, fracture, or pain. Other, less frequent causes include implant wear, implant fracture, or component dissociation. Infection is a major cause of failure in total knee arthroplasty and is discussed in detail in Chapter 72.

Loosening is the most common reason for failure of first-generation knee replacements at 10 years' and longer follow-up.[5, 10, 17] The surgeon must evaluate the patient's clinical and radiographic course prior to failure to determine the cause of loosening. Inability to achieve initial stable fixation is an important mechanism of failure. Another is overload of the cancellous bone due to body weight, activity level, and number of cycles (i.e., the length of time the implant is in). Eccentric load is particularly problematic and is increased by malalignment and instability.[2] Poor-quality bone and ligamentous instability may also lead to malfunctioning of the knee. Increased prosthetic constraint also increases the risk of loosening by stressing the interface, as results of hinged TKRs demonstrate. The revision must correct the underlying problem.

Patellar complications are the most common reason for revision in second-generation TKRs (1980–1990). Merkow et al.[16] have shown that surgical error in placing the components is the most common reason for these problems. The frontal and axial alignment of the components must be identified, and revision surgery must correct the malalignment. Shallow or nonconforming design of the prosthetic patellofemoral joint may also increase the risk of patellar subluxation or dislocation. Patellar strain increases when the height of the patellar construct increases, and particularly when the bony portion of the patella is less than 15 mm,[21] or when the femoral component is oversized. Increased strain can lead to fracture or decreased range of motion (ROM), as well as anterior knee pain.

Revision for instability is slightly less common. Instability at the tibiofemoral joint may be anteroposterior (AP) or mediolateral. Theoretically, anterior instability is present in any arthroplasty because the ACL is sacrificed or deficient, but clinically this is not a problem. Posterior instability may occur in cruciate-substituting arthroplasties when the peg is not high enough, when the flexion gap is mismatched with the extension gap, or when the knee is in extreme flexion (associated with rotatory imbalance). Most designs now have a sufficiently tall peg so that the first cause is less likely, although it has been re-

1297

ported.[11,12] Mismatched flexion gaps must be recognized and corrected in revision surgery. Knee prostheses are not designed for normal extremes of flexion, and patients must be aware of this.

Subluxation or posterior sag may also occur in posterior cruciate ligament (PCL)–sparing designs, if the PCL is cut, overlengthened, or becomes incompetent postoperatively. These knees should be revised to a substituting design if symptomatic.

Mediolateral instability is probably more common, and is closely related to malalignment and loosening. Failure to properly balance the knee at primary surgery may lead to instability, which then eccentrically increases the tibial load. This results in functional malalignment, which leads to loosening. Alternatively, malalignment at surgery leads to increased load and loosening which can then lead to instability via ligament insufficiency. Each of these factors must be considered by the surgeon if instability is the reason for revision. Occasionally, absorption or fracture may cause or aggravate ligamentous instability.

Fracture around a prosthesis may also require revision. Supracondylar femur fractures, proximal tibial fractures, and patella fractures can sometimes be managed with open reduction and internal fixation around a TKR, (ORIF), but often a revision is required.[4,9] Special attention must be paid to alignment and fixation in these cases. Some fractures are largely preventable—those caused by notching of the anterior femur or excessive resection of the patella or devascularization of the patella.[4,9,21]

Perhaps the most uncertain indication for revision is unexplained pain in the TKR. This is responsible for about 2% to 3% of revisions,[10,17] and results in these cases are often less than satisfactory. Sympathetic dystrophies may play a role, as may arthritis in the spine or ipsilateral hip. Arthritis can be managed, but dystrophies are frequently exacerbated by more surgery. Very careful evaluation must be carried out preoperatively, and patients must be made aware of the possibility of an unreliable result.

Decreased ROM is rarely a reason for revision, although less than 90 degrees of flexion tends to diminish function. If manipulation does not improve motion, one should consider the possibility of reflex sympathetic dystrophy (RSD). Prosthetic factors, such as thickness of the tibial or patellar components, and placement and AP dimension of the femoral component, may also impede flexion. If prosthetic factors seem to be the cause for decreased ROM, then revision may be indicated.[19]

Other uncommon but reported reasons for revision are wear synovitis, prosthetic fracture, and component dissociation. Wear is not as problematic in the knee as in the hip, but heat-treated, thin (<6mm) polyethylene tibial inserts with small contact areas have shown delamination and catastrophic failure.[13,14] Fractures of cobolt-chromium porous-coated tibial trays have been reported,[18,22] as have fractures or dissociations of metal-backed patellae.[20]

GENERAL CONSIDERATIONS

The overall condition of the patient must also be carefully evaluated. Revision surgery can be extensive and involve significant blood loss. Patients with cardiopulmonary problems must be evaluated before surgery. Patients with a history of infection, diabetes, psoriasis, immune system compromise, and rheumatoid arthritis (RA) have an increased risk of infection, and any potential sources (oral, urinary, gastrointestinal, skin, etc.) must be eliminated preoperatively. Any neurologic or vascular problems should also be investigated prior to surgery. Obese patients should be encouraged to lose weight if possible: this will make the operation technically easier, allow for easier rehabilitation, and potentially prolong the lifetime of the implant. Other causes of pain, including spinal and hip abnormalities, must be ruled out.

When feasible, patients donate 3 to 4 units of autologous blood preoperatively. If this is not possible, bank blood is used. Reinfusion of drained blood may also be used, but it has limitations, including hematologic reactions. Cell Saver (Haemonetics, Braintree, Mass.) is usually not an option because the surgery is done under tourniquet. In addition, Cell Saver or reinfusion cannot be used in patients with infection.

PREOPERATIVE SURGICAL ASSESSMENT AND PLANNING

Once the reason for revision has been determined, and the patient's condition optimized, surgical planning can begin. The surgeon must first consider patient factors. The skin must be examined for previous incisions and any evidence of poor blood supply. The stability of the ligaments must be assessed as well as the presence and strength of the quadriceps mechanism. ROM must be documented. The surgeon must determine the alignment of the ipsilateral hip and foot, and decide if there are disabilities of the opposite lower extremity.

Adequate radiographs must be available to evaluate the prosthesis, including AP, lateral, and patellar views. Full-length films showing the hip, knee, and ankle joints allow more accurate determination of the mechanical axis.

The surgeon must then consider the type of implant that is to be removed or revised. Is it cemented or noncemented? Is it well-fixed or loose? Have stems, screws, or other supplementary fixation devices been used? Are the tibial and patellar components all-polyethylene or metal-backed? Is the TKR a hinge design or semi- or unconstrained? What will be the expected extent of longitudinal and central bone loss? Finally, what are the surgeon's and the patient's expectations regarding revision?

SURGICAL CONSIDERATIONS

The surgeon must consider the type of surgery contemplated. Because infected TKR is discussed in Chapter 72, we confine this section to revision for other reasons. Considerations include prosthesis selection, the surgical approach used, and the method of implant removal and revision fixation.

Prosthesis Selection

The surgeon should decide before surgery which implant he or she wishes to use for revision, as well as which other implants *may* be required if complications arise. These must be immediately available, along with any specialized tools required for prosthesis removal. Today's modular knee systems can accommodate many potential deformities and problems, and the surgeon should become familiar with at least one of these systems. However, even these extensive systems cannot cover all possibilities so their availability *does not* substitute for planning. Table 74–1 lists modular systems. Custom components may be required for: (1) knees with an AP femoral dimension of less than 50 mm or greater than 70 mm; (2) knees with extensive bone loss; and (3) technical considerations such as offset canal, or fracture with need for longer stems.

Approach

The surgical approach depends on the soft tissue coverage of the knee and the preoperative alignment and ROM. Generally, a midline or slightly paramedian incision is used, incorporating previous incisions. The sinus tract should be excised if present. The surgeon must avoid parallel incisions less than 5 cm apart. The approach should allow proximal and distal access to the joint as well as mediolateral access. In first revisions, one can generally use the incision from the primary arthroplasty. If there is a question about the viability of the skin, the incision can be made without a tourniquet. If the edges of the flap show an adequate blood supply, then the tourniquet is inflated and the operation continued. In cases with preexisting soft tissue loss or in those where soft tissue excision is contemplated, a plastic surgeon may be consulted for the possibility of flap coverage of the defect, usually with a gastrocnemius flap.

If preoperative ROM is good, there is generally minimal difficulty exposing the joint. In a stiff knee there are three areas which may need correction: (1) contracture of the quadriceps mechanism, (2) intraarticular adhesions, and (3) contracture of the capsular and ligamentous structures. Often, two or all three are present, and the surgical approach must allow correction of all. One approach is the V-Y quadricepsplasty described by Coonse and Adams,[7] and modified by others. This approach allows lengthening of the quadriceps mechanism and release of the adhesions, capsule, and ligaments. Tibial tubercle osteotomy allows excellent exposure and release of contracted structures, but does not really allow lengthening of the quadriceps mechanism. Fixation can be a problem with minimal osteotomy, and more extensive osteotomies can create soft tissue problems and vascular compromise. We prefer subperiosteal exposure.

A long straight incision is used. Subperiosteally, the superficial and deep medial collateral ligament (MCL), the medial quadriceps and retinaculum, and the medial capsule are elevated as a sleeve. A long, inside-out, lateral release is performed. If there is bony ankylosis, an intraarticular osteotomy is performed. Otherwise, the fibrous tissue causing the ankylosis is removed. The lateral quadriceps, lateral retinaculum, iliotibial band, popliteus, and lateral collateral ligament (LCL) are elevated subperiosteally in succession, enucleating the femur. As this is being performed, the knee is flexed, with gradually increasing external rotation of the tibia, which relieves the stress at the insertion of the patellar tendon. After the appropriate bone cuts are made, and the trial prosthesis is implanted, tension in the quadriceps is adjusted by releasing the vastus intermedius from the rectus femoris. The knee is flexed to produce tension in the quadriceps mechanism, and the rectus is released by controlled multiple Z lengthenings until 80 to 90 degrees of flexion is possible. This approach therefore allows for release of fibrous or bony ankylosis, release of contracted capsular and ligamentous structures, and selective lengthening of the quadriceps mechanism, as opposed to the excess lengthening which can occur with V-Y plasty.

Once the knee joint has been satisfactorily exposed, the prosthetic margins are cleared, and preparations for removal are begun.

TABLE 74–1.
Modular Systems

		PFC	Insall-Burstein II	Genesis	Miller-Galante II	AGC	Omnifit	Kinemax+
I N S E R T	Retain	Yes	No	Yes	Yes	Yes	Yes	Yes
	Sacrifice	Yes	Yes	Yes			Yes	Yes
	Constrain	Yes	Yes	Yes			Yes	Yes
F E M U R	Distal	4,6,8 mm	5,10 mm	4,8 mm	Not modular	Combined 5 mm	4 mm	Combined 4 mm
	Posterior	4,6,8, combined	Combined distal	4,8 mm		5 mm	4 mm × 8 distal	4 mm
	Fixation	Mechanical + cement	Screw	Distal—lug nut, posterior cement		Cement	Mechanical	
T I B I A	Wedge		7,13,20 degrees	5,10 mm				
	Hemiwedge	10,15 degrees mediolateral	16,26 degrees	10 mm	16,26 degrees, not modular	10 mm mediolateral	5,10 mm mediolateral	7.5 mm mediolateral
	Fixation	Mechanical + cement	Screw	Mechanical + cement		Cement	Cement	Cement
F E M O R	Length	75 (15,25 × 15) mm	75 (15,25 × 15) mm	100,150,200 mm	23,43,67,145,200 mm	40,80,120 mm	Not modular 85,93,100,108,115, 124 mm	40,80 155 mm
	Diameter	13,15,17,19 mm	10–24 mm	12,14,16,18,20,22 mm	10,12,14,16,18, for 145 and 200	10,12,14,16,18,20,22,24 mm		
	Fixation	Taper, Spiralock	Morse taper, screw	Morse taper, spiralock	Screw	Morse taper, screw		
T I B I A	Length	75 (15,25 × 15) mm	75 (15,25 × 15) mm	41–91 mm		40,80,120,160 mm	Not modular 85,93,100,108,115, 124 mm	40,80,155 mm
	Diameter	13,15,17,19 mm	10–24 mm	10,12 mm				
	Fixation	Taper, Spiralock	Morse taper, screw	Morse taper, Spiralock				

PFC (Press Fit Condylar, Johnson & Johnson Orthopaedics, Braintree, Mass.); Insall-Burstein II (Zimmer, Warsaw, Ind.); Genesis (Richards.); Miller-Galante II (Zimmer): AGC (Anatomically Graduated Components, Biomet, Omnifit (Osteonics, Kinemax + (Howmedica, Rutherford, N.J.).

Implant Removal

There are many ways to remove the components of a knee arthroplasty. Those which are grossly loose may be removed by hand or with the minimal use of thin osteotomes. Prostheses, which are better fixed, may be removed with a slap-hammer device after the interfaces have been disrupted with thin osteotomes. This generally results in little bone loss, unless the prosthesis has fixation pegs with grooves. All-polyethylene components may be easily removed with a saw, and the pegs with a curette or Midas Rex type of tool (Midas Rex Pneumatic Tools). Prostheses with long stems must be removed carefully to avoid fracturing the tibial or femoral shaft. Removal is followed by debridement and then by implantation of the new components.

Final Implant Selection and Fixation

Prior to, and at the time of surgery, careful assessment of the bony, ligamentous, and extensor deficiencies must be carried out before any revision prosthesis is implanted.

Bone loss may be extensive, and assymetric. For revision surgery to be successful, anatomy must be restored to as near to normal as possible. This includes overall limb alignment, patellar tracking, and height of the joint. Bone graft, either autograft or allograft, or mechanical grafts (cement, wedge augments, custom components) may be used: an in-depth discussion of this area is available in Chapter 77.

Autograft has advantages compared to mechanical augmentation. Once a graft becomes incorporated, it may transfer load in a more physiologic manner. In addition, incorporated bone graft means more bone stock if another revision is required. However, grafts that are heavily loaded may resorb,[8] and so morselized grafts or small allografts are best reserved for small to moderate, contained defects. Generally, if there is more than 1.5 to 2.0 cm of bone loss in a given area, cancellous graft, modular wedges, hemiwedges, and augments will not be sufficient and custom components will be necessary. These components are expensive, but provide the strongest construct available. Large allografts can replace larger bone defects, but are associated with higher rates of infection, absorption, and other complications.[3, 15]

In situations with less bone loss, today's modular knee systems provide an excellent solution. Tibial defects may be compensated for by full wedges or hemiwedges, or augmented tibial components. Distal femoral and posterior femoral augments are also available with many systems. These augments may be particularly important, because they allow the surgeon to match the flexion gap to the extension gap. In addition, distal augments allow the joint line to be restored close to its original position, which minimizes patella baja and extensor mechanism dysfunction. There is no good long-term follow-up on the use of modular components as yet, and there are some theoretic disadvantages. Fretting between augments and main components could lead to particulate wear and subsequent resorption. Alternatively, augments could become separated from the main component.

In situations with a small amount of bone loss (2–5 mm in contained defects), cement can be used as a filler.

Ligamentous loss may also be extensive, but can generally be compensated for with the modular tibial inserts currently available. Patients with cruciate-deficient knees require a Posterior Stabilized or Total Condylar III type of insert to substitute function and allow controlled, reproducible rollback. Those with collateral ligament deficiencies present a more difficult problem. In general, the surgeon should try to use the least constrained implant which allows stability in order to minimize stress on the interface. For patients with collateral insufficiency, this usually means a Total Condylar III type of insert, which is available in many systems. In some systems, no change is required in the femoral component in order to use a constrained insert. This is clearly an advantage in prosthetic design that allows for easier revision.

The combination of a Total Condylar III type of insert and postoperative bracing will allow a stable knee in most patients. Some with more severe instability may require a hinged implant, which is clearly suboptimal. An alternative is arthrodesis.

Most systems also have a large number of tibial implant thicknesses to compensate for joint height loss on the tibial side: a minimum of 6 mm polyethylene should be used.[23]

Extensor mechanism loss or insufficiency can be a major problem. Care must be taken not to injure or avulse the extensor mechanism during the exposure. It is sometimes possible to reconstruct or reattach the extensor mechanism, but results are uncertain. It should be noted that patients with very large flexion contractures preoperatively often develop extensor lag postoperatively, which can hinder ambulation. Allowing these patients to ambulate with the knee extended in a brace will often improve the lag as the quadriceps adjusts to a new length. Patients who have a neurologic or myopathic deficiency of the extensor mechanism should be advised to have an arthrodesis, or be managed in a long leg brace.

Alignment of the revision prosthesis is crucial, particularly for those patients who failed by loosening or malalignment. Alignment can be difficult to judge because of bone loss, although intramedullary devices are a great aid. It is important to place the implants in the proper position in the mediolateral plane and to rotate them correctly to allow proper function of the quadriceps mechanism. Alignment should generally be in the range of 3 to 8 degrees of overall valgus alignment.

Fixation of the revision components is also critical. Generally, all components are cemented with antibiotic-impregnated cement. Pulsatile lavage is used, sclerotic areas are drilled, and the cement is finger-pressurized to ensure microinterlock. Noncemented fixation can also be utilized, but bone loss generally makes a good press fit impossible. In patients with poor-quality cancellous bone, the surgeon should consider the use of a *stem* on the tibia, femur, or on both. Longer stems aid immediate fixation, distribute the load, and restore the mechanical axis of the knee.[1] They may cause stress shielding, and patients may be at slightly increased risk for fracture (at the tip of the stem), but the advantages outweigh the disadvantages in these situations. *Do not cement the stems distally* in case further revision is required at a later date. Stems should also be considered if a constrained prosthesis is used, so as to share the increased load.

Special considerations are present in certain cases. In patients with a previous fracture or osteotomy, the femoral or tibial canal may be malaligned with the joint. This can lead to errors if intramedullary instrumentation is used solely. In addition, if the canal is "offset" from the joint, standard modular stems will place the prosthesis in an incorrect position; custom components with offset stems should be used.

In cases with fracture around a well-fixed TKR, open reduction and internal fixation (ORIF) may be the appropriate procedure. If there is any concern about the fixation of the prosthesis, a revision should be carried out with stems used to fix the fracture via the intramedullary canal. Customized, longer stems may be necessary to adequately bypass the fracture site. If there is concern about rotational stability, additional fixation may be obtained at the fracture site with a plate, wires, screws, or a combination of these.

In cases with old, malaligned fracture, or with other bone deformity, revision plus osteotomy should be considered. If properly planned and executed, this will allow more normal mechanics and stresses on the joint. Fixation is generally accomplished using fluted intramedullary stems, with additional rotational control by step-cut or other fixation if necessary.

Careful preoperative planning and evaluation will allow the surgeon to avoid many potential problems with revision TKR. However, results of revisions are not so good as those of primary arthroplasty, and the complication rate is higher. The surgeon must have realistic expectations and these must be clearly conveyed to the patient before surgery.

REFERENCES

1. Albrektsson BE, et al: The effect of a stem on the tibial component of knee arthroplasty. A roentgen stereophotogrammetric study of uncemented tibial components in the Freeman-Samuelson knee arthroplasty, *J Bone Joint Surg [Br]* 72:252–258, 1990.
2. Bargren JH, Blaha JD, Freeman MAR: Alignment in total knee arthroplasty. Correlated biomechanical and clinical observations, *Clin Orthop* 173:178, 1983.
3. Berrey BH Jr, et al: Fractures of allografts. Frequency, treatment and end-results, *J Bone Joint Surg* 72:825–833, 1990.
4. Cain PR, et al: Periprosthetic femoral fractures following total knee arthroplasty, *Clin Orthop* 208:205, 1986.
5. Cameron HU, Hunter GA: Failure in total knee arthroplasty: Mechanisms, revisions and results, *Clin Orthop* 170:141, 1982.
6. Cameron HU, Turner DG, Cameron GM: Results of bone grafting of tibial defects in uncemented total knee replacements, *Can J Surg* 31:30, 1988.
7. Coonse K, Adams JD: A new operative approach to the knee joint, *Surg Gynecol Obstet* 77:344, 1943.
8. Dorr LD, et al: Bone graft for tibial defects in total knee arthroplasty, *Clin Orthop* 205:153–165, 1986.
9. Figgie MP, et al: The results of treatment of supracondylar fracture above total knee arthroplasty, *J Arthroplasty* 5:267, 1990.
10. Friedman RJ, et al: Results of revision total knee arthroplasty performed for aseptic loosening, *Clin Orthop* 255:235, 1990.
11. Galinat BJ, et al: Dislocation of the Posterior Stabilized total knee arthroplasty. A report of 2 cases, *J Arthroplasty* 3:363–367, 1988.
12. Gebhard JS, Kilgus DJ: Dislocation of a Posterior Stabilized knee prosthesis. A report of two cases, *Clin Orthop* 254:225–229, 1990.
13. Heck DA, Clingman JK, Kettelkamp DG: Gross polyethylene failure in total knee arthroplasty, *Orthopedics* 15:23, 1992.
14. Kilgus DJ, et al: Catastrophic wear of tibial polyethylene inserts, *Clin Orthop* 273:223, 1991.
15. Lord CF, et al: Infection in bone allografts Incidence, nature and treatment, *J Bone Joint Surg* 70:369–376, 1988.

16. Merkow RL, Soudry M, Insall JN: Patellar dislocations following total knee replacement, *J Bone Joint Surg [Am]* 67:1321, 1985.
17. Moreland JR: Mechanisms of failure in total knee arthroplasty, *Clin Orthop* 226:49, 1988.
18. Morrey BF, Chao EY: Fracture of the porous coated tray of a biologically fixed knee prosthesis. Report of a case, *Clin Orthop* 228:182–189, 1988.
19. Nicholls DW, Dorr LD: Revision surgery for stiff total knee arthroplasty, *J Arthroplasty* 5(suppl):73, 1990.
20. Peters JD, Engh GA, Corpe RS: The metal backed patella. An invitation for failure?, *J Arthroplasty* 6:221, 1991.
21. Reuben JD, et al: Effect of patella thickness on patella strain following total knee arthroplasty, *J Arthroplasty* 6:251, 1991.
22. Scott RD, Ewald FC, Walker PS: Fracture of the metallic tibial tray following total knee replacement. Report of two cases, *J Bone Joint Surg [Am]* 66:780–782, 1984.
23. Wright TM, Bartel DL: The problem of surface damage in polyethylene total knee components, *Clin Orthop* 205:67–74, 1986.

75

Constrained Knee Arthroplasty

ADOLPH V. LOMBARDI, JR., M.D.
THOMAS H. MALLORY, M.D.
ROBERT W. EBERLE

History
Indications
   Rigid-hinge prostheses
   Rotating-hinge prostheses
   Constrained condylar prostheses
   Posterior-stabilized prostheses
   Conforming condylar prostheses
   Posterior cruciate ligament–retaining prostheses
Surgical techniques
   Exposure
   Prosthesis removal
   Debridement of bone and soft tissue
   Assessment of bone stock
   Assessment of ligamentous competence
   Preparation of bone stock for prosthetic implantation
   Trial reduction
   Implantation
   Closure
   Postoperative management
Clinical review
Conclusion

Throughout the evolution of total knee arthroplasty, a prosthetic design that would mimic the sophistication of knee function has been the foremost aim. The early prosthetic designs more or less created interpositional surfaces that eventually failed because of improper balance between the mobility and stability of the joint.[64] Single-unit, hinged devices were developed to improve stability, but only allowed for unidirectional motion. These devices were characterized by short-term relief of pain, but owing to their extreme constraints (i.e., no allowance for rotation or anteroposterior displacement), they eventually succumbed to the effects of severe interface shear forces. Recurrence of pain, bone loss, and implant loosening were the frequent consequences.*

We have learned that the soft tissues do not fully restrain knee motion, and thus surface contours and soft tissues must act in unison.[15, 17, 27, 32, 67, 68, 72] As a result, we have witnessed the development of more sophisticated prosthetic components. These particular devices have characteristics allowing for varus-valgus angulation, anteroposterior translation, rotation, rolling, and gliding within normal ranges of knee joint flexion and extension. This has given rise to a large and varied prosthetic nomenclature, loosely defined degrees of constraint,[76] and multiple indications for the use of such devices. Therefore, it is in this particular regard that the definition of all levels of constrained prosthetic knee design be standardized and the indications for each type of device be clearly identified.

HISTORY

The concept of surgically substituting knee function by prosthetic devices began in the 1800s with the work of Verneuil.[85] It was suggested that the surgical interposition of soft tissue could restore the articular surfaces of various joints. Because of the limited application of simple surface contact, in combination with the complexities of knee joint function, these early interpositional arthroplasties yielded discouraging results. Not until the advancement of mold hip arthroplasty in the early to mid-1900s was the concept of prosthetic replacement for the knee revisited.[2, 7, 53, 58, 80] Incorporating the perceptions for hip prosthetic materials, condylar inserts were designed in an attempt to resurface the knee utilizing the surrounding soft tissue envelope for stability.[2, 36, 50, 53–55]

*References 3, 12, 22, 27, 33, 35, 37, 89, 90.

In the 1950s, Shiers, Waldius and others began to develop knee prosthetics that would transfer, restrict, direct, and stabilize surface joint loads by simple mechanical principles.[56, 65, 66, 68, 87, 89, 90] These early totally constrained hinged prosthetic designs were unidirectional in nature and offered no capacity to dampen or decrease rotational joint forces between the prosthetic device and the host bone.[5] Short-term results of the totally constrained devices were promising in relieving joint pain and reestablishing joint stability. While these prosthetic devices filled a clinical need, many severe problems were encountered, including limited motion, patellar pain, bone resorption, loosening, bone fracture around the stem tips, deep infection, and metallic wear debris within the joint capsule.[25, 26, 33, 34, 73, 86] Hence, from these results emerged limitations for the use of totally constrained prosthetic knee devices including the finding that the hinged device is only of value in extreme desperate situations to correct severe joint deformity.[3, 6, 33, 78, 80]

The basic problem with rigid-hinged designs was that they did not permit rotation of the knee.[16, 63, 81] Rotational torque stresses were therefore transmitted either to the hinge pin or to the interface, leading to the above-noted complications. In response to the dilemma posed by rigid-hinge devices, designers sought the incorporation of rotation into hinged devices.[16, 63, 81] Hence, the genesis of designs such as the Spherocentric (Howmedica, Rutherford, N.J.) and Attenborough (Zimmer, Warsaw, Ind.) total knee arthroplasty systems, both of which required excessive bone removal for implantation, thereby complicating revision arthroplasty.

Concurrent with the development of linked prostheses was the introduction of a series of nonlinked knee designs. Following the advancement of the low-friction principles of the Charnley total hip replacement,[2, 8, 36, 80] a variety of designs were offered to address the increased implications on the biomechanics of the knee joint[51, 52, 57, 71]; these prosthetic devices include the four-part Polycentric (Howmedica) and modular knee systems, followed by the bicompartmental knee replacement systems such as the Geomedic (Howmedica, Inc.) and Duocondylar (Johnson & Johnson Orthopaedics, Brockton, Mass.). Finally, a number of tricompartmental knee arthroplasty systems were introduced. The tricompartmental knee arthroplasty systems essentially followed two developmental paths: the posterior cruciate ligament (PCL)–retaining designs and the PCL-substituting designs, with the latter being further subdivided into designs which provide posterior stabilization only and designs which provide posterior stabilization as well as varus-valgus stabilization.

Upon reviewing the historical developments in total knee arthroplasty, it becomes apparent that there are innumerable designs of knee arthroplasty systems. Classification of knee prostheses is vaguely defined. Generally, however, all prosthetic knee devices are grouped into two major categories, linked and nonlinked. The linked devices (femoral and tibial components physically connected by a bolt, or ball or post and socket) are then subdivided into two groups, *constrained rigid-hinge* prostheses (Fig 75–1), e.g., the GUEPAR (Howmedica), the St. Georg (Waldemar Link), and the Walldius (Howmedica), and the *constrained rotating-hinge* prostheses (Fig 75–2), including the Finn Knee System (Biomet), Kinematic Rotating Hinge (Howmedica), the Link Endo-Model Rotational Knee (Waldemar Link), and the Noiles Modular Rotating Hinge Knee (Joint Medical Products). The nonlinked devices are subdivided into four groups, the *constrained condylar* prostheses (Fig 75–3) which provide inherent varus-valgus stability as well as anteroposterior stability. Such devices include the Total Condylar III (TC-III) (Johnson & Johnson Orthopaedics), Insall-Burstein Posterior Stabilized Constrained (Zimmer), and the Maxim Posterior Stabilized Constrained (Biomet). Semiconstrained, *posterior-stabilized* prostheses (Fig 75–4) incorporate varus-valgus freedom and prevent posterior subluxation. Such designs include the Insall-Burstein Posterior Stabilized (Zimmer) and the Kinematic Stabilizer (Howmedica). Semiconstrained *conforming condylar* prostheses incorporate varus-valgus freedom and prevent posterior subluxation by virtue of a roller-in-trough design (Fig 75–5). Perhaps the best-known design of this type is the Total Condylar prosthesis (Johnson & Johnson Orthopaedics). *Posterior cruciate–retaining* prostheses (Fig 75–6) retain the PCL and allow significant degrees of freedom in all planes of motion. These designs include, but are not limited to the AGC (Anatomically Graduated Components, Biomet), the AMK (Anatomic Modular Knee, (DePuy), the Genesis (Richards, Memphis TN), the Maxim Knee (Biomet), the Miller-Galante Total Knee Arthroplasty System (Zimmer), the PCA (Porous Coated Anatomic, Howmedica), the Press Fit Condylar (Johnson & Johnson Orthopaedics), and the Whiteside Ortholoc Modular Knee System (Dow Corning Wright, Arlington, TN).

The evolution of knee joint prostheses was wrought by many technical and engineering changes. The orthopaedic surgeon involved in total joint arthroplasty today has an overwhelming selection of devices, each with various features from which to

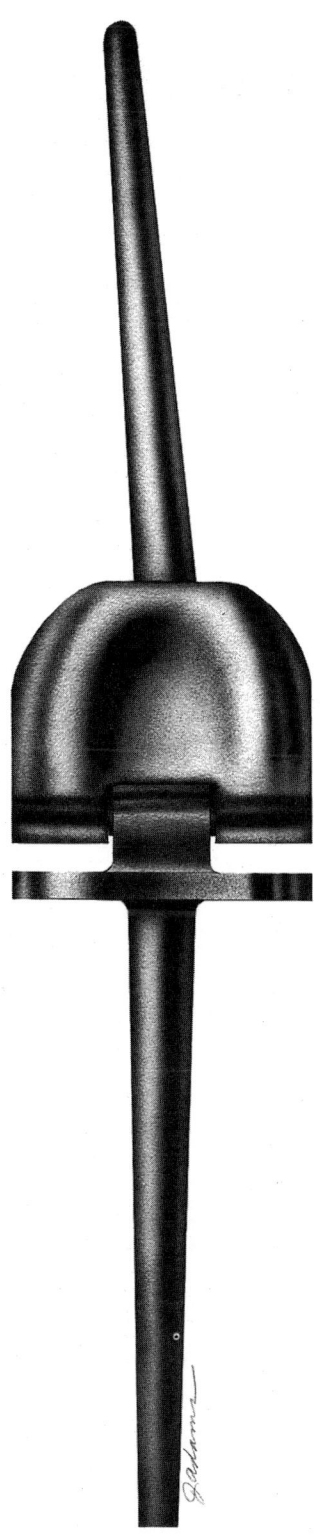

FIG 75–1.
Rigid-hinge device is a constrained linked design which allows only flexion and extension. All other degrees of freedom are restricted by these devices.

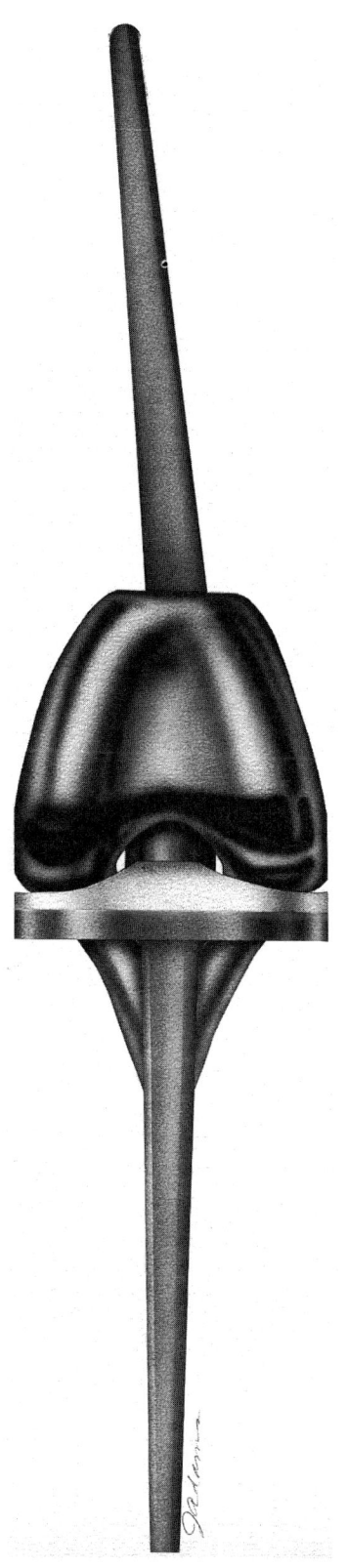

FIG 75–2.
Rotating-hinge device is a constrained linked design which allows rotation within the flexion-extension axis of the knee. Varus-valgus deflection and anteroposterior displacement are prohibited by virtue of the linkage.

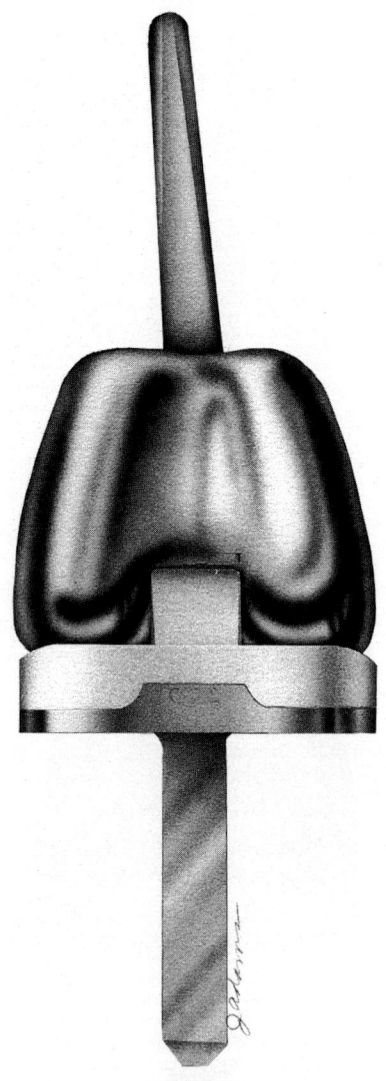

FIG 75–3.
The constrained condylar device is an unlinked constrained design which places limitations on varus-valgus deflection, anteroposterior displacement, and rotation within the flexion-extension axis of the knee. Restriction of varus-valgus deflection and rotation is provided by a large tibial spine within an intracondylar femoral box, while posterior subluxation is prevented by engagement of the spine upon the femoral cam.

choose. It behooves the orthopaedic surgeon to be familiar with each category of knee prosthesis, the indications for these devices, and the short- to long-term results to be expected from them.

INDICATIONS

Within the preoperative planning scheme for total knee replacement, the surgeon must evaluate and determine the basis for the progressive degenerative joint disorder, degree of related pain, the compromising adjustments made within the patient's normal activities of daily living, and the potential benefit of the

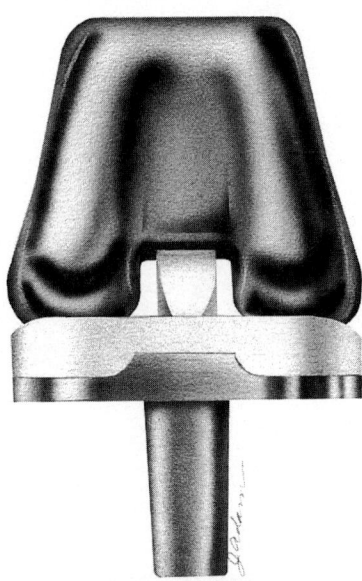

FIG 75–4.
Posterior-stabilized device. Nonlinked semiconstrained posterior stabilized devices prevent posterior subluxation via a tibial spine which engages a femoral cam. Slight rotational constraint is afforded by the degree of conformity of the femorotibial articulation.

surgical procedure in restoring joint normalcy.[82] Once the criteria for surgery have been met, physical and roentgenographic evaluations of the knee joint are of paramount importance in determining the type of device that should be used for the scheduled arthroplasty.

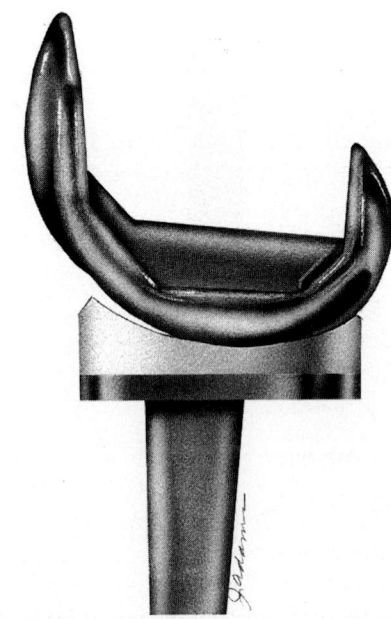

FIG 75–5.
Conforming condylar device. Nonlinked conforming condylar devices are essentially roller-in-trough designs which provide anteroposterior stability by virtue of the degree of conforming femorotibial articulation. As a result, slight rotational constraint also occurs.

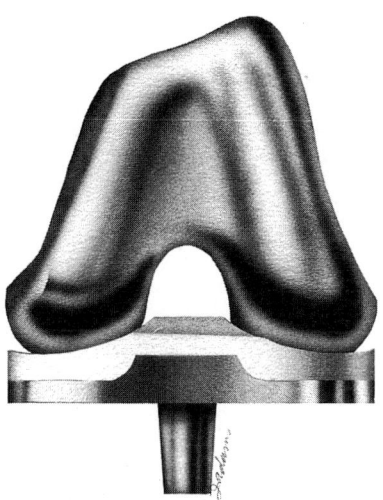

FIG 75–6.
Posterior cruciate ligament–retaining device. Nonlinked posterior cruciate–retaining devices are totally nonconstrained surface replacements with very little conformity with respect to the femortibial articulation.

Rigid-Hinge Prostheses

While the reported results of the early trials of rigid-hinge replacement knee arthroplasty were deemed unacceptable,[3] a more clearly defined set of indications were subsequently developed. A current primary indication for the rigid-hinge device is the patient who presents with incompetence of both collateral ligaments and associated weakness or deficiency of the extensor mechanism.[16, 63, 81]

This category typically includes patients who have undergone extensive resection of the quadriceps mechanism secondary to limb salvage procedures,[79] patients with associated neuromuscular disease such as poliomyelitis, and multiply revised patients whose only other option is arthrodesis. These patient categories represent a very desperate group. The lack of acceptance of arthrodesis and its functional limitations and long-term sequelae led to the rigid-hinged device.

Rotating-Hinge Prostheses

Cognizant of the extreme rotatory torque stresses in rigid-hinge arthroplasty, rotating-hinge designs were developed.[16, 63, 81] The indications for these designs are similar to those previously mentioned for the rigid-hinge, with the exception that these patients have intact and well-functioning extensor mechanisms.

Patients in this category include multiply revised patients with attenuated collateral ligament systems but intact extensor mechanisms, and patients undergoing total knee reimplantation for sepsis who, by virtue of the destruction caused by sepsis and the need for radical debridement, have attenuated collateral ligament systems and, again, intact extensor mechanisms. Rotating-hinge prostheses are indicated for the following:

1. Patients undergoing revision knee arthroplasty secondary to supracondylar fracture about a total knee arthroplasty. Elderly and compromised patients with periprosthetic fractures that are associated with multiple comminution and significant osteopenia can be managed with a large-segment distal femoral allograft and with a long-stem rotating-hinge device to satisfactorily restore function[13, 42] (Fig 75–7, A–E).

2. Patients who suffer from an extremely "stiff knee."[62] This may be encountered in both primary and revision situations. In these cases, exposure is best afforded by the "femoral peel" approach described by Windsor and Insall.[91] The technique involves stripping of the entire ligamentous complex from the distal femur to allow for correction of the deformity and adequate exposure of the knee joint. Reconstruction is then carried out with either the constrained condylar prosthesis or the rotating-hinged prosthetic device based on the degree of stability and the flexion-extension gap balance.

3. The reconstructive orthopaedic surgeon should contemplate the use of a rotating-hinge design in revisional surgery in which there is extreme imbalance of the flexion-extension gaps, especially in light of reports of dislocation of constrained condylar designs[83] (Fig 75–8, A and B).

Constrained Condylar Prostheses

Constrained condylar prostheses are nonlinked devices with a significant degree of constraint.[30, 31, 67] By virtue of an extended tibial spine which fits snugly within the intracondylar notch of the femoral component, these designs place restriction on motion in three planes: anteroposterior, varus-valgus, and rotational. However, these designs are not as rigid in constraint as hinged devices, since they are unlinked. Several degrees of varus-valgus and rotational deflection are inherent in the design as well as anteroposterior displacement. The earliest of these designs is the Total Condylar III, which has evolved into the current Insall-Burstein Constrained Condylar system. The most significant modifications are the incorporation of modularity and conversion from cemented stems to press-fit stems. Several other posterior-stabilized constrained systems have emerged to offer

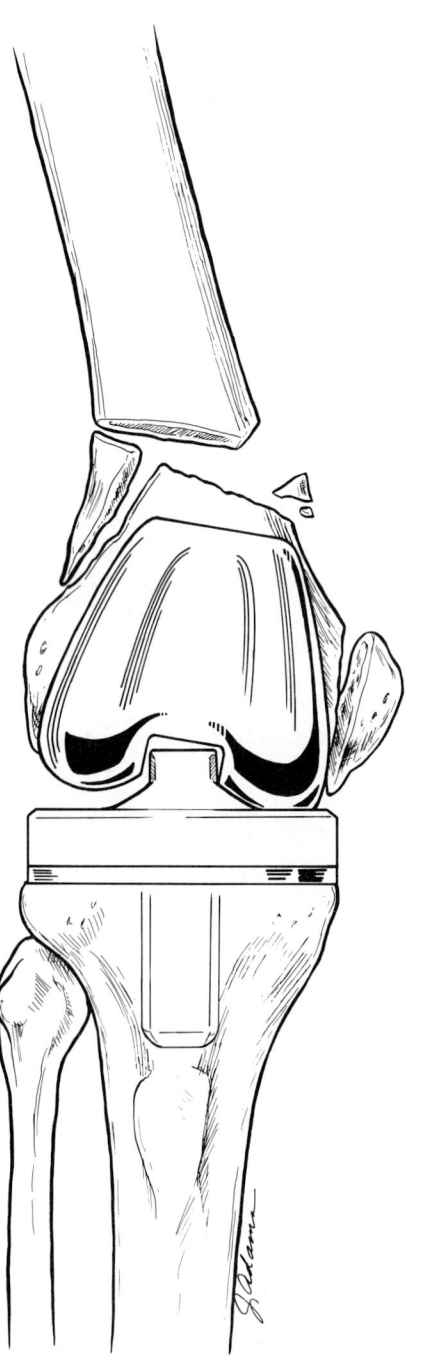
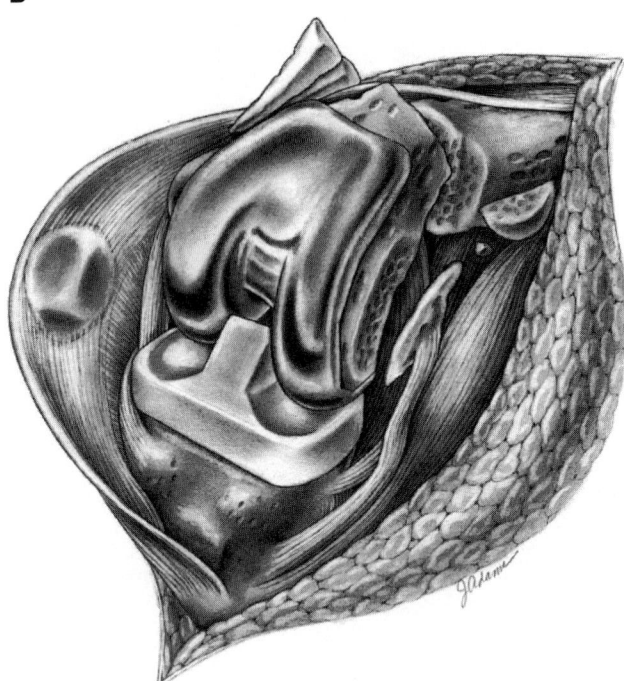
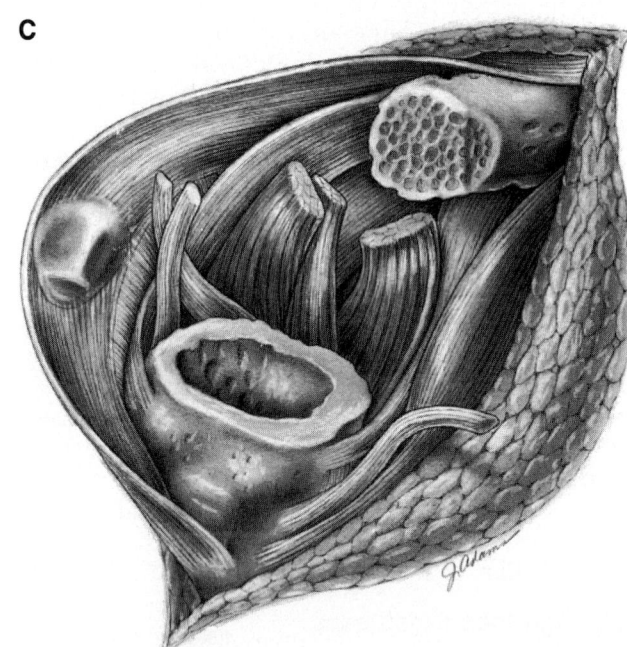

FIG 75–7.
A, comminuted periprosthetic fracture complicated by significant osteopenia. **B,** intraoperatively, multiple fracture fragments are identified. Significant osteopenia is noted. Attenuation of the collateral ligament systems is found. **C,** the prosthesis and multiple fragments of bone have been removed with resultant deficiency of the distal femur and associated ligamentous incompetence of the medial and lateral collateral ligaments as well as the posterior cruciate ligament.

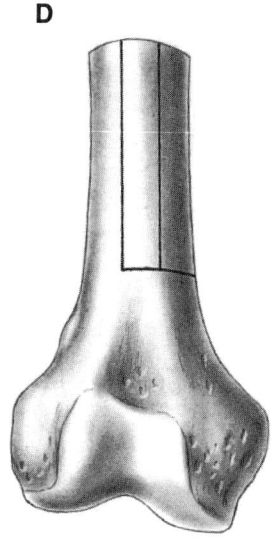
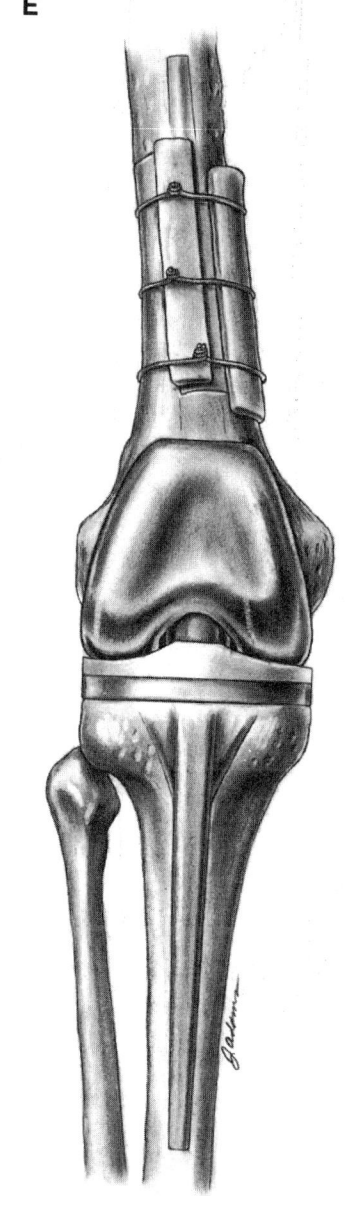

FIG 75-7 (cont.).
D and **E,** reconstruction is accomplished with a large-segment distal femoral allograft in conjunction with a long-stemmed rotating-hinge design.

the surgeon the enhanced ability of intraoperative customization of the prosthesis via modular stems, wedges, augments, and an increased inventory of sizes. Constrained condylar prostheses represent the most frequently used constrained knee replacement systems.* They are indicated in primary and revision arthroplasty that is complicated by ligamentous deficiency.

Constrained condylar prostheses are indicated in the patient undergoing primary arthroplasty who presents with a significant valgus deformity and asso-

*References 1, 9, 14, 17, 24, 28–30, 39–41, 44, 46, 48, 49, 61, 70, 74, 77.

ciated flexion contracture. This has been classified by Krackow[43] as a type II valgus deformity. Therefore, these patients have a significantly stretched medial collateral ligament (MCL). In these patients, the reconstructive orthopaedic surgeon has three choices. The first is reconstruction using nonconstrained or semiconstrained devices following appropriate bony resections (Fig 75–9) and release of lateral structures (Fig 75–10) to obtain normal alignment and therefore restore the mechanical axis. This must be accompanied by reconstruction of the MCL as described by Krackow[43] (Fig 75–11). The primary advantage is the minimal degree of constraint. Disadvantages are the requirement for extended bracing postoperatively

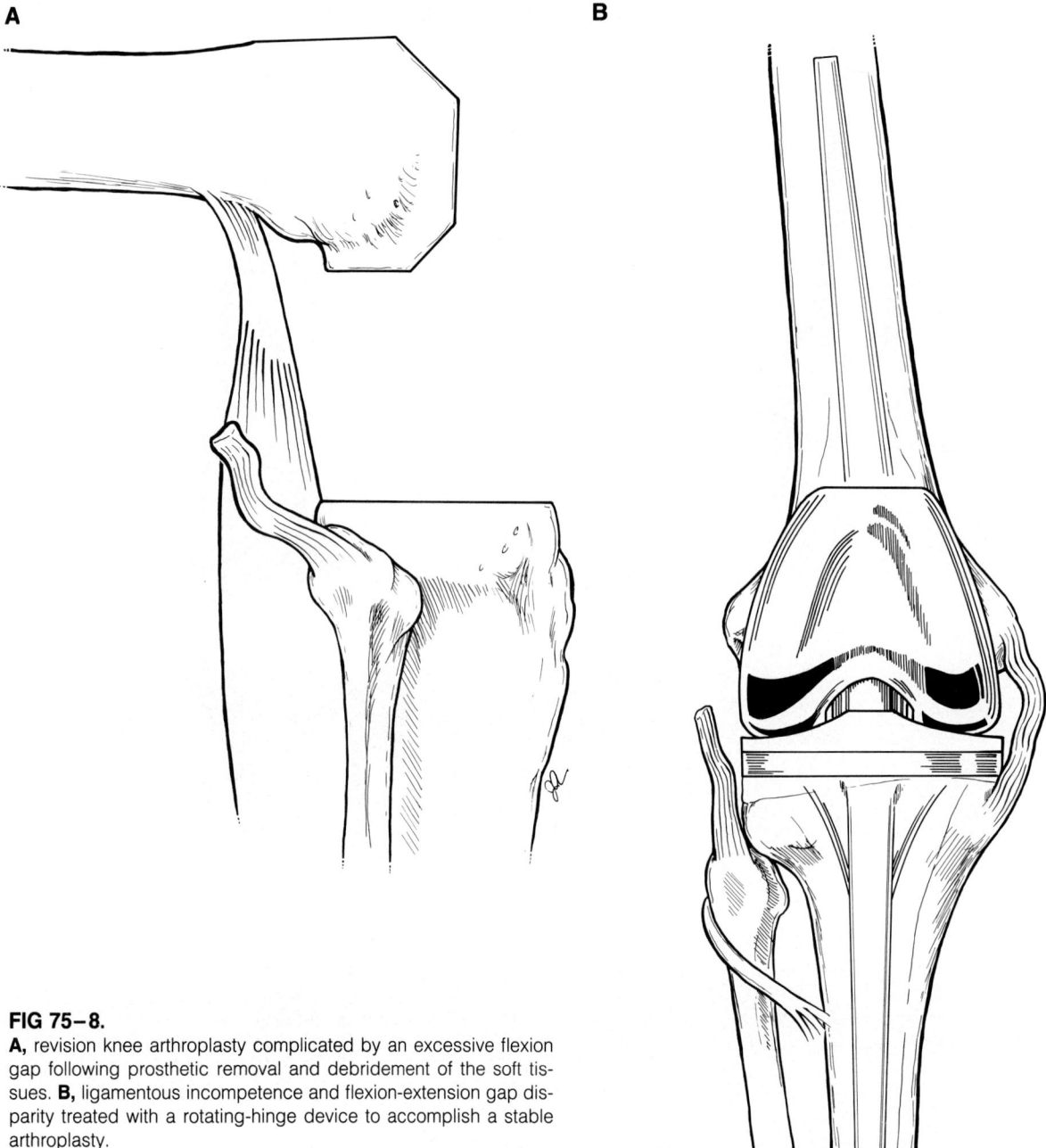

FIG 75–8.
A, revision knee arthroplasty complicated by an excessive flexion gap following prosthetic removal and debridement of the soft tissues. **B,** ligamentous incompetence and flexion-extension gap disparity treated with a rotating-hinge device to accomplish a stable arthroplasty.

and modification of the physical therapy and rehabilitation programs in order to protect the reconstruction of the MCL.

A second option is reconstruction using nonconstrained or semiconstrained devices with appropriate bony resections (see Fig 75–9) and extensive lateral release (Fig 75–10) in order to obtain balance of the knee with an excessively thick tibial polyethylene spacer (Fig 75–12). The advantage is avoidance of constraint, while the disadvantages are the difficulty in obtaining satisfactory balance between flexion-extension gaps and significant alteration of the joint

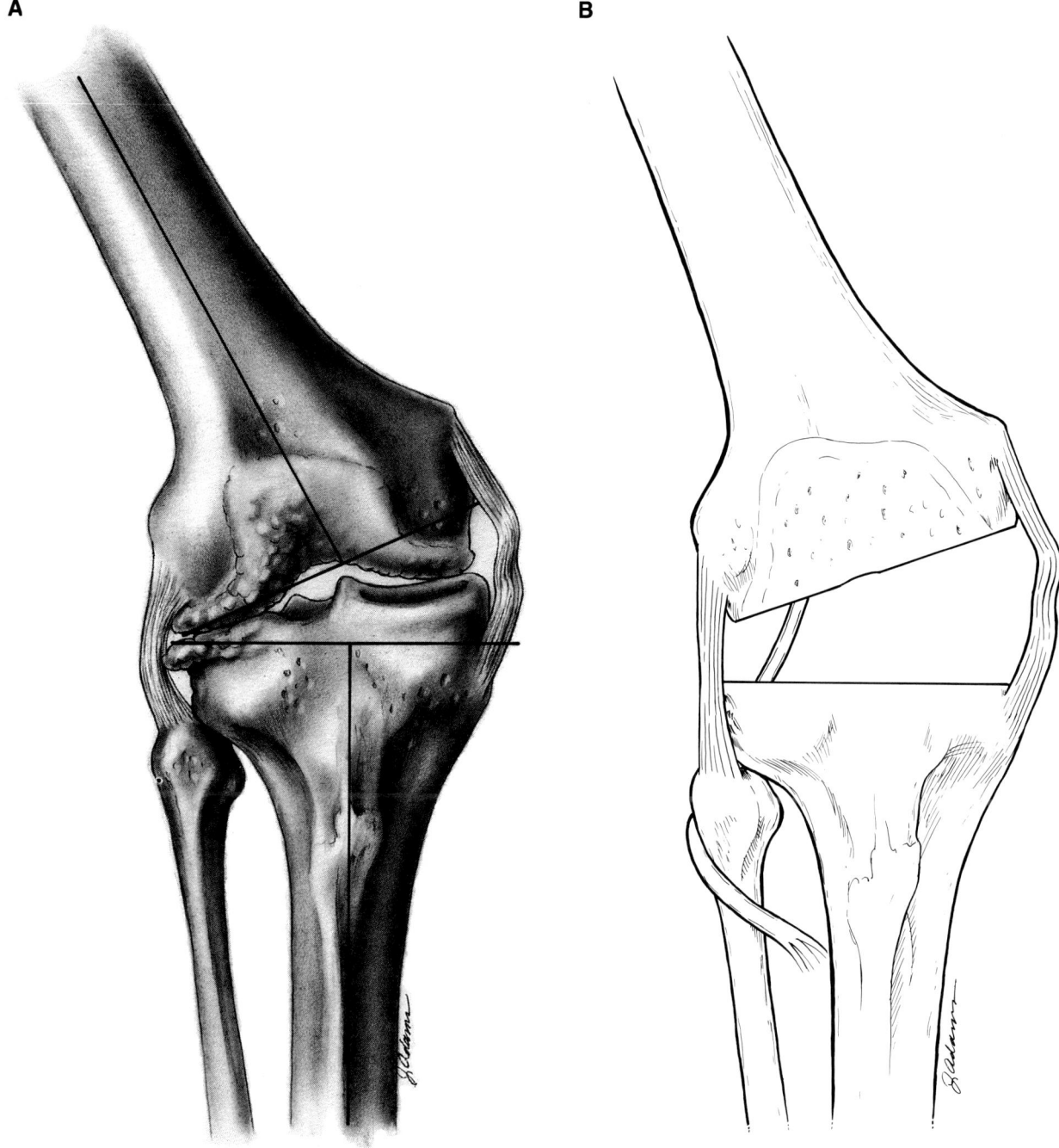

FIG 75-9.
A, preoperative planning in a type II valgus knee. Bony resections are planned so that the femoral resection is accomplished at 5 to 7 degrees of valgus alignment and the tibial resection at 90 degrees to the tibial axis. These bony resections allow for reconstruction of the mechanical axis. **B,** appropriate bony resections accomplished in a type II valgus deformity. Note significant contracture of the lateral soft tissue structures.

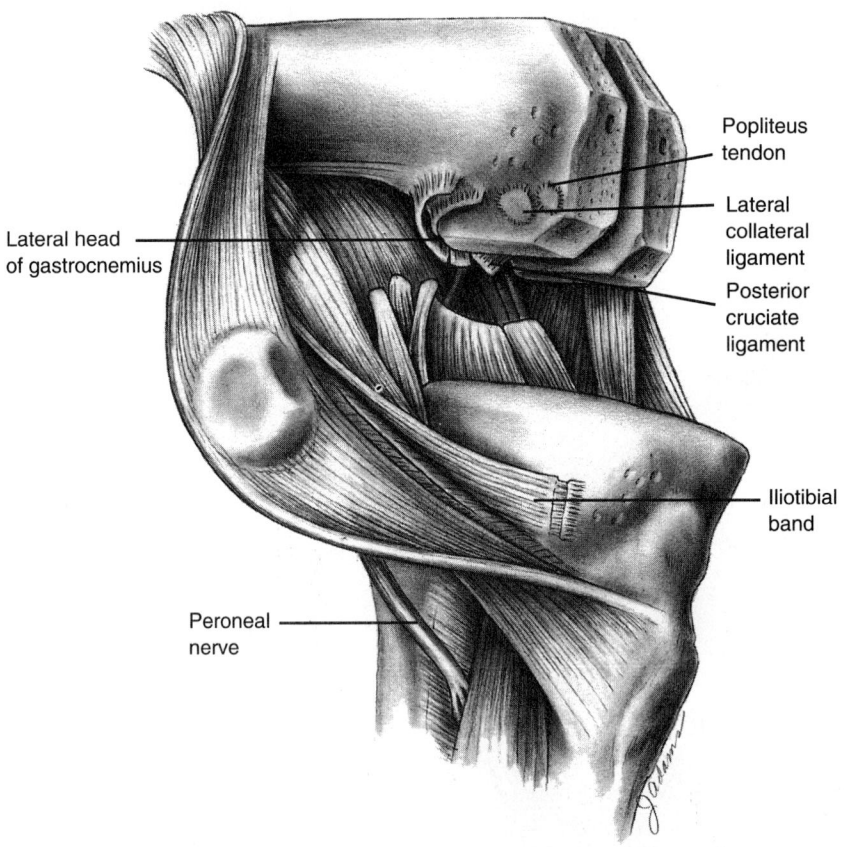

FIG 75–10.
Sequential release of contracted lateral structures in a type II valgus deformity including release of the illiotibial band, popliteus tendon, lateral collateral ligament, posterior capsule, and lateral head of the gastrocnemius.

line (see Fig 75–12), and therefore associated alteration of the tibial-patellofemoral dynamics.[17, 67]

The final option is the use of a constrained condylar prosthesis in which appropriate bony resections (see Fig 75–9) and sufficient lateral releases (see Fig 74–10) are performed to reconstruct the mechanical axis (Fig 75–13). The advantages of this approach are the inherent stability without the need for postoperative bracing, maintenance of the joint line, and therefore little or no alteration of the patellotibial-femoral dynamics, and a lower probability of peroneal palsy secondary to stretch. The potential disadvantage is the use of constraint.

Posterior-Stabilized Prostheses

Posterior-stabilized devices are nonlinked devices with a minimal degree of constraint. These designs have their origin with the Insall-Burstein Posterior Stabilized Condylar prosthesis, which was designed and developed at The Hospital for Special Surgery in New York City in 1978.[29] The design incorporates a tibial spine and femoral cam. The tibial spine engages the femoral cam and prevents posterior subluxation. The indications for these devices are extremely controversial. Laskin et al.[46] reported that PCL–substituting designs were indicated in patients with combined varus-valgus deformities and associated flexion contractures. In patients with excessive deformity in which the PCL was retained, flexion contractures and malalignment persisted postoperatively.

Conforming Condylar Prostheses

Conforming condylar devices are nonlinked devices in which the degree of constraint is derived from the conformity between the femoral and tibial components in the sagittal plane. The articulation in conjunction with collateral ligament tension provides anteroposterior stability in these roller-in-trough designs.[43] Furthermore, the degree of conformity of the articulating surfaces places some constraint on the rotation of the femoral device

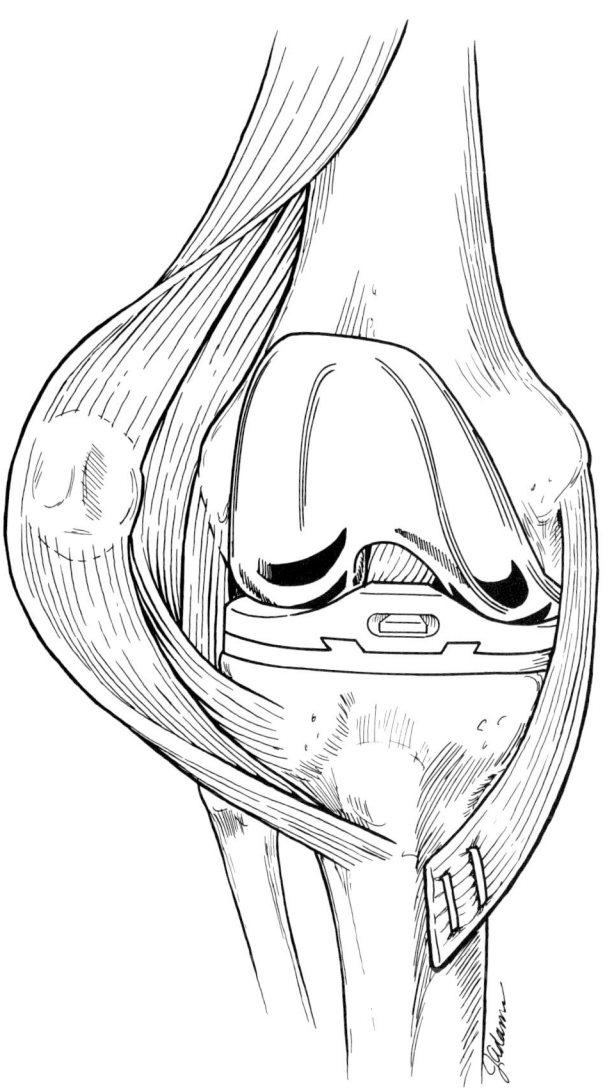

FIG 75–11.
Reconstruction of a type II valgus deformity using a nonconstrained device and medial collateral ligament advancement.

upon the tibial component. The Total Condylar prosthesis was developed with this design rationale. Concerns regarding inadequate flexion, posterior subluxation, and difficulty with stair climbing led to the development of the Insall-Burstein Posterior Stabilized device.[29]

Posterior Cruciate Ligament–Retaining Prostheses

The final category of nonlinked prosthetic devices are the PCL-retaining devices. These devices are indicated in patients with mild to moderate joint destruction and deformity, and with intact collateral and posterior cruciate ligaments. The 1980s have wit-

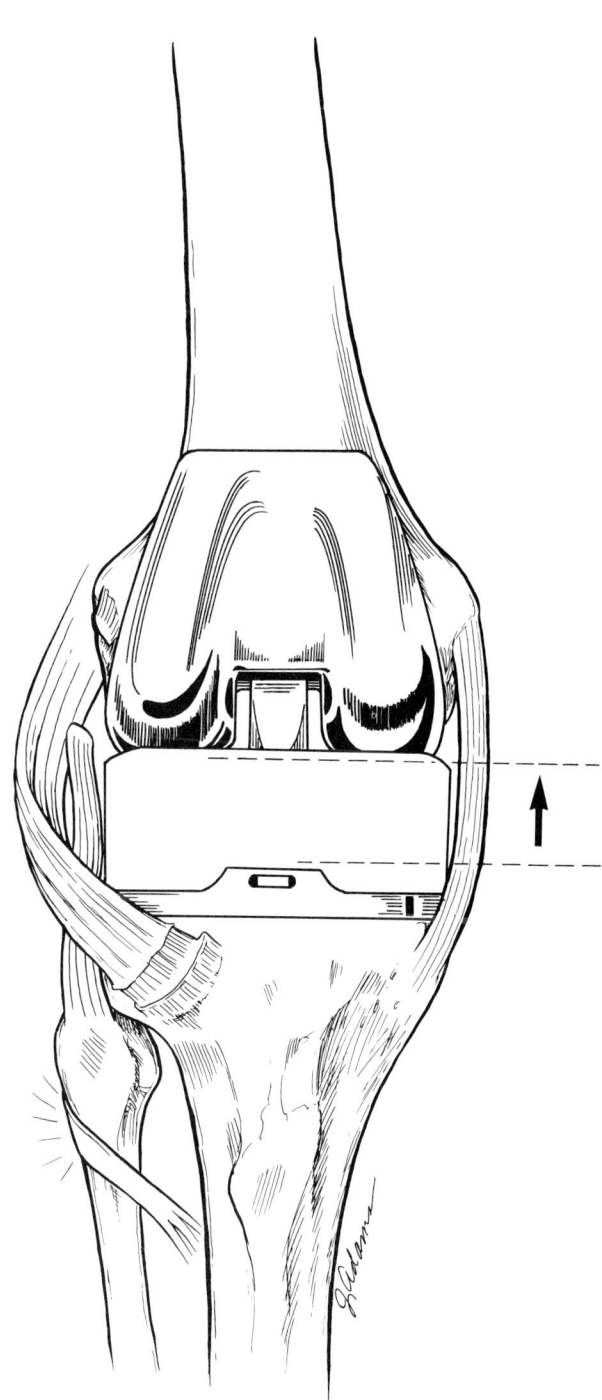

FIG 75–12.
Reconstruction of type II valgus deformity using a nonconstrained device. Stability of the arthroplasty is accomplished by tensing of the medial collateral ligament with a thick tibial component. Joint line alteration occurs with associated alteration of the patellotibial-femoral dynamics. Additionally, peroneal palsy may occur as a result of tension on the peroneal nerve.

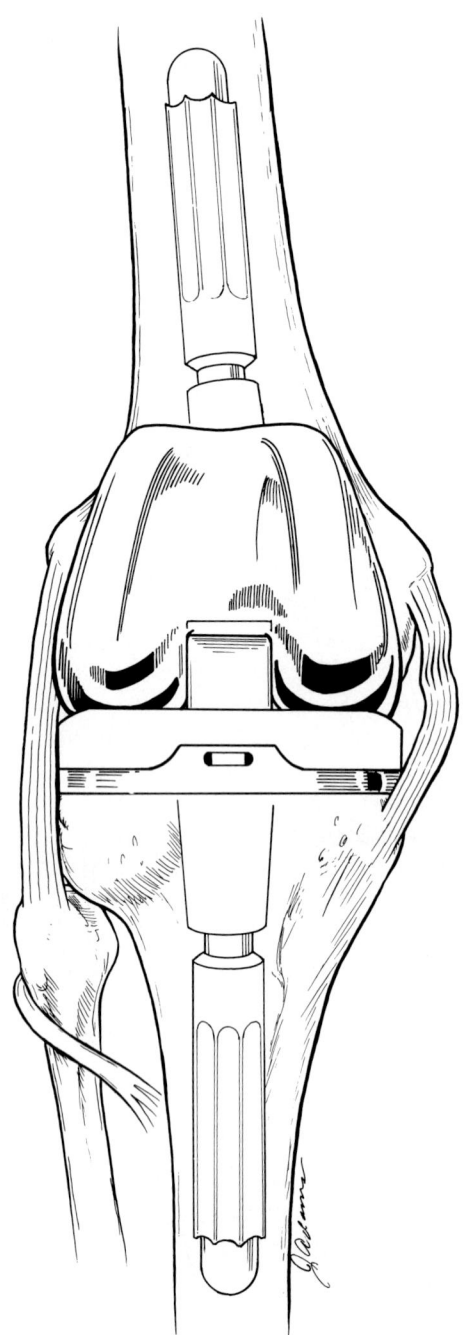

FIG 75–13.
Reconstruction of the type II valgus deformity using a constrained condylar device. Note that the joint line is maintained and that inherent stability is provided by the prosthetic design.

nessed a significant increase in the number of posterior cruciate–retaining designs. These designs are essentially variations of a generic condylar total knee arthroplasty design.

SURGICAL TECHNIQUES

The surgical technique for constrained total knee arthroplasty is essentially no different from that for nonconstrained knee arthroplasty. When confronting a complex primary or revision total knee arthroplasty, the reconstructive surgeon must understand the degree of constraint required for the patient and afforded by the various prosthetic designs. The surgical technique for constrained total knee arthroplasty is described here with respect to revision total knee arthroplasty, since a higher percentage of revision arthroplasties will require constrained designs. In order to accomplish successful revision, the surgeon must use an ordered and progressive procedural algorithm (Fig 75–14).

Exposure

Patients who require constrained total knee arthroplasty will often have undergone a number of previous operative interventions. To minimize postoperative wound complications, previous incisions should be used or incorporated into the incision. If there are multiple incisions across the anterior aspect of the knee, the new incision should favor the shortest of the previous incisions. If the previous parapatellar incisions are of equal length, then either one can be used.[11] In the stiff or contracted knee, exposure via the straight midline skin approach and standard medial peripatellar arthrotomy may not be adequate. A modification of the Coonse-Adams[10] or V-Y turndown may assist with exposure.[61, 78] Another approach may be the tibial tubercle slide osteotomy described by Whiteside and Ohl.[88]

Prosthesis Removal

Exposure of the interfaces is mandatory for successful removal of the implants with preservation of bone stock. In the case of cemented devices, the prosthesis-cement interface should be violated. In the case of a cemented all-polyethylene patella, the reciprocating saw can be used to disrupt the prosthesis-cement interface. The surgeon should proceed through the patellar peg or pegs. These can then be removed either with a small osteotome and mallet or a dental burr. With respect to a metal-backed cementless patella, a flexible osteotome can be utilized at the prosthesis-bone interface. A cemented femoral component can be removed using a combination of reciprocating saw, flexible osteotomes, and pencil-tip AM-10 Midas Rex instrumentation (Midas Rex Pneu-

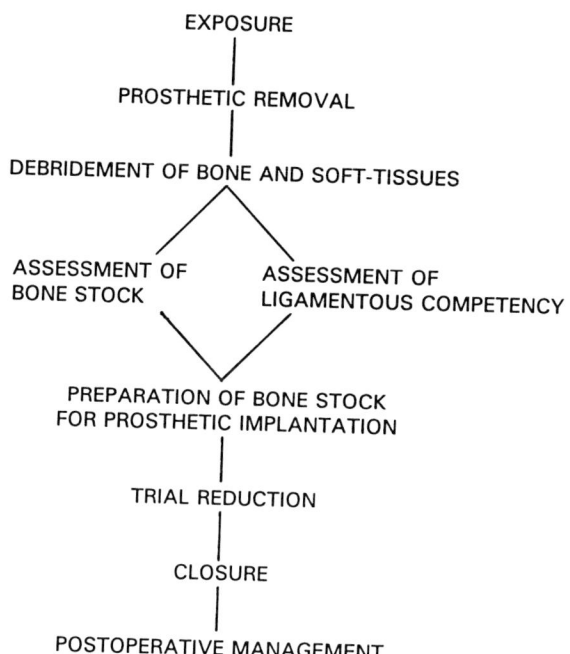

FIG 75-14.
Revision algorithm.

matic Tools, Fort Worth, TX). For cementless devices, Firestone and Krackow[19] have described a method of using a giggly-saw to separate the prosthesis-bone interface. Cemented all-polyethylene tibial components can be removed by using a reciprocating saw violating the prosthetic bone interface and severing the stem from the remainder of the component. Flexible osteotomes and the pencil-tipped AM-10 Midas Rex instrumentation can then be used to remove the stem from the proximal tibia. Cement tools or high-speed burrs can then be used to remove the remainder of the polymethylmethacrylate. Cemented, metal backed tibial components can be removed by disrupting the prosthesis-cement interface with a reciprocating saw. A mallet and retrodriver is then used to remove the component. Cementless tibial components are dealt with in much the same way. After removal of any screws, the reciprocating saw interrupts the prosthesis-bone interface and a mallet or retrodriver is used to remove the component.

Debridement of Bone and Soft Tissue

Once the prosthetic devices have been removed, the femur, tibia, and patella must be debrided of the remaining polymethylmethacrylate and fibrinous material. The surgeon may elect to use hand tools, high-speed burrs, or ultrasound. Additionally, any remaining periarticular scar tissue, especially in the posterior recess of the knee, should be thoroughly excised.

Assessment of Bone Stock

Upon successful removal of the prosthetic components and complete debridement of bone and soft tissues, the surgeon must assess the remaining bone stock. Issues which need to be addressed are the quantity of bone loss from both the distal femur and proximal tibia and the presence of any disparity in bone loss from either the medial or lateral femoral condyle or mediolateral tibial plateau.[43] The presence and degree of these deficiencies will dictate the requirement for use of stems and augments or bone grafts, individually or severally.

Assessment of Ligamentous Competence

In conjunction with assessing the status of the remaining bone stock, the surgeon must assess ligamentous competence. The status of the MCL and lateral collateral ligament (LCL) must be noted. Additionally, the competence of the bone stock to which they are attached should be evaluated. If there is a significant deficiency of the medial or lateral epicondyle with associated osteopenia, fracture of either epicondyle may occur with associated collateral ligament incompetence if the arthroplasty is performed with a nonconstrained device.

Preparation of Bone Stock for Prosthesis Implantation

Based on the assessments of bone stock and ligamentous competence, the surgeon then selects the appropriate implant. The goal is construction of the implant to accommodate deficiencies in bone stock and ligamentous structures. Bone stock deficiencies are dealt with by incorporation of stems, metallic augments, wedges, or bone grafts, while ligamentous deficiency is handled with varying degrees of constraint. With intact MCL, LCL, PCL, and extensor mechanism, a PCL-retaining arthroplasty can be performed. When there is a deficiency only with the PCL, but the remaining structures are intact, a PCL-substituting arthroplasty should be performed. When there is a deficiency of the PCL and one of the collateral ligament complexes, a constrained condylar arthroplasty should be performed. When there is a deficiency of the PCL and both collateral ligament structures, but an intact extensor mechanism, a rotating-hinge arthroplasty should be performed. When there

TABLE 75-1.
Musculotendinous and Ligamentous Assessment*

Prosthesis	Quadriceps Mechanism	MCL	LCL	PCL
Rigid-hinge	D	D	D	D
Rotating-hinge	I	D	D	D
Constrained condylar	I	D	I	D
	I	I	D	D
Posterior-stabilized	I	I	I	D
Conforming Condylar	I	I	I	D
PCL-retaining	I	I	I	I

*MCL = medial collateral ligament; LCL = lateral collateral ligament; PCL = posterior cruciate ligament; D = deficient; I = intact.

is a deficiency of the PCL, mediolateral collaterals, and the extensor mechanism, a rigid-hinge arthroplasty should be performed. Using this algorithm (Table 75-1), the surgeon can reconstruct from the simplest to the most difficult arthroplasty.

Trial Reduction

As with primary total knee arthroplasty, once the prosthesis has been selected and bony preparation has been performed, a trial reduction must be accomplished to assess the competence of the prosthetic complex.

Implantation

Controversy exists as to whether these arthroplasties should be performed with cementless techniques or with polymethylmethacrylate.[20] A combined technique has been reported in the literature[59] and remains our preferred technique. The technique involves implantation of the prosthesis using press-fit femoral and tibial stems, metallic augments to accommodate bony deficiencies, and surface cement fixation.

Closure

Closure is accomplished in the traditional manner. Special attention, however, must be directed to arthrotomies performed using the Coonse-Adams or modified V-Y quadricepsplasty. In these cases, closures should be accomplished with the knee flexed to about 30 degrees.[78] Once the extensor mechanism is approximated, the surgeon should flex the knee to the point of suture disruption. This should be noted, and no flexion beyond this point is advisable for the first 10 to 12 weeks postoperatively. An extensive quadriceps rehabilitation is imperative to avoid a quadriceps lag.

Postoperative Management

The postoperative physical therapy and rehabilitation course should be individualized for the specific operative procedure. The vast majority of these constrained arthroplasties will follow a very routine operative approach and therefore require routine postoperative management. However, in those situations in which there is evidence of wound compromise secondary to extensive surgical dissection or in which a modified approach is used, such as the V-Y quadricepsplasty or the tibial tubercle osteotomy, postoperative patient management must be modified accordingly. Immobilization in a long leg cast for a period of 4 to 6 weeks may be required to allow for satisfactory wound healing.

CLINICAL REVIEW

The evaluation of reported results affords the clinician a mechanism to assess prosthetic devices and the surgical techniques associated with each. While true META analyses are difficult to perform within the realm of current orthopaedic literature, published studies can be compared so that an understanding of trends can be inferred. A review of our records from 1980 to the present reveal that 4,233 total knee arthroplasties have been performed, comprising 3,510 primary and 723 revision total knee arthroplasties. Table 75-2 lists the number of arthroplasties and the particular type of arthroplasty performed according to prosthetic category. Rigid-hinge, rotating-hinge, and constrained condylar devices were used in both primary and revision total knee arthroplasties according to the indications outlined in the previous discussion.

In published results of various rigid-hinge arthroplasty devices (Table 75-3), complications included septic and aseptic loosening, patellar subluxation and fracture, femoral and tibial fracture, and implant failure.[3, 6, 12, 23, 33] Revision rates ranged from 6% to 22%

TABLE 75-2.
Total Knee Arthroplasties Performed by Category, 1980–1992*

Prosthesis	Primary	Revision
Linked		
Rigid-hinge	0	4
Rotating-hinge	15	103
Nonlinked		
Constrained condylar	205	279
Posterior-stabilized	2,366	319
Conforming condylar	0	0
Posterior cruciate ligament–retaining	924	18
Total	3,510	723

*Data from Joint Implant Surgeons, Inc., Columbus, Ohio.

TABLE 75-3.
Results of Rigid-Hinge Arthroplasty*

Authors	Primary/Revision	No. of Knees	Follow-up (yr)	Good–Excellent (%)	Revised (%)	No. Revised—Reason
Bargar et al.[3]†	P	39	2–4	NA	16	4—Eroded patella
	R	17	2–4	NA		3—Wear debris
						2—Deep sepsis
Cameron & Jung[6]†	P	8	1–7	NA	22	4—Patellar complications
	P	19	1–7	NA		1—Aseptic loosening
						1—Tibial shaft fracture
Deburge & GUEPAR[12]	P	103	≥2 years	NA	6	6—Aseptic loosening
Haberman et al.[23]	P	18	1.0–3.5	NA	11	1—Deep infection
						1—Penetration of femoral cortex
Jones et al.[33]	P	45	1–7	NA	7	3—Deep infection

*NA = not available; no HSS scores available.
†Percentage revised and reasons are combined for primary and revision cases.

in follow-up from 1 to 7 years. Many authors* recommend that rigid-hinge arthroplasty be used in only severely disabled patients with major fixed deformities and in extreme salvage situations when arthrodesis represents the only alternative. Engelbrecht and Heinert,[16] however, reporting on both the St. Georg rigid-hinge arthroplasty and the Link Endo-Model Rotational Knee arthroplasty, present favorable results with both implants. They conclude that implants with varying degrees of constraint are required to accommodate various patient profiles. Upon reviewing other published reports of rotating-hinge devices (Table 75-4), revision rates range from 0% to as high as 43%, as reported by Rand et al.[71] The consensus from the literature is that rotating-hinge devices should be used in patients with severe soft tissue deficits.*

Table 75-5 outlines the published results of the Total Condylar III prosthesis. With a follow-up range of 2 to 12 years, 102 primary Total Condylar III knee arthroplasties were reported with revision rate of 0% and 204 revision Total Condylar III knee arthroplasties yielding revision rates from 0% to 36%. The consensus from these studies is that a place does exist in the surgical armamentarium for the constrained condylar designs.† Montgomery et al.[59] and Rand[70] describe the potential for improvement in results with constrained condylar designs which are modular so that press-fit noncemented intramedullary rods

*See references, 3, 4, 12, 21–23, 25, 26, 31, 33–35, 37, 45, 47, 56, 57, 60, 73, 75, 84, 87, 90.

*References 5, 16, 18, 38, 42, 45, 51, 52, 57, 63, 71, 81.
†References 9, 14, 17, 24, 28, 29, 39, 41, 44, 46, 48, 49, 70, 74, 77.

TABLE 75-4.
Results of Rotating-Hinge Arthroplasty*

Authors	Primary/Revision	No. of Knees	Follow-up (yr)	Good–Excellent	Revised (%)	No. Revised—Reason
Engelbrecht & Heinert[16]	P	1,075	1–8	NA	1	6—Aseptic loosening
						3—Bone fracture
						4—Dislocation of component
						2—Material fracture
Finn et al.[18]	P/R	23	1	NA	0	
Kaufer & Matthews[38]	P	82	2–6	NA	4	3—Loosening
Matthews et al.[51]	P	58	2–6	NA	21	8—Loosening
						4—Deep infection
Murray et al.[60]	P	23	1–2	NA	17	4—Material breakage
Rand et al.[71]	P	15	2–6	33%	20	3—Material breakage
	R	23	2–6	70%	43	5—Material breakage
						3—Aseptic loosening
						2—Femoral fracture
Sonstegard et al.[81]	P	25	2–3	NA	0	

*NA = not available; no HSS scores available.

TABLE 75-5.

Results of Total Condylar III Arthroplasty*

Authors	Primary/Revision	No. of Knees	Follow-up (yr)	Preoperative HSS	Postoperative HSS	Good–Excellent (%)	Revised (%)	No. Revised—Reason
Chotivichit et al.[9]	P	9	2–8	45.0	77.0	89	0	
	R	18	2–8	51.0	74.0	78	0	
Donaldson et al.[14]	P	17	2–8	28.5	82.5	100	0	
	R	14	2–8	44.8	51.2	50	36	3—Deep infection 2—Aseptic loosening
Hohl et al.[24]	P	6	2–12	16.2	73.3	66	0	
	R	29	2–12	23.1	73.8	72	10	2—Deep infection 1—Aseptic loosening
Insall et al.[30]	P	220	3–5	43.0	84.0	9	4	3—Infection 2—Subluxation 2—Patellar replacement
Kavolus et al.[39]	P	5	5	NA	93.4	100	0	
	R	11	4	NA	84.0	91	0	
Kim[40]	R	14	2–6	58.0	81.0	NA	0	
Lombardi et al.[48]	P	65	3–10	47.0	88.0	98	0	
Lombardi et al.[49]	R	62	2–5	NA	NA	77	8	3—Deep infection 1—Supracondylar fracture 1—Aseptic loosening
Rand[70]	R	20	2–7	41.0	73.0	50	10	1—Deep infection 1—Preexisting supracondylar fixation
Rosenberg et al.[74]	R	36	2–8	36.0	77.0	69	3	1—Patellar wear

*HSS = The Hospital for Special Surgery scoring system; NA = not available.

can be used in combination with metallic augments and wedges.

CONCLUSION

The current practice of total knee arthroplasty has its basis in a large and diverse evolution of concepts and designs. Design convergence has led to a condylar type of knee arthroplasty system (Fig 75-15). These condylar designs have enjoyed great clinical success in both the PCL-retaining design as well as the PCL-substituting design, with long-term studies demonstrating greater than 90% survivorship at 10 or more years.[14, 28, 68, 69, 76]

Despite the fact that these two designs are used in the vast majority of total knee arthroplasties per-

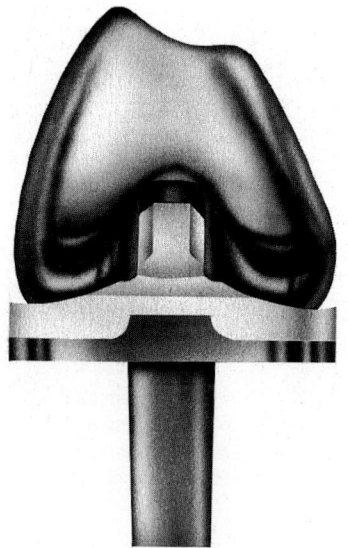
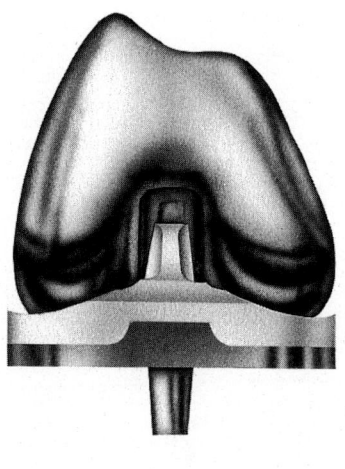
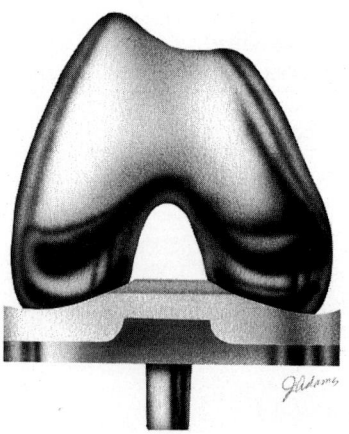

FIG 75-15.
A condylar total knee system offering components with varying degrees of constraint from the constrained condylar to the posterior-stabilized to the posterior cruciate–retaining design.

formed, there continues to be a need in individual cases for constrained total knee arthroplasty. The indications have been outlined in this chapter. The results have been presented and certainly are inferior to the results of primary PCL-retaining and PCL-substituting knee arthroplasties. However, it should be noted that constrained arthroplasties are used in complex primary and revision knee arthroplasty in which there is compromise of the bony anatomy and soft tissue structures. With a clear understanding of the specific indications, improved knowledge of the kinematics of the knee, refined modular designs, and sophisticated instrument systems, the orthopaedic surgeon can rationally and consistently address a wide spectrum of knee reconstructions.

REFERENCES

1. Aglietti P, Rinonapoli E: Total condylar knee arthroplasty: A five-year follow-up study of 33 knees, *Clin Orthop* 186:104–111, 1984.
2. Aufranc OE: Arthroplasty: Constructive hip surgery with mold arthroplasty, *Instr Course Lect* 11:163–187, 1954.
3. Bargar WL, Cracchiolo A, Amstutz HC: Results with the constrained total knee prosthesis in treating severely disabled patients and patients with failed total knee replacements, *J Bone Joint Surg [Am]* 62:504–512, 1980.
4. Besser MIB: Bilateral Attenborough total knee replacement as a single procedure, *Arch Orthop Trauma Surg* 101:271–272, 1983.
5. Blauth W, Hassenpflug J: Are unconstrained components essential in total knee arthroplasty? Long-term results of the Blauth knee prosthesis, *Clin Orthop* 258:86–94, 1990.
6. Cameron HU, Jung YB: Hinged total knee replacement: Indications and results, *Can J Surg* 33:53–57, 1990.
7. Campbell W: Arthroplasty of the knee, *J Orthop Surg* 3:430, 1921.
8. In Charnley J, editor: *Friction arthroplasty: Theory and practice,* New York, 1979, Springer-Verlag.
9. Chotivichit AL, et al: Total knee arthroplasty using the Total Condylar III prosthesis, *J Arthroplasty* 6:341–350, 1991.
10. Coonse K, Adams JD: A new operative approach to the knee joint, *Surg Gynecol Obstet* 77:344, 1943.
11. Craig SM: Soft tissue considerations. In Scott NW, editor: *Total knee revision arthroplasty,* Orlando, Fla, 1987, Grune & Stratton, pp 99–112.
12. Deburge A, GUEPAR: Guepar hinge prosthesis: Complications and results with two years' follow-up, *Clin Orthop* 120:47–53, 1976.
13. DiGioia AM, Rubash HE: Periprosthetic fractures after total knee arthroplasty, *Clin Orthop* 271:135–142, 1991.
14. Donaldson WF, et al: Total Condylar III knee prosthesis: Long-term follow-up study, *Clin Orthop* 226:21–28, 1988.
15. Dorr LD, Boiardo RA: Technical considerations in total knee arthroplasty, *Clin Orthop* 205:5–11, 1986.
16. Engelbrecht E, Heinert K: Experience with a surface and total knee replacement: Further development of the model St. Georg. In Niwa S, Paul JP, Yamamoto S, editors: *Total knee replacement,* Tokyo, Springer-Verlag, pp 257–273, 1988.
17. Figgie HE, et al: The influence of tibial-patellofemoral location on function of the knee in patients with the posterior stabilized condylar knee prosthesis, *J Bone Joint Surg [Am]* 68:1035–1040, 1986.
18. Finn HA, et al: Constrained endoprosthetic replacement of the knee, *Sixth International Symposium on Limb Salvage.* Montreal, Sept 10, 1991.
19. Firestone TP, Krackow KA: Removal of femoral components during revision knee arthroplasty, *J Bone Joint Surg [Br]* 73:514, 1991.
20. Freeman MAR, Tennant R: The scientific basis of cemented versus cementless fixation, *Clin Orthop* 276:19–25, 1992.
21. Freeman PA: Walldius arthroplasty: A review of 80 cases, *Clin Orthop* 94:85–91, 1973.
22. Grimer RJ, Karpinski MRK, Edwards AN: The long-term results of Stanmore total knee replacements, *J Bone Joint Surg [Br]* 66:55–62, 1984.
23. Habermann ET, Deutsch SD, Rovere GD: Knee arthroplasty with the use of the Walldius total knee prosthesis, *Clin Orthop* 94:72–84, 1973.
24. Hohl WM, et al: The Total Condylar III prothesis in complex knee reconstruction, *Clin Orthop* 273:91–97, 1991.
25. Hoikka V, et al: Results and complications after arthroplasty with a totally constrained knee prosthesis (GUEPAR), *Ann Chir Gynaecol* 78:94–96, 1989.
26. Hui FC, Fitzgerald RH Jr: Hinged total knee arthroplasty, *J Bone Joint Surg [Am]* 62:513–519, 1980.
27. Insall JN: Total knee replacement. In Insall JN, editor: *Surgery of the knee,* New York, 1984, Churchill Livingstone, pp 587–695.
28. Insall JN, Kelly M: The total condylar prosthesis, *Clin Orthop* 205:43–48, 1986.
29. Insall JN, Lachiewicz PF, Burstein AH: The posterior stabilized condylar prosthesis: A modification of the total condylar design, *J Bone Joint Surg [Am]* 64:1317–1323, 1982.
30. Insall JN, Scott WN, Ranawat CS: The Total Condylar knee prosthesis: A report of two-hundred and twenty cases, *J Bone Joint Surg [Am]* 61:173–180, 1979.
31. Insall JN, et al: A comparison of four models of total-knee replacement prostheses, *J Bone Joint Surg [Am]* 58:754–765, 1976.
32. Insall JN, et al: Total knee arthroplasty, *Clin Orthop* 192:13–22, 1985.
33. Jones EC, et al: GUEPAR knee arthroplasty results and late complications, *Clin Orthop* 140:145–152, 1979.

34. Jones GB: Arthroplasty of the knee by the Walldius prosthesis, *J Bone Joint Surg [Br]* 50:505–510, 1968.
35. Jones GB: Total knee replacement—The Walldius hinge, *Clin Orthop* 94:50–57, 1973.
36. Jones WN, Aufranc OE, Kermond WL: Mould arthroplasty of the knee. *J Bone Joint Surg [Am]* 49:1022, 1967.
37. Karpinski MRK, Grimer RJ: Hinged knee replacement in revision arthroplasty, *Clin Orthop* 220:185–191, 1987.
38. Kaufer H, Matthews LS: Spherocentric arthroplasty of the knee: Clinical experience with an average four-year follow-up, *J Bone Joint Surg [Am]* 63:545–559, 1981.
39. Kavolus CH, et al: The Total Condylar III knee prosthesis in elderly patients, *J Arthroplasty* 6:39–43, 1991.
40. Kim YH: Salvage of failed knee arthroplasty with a Total Condylar III type prosthesis, *Clin Orthop* 221:272–277, 1987.
41. Kraay M, et al: Technical factors influencing the results of Total Condylar III knee arthroplasty, *Am J Knee Surg* 1:125–133, 1988.
42. Kraay MJ, et al: Distal femoral replacement with allograft/prosthetic reconstruction of supracondylar fractures in patients with total knee arthroplasty, *J Arthroplasty* 7:7–16, 1992.
43. Krackow KA, editor: *The technique of total knee arthroplasty,* St Louis, 1990, Mosby–Year Book.
44. Laskin RS: Total condylar knee replacement in rheumatoid arthritis: A review of one hundred and seventeen knees, *J Bone Joint Surg [Am]* 63:29–35, 1981.
45. Laskin RS: The spectrum of total knee replacement. In Laskin RS, Denham RA, Apley AG, editors: *Replacement of the knee,* New York, 1984, Springer-Verlag, pp 11–45.
46. Laskin RS, et al: The posterior stabilized total knee prosthesis in the knee with severe fixed deformity, *Am J Knee Surg* 1:199–203, 1988.
47. Lettin AWF, et al: Assessment of the survival and the clinical results of Stanmore total knee replacements, *J Bone Joint Surg [Br]* 66:355–361, 1984.
48. Lombardi AV, et al: The Total Condylar III prosthesis in complex primary total knee arthroplasty: A three-to-ten year clinical and radiographic evaluation, *Ninth Combined Meeting of the Orthopaedic Associations of the English-Speaking World,* Toronto, June, 1992.
49. Lombardi AV, et al: Total Condylar III prosthesis in revision total knee arthroplasty. *Mid-American Orthopaedic Association,* Hilton Head Island, SC, April 28–May 2, 1993.
50. MacIntosh DL: Hemiarthroplasty of knee using space occupying prosthesis for painful varus and valgus deformities, *J Bone Joint Surg [Am]* 40:1431, 1958.
51. Matthews LS, Goldstein SA, Kaufer H: Experiences with three distinct types of total knee arthroplasty, *Clin Orthop* 192:97–107, 1985.
52. Matthews LS, et al: Spherocentric arthroplasty of the knee: A long-term and final follow-up evaluation, *Clin Orthop* 205:58–66, 1986.
53. McElfresh E: History of arthroplasty. In Petty W, editor: *Total joint replacement,* Philadelphia, 1991, WB Saunders, pp 3–18.
54. McKeever DC: Patellar prosthesis, *J Bone Joint Surg [Am]* 37:1074–1084, 1955; In Petty W, editor: *Total joint replacement,* Philadelphia, 1991, WB Saunders, pp 3–18.
55. McKeever DC: Tibial plateau prosthesis, *Clin Orthop* 18:86–95, 1960.
56. Merryweather R, Jones GB: Total knee replacement: The Walldius arthroplasty, *Orthop Clin North Am* 4:585–596, 1973.
57. Milicic M: Indications for total knee replacement: Early experience with polycentric and geometric implants, In Ingwersen OS, et al, editors: *The knee joint,* New York, 1974, Elsevier, pp 277–283.
58. Moore AT: Hip joint surgery: An outline of progress made in the past forty years. Columbia, 1963; In Petty W, editor: *Total joint replacement,* Philadelphia, 1991, WB Saunders, pp 3–18.
59. Montgomery WH, et al: Revision total knee arthroplasty for aseptic failure using metal-backed tibial and custom implants. *The Knee Society: Scientific Meeting,* Washington, DC, Feb 23, 1992.
60. Murray DG, et al: D. Herbert total knee prosthesis: Combined laboratory and clinical assessment, *J Bone Joint Surg [Am]* 59:1026–1032, 1977.
61. Nelissen RGHH, Brand R, Rozing PM: Survivorship analysis in total condylar knee arthroplasty: A statistical review, *J Bone Joint Surg [Am]* 74:383–389, 1992.
62. Nichols DW, Dorr LD: Revision surgery for stiff total knee arthroplasty, *J Arthroplasty* 5(suppl):S73–S77, 1990.
63. Nieder E: Schnittenprothese, Rotationsknie und Scharnierprothese Modell St. Georg und Endo-Modell: Differentialtherapie in der priären Kniegelenkalloarthroplastik, *Orthopade* 20:170–180, 1991.
64. Oglesby JW, Wilson FC: The evolution of knee arthroplasty, *Clin Orthop* 186:96–103, 1984.
65. Phillips H, Taylor JG: The Walldius hinge arthroplasty, *J Bone Joint Surg [Br]* 57:59–62, 1975.
66. Phillips RS: Shiers' alloplasty of the knee, *Clin Orthop* 94:122–127, 1973.
67. Ranawat CS, editor: *Total condylar knee arthroplasty,* New York, 1985, Springer-Verlag.
68. Ranawat CS: The patellofemoral joint in total condylar knee arthroplasty: Pros and cons based on five- to ten-year follow-up evaluations, *Clin Orthop* 205:93–99, 1986.
69. Ranawat CS, Hansraj KH: Effect of posterior cruciate sacrificing on durability of the cement-bone interface: A nine-year survivorship study of 100 total condylar knee arthroplasties, *Orthop Clin North Am* 20:63–69, 1989.
70. Rand JA: Revision total knee arthroplasty using the Total Condylar III prosthesis, *J Arthroplasty* 6:279–284, 1991.
71. Rand JA, Chao EYS, Stauffer RN: Kinematic rotating-hinge total knee arthroplasty, *J Bone Joint Surg [Am]* 69:489–497, 1987.

72. Riley LH: Total knee arthroplasty, *Clin Orthop* 192:34–39, 1985.
73. Roscoe MW, Goodman SB, Schatzker J: Supracondylar fracture of the femur after GUEPAR total knee arthroplasty: A new treatment method, *Clin Orthop* 241:221–223, 1989.
74. Rosenberg AG, Verner JJ, Galante JO: Clinical results of total knee revision using the Total Condylar III prosthesis, *Clin Orthop* 273:83–90, 1991.
75. Schurman DJ: Functional outcome of GUEPAR hinge knee arthroplasty evaluated with ARAMIS, *Clin Orthop* 155:118–132, 1981.
76. Scott WN: Constraint in total knee arthroplasty. In Goldberg, VM, editor: *Controversies in total knee arthroplasty,* New York, 1991, Raven Press, pp 19–25.
77. Sculco TP: Total Condylar III in ligament instability, *Orthop Clin North Am* 20:221–226, 1989.
78. Sculco TP, Faris PM: Total knee replacement in the stiff knee, *Tech Orthop* 3:5–8, 1988.
79. Sim FK, Chao EYS: Prosthetic replacement of the knee and large segment of the femur or tibia, *J Bone Joint Surg [Am]* 61:887–892, 1979.
80. Smith-Petersen, MN: Evolution of mould arthroplasty of hip joint, *J Bone Joint Surg [Br]* 30:59–75, 1948;
81. Sonstegard DA, Kaufer H, Matthews LS: The Spherocentric knee: Biomechanical testing and clinical trials, *J Bone Joint Surg [Am]* 59:602–616, 1977.
82. Stulberg BN, Hupfer T: Indications and preoperative planning for total knee arthroplasty. In Petty W, editor: *Total joint replacement,* Philadelphia, 1991, WB Saunders, pp 3–18.
83. Sydney SV, Mallory TH: Dislocation of a constrained knee prosthesis: Two case reports, *Complications Orthop* 4:93–97, 1989.
84. Tew M, Waugh W, Forster IW: Comparing the results of different types of knee replacement: A method proposed and applied, *J Bone Joint Surg [Br]* 67:775–779, 1985.
85. Verneuil A: De la création d'une fausse articulation par section ou résection partielle de l'os maxillaire inférieur, comme moyen de remédier a l'ankylose vraie ou fausse de la mâchoire inférieure, *Arch Gen Med* 15:174, 1860.
86. Walker PS: Requirements for successful total knee replacements: Design considerations, *Orthop Clin North Am* 20:15–29, 1989.
87. Watson JR, Wood H, Hill RCJ: The Shiers arthroplasty of the knee, *J Bone Joint Surg [Br]* 58:300–304, 1976.
88. Whiteside LA, Ohl MD: Tibial tubercle osteotomy for exposure of the difficult total knee arthroplasty, *Clin Orthop* 260:6–9, 1990.
89. Wilson FC, Fajgenbaum DM, Venters GC: Results of knee replacement with the Walldius and Geometric prostheses, *J Bone Joint Surg [Br]* 62:497–503, 1980.
90. Windsor RE, Insall JN: Exposure in revision total knee arthroplasty: The femoral peel, *Tech Orthop* 3:1–4, 1988.
91. Wilson FC, Venters GC: Results of knee replacement with the Walldius prosthesis: An interim report, *Clin Orthop* 120:39–46, 1976.

76

Patellar Complications in Total Knee Arthroplasty

ROBERT E. BOOTH, JR., M.D.

Patellar loosening
Patellar component failure
Patellar clunk syndrome

Patellofemoral instability
Extensor disruptions
Surgical technique

Total knee arthroplasty, by virtue of its long-term survivorship and superlative success rates, has in recent years surpassed total hip surgery in the United States. Reliable pain relief, extended durability, and improved joint function have made it the most frequently performed arthroplasty procedure. The earliest total knee designs addressed only the tibiofemoral articulation and did not provide for patellofemoral resurfacing, which was often considered an isolated procedure. Without patellar resurfacing, anterior knee pain has had a reported incidence as high as 50%.* The extension of the femoral component to include a flange did not materially improve the result.[18, 46] Because of this experience, a patellofemoral component was added to most modern total knee designs, with an attendant decrease in pain and an improvement in function.[18, 27, 28, 29, 36, 37, 48, 50, 52, 65, 71]

While few joint surgeons would dispute patellar resurfacing in patients with rheumatoid arthritis to avoid the antigenic response to retained cartilage, there remains some controversy over its use in pure degenerative disease. Most contemporary series still reveal increased problems without patellar resurfacing, generally producing anterior knee pain in up to 30% of patients.[4, 12, 27, 49, 52] Boyd et al.[4] reported patellar complication rates of 4% with and 12% without patellar arthroplasty. Soudry et al.[71] found little difference in pain symptoms between resurfaced and unresurfaced populations, with progressive cartilage erosion in 65% being unrelated to deteriorating pain scores.

*References 8, 11, 13, 16, 18, 27, 28, 33, 35, 39, 43, 44, 46, 61, 69, 70, 74.

As is so often the case with orthopaedic innovation, however, the solution has become the problem. While the overall result may be improved, a new group of complications has emerged, all related to extensor resurfacing and its attendant problems. Patellar loosening, prosthetic failure, extensor rupture, patellar clunk, and chronic instability are among these, with a reported incidence of up to 55%.[8, 10, 17, 23, 26, 30, 40, 42, 55, 68, 75] In several series, patellofemoral complications are responsible for as much as 50% of revisional knee arthroplasty.[2, 5, 73]

PATELLAR LOOSENING

For most of the history of patellar resurfacing as part of total knee arthroplasty, polymethylmethacrylate fixation has been employed. The results have been uniformly excellent, with loosening rates of less than 2% on average.[8, 10, 38, 48, 49] Domical buttons have been the rule, with single-peg stabilization. While even successful patellar implants have generally shown some wear over time, the "particle disease" implications of patellar wear alone appear to be relatively benign when compared with the volume of tibial polyethylene debris.

Nonetheless, in a response to this as well as other problems more theoretic than real-such as cement fragmentation, durability, bioactivity, and thermal necrosis-porous ingrowth technology was applied to patellar fixation. Metal backing to reduce stress on the polyethylene has left insufficient plastic, with attendant rates of wear and dissociation far worse than pure plastic patellae.[5, 54] In addition, component-dissociating metallic synovitis and gouging of femoral components have been reported. Ingrowth of patellar bone around anchoring pegs has been quite reproducible,[9] but ingrowth into patellar surfaces has been unreliable. This partial ingrowth pattern has led to peg shear failure and component dissociation, usually with disastrous implications. Even radiographically or clinically, loose patellae may be asymptomatic, retained in their appropriate position by a "patellar meniscus" or rim of confining fibrous tissue. Indeed, it would appear that the avoidance of patellar loosening is related less to design and is more dependant upon proper bone cuts, soft tissue balancing, bone quality, cementation techniques, and component sizing. When symptomatic patellar loosening does occur, therapeutic options range from pure patellar revision to component excision, to a full total knee revision if other mechanical factors are at fault. While most loose patellae are asymptomatic, Brick and Scott[5] have suggested that as many as 75% will eventually require revision surgery.

PATELLAR COMPONENT FAILURE

The primary concern in patellar component design is the distribution of stress and strain. A brief look at the patellofemoral forces generated in daily activities makes this obvious. During level gait, the patellofemoral joint reaction forces reach 0.5 to 1.0 times body weight. These rise to 3 to 4 times body weight on stair climbing, and as high as 7 to 8 times body weight in a deep squat.[25, 45, 56, 61]

The original domical prosthetic implant designed by Aglietti et al.[1] was intended as a "universal" isolated patellar resurfacing. Its advantages, both then and now, were to eliminate concerns about rotational alignment, to fit all shapes and sizes of natural knees, and to maintain roughly the same contact area despite various twists or tilts in its altitude relative to the femur. It has worked extremely well, and the pendulum of prejudice appears to be swinging back to simple domical patellae at this writing.

The primary disadvantage of the domical patellar design was a point or line contact area on the femur as well as greater strain when compared with anatomic conforming patellar designs.[19] This generation of implants was intended to create area contact and decrease polyethylene wear. Unfortunately, the thin plastic on the congruous lateral facet, particularly when combined with a metal backing, has exposed the great weakness of thin polyethylene and actually increased the incidence of wear and failure. Additionally, the implant is quite sensitive to rotational alignment and requires significant attention at implantation.[26, 46] (Fig 76-1).

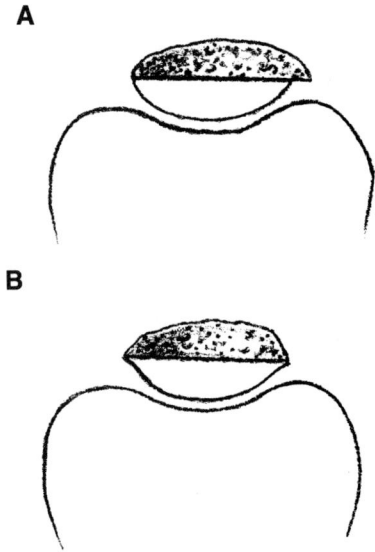

FIG 76-1.
A, medialized domical patellar button. **B,** conforming full-coverage patellar button.

Finally, the lure of greater patellofemoral stability appears to be related more to the geometry of the femoral prosthesis than to the conformity of the patellar design. Acute changes in the radii of curvature will produce excessive forces or patellar impingement as the knee passes from flexion into extension.[23] Handed femoral components with an oblique groove, higher on the lateral side, appear to improve tracking and stability.[8] The greater the slope of the groove, the more patellar containment can be generated, as long as there is slight external rotation of the femur to avoid excessive patellofemoral stress.[7] Merely increasing the conformity of the components does not necessarily enhance the stability of the construct.[7] Soft tissue balance and a certain natural laxity in the extensor mechanism are required in either conforming or domical patellar designs.

PATELLAR CLUNK SYNDROME

The intimate relationship between the patella and the femoral component, both in terms of prosthetic design and surgical technique, is beautifully illustrated by the patellar clunk syndrome.[22, 23] In this complication of total knee arthroplasty, a fibrous nodule develops on the posterior surface of the quadriceps tendon, just superior to the proximal pole of the patella. With deep knee flexion, this fibrosynovial mass becomes entrapped in the intercondylar femoral notch. As the knee is extended, the nodule pops out of the notch, producing a "clunk," usually accompanied by pain. This occurs most frequently at 30 to 45 degrees short of full extension, creating a hazard to stair climbing or rising from a seated position. It is never symptomatic in level gait (Fig 76–2).

Although two general pathogenic patterns have been described, their common etiologic factor is the abrupt change in the radius of curvature of certain femoral components. These are almost exclusively posterior cruciate ligament–substituting designs in which an abrupt anterior transition was necessary to accommodate the peg-in-box stabilizer. In this setting, therefore, the quadriceps tendon may rub over the anterosuperior edge of the intercondylar notch, especially when a small patellar prosthesis is insufficient to elevate the quadriceps tendon from the femoral component. These forces are not inconsiderable, as the quadriceps tendon shares almost 50% of the patellofemoral load at high degrees of flexion.[24] In a second mechanism, a patellar button that is placed beyond the proximal border of the patella may itself irritate the quadriceps tendon and produce the offending clunk.

Conservative treatment, consisting of a vigorous quadriceps exercise program, is occasionally successful, particularly in cases where there is more noise than pain. Invasive therapy consists of either arthroscopic or open debridement of the nodule, and is quite effective.[75] When open debridement is chosen, strong consideration should be given to exchange of patellar implants which are either undersized or malpositioned.

PATELLOFEMORAL INSTABILITY

It is difficult to underestimate the importance of proper tracking and alignment of the patellofemoral articulation to the success of a total knee arthroplasty.

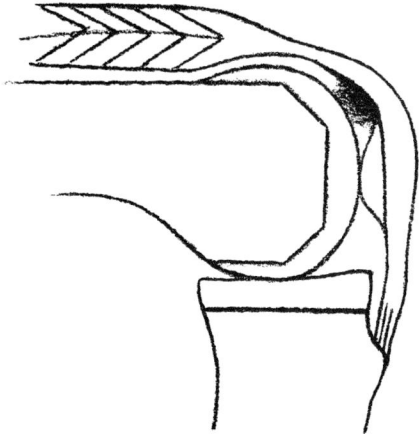

FIG 76–2.
Suprapatellar fibrous nodule of patellar clunk syndrome.

Much like the retained posterior cruciate ligament, it is a primary anatomic structure whose kinematics must be mated with an artificial and necessarily nonanatomic prosthetic device, usually without benefit of sophisticated instrumentation. Almost all the potential patellofemoral complications can be related to improper extensor kinematics, including unexplained pain and crepitus, extensor ruptures, premature component failure, loosening, and particle disease.* Despite this significance, and despite reported rates of extensor subluxation as high as 29%,[6] balancing the patella is usually relegated to terminal importance in a total knee arthroplasty.

Patellofemoral instability is usually multifactorial, and is rarely attributable to a single error. Nonetheless, the most common cause of extensor subluxation remains weakness of the vastus medialis musculature with attendant uncorrected contracture of the lateral retinaculum.[10, 44, 49] Often, this can be predicted preoperatively, from a lateral patella on radiograph to a palpably contracted lateral extensor on physical examination. Uncorrected genu valgum with an attendant Q (quadriceps) angle greater than 15 degrees perpetuates the lateral forces on the extensor and increases the likelihood of subluxation.[10, 36, 42, 54] Last, any biologic dehiscence or attenuation of the medial capsular structures, as from poor extensor repair, early hematoma, or excessive early range of motion will cause patellofemoral instability.[27]

The orientation of the tibial and femoral components in a total knee arthroplasty is well directed in the sagittal and coronal axes by existing intramedullary instrumentation. The only common malalignment error using these systems is flexion of an undersized femoral component to avoid notching the anterior femoral cortex, but at the same time significantly increasing the force on the patellofemoral joint. Rotational orientation of the components is largely subjective and left to surgical discretion. Because most knees are exposed through a medial approach, the surgeon's visual orientation influences an internal rotation of both the femoral and tibial components. On the tibial side, this induces an external rotation of the tibial tuberosity with a concomitant increase in the Q angle. A similar result is generated from medial placement of an undersized tibial component or inadequate resection of medial osteophytes. Floating tibial trials will often expose this error, but their use is not uniform.

On the femoral side, the same tendencies to medial displacement and internal rotation are present,

*References 5, 8, 10, 38, 40, 42–44, 49, 54, 58, 61, 72.

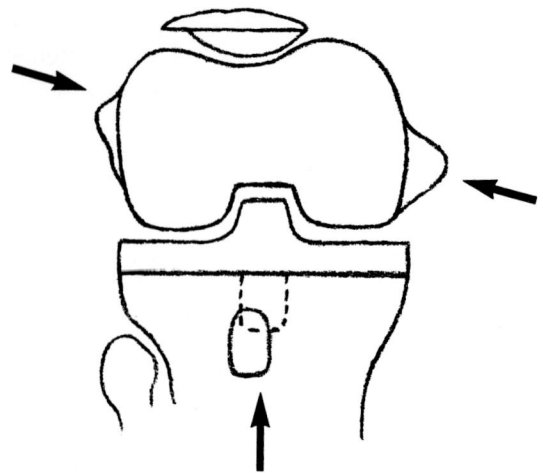

FIG 76-3.
Slight external rotation of the tibial component relative to the tibial tuberosity and the femoral component relative to the epicondylar axis are desirable.

largely because of the medial approach and visual dominance of the broad medial femoral condyle with its adductor tubercle. Internal rotation of the femoral flange forces the extensor more medially, increasing stresses and facilitating subluxation. Indeed a conscious 5-degree *external* rotation of the femoral implant is currently recommended to present the trochlear groove to the patella (Fig 76-3).

Last, the position of the patellar button is crucial to the kinematics of the extensor. The normal posterior patellar surface is irregular, thicker on the medial than on the lateral side. Bony resection should therefore remove more medial than lateral bone, and the axial bone resection should also be symmetric.[21, 38, 54] The residual surface is often oval, and one should *not* replace the entire exposed bone with prosthesis, lest the lateral side be made too thick. The patellar button, indeed, should be shifted medially, and in most knee systems slightly proximally, to preserve normal patellofemoral kinematics. Since femoral components tend to augment the normal distal femoral bone, one should also slightly downsize patellar components to maintain a constant radius about the knee's variable axes of rotation. The safest policy is to measure the medial patellar thickness and to replace only what is resected. Excessively thick or thin patellae predispose to fracture and respective limitation of flexion or extension.

Even the choice of implant design can influence patellar instability. Components without rotatory constraint may allow external tibial rotation and extensor subluxation. Rand et al.,[53] for example, have reported a 22% incidence of patellar instability with the kinematic rotating-hinge prosthesis. At the other end of the spectrum, rigid prosthetic designs without the normal tibial rotation during flexion may also predispose to subluxation.[31, 43, 67] Lastly, cruciate-deficient total knees with attendant collateral or rotational instability may also increase the chances of patellar subluxation.[62, 63]

The treatment of patellofemoral instability is dependent on clearly identifying the cause of the problem. Often a simple retinacular release, either arthroscopic or open, with a medial reefing will suffice. Capsular imbrication, tibial tuberosity transfer, or even component exchange may also be necessary.

EXTENSOR DISRUPTIONS

Perhaps the most devastating complication of total knee arthroplasty is disruption of the extensor mechanism, which condemns the knee to dysfunction and failure. As a general rule, the more distal the lesion, the more difficult the repair. The primary reason for this principle is that most extensor complications share a vascular etiology, and the blood supply of the extensor mechanism is now fairly well defined. Patellar vascularity studies have identified both extraosseous and intraosseous systems.[3, 34, 59, 60] The extraosseous system consists of a peripatellar anastomotic circuit served by six main arteries. Superiorly, the vessels penetrate the anterior aspect of the quadriceps tendon, while inferiorly they pass through the infrapatellar fat pad. The intraosseous system consists of polar, midpatellar, and quadriceps sources. The midpatellar vessels are the most abundant, and are probably the most important (Fig 76-4).

A standard medial arthrotomy compromises the entire medial supply, and should be kept 1 cm medial to the patella to avoid the anastomotic ring itself. Lateral meniscectomy and partial fat pad dissection disrupt the lateral supply, which may be further violated by a lateral retinacular release with disturbance of the superior lateral genicular vessels.[66, 76] The intraosseous supply is at greatest risk from a large single central patellar peg, and multiple small pegs are now popular for this and other reasons.[54] Most postoperative scan studies show decreased vascularity after lateral release,[66, 76] and avascular necrosis has been observed in patellar specimens after stress fractures.[28, 64]

Quadriceps tendon rupture is relatively rare after primary total knee arthroplasty, with a reported incidence of about 1%.[38] It is definitely related to lateral retinacular releases, quadriceps turndown approaches, and revision surgeries.[38] Repair techniques are reasonably successful, although residual extensor

remains the best cure. Recent experience with extensor allografts has been promising, both in the literature and in our own experience, but long-term results are still awaited[12] (Fig 76–5).

Patellar fractures represent the most common extensor disruption, with an incidence as high as 21%.[6, 19, 21] There appears to be an optimal level of patellar bone resection for prosthetic resurfacing, leaving a residual bone fragment of at least 15 mm.[57] If excessive bone is resected, fractures are more common in the avascular residual fragment, particularly if below the subchondral bone level.[32] If insufficient

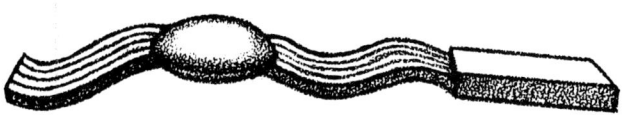

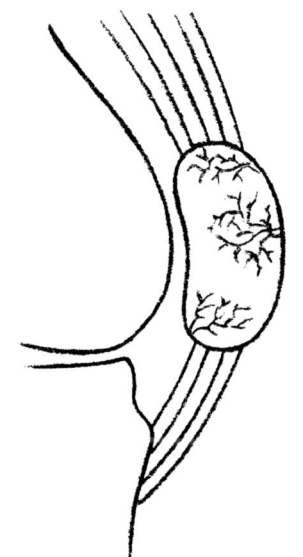

FIG 76–4.
A, peripatellar arterial arcade: *SG* = supreme genicular; *MSG* = medial superior genicular; *MIG* = medial inferior genicular; *LSG* = lateral superior genicular; *LIG* = lateral inferior genicular; *ATR* = anterior tibial recurrent. **B,** intraosseous patellar blood supply, including quadriceps tendon, midpatellar, and polar arborizations.

lags and diminished passive flexion are generally experienced.

Isolated patellar tendon rupture occurs with about the same frequency as quadriceps tendon rupture, but is far more devastating. Ruptures are most common after distal realignment procedures involving the tibial tuberosity.[55] Many biologic and prosthetic repair techniques have been proposed, but the irreparable vascular deficiency that underlies most ruptures dooms even the most clever reconstructive techniques. Rand et al.[55] reported a 60% failure rate despite multiple attempts at repair, and prevention

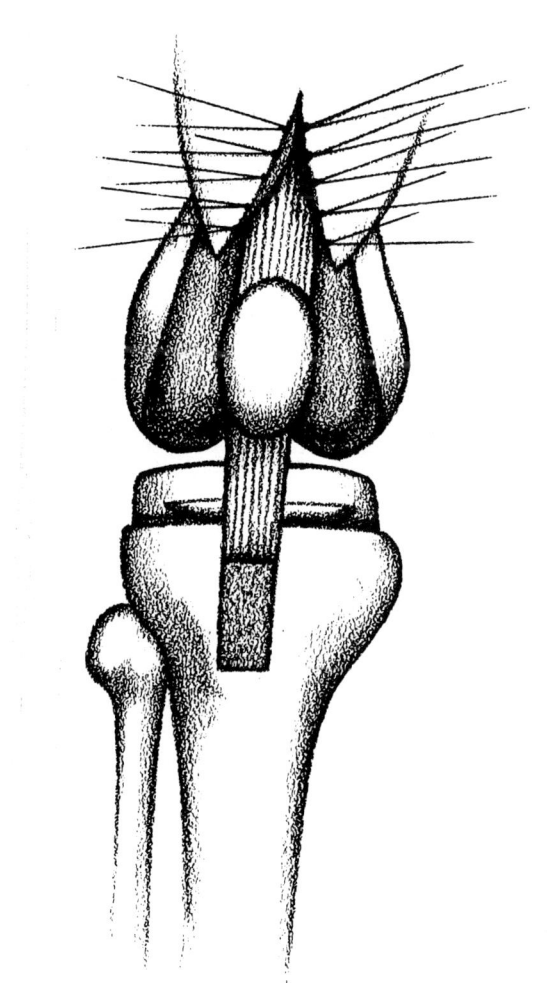

FIG 76–5.
Patellar tendon allograft for extensor deficiency.

bone is resected or too thick a patellar prosthesis is applied, fractures will also occur because of the increased patellofemoral joint forces. The "overstuffed" knee will not flex without patellar disruption.

Recent enthusiasts for circumferential "patellar neurolysis" with an electrocautery to reduce anterior knee pain are also probably ill-advised, as the potential for fracture and patellar fragmentation is also elevated in neurotrophic joints. Indeed, many patellar fractures are asymptomatic, identified only on follow-up radiographs.

The treatment of patellar fractures about a total knee arthroplasty is largely nonoperative except for displaced components, complete extensor incompetence, and free fragments. The outcome of therapy and the restoration of full knee extension are more dependent on the degree of extensor loss at the time of fracture than they are on the type or quality of the repair.

SURGICAL TECHNIQUE

An approach to total knee arthroplasty intended to minimize patellofemoral complications must be supported by the literature and conventional wisdom. An attempt should be made preoperatively to identify appropriate component sizes as well as tight lateral retinacular tissues. A medial parapatellar approach should consciously avoid the peripatellar vascular arcade. Sufficient exposure should be created so that one may avoid medialization or internal rotation of femoral or tibial components. The size of the components selected should be kept in mind, so that the composite of the patellar button and the femoral prosthesis approaches the normal anatomic ratio. Alignment should reduce the Q angle to less than 10 degrees, and conscious slight external rotation of both femoral and tibial implants should be attempted. The use of floating tibial trials and the "no thumbs" assessment of patellar tracking after tourniquet release should confirm the wisdom of these choices.

A domical multipegged all-polyethylene patellar implant would seem to be most appropriate, secured by good cement technique into a symmetric patellar fragment. A slightly downsized patellar button should sit on the superomedial aspect of the exposed oval of patellar bone. Thickness should usually equal that of the premorbid patella, but the relative proportions of the femoral contribution to this equation must be considered (Fig 76–6).

In general, cruciate-sparing implants lower the joint line and cruciate-sacrificing implants elevate it. The patellar height may therefore require some ad-

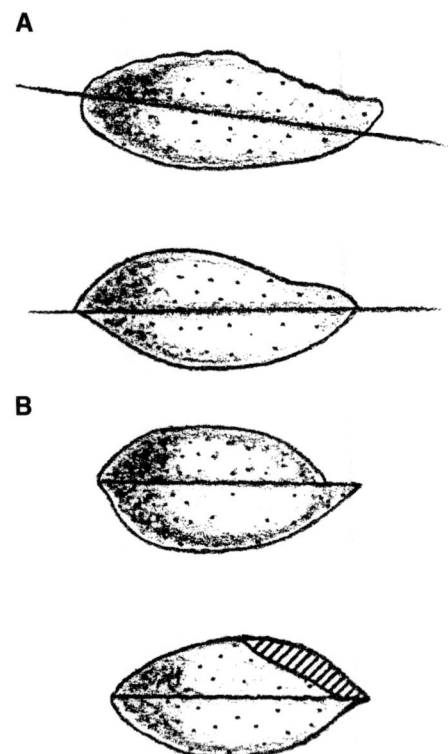

FIG 76–6.
A, common asymmetric patellar resection. **B,** correct symmetric patellar resection.

justment before final cementation. In patella baja, as in conversion of a high tibial osteotomy, a large anterior tibial tuberosity slide should be considered to preclude excessive stress in flexion.

If a lateral retinacular release is necessary, it should be performed 2 cm posterior to the patella to preserve vascularity, and it should be done in stages for similar reasons. Closure should secure the medial capsular arthrotomy, and excessive early motion should be pursued with moderation. With care and consideration, the complications of patellofemoral resurfacing need not compromise the quality and durability of a total knee arthroplasty.

REFERENCES

1. Aglietti P et al: A new patella prosthesis, *Clin Orthop* 107:175–187, 1975.
2. Bayley JC, et al: Failure of the metal-backed patella component after total knee replacement, *J Bone Joint Surg [Am]* 70:674–688, 1988.
3. Bjorkstrom S, Goldie IF: A study of the arterial supply of the patella in the normal state, in chondromalacia patellae and in osteoarthrosis, *Acta Orthop Scand* 51:63–70, 1980.
4. Boyd AD, et al: Long term complications of the resur-

faced and unresurfaced patella in total knee arthroplasty, American Academy of Orthopaedic Surgeons, Anaheim, Calif, March 7–11, 1991.
5. Brick, GW, Scott RD: The patellofemoral component of total knee arthroplasty, *Clin Orthop* 231:163–178, 1988.
6. Cameron HU, Fedorkow DM: The patella in total knee arthroplasty. *Clin Orthop* 165:197–199, 1982.
7. Cepulo AJ, et al: Mechanical characteristics of patellofemoral replacement, *Trans Orthop Res Soc* 8:41, 1983.
8. Clayton ML, Thirupathi R: Patellar complications after total condylar arthroplasty, *Clin Orthop* 170:152–155, 1982.
9. Dennis DA: Removal of well-fixed cementless metal-backed patellar components, *J Arthroplasty* 7:217–220, 1992.
10. Doolittle KH, Turner RH: Patellofemoral problems following total knee arthroplasty. *Orthop Rev* 17:696–702, 1988.
11. Eftekhar NS: Total knee-replacement arthroplasty. Results with the intramedullary adjustable total knee prosthesis, *J Bone Joint Surg [Am]* 65:293–309, 1985.
12. Emerson RH Jr, Head WC, Malinin TI: Reconstruction of patellar tendon rupture after total knee arthroplasty with an extensor mechanism allograft, *Clin Orthop* 260:154–161, 1990.
13. Enis JE, et al: Comparison of patellar resurfacing versus nonresurfacing in bilateral total knee arthroplasty, *Clin Orthop* 260:38–42, 1990.
14. Evanski PM, et al: UCI knee replacement, *Clin Orthop* 120:33–38, 1976.
15. Ewald FC, et al: Duopatella total knee arthroplasty in rheumatoid arthritis, *Orthop Trans* 2:202, 1978.
16. Ficat RP, Hungerford DS: *Disorders of the patellofemoral joint*, Baltimore, 1979, Williams & Wilkins.
17. Freeman MA, Samuelson KM, Bertin KC: Freeman-Samuelson total arthroplasty of the knee, *Clin Orthop* 192:46–58, 1985.
18. Freeman MA, et al: ICLP arthroplasty of the knee 1968–1977, *J Bone Joint Surg [Br]* 60:339–344, 1978.
19. Goldberg VM, et al: Patellar fracture type and prognosis in condylar total knee arthroplasty, *Clin Orthop* 236:115–122, 1988.
20. Goldstein SA, et al: Patellar surface strain, *J Orthop Res* 4:372–377, 1986.
21. Gomes LSM, Bechtold JE, Gustilo RB: Patellar prosthesis positioning in total knee arthroplasty. A roentgenographic study, *Clin Orthop* 236:72–81, 1988.
22. Hozack WJ, et al: The treatment of patellar fractures after total knee arthroplasty, *Clin Orthop* 236:123–127, 1988.
23. Hozack WJ, et al: The patellar clunk syndrome. A complication of posterior stabilized total knee arthroplasty, *Clin Orthop* 241:203–208, 1989.
24. Huberti HH, Hayes WC: Patellofemoral contact pressure: The influence of Q angle and tendofemoral contact, *J Bone Joint Surg [Am]* 66:715–724, 1984.
25. Hungerford DS, Barry M: Biomechanics of the patellofemoral joint, *Clin Orthop* 144:9–15, 1979.
26. Hungerford DS Krackow KA: Total joint arthroplast of the knee, *Clin Orthop* 192:23–33, 1985.
27. Insall JN, Lachiewicz P, Burstein A: The posterior stabilized condylar prosthesis; a modification of the total-condylar design. Two and four year clinical experience, *J Bone Joint Surg [Am]* 64:1317–1323, 1982.
28. Insall JN, Scott WN, Ranawat CS: The total condylar knee prosthesis: A report of 220 cases, *J Bone Joint Surg [Am]* 61:173–180, 1979.
29. Insall JN, Tria AJ, Aglietti P: Resurfacing of the patella, *J Bone Joint Surg [Am]* 62:933–936, 1980.
30. Insall J, Tria AJ, Scott WN: The total condylar knee prosthesis. The first 5 years, *Clin Orthop* 145:68–77, 1979.
31. Jones EC, et al: GUEPAR knee arthroplasty results and late complications, *Clin Orthop* 140:145–152, 1979.
32. Josefchak RG, et al: Cancellous bone support for patellar resurfacing, *Clin Orthop* 220:192–199, 1987.
33. Kaufer H. Matthews L: Spherocentric arthroplasty of the knee, *J Bone Joint Surg [Am]* 63:545–559, 1981.
34. Kayler DE, Lyttle D: Surgical interruption of patellar blood supply by total knee arthroplasty, *Clin Orthop* 229:221–227, 1988.
35. Kettlekamp DB, Pryor P, Brady TA: A selective use of the variable axis knee, *Orthop Trans* 3:543.
36. Leblanc JM: Patellar complications in total knee arthroplasty: A literature review, *Orthop Rev* 18:296–304, 1989.
37. Levai JP, McLeod HC, Freeman MAR: Why not resurface the patella?, *J Bone Joint Surg [Br]* 65:448–451, 1983.
38. Lynch AF, Rorabeck CH, Bourne RB: Extensor mechanism complications following total knee arthroplasty, *J Arthroplasty* 2:135–140, 1987.
39. Matthews L, Sonstegard DA, Henke JA: Load bearing characteristics of the patellofemoral joint, *Acta Orthop Scand* 48:511–516.
40. Mazas FB, GUEPAR: Guepar total knee prosthesis, *Clin Orthop* 94:211–221, 1973.
41. McMahon MS, et al: Scintigraphic determination of patellar viability after excision of infrapatellar fat pad and/or lateral retinacular release in total knee arthroplasty, *Clin Orthop* 260:10–16, 1990.
42. Merkow RL, Soudry M, Insall JN: Patellar dislocation following total knee replacement, *J Bone Joint Surg [Am]* 67:1321–1327, 1985.
43. Mochizuki RM, Schurman DJ: Patellar complications following total joint arthroplasty, *J Bone Joint Surg [Am]* 61:879–883, 1979.
44. Moreland JR, Thomas RJ, Freeman MAR: ICLH replacement of the knee. 1977 and 1978, *Clin Orthop* 145:47–59, 1979.
45. Morrison JB: The forces transmitted by the human knee joint during activity (thesis), Strathclyde, Scotland, University of Strathclyde, 1967.
46. Murray DG, Webster PA: Variable axis knee prosthe-

sis. Two year follow-up study, *J Bone Joint Surg [Am]* 63:687–694, 1981.
47. Picatti GD, McGann WA, Welch RB: The patellofemoral joint after total knee arthroplasty without patellar resurfacing, *J Bone Joint Surg [Am]* 72:1379–1382, 1990.
48. Rae PJ, Noble J, Hodgkinson JP: Patellar resurfacing in total condylar knee arthroplasty. Technique and results, *J Arthroplasty* 5:259–265, 1990.
49. Ranawat CS: The patellofemoral joint in total condylar knee arthroplasty. Pros and cons based on 5–10 year follow-up observations, *Clin Orthop* 205:93–99, 1986.
50. Ranawat CS, Insall J, Shine J: Duo-condylar knee arthroplasty, *Clin Orthop* 120:76–82, 1976.
51. Ranawat CS, Rose HA: Total-condylar knee arthroplasty: A three to eight year follow-up, American Academy of Orthopaedic Surgeons Annual Meeting, Los Angeles, 1983.
52. Ranawat CS, Rose HA, Bryan JW: Technique and results of patellofemoral joint with total-condylar knee arthroplasty, *Orthop Trans* 6:88, 1982.
53. Rand JA, Chao EY, Stauffer RN: Kinematic rotating hinge total knee arthroplasty, *J Bone Joint Surg [Am]* 69:489–497, 1987.
54. Rand JA, Gustilo RB: Technique of patellar resurfacing in total knee arthroplasty, *Tech Orthop* 133:57, 1988.
55. Rand JA, Morrey BF, Bryan AS: Patellar tendon rupture after total knee arthroplasty, *Clin Orthop* 244:233–238, 1989.
56. Reilly TR, Martens M: Experimental analysis of the quadriceps muscle force and patellofemoral joint reaction force for various activities, *Acta Orthop Scand* 43:126–137, 1972.
57. Reuben, JD, et al: The effect of patella thickness on patella strain following total arthroplasty, *J Arthroplasty* 6:251–258, 1991.
58. Rosenberg AG, et al: Patellar component failure in cementless total knee arthroplasty, *Clin Orthop* 236:106–114, 1988.
59. Scapinelli R: Blood supply of the human patella, *J Bone Joint Surg [Br]* 49:563–570, 1967.
60. Scapinelli R: Studies on the vasculature of the human knee joint, *Acta Anat (Basel)* 70:305–331, 1968.
61. Scott RD: Prosthetic replacement of the patellofemoral joint, *Orthop Clin North Am* 10:129–137, 1979.
62. Scott WN, Rubinstein M: Posterior stabilized knee arthroplasty. Six years experience, *Clin Orthop* 205:138–148, 1986.
63. Scott WN, Rubinstein M, Scuderi G: Results after knee replacement with a posterior cruciate-substituting prosthesis, *J Bone Joint Surg* 70:1163–1173, 1988.
64. Scott RD, Turoff N, Ewald FC: Stress fracture of the patella following duopatellar total knee arthroplasty with patellar resurfacing. *Clin Orthop* 170:147–151, 1982.
65. Scott WN, et al: Clinical and biomechanical evaluation of patella replacement in total knee arthroplasty, *Orthop Trans* 2:203, 1978.
66. Scuderi G, et al: The relationship of lateral releases to patella viability in total knee arthroplasty, *J Arthroplasty* 2:209–214, 1987.
67. Sheehan J: Arthroplasty of the knee, *Clin Orthop* 145:101–109, 1979.
68. Simison AJM, Noble J, Hardinge K: Complications of the Attenborough knee replacement, *J Bone Joint Surg [Br]* 68:100–105, 1986.
69. Sledge CB, Ewald FC: Total knee arthroplasty: experience at the Robert Breck Brigham Hospital, *Clin Orthop* 145:78–84, 1979.
70. Sledge CB, et al: Two year follow-up of the duocondylar total knee replacement, *Orthop Trans* 2:193, 1978.
71. Soudry M, et al: Total knee replacement without patella resurfacing, *Clin Orthop* 205:166–170, 1986.
72. Stulberg SD, et al: Failure mechanisms of metal-backed patellar components, *Clin Orthop* 236:88–105, 1988.
73. Thomas WH, et al: Duopatella total knee arthroplasty, *Orthop Trans* 4:329, 1980.
74. Vanhegan J, Dabrowski W. Arden GP: A review of 100 Attenborough stabilized gliding knee prosthesis, *J Bone Joint Surg [Br]* 61:445, 1979.
75. Vernace JA, et al: Arthroscopic management of the patellar clunk syndrome following posterior stabilized total knee arthroplasty, *J Arthroplasty* 4:179–182, 1989.
76. Wetzner SM, et al: Bone scanning in the assessment of patellar viability following knee replacement, *Clin Orthop* 199:215–219, 1985.

77

Bone Grafting in Total Knee Arthroplasty

THOMAS P. SCULCO, M.D.

Tibial bone loss
   Defects 6 to 12 mm deep
   Defects greater than 12 mm deep
      Autogenous bone grafting for tibial deficiency
Femoral bone loss

Bone grafting in revision total knee arthroplasty
   Cystic deficiencies
   Central medullary deficiency
   Peripheral tibial plateau or condylar bone loss

Over the past two decades, total knee replacement has evolved into one of the most successful of orthopaedic procedures. The quality of the clinical result has become predictable and reproducible, pain is relieved, and function is improved. With excellent results in the less complex cases and increased surgical experience, more severely damaged knees have been addressed. It is in these more complex knees that combinations of soft tissue and bone deficiency exist and these present challenging reconstructive dilemmas to the operating surgeon. This chapter concerns itself with those more complicated knees with marked angular deformities in the varus-valgus, flexion-extension, or rotatory planes associated with bone defects.

Bone loss in knees with angular deformity occurs most frequently on the tibial side of the joint. The defects are usually localized posteriorly on the tibial plateau due to the frequently associated flexion deformity in these knees. There may be associated fragmentation of the tibial surface, but as a rule the tibial surface is concave, extremely sclerotic, and completely devoid of cartilage. (Fig 77-1). Because there is often frank subluxation of the femur on the tibia, there tends to be little, if any, peripheral tibial rim remaining. The deficiency occurs as a result of the progression of deformity and the forces driving the femur into the tibial surface. Consequently there is a steep descent from the middle of the tibial surface to the periphery.

Femoral bone loss on the concave side of the deformity of an angular deformity occurs with much less frequency than does tibial bone loss. An exception to this is the valgus knee where combinations of both tibial and femoral bone loss are seen. The sclerotic quality of the femoral subchondral bone and the ram's-horn configuration of the distal femoral condyle favor the tibia collapsing rather than the femur. When femoral condylar collapse does occur there may be an element of osteonecrosis present which facilitates the destruction.

If severe degrees of bone loss are associated with marked fragmentation and disorganization of the joint, one must suspect an underlying neuropathic process. In this instance, severe degrees of deformity with marked loss of joint stability and bone destruction are present which are out of proportion to the mild degree of pain perceived by the patient. A careful history and neurologic examination is important in these patients. The most common cause of a neuropathic joint is diabetes mellitus and although more distal lower extremity joints are affected, the knee may be involved in some patients. Successful total knee arthroplasty in the neuropathic knee is unlikely. The underlying pathologic environment for knee joint destruction remains, and therefore this entity should be viewed as a contraindication to total knee replacement.

The management of bone deficiency in total knee arthroplasty will vary depending upon the location and degree of the bone loss. Various methods have been employed with success including the use of polymethyl methacrylate alone,[4, 5] polymethyl methacrylate reinforced with mesh or screws,[6] bone

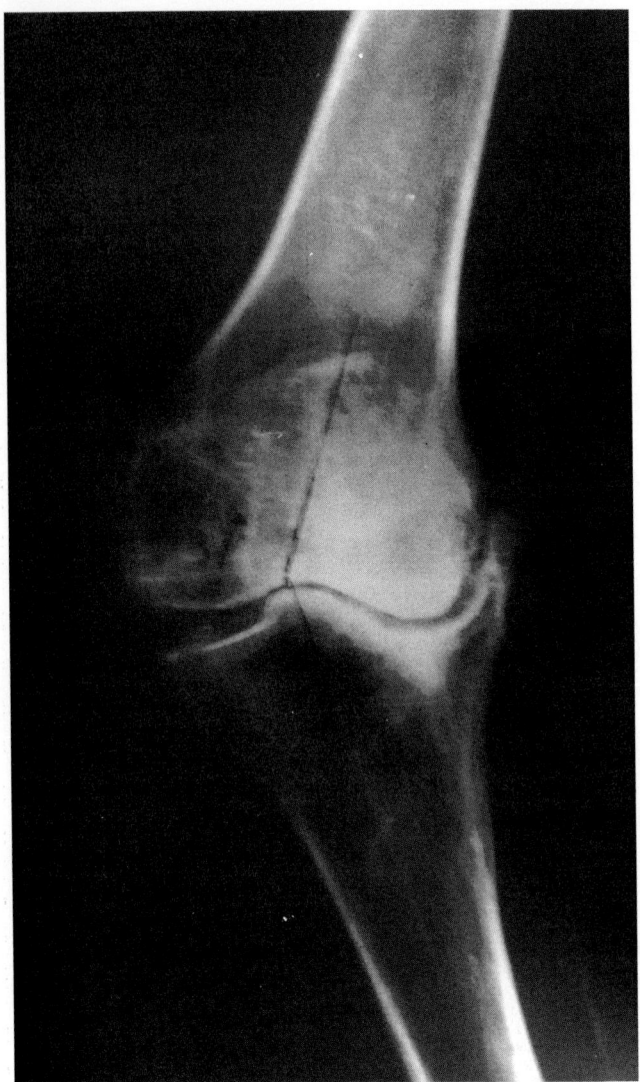

FIG 77-1.
Severe tibial bone loss in a valgus knee with marked sclerosis on the lateral tibial plateau surface.

grafting,[1, 2, 4, 7, 8] and the use of custom or augmented modular knee implants.[3]

Except in the mildest of bone defects (less than 8 mm) the tendency to resect to the floor of the defect must be resisted. A series of problems arises when bone is resected too far distally into the tibia and these will further complicate the technique of the arthroplasty and any necessary subsequent revision surgery. A basic tenet of reconstructive joint surgery is to preserve bone stock at all times and this is particularly important in the proximal tibia. If excess bone is removed to level the tibia at the base of a significant bone defect, the flexion gap is increased requiring a thicker tibial implant for stability in flexion and extension. This will alter the patellofemoral kinematics as the patella, tethered by the patellar tendon, will descend and come into frank contact with the tibial implant itself. Furthermore, the tibial component becomes seated on poorer-quality cancellous bone the further into the metaphysis it is placed. Sizing problems will likewise occur because the cross-sectional area available for prosthetic seating becomes smaller. The patient may require a larger femoral component for the anteroposterior and mediolateral dimensions of the femur, but the corresponding tibial component may be too large for the tibial surface available after a larger tibial bone resection.

TIBIAL BONE LOSS

Defects 6 to 12 mm Deep

There are several techniques to deal with bone loss on the tibial side which is less than 12 mm in depth and encompassing less than one half of the tibial plateau surface. In those patients with less than 5 or 6 mm of deficiency on the medial side of the joint, the tibial osteotomy can be performed to the base of the defect. If there is a slightly greater deficit, there may remain a small defect after tibial resection. In these cases, the remaining sclerotic bed is fenestrated with an 1/8-in. drill to allow penetration of bone cement into the subchondral bone. Up to 2 to 3 mm of remaining void can be filled with polymethyl methacrylate. Small amounts of unsupported polymethyl methacrylate have remained intact without evidence of fatigue fracture or fragmentation. Larger columns of polymethyl methacrylate, however, may fracture and initial implant support may be lost. This is particularly true in the patient in whom optimal alignment has not been achieved at the time of arthroplasty.

If after tibial resection a defect of 4 to 6 mm remains, screws can be used to reinforce the polymethyl methacrylate column (Fig 77-2). One or two cortical screws are placed into the tibial defect so that they are just below the metal tibial component. Acrylic cement is used surrounding the screws to fill the bone deficit. In order to avoid electrolytic interaction of metals, synergistic metals must be used for the screws and the metal base plate of the tibial component.

Defects Greater Than 12 mm Deep

For defects greater than 12 mm in depth and those encompassing more than 30% of the upper tibial surface, an implant with a metallic wedge filler may be used.[3] Initially these implants had to be fabricated on a custom basis. This was costly, required consider-

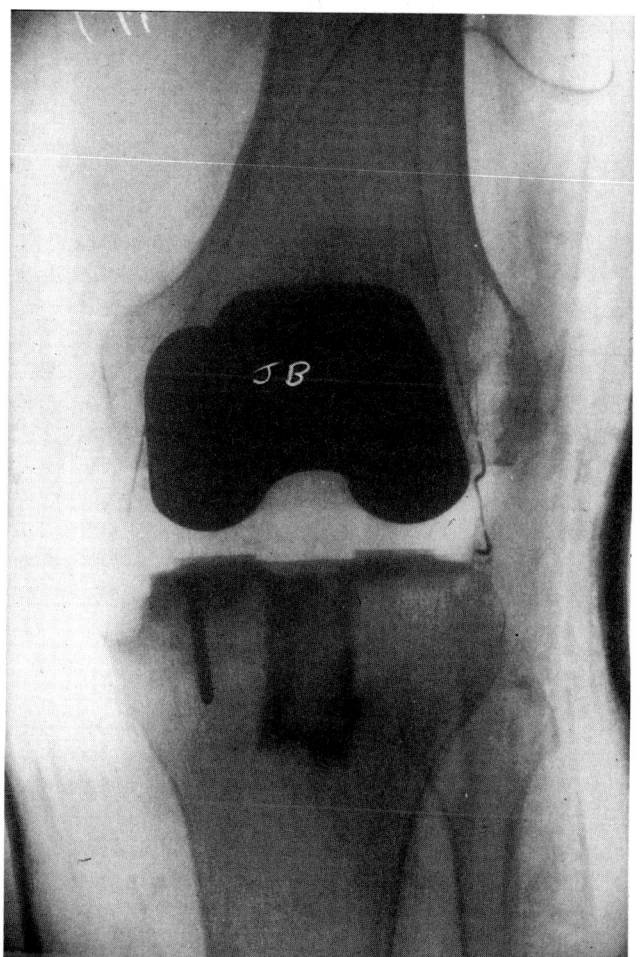

FIG 77–2.
Screw polymethyl methacrylate augmentation for a minor tibial defect.

able time for the implant to be made, and at times the fit of the custom implant to the deficit was suboptimal (Fig 77–3). The metal wedge was then placed on an unsupported column of polymethyl methacrylate and fragmentation and shift of implant position could occur.

More recent advances in implant design have led to the evolution of the modular component systems. These systems allow alteration in the implant by augmenting the components with metal wedges and blocks of various thicknesses which can be added directly to the surface of the tibial and femoral components. Bone deficiency can be corrected by these augmented components and the advantage of these devices over the custom devices is providing the surgeon with the ability to essentially build the component that is needed at the operating table. However, in my experience, bone grafting is a better option in these larger tibial defects in the primary arthritic knee. The use of autogenous bone allows pres-

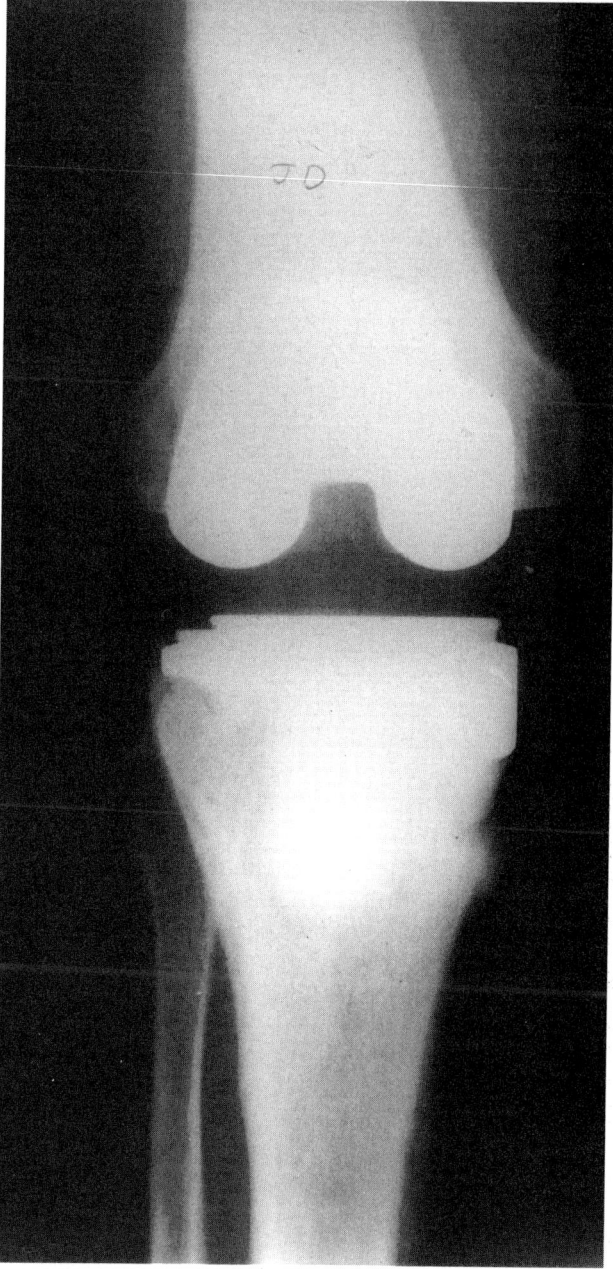

FIG 77–3.
Custom-fabricated tibial component with imperfect coaptation of implant to defect.

ervation of bone stock and consolidation will occur at the donor-recipient bed site. Autogenous bone is readily available at the time of primary total knee arthroplasty and can be harvested from a number of areas. Laskin[4] has reported on bone utilized from the posterior femoral condyle to fill these tibial defects. Although this is a useful technique, the bone is often deficient if reconstruction of large defects is needed. The bone is also primarily cortical and subchondral and the cancellous substrate is quite meager. The following technique, which I have used for the past 14 years in over 35 patients, utilizes bone resected from the distal femur.[1, 8]

Autogenous Bone Grafting for Tibial Deficiency

The initial tibial proximal cut is made perpendicular to the long axis of a line drawn from the midpoint of the tibial surface to the midpoint of the ankle joint. This proximal tibial cut should be conservative, resecting no more than 8 mm of bone. An oscillating saw is then used to create an oblique osteotomy on the side of the tibial defect. The concave surface of the defect should be resected as it will be filled with sclerotic, arthritic bone. The deep surface of the bed, once the osteotomy has been performed through the bed of the defect, should be 80% to 90% cancellous. There may be cystic areas in this bed once the sclerotic surface has been removed, and these may be curetted and filled with cancellous bone. It is important not to be timid in the removal of this sclerotic bed as consolidation of the graft will be greatly impeded if there is not a cancellous bed onto which to place the donor bone. The cut should be planar and smooth so that a flattened graft will fit intimately with the bed (Fig 77–4).

The tibial surface should then be gauged and prepared for the tibial component. Peg, keel, or other fixation surfaces should be made to ensure that the pin and screw stabilization of the bone graft do not compromise tibial component seating.

Attention is then drawn to the femur where distal femoral bone is resected in the standard manner. The resected distal medial femoral condyle is larger than the lateral condyle and therefore it tends to be better graft material. Having resected the distal femoral condyle, this segment of bone is then rotated so that its cancellous surface fills the defect on the upper tibia and there is intimate coaptation between graft and underlying bed (Fig 77–5). The defect should be completely filled with the graft. There will often be an overhanging segment of bone which protrudes above the surface of the tibia. If there is any rocking of the graft or irregular surfaces on the tibial bed, these must be shaved until the surface is planar. Once coaptation is precise, two Kirschner-wires may be used to stabilize the graft to the proximal tibia. The wires should be inserted peripherally so that when the overhanging portion of the bone graft is resected these pins do not prevent a complete osteotomy. Once this graft has been fixed, the excess graft bone is resected using the tibial cut of the opposite of the tibial plateau as a guide. At this point the proximal tibia will be reconstituted. On looking at the upper surface of the tibia the subchondral bone of the femoral condylar bone when resected will act as the peripheral tibial rim of the upper tibia.

The Kirschner-wires are then individually removed and replaced with screws. Cancellous malleolar screws may be used for fixation. As an alternative, cortical screws can be used and the screw hole can be overdrilled at its entrance point to allow compression of the graft. The fixation hole of the prosthesis should be examined when the holes are being drilled and the screw length determined with a gauge to avoid inserting a screw that will contact the tibial prosthesis. This is particularly important if stainless steel screws are used. Therefore vitallium or titanium screws should be used (Fig 77–6).

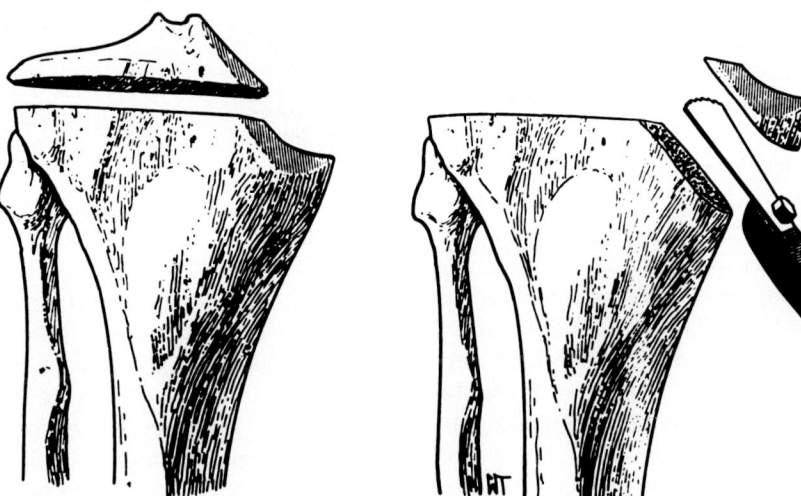

FIG 77–4.
Upper tibial osteotomy has been made with planar excision of the sclerotic bed of the bone defect.

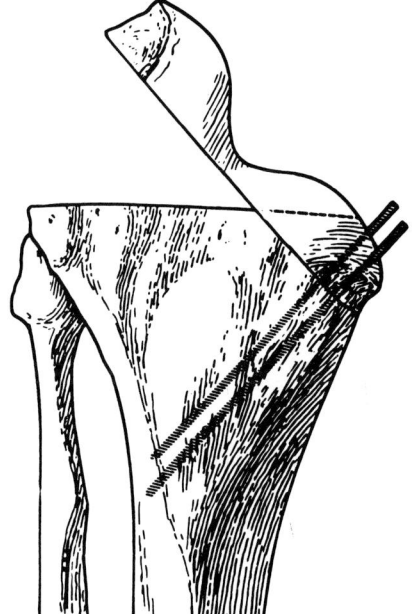
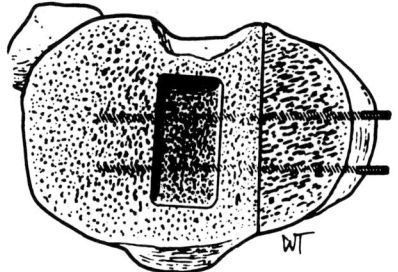

FIG 77–5.
Femoral condyle is used to fill the defect with cancellous-to-cancellous coaptation. Note reconstitution of the tibial peripheral rim on the view of the top surface of the tibia *(right)*.

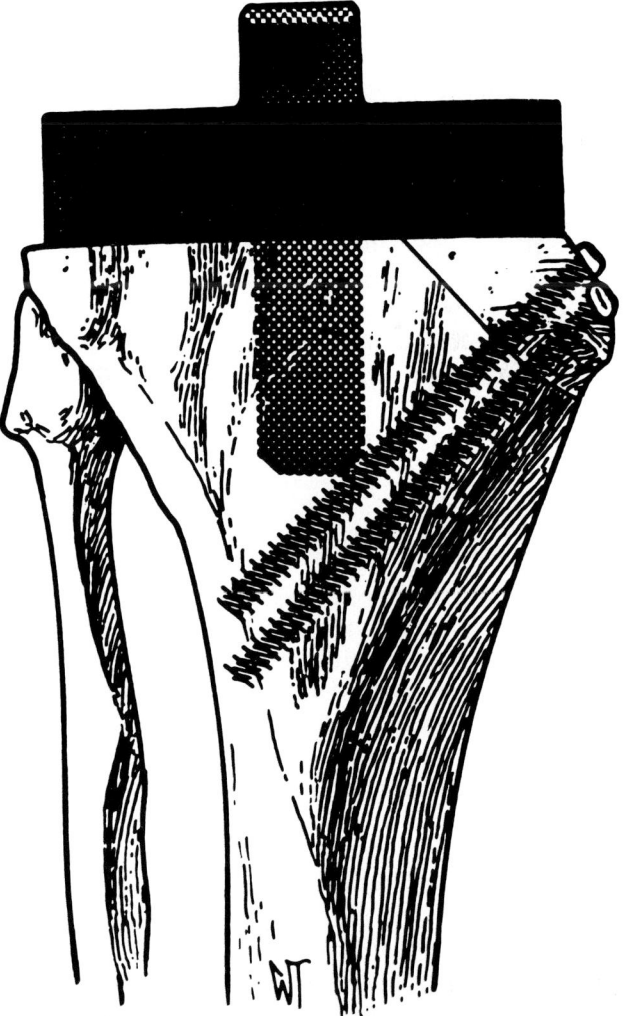

FIG 77–6.
Bone graft is fixed with cortical screws and the implant is seated.

It is important that cement not be allowed to enter the interval between the graft and the recipient bed. This can be prevented by cementing the femoral and patellar components first. A small portion of cement can be used to caulk the interface between the graft and the underlying tibia by applying it to the upper surface of the tibia at the graft-tibia interface. This will harden so that when the lower-viscosity tibial cement is inserted it will not penetrate into the graft interface. Initially this was not appreciated and in the first patient undergoing this technique the graft became sclerotic. However, in follow-up at 13 years the graft had not resorbed or collapsed and there has been no shift in implant position (Fig 77-7).

Postoperative rehabilitation for these patients is the same as for patients without bone grafting. Because the tibial implant support is maintained on the more normal side of the tibia and because of the excellent fixation of the graft, modification of weight-bearing has not been necessary. Continuous passive motion is employed on the first postoperative day and most patients are discharged with a cane.

This technique has been used in 35 patients over the past 14 years. The results to date have been excellent with radiographic evidence of graft consolidation and no patient experiencing collapse of the graft (Fig 77-8). In two patients reoperation has been necessary (one patient for infection, one for ligamentous instability after a fall). Examination of the graft site revealed in both patients evidence of trabecular incorporation at the graft-tibia interface.

Because of the complex nature of the deformities in this series of patients, a more constrained prosthesis (the Total Condylar III, Howmedica, Rutherford, N.J.) was used in five of the knees. The greatest deformities treated included patients with 25 degrees of varus and 30 degrees of valgus deformity.

FEMORAL BONE LOSS

Femoral bone loss occurs less commonly than tibial bone loss. It may be seen in posttraumatic arthritis or in inflammatory arthritis associated with osteonecrosis. It occurs most frequently in my experience in the valgus knee. It is almost always associated with bone loss on the tibial side as well. The concepts of management of femoral bone loss are similar to those for tibial bone loss and include developing a suitable cancellous bed for the graft, achieving optimal coaptation of the graft to the bed, maintaining position of the graft with internal fixation devices, and reestablishing the joint line to its proper height.

The surgeon must adequately expose the distal femoral condyles in order to visualize the anterior and posterior margins of the femoral bone. All soft tissue at the interface between the collapsed and normal bone must be debrided from the bony surface of the femur to allow thorough evaluation of the defect. In many instances the femoral bone loss may be cystic, especially in inflammatory arthritis, and these are easily grafted using bone from the intercondylar area or from the tibia during preparation of the tibial implant seating hole. This cancellous bone can be impacted into these cystic areas and a deficient surface can be completely filled with this bone.

For extensive defects where there has been complete loss of the condylar surface, more formal grafting will be necessary. Bone can be used from the intercondylar area and fixation screws can be inserted directly into the graft and advanced into the underlying femoral bone along the longitudinal axis of the femur. Since contact may occur between femoral component and screw, compatible metals must be used. Precise coaptation must be achieved between the graft and the underlying bed and both surfaces must be cancellous where bone-to-bone contact occurs. For smaller grafts in this area, Kirschner-wire fixation alone may be sufficient.

When grafting the distal femur it is important to reestablish the joint line at a location close to its anatomic origin. The distal articular surface of the femoral condyle was measured in a series of 30 knees at surgical reconstruction. Its location was determined by using the anterior margin of the collateral ligament at its origin from the femur. This is a constant landmark and is generally present except in the most severe cases of femoral condylar bone loss. The distance from the anterior margin of the ligament to the articular surface was 17 to 20 mm in this series of knees evaluated. Therefore the articular surface of the femoral component should be placed at this distance from the collateral ligament origin to approximate the normal location of the joint line. The graft must allow seating of the femoral component to reproduce this measurement if the joint line is to be maintained in the replaced knee.

BONE GRAFTING IN REVISION TOTAL KNEE ARTHROPLASTY

Bone deficiency is a common finding in revision knee replacement surgery. Bone loss may at times be the cause of the total knee replacement failing, but more commonly it is produced when the implants themselves loosen. The inflammatory environment produced by polymethyl methacrylate fragmentation, wear debris, and other factors not fully understood can produce a progressive and injurious loss of bony

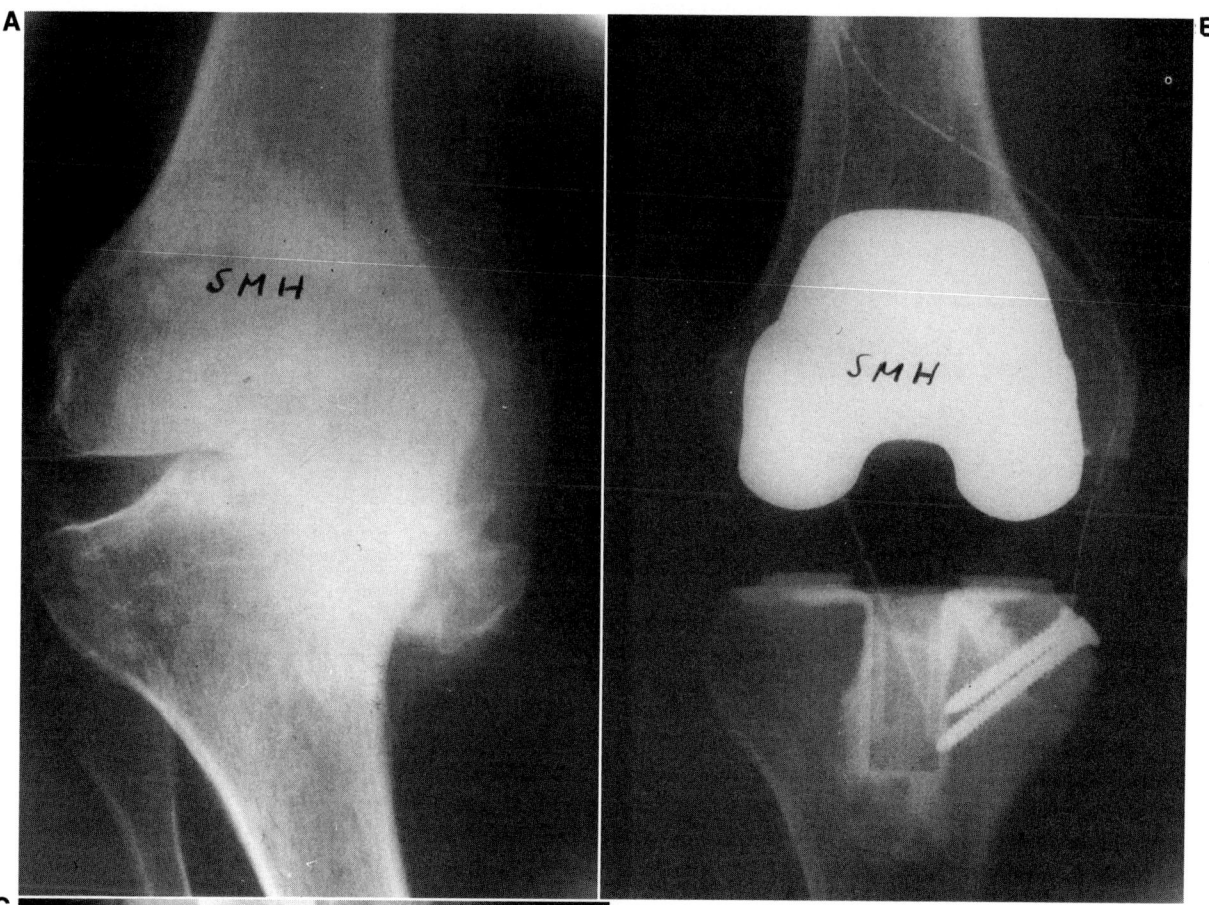
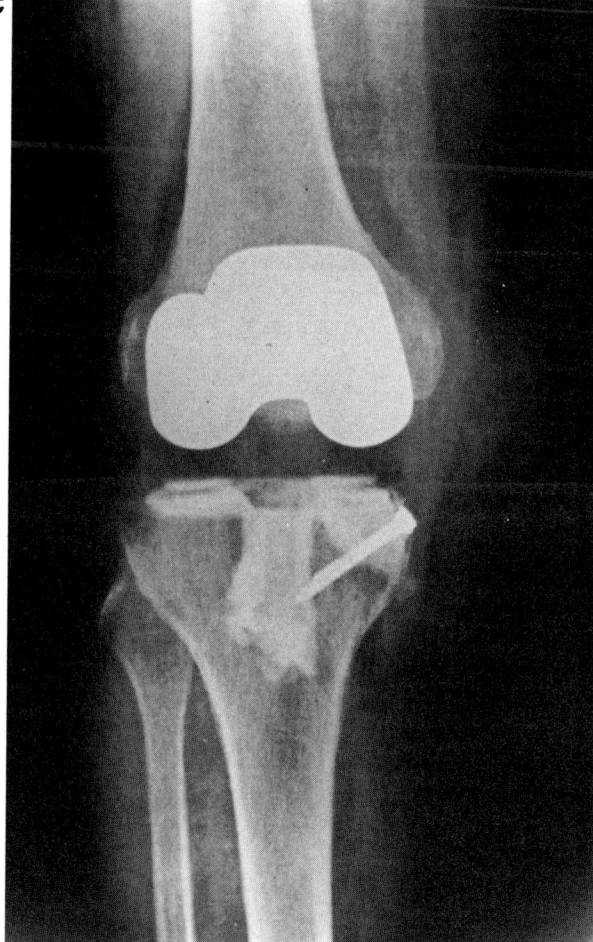

FIG 77–7.
A, a marked varus deformity with tibial bone loss in a 70-year-old patient. **B,** the first autogenous bone graft was performed in 1978. Note polymethyl methacrylate in the graft-tibial interface. **C,** at 13-year follow-up, sclerosis of the graft is noted, but there is no evidence of resorption or collapse.

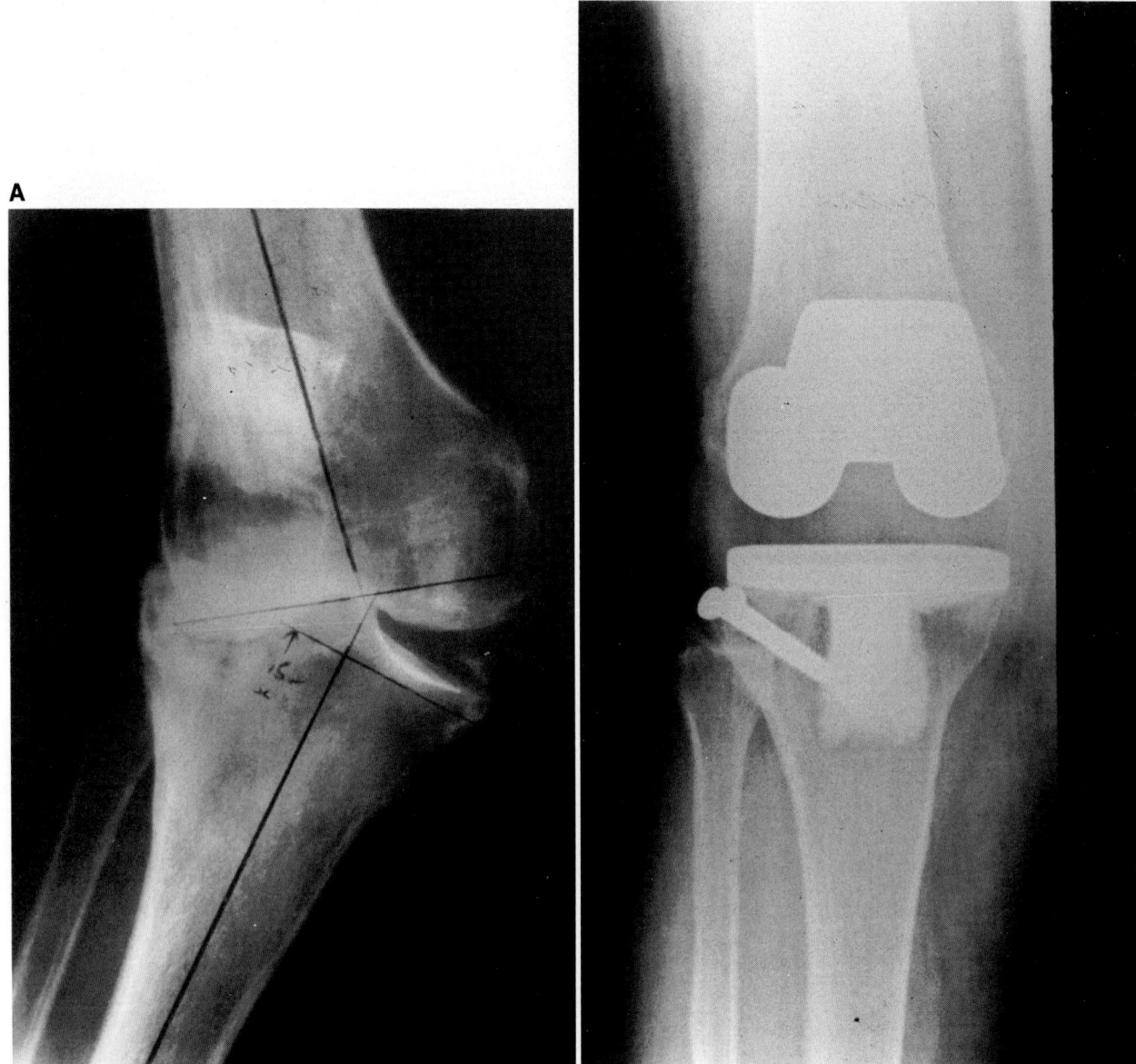

FIG 77-8.
A, a severe valgus deformity with a severe lateral bone deficit. **B,** 8-year follow-up radiograph showing graft incorporation without evidence of resorption or collapse.

support to the implant. Additionally, levering the component from the underlying bone at the time of revision surgery may cause further bony collapse and fracture. Axial distraction is preferred, but even this may cause bone adhering to the component to avulse from the underlying substrate. It is crucial to disrupt the interface between the prosthesis and the bone as much as possible before attempting to extract the implant.

In the revision knee replacement three major types of bone defects may be present, and each is managed in a different manner. There may be variations or combinations of these three general types of bone loss, but cystic deficiencies, central medullary deficiencies, and peripheral plateau or condylar bone loss remain the generic categories of bone loss in revision knee replacement surgery.

Cystic Deficiencies

Cystic deficiencies are generally encountered on the surfaces of the tibia and femur after removal of the total knee implant. They may be the result of acrylic which has penetrated into the subchondral bone and

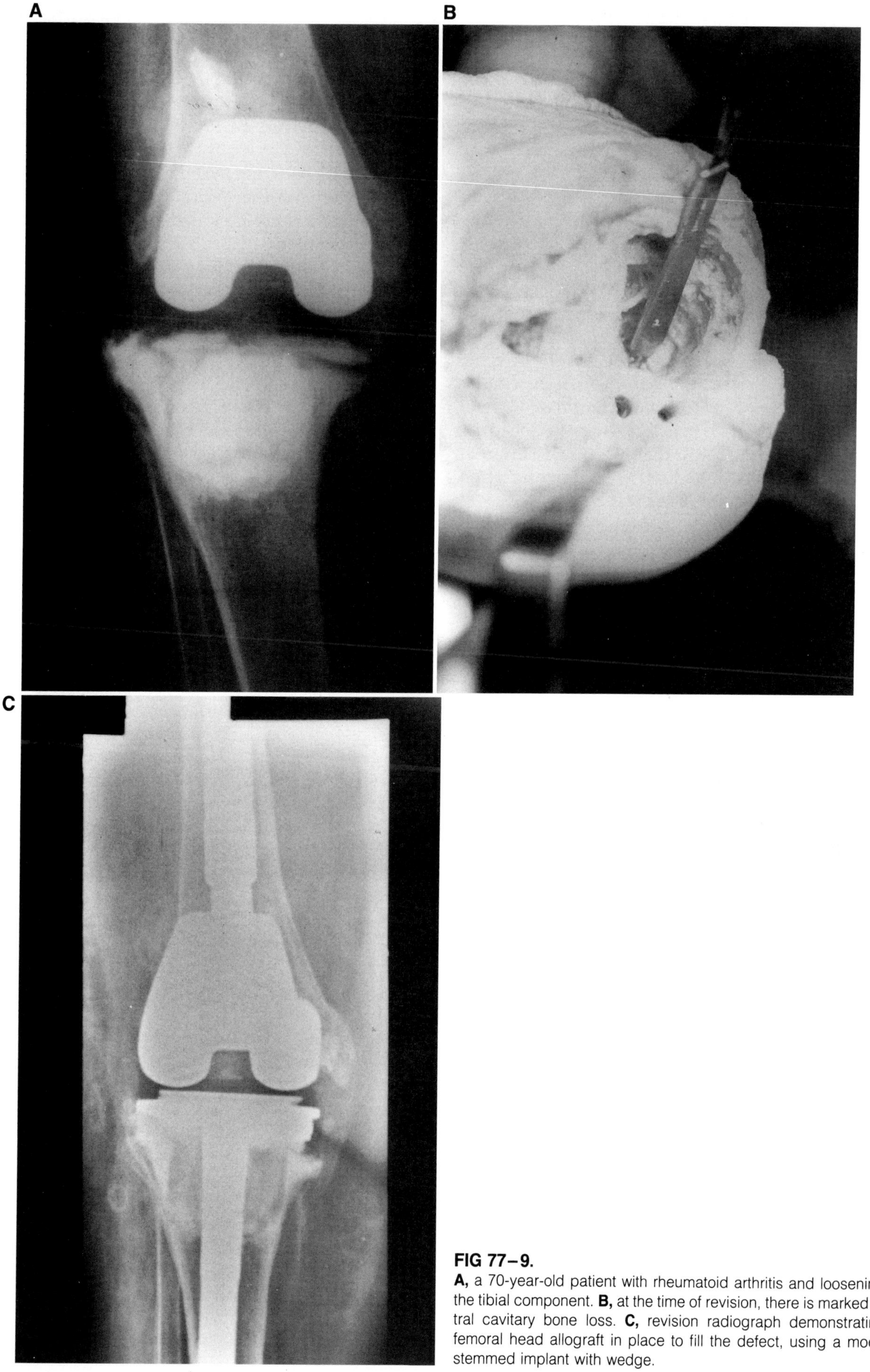

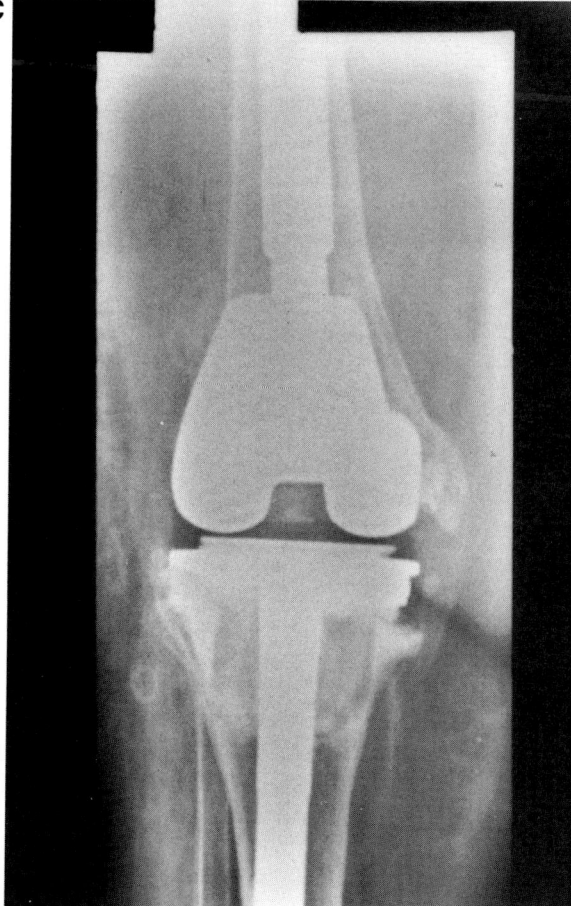

FIG 77–9.
A, a 70-year-old patient with rheumatoid arthritis and loosening of the tibial component. **B,** at the time of revision, there is marked central cavitary bone loss. **C,** revision radiograph demonstrating a femoral head allograft in place to fill the defect, using a modular stemmed implant with wedge.

produced a punctate crater. They also may occur when the implant itself is removed from the bone and portions of bone adhere to the implant. If the femoral component has condylar fixation pegs, these may produce cystic areas of bone loss in the underlying bone. Usually these cystic areas are associated with larger plateau or condylar deficiencies and therefore combined techniques to handle both problems must be employed.

Cystic defects are easily filled with cancellous bone available locally at the time of the revision. The base of the deficiency should be cleared of any adherent cement and soft tissue. The cancellous bone should be driven deep into the depression with an impactor. The bone will usually compress without problem into these areas and a significantly improved surface will be available to the implant. If sufficient bone is not available from local bone removed at revision surgery, iliac crest bone can be used.

Central Medullary Deficiency

Central medullary bone deficiencies may be present on the femur or tibia during revision surgery. These most often occur if the primary implants used had central intramedullary stems. The deficiency on the tibial surface is funnel-shaped and can be quite large. Often only the cortical rim is left without any cancellous plateau support on the medial or lateral side. If one is revising a hinged implant with a bulky femoral axle, there will also be a large amount of femoral bone loss. In some cases, the entire femoral condylar bone may be absent.

Because of the poor quality of supporting bone of the surface faces of the femur and tibia in these cases, the surgeon must add bone to the deficient areas and then transfer load and stress distal to the deficient proximal tibia and femur by utilizing an intramedullary stem. Usually autogenous bone is inadequate to deal with these larger defects even if the entire iliac crest is used. Femoral head allograft bone is often needed. The femoral head can be shaped to fill these large cavitary defects and a hole placed through the graft once the head has been impacted into place. The stem can then be passed through this fenestration and gain fixation beyond it (Fig 77–9). Autogenous bone, which is available, can be placed around the allograft in an attempt to augment incorporation of the periphery of the graft. There is concern that in using these large allografts resorption may occur with time, but this tendency may be lessened by unloading the graft with the use of intramedullary stems.

The availability of modular revision systems allows for variation in the length and thickness of the tibial and femoral stems. The length of the stem is determined by the quality of the proximal femoral and tibial bone. Currently the stems are not being cemented but rather are fluted rods which are sized to gain purchase on the cortical bone of the femur and tibia. The stems are press-fitted into the canals, and the upper portion of the stem and implant are cemented in place. Careful preoperative planning is mandatory in these cases so that implants of the proper length and diameter are available.

Peripheral Tibial Plateau or Condylar Bone Loss

Peripheral rather than intramedullary loss can occur in those cases in which the previous implant has been malaligned or where there has been an overload of one femoral condyle or tibial plateau. Bone collapse occurs on the overloaded side of the implant with tension forces on the opposite side causing liftoff of the implant from the bone. At times the entire plateau or condyle may collapse.

The tendency to resect further bone to get below the base of the defect must be avoided. These defects can be handled either by bone grafting or autogenous bone graft from the iliac crest. Bone loss on the tibial side can be replaced by taking an iliac crest graft and using the cancellous surface against the cancellous bone and allowing the cortical surface to provide support to the implant. A stemmed component must be used in these cases to transfer load to the more distal tibia.

Alternatively, modular augments can be used on the distal femur or proximal tibia to fill these defects. Distal femoral augments can replace lost distal femoral bone and restore alignment (Fig 77–10). On the tibial side wedge augments can be attached to the tibial surface to accomodate both partial and full plateau loss (Fig 77–11). Augments can also be used to fill deficiency of bone on the posterior femoral surface.

In summary, bone grafting provides the surgeon with a biologic approach to the management of bone deficiency either in primary or revision total knee arthroplasty. Whenever possible, preservation of the underlying bone is vital to long-term success of the replacement. In primary knee replacement with autogenous bone readily available, grafting should be used. In revision total knee replacement, the long-term results of allografts are still unclear and follow-up is short-term. Modular revision total knee systems in combination with both allograft and autograft in these more difficult cases seems the best solution at this time. Modular systems provide the flex-

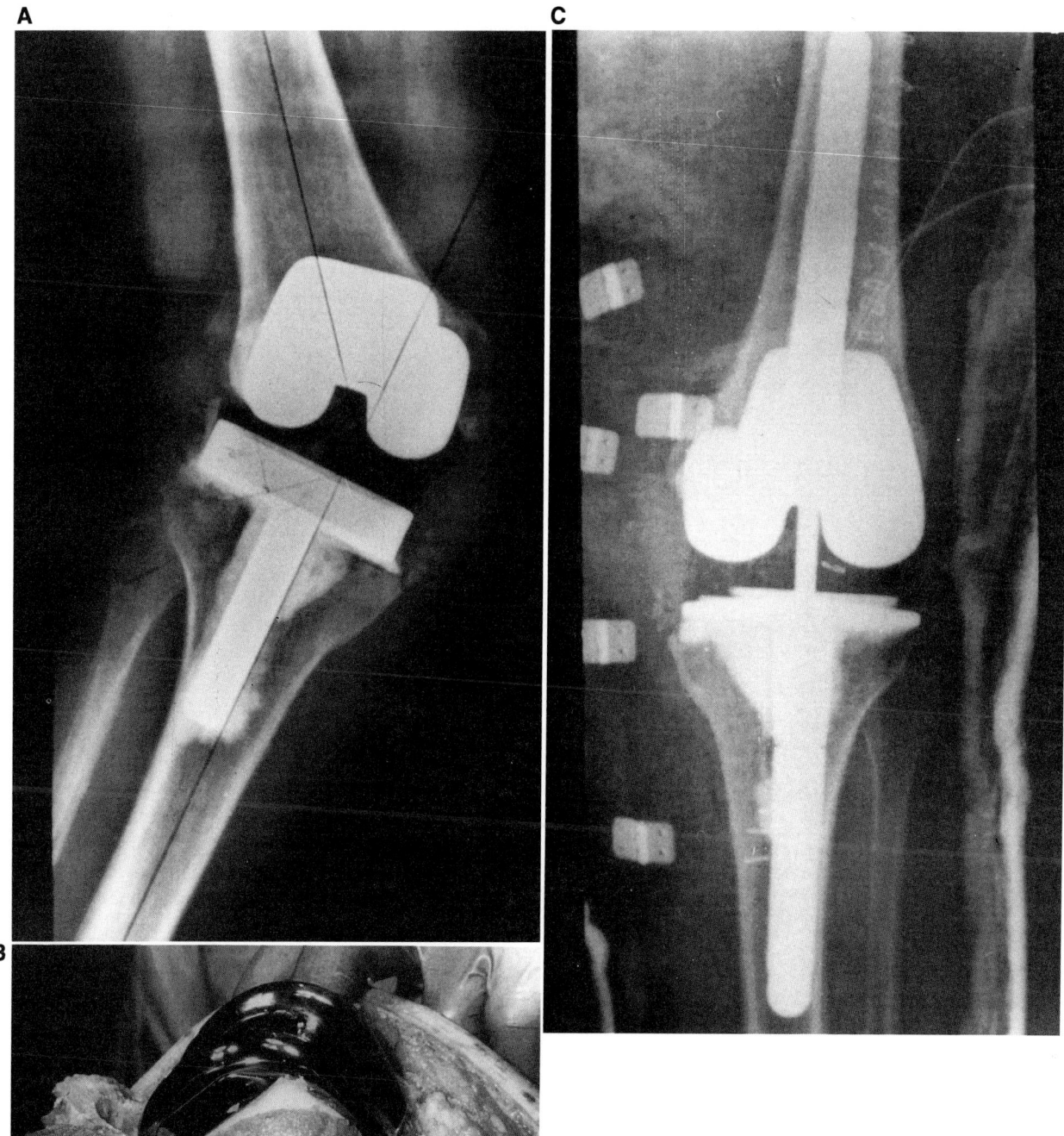

FIG 77-10.
A, marked lateral femoral condylar collapse and severe valgus deformity. **B,** a lateral femoral augment used to correct the condylar deficit. **C,** postoperative radiograph demonstrating restoration of alignment.

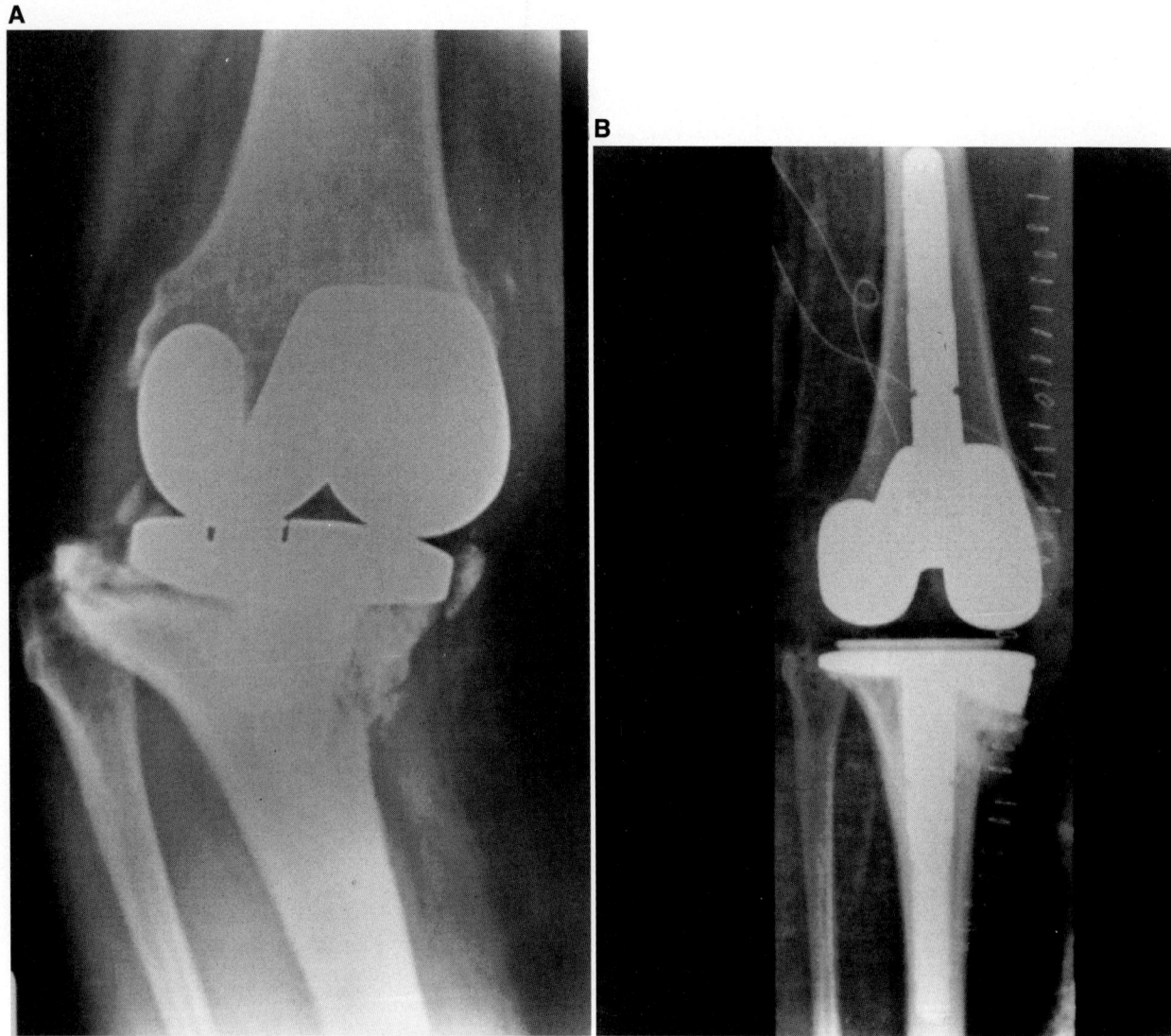

FIG 77-11.
A, severe medial bone loss and tibial component loosening. **B,** revision radiograph demonstrating an autogenous bone graft from revision and the modular wedge tibial component.

ibility needed to augment bone deficiency and also transfer load away from deficient areas to more distal sites. The long-term results with these systems, however, await the passage of time.

REFERENCES

1. Altchek D, Sculco TP, Rawling B: Autogenous bone grafting for severe angular deformity in total knee arthroplasty, *J Arthroplasty* 4:151–156, 1989.
2. Dorr, et al: Bone graft for tibial defects in total knee arthroplasty, *Clin Orthop* 205:153–165, 1986.
3. Insall JN: Total knee replacement. In Insall JN, editor: *Surgery of the knee,* New York, 1984, Churchill Livingstone.
4. Laskin RS: Total knee replacement in the presence of large bony defects of the tibia and marked knee instability, *Clin Orthop* 248:66–70, 1989.
5. Lotke PA, Wong R, Ecker ML: The management of large tibial defects in primary total knee replacement, 52nd Annual Meeting of the American Academy of Orthopaedic Surgeons, Las Vegas, 1985.
6. Ritter MA: Screw and cement fixation of large defects in total knee arthroplasty, *J Arthroplasty* 1:125–130, 1986.
7. Sculco TP: Bone grafting in revision total knee replacement. In Scott WN, editor: *Total knee revision arthroplasty,* Orlando, Fla, 1987, Grune & Stratton.
8. Windsor RE, Insall JN, Sculco TP: Bone grafting of tibial defects in primary and revision total knee arthroplasty, *Clin Orthop* 205:132–137, 1987.

78

Arthrodesis and Resection Arthroplasty for the Failed Total Knee Replacement

DOUGLAS A. DENNIS, M.D.

Knee arthrodesis
  Surgical techniques
    General principles
    External fixation

Internal fixation
Intramedullary nail fixation
Resection arthroplasty
Summary

Cemented total knee arthroplasty (TKA) has proved to be a successful and durable surgical procedure with over 90% success reported by numerous investigators at follow-up periods of 10 years or longer.[17, 58, 61, 74] Despite the success of TKA, numerous failure modes have been identified, including aseptic loosening, infection, instability, prosthetic wear or failure, patellofemoral complications, and persistent pain.[33, 54, 77] Treatment options for failed TKA include revision TKA, arthrodesis, and resection arthroplasty.

Factors influencing the preferred treatment option for the failed TKA are the patient's age, weight, activity level, diagnosis, and general health; the status of the soft tissues and adjacent joints; the amount of bone loss; and the bacterial virulence and sensitivity in those cases which are infected.[45, 70] In cases with extensive bone loss, infection with highly virulent and less sensitive organisms, or poor soft tissues, knee arthrodesis is often the favored method of treatment.

KNEE ARTHRODESIS

Indications for knee arthrodesis include septic arthritis, traumatic osteoarthritis in a young person, painful ankylosis, paralytic conditions, Charcot joint neuropathy, and an incompetent extensor mechanism.[38] In the last two decades, failed TKA has become the most common indication for arthrodesis, particularly if secondary to deep sepsis.*

For conditions other than failed TKA, the rates of union following knee arthrodesis have been as high as 95% to 100%.[5, 11, 13, 15, 30, 52, 68, 71] Reports of union for cases of failed TKA have been extremely variable, with rates ranging from 0% to 100%.† Nonunion has been associated with factors such as extensive bone loss,‡ poor quality of remaining bone,[5, 69] an inability to obtain rigid fixation,[25, 33, 45, 54, 60, 69, 77] and persistent sepsis.[2, 25, 33, 42, 53, 54, 69] Others have observed that infection, if controlled, has little effect on the rate of union,[3, 33, 47, 69, 73, 77] although time to union may be prolonged.[77]

There have been numerous reports of superior rates of union in cases of knee arthrodesis following failure of less constrained prosthetic designs as opposed to more highly constrained designs.* Broderson et al.,[8] in a review of attempted knee arthrodeses in 45 cases of failed TKA, obtained union in 81% of failed resurfacing TKA vs. 56% union with failed hinge designs. Rand et al.,[60] in a similar review, noted union in only 43% with failed hinge TKAs in comparison to an 85% rate of union with knee arthrodeses for failed resurfacing designs.

Hankin et al.[34] have measured the volume of bone removal and remaining interface areas available for knee arthrodesis with various types of TKA. They observed increased volumetric bone loss and a subsequent reduction in interface contact areas with more constrained prostheses, particularly hinge de-

---

*References 8, 10, 28, 29, 31, 33, 40, 41, 48, 49, 56, 57, 64, 66, 67, 69.

†References 2, 13, 16, 21, 24, 25, 31, 33, 45, 47, 54, 59, 60, 63, 70, 73, 76, 77.

‡References 4, 8, 11, 19, 27, 33, 37, 39, 46, 47, 56, 59, 60, 69, 70, 72.

*References 2, 4, 5, 8, 31, 47, 54, 60, 69, 70.

signs with bulky stems and protrusions. Condylar resurfacing designs proved to be bone-preserving with superior interface contact areas.

Surgical Techniques

While numerous methods of knee arthrodesis have been developed, techniques utilizing external fixation, internal fixation (dual compression plating), and intramedullary nailing are predominately utilized. Bigliani et al.[5] obtained union in 85% of cases by utilizing adjunctive electrical stimulation in 20 cases of attempted knee arthrodeses following failed TKA which had progressed to nonunion. Regardless of the surgical technique chosen, adherence to certain general principles is necessary to obtain optimal results.

General Principles

When performing arthrodesis following a failed TKA, the skin and underlying soft tissues are often heavily scarred and inelastic, as well as hypovascular. The previous skin incision should be utilized whenever possible and carried directly to the bone to avoid thin skin flaps.[69] Prosthetic components must be carefully removed, both to preserve remaining cancellous bone and avoid fracture, as the remaining cortical shells are often thinned and brittle.

Radical debridement of all necrotic tissue and total removal of polymethyl methacrylate (PMMA) is mandatory in infected cases. In noninfected cases, distant PMMA remaining within the intramedullary canals may augment fixation of external fixation pins or compression plate screws in patients with extremely thin and osteopenic bone.

Alignment jigs utilized for TKA are useful to ensure proper orientation of bone cuts.[69] The recommended position of knee arthrodesis has been debated. In a series of patients with rheumatoid arthritis, Figgie et al.[25] reported a fusion in 7 ± 5 degrees of valgus alignment, and 15 ± 15 degrees of knee flexion was associated with the highest rate of union and functional score and the lowest rate of rheumatoid disease progression in adjacent joints. Others[9, 57, 72] have advocated fusing the knee in full extension to avoid extensive shortening which so commonly occurs with knee arthrodesis following a failed TKA.

In cases with substantial femoral or tibial bone loss, resection of the fibular head may be required to allow compression of the bone surfaces. In such cases, the fibular head as well as the patella or any bone resected during preparation of the condylar surfaces may be utilized as autogenous bone graft. Rand et al.[60] recommend adjunctive bone grafting at the time of knee arthrodesis if the femorotibial contact area is reduced to 70% or less. Placement of the graft at the periphery of the arthrodesis site, rather than within the medullary canals, is preferred to allow revascularization from the surrounding soft tissues.[60, 69]

Owing to the reduced elasticity and mobility of skin flaps from previous surgical procedures, skin closure without excessive tension may be difficult. Utilization of relaxing skin incisions, myocutaneous flaps (rotational vs. free), or delayed primary closure should be considered in these cases. Patellectomy may also be required to decrease bulk and facilitate wound closure.[70]

In infected cases, if internal fixation or intramedullary nailing is the desired method of fixation, a two-stage arthrodesis technique utilized by Knutson et al.[45, 47] and others[23, 54, 55, 57, 76, 77] is recommended. During the initial operative stage, the prosthesis and PMMA are removed, soft tissues are aggressively debrided, and antibiotic-impregnated PMMA beads are inserted. Temporary fixation is provided by external fixation or cast immobilization. Intravenous antibiotics are then administered. When the wound is healed and quiescent (typically 4–6 weeks), a second surgical procedure is performed to remove the beads, redebride the wound, apply the final fixation device, and bone graft, if indicated.

External Fixation

External fixation as a method of compression knee arthrodesis was first performed by Key[42] in 1932, utilizing a turnbuckle apparatus, and later refined and popularized by Charnley.[13, 14] It is the favored technique when active infection is present, as fixation pins may be placed distant from the knee joint while providing the rigid immobilization so beneficial in the management of infection. Rigid fixation may be difficult to obtain in cases with advanced bone loss, particularly in the anteroposteior plane, owing to poor contact between the opposing bone surfaces.[33, 60, 69] Other disadvantages include the need for the patient to remain nonweightbearing to avoid excessive load on the pins and subsequent loosening, as well as the prolonged period of treatment. Most authors recommend maintenance of the external fixation device for 3 to 4 months followed by cast immobilization until union is evident, often for another 3 to 4 months.[60, 69]

Biomechanical evaluations of uniplanar external fixation devices, such as the Hoffmann-Vidal quadrilateral frame, have found diminished stability in the anteroposterior plane, with anteroposterior bending stiffness measuring as low as 20% of lateral bending stiffness levels.[7, 9, 26, 44, 51] The addition of an anterior frame with sagittal pins to provide biplanar fixation

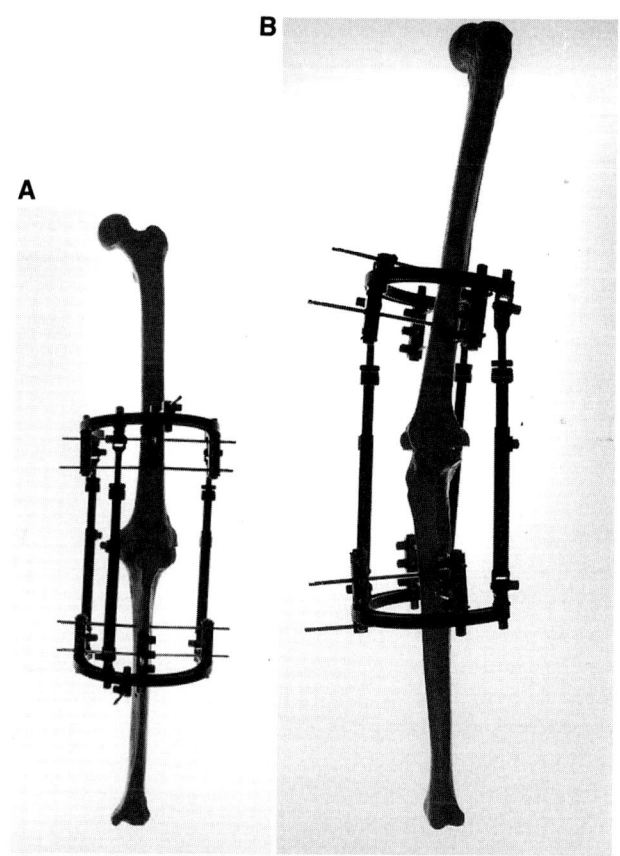

FIG 78–1.
Frontal **(A)** and lateral **(B)** views of a recommended external fixation configuration with the addition of anteriorly placed sagittal pins to provide biplanar fixation.

has been shown to significantly improve anteroposterior stability of the external fixation apparatus,[44, 50] and has been noted in numerous reports to improve the rate of union in knee arthrodesis[9, 24, 26, 44, 47, 62] (Fig 78–1). The stability of an external fixation device can also be enhanced by using one of several techniques: (1) utilizing threaded vs. smooth pins; (2) selecting pins with a larger diameter; (3) ensuring wider pin separation within each group of pins; (4) increasing the number of pins; and (5) minimizing the distance of sidebar separation.[7] Greatly improved bending and torsional stability is also obtained when compression is applied secondary to static friction between opposing bone surfaces.[7, 36]

The results of knee arthrodesis with external fixation following a failed TKA have been widely variable.* A literature review by Stulberg[69] reported union rates between 25% and 100% when external fixation was utilized. The majority of reports note higher rates of union with arthrodesis of a failed con-

*References 8, 16, 24, 33, 41, 47, 60, 62, 66, 67, 75.

dylar vs. hinge TKA, as well as superior results with biplanar external fixation devices. Reported complications include pin tract infection[11, 20, 47, 60, 65] (as high as 35%[31]), pin fracture or loosening,[47] and osseous fracture through a pin hole.[31, 45, 55, 60]

Pin tract complications may be minimized by utilizing one of the following techniques: (1) predrilling to lessen thermal necrosis[47]; (2) use of a drill sleeve to protect adjacent soft tissues; (3) utilization of threaded pins to enhance pin anchorage[6, 7, 44]; and (4) diligent pin care.[32] Titanium pins are recommended for their superior biocompatability with bone.[1] However, Briggs and Chao[7] reported a 41% decrease in stiffness of a Hoffmann-Vidal type of external fixation apparatus when titanium pins were used with a titanium frame. When the titanium frame was used in conjunction with stainless steel pins, only a minimal reduction in stability of the external fixation device was observed.

Internal Fixation

Internal fixation, typically two dynamic compression plates, is a favorable technique when presented with porotic bone, and usually provides an opportunity for secure fixation. Little or no external immobilization is required if rigid fixation is obtained. The plates may be left in place indefinitely, an advantage when the time to fusion is prolonged.

Wound closure difficulties may be encountered owing to the bulkiness of the plates, especially if an anterior plate is used.[25, 55] Sustained plate use creates a potential for stress shielding which may later require plate removal if weakening of the bone is substantial. Femoral fracture at the proximal end of the plates has been reported.[54, 55, 69] As with external fixation, extended limited weightbearing is recommended, a disadvantage for obese patients and those with an upper extremity weakness such as rheumatoid arthritis. Nichols et al.[54] allowed weightbearing as tolerated, although a long leg cast was also utilized. Utilization of dual compression plates is not recommended in the presence of active infection,[54, 69] although successful single-stage use of this technique has been reported in cases infected with organisms of low virulence.[54] If a more virulent infecting organism or active drainage is encountered, a two-stage technique, as previously discussed, is favored.

A double-plating technique utilizing dynamic compression plates is preferred, placing plates medially and laterally (Fig 78–2), or on one side and anteriorly.[55] The plates must be carefully contoured to the periphery of the femur to enhance fixation and minimize bulk. Placement of the plates in a staggered fashion can lessen stress shielding and the risk of os-

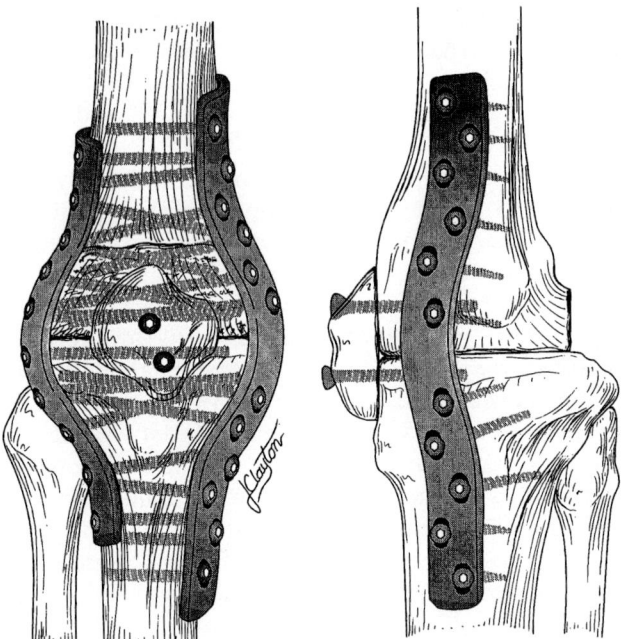

FIG 78–2.
Diagram demonstrating the internal fixation technique with staggered, dual, dynamic compression plates.

seous fracture at the plate ends.[54] A minimum of four bicortical screws are necessary, both proximal and distal to the arthrodesis site (16 engaged cortices). Use of the AO/ASIF compression apparatus is beneficial when bone quality of the opposing bone surfaces is adequate.

Results of the internal fixation method with compression plates have generally been superior to those utilizing external fixation. Nichols et al.[54] reported on 11 cases of attempted knee arthrodesis following failed TKA and obtained solid fusion in all cases in an average of 5.6 months. In a similar series of 44 failed TKAs, Munzinger and co-workers[53] obtained fusion in 100% of 34 cases treated with compression plating, but in only 60% of 10 cases managed with external fixation.

Intramedullary Nail Fixation

The use of intramedullary (IM) nail fixation for knee arthrodesis was initially reported by Chapchal in 1948.[12] Stability is provided through three-point fixation within the diaphyses of femur and tibia.[76] Early weightbearing without external immobilization is permitted providing longitudinal compression across the arthrodesis (Fig 78–3). Later removal of the IM nail is usually not required. This method is often more technically demanding as evidenced by the extended operative time (average, 4.1 hours) and increased blood loss (average, 1,574 mL) reported by Donley et al.[18] All PMMA must be removed to allow for nail passage. Contraindications include ipsilateral total hip arthroplasty and deformity secondary to femoral or tibial malunion or excessive bowing. In cases with active infection, a two-stage technique is preferred,[23, 35, 57, 76] obtaining control of the infection before IM nail insertion. However, successful single-stage use in the presence of infection has been reported,[23] and fusion may still occur in the presence of an IM nail and persistent infection.[76]

Preoperative planning includes templating of roentgenograms to determine nail length and diameter and to assess the magnitude of femoral and tibial bowing. Curved nails are preferred. By placing the convexity of the nail anteromedially, some degree of knee flexion and valgus alignment may be obtained. Fluted nail designs offer improved rotational stability. The IM nail may be inserted antegrade through the greater trochanter or retrograde through the knee joint. Some intramedullary reaming, particularly of the tibia, is usually necessary to allow for use of a larger-diameter nail, thereby filling the femur more completely. The distal end of the nail should extend beyond the tibial isthmus. To reduce the risk of proximal nail migration, wire loop fixation through the greater trochanter[18] or a proximal interlocking nail[43] may be utilized. If satisfactory stability is not obtained following IM nail insertion, supplementary staples[57] or a single compression clamp[35] may be added.

The success of IM nail fixation for arthrodesis of the failed TKA has ranged from 66.6% to 100%.[18, 35, 43, 57, 76] In a review of the literature with this technique for failed, infected TKA, Wilde and Stearns[76] noted a combined average fusion rate of 84%, which was superior to the use of external fixation. This technique has often provided successful results when attempted knee arthrodesis using other methods has failed.[45]

Reported complications include proximal nail migration,[18] IM nail fracture in cases of persistent nonunion,[57] and tibial perforation or fracture during nail insertion.[18, 47] Donley and associates[18] observed that intraoperative tibial fracture enhances the risk of later nonunion and infection.

RESECTION ARTHROPLASTY

Resection arthroplasty plays a limited role in the management of the failed TKA. Indications include patients who are limited ambulators even before TKA failure and those with severe polyarticular rheumatoid arthritis in whom even limited knee motion will enhance functional capabilities.[18, 69, 70]

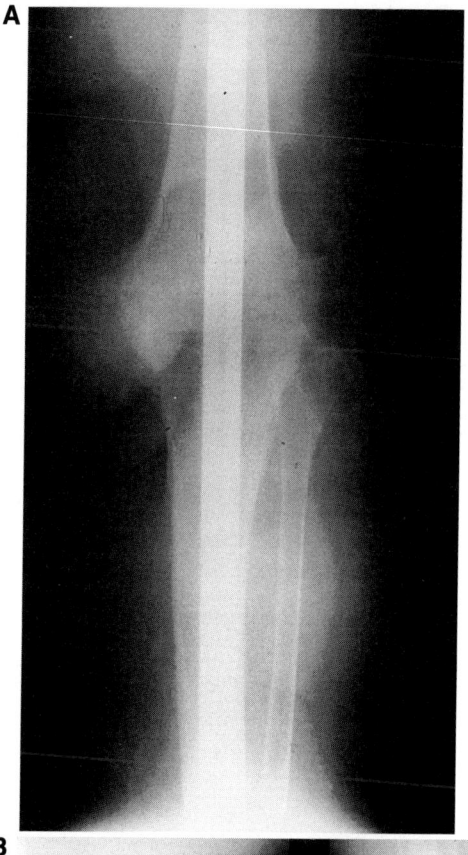
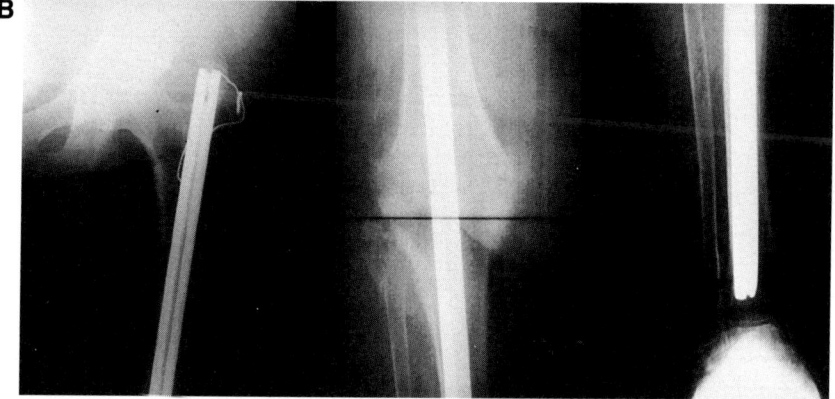

FIG 78–3.
A and **B**, postoperative radiographs following arthrodesis with intramedullary nail fixation. (Courtesy of Larry Matthews, M.D.)

The surgical technique involves initial prosthesis removal and debridement. The articular ends are then shaped to obtain maximum contact with the leg in full extension.[18] A key to success is prolonged postoperative immobilization for 6 to 9 months to allow stabilization of the resection arthroplasty.[18, 69] Additional external support (universal knee splint, knee-ankle-foot orthosis) is utilized if sufficient stability to allow weightbearing is not obtained.[18]

In reviewing results of resection arthroplasty, one must differentiate between those cases in which a pseudarthrosis results from an attempted knee arthrodesis and cases in which a resection arthroplasty was performed primarily without any attempt at obtaining fusion. Results of pseudarthrosis following attempted knee arthrodesis are often poor owing to chronic pain and instability, leading some authors to recommend repeated attempts to obtain a solid fusion.[25, 59] Falahee et al.[22] reported their results with resection arthroplasty as the primary salvage procedure for 26 patients with failed, infected TKAs. Fifteen of the 26 patients were able to walk without the

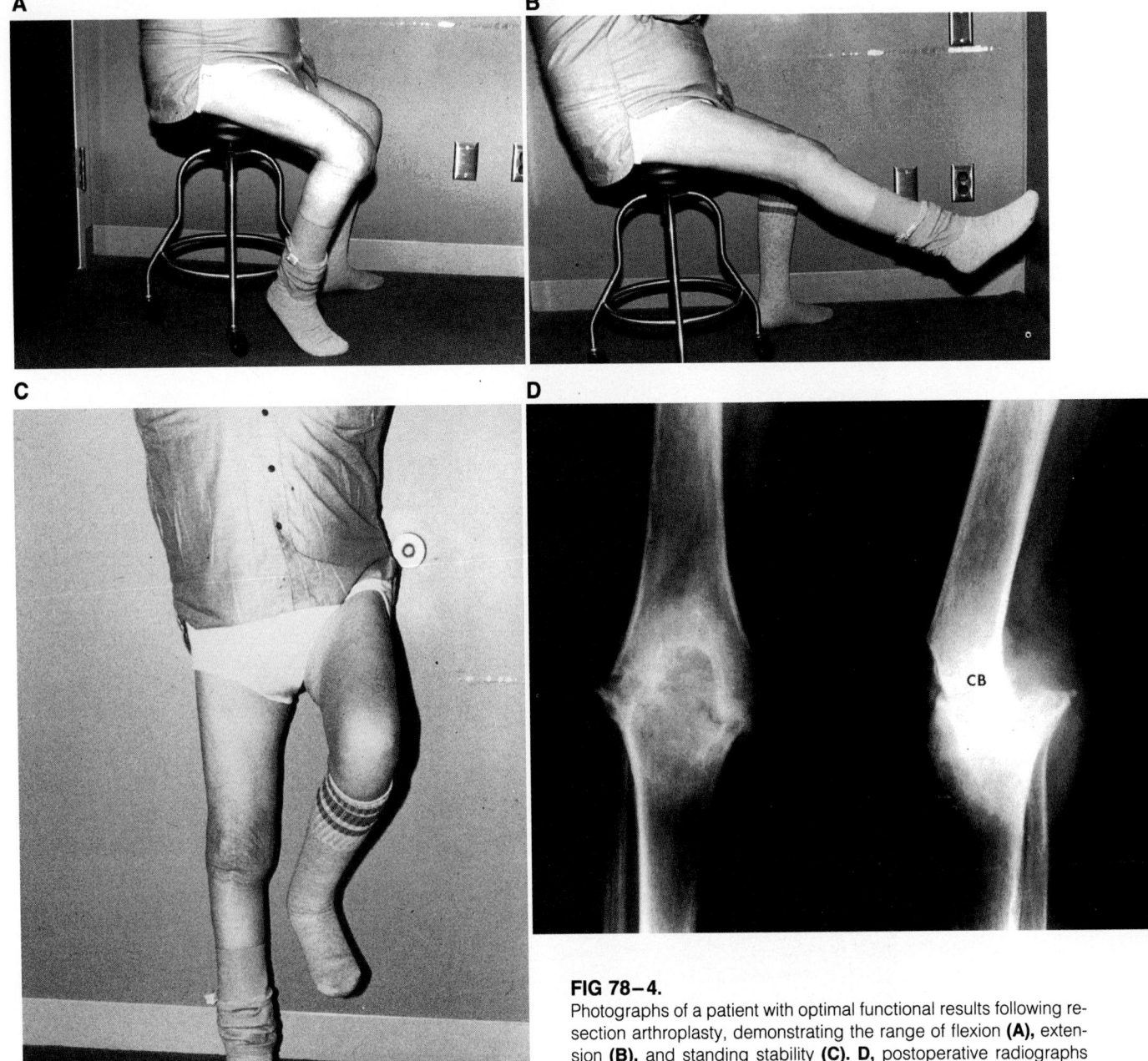

FIG 78-4.
Photographs of a patient with optimal functional results following resection arthroplasty, demonstrating the range of flexion **(A)**, extension **(B)**, and standing stability **(C)**. **D**, postoperative radiographs of the same patient following removal of an infected total condylar arthroplasty and subsequent resection arthroplasty. (Courtesy of Herbert Kaufer, M.D., Lexington, Ky.)

aid of another person, but all required some type of ambulatory aid. Only one third of patients could walk without bracing. An average flexion arc of 36 degrees (range, 10 degrees of hyperextension to 90 degrees of flexion) and an average of 3 degrees of both varus and valgus instability (range, 20 degrees of varus angulation to 20 degrees of valgus angulation) were observed (Fig 78-4). Overall, 56% of patients were satisfied with the result of the resection arthroplasty.

The authors found resection arthroplasty to be most suitable for patients with severe disability before TKA, typically due to polyarticular joint involvement, by providing a useful range of motion for the disabled sedentary patient.

A resection arthroplasty may be converted to knee arthrodesis if an unsatisfactory result occurs. Spontaneous fusion may also occur following resection arthroplasty.[18]

SUMMARY

The failed TKA, particularly if infected, now serves as the most common indication for knee arthrodesis. The most important factor influencing the rate of union of knee arthrodesis is the surgeon's ability to obtain sustained rigid fixation.[69] With improved treatment of the infected TKA, including better management of excessive bone loss and ligamentous instability as well as improved prosthetic design, the number of patients requiring knee arthrodesis will continue to decrease. Resection arthroplasty should be reserved for those patients with limited ambulatory capacity and those with severe polyarticular joint disease.

REFERENCES

1. Albrektsson T, et al: Osseointegrated titanium implants, *Acta Orthop Scand* 52:155–170, 1981.
2. Andersen MP, et al: Arthrodesis of the knee following failed total knee arthroplasty, *J Bone Joint Surg [Am]* 61:181–185, 1979.
3. Arden GP: Total knee replacement, *Clin Orthop* 94:92–103, 1973.
4. Behr JT, Chmell SJ, Schwartz CM: Knee arthrodesis for failed total knee arthroplasty. *Arch Surg* 120:350–354, 1985.
5. Bigliani LU, et al: The use of pulsing electromagnetic fields to achieve arthrodesis of the knee following failed total knee arthroplasty: A preliminary report, *J Bone Joint Surg [Am]* 65A:480–485, 1983.
6. Bonnel, F.: Augmentation de la stabilité du fixateur externe d'Hoffmann par fiches à filetage médian, *Nouv Presse Med* 3:2249, 1974.
7. Briggs BT, Chao EYS: The mechanical performance of the standard Hoffmann-Vidal external fixation apparatus, *J Bone Joint Surg [Am]* 64:566–573, 1982.
8. Broderson MP, et al: Arthrodesis of the knee following failed total knee arthroplasty, *J Bone Joint Surg [Am]* 61:181–185, 1979.
9. Brooker AF Jr, Hansen NM Jr: The biplane frame: Modified compression arthrodesis of the knee, *Clin Orthop* 160:163–167, 1981.
10. Bryan RS, Brodersen MP: Arthrodesis of the knee. In Evarts CM, (editor): *Surgery of the musculoskeletal system*, ed 2, vol 4, New York, 1990, Churchill Livingstone, pp 3692–3723.
11. Burny F: Elastic external fixation of tibial fractures: Study of 1,421 cases. In Brooker AF Jr, Edwards CC, (editors): *External fixation: The current state of the art*, Baltimore, 1979, Williams & Wilkins.
12. Chapchal G: Intramedullary pinning for arthrodesis of the knee joint, *J Bone Joint Surg [Am]* 30:728–734, 1948.
13. Charnley J: Positive pressure in arthrodesis of the knee joint, *J Bone Joint Surg [Br]* 30:478–486, 1948.
14. Charnley J: Arthrodesis of the knee, *Clin Orthop* 18:37–42, 1960.
15. Charnley J, Lowe HG: A study of the end results of compression arthrodesis of the knee, *J Bone Joint Surg [Br]* 40:633–635, 1958.
16. Deburge A, GUEPAR: GUEPAR hinge prosthesis. Complications and results with two years' follow-up, *Clin Orthop* 120:47–53, 1976.
17. Dennis DA, et al: Posterior cruciate condylar total knee arthroplasty: Average 11-year-follow-up, *Clin Orthop* 281:168-176, 1992.
18. Donley BG, Matthews LS, Kaufer H: Arthrodesis of the knee with an intramedullary nail, *J Bone Joint Surg [Am]* 73:907–913, 1991.
19. Drinker H, et al: Arthrodesis for failed knee arthroplasty (abstract), *Orthop Trans* 3:302, 1979.
20. Edwards CC: Management of the polytrauma patient in a major US center. In Brooker AF Jr, Edwards CC, (editors): *External fixation: The current state of the art*, Baltimore, 1979, Williams & Wilkins.
21. Fahmy NRM, Barnes KL, Noble J: A technique for difficult arthrodesis of the knee, *J Bone Joint Surg [Br]* 66:367–370, 1984.
22. Falahee MH, Matthews LS, Kaufer H: Resection arthroplasty as a salvage procedure for a knee with infection after a total arthroplasty, *J Bone Joint Surg [Am]* 69:1013–1021, 1987.
23. Fern ED, Stewart HD, Newton G: Curved Kuntscher nail arthrodesis after failure of knee replacement, *J Bone Joint Surg [Br]* 71:588–590, 1989.
24. Fidler MW: Knee arthrodesis following prosthesis removal: Use of the Wagner apparatus, *J Bone Joint Surg [Br]* 65:29–31, 1983.
25. Figgie HE III, et al: Knee arthrodesis following total knee arthroplasty in rheumatoid arthritis, *Clin Orthop* 224:237–243, 1987.
26. Fischer DA: Skeletal stabilization with a multiplane external fixation device: Design rationale and preliminary clinical experience, *Clin Orthop* 180:50–62, 1983.
27. Freeman MAR, Charnley J: Arthrodesis. In Freeman MAR, (editor): *Arthritis of the knee: Clinical features and surgical management*. Berlin, Springer-Verlag, 1980, pp 142–147.
28. Freeman PA: Walldius arthroplasty. A review of 80 cases, *Clin Orthop* 94:85–91, 1973.
29. Frymoyer JW, Hoaglund FT: The role of arthrodesis in reconstruction of the knee, *Clin Orthop* 101:82–92, 1974.
30. Green DP, Parkes JC, Stinchfield FE: Arthrodesis of the knee. A follow-up study, *J Bone Joint Surg [Am]* 49:1065–1078, 1967.
31. Green SA, Kolsnick R: Arthrodesis of the knee, *Orthopedics* 8:1514–1518, 1985.
32. Green SA: Complications of external skeletal fixation, *Clin Orthop* 180:109, 1983.
33. Hagemann WF, Woods GW, Tullos HS: Arthrodesis in failed total knee replacement, *J Bone Joint Surg [Am]* 60:790–794, 1978.
34. Hankin F, Louie DW, Matthews LS: The effect of total knee arthroplasty prosthesis design on the potential for

salvage arthrodesis: Measurements of volumes, lengths and trabecular bone contact areas, *Clin Orthop* 155:52–58, 1981.
35. Harris CM, Froehlich J: Knee fusion with intramedullary rods for failed total knee arthroplasty, *Clin Orthop* 197:209–216, 1985.
36. Hayes WC: Biomechanics of fracture treatment. In Heppenstall RB, (editor): *Fracture treatment and healing,* Philadelphia, 1980, WB Saunders, pp 124–172.
37. Hui FC, Fitzgerald RH Jr: Hinged total knee arthroplasty, *J Bone Joint Surg [Am]* 62:513–519, 1980.
38. Insall JN: Miscellaneous items: Arthrodesis, the stiff knee, synovectomy, and popliteal cysts. In Insall JN, (editor): *Surgery of the knee,* New York, 1984, Churchill Livingstone, pp 729–731.
39. Irvine G, Kaufer H, Matthews LS: Intramedullary arthrodesis of the knee, *Orthop Trans* 7:416, 1983.
40. Jones EC, et al: GUEPAR knee arthroplasty results and late complications, *Clin Orthop* 140:145–152, 1979.
41. Jones GB: Total knee replacement. The Walldius hinge, *Clin Orthop* 94:50–57, 1973.
42. Key JA: Positive pressure in arthrodesis for tuberculosis of the knee joint, *South Med J* 25:909–915, 1932.
43. Klemm K: Die Verriegelungsnagelung. Entwicklung und Behandlungsprinzip der Verriegelungsnagelung. In Vécsei V, (editor): *Verriegelungsnagelung, Symposium am 3. Februar 1978.* Vienna, 1978, Verlag Wilhelm Mandrich, pp 31–39.
44. Knutson K, Bodelind B, Lidgren L: Stability of external fixators used for knee arthrodesis after failed knee arthroplasty, *Clin Orthop* 186:90–95, 1984.
45. Knutson K, Lindstrand A, Lidgren L: Arthrodesis for failed knee arthroplasty. A report of 20 cases, *J Bone Joint Surg [Br]* 67:47–52, 1985.
46. Knutson K, et al: Eighty-five knee arthrodeses after failed knee arthroplasty: A multicenter investigation, 49th Annual Meeting of the American Academy of Orthopaedic Surgeons, New Orleans, Jan 21–26, 1982.
47. Knutson K, et al: Arthrodesis after failed knee arthroplasty. A nationwide multicenter investigation of 91 cases, *Clin Orthop* 191:202–211, 1984.
48. Laskin RS: Total knee replacement, *Orthop Clin North Am* 10:223–247, 1979.
49. Locht RC, Hunter GA: Deep sepsis after cemented total knee replacement, *Infect Surg* 2:219–224, 1983.
50. Matthews LS, Hirsch C: Temperatures measured in human cortical bone when drilling, *J Bone Joint Surg [Am]* 54:297–308, 1972.
51. McCoy MT, Chao EYS, Kasman RA: Comparison of mechanical performance in four types of external fixators, *Clin Orthop* 180:23–33, 1983.
52. Morris HD, Mosiman RS: Arthrodesis of the knee. A comparison of the compression method with the non-compression method, *J Bone Joint Surg [Am]* 33:982–987, 1951.
53. Munzinger U, Knessl J, Gschwend N: Arthrodese nach Knie-Arthroplastik, *Orthopade* 16:301–309, 1987.
54. Nichols SJ, Landon GC, Tullos HS: Arthrodesis with dual plates after failed total knee arthroplasty, *J Bone Joint Surg [Am]* 73:1020–1024, 1991.
55. Petty W: Knee arthrodesis for failed total knee arthroplasty. In Petty W, (editor): *Total joint replacement,* Philadelphia, 1991, WB Saunders, pp 587–592.
56. Phillips HT, Mears DC: Knee fusion with external skeletal fixation after an infected hinge prosthesis: A case report, *Clin Orthop* 151:147–152, 1980.
57. Puranen J, Kortelainen P, Jalovaara P: Arthrodesis of the knee with intramedullary nail fixation, *J Bone Joint Surg [Am]* 72:433–442, 1990.
58. Ranawat CS, Boachie-Adjei O: Survivorship analysis and results of total condylar knee arthroplasty. Eight to 11-year follow-up period, *Clin Orthop* 226:6, 1988.
59. Rand JA, Bryan RS: The outcome of failed knee arthrodesis following total knee arthroplasty, *Clin Orthop* 205:86–92, 1986.
60. Rand JA, Bryan RS, Chao EYS: Failed total knee arthroplasty treated by arthrodesis of the knee using the Ace-Fischer apparatus, *J Bone Joint Surg [Am]* 69:39–45, 1987.
61. Ritter MA, et al: Long-term survival analysis of the posterior cruciate condylar total knee arthroplasty: A 10-year evaluation, *J Arthroplasty* 4:293–296, 1989.
62. Rothacker GW Jr, Cabanela ME: External fixation for arthrodesis of the knee and ankle, *Clin Orthop* 180:101–108, 1983.
63. Shea JG, Wynn Jones CH, Arden GP: A study of the results of the removal of total knee arthroplasty. A two-year follow-up study (abstract), *J Bone Joint Surg [Br[* 63:287, 1981.
64. Shoji H, D'Ambrosia RD, Lipscomb PR: Failed polycentric total knee prostheses, *J Bone Joint Surg [Am]* 58:773–777, 1976.
65. Siris I: External pin transfixion of fractures: An analysis of 80 cases, *Ann Surg* 120:911, 1944.
66. Skolnick MD, Coventry MB, Ilstrup DM: Geometric total knee arthroplasty: A two-year follow-up study, *J Bone Joint Surg [Am]* 58:749–753, 1976.
67. Skolnick MD, et al: Polycentric total knee arthroplasty: A two-year follow-up study, *J Bone Joint Surg [Am]* 58:743–748, 1976.
68. Stewart MJ, Bland WG: Compression in arthrodesis. A comparative study of methods of fusion of the knee in 93 cases, *J Bone Joint Surg [Am]* 40:585–606, 1958.
69. Stulberg SD: Arthrodesis in failed total knee replacements, *Orthop Clin North Am* 13:213–224, 1982.
70. Thornhill TS, Dalziel RW, Sledge CB: Alternatives to arthrodesis for the failed total knee arthroplasty, *Clin Orthop* 170:131–140, 1982.
71. Toumey JW Jr: Knee joint tuberculosis. Two hundred twenty-two patients treated by operative fusion, *Surg Gynecol Obstet* 68:1029–1037, 1939.
72. Vahvanen V: Arthrodesis in failed knee replacement in eight rheumatoid patients, *Ann Chir Gynaecol* 68:57–62, 1979.
73. Wade PJF, Denham RA: Arthrodesis of the knee after failed knee replacement, *J Bone Joint Surg [Br]* 66:362–366, 1984.

74. Walker PS, et al: Fixation of tibial components of knee prostheses, *J Bone Joint Surg [Am]* 63:258–267, 1981.
75. Walldius B: Arthroplasty of the knee using an endoprosthesis: Eight years experience, *Acta Orthop Scand* 30:137–148, 1960.
76. Wilde AH, Stearns KL: Intramedullary fixation for arthrodesis of the knee after infected total knee arthroplasty, *Clin Orthop* 248:87–92, 1989.
77. Woods GW, Lionberger DR, Tullos HS: Failed total knee arthroplasty. Revision and arthrodesis for infection and noninfectious complications, *Clin Orthop* 173:184–190, 1983.

PART XVI

Fractures About the Knee

79

Supracondylar and Intercondylar Distal Femoral Fractures

DAVID TEMPLEMAN, M.D.

Clinical evaluation
Classification
Operative vs. nonoperative management
   Operative management
   Nonoperative management
Open reduction and internal fixation
   Surgical planning

Unicondylar fractures
Surgical implants
   Blade plate or condylar screw
   Bone grafting
   Author's preferred technique for insertion of dynamic condylar screw
Distal femoral fractures after total knee replacement

Supracondylar and intercondylar fractures of the femur are complex injuries that are difficult to treat. The goals of treatment are: (1) to achieve fracture union, and (2) to restore knee motion.[20–22] Failure to achieve these goals frequently results in a stiff and painful knee. Knee pain is secondary to posttraumatic arthritis, the end result of intraarticular incongruities or axial malalignment that leads to uneven loading of joint surfaces.[9] Capsular and periarticular fibrosis is caused by the initial injury, surgical dissection, or prolonged immobilization, all of which may lead to limited knee motion.

In the last two decades, there has been an evolution from nonoperative to operative treatment of distal femoral fractures. In the 1960s and 1970s, publications by Connolly et al.,[6] Mooney et al.,[14] Neer et al.,[15] and Stewart et al.[25] documented that the results of nonoperative treatment were superior to the results of operative treatment. Surgical care was complicated by high rates of infection (25%) and nonunion (10%), which led to dismal results. However, a critical study of these reports indicates that the surgical techniques and implants used in these series were inferior to current methods. The Association for Osteosynthesis (AO), believing in stable fixation to allow early motion, proceeded to develop surgical techniques and implants that have become today's standard of care. Successful operative treatment requires that the following goals be achieved: (1) anatomic reduction of joint surfaces; (2) restoration of limb length and alignment; (3) rigid fixation; and (4) early knee motion.[16, 19, 20]

CLINICAL EVALUATION

The strength of bone in the distal femur defines two different types of patient that suffer distal femoral fractures. Young patients are usually injured in motor vehicle accidents or other high energy injuries. In contrast, elderly patients with osteoporosis may suffer distal femoral fractures from simple falls, or other low velocity injuries.[2, 3] Defining the difference between these two groups of patients is the quality of bone. In osteoporotic patients, little force is necessary to create a distal femoral fracture.[23]

The goal of the initial examination is to classify the fracture type and to detect associated injuries. The first priority is to confirm that the circulation is intact. Absent or asymmetric pulses require immediate action. When there is marked deformity of the limb, gentle traction will usually restore alignment and may restore the pulses. Medial displacement of the proximal shaft is viewed with concern, as a proximal fragment can injure the vessels in the femoral canal. In addition to asymmetric pulses, other indications for arteriography include active swelling, hemorrhage, and penetrating wounds close to the vessels.

Next, the motor function and sensation of the lower extremity are assessed and documented. The soft tissues are inspected to look for wounds and palpation is done to diagnose compartmental syndromes. The presence of an open soft tissue wound in the distal femur is considered to be an open fracture until proved otherwise.

The diagnosis of a distal femoral fracture is made from roentgenograms which are ordered to evaluate pain, swelling, or deformity about the knee. Anteroposterior (AP) and lateral views that include the distal femoral epiphysis, metaphysis, and diaphysis are recommended. High energy injuries require roentgenograms of the pelvis, hip, and tibia to exclude ipsilateral fractures.

After the initial examination, the leg is splinted to prevent excessive motion at the fracture site. When surgery is being delayed, skeletal traction is recommended to maintain the length and the alignment of the fracture. Great care must be taken in the placement of the skeletal traction pin so that it does not compromise the planned surgical incision.

CLASSIFICATION

The AO classification system, the system used most, is divided into three types: A, B, and C. Each group has a subset that defines increasing degrees of fracture comminution (Fig 79–1). Type A fractures are extraarticular, with type A3 fractures describing severe supracondylar comminution. Type B fractures separate varying amounts of one condyle. A careful study is necessary to detect the type B3 fracture, which is a coronal split that separates the posterior aspect of the condyle. Type B3 fractures are sometimes referred to by their eponym, the Hoffa fracture. Recognition of this fracture is important because the fracture requires fixation in a plane different from that done with the usual laterally applied plate and screw devices. Type C injuries define intercondylar fractures that separate the two condyles from one another and from the metaphysis. The condyles are usually rotated relative to one another by the gastrocnemius muscles.

OPERATIVE VS. NONOPERATIVE MANAGEMENT

The relative roles of nonoperative and operative treatment of distal femoral fractures continue to be debated. Nonunions and joint stiffness frequently complicate closed treatment. When encountered, technical problems and infection frequently complicate open reduction and internal fixation. Deciding between operative and nonoperative treatment requires a careful study of patient and fracture site characteristics. Factors affecting the patient's care include age, activity level, health problems, associated injuries, and the ability to tolerate traction or surgery as a method of treatment. Fracture site features include the degree of soft tissue damage, bony comminution, osteoporosis, and articular surface injury.

Operative Management

Advances in surgical technique and implants continue to increase the number of distal femoral fractures that are successfully treated by open reduction and internal fixation. It must be remembered that successful operative treatment requires achieving the following goals: (1) anatomic reduction of joint surfaces; (2) restoration of limb length and alignment; (3) rigid fixation; and (4) early range of motion of the knee. Schatzker and associates[20, 21] documented the importance of accomplishing these principles. When these goals were achieved, 71% of the patients had a good or excellent result. However, in patients in whom there was a failure to achieve anatomic reduction or stable fixation, only 21% of the patients had a good or excellent result. This study found that most failures after internal fixation occurred in patients older than 50 years (nine failures in 19 cases), in contrast to a higher success rate in patients younger than 50 years (one failure in 17 cases).[20, 21] Schatzker et al. concluded that the presence of significant comminution and severe osteoporosis in many instances precludes an anatomic fixation and stable fixation. Therefore, prior to surgery the surgeon must determine whether or not these goals can be predictably attained. A widely accepted indication for open reduction and internal fixation is 3 mm of intraarticular displacement that is not reduced by closed manipulation. Schatzker et al.[22] have outlined the following as relative indications for open reduction and internal fixation: displaced intercondylar fractures, condylar fractures in the coronal plane, T or Y bicondylar fractures with rotational displacement of the condyles, open intraarticular fractures, associated neurovascular injuries, ipsilateral tibial plateau or shaft fractures, patients with multiple system injuries where the patient needs to be mobilized, and pathologic fractures.

Nonoperative Management

Most protocols that describe nonoperative management of distal femoral fractures use a period of skeletal traction and some form of early motion, usually with a cast brace.[6, 14] Varus deformities, internal rotation, and apex-posterior angulation are common deformities. Neer et al.[15] performed clinical and ca-

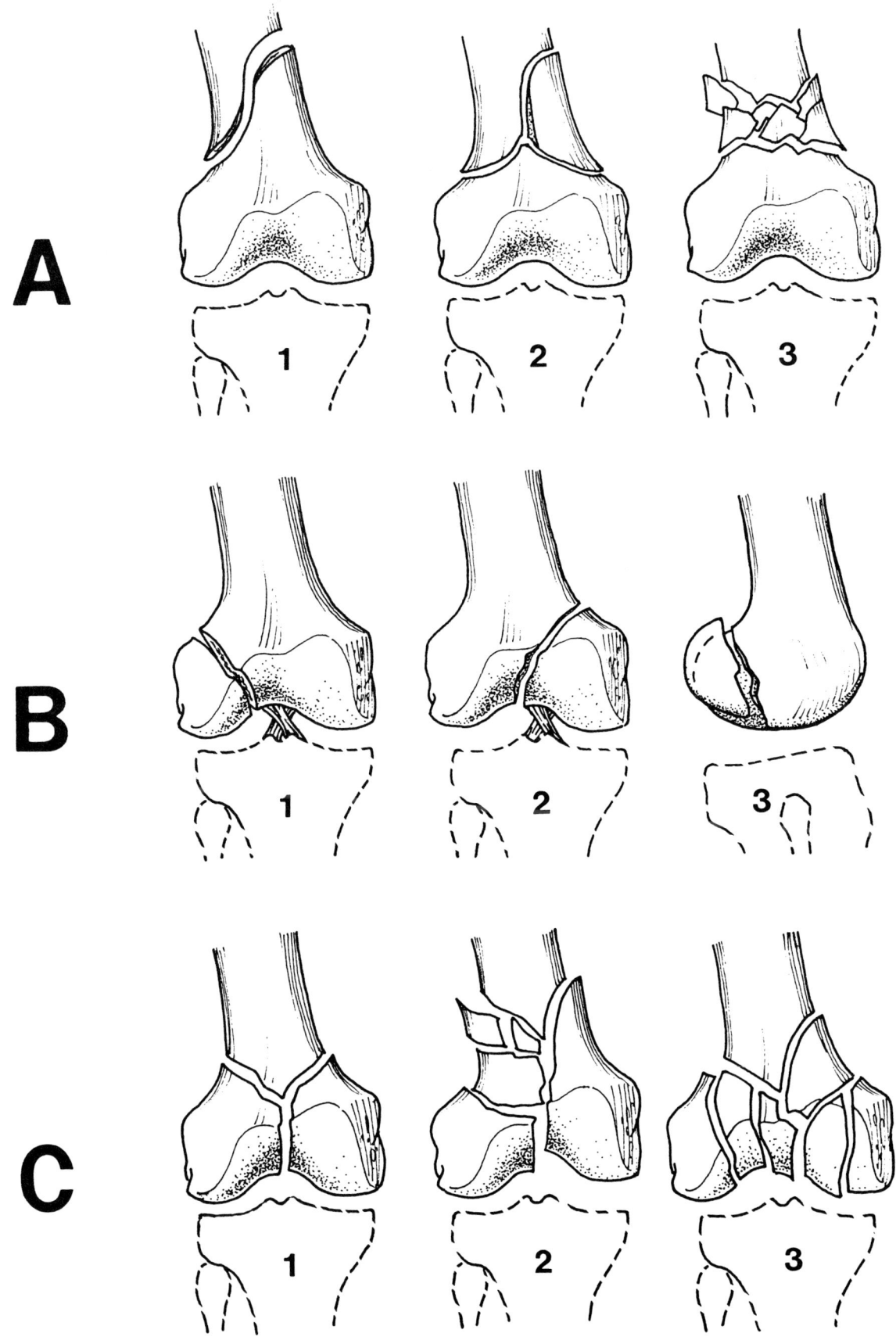

FIG 79–1.
The AO classification of supracondylar and intercondylar fractures of the distal femur. Fractures are divided into three types: A, B, and C. Each type is further divided into three subgroups, 1, 2, and 3, which indicate increasing degree of fracture complexity. The classification of fractures is thus organized in terms of increasing severity relating to the complexity of the fracture, the difficulty of treatment, and the prognosis. (From Gustilo RB, Kyle RF, Templeman D, eds: *Fractures and Dislocations*. St Louis, 1993, Mosby.)

daver studies and identified what they termed "prevalent errors" in traction management. They recommended the following: to avoid posterior angulation, knee flexion was limited to approximately 20 degrees while traction was applied in the axis of the femoral shaft; to avoid apex-posterior angulation, overriding of the proximal fragment should be avoided because this displaces the distal fragment posteriorly; and excessive flexion of the knee is avoided because this displaces the distal fragment posterior to the proximal fragment. This study noted that medial displacement and internal rotation of the distal fragment also gave a false roentgenographic appearance of posterior angulation.[15]

Varus and internal rotation is a common deformity after traction and is thought to be secondary to external rotation of the hip joint and the femoral shaft relative to the distal fragment.[15] The distal fragment is held in relative neutral position by the traction pin. When union occurs between these two fragments, the distal fragment appears to be in relative varus and neutral rotation in relationship to the proximal fragment. This problem can be corrected by modifying the insertion of the tibial traction pin to place the distal fragment in a similar rotational alignment to the proximal fragment.[15]

The final "prevalent error" of traction is prolonged immobilization.[15] Early quadriceps exercises and knee motion are necessary to prevent adherence of the quadriceps mechanism to the fracture hematoma and subsequent site of callus formation. Complete fracture union, defined by roentgenograms, usually takes several months. However, clinical union, defined by the absence of tenderness and evident by the formation of callus, may be seen as early as the fifth week after injury. At this time, passive motion can be begun, with the patient controlling the position of the Thomas splint.

An alternative technique is the application of a cast brace.[6, 14] The cast brace is used until solid union is present by radiographic examination. Close radiographic follow-up is recommended after the discontinuation of traction and the cast brace is applied, to ensure that a deformity does not develop. Most distal femoral fractures heal between 3 and 4 months after injury. This method of treatment also implies careful physical therapy to regain knee motion and quadriceps strength.

OPEN REDUCTION AND INTERNAL FIXATION

Surgical reconstruction of distal femoral fractures is demanding. Successful internal fixation requires: (1) anatomic reduction of joint surfaces; (2) acceptable axial alignment; and (3) stable fixation to provide for early motion of the knee.[13, 16, 18, 19, 22] A detailed preoperative plan assists the surgeon in accomplishing these goals. The preoperative plan outlines the fracture patterns, determines the sequential steps of the reduction, selects the appropriate implants, and outlines the application of the implants.

Surgical Planning

The use of a preoperative planner, such as the one developed by Mast and Müller, is a reproducible way to plan the proposed surgery. This method allows the surgery to be done on paper, prior to the actual operation. This surgical "dry run" is helpful in planning the exact sequence of the surgery and identifies potential problems that can be anticipated.

To plan the open reduction and internal fixation of a distal femoral fracture, AP and lateral roentgenograms of the fractured and uninjured limbs are obtained. The entire distal femur and distal diaphysis should be included on these films. First, a tracing of the uninjured limb is made to define the patient's anatomic axis. Next, this tracing is placed over the roentgenogram of the fractured limb. The fracture fragments are traced within the original tracing. This shows the fractured fragments in a reduced position. Next, the templates of the appropriate implant are used to indicate the final fixation of the fracture. This step determines the appropriate implant size, screw length, and number of screws that are needed. The plan should also number the different fracture fragments and incorporate the sequence and method of their reduction. This is a key element of the plan that is necessary to minimize soft tissue dissection. Meticulous planning benefits the treatment of fractures of the distal femur, which are uncommon injuries that require a demanding operation.

Unicondylar Fractures

Unicondylar fractures define separation of the medial or lateral femoral condyles from the metaphysis. The separated condyle is subjected to rotational forces from the knee ligaments and gastrocnemius muscles, forces which usually prevent acceptable closed reduction of the intraarticular displacement. Open reduction and internal fixation with large cancellous screws provide rigid fixation and allow early knee motion. Fractures in the coronal plane, which separate the posterior portion of the condyles, require careful

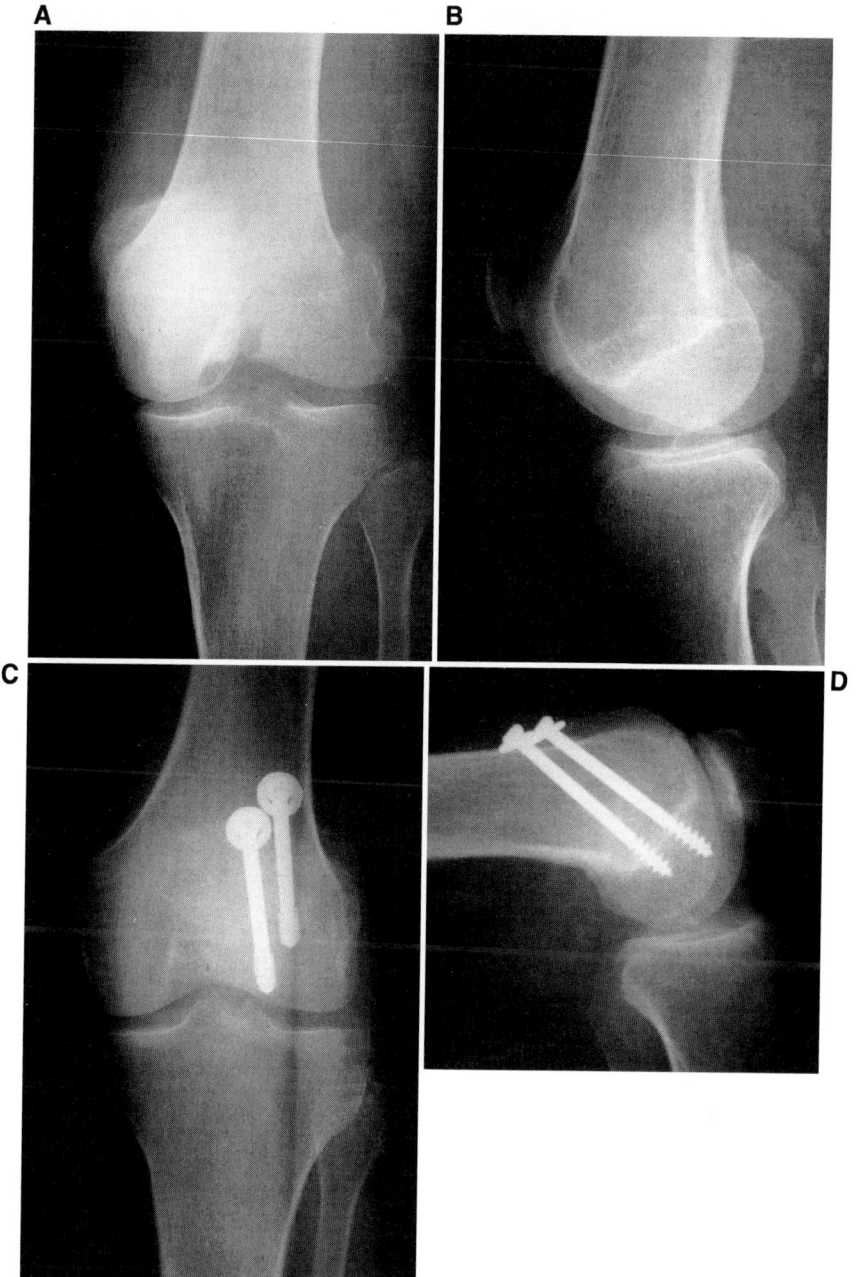

FIG 79-2.
A and **B,** this 42-year-old man was injured in a fall and sustained a lateral condylar fracture in the coronal plane. This is a type B3 injury. **C** and **D,** AP and lateral roentgenograms taken 1 year after open reduction and interfragmentary fixation with two 6.5 cancellous screws. Note the shorter 16-mm thread length was used. (From Gustilo RB, Kyle RF, Templeman D, eds: *Fractures and Dislocations.* St Louis, 1993, Mosby.)

countersinking of the screwheads when screw placement is close to the patellofemoral joint (Fig 79–2,A–D). In most cases, broad cancellous bone surfaces are stable after rigid internal fixation, which allows early range of motion after surgery. However, when there is osteoporosis, a buttress plate is needed. Usually, a large-fragment T plate is best.

Surgical Implants

Current implants for distal femoral fractures are divided into two groups: (1) forms of intramedullary fixation,[4, 12, 23] and (2) screw plate devices.[18–20] Intramedullary appliances include interlocking femoral nails, Rush pins, the Zickel device, and the GSH intramedullary nail. The GSH intramedullary nail is a new device that is inserted through the intercondylar notch. The GSH nail contains multiple slots for interlocking bolts. Only preliminary reports are available, and more information is needed before the device can be recommended.

Plate and screw assemblies, primarily developed by the AO, are the supracondylar blade plate, dynamic condylar screw, and condylar buttress plate[18-22] (Fig 79-3,A-D). Open reduction and internal fixation with various forms of plates are the more widely accepted philosophy of surgical treatment of distal femoral fractures. However, given the number of complex variables associated with this in-

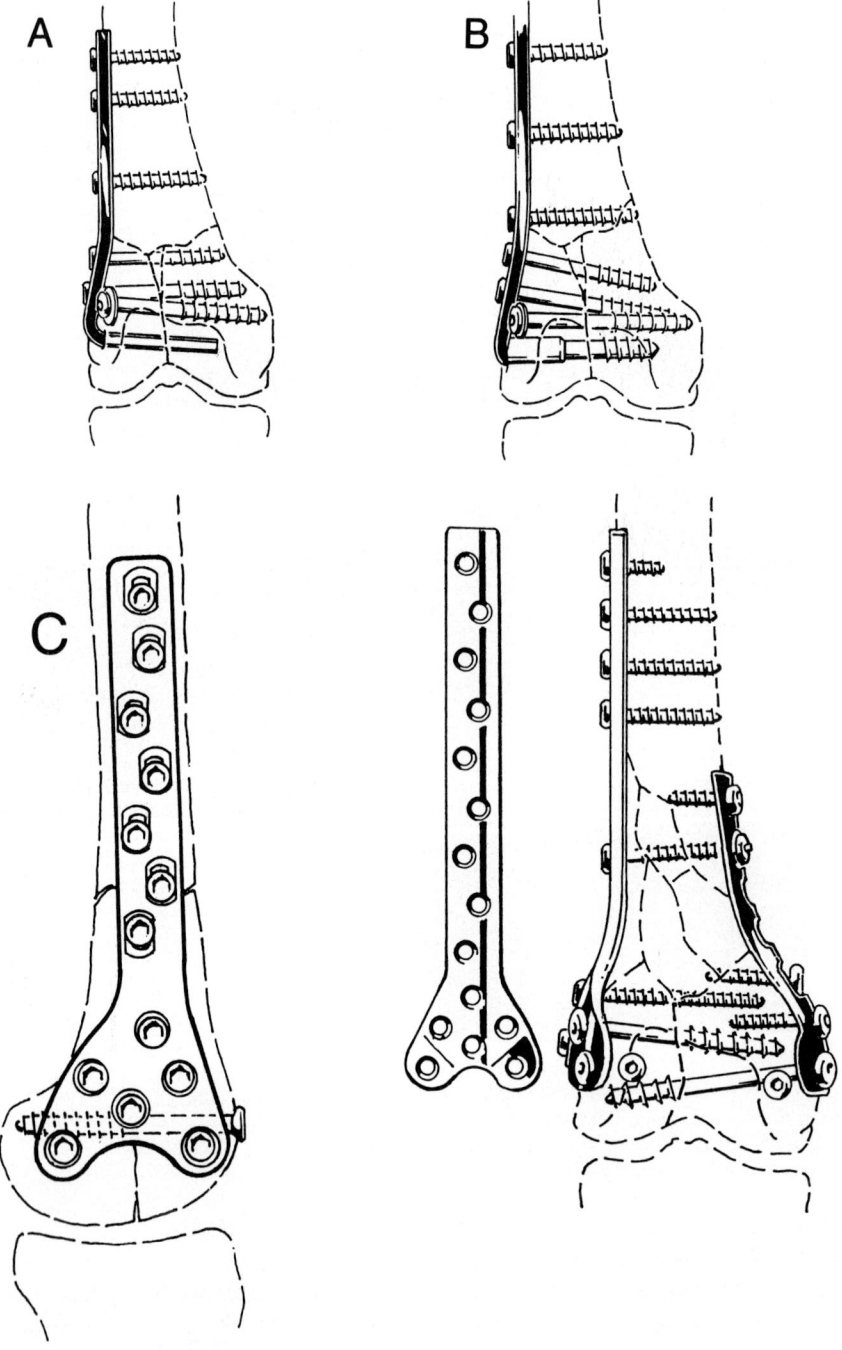

FIG 79-3.
A, condylar blade plate. **B,** dynamic compression screw. **C,** condylar buttress plate. **D,** condylar buttress plate with an accessory medial T buttress plate to restore stable medial buttress. (From Gustilo RB, Kyle RF, Templeman D, eds: *Fractures and Dislocations.* St Louis, 1993, Mosby.)

jury, it is unlikely that one implant or philosophy of treatment will become either appropriate or universally accepted.

Intramedullary fixation has the advantage of being a closed technique which decreases the risk of infection. Since the fracture hematoma is not disturbed, periosteal healing is likely and there is less need for a bone graft. Since closed intramedullary nailing does not address intraarticular fracture displacements, this form of treatment is most appropriate for the extraarticular (type A) fractures. Supracondylar femur fractures, 6 to 8 cm proximal to the intercondylar notch, can be managed with interlocking femoral nails. The use of two distal locking bolts is needed to avoid rotation in the sagittal plane. The use of an intramedullary nail for these distal fractures requires careful preoperative planning. The exact length of the nail needs to judged carefully, so that both interlocking bolts gain fixation in the distal fragment. The various forms of intramedullary fixation are not recommended for displaced intraarticular fractures. Open reduction is usually required to achieve anatomic reduction of joint surfaces that are best secured with interfragmentary screws. The use of cerclage wire, as described for associated fixation with Rush rods and the Zickel device, provides less rigid fixation than that achieved by AO principles.[23] However, selected intraarticular distal femoral fractures, especially those with nondisplaced intraarticular extension, can be successfully treated with a combination of interfragmentary screws and intramedullary nails.[12] Prior to insertion of the intramedullary nail, the intraarticular portion of the fracture is fixed with interfragmentary screws. The screws must be positioned so that they do not block the subsequent insertion of the intramedullary device.

A problem inherent to closed femoral nailing of distal femoral fractures is the development of valgus deformities after the patient is positioned in the lateral decubitus position. Apex-posterior angulation is a common deformity after supine nailing. Both of these malalignments relate to the sag of the leg caused by gravity. Careful attention to the technique of closed reduction is necessary to prevent these malreductions and subsequent malunions.

Bucholz et al.[4] have shown that fatigue failure of femoral nails can occur when the fracture is within 5 cm of the distal locking bolts. To prevent fatigue fracture of the intramedullary nail, the patient should be kept nonweightbearing until there is evidence of fracture callus. In addition, nails as large as possible should be used and the distal tip of the nail should be impacted into the epiphyseal scar.

When open reduction and internal fixation are indicated, the geometry of the fracture determines which implant is best to use. The use of a preoperative planner is invaluable in determining the best implant.

Blade Plate or Condylar Screw

After the distal fragment has been stabilized by interfragmentary screws, there should be a minimum of 4 cm of intact bone in the distal fragment of the femur. This is necessary if either the condylar blade plate or the condylar buttress plate is used. If there is less than 4 cm of the distal fragment present and either of these two devices is used, it may be cut out of the small distal fragment. Therefore, there must be enough distal metaphyseal bone to allow adequate seating and purchase by either the condylar buttress plate, or the dynamic condylar screw (see Fig 79-3, A and B).

The most important factor in deciding between the condylar blade plate or the dynamic condylar screw is the surgeon's proficiency. Arguments supporting the use of the blade plate are, reportedly, improved rotational stability in the sagittal plane, and a smaller bony defect after removal of the blade plate. However, because of familiarity with the compression hip screw, many surgeons find this device easier to use and safer to insert in comminuted and osteoporotic bone. Since distal femoral fractures are uncommon injuries and surgical reconstruction is technically demanding, the physician should select either a blade plate or compression screw and become proficient with its use. The merits of the dynamic condylar screw are its ease of insertion and similarity to the compression hip screw. Because the dynamic condylar screw is a two-piece system, insertion requires alignment in the frontal and axial planes. This is in contrast to fixed-angle blade plates, which must be simultaneously aligned in three planes, reducing the margin for error during insertion. In addition to more difficult placement, the blade plate requires impaction by a seating chisel, which can disrupt the reduction of the distal fragment. This is especially true in osteoporotic bone.[18, 22]

The condylar buttress plate is used for very distal condylar fractures and when there is marked comminution of the condyles. However, the use of this implant requires the presence of a stable medial buttress. In the absence of a stable medial buttress due to either comminution or segmental bone loss, Sanders and colleagues[19] recommend the use of a second plate to act as an accessory medial buttress (see Fig 79-3,D). Although the condylar buttress plate achieves fixation in most cases, the bone-plate interface should be examined for motion during flexion, extension, and varus-valgus stresses to ensure sufficient fixation. The presence of motion during this examination defines an unstable fixation and usually indicates an inadequate medial buttress. If this is the case, insertion of a medial buttress plate is recommended. This is done through a separate medial incision. Usually, a T plate is used to buttress the medial column of the distal femur.

Bone Grafting

Nonunions after supracondylar femoral fractures usually occur at the metaphyseal-diaphyseal junction. Fractures with extensive comminution at this site are prone to nonunion. There is a trend for the increased use of bone grafting when performing internal fixation.[11, 18, 22] Bone grafting assists with two goals: prevention of nonunion, and promotion of earlier fracture union to avoid fixation failures and angulation malunions. Bone grafting is beneficial when extensive comminution is present at the metaphyseal-diaphyseal junction, which precludes anatomic reduction at this site. In these cases, avoiding extensive stripping of the small bone fragments, the use of the plate to achieve indirect reduction by bridging the fracture site, and placement of bone graft at the defect helps secure union (Fig 79–4, A–D).

Author's Preferred Technique for Insertion of Dynamic Condylar Screw

The patient is placed supine on a table, where the distal end of the femur can be imaged by either fluoroscopy or roentgenograms. I prefer to use a total hip pack for draping. This leaves the limb free for manipulation and also provides access to the iliac crest, when a bone graft is needed. The distal femur is exposed via a straight lateral approach that begins to curve anteriorly at the distal end of the lateral femoral condyle. When an extensile approach is needed, it extends along the lateral aspect of the patellar ligament to the level of the tibial tubercle. An osteotomy of the tibial tubercle is avoided. If additional exposure of the medial condyle is necessary, a second medial incision can be made at the level of the medial intermuscular septum.

The lateral approach is made by dividing the iliotibial band in line with its fibers. The vastus lateralis is swept over the anterior cortex of the femur with blunt retraction. Great care is given to identifying and dividing perforating vessels posterior to the lateral intermuscular septum. These vessels should be either cauterized or ligated by suture prior to their transection; otherwise, troublesome bleeding may occur after their retraction behind the intermuscular septum. Dissection is next undertaken to identify fracture surfaces. An attempt should be made to maintain the soft tissue attachments of bony fragments. A special effort is made to preserve the soft tissue attachments on the posterior aspect of the femoral shaft and metaphysis which preserve the blood supply of these fragments. For better exposure, the patella can be pushed medially to expose distal interarticular fracture lines. After the interarticular fracture is exposed, large reduction forceps of Kirschner-wires can be used for provisional fixation. In highly comminuted fractures, one begins by reconstructing the intercondylar notch. Next, definitive fixation is achieved with cancellous lag screws (Fig 79–5,A–C). Care should be made when selecting between screws with either 32-mm or 16-mm threads, so that the threads do not cross the fracture site. This is necessary to achieve interfragmentary compression. Placement of the interfragmentary screws must be done so that the screws do not interfere with the subsequent insertion of the dynamic condylar screw (Fig 79–6,A and B).

DISTAL FEMORAL FRACTURES AFTER TOTAL KNEE REPLACEMENT

Distal femoral fractures after total knee replacement are uncommon. The incidence of this complication is estimated to be between 0.6% and 2.5%.[1, 18] Fractures have been observed to occur at the time of surgery and as late as 10 years after the total knee replacement.

In most instances, the fracture is caused by a fall, or other low energy injury. Conditions that weaken the distal femur are associated with periprosthetic fractures. These conditions include notching of the femoral cortex during total knee replacement, osteoporosis, revision total knee replacement, and neurologic disorders.[5, 7, 8, 10] Notching of the femoral cortex during replacement arthroplasty is iatrogenic. It is thought that the notching of the femoral cortex weakens the transition of the cortical to the cancellous bone at the diaphyseal-metaphyseal junction, and results in a potential stress riser.[1] Calculations estimate that the removal of as little as 3 mm of bone causes a 29% reduction in the torsional strength of the femur where the notching occurs. This is due to reduction in the polar moment of inertia, which is proportional to the fourth power of the radius. Although disputed in one report, notching is cited as a cause of fractures by most authors, and in one series was observed in 40% of patients that developed a distal femoral fracture after total knee replacement.[1, 17]

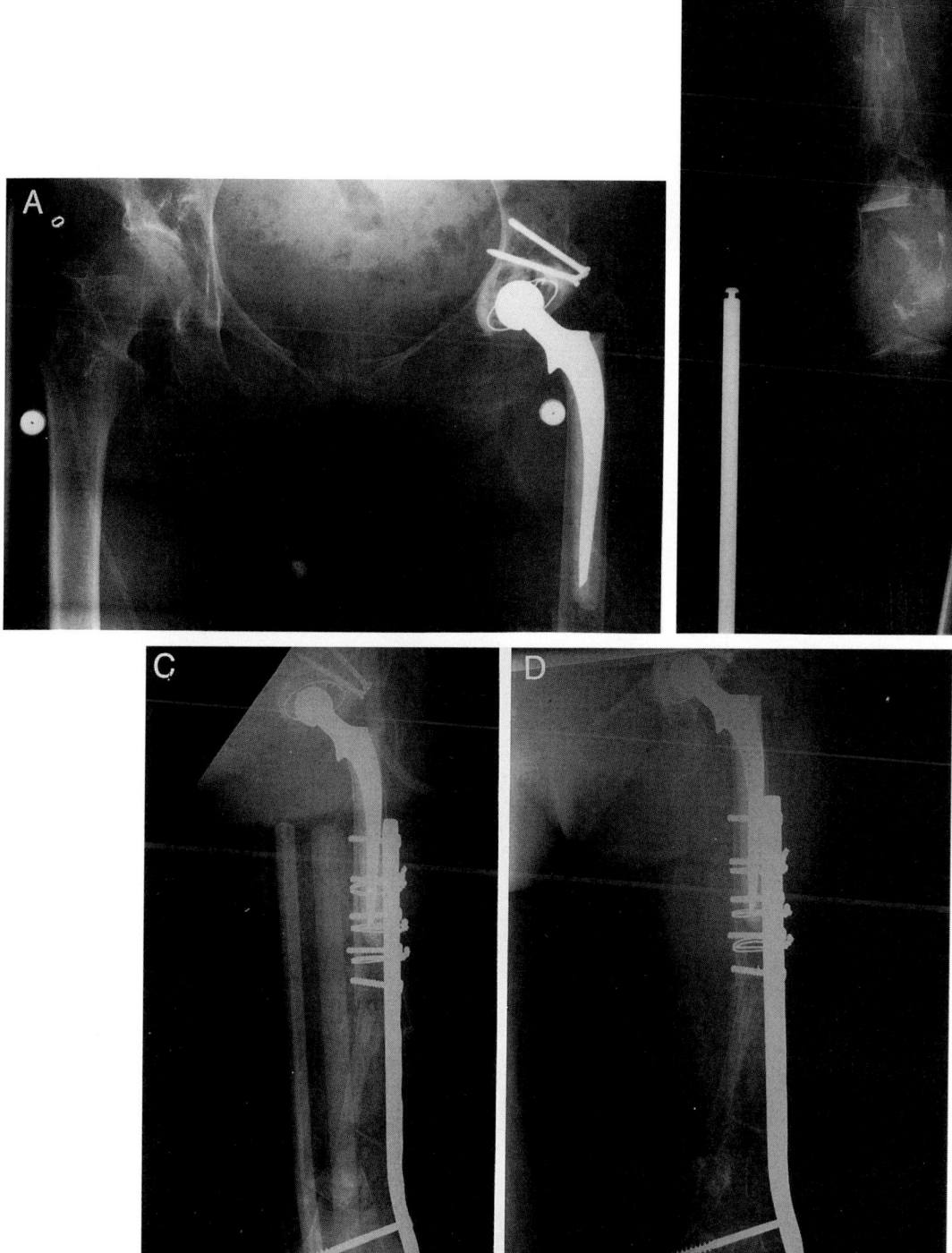

FIG 79–4.
A and **B**, this 79-year-old woman was struck by a bus. She had a prior successful total hip revision. Preoperative arteriogram indicated an intact femoral artery. These preoperative films show extensive comminution of the distal femur. Open reduction and internal fixation was undertaken with a plate spanning the area of comminution, with no attempt made to achieve anatomic reduction of multiple comminuted fracture fragments. The plate was used to recreate the length of the femur and thereby indirectly reduce fracture fragments according to the principles of indirect reduction. Additional bone graft was inserted at the time of surgery. **C**, postoperative films indicate the fixation montage. **D**, union has been achieved at 9 months after surgery. The patient is walking with the use of a cane at the time of this film. (From Gustilo RB, Kyle RF, Templeman D, eds: *Fractures and Dislocations*. St Louis, 1993, Mosby.)

Supracondylar femoral fractures after total knee replacements are difficult to treat and the best method of management is not established. Current treatment recommendations include: cast immobilization; traction, followed by cast bracing; open reduction and internal fixation, usually with plate and screw combinations; and revision of the components with the use of an intramedullary stem for the femoral component.[5, 7, 10, 24]

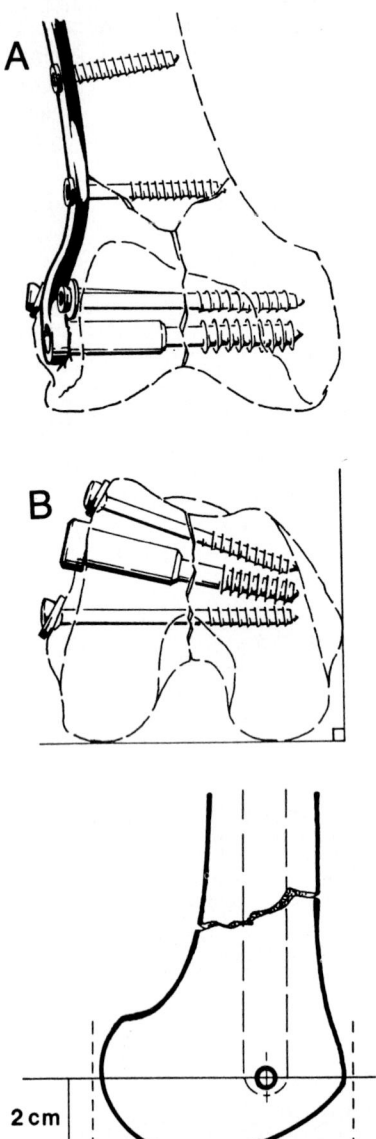

FIG 79–5.
A, internal fixation of a type C1 intercondylar distal femoral fracture with a compression screw and cancellous lag screws. Note that on the AP projection the lag screw and cancellous threads cross the fracture line and the length of the screws appears approximately 1 cm short of the medial cortex. **B,** axial projection of the distal one-third of the femur. Note the oblique orientation of the cancellous screws and lag screw. Because of the trapezoid shape of the distal end of the femur, the posterior width of the femur is greater than the anterior width. This shape accounts for the apparent shortness of the screws when an AP roentgenogram is taken. Appropriate screw length should appear approximately 1 cm short of the medial cortex when verified on an AP x-ray film. **C,** the appropriate entry site for the dynamic condylar screw. Posterior displacement of the screw will translate the distal fragment medially. This is because of the greater width of the femur in its half, as noted in **B**. (From Gustilo RB, Kyle RF, Templeman D, eds: *Fractures and Dislocations.* St Louis, 1993, Mosby.)

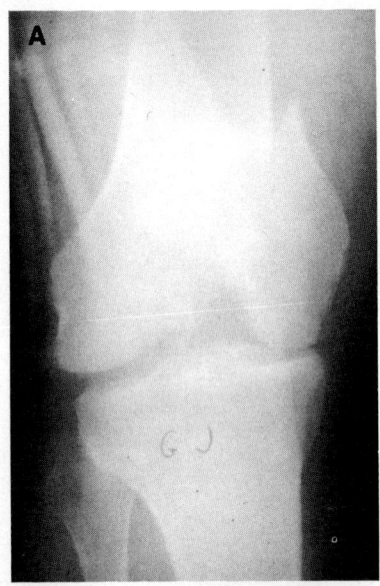

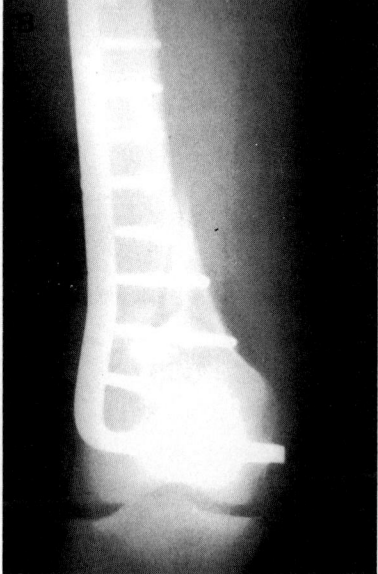

FIG 79–6.
A and **B,** example of a blade plat used to stabilize a supracondylar femoral fracture. Note that the blade is too long and has penetrated the medial cortex. Appropriate blade length would appear to be approximately 1 cm short of the medial cortex. (From Gustilo RB, Kyle RF, Templeman D, eds: *Fractures and Dislocations.* St Louis, 1993, Mosby.)

Precise indications for the best treatment methods are not established. However, the goals of treatment are union, acceptable alignment, knee motion of 90 degrees or greater, and restoration of knee motion to maintain the prefracture walking ability.[5, 8]

In most series, the complications of open reduction and internal fixation are more serious than those of nonoperative treatment. These operative complications include death, infection, above-knee amputations, nonunions, and the need for secondary surgeries to achieve union. Despite these complications, nonoperative treatment more frequently results in malunions and limited motion of the knee. Varus malunion is a frequent complication of nonoperative management. This varus malalignment promotes later loosening of the tibial components.[10] Limited motion and poor knee function after nonoperative treatment are common, and in one series, 15 of 30 patients had increased pain after nonoperative treatment. In the same series, only 4 of 30 patients had decreased function after operative treatment.[7] However, the surgical complications in this series were three malunions, one nonunion, and two above-knee amputations after open reduction and internal fixation of these fractures.[7] These poor results after operative treatment are not significantly different from the low rate of 21% acceptable results achieved by Schatzker and Lambert[21] in the treatment of older patients with osteoporosis and comminution. It should be noted that in one series, 80% of the patients that developed this fracture were postmenopausal women.

Current recommendations for treatment include the use of cast or traction and cast bracing, when the alignment is acceptable.[1, 5, 7, 8, 10] When an adequate reduction cannot be achieved or maintained, operative treatment is justified. The decision between open reduction and internal fixation vs. revision of the components is determined by whether or not the fracture involves the prosthesis, or if loosening of the prosthesis was evident prior to the fracture.[1, 7, 10]

Most series reporting on the complications of distal femoral fractures after total knee replacements outline the multiple problems of a weakened distal femur, an elderly patient, and problems in achieving early motion and weightbearing. Future improvements are needed to manage this difficult fracture problem.

REFERENCES

1. Aaron RK, Scott R: Supracondylar fracture of the femur after total knee arthroplasty, *Clin Orthop* 219:136–139, 1987.
2. Benum P: The use of bone cement as an adjunct to internal fixation of supracondylar fractures of osteoporotic femurs, *Acta Orthop Scand* 48:52–56, 1977.
3. Brown A, D'Arcy JC: Internal fixation for supracondylar fractures of the femur in the elderly patient, *J Bone Joint Surg [Br]* 53:420–424, 1973.
4. Bucholz RW, Ross SE, Lawrence KL: Fatigue fracture of the interlocking nail in the treatment of fractures of the distal part of the femoral shaft, *J Bone Joint Surg [Am]* 69:1391, 1987.
5. Cain PR, et al: Periprosthetic femoral fractures following total knee replacement, *Clin Orthop* 208:205–214, 1986.
6. Connolly JF, Dehne E, LaFollette B: Closed reduction and early brace ambulation treatment of fractures. Part II. Results in 143 fractures, *Acta Orthop Scand* 53:963–974, 1982.
7. Culp RW, et al: Supracondylar fracture of the femur following prosthetic knee arthroplasty, *Clin Orthop* 222:212–222, 1987.
8. DiGioia AM III, Rubash HE: Periprosthetic fractures of the femur after total knee arthroplasty, *Clin Orthop* 271:135–142, 1991.
9. Egund N, Kolmert L: Deformities, gonarthrosis and function after distal femoral fractures, *Acta Orthop Scand* 53:963–974, 1982.
10. Figgie MP, et al: The results of treatment of supracondylar fracture above total knee arthroplasty, *J Arthroplasty* 5:267–276, 1990.
11. Giles JB, et al: Supracondylar-intercondylar fractures of the femur treated with a supracondylar plate and lag screw, *J Bone Joint Surg [Am]* 64:864–870, 1982.
12. Leung KS, et al: Interlocking intramedullary nailing for supracondylar and intercondylar fractures of the distal part of the femur, *J Bone Joint Surg [Am]* 73:332–340, 1991.
13. Mize RD, Bucholz RW, Grogan DP: Surgical treatment of displaced, comminuted fractures of the distal end of the femur, *J Bone Joint Surg* 64:871–879, 1982.
14. Mooney V, et al: Cast brace treatment for fractures of the distal part of the femur, *J Bone Joint Surg [Am]* 52:1563–1578, 1970.
15. Neer CS III, Grantham SA, Shelton ML: Supracondylar fracture of the adult femur. A study of 110 cases, *J Bone Joint Surg [Am]* 49:591–693, 1967.
16. Olerud S: Operative treatment of supracondylar fractures of the femur, *J Bone Joint Surg [Am]* 54:1015–1032, 1972.
17. Ritter MA, Faris PM, Keating EM: Anterior femoral notching and ipsilateral supracondylar femur fracture in total knee arthroplasty, *J Arthroplasty* 3:185–187, 1988.
18. Sanders R, Regazonni P, Reudi T: Treatment of supracondylar-intercondylar fractures of the femur using the dynamic condylar screw, *J Orthop Trauma* 3:214–222, 1989.
19. Sanders R, et al: Double plating of comminuted, unstable fracture of the distal part of the femur, *J Bone Joint Surg [Am]* 73:341–346, 1991.

20. Schatzker J, Horn G, Waddell J: The Toronto experience with supracondylar fracture of the femur: 1966–1972, *Injury* 6:113–128, 1975.
21. Schatzker J, Lambert DC: Supracondylar fractures of the femur, *Clin Orthop* 138:77–83, 1979.
22. Schatzker J, et al: Dynamic condylar screw: A new device. A preliminary report, *J Orthop Trauma* 3:124–132, 1989.
23. Shelbourne KD, Brueckmann FR: Rush pin fixation of supracondylar and intercondylar fractures of the femur, *J Bone Joint Surg [Am]* 64:161–169, 1982.
24. Sisto DJ, Lichiewicz PF, Insall JN: Treatment of supracondylar fractures following prosthetic arthroplasty of the knee, *Clin Orthop* 196:265–272, 1985.
25. Stewart MJ, Sisk TD, Wallace SL Jr: Fractures of the distal one-third of the femur. A comparison of method of treatment, *J Bone Joint Surg [Am]* 48:784–807, 1966.

80

Tibial Plateau Fractures

JOHN P. REILLY, M.D.

Anatomy
Mechanism of injury
Classification
Clinical findings
Radiographic evaluation
Conservative management
    Early range-of-motion mobilization
    Cast immobilization
    Skeletal traction and early mobilization
    Cast bracing
Operative management
    Surgical approaches to tibial plateau

Open reduction and internal fixation
    Cleavage fracture
    Depression fracture
    Cleavage with depression fracture
    Medial condyle fracture
    Bicondylar fracture
    Complex fracture
    Fracture fixation and arthroscopy
Complications
Postoperative care
Summary and conclusions

This chapter explores, in some detail, numerous aspects concerning the diagnosis and treatment of proximal tibial fractures that involve the articular surface. The discussion is limited to the tibial plateau and the proximal metaphysis. Management and discussion relevant to injuries involving the tibial spine, anterior tibial tubercle, or epiphyseal injuries are not presented.

The tibial plateau is one of the most critical load-bearing joints in the human body. Because of this fact, articular fractures remain, to this day, a difficult, frustrating, and challenging area of fracture care for the orthopaedic surgeon. The fracture is quite common and may result in disability with upward of 50% unacceptable results.[84] Although management may be controversial, the goals of treatment are not. In view of the often unpredictable and sometimes dismal functional results, there are still many active proponents of nonoperative treatment.[12, 14, 15, 21, 45, 51, 61] In recent years technologic progress and long-term assessment of surgical treatment have made a strong argument for operative care of these fractures.[5, 35, 43, 48, 78, 87] Both will be explored in greater detail.

The goals of treating this fracture, similar to any other intraarticular fracture, are to obtain a stable and mobile joint and restore the articular surface to its preinjury contour. This will restore the biomechanical axis of the extremity. Within the limitations of the treatment venue selected, acknowledging the severity of the articular injury, effort is directed to minimize surface irregularities such as step-offs or gaps. Healing of the various soft tissues, including those associated with the trauma, such as the knee ligaments and the surgical wound, is imperative. The initial assessment and treatment should therefore try to minimize the known early and late complications, especially traumatic degenerative arthritis.[39]

The proximal tibia has specific features which make the operation particularly difficult. Because of the lower extremity biomechanics, its return to preinjury function is critical. The literature as far back as the mid-19th century acknowledges these problems, some of which are medicolegal.[26] In our own time, Hohl[28] and Schatzker and Tile,[80] speaking from decades of experience, have further substantiated the reasons to approach even the simplest of these fractures with caution and thorough preparation.

ANATOMY

An understanding of the anatomy of the proximal tibia provides insight into the reasons why certain fracture patterns exist and occur with such regularity. The proximal tibia expands from the diaphysis through a metaphyseal flare. In the posterolateral quadrant contact is made with the head of the fibula. The surface of the tibia has a medial and lateral weightbearing portion and an intercondylar eminence which is both nonarticular and nonweight bearing (Fig 80–1). The medial and lateral condylar surfaces have some differences which must be distinguished. The medial plateau is generally larger than the lateral plateau and is concave in both the sagittal and coronal plane. The lateral plateau is shaped more like a saddle: convex in the sagittal plane and mildly concave in the coronal plane.

The frontal plane of the proximal tibia is basically perpendicular to the tibial shaft, whereas in the sagittal plane there is usually a 10- to 15-degree posteroinferior slope.[6] This fact is well known to surgeons familiar with total knee arthroplasty. The intercondylar eminence provides an area of attachment to both the medial and lateral menisci as well as both cruciate ligaments.

In the normal person the majority of the load transmitted across the knee is medial to the eminence.[36, 62] Cadaver studies have demonstrated stronger trabecular cancellous bone in this region. The lateral "bands" are weaker, particularly in the anterior one half to two thirds of the lateral portion of the tibia. This results in what has been described as "weak spots" or faults. One is in a horizontal plane crossing the metaphysis and the second is an inverted V with its apex at the intercondylar eminence (Fig 80–2).

Biomechanical studies have indicated clearly what many had believed: the menisci increase the contact area available for femorotibial weightbearing and more evenly distribute the stresses between both plateaus. This contact area moves posteriorly as the degree of flexion increases at the knee. Removal of menisci decreases the contact area and increases the stress on the articular cartilage and underlying subchondral bone of the proximal tibia.[42]

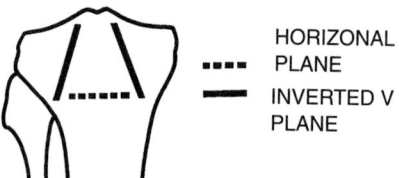

FIG 80–2.
Orientation of proximal metaphyseal fault lines.

A final lesson to be drawn from knee anatomy has to do with the shape of the femoral condyles. The anterior transverse width of the condyles is less than the posterior width. Furthermore, the medial condyle is more "round" as opposed to the lateral condyle, which has a flatter appearance. This allows, especially in extension, some of the anterior articular surface of the lateral plateau to be exposed, and offers an insight into understanding the patterns of fracture.

MECHANISM OF INJURY

Tibial plateau fractures can occur at any age, but for certain reasons, such as osteoporosis, tend to occur more frequently later in adult life. They occur with similar frequency in either sex. These injuries may be the result of:

1. Bumper strike (pedestrian vs. automobile).
2. Motor vehicle accidents (driver or passenger).
3. Fall from a height.
4. Sports.[53, 54]
5. Miscellaneous injuries (gunshots, industrial, crush).[30, 92]

Fifty-five percent to 70% of these fractures involving the tibial plateau are isolated to the lateral condyle.

Ligamentous injury may occur with the tibial plateau fracture. The ligament considered most at risk is the medial collateral ligament. This is due to the frequent valgus stress at the moment of impact. The incidence of ligamentous injuries varies from study to study, ranging between 0% and 15%.[5, 9, 16, 60, 78]

Along with knowing the causes and demographics of this fracture is the importance of knowing the pathomechanics which produce the injury. It is essential to apply understanding of normal anatomy and biomechanics to treatment of these fractures.

Kennedy and Bailey[38] created tibial plateau fractures in 44 cadaver knees, and confirmed that the forces involved in producing these fracture patterns are valgus stress (abduction), compression, or a combination of the two. The fracture pattern produced

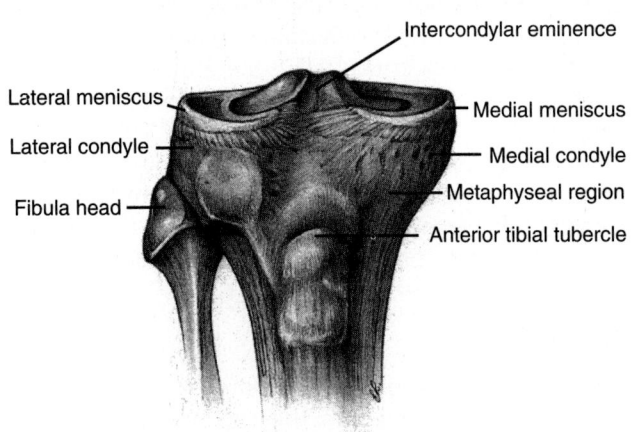

FIG 80–1.
Proximal tibia anatomy.

depends on the magnitude of force exerted as well as the amount of knee flexion at the moment of impact. The authors' studies indicate that with an abduction force applied, a split or cleavage fracture pattern occurs. When a compressive force is applied, typically compression fractures occur with an area of depression, producing an area of articular damage resembling a mosaic pattern. As the amount of flexion increases, the fracture line, in many cases, moves posteriorly.

Biomechanical analysis confirms that during abduction at the knee the center of rotation is medial to the intercondylar eminence and the hinge in this mechanism is the medial collateral ligament, which is taut in full extension. In full extension the contact zone between the femoral and tibial condyles is anterior. As the degree of flexion increases, the contact zone moves posteriorly. However, because the medial collateral ligament becomes increasingly lax, the effectiveness of this hinge to produce a pure wedge decreases, making the outcome less predictable. It may be that some of the force (energy) at the moment of impact is dissipated in the knee through a rotatory motion.

Osteoporosis and high velocity (energy) both contribute to the occurrence of this fracture and to the fracture pattern that results. The knee has a normal physiologic valgus alignment and for this reason injury is more likely to result in a lateral condylar fracture. This is supported by observations from many sources. Varus forces can be experienced by the knee but are not observed with nearly the same frequency.

Weis et al.[90] in studies on cadavers, assessed the mechanism of injury in the pedestrian-automobile injury. Fifteen cadavers were studied to assess the types of injury that occur when a pedestrian is struck by the bumper of a vehicle imparting valgus stress to the fully extended knee. They analyzed crash data with standard bumper height and a nose-dive position to mimic a deceleration injury. They also assessed injuries sustained with hard and soft bumpers. The authors concluded that lateral tibial plateau fracture is the most frequent bony injury. Further, the magnitude of injury is directly related to the velocity of the vehicle and that severe valgus forces with up to 6 in. of deformation may result.[90]

Basic science researchers have studied normal knee biomechanics with the use of mathematical models and computer-assisted finite element analysis. Struben[85] developed a sophisticated model to analyze motion in the knee joint. He proposed that the knee acts like a closed kinematic chain and therefore conforms to an exact mathematical formula. The linkages in a closed kinematic chain can only move in a fashion or direction that is defined by the other parts. In the knee this system includes the femoral condyles, the tibial plateau, and the ligamentous attachments which connect the first two structures. To allow the knee its particular range of motion, the respective joint surfaces must display an appropriate shape. Although the surfaces of the tibia and femur appear to be incongruous, this is a static view and is incorrect. Struben further states that if one of the parts in the chain is removed, the resulting pattern of movement will be altered unless its replacement is of identical geometric shape. If not, the replacement must be able to be molded into the correct shape.[85] The implication of Struben's model for treatment of tibial plateau fractures suggests that early range of motion in flexion and extension while protecting the knee from rotatory motion or varus-valgus stress may help the joint to remold to its proper shape. This concept may be extremely helpful, particularly when the reduction is less than perfect. Interestingly, tibial traction in conjunction with early range-of-motion exercises, as proposed by Apley,[2] and to be discussed in more detail later, achieves this combination. More detailed study of the articular alignment of these fractures has been performed to assess the degree of accuracy required in reducing these fractures.

Damaged articular surface has only limited capacity to heal. The fracture will produce injury to the subchondral bone and its associated blood supply. Observers have noted that this results in defects filling in with fibrocartilage whose mechanical properties are poorer than those of hyaline cartilage.

Mathematical models using contact finite element analysis can assess the stress aberrations which occur when a step-off is created by an incongruous (imprecise) reduction of the tibial plateau.[7, 29] These increases in stress locally depend obviously on the magnitude of the step-off.

Recognizing the limitations of the mathematical model, it has been observed that in addition to the magnitude of step-off (in millimeters), factors such as cartilage thickness and subchondral bone stiffness will contribute to increases in the recorded stress. Studies also reaffirm the importance of preserving the meniscus since meniscectomy increases the locally perceived contact stress.

With regard to treatment and long-term outcome this provides us with interesting information. We can assume that increases in contact stress will alter normal cartilage metabolism. The question is, What amount of increase stress equating to an upper limit of step-off can be deemed acceptable? Statistically significant departure from normal anatomic stress levels are not seen until the step-off is 1.5 mm. At 3 mm the increase in stress is still not increased by more than a factor of 2.

Given the prevailing clinical opinion of accepting 5 to 10 mm of step-off, current laboratory data predict that as long as the region in which the articular noncontact is small, it will be within the long-term tolerances of the articular cartilage.

While late degenerative changes occur, it is acknowledged that they do so slowly—even up to 20 years after the injury. This supports the premise that long-term tolerances of cartilage are higher than has been believed. An alternative hypothesis is that the bone-cartilage remodels to restore local congruity, thereby decreasing the local contact stress and restoring the closed kinematic chain.

CLASSIFICATION

Anatomically, tibial plateau fractures can be divided into fractures isolated to the lateral plateau, the medial plateau, and those involving both plateaus (bicondylar fractures). A concise classification system should evolve with our overall understanding of specific fractures. A method must be available to identify which fractures require surgical intervention and also serve the purpose of assessing the long-term results of treatment. Structurally, tibial plateau fractures can be subdivided into:

1. Split fracture, in which a separation or cleavage is produced.
2. Compression fracture, in which there is compression of the metaphyseal trabecular bone underlying the articular surface. There is an associated area of depression in the articular surface with some degree of comminution.
3. Split compression fracture, which combines elements of the first two categories. Numerous researchers have attempted to correlate these patterns with their understanding of the mechanics of the injury.

A variety of classification systems have been proposed, but have caused problems when attempting to compare results between series in which different classification systems have been used. This is compounded when an attempt is made to evaluate differences between series with different treatment modalities.

The reader should be familiar with some of the many classifications proposed over the years.[27, 58, 63, 72, 78] The classification of Schatzker and associates[78] is the result of an exhaustive study of 94 fractures treated in Toronto between 1968 and 1975. The authors divided fractures into the following six categories (Fig 80–3):

I. Cleavage.
II. Cleavage with depression.
III. Pure depression.
IV. Medial condyle.
V. Bicondylar.
VI. Plateau fracture with dissociation of the metaphysis and diaphysis.

In the type I injury the lateral femoral condyle impacts the tibial surface creating a wedge-shaped fragment, which may displace laterally or distally. A type II fracture creates a wedge-type fracture as in type 1, but additionally some portion of the remaining plateau and articular surface is depressed distally. There is usually some degree of comminution to the articular surface. A type III fracture is a pure depression injury in which there is a central compression of the articular surface and underlying subchondral bone, but no split, and the lateral tibial cortex remains intact. The type IV injury recognizes the less often observed fractures to the medial plateau. Two subtypes are observed: a pure split similar to type I or a depressed fracture similar to type III. Type V fractures are more complex and involve both the medial and lateral plateaus. As previously discussed, the fracture pattern follows the fault lines in the region giving the appearance of an inverted Y or V. The intercondylar eminence may have an associated fracture. In the type VI fracture the injury pattern is more severe. A transverse or oblique fracture in the proximal tibia produce separation of the metaphysis and diaphysis. In addition, there are varying degrees of fracture to one or both tibial condyles.

Recent modification of the classification system has been suggested by the Association for the Study of Internal Fixation (ASIF) to more completely define all possible types of fracture configuration.[63] Mueller et al.[63] have provided an exhaustive classification system which is applicable to the proximal end of the tibia. The authors state: "A classification is useful only if it considers the severity of the bone lesion and serves as a basis for treatment and for evaluation of the results."[63] Their system acknowledges all previous work on the types of fractures of the proximal tibia. It then is subdivided into groups and subgroups (Fig 80–4) arranged in numeric order based on the acknowledged complexities of the fracture, the difficulties recognized in treatment, and to some extent on experience, i.e., the authors' prognosis. Thus A1 pertains to a simple fracture with a good prognosis and C3 pertains to the most difficult type of fracture with the worst prognosis. The classification thus in-

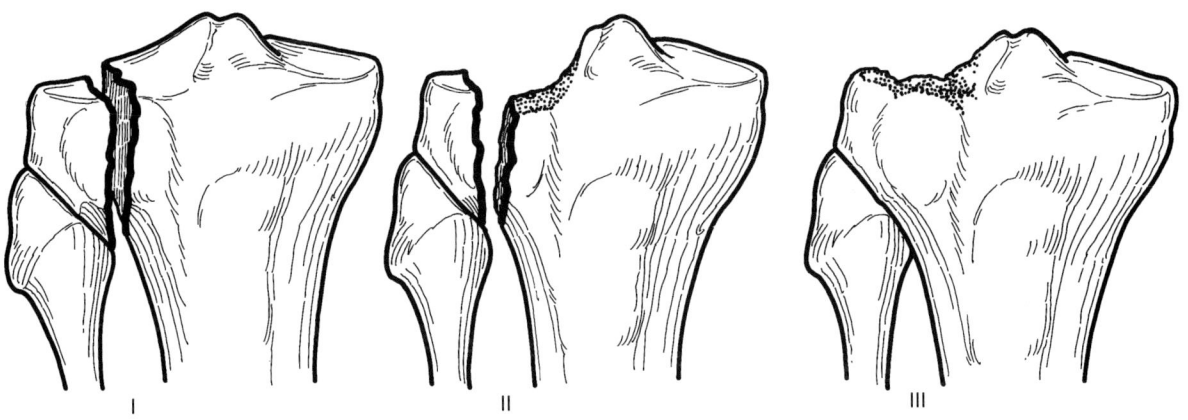

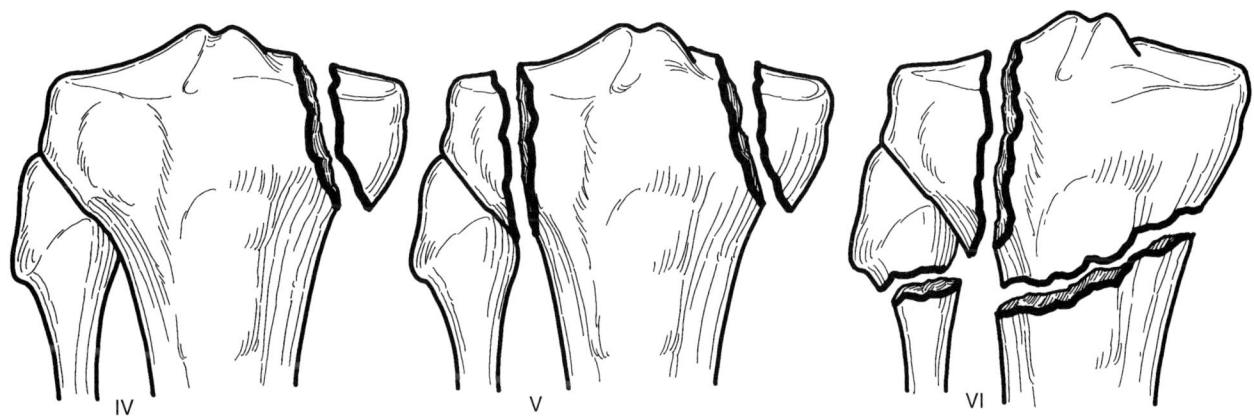

FIG 80–3.
Classification of tibial plateau fractures: *I*, cleavage; *II*, cleavage with depression; *III*, pure depression; *IV*, medial condyle; *V*, bicondylar; *VI*, plateau with dissociation of the metaphysis and diaphysis.

corporates an anatomic understanding of the injury as well as an expectation as to the ultimate result. The classification of proximal tibial and fibular fractures, according to Mueller et al.,[63] follows:

A. Extraarticular fracture.
    A1. Extraarticular fracture, avulsion.
        1. Of the fibular head.
        2. Of the tibial tuberosity.
        3. Of the cruciate insertion.
    A2. Extraarticular fracture, metaphyseal simple.
        1. Oblique in the frontal plane.
        2. Oblique in the sagittal plane.
        3. Transverse.
    A3. Extraarticular fracture, metaphyseal multifragmentary.
        1. Intact wedge.
        2. Fragmented wedge.
        3. Complex.
B. Partial articular fracture.
    B1. Partial articular fracture, pure split.
        1. Of the lateral surface.
        2. Of the medial surface.
        3. Oblique, involving the tibial spines and one of the surfaces.
    B2. Partial articular fracture, pure depression.
        1. Lateral total.
        2. Lateral limited.
        3. Medial.
    B3. Partial articular fracture, split-depression.
        1. Lateral.
        2. Medial.
        3. Oblique, involving the tibial spines and one of the surfaces.
C. Complete articular fracture.
    C1. Complete articular fracture, articular simple, metaphyseal simple.
        1. Slight displacement.

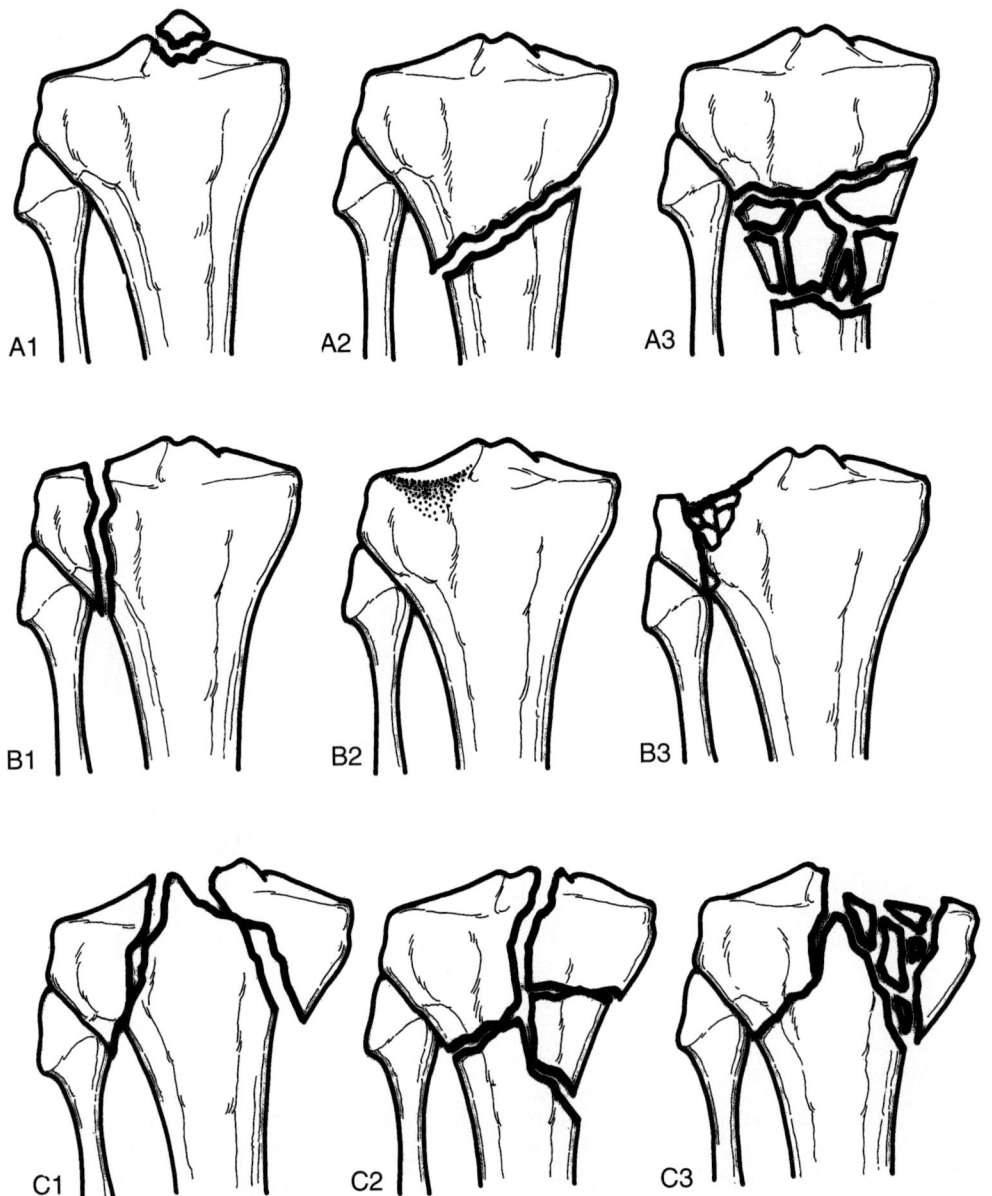

FIG 80–4.
Classification of tibial plateau fractures according to Mueller et al.[64] *A1*, cruciate insertion; *A2*, transverse; *A3*, complex; *B1*, lateral pure split; *B2*, lateral limited depression; *B3*, lateral split-depression; *C1*, both condyles; *C2*, intact wedge; *C3*, medial. (Redrawn from Mueller ME, et al: *Manual of internal fixation*, ed 3, Berlin, 1991, Springer-Verlag. Used by permission.)

  2. One condyle displaced.
  3. Both condyles displaced.
 C2. Complete articular fracture, articular simple, metaphyseal multifragmentary.
  1. Intact wedge.
  2. Fragmented wedge.
  3. Complex.
 C3. Complete articular fracture, multifragmentary.
  1. Lateral.
  2. Medial.
  3. Lateral and medial.

CLINICAL FINDINGS

There will routinely be a large hemarthrosis observed in patients sustaining fractures to the proximal tibia with articular extension. This collection may not occur if there is an associated tear in the capsule allowing the blood to dissipate into the surrounding soft tissue. The knee will be swollen, boggy, and often ecchymotic. There will be tenderness on the plateau involved and depending on the exact mechanism producing the injury the ligament on the opposite side of the knee may also be tender.

The range of motion of the knee should be assessed, if possible, and a straight leg raise test performed to assess patellar tendon function. These maneuvers may, however, be too painful for the unanesthesized patient. An assessment of the collateral ligaments may be done by aspirating the hemarthrosis and infiltrating the joint with local anesthetic. The ligaments should be compared with those of the uninjured knee. The injured leg should be examined for associated soft tissue injuries or other distant fractures, particularly in the patient with multiple trauma. Neurovascular complications should be anticipated. Peroneal nerve and major vascular injuries are rare, but are more frequent in high-energy injuries and with fracture-dislocations. Inspection of the knee and assessment for open wounds in the vicinity of the knee should alert the surgeon to the possibility of the injury being an open fracture. As always, one should be cognizant of the possibility of a compartmental syndrome, even with open fractures. Compartmental pressures should be documented if there is a clinical suspicion of same.

RADIOGRAPHIC EVALUATION

Plain films of the knee should always be obtained in patients suspected of having a tibial plateau fracture. Management of the fracture will in large part be determined by what information can be obtained from radiographic studies. Without adequate information the final result may be compromised. When considering a diagnostic study one must be critical and ask, What information can this test provide? Will the information in the format received be adequate to formulate a treatment plan? What studies can be used to follow these fractures during the acute treatment course and also for the long-term follow-up?[33] These have become more important questions today when we consider the diversity of tests currently available to the orthopaedic surgeon, including computed tomography (CT) and magnetic resonance imaging (MRI). Selection is critical when one recognizes their associated costs. Plain radiographs remain an easy and rapid way to locate these fractures, classify them, and communicate this information to the other physicians involved with the patient's care.

Routine frontal and lateral views of the knee will identify most fractures easily and accurately. There are certain fractures which can only be detected with an oblique or tunnel view. Trauma oblique views (medial and lateral) are obtained with the x-ray tube at an angle of 45 degrees and making two exposures.[13] This provides an elongated view of the tibial plateau in the horizontal plane.

Certain depressed areas may be subtle or can be obscured by other portions of the tibial plateau, the opposing femoral condyle, or the patella. One of the basic criteria for treatment is the amount of articular depression. One must be very certain that what the radiographs indicate is neither over- or underestimated. Anatomic analysis of the knee by Böhler[6] shows that the tibial plateau has a normal posterior slope of 10 to 15 degrees. This fact may contribute to incorrect estimation of the articular depression by distorting the anteroposterior projection. As investigation suggests, the amount of acceptable depression may be only a few millimeters, and therefore accuracy in this measurement is important.

The tibial plateau angle view is a means to more accurately determine the amount of depression.[59] It is obtained by tilting the x-ray tube 15 degrees caudad (Fig 80-5). Besides assessing the radiographic views for the amount of depression (in millimeters), careful evaluation should determine the amount of articular surface involved, how much comminution has occurred, and what damage may have occurred in the area of the various ligament attachments, often indicated by an avulsion fragment. Here, a lateral view may be invaluable. All this necessary information may not be clearly found with routine plain films. Although controversial, stress views in varus and valgus angulation can be performed to identify associated collateral ligament damage. There is no consensus today that stress studies are of significant clinical value.

Conventional tomography is the procedure of choice after plain films are performed (Fig 80-6). As the indications for surgical treatment have become better defined, tomograms have become a valuable preoperative tool. In one study, 9 of 21 patients had depression or displacement that was significantly underestimated by plain films.[21] Tomography eliminates superimposition of other structures, providing excellent assessment of the comminuted depression and fragment displacement. This information affords the surgeon a better three-dimensional image of the anatomy and fracture pattern. Tomograms may be done in the anteroposterior and lateral projections. All temporary dressings and splints must be removed. Exposures are routinely provided at 0.5-cm intervals.[65]

CT scans were previously applied to spinal and pelvic fractures. They were received enthusiastically by the orthopaedic community because of the difficulty in understanding and assessing these complex three-dimensional structures. It became a natural transition to apply the technology to the knee, not necessarily because of its complex geometry or

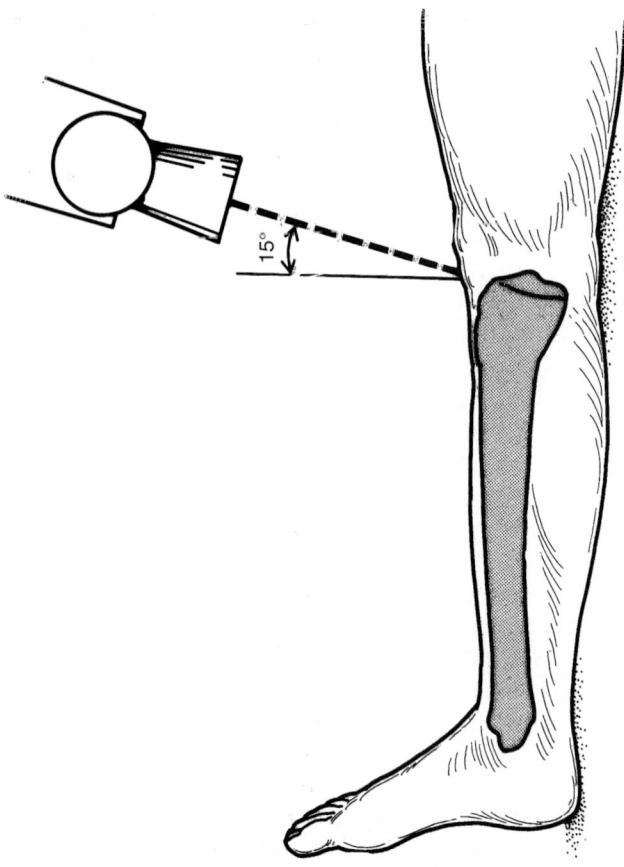

FIG 80–5.
Tibial plateau angle obtained by tilting the x-ray tube 15 degrees caudad.

anatomy, but rather because of the complexity of some resulting fracture patterns. Its application to joint injury can be quick and accurate. The CT scan provides a new and more detailed view of the fracture pattern and articular surface.[18, 64, 70, 71] By providing an axial view of the knee and using sagittal reconstruction, the CT scan gives detailed information as to the exact amount of depression and displacement. It also presents the anatomy in a manner that the surgeon will see when surgery is performed. With the use of more sophisticated software, a three-dimensional reconstruction may be generated using the original information, thus allowing the surgeon to see the plateau as he or she would intraoperatively, and facilitating the choice of surgical approach.[44]

Conventional tomograms have certain weaknesses. For optimal evaluation they need to be done in both the anteroposterior and lateral planes. Casts and splints must be removed for adequate visualization and they may not visualize certain damage to the tibial rim. They are also magnified by 15%. The CT scan is more rapid and more convenient for older patients and those sustaining multiple trauma. Casts and splints need not be removed, allowing the patient to be more comfortable and receive less radiation.

The use of MRI for knee injuries occurred after improvements were made in the surface coils necessary for the extremities and improved scanning tech-

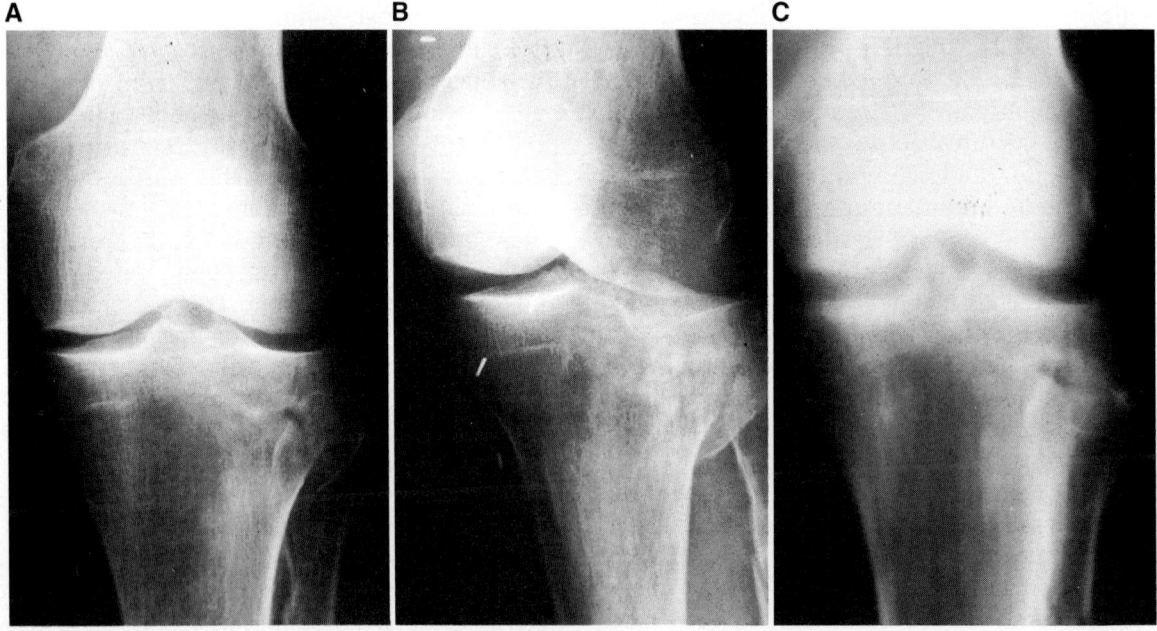

FIG 80–6.
This 62-year-old male pedestrian was struck by a car. He sustained a type III fracture and a contralateral bimalleolar ankle fracture. **A** and **B**, original radiographs could not adequately determine the amount of displacement. **C**, tomograms indicated that there was minimal displacement. The patient was treated conservatively.

niques became available.[44, 50] MRI is acknowledged as a reliable and accurate tool to assess meniscal and collateral and cruciate ligamentous injury. Recent reports have suggested that it may be valuable in identifying certain occult injuries to the osteochondral surface of the supracondylar femur and tibial plateau. Certain patterns of occult injuries have been identified by MRI.[17] A bone bruise is indicated by epiphyseal and metaphyseal changes in T1- and T2-weighted images. These signals indicate normal articular and cortical bone surfaces. They do reflect changes in marrow content. They are thought to represent edema, hyperemia, hemorrhage, and microfracture. No associated changes are seen on plain films. Plateau fractures are identified with MRI when radiographs are normal, even when reviewed retrospectively (Fig 80–7). Some authors acknowledge that there may not be much additional benefit managing these fractures with this modality since none of their patients had either plain tomograms or a CT scan.[57] One advantage of MRI is that it does not utilize ionizing radiation. Disadvantages include its cost and the time necessary to complete the study. Mostion artifact will occur if the patient moves during the scan. There is a distinct subset of patients who present with an abnormal signal to the tibial plateau with associated anterior cruciate ligament injury, but there is hesitation to use the term "fracture" since biopsies from these sites have not shown evidence of trabecular compression.[76]

One recent report suggests an interesting use for MRI in distinguishing what type of tissue occupies the bony defects seen in fractures with persistent radiographic depression.[34] The amount of fibrous tissue present may explain the apparent discrepancy between persistent defects and good knee function. Arthrography,[1] radionuclide bone scans,[49] and ultrasound have little application to the routine management of tibial plateau fractures. Arteriography may be employed on a case-by-case basis when there is a knee dislocation, which has a higher risk of an associated popliteal artery injury (Fig 80–8).

CONSERVATIVE MANAGEMENT

Traditional care of tibial plateau fractures has been by various closed methods. Even though many tibial plateau fractures have a significant degree of displacement or articular damage, there remain a significant group of surgeons who propose conservative nonoperative treatment in many instances. This philosophy stems in part from the poor results obtained in the early series on open reduction and internal fixation, (ORIF).[81, 91] Nonoperative include early mobilization with active exercise, cast immobilization, traction immobilization, and cast bracing. Closed reduction to manipulate the fracture may be utilized in conjunction with any of these methods.

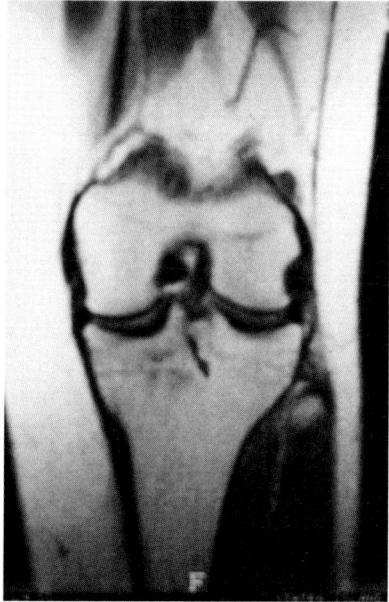

FIG 80–7.
This 32-year-old woman fell down some steps. She complained of pain in her knee. Except for a minimal effusion her clinical examination was normal. Radiographs were normal. Subsequent MRI indicated a fracture in the tibial plateau.

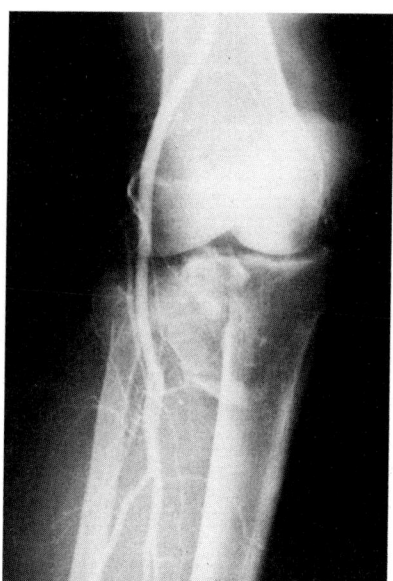

FIG 80–8.
This pedestrian was struck by a car and sustained a closed type III fracture. Pulses in the foot were not palpable. An arteriogram was performed to rule out an arterial injury. Compartment pressures were normal.

Early Range-of-Motion Mobilization

Early mobilization with active exercise can be utilized for minimally displaced stable fractures. It requires a period of nonweightbearing for 2 to 8 weeks. Often a soft compressive dressing can be added to the initial regimen for pain management and control of soft tissue swelling. This method is often used in patients whose advanced age or other medical conditions preclude other, and certainly other more aggressive, types of treatment. After an initial period of rest, range-of-motion exercises are initiated. Although routinely considered for a stable fracture, serial follow-up radiographs should be routine during the healing period. Weightbearing should be restricted until there is adequate radiographic evidence of fracture healing. Early range-of-motion exercises have been employed by many to reduce the loss of knee motion which often complicates the treatment of this and other articular fractures. The benefits of this treatment include decreased stiffness and possible benefit to the cartilage cells by stimulating the healing process.[77] The potential improvements of early mobilization must be balanced against a possible loss of reduction, and when used with internal fixation early range of motion may, if the fracture is unstable and poorly secured, contribute to loss of implant fixation and compromise soft tissue and ligament healing. To try to minimize these risks a period of immediate immobilization has been suggested, although its duration remains controversial, varying anywhere from 2 to 8 weeks. Gausewitz and Hohl[23] report that immediate range-of-motion therapy is recommended, but actual benefit is only seen statistically in those displaced fractures that were treated operatively.

Cast Immobilization

Cast immobilization is another time-honored method of treatment and is done by applying a long leg cast or cylinder cast in full extension. Spica cast treatment has also been reported.[19] This cast can be used for undisplaced or minimally displaced fractures of many types. Using a single hip spica cast, Drennan et al.[19] reported 85% good to excellent results. The basic cylinder casts can be used for 4 to 6 weeks, after which early range-of-motion exercises can be started. Closed reduction and good molding of the cast are beneficial (Fig 80–9). Care should be taken to provide adequate padding around the head of the fibula because of its proximity to the peroneal nerve. Partial weightbearing is recommended at between 9 and 12 weeks depending on the fracture type, the initial amount of comminution, and radiographic evidence of callus formation. Cast management can maintain correct alignment, but displacement can still occur, especially in unstable fracture configurations.

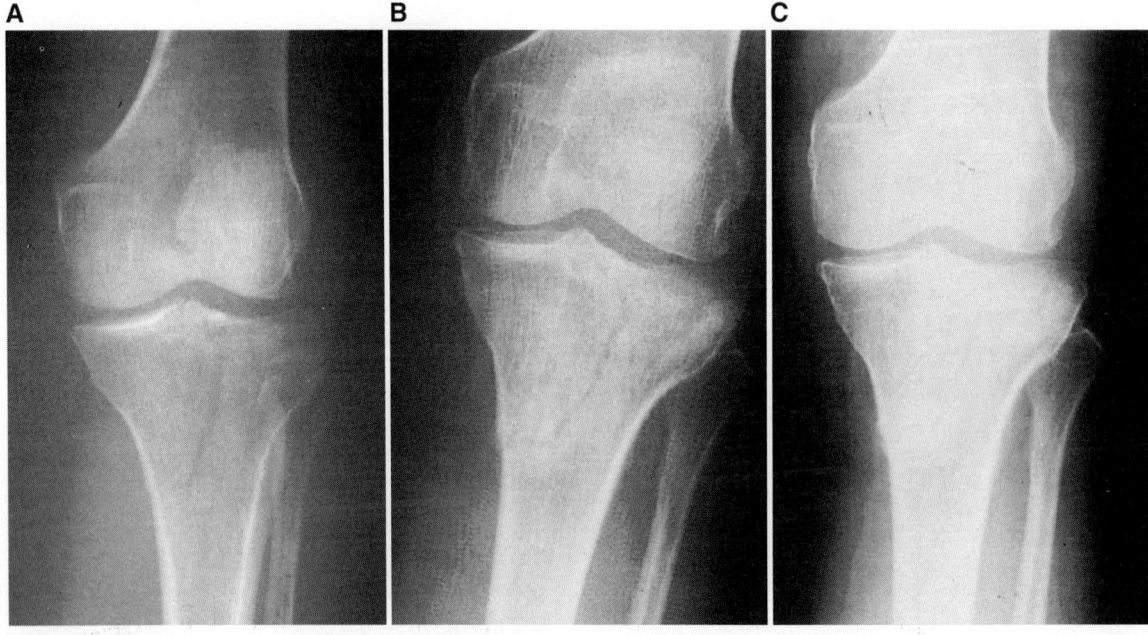

FIG 80–9.
This 65-year-old woman fell off a stool. She sustained a nondisplaced type IV fracture. **A,** original radiograph. **B,** the patient was treated in a cast for 4 weeks and started on range-of-motion therapy. **C,** the fracture healed uneventfully.

Skeletal Traction and Early Mobilization

Marwah et al.[51] and others report good results using skeletal traction and early mobilization. It can produce and maintain the reduction as well as the alignment. In skeletal traction, as the acute symptoms resolve, early range-of-motion activity may be permitted. It can be used for the entire spectrum of fractures—nondisplaced, minimally displaced of various types, as well as pure compression and bicondylar fractures. Since the lateral meniscus covers most of the load-bearing surface, some authors believe that as long as it is preserved good results are obtainable unless there is meniscal detachment or a tear. Traction can be used for the entire length of treatment or, in a stable situation, for 3 to 8 weeks in conjunction with cast bracing, which is discussed below. Various schemes are proposed. Moore et al.[61] report on the use of traction using either skeletal traction with a "knee exerciser" consisting of a Hodgson-Person apparatus, or Buck's traction. For the majority of fractures, which do not require ORIF, their complication rate was 8% compared with 19% in the operative group.[61] Skeletal traction may be useful in certain open fractures with associated contaminated wounds. Traction is applied with a Steinmann pin threaded through the calcaneus, and the leg is elevated. A Böhler-Braun frame can be helpful in this regard. The difficulty with this method of treatment centers around problems with pin tract irritation, inflammation and infection, possible rotational instability of the tibia, development of an equinus deformity, knee stiffness, and systemic difficulty such as deep venous thrombosis. Although traction with early mobilization has shown promise, there remain many drawbacks. In today's medical environment with fiscal restraints, diagnostic relation groups (DRGs), and so forth, the rationale for selecting this treatment is less compelling.

Cast Bracing

The most recent development in nonoperative care is cast bracing.[12, 14, 15, 82] Bracing has the advantage of maintaining fragment position (after reduction) while allowing better range of motion to the knee and ankle. Duwelius and Connolly[20] state that most fracture configurations can be treated this way. Less than satisfactory radiographic results still have good to excellent long-term functional results. The authors express concern that ORIF may add to devascularizing bone fragments.[19] Bracing still needs the radiographic follow-up required with all conservative methods of treatment. Critics of this treatment abound, and to some extent general orthopaedic experience with this method is somewhat limited. Its use requires skillful application of the cast brace and frequent follow-up visits to ensure that the position of the fracture remains acceptable. The stability of the fibula is critical to the success of this treatment and as has been suggested by many authors, patients with certain unstable fractures may not be good candidates.

Lansinger et al.[45] have reported on a large number of the patients initially treated conservatively by Rasmussen. The authors concluded that is was not the radiographic displacement but rather that 10-mm instability to varus-valgus stress in full extension would be the only indications for operative consideration. Some authors have demonstrated that conservative treatment is a satisfactory alternative despite the imperfect radiographic appearance of the fracture upon completion of treatment. Cast bracing can be applied to all fractures regardless of whether these fractures are treated primarily with surgery or by traction. It allows for earlier weightbearing and earlier hospital discharge. Early mobilization of the patient is also beneficial.

Finally, early protected weightbearing may, by dissipating the forces away from the area of the fracture, promote restoration of normal muscle function and better blood flow to the affected leg. Some results indicate that the cast brace can control varus and valgus malalignment within acceptable limits.[82] A 10-year follow-up study indicates that the cast brace provides satisfactory results for minimally displaced fractures.[14] Treatment of complex fractures has yielded many more variable results.

OPERATIVE MANAGEMENT

Surgical Approaches to Tibial Plateau

Open reduction and internal fixation can be approached by a straight midline incision, or in simpler cases which involve the lateral plateau only, by a curved incision starting proximally 1 cm lateral to the proximal pole of the patella midway between the patella and the plateau, and curving distally for about 10 cm to the lateral anterior crest of the tibia.[63] The traditional use of a transverse incision, which was often suggested to conform to the transversely oriented Langer's lines in order to obtain a better cosmetic result, has fallen into disfavor. This is primarily because many of these complex injuries to the proximal tibia may require late reconstructive surgery, such as a total knee replacement. The use of a transverse incision would risk wound healing in this situation. The Mercedes Y incision, once popular for extensile approaches, has been discouraged because of problems with the vascular supply to the flaps and subsequent infection. Regardless of the incision selected, the surgeon has to be aware of the associated neurovascular structures. Respect must be given to the soft tissues since they often are already compromised by the injury. Soft tissue dissection and excessive periosteal stripping should be avoided. A thigh tourniquet may routinely be applied, but often need not be inflated.

The incision is carried into the extensor retinaculum and crural fascia. As most authors have stressed, skin flaps are not raised. A lateral parapatellar arthrotomy incision is then made. Some of the prepatellar fat pad may be removed distally, and the muscles and periosteum of the anterior compartment are raised to expose the anterolateral aspect of the proximal tibia. At this time the surgeon should be able to see much of the fracture, although the articular surface along with the amount and location of any depressed articular fracture fragments is not yet seen.

At this point adequate exposure of the joint surface is necessary, which often necessitates raising some of the lateral meniscus from the tibial surface to provide appropriate visualization. A different approach has been described in which the anterior portion of the lateral meniscus, which attaches to the coronary ligaments, is incised and the fracture is hinged open.[69] At the completion of the reduction the anterior horn of the lateral meniscus with the coronary ligament is repaired with a fine absorbable suture (Fig 80–10). Excellent exposure is necessary to reduce articular deformity as well as to thoroughly inspect the joint for additional meniscal or ligamentous injury.

When dealing with the more serious bicondylar fracture patterns (Schatzker grade V or Mueller C1–3; see above) or a complex fracture-dislocation, a more extensile approach is required. Some manage this with two incisions, but recent sports suggest excellent results with an anterior approach combined with a tibial tubercle osteotomy.[22] This allows for complete exposure of both the medial and lateral condyles. It will also allow for replacing the patellar tendon securely and provide opportunity for early range of motion with a continuous passive motion (CPM) machine. Elevation of the patellar tendon off the tubercle, or Z plasty, has been suggested, but is not routinely utilized.[80] The main advantage of the extensile approach is that the quality of reduction achieved is greater and exposure is more complete for the pla-

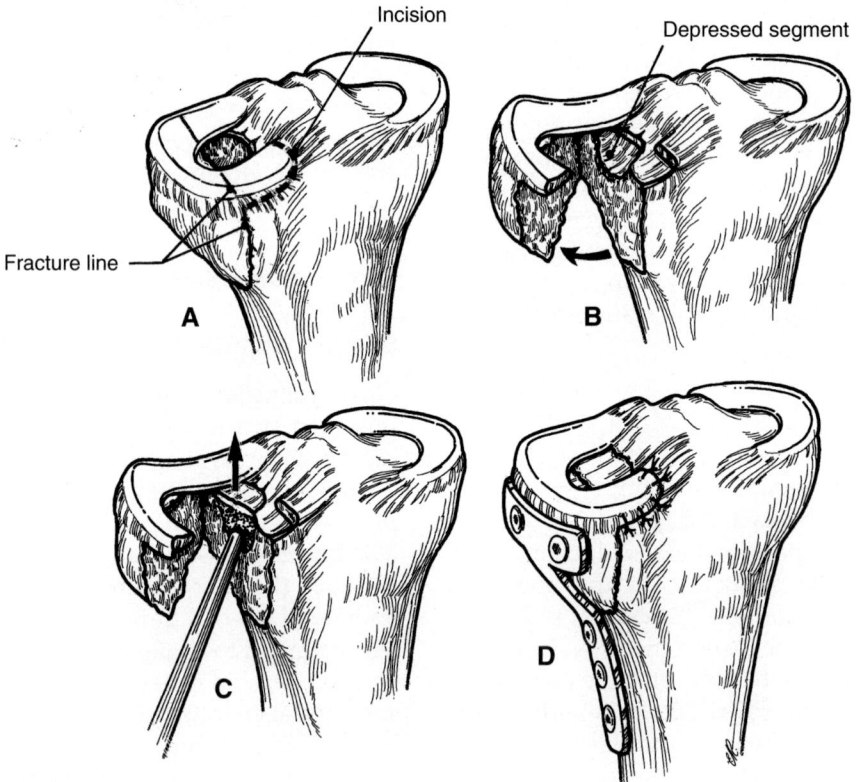

FIG 80–10.
A–D, surgical exposure to visualize the lateral tibial plateau.

teau and intercondylar notch. Efforts should always be made to maintain and preserve the menisci.

Open Reduction and Internal Fixation

The evolution of surgical treatment of fractures of the tibial plateau has been furthered by the ASIF.[63, 80] The ASIF has developed implants based on anatomic and biomechanical principles, the biology of fracture healing, and on a thorough metallurgic foundation. Use of these implants is based on results which match or exceed those of more conservative nonoperative means. Improving range of motion and return to early function lead to improved long-term results. The surgical approaches and classification have been discussed. Here we present the fixation options.

Opinion varies as to what constitutes significant displacement or depression. Some authors accept 10-mm displacement,[88] some 5 mm,[5, 27] some none.[9] All utilize the same instrumentation and implants. Implants that are now available include cortical and cancellous screws and assorted plates which act as a buttress to shore up unstable fragments. All implants are made of stainless steel. Cannulated screws are now available and are compatible with currently available implants. These screws afford the surgeon many benefits. Instead of having to remove Kirschner-wires, and then drill and secure the screws, one can simply drill over the wire. In this way the surgeon does not risk disturbing or losing a reduction which may have been difficult to obtain and tenuous to maintain. These screws may also be used to minimize or reduce the need for excessive soft tissue dissection by percutaneous placement either through a stab wound in an open fixation setting or with the assistance of fluoroscopic control, often now in conjunction with the arthroscope. New metallurgy continues to evolve with the recent development of titanium implants, which are designed with more consideration of the biology of fracture healing.[67]

Cleavage Fracture

Cleavage fractures (type I) that have significant displacement requiring reduction and fixation can be secured with one or more large-fragment AO cancellous screws. Screw length should be carefully selected in order to avoid an unnecessary prominence on the side opposite the fracture. Washers may be used to increase the surface area over which to obtain compression and also to effectively act as a buttress. The use of cannulated screws with this fracture pattern is an appropriate option and may be of value to minimize dissection of the soft tissues (Fig 80–11). The use of the washer can be especially helpful in osteopenic bone. In addition to a screw placed more proximally in the fracture, a cancellous screw with washer can be placed at the axilla of the fracture to act as a one-hole buttress plate. An anteriorly placed

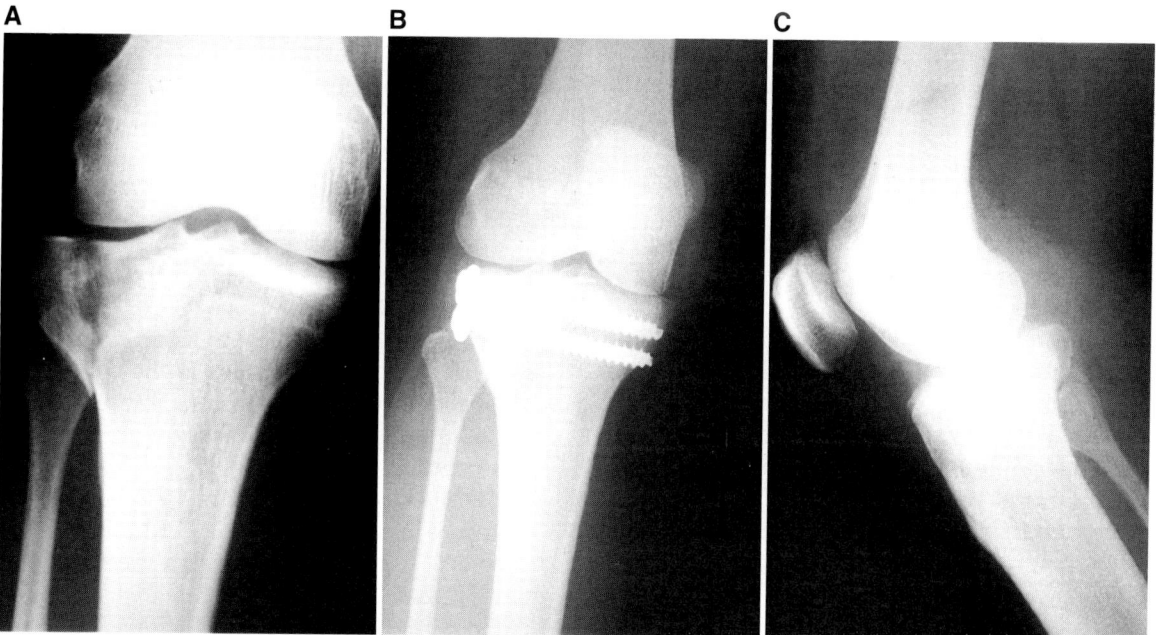

FIG 80–11.
This 25-year-old woman sustained a type I fracture and a comminuted humeral shaft fracture after being struck by a car. **A,** original radiograph. The fracture was reduced and fixed with cannulated large-fragment screws with washers. **B** and **C,** radiographs 4 months postoperatively.

one-third tubular plate can be utilized with difficult transverse fractures to facilitate reduction and be used as a tension band.[52] If there is significant comminution to the split, either from trauma, or as may occasionally occur, from intraoperative manipulation, buttress plates are available in a T or L configuration to maintain the position of the split fragment. Owing to the posterior position of the fibula head, the L plate is usually easier to apply. These plates may be shaped with contouring templates and plate benders. The split, however, must be adequately reduced since the plate cannot be considered an appropriate method of securing and maintaining the reduction. At this time the use of wire loops, Kirschner-wires, bolts, or Knowles pins cannot be considered appropriate when currently available implants provide more biomechanically secure fixation.

Depression Fracture

The important part of treatment with regard to the depression fracture (type III) is the effort that must be made to restore the articular surface of the lateral tibial condyle to its original level and contour. What must be understood is that (1) the degree of comminution and underlying damage to the depressed segment may be quite extensive; (2) there may actually be some of the surface missing or beyond salvage; and (3) when the surface is elevated it should be raised slightly higher than what would appear to be appropriate in order to anticipate some eventual settling and compression when the normal biomechanical forces are again transmitted across the knee joint. Because the compression injury reduces the volume of trabecular bone, when the surface is adequately elevated there will be a substantial void underneath. This surface is visualized fully through the surgical approach, while through a separate metaphyseal window in the appropriate condyle the surface is elevated with either bone tamps or elevators with varying radii of curvature (Fig 80–12). A graft must be placed in the defect created below the restored articular surface. A cortical-cancellous graft harvested from the iliac crest is the best source for this bone which acts as a strut while the fracture heals. Other options are available including cadaver sources, and more recently, synthetic hydroxyapatite.[8] The fibula has been advocated as a source of bone graft for cortical support, but currently cannot be considered as an initial choice.[31]

If very little bone is necessary, occasionally the graft may be obtained from the adjacent femoral condyle. The graft should further be secured with a large AO screw to prevent settling and loss of articular congruence.

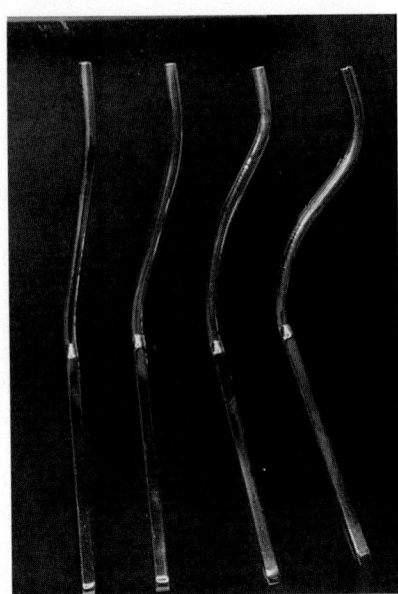

FIG 80–12.
Bone tamps for elevation of depressed tibial plateau fractures. Note the various radii of curvature available.

Cleavage With Depression Fracture

The more extensive cleavage with depression fracture (type II) requires more dissection, more attention to detail, and usually more fixation (Figs 80–13 and 80–14). There is not only a split, which is easily reapproximated, but a distorted area of articular surface which must be matched to the stable side of the fracture. Since there are elements of both previously mentioned fracture types to manage, a more extensive exposure is necessary. In order to visualize the compression the split fragment is opened like a book on its typically intact posterior hinge. The articular surface is now seen clearly. After curettage and debridement of clot and other debris with a dental pick, the articular surface is elevated, most often involving the intact medial portion. Provisional fixation of some type is often necessary with Kirschner-wires. The split portion is raised cephalad from its distally displaced position. One observation, which is often made but rarely mentioned, is the phenomenon of plastic deformation. This occurs when there has been permanent deformation in the contour of one or more of the cortical fragments. This may explain why the pieces "should fit but don't." With care it is sometimes possible to reshape the deformed portion. It is necessary sometimes to discard free articular fragments rather than let them remain, since they may float loose and become a joint irritant. The bone graft is then inserted into the void under the depressed segment, but emphasis should be placed on avoiding the insertion of an excessive amount of graft in the defect lest the split fragment cannot be anatomi-

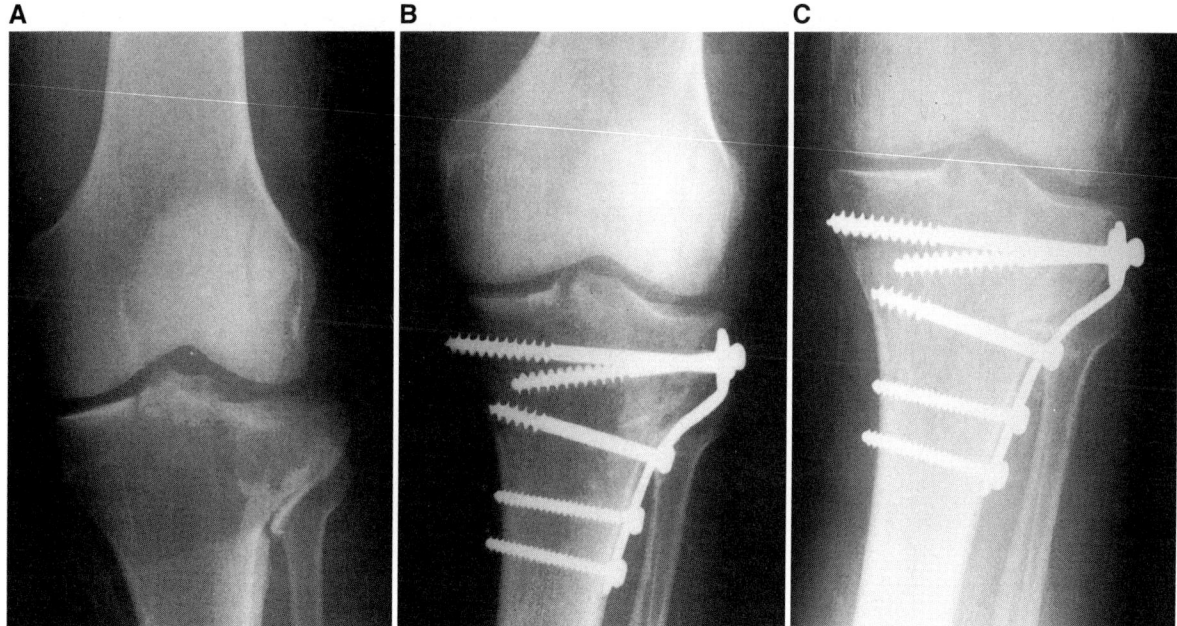

FIG 80–13.
This 55-year-old man sustained a type III fracture and an ipsilateral posterior column acetabulum fracture in a motor vehicle accident. **A,** original radiograph. **B,** 2 months postoperatively. Note the area of the bone graft. **C,** healed fracture 6 months postoperatively.

cally reduced. If this happens it may leave a gap at the articular surface. Internal fixation should be utilized to rigidly fix the reconstructed articular elements. Fixation can include T or L buttress plates. Fixation should be adequate to allow at least protected early range of motion.

Medial Condyle Fracture

Medial plateau fractures (type IV) occur less frequently. This fracture is observed in elderly patients with osteporotic bone and in younger patients as a result of a high velocity trauma. It is produced by a less often observed varus force on the knee. A medial parapatella incision and arthrotomy are utilized. Similar concern and attention is directed toward restoring articular congruence. When the bone is strong enough, lag screw fixation alone is adequate. If buttressing is necessary, the T plate is usually more appropriate. This fracture may extend into the intercondylar eminence. If the spine is avulsed with the cruciate ligaments, they should be replaced with either a lag screw or wire.

Bicondylar Fracture

When both condyles of the tibia are involved (type V fracture) a more extensive exposure may be necessary as described above in the discussion on surgical approaches. The philosophy for fixation remains the same. Restoration of the articular surface and congruence must be followed by securing the articular-metaphyseal fragments to the more distal intact tibia. Often with this type of fracture there is an associated bony avulsion of the anterior cruciate ligament which should be repaired concurrently. Use of one or possibly two buttress plates may be required (Fig 80–15). The use of a second buttress plate should be considered with some caution because of the additional dissection necessary to secure it. Various uses of external fixation have been indicated recently, sometimes in conjunction with limited internal fixation of the articular surface to minimize the amount of soft tissue disruption.[4, 11, 41, 52, 89]

Complex Fracture

There are certain fracture patterns that are often associated with high velocity injuries in which more extensive bone and soft tissue injury occurs. These complex type VI injuries require more thought, and demand extraordinary surgical skills and innovative treatment modalities in order to achieve good results (Fig 80–16). Complex fractures involving not only the articular surface but the diaphysis as well present such a challenge. Lateral tibial buttress plates are now available which can stabilize the entire fracture configuration with a single plate.[67] This implant blends the buttress element of the traditional buttress plate with the strength and compression capabilities of the dynamic compression plate (Fig 80–17). Owing to the complexity of these fractures and the subtle and often underestimated soft tissue injury, efforts have

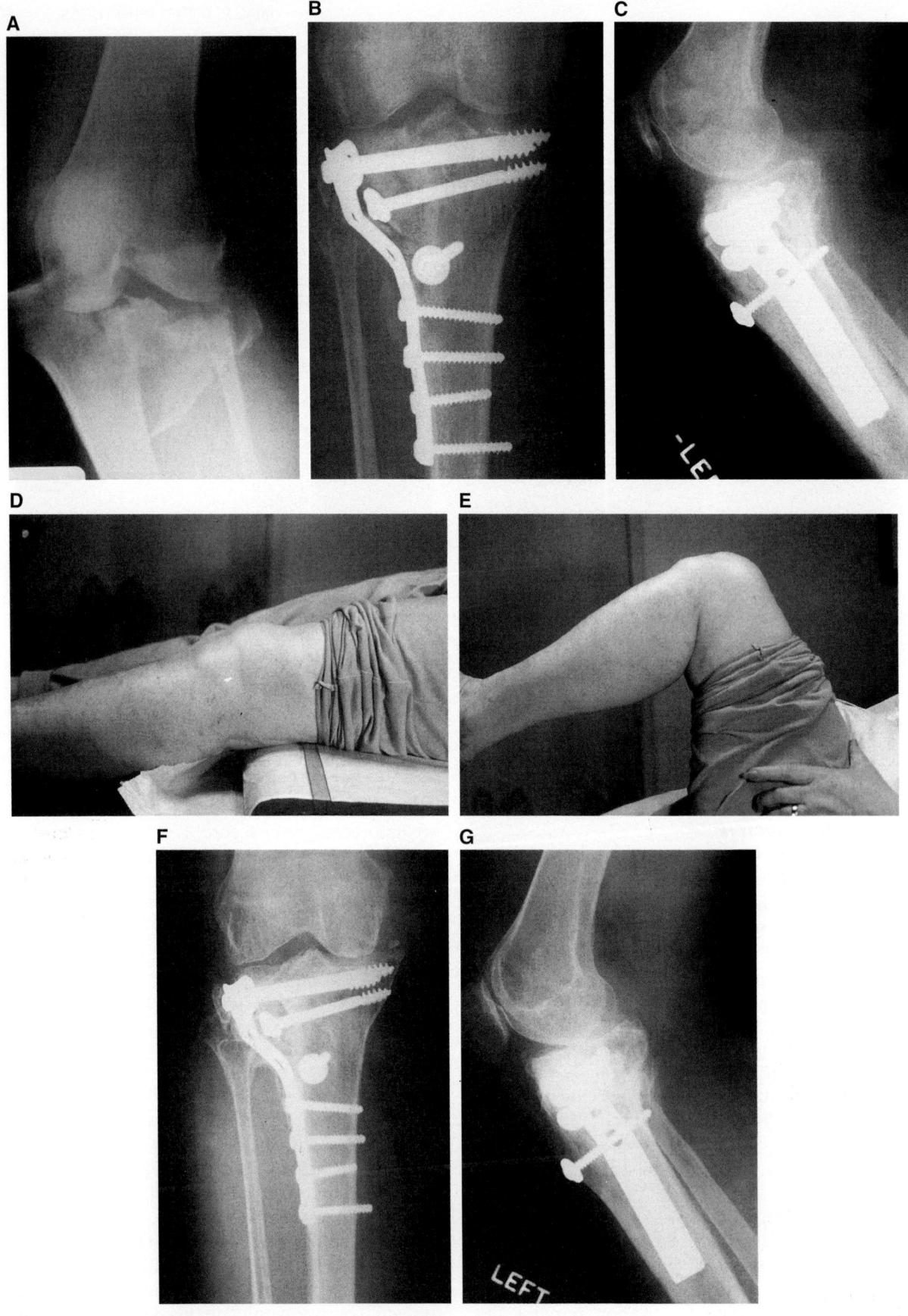

FIG 80–14.
A, preoperative radiograph of a 50-year-old woman who was struck by a car. **B** and **C,** postoperative radiographs. The severe degree of comminution influenced the need to do an anterior tibial tubercle osteotomy. **D** and **E,** clinical examination 4 years after injury reveals a range of motion from 0 to 110 degrees. The patient ambulates without pain or assistance. **F** and **G,** radiographs 4 years postoperatively.

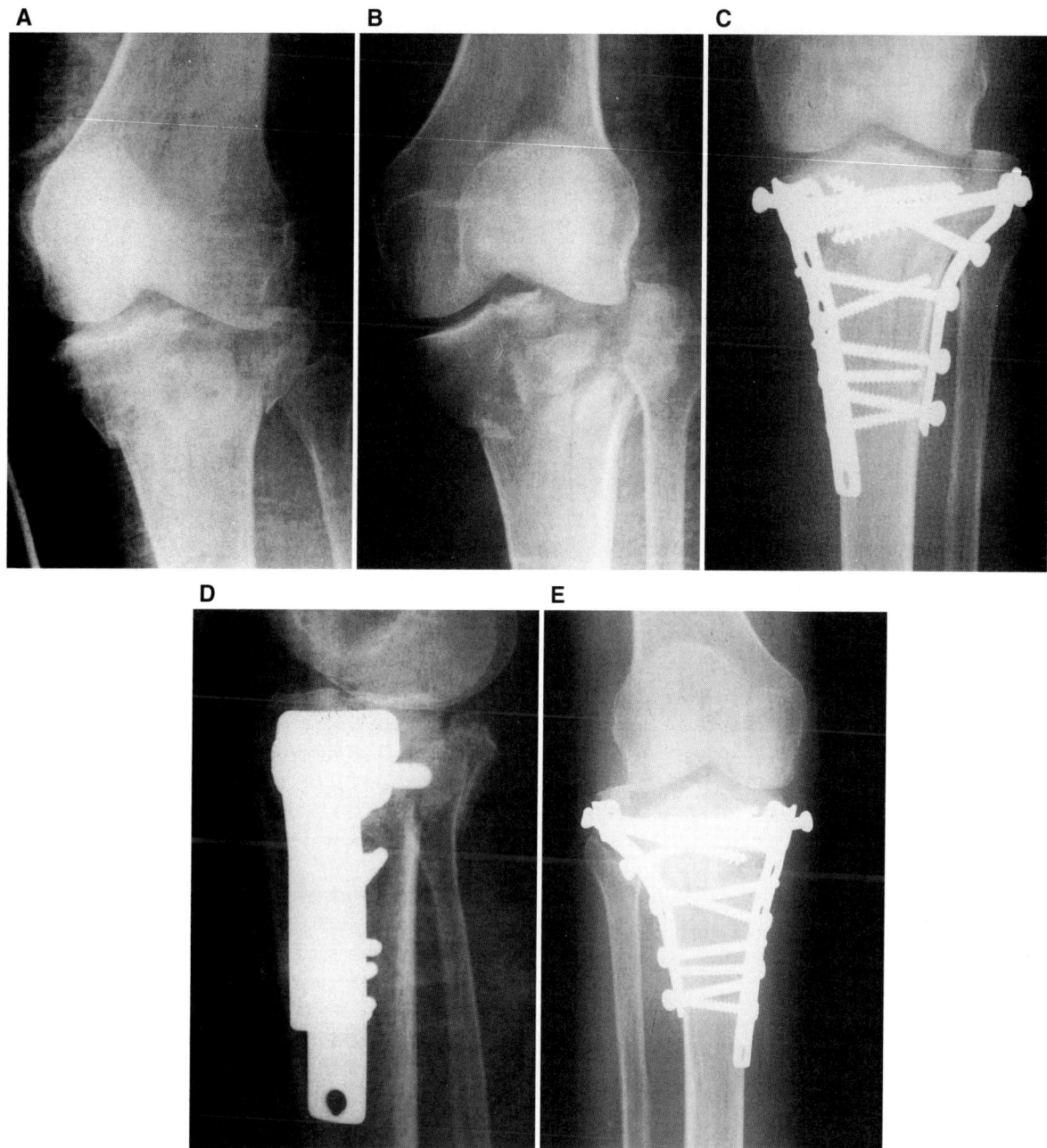

FIG 80–15.
This 58-year-old woman with a history of alcohol abuse fell down a flight of stairs. She sustained a comminuted type V fracture. **A** and **B**, original radiographs. **C** and **D**, the fracture was stabilized with two plates. There was early evidence of articular collapse even with cortical-cancellous grafting. The patient developed a wound slough which required a small split-thickness skin graft. **E**, the patient was kept in a cast for 8 weeks and was nonweightbearing for 12 weeks. Range of motion is now 0 to 115 degrees. She is pain-free and rides a bicycle.

been made to further limit the amount of internal fixation, thereby limiting surgical dissection to an already traumatized region. The stability is then supplemented with external fixation applied below the knee joint (Fig 80–18).

Open fractures are reported in large series as ranging from 0% to 27%.[3, 5, 61] Owing to the open wounds and potential for infection, internal fixation often had not been considered an appropriate method of treatment at least not initially. The open joint injury can be further complicated by damage to the articular cartilage. To allow for management of wound and soft tissue loss, external fixation occasionally constructed across the knee initially will maintain

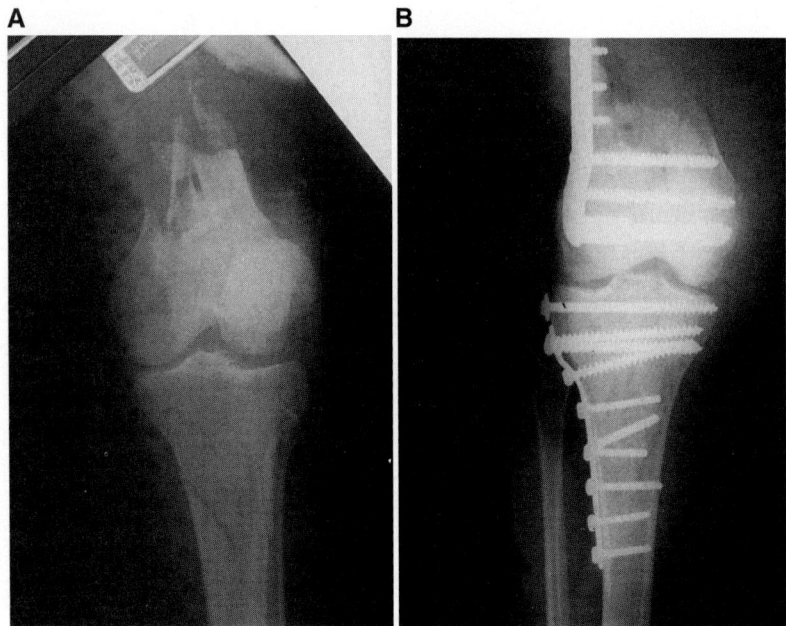

FIG 80–16.
This 27-year-old man sustained a complex intraarticular knee injury when he fell off a motorcycle. **A,** radiograph shows a grade III open distal femur fracture and a type VI tibial plateau fracture. **B,** postoperative radiograph.

an acceptable alignment and length as well as position of the fracture fragments until a more definitive fracture fixation can be provided. This will provide a stable platform for associated trauma specialists to do vascular repairs or perform muscle flaps to cover exposed bone. At the earliest possible time the frame should be reduced, at least to free the knee joint. The current management methods for open tibial fractures support this concept. In a recent review, however, 14 Schatzker grade V and VI fractures, which were grade II or III open injuries and had immediate rigid fixation with delayed wound closure, were analyzed (Fig 80–19). Benirschke et al.[3] reported acceptable functional results with no acute deep infections.

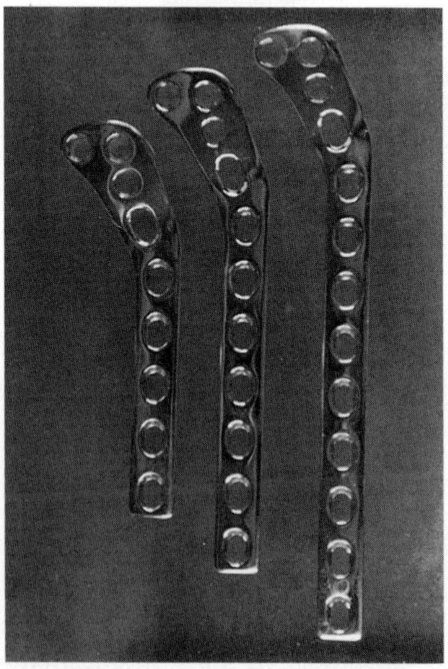

Fracture Fixation and Arthroscopy

As familiarity and skill with the use of the arthroscope has progressed, it is natural that an attempt be made to extend the role of arthroscopy into the setting of fracture fixation. While it may not be for every surgeon or for every fracture, there are some benefits to arthroscopy that can be considered appropriate to the treatment of tibial plateau fractures, including minimal soft tissue dissection and, as a direct consequence, less potential for postoperative knee stiffness. As with more traditional open means of treatment, malreduction and loss of reduction are to be avoided by understanding the relative indications for the use of this comparatively new modality.[10, 32, 46, 66, 73, 74, 86]

COMPLICATIONS

Complications are seen in the treatment of the tibial plateau fracture. Infection has been reported in some operative series to occur in up to 19% of cases, particularly when more extensive dissection is performed.[61] Deep vein thrombosis occurs in 6% to 14%

FIG 80–17.
Lateral tibial buttress plates.

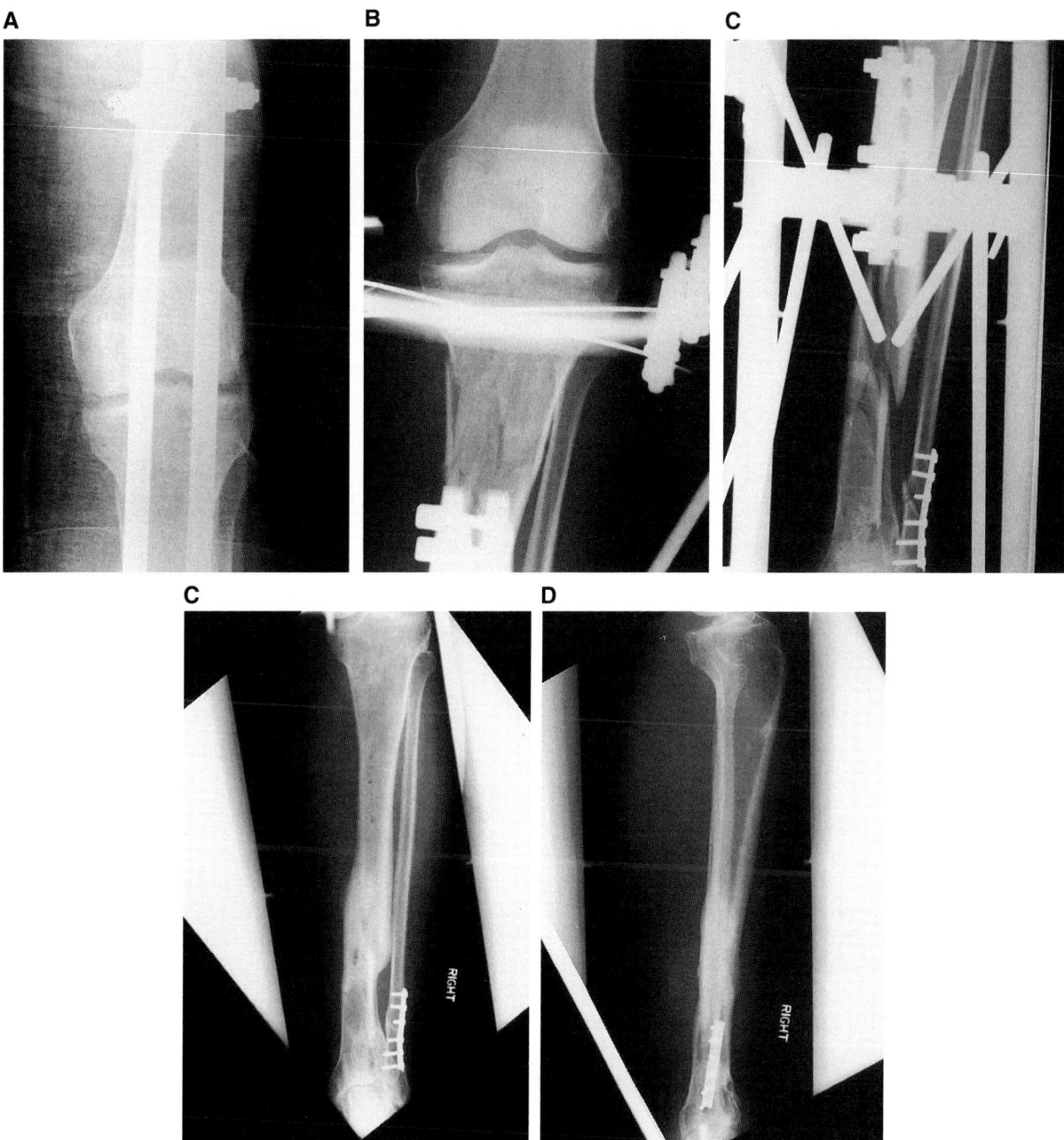

FIG 80-18.
This 52-year-old man sustained a complex tibial injury in a motor vehicle accident. The tibial plateau was nondisplaced. The shaft fracture was grade III open, complicated by a compartmental syndrome. **A,** he was initially placed in an external fixator across the knee and ankle. **B** and **C,** when the wound and fasciotomy incisions were closed, the frame was shortened to allow knee motion. **D** and **E,** final radiographs at 13 months. Knee motion now is 0 to 130 degrees. The tibial shaft healed without bone grafting. A mild varus angulation of the ankle was accepted.

of patients during the treatment period.[81] Myers et al.[56] report that most arterial injuries occur with the more severe fracture dislocations. Burri et al.[9] correlated complications, in particular hematoma and deep or superficial infection, with the experience of the surgeon.

Peroneal nerve palsy occurs as well, although the literature would suggest that most, if not all, eventually resolve. Peroneal injury may have multiple origins, including the initial injury or retraction during surgery (Fig 80-20). There have been occasional reports of pseudarthrosis involving tibial plateau fractures.[40, 61, 79]

The compartmental syndrome can occur as a re-

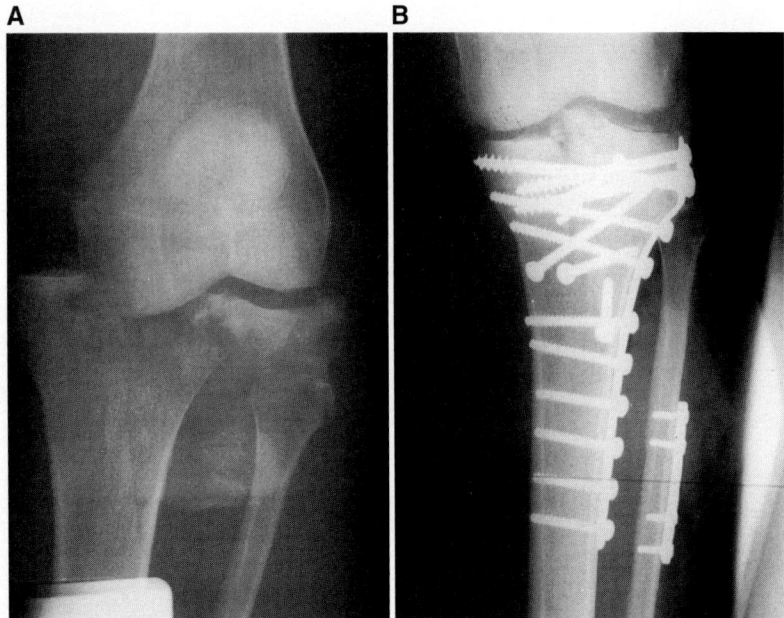

FIG 80–19.
This 37-year-old man sustained a comminuted type III tibial plateau fracture in a motorcycle accident. **A,** original radiograph. Compartment pressures in the calf were elevated. Fasciotomies were done. **B,** open reduction with internal fixation was performed as well. The wounds were treated as an open fracture and closed at 5 days.

sult of the injury and has been reported as a postoperative complication in a patient in whom anticoagulants and early range-of-motion exercises were utilized.[24] In both the initial injury assessment and postoperative period one should always be concerned with the development of a compartmental syndrome, especially when one considers the potential for disastrous consequences. Poor results occasionally occur when highly comminuted or severely osteopenic bone is involved. In these instances both the lateral patellar facet[37] and iliac crest[83] have been used as a reconstructive substitute for the severely comminuted fracture. A replacement for the area of damage is created with the goal of reapproximating the original contour of the tibial plateau surface. In patients who have had secondary degenerative changes, residual structural deformities, or an incomplete reduction, this may result in accelerated degenerative arthritis. Many less-than-optimal options are available to salvage the situation. Reports of osteochondral allograft resurfacing have indicated some success.[25, 47, 55] It may be considered in patients who are young and have minimal degenerative changes in the rest of the knee. The patient must be well motivated and someone for whom the more conventional procedures, such as arthrodesis or arthroplasty, are not considered reasonable options. The rationale for using fresh allograft is that some of the cartilage cells may remain viable and thus act as a functional articular surface. As a final option, total knee arthroplasty is an alternative in a knee that has significant posttraumatic arthritis.[75]

POSTOPERATIVE CARE

Postoperative care is as important, if not more so, than the operative treatment. Perioperative antibiotics, suction drainage, elevation, and deep venous thrombosis prophylaxis help in avoiding complications and preparing the patient's knee for initial mobilization.

The regimen of immediate postoperative care has evolved toward early immobilization. Reports suggest that the period of immobilization can affect the range of motion achieved as a final outcome no matter which modality for treatment is utilized. Salter et al.[77] and others have reported the positive effect that range of motion has on cartilage metabolism and healing. As this becomes more obvious with additional studies, it is now more critical for the surgeon to obtain maximum rigid internal fixation. Schatzker et al.[78] reported better results with less than 4 weeks' immobilization. Other reports vary from 2 to 12 weeks. It is unaminous that more than 6 weeks of immobilization increases the risk of permanent joint stiffness. A CPM machine may be used with the uncomplicated fracture in which solid fixation is achieved and there has been no overwhelming soft

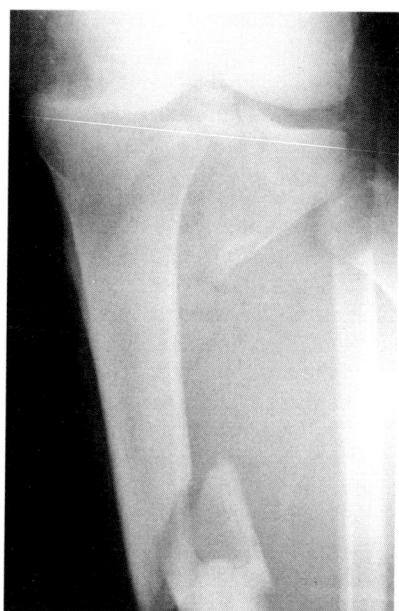

FIG 80–20.
This 22-year-old-man was struck by a car. He sustained a type I fracture with an associated knee dislocation. He also sustained a contralateral midshaft tibial fracture. A complete peroneal nerve palsy was documented on arrival at the emergency room.

tissue injury or dissection. It may be applied postoperatively with an initial range of full extension to 30 degrees of flexion at a slow rate. The range should be increased slowly over the first postoperative week. This may be modified in instances in which additional ligamentous reconstruction was required, such as repair of the medial collateral ligament, anterior cruciate ligament, or patellar tendon.

Weightbearing must be delayed until there is adequate bony union at the fracture site. This period of time must be gauged by the type of fracture, amount of osteopenia, and type of fixation. The more comminuted the fracture, the longer the period of nonweightbearing required. Fractures requiring a bone graft may require a more lengthy time of nonweightbearing to allow full consolidation of the graft construct. Toe-touch weightbearing can be initiated at 6 weeks' post surgery and full weightbearing at between 12 and 16 weeks' post surgical fixation.[5, 43] Fracture bracing may, in certain hands, decrease the total length of time required to be nonweightbearing. During this period of immobilization, exercise to rehabilitate and retrain the quadriceps and hamstrings is also beneficial.

SUMMARY AND CONCLUSIONS

Despite some unresolved controversies, this much is clear: the knee joint is a large weightbearing joint whose function relies on the congruence, alignment, and stability of bones and soft tissues, and adequate range of motion. Whichever treatment is selected, it must first restore knee function. Range of motion must be restored. Weightbearing must be delayed, regardless of which treatment was selected, until adequate fracture healing has occurred.

The past 20 years have brought many changes to the treatment of fractures, including fractures of the tibial plateau. Achieving good results with this injury clearly remains a challenge to the orthopaedist, since some disability often persists after completion of treatment. Numerous protocols have been put forth by respected authors. Many view the same fracture differently and attempt to achieve satisfactory results with modalities that may appear on the surface as being diametric to each other. These differences are obvious when one reviews the numerous classification systems that have been proposed as well as the schemes for assessing the results.

Surgical treatment, though promising and more recently achieving good results, clearly has risks and complications not previously reported. Although the operative results are encouraging, judgment is required lest technology triumph over reason. If one is considering surgery, these goals and principles should be followed:

1. Anatomic reduction.
2. Restoration of articular congruence.
3. Stable *and* adequate fixation.
4. Metaphyseal bone grafting when necessary.
5. Treatment of associated ligamentous injuries.
6. Preservation of menisci.
7. Initiation of early motion.

All these goals should be met or one risks disaster. For, as Schatzker and Tile say, "the result of a failed open reduction and internal fixation is always worse than the result of a failed closed treatment."[80]

Some historical perspective is necessary when attempting to predict the future. Certain factors outside the direct realm of medicine have influenced both treatment selections and future avenues of development. The financial impact of the DRG system has reduced the desirability of modalities that require a lengthy hospital stay, such as skeletal traction. The increasing severity of soft tissue damage associated with motor vehicle accidents has also influenced the use of arthroscopically assisted fixation as well as consideration of minimal ORIF with external fixation. All is not perfect. What is still lacking? Certainly a consensus on a classification system, which may ultimately be the one proposed by Mueller et al.[63] There is also a need for more prospective studies as well as outcome studies. Agreement on objective criteria in order to define a good result is necessary. Subjective symptoms remain elusive to quantitate. Many cases are either work-related or are involved in the litigation process. These issues can blur the results because of secondary gain. Observing these fundamental principles will help to provide patients with optimal results no matter which method is selected. If the last two decades provide us with a glimpse into the future, more new, exciting, and potentially innovative ideas and treatments lie ahead.

REFERENCES

1. Anderson PW, Harley JD, Maslin PU: Arthrographic evaluation of problems with united tibial plateau fractures, *Radiology* 119:75–78, 1976.
2. Apley AG: Fractures of the tibial plateau, *Orthop Clin North Am* 10:61–74, 1979.
3. Benirschke SK, et al: Immediate internal fixation of open, complex tibial plateau fractures: Treatment by a standard protocol, *J. Orthop Trauma* 6:78–86, 1992.
4. Blackburn JE: Maintenance of reduction of tibial plateau fractures with Charnley compression device, *Clin Orthop* 123:112–113, 1977.
5. Blokker CP, Rorabeck CH, Bourne RB: Tibial plateau fractures. An analysis of the results of treatment in 60 patients, *Clin Orthop* 182:193–199, 1984.
6. Böhler L: *The treatment of fractures,* vol 3. New York, 1958, Grune & Stratton.
7. Brown TD, et al: Contact stress aberrations following imprecise reduction of simple tibial plateau fractures, *J Orthop Res* 6:851–862, 1988.
8. Bucholz RW, Carlton A, Holmes R: Interporous hydroxyapatite as a bone graft substitute in tibial plateau fractures, *Clin Orthop* 240:53–62, 1989.
9. Burri C, et al: Fractures of the tibial plateau, *Clin Orthop* 138:84–93, 1979.
10. Caspari RB, et al: The role of arthroscopy in the management of tibial plateau fractures, *Arthroscopy* 1:76–82, 1985.
11. Christensen KP, et al: Early results of a new technique for the treatment of high grade tibial plateau fractures, *J Orthop Trauma* 4:226, 1990.
12. Connolly JF: Closed treatment of pelvic and lower extremity fractures, *Clin Orthop* 240:115–128, 1989.
13. Daffner RH, Tabas JH: Trauma oblique radiographs of the knee, *J Bone Joint Surg [Am]* 69:568–572, 1987.
14. DeCoster TA, Nepola JV, El-Khoury GY: Cast brace treatment of proximal tibia fractures, *Clin Orthop* 231:196–204, 1988.
15. Delamarter RB, Hohl M: The cast brace and tibial plateau fractures, *Clin Orthop* 242:26–31, 1989.
16. Delamarter RB, Hohl M, Hopp E Jr: Ligament injuries associated with tibial plateau fractures, *Clin Orthop* 250:226–233, 1990.
17. Deutsch AL, Mink JH, Shellock FG: Magnetic resonance imaging of injuries to bone and articular cartilage. Emphasis on radiologically occult abnormalities, *Orthop Rev* 19:66–75, 1990.
18. Dias JJ, et al: Computerized axial tomography for tibial plateau fractures, *J Bone Joint Surg [Br]* 69:84–88, 1987.
19. Drennan DB, Locher FG, Maylahn DJ: Fractures of the tibial plateau treatment by closed reduction and spica cast, *J Bone Joint Surg [Am]* 61:989–995, 1979.
20. Duwelius PJ, Connolly JF: Closed reduction of tibial plateau fractures, *Clin Orthop* 230:116–126, 1988.
21. Elstrom J, Pankovich AM, Sassoon H: The use of tomography in the assessment of fractures of the tibial plateau, *J Bone Joint Surg [Am]* 58:551–555, 1976.
22. Fernandez DL: Anterior approach to the knee with osteotomy of the tibial tubercle for bicondylar tibial fractures, *J Bone Joint Surg [Am]* 70:208–219, 1988.
23. Gausewitz S, Hohl M: The significance of early motion in the treatment of tibial plateau fractures, *Clin Orthop* 202:135–138, 1986.
24. Graham B, Loomer RL: Anterior compartment syndrome in a patient with fracture of the tibial plateau treated by continuous passive motion and anticoagulants. Report of a case, *Clin Orthop* 195:197–199, 1985.
25. Gross AE, et al: Reconstruction of skeletal deficits at the knee, *Clin Orthop* 174:96–106, 1983.
26. Hamilton FH: *A practical treatise on fractures and dislocations,* Philadelphia, 1860, Blanchard & Lea.
27. Hohl M: Tibial condylar fractures, *J Bone Joint Surg [Am]* 49:1455–1467, 1967.
28. Hohl M: President's guest lecturer, Chicago Orthopedic Society May 12, 1978.
29. Huber-Betzer H, Brown TD, Mattheck C: Some effects of global joint morphology and local stress aberrations near imprecisely reduced intra-articular fractures, *J Biomech* 23:811–822, 1990.
30. Ivey M, Cantrell JS: Lateral tibial plateau fractures as a post operative complication of high tibial osteotomy, *Orthopedics* 8:1009–1013, 1985.
31. Jackson DW: The use of autologous fibula for a prop graft in depressed lateral tibial plateau fractures, *Clin Orthop* 87:110–115, 1972.
32. Jennings JE: Arthroscopic management of tibial plateau fractures, *Arthroscopy* 1:160–168, 1985.
33. Jensen DB, Bjerg-Nielsen A, Laursen N: Conventional radiographic examination in the evaluation of sequelae after tibial plateau fractures, *Skeletal Radiol* 17:330–332, 1988.
34. Jensen DB, et al: Magnetic resonance imaging in the evaluation of sequelae after tibial plateau fractures, *Skeletal Radiol* 19:127–129, 1990.
35. Jensen DB, et al: Tibial plateau fractures. A comparison of conservative and surgical treatment, *J Bone Joint Surg [Br]* 72:49–52, 1990.
36. Johnson F, Leitl S, Waugh W: The distribution of load across the knee. A comparison of static and dynamic measurements, *J Bone Joint Surg [Br]* 62:346–349, 1980.

37. Karpinski MRK: Patellar graft for late disability following tibial plateau fractures, *Injury* 15:197–202, 1983.
38. Kennedy JC, Bailey WH: Experimental tibial plateau fractures. Studies of the mechanism and a classification, *J Bone Joint Surg* 50:1522–1534, 1968.
39. Kettelkamp DB, et al: Degenerative arthritis of the knee secondary to fracture malunion, *Clin Orthop* 234:159–169, 1988.
40. King GJW, Schatzker J: Case report. Nonunion of a complex tibial plateau fracture, *J Orthop Trauma* 5:209–212, 1991.
41. Koval K, et al: Indirect reduction and percutaneous screw fixation of displaced tibial plateau fractures, *J Orthop Trauma* 5:237, 1991.
42. Krause WR, et al: Mechanical changes in the knee After meniscectomy *J Bone Joint Surg* 58:599–604, 1976.
43. Lachiewicz PF, Funcik T: Factors influencing the results of open reduction and internal fixation of tibial plateau fractures, *Clin Orthop* 259:210–215, 1990.
44. Langer JE, Meyer SJF, Dalinka MK: Imaging of the knee, *Radiol Clin North Am* 28:975–990, 1990.
45. Lansinger O, et al: Tibial condylar fractures. A twenty-year follow-up, *J Bone Joint Surg* 68:13–19, 1986.
46. Lemon RA, Bartlett DH: Arthroscopic assisted internal fixation of certain fractures about the knee, *J Trauma* 25:355–358, 1985.
47. Locht RC, Gross AE, Langer F: Late osteochondral allograft resurfacing for tibial plateau fractures, *J Bone Joint Surg [Am]* 66:328–335, 1984.
48. Maheson M, Colton CL: Fractures of the tibial plateau in Nottingham, *Injury* 19:324–328, 1988.
49. Manco LG, Schneider R, Pavlov H: Insufficiency fractures of the tibial plateau, *Am J. Radiol* 140:1211–1215, 1983.
50. Mandelbaum BR, Finerman GAM, Reicher MA: Magnetic resonance imaging as a tool for evaluation of traumatic knee injuries. Anatomical and pathoanatomical correlation, *Am J Sports Med* 14:361–370, 1986.
51. Marwah V, Gadegone WM, Magarkar DS: The treatment of fractures of the tibial plateau by skeletal traction and early mobilization, *Int Orthop* 9:217–221, 1985.
52. Mast J, Jakob R, Ganz R: *Planning and reduction technique in fracture surgery,* Berlin, 1989, Springer Verlag.
53. McConkey JP, Meeuwisse W: Tibial plateau fractures in Alpine skiing, *Am Sports Med* 16:159–164, 1988.
54. McDonnell MF, Butler JE: Osteochondral fracture of the tibial plateau in a ballerina, *Am J Sports Med* 16:417–418, 1988.
55. Meyers MH, Akeson W, Convery FR: Resurfacing of the knee with fresh osteochondral allograft, *J Bone Joint Surg [Am]* 71:704–713, 1989.
56. Meyers MH, Moore TM, Harvey JP: Follow-up notes on articles previously published in the journal. Traumatic dislocation of the knee joint, *J Bone Joint Surg [Am]* 57:430–433, 1975.
57. Mink JH, Deutsch AL: Occult cartilage and bone injuries of the knee: Detection, classification, and assessment with MR imaging, *Radiology* 170:823–829, 1989.
58. Moore TM: Fracture-dislocation of the knee, *Clin Orthop* 156:128–140, 1981.
59. Moore TM, Harvey JP: Roentgenographic measurement of tibial plateau depression due to fracture, *J Bone Joint Surg [Am]* 56:155–160, 1974.
60. Moore TM, Meyers MH, Harvey JP: Collateral ligament laxity of the knee, *J Bone Joint Surg [Am]* 58:594–598, 1976.
61. Moore TM, Patzakis MJ, Harvey JP: Tibial plateau fractures: Definition, demographics, treatment rationale, and long-term results of closed traction management or operative reduction, *J Orthop Trauma* 1:97–119, 1987.
62. Morrison JB: The mechanics of the knee joint in relation to normal walking, *J Biomech* 3:51–61, 1970.
63. Mueller ME, Allgower M, Schneider R, et al: *Manual of internal fixation,* ed 3, Berlin, 1991, Springer-Verlag.
64. Newberg AH: Computer tomography of joint injuries, *Radiol Clin North Am* 28:445–460, 1990.
65. Newberg AH, Greenstein R: Radiographic evaluation of tibial plateau fractures, *Radiology* 126:319–323, 1978.
66. Pankovich AM: Arthroscopic management of tibial plateau fractures (letter), *Arthroscopy* 2:132–134, 1986.
67. Paloin PA. Buttress plates for the lateral tibial head, Synthes [USA]—update bull 89-11, July 31, 1989.
68. Perren SM, et al: The concept of biological plating using the limited contact–dynamic compression plate (LC-DCP), *Injury* 225:1–41, 1991.
69. Perry CR, et al: A new surgical approach to fractures of the lateral tibial plateau, *J Bone Joint Surg [Am]* 66:1236–1240, 1984.
70. Rafii M, Lamont JG, Firooznia H: Tibial plateau fractures: CT evaluation and classification, *Crit Rev Diagn Imaging* 27:91–112, 1987.
71. Rafii M, et al: Computed tomography of tibial plateau fractures, *Am J Radiol* 142:1181–1186, 1984.
72. Rasmussen PS: Tibial condylar fractures. Impairment of knee joint stability as an indication for surgical treatment, *J Bone Joint Surg [Am]* 55:1331–1350, 1973.
73. Reilly JP, Accettola AB: Arthroscopic diagnosis and treatment of intra-articular fractures. In Scott WN, editor: *Arthroscopy of the knee,* Philadelphia, 1990, WB Saunders.
74. Reiner MJ: The arthroscope in tibial plateau fractures: Its use in evaluation of soft tissue and bony injury, *J Am Osteopath Assoc* 81:704–707, 1982.
75. Roffi RP, Merritt PO: Total knee replacement after fractures about the knee, *Orthop Rev* 19:614–620, 1990.
76. Rosen MA, Jackson DW, Berger PE: Occult osseous lesions documented by magnetic resonance imaging associated with anterior cruciate ligament ruptures, *Arthroscopy* 7:45–51, 1991.
77. Salter RB, et al. The biological effect on continuous passive motion on the healing of full-thickness defects

in articular cartilage, *J Bone Joint Surg [Am]* 62:1232–1251, 1980.
78. Schatzker J, McBroom R, Bruce D: The tibial plateau fracture. The Toronto experience 1968–1975, *Clin Orthop* 138:94–104, 1979.
79. Schatzker J, Schulak DJ: Pseudarthrosis of a tibial plateau fracture: Report of a case, *Clin Orthop* 145:146–149, 1979.
80. Schatzker J, Tile M: *The rationale of operative fracture care,* Berlin, 1987, Springer-Verlag.
81. Schulak DJ, Gunn DR: Fractures of the tibial plateaus. A review of the literature, *Clin Orthop* 109:166–177, 1975.
82. Scotland T, Wardlaw D: The use of cast bracing as treatment for fractures of the tibial plateau, *J Bone Joint Surg [Br]* 63:575–578, 1981.
83. Segal D, Franchi AV, Campanile J: Iliac autograft for reconstruction of severely depressed fractures of a lateral tibial plateau, *J Bone Joint Surg* 67:1270–1272, 1985.
84. Shybut GT, Spiegel PT: Tibial plateau fractures, *Clin Orthop* 138:12–17, 1979.
85. Struben PJ: The tibial plateau, *J Bone Joint Surg [Br]* 64:336–339, 1982.
86. Uppal G, et al. Arthroscopic guided tibial plateau reconstruction, *J Orthop Trauma* 5:237, 1991.
87. Waddell JP, Johnston DWC, Neidre A: Fractures of the tibial plateau: A review of ninety-five patients and comparison of treatment methods, *J Trauma* 21:376–381, 1981.
88. Waldrop JI, Macey TI, Tettin JC: Fractures of the posterolateral tibial plateau, *Am J Sports Med* 16:492–498, 1988.
89. Weiner LS, et al. Treatment of severe proximal tibia fractures with minimal internal and external fixation, *J Orthop Trauma* 5:236, 1991.
90. Weis EB, Pritz HB, Hassler CR: Experimental automobile-pedestrian injuries, *J Trauma* 17:823–827, 1977.
91. Weissman SL, Herold ZH: Fractures of the tibial plateau, *Clin Orthop* 33:194–200, 1964.
92. Yao L, Lee JK: Avulsion of the posteromedial tibial plateau by the semimembranosus tendon: Diagnosis with MR imaging, *Radiology* 172:513–514, 1989.

81

Fractures of the Patella

ROBERT R. SCHEINBERG, M.D.
ROBERT W. BUCHOLZ, M.D.

Mechanisms of injury
Classification
Diagnosis
Treatment
   Open fractures

Marginal and osteochondral fractures
Complications
Prognosis

The perceived role of the patella in knee function has profoundly influenced the preferred treatment of patellar fractures over the last century. Brooke,[8] Hey Groves,[25] Watson-Jones,[67] and other early authors believed that the patella inhibited the action of the quadriceps tendon and that patellectomy improved the strength of the knee. They therefore recommended complete patellectomy for the treatment of fractures of the patella. DePalma and Flynn,[15] Kaufer,[32] Smillie,[58] McKeever,[44] Scott,[57] Sutton et al.,[62] Haxton,[24] Thomson,[65] and more recent investigators have appreciated the fact that the patella is an important functional component of the extensor mechanism of the knee and that every effort should be made to preserve the patella following fracture.

Total patellectomy results in permanent dysfunction of the knee with decreased extensor strength, extensor lag, quadriceps atrophy, ligamentous instability, and reduced stance-phase flexion during walking.* These functional problems are of sufficient magnitude to warrant surgical reconstruction of the patella or partial excision of the patella, even in the presence of extensive fracture comminution, whenever technically possible.†

The first open reduction of a fracture of the patella was performed in 1877 by both Cameron[10] and Lister[35] using silver thread through drill holes in the bone. Over the following 20 years, several surgeons including Trendelenburg, Dennis,[13] and Stimson,[61] reported good results using similar treatment methods. Prior to this period, fractures of the patella were treated by splinting the extremity in extension, thus relaxing the quadriceps muscle and minimizing the fracture displacement. This closed method often resulted in poor knee function from contractures, decreased extensor mechanism strength, and delayed union or nonunion. These poor results stimulated the application of percutaneous pins or clamps to displaced fractures of the patella.[41] These percutaneous methods were successful in obtaining fracture union, but were abandoned because of an unacceptably high incidence of wound infection or joint sepsis.

The popularity of open reduction increased in the 1900s as aseptic surgical techniques improved. Many investigators described passing various suture materials, including stainless steel, silver thread, tendon, or catgut, through drill holes in the fracture fragments.[10,35] Others used either cerclage of the major fracture fragments or partial patellectomy with repair of the quadriceps or patellar tendon to the remaining patellar fragments.[63,64] More recently, the Association for the Study of Internal Fixation (ASIF) group has popularized the tension band wire technique originally described by Pauwels, which allows early knee motion without compromising fracture stabilization.[47]

MECHANISMS OF INJURY

The majority of fractures of the patella occur in patients between 20 and 50 years of age, with the incidence in males being nearly twice that in females.[4,7,29,31,48] These fractures constitute approxi-

---

*References 9, 11, 14, 17, 18, 21, 30, 54, 57, 69, 70.
†References 5, 6, 18, 22, 26, 37, 47, 48, 68.

mately 1% of all fractures.[7, 29, 31, 56, 66] The subcutaneous location of the patella on the anterior aspect of the knee makes it vulnerable to direct trauma such as a fall on the knee or a direct blow from the knee striking the dashboard during a motor vehicle accident. Such fractures from direct trauma may be associated with posterior hip dislocations, fractures of the hip, or ipsilateral femoral shaft fractures. Fractures from direct trauma are usually comminuted or minimally displaced or both.[45, 48] There is typically little damage to the extensor retinaculum, and therefore active extension of the knee may still be possible.

Fractures from indirect forces occur when the pull of the extensor mechanism exceeds the intrinsic strength of the patella.[45, 48] Eccentric loading of the knee during the act of stumbling, partially falling, or during various athletic activities results in failure of the patella in tension. Such fractures are usually transverse with little comminution but wide separation of the major fracture fragments. The extensor retinaculum is commonly disrupted, and active knee extension is impossible.

CLASSIFICATION

Fractures of the patella are commonly classified according to their fracture configuration and their degree of displacement (Fig 81–1). Transverse fractures are the most common (50%–80%) and usually occur in the middle and lower third of the patella.[29, 48] Comminuted or stellate fractures are the next most common (30%–35%); vertical or marginal fractures and osteochondral fractures are the least common (12%–17%).[29, 48] Vertical fractures are usually the result of direct trauma to the lateral facet of the patella, while osteochondral fractures are usually sustained by adolescents during traumatic subluxation or dislocation of the patella.[16, 29, 34, 48] (Fig 81–2). Osteochondral fractures usually involve the medial facet of the patella and occur as the patella relocates following a dislocation.* These fractures may or may not be identified on routine radiographs, as the fracture fragment may be primarily cartilaginous.

Fracture displacement can be assessed most accurately on the lateral radiograph by measuring the gap in the subchondral bone. Most frequently this displacement is due to a diastasis of the major fracture fragments in the axial plane, but horizontal translation of the fracture fragments may also be present.

DIAGNOSIS

Because of its subcutaneous location, the clinical detection of a fracture of the patella is usually easy. Palpation reveals an effusion or a hemarthrosis of the knee with tenderness directly over the patella. A palpable defect or crepitus of the patella may be present.

*References 3, 20, 23, 27, 31, 33, 40, 46, 48, 51, 52.

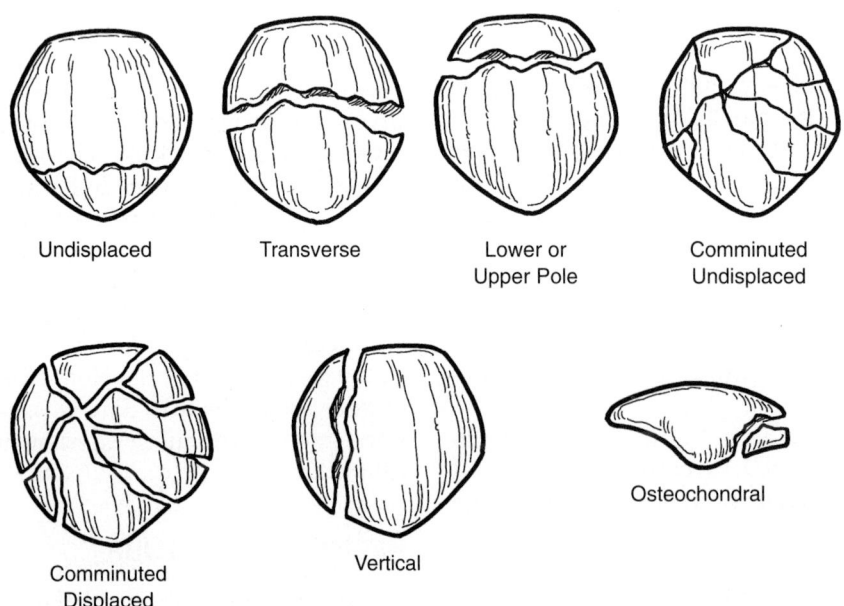

FIG 81–1.
Classification of patellar fractures. (From Johnson EE: Fractures of the patella. In Rockwood C, Green D, Bucholz, RW, editors: *Rockwood and Green's fractures in adults* ed 3, Philadelphia, 1991, JB Lippincott Company.)

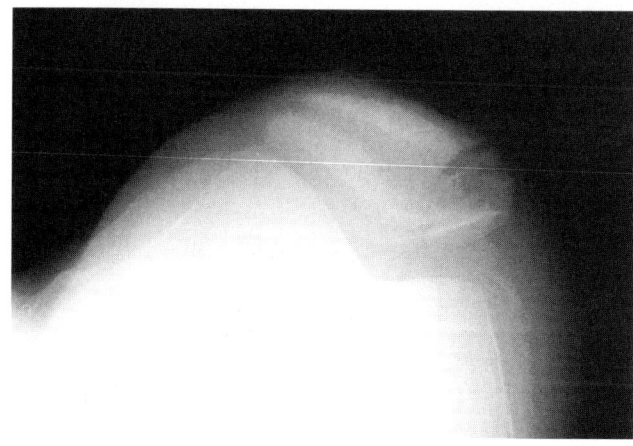

FIG 81-2.
A nondisplaced vertical fracture through the medial facet of the patella. This type of injury is most commonly due to direct trauma.

Any passive movement of the patella results in pain.

Anteroposterior and lateral radiographs usually suffice for the diagnosis and classification of most fractures of the patella. Sunrise views with the knee in varying degrees of flexion may be necessary to diagnose marginal or osteochondral fractures.[3, 20, 33, 46] Occasionally, arthrography or magnetic resonance imaging may be needed to identify free chondral or osteochondral fragments.

Once the diagnosis of a patella fracture is confirmed, it is helpful to determine the effect of the fracture on the integrity of the extensor mechanism. A gap of 5 mm or more in major fractures implies major disruption of the extensor retinaculum and incompetence of the extensor mechanism. In fractures with less than 5 mm of displacement, the patient should be asked to extend the leg against gravity. Full active extension of the leg indicates preservation of the soft tissue components of the extensor mechanism, whereas inability to extend the leg implies extensor insufficiency. Local anesthesia injected into the knee joint following aspiration of the hemarthrosis makes this test of active extension less painful in the apprehensive patient.

TREATMENT

The goals of management of fractures of the patella are restoration of full active knee motion, repair of the extensor mechanism, and anatomic reduction of the articular surface of the patella. These goals are most easily achieved when anatomic reduction and fixation of all major fracture fragments is technically possible. The decision for operative or nonoperative care is based on multiple factors, including the fracture configuration and displacement, the amount of disruption of the extensor mechanism, the age of the patient, the bone quality, and the patient's general medical condition.

Nonoperative treatment is indicated if the extensor mechanism is sufficiently preserved to allow full active knee extension and the fracture is displaced less than 3 mm on any radiographic view.[4, 14, 31, 48, 58, 59] These requisites for nonoperative care may be relaxed somewhat in severely debilitated patients or patients with soft tissue injuries which might increase the risk of surgery.

Nonoperative treatment should include immobilization of the leg in a cylinder or long leg cast with the knee in full extension for 4 to 6 weeks, with quadriceps setting exercises and straight leg raising exercises beginning a few days after casting.[7, 14, 48, 58] Aspiration of any tense hemarthrosis of the knee at the time of presentation and prior to cast application may lessen patient discomfort.[7, 14, 58] A compressive dressing should be applied to the leg for a few days prior to casting to help control edema. Partial to full weightbearing as tolerated with crutches may be commenced following cast application.[4, 7, 14, 58] Radiographic monitoring of the fracture is important to check the alignment of the fracture and the status of fracture healing.

Operative treatment of fractures of the patella is indicated if there is an articular step-off greater than 3 mm, fracture fragment displacement greater than 3 mm, or extensor mechanism insufficiency.[5, 14, 31, 47, 48, 51] Since the inferior quarter of the patella is extraarticular, greater degrees of fracture displacement are acceptable in this area as long as full active extension of the knee is possible. Displacement of fracture fragments on the superficial, nonarticular surface of the patella is less important than displacement of the articular surface. Arthroscopy or arthrotomy, or both, are indicated for osteochondral fragments displaced into the joint or of sufficient size to permit operative repair and fixation.[23, 27, 33, 40, 51, 52]

Surgery should be performed as soon as the patient's condition and skin permit. Abrasions over the patella are common, and do not contraindicate surgery unless they are greater than 24 hours old or grossly contaminated. Extensive or colonized abrasions may necessitate a delay of surgery of 7 to 10 days until the risk of contaminating the operative wound is minimal.[1, 31] There are essentially three surgical options for the treatment of fractures of the patella: (1) open reduction and internal fixation, (2) partial patellectomy with suture of the quadriceps or patellar tendon to the remaining patella, and (3) total patellectomy with soft tissue repair of the extensor mechanism. Patellar prostheses have been designed

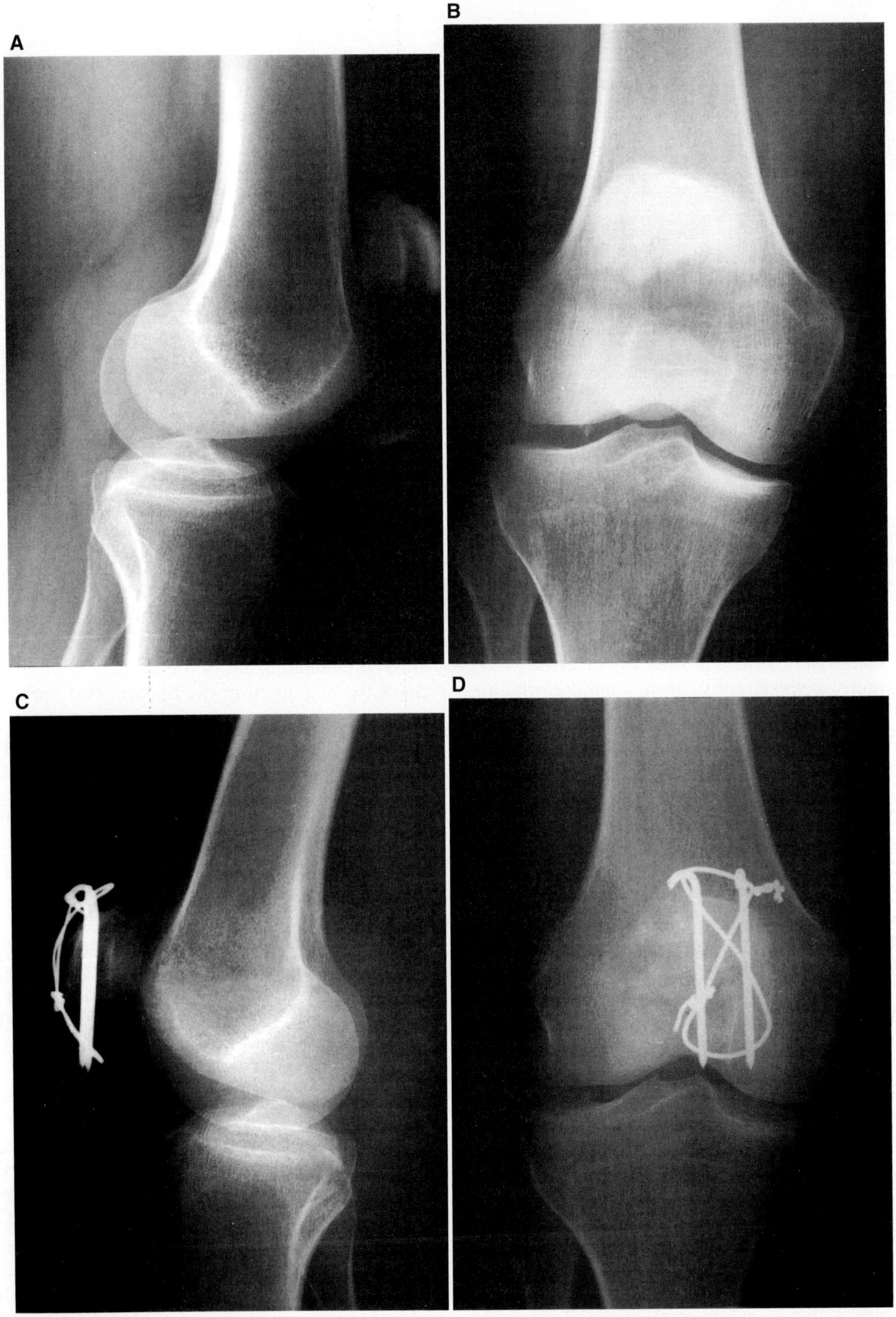

FIG 81–3.
A and **B,** lateral and anteroposterior radiographs of a simple transverse displaced patellar fracture. **C** and **D,** postoperative lateral and anteroposterior radiographs showing anatomic reduction and fixation with two parallel Steinmann pins and a figure-eight tension band wire.

by McKeever[44] but are not indicated in modern fracture care.

The goals of open reduction and internal fixation are reconstruction of the normal architecture of the patella, restoration of its articular surface, and repair of the extensor mechanism (Fig 81–3). A straight midline or peripatellar incision with the development of medial and lateral soft tissue flaps gives excellent exposure to the patella fracture fragments, the knee joint, and the extensor retinaculum. This approach also simplifies any future exposure of the knee joint should reconstructive surgery become necessary. Following debridement of the fracture hematoma, the fracture fragments are identified and assessed. Nondisplaced vertical fractures of the major fragments are common. The knee joint is inspected for any associated intraarticular injuries or loose fracture fragments.

The major fracture fragments are reduced with a tenaculum clamp or towel clip, and the articular surface is assessed under direct visualization.

Internal fixation may be achieved in several ways: a circumferential wire loop, intrafragmentary wiring or pinning as described by Payr,[49] Magnusen,[39] and Anderson,[1] or screw fixation as described by DePalma,[14] Müller et al.[47] and Smillie.[58] All of these methods of fixation should be supplemented with a tension band wire (Fig 81–4). Weber et al.[68] noted in

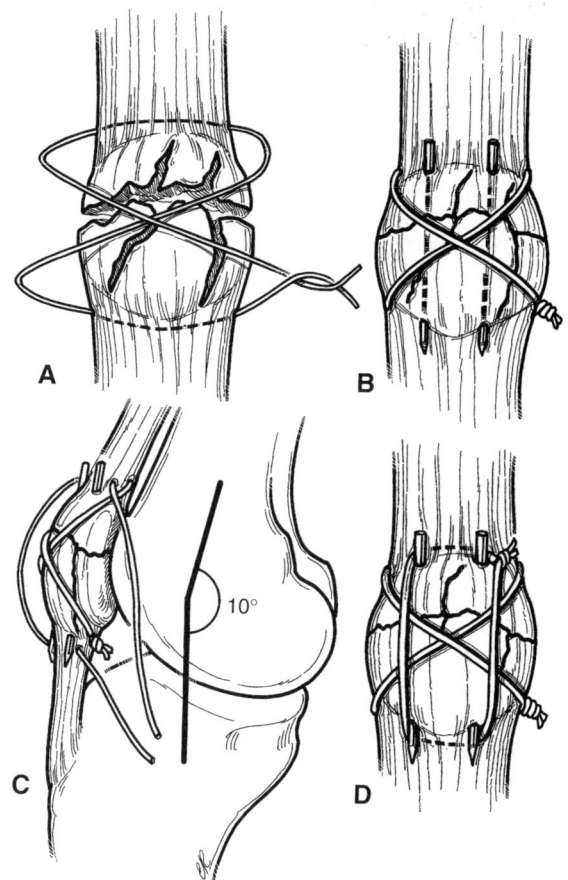

FIG 81–5.
Technique for indirect reduction of comminuted patellar fractures. (From Johnson EE: Fractures of the patella. In Rockwood C, Green D, Bucholz RW, editors: *Rockwood and Green's fractures in adults*, ed 3, Philadelphia, 1991, JB Lippincott Company.)

their mechanical studies that the most secure fixation was achieved with a modified tension band and two parallel vertical pins. If early motion of the knee is planned, the tension wiring should be anchored directly in the bone rather than threaded through the soft tissues about the patella. All slack must be removed from the wire prior to its tightening. A double twist loop technique is useful to ensure an effective tension band construct.[47] Tension band wiring converts the tension forces generated by the extensor mechanism to compressive forces resulting in dynamic compression of the fracture site with knee flexion. Indirect reduction techniques with placement of an anterior figure-eight tension band wire through the quadriceps tendon and the patellar tendon near the bone-tendon junction can be used to salvage severely comminuted fractures not amenable to direct anatomic reduction[31] (Fig 81–5).

Regardless of the method chosen for internal fixation, it is essential that the extent of the injury to the

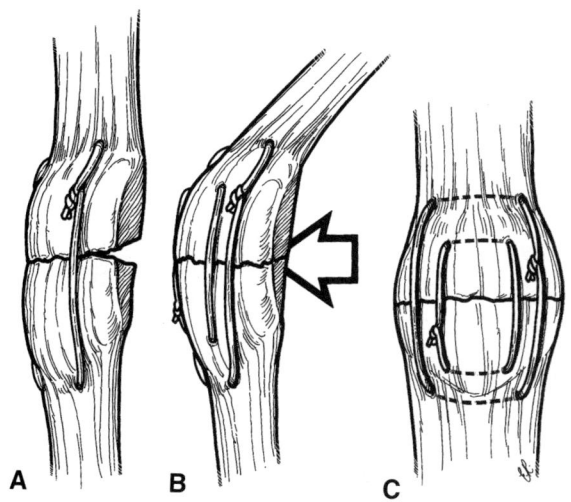

FIG 81–4.
A–C, the principle of tension band wiring of the patella. The first wire should be passed around the insertion of the patellar tendon and the quadriceps tendon so as to tighten the fracture into a slightly overcorrected position. The second wire is passed at a more superficial location through the bony fragments. Flexion of the knee results in pressure of the condyles against the patella, compressing the bony fragments. (Müller ME, Allgöwer M, Willenegger H: *Manual of internal fixation: technique recommended by the AO group*, New York, 1979, Springer-Verlag, pp 249–250.)

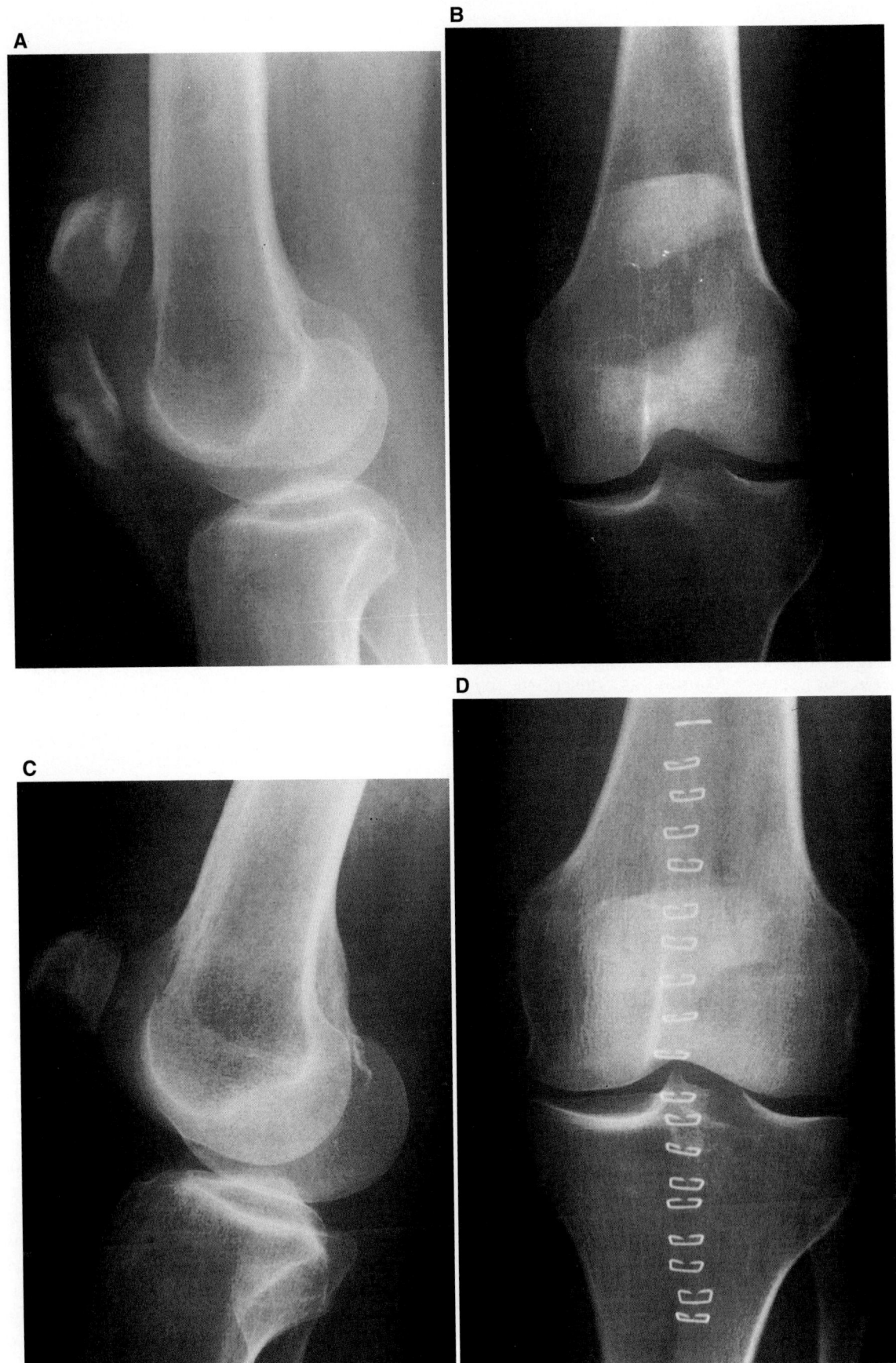

FIG 81–6.
A and **B,** lateral and anteroposterior radiographs of a displaced patellar fracture with obvious comminution of the inferior pole. **C** and **D,** at the time of surgery extensive irreparable comminution of the inferior pole of the patella was noted. A partial patellectomy was performed with reattachment of the patellar tendon to the proximal fragment.

medial and lateral retinaculum be recognized and repaired anatomically. Multiple, interrupted, nonabsorbable sutures are preferred for this repair.

Prior to wound closure, the knee should be placed through a near full range of motion. Any residual instability can be addressed at that time. The subcutaneous dead space should be drained to minimize the development of a postoperative hematoma.

Active knee motion is commenced soon after surgery if rigid fixation of the fracture is achieved.[47] The presence of residual fracture instability, marked comminution, poor bone stock, or associated limb injuries may preclude early motion.[14, 57, 67]

Partial patellectomy with repair of the extensor mechanism to the remaining patella, as first described by Thomson,[64] is indicated in severely comminuted fractures or in transverse fractures in which it is impossible to restore a congruent articular surface.[1, 2, 4, 14, 61] The quadriceps tendon should be sutured to the retained fragment through drill holes near its articular surface. Superficial reattachment will result in tilting of the fragment during knee flexion and possible damage to the femoral articular surface[2, 17] (Fig 81–6). Lag screw fixation of vertical fractures within the retained fragment may be necessary to preserve either the proximal or distal pole. Scapinelli[55] recommended saving the distal pole if possible to avoid avascular necrosis of the remaining patella, while other authors recommend salvage of the proximal pole.[15, 58, 65] The torn retinaculum is repaired in all partial patellectomies (Fig 81–7). Immobilization with a cylinder or long leg cast is necessary for a minimum of 3 to 4 weeks to allow soft tissue healing to the bone. If the suture repair is tenuous, a cerclage wire or nonabsorbable (Mersilene) tape may be drawn around the superior pole of the patella to the tibial tuberosity to reinforce the ligament repair.

Total patellectomy is recommended only in comminuted fractures where no large fragments are present and in severe knee injuries with extensive damage to the cartilage of the distal femur.[8, 28, 50, 66, 67, 69] The fragments of the patella should be completely shelled out from the quadriceps tendon and patellar ligament, preserving as much of the soft tissue as possible. Tensioning of the suture repair of the extensor mechanism is critical. Some authors recommend suturing the quadriceps tendon to the patellar tendon in an end-to-end fashion, while others suture the tendon with mattress sutures to avoid an extension lag.[14, 57, 67] Excessive tension on the repair implies a marked shortening of the extensor mechanism and the potential risk of an extension contracture. Cast immobilization is generally needed for 3 to 6 weeks. Despite intensive rehabilitation, loss of 5% to 30% of knee extension strength should be expected[32] (Fig 81–8).

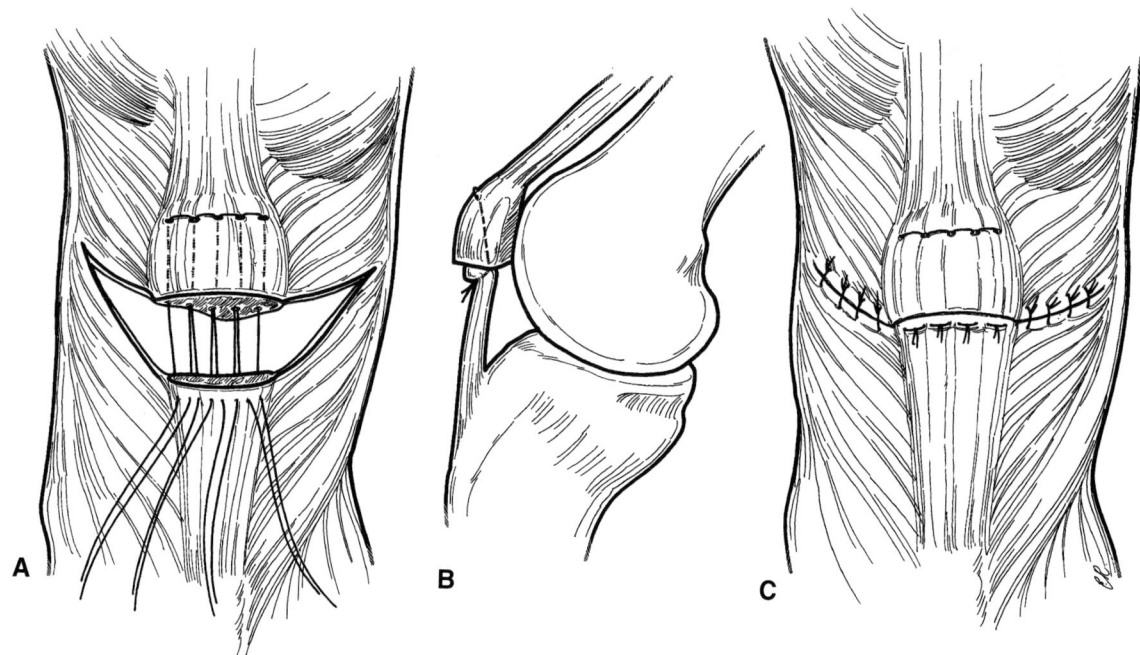

FIG 81–7.
A–C, technique of partial patellectomy. (From Saltzman CL, et al: *J Bone Joint Surg [Am]* 72:1279–1285, 1990.)

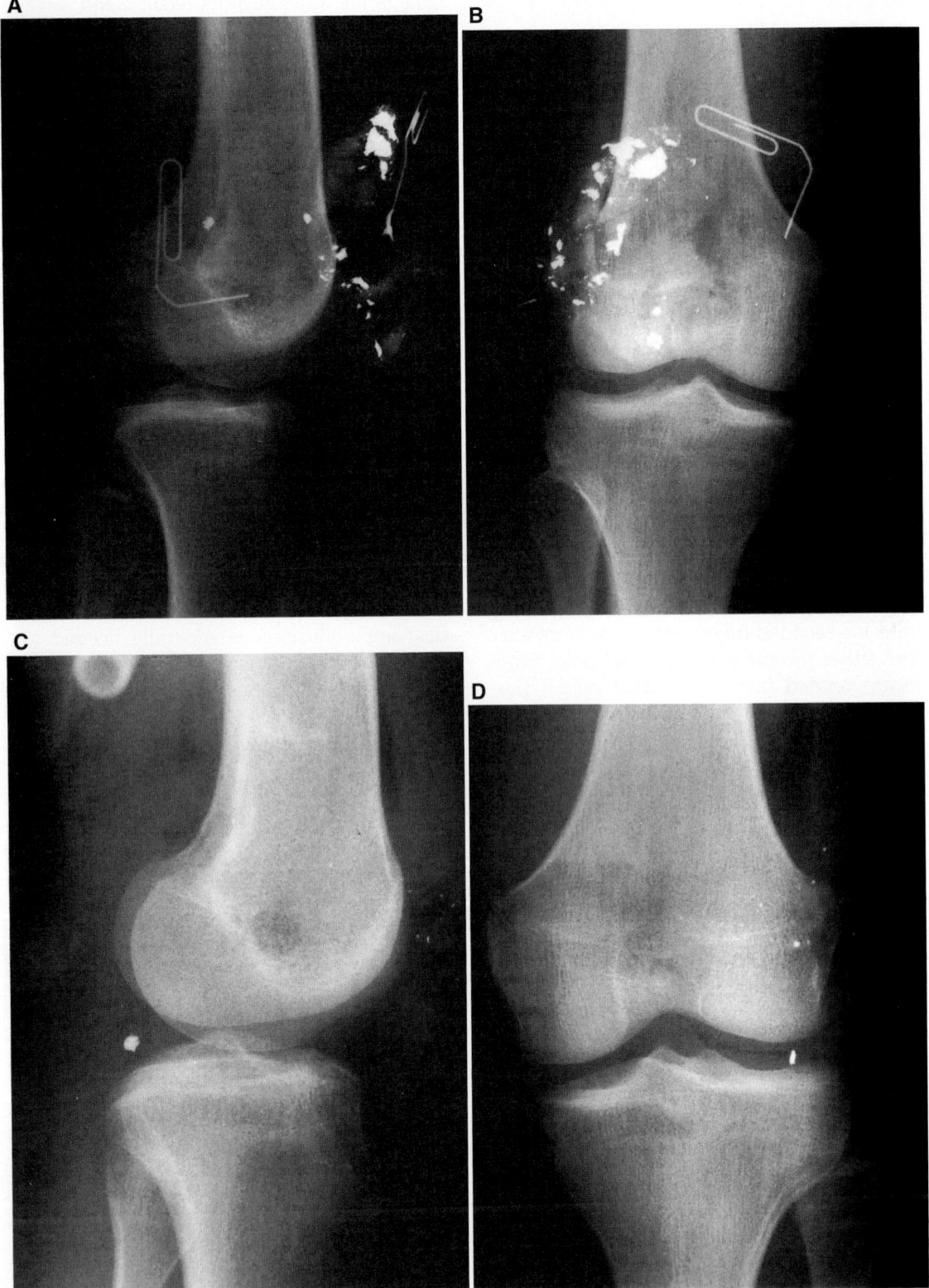

FIG 81-8.
A and **B,** lateral and anteroposterior radiographs of a severely comminuted patellar fracture secondary to a low-velocity gunshot wound. The degree of comminution precluded open reduction and internal fixation of the multiple fragments. **C** and **D,** postoperative lateral and anteroposterior radiographs demonstrating complete patellectomy. Repair of the extensor mechanism was possible.

Open Fractures

Open fractures should be treated by extensive irrigation and debridement of the wound and the knee joint. All completely devitalized fragments of bone are excised. Internal fixation should not be performed unless the wound is clean and free of all devitalized tissue. Soft tissue coverage of all fixation implants is desirable. Delayed repair is indicated if the wound is contaminated or if it is deemed that multiple debridements will be needed to provide adequate soft tissue closure.

Marginal and Osteochondral Fractures

Nondisplaced vertical fractures and nondisplaced marginal fractures of the lateral or medial facet can usually be managed nonoperatively with early range-of-motion exercises. Displaced vertical fractures occasionally require fixation with interfragmental screws and a tension band wire. Osteochondral fractures can usually be managed by arthroscopic removal of the loose fragment, but if the fragment is large and noncomminuted it may be reduced to its bed on the patella using Kirschner wires, lag screws, or bioabsorbable pins.[23, 31, 33, 40, 51, 52]

COMPLICATIONS

Posttraumatic patellofemoral arthritis is the most common major sequela of fractures of the patella. Most cases, however, are mild and cause few symptoms.[7, 15, 48] The initial impact to the articular surface at the time of fracture leads to articular cartilage degeneration that may be aggravated by an incongruent reduction.[11, 15, 58] Slow or rapid progression to patellofemoral arthritis and the classic findings of decreased joint space, eburnated bone, and spur formation may occur. The majority of patients with posttraumatic arthritis can be treated conservatively with physical therapy and nonsteroidal anti-inflammatory medications. In young patients with intractable pain, a tibial tuberosity advancement (Maquet procedure[42, 43]) may provide symptomatic relief.[19, 48] Patellofemoral osteoarthritis also develops in some patients following total patellectomy, but has been shown to be attributable to the impact injury of the femoral condyles at the time of fracture of the patella rather than to patellectomy per se.[11, 58]

Painful retained hardware is a very common minor complication of internal fixation of fractures of the patella. Subcutaneous Kirschner wires, screws, or tension band wires may irritate the adjacent tendons or retinaculum as motion returns to the knee. This problem is easily managed by hardware removal after union of the fracture has occurred.

The incidence of refracture of the patella varies from 1% to 5%.[7, 48] Repeat osteosynthesis is indicated only if the extensor mechanism is disrupted or if there is moderate displacement of the fracture fragments. Loss of reduction of one or more of the fracture fragments following open reduction and internal fixation is more common, with a prevalence of approximately 10%. Refracture and fracture fragment separation are generally the result of inadequate internal fixation or an inadequate period of immobilization.

Traumatic avascular necrosis of the patella usually involves the upper half of the bone, or more rarely, an intermediate fragment.[55] The incidence of radiographically evident avascular necrosis is approximately 25%, although complaints attributable to this finding are much less and are usually related to varying degrees of patellofemoral arthritis.[31, 48, 55] Avascular necrosis is evident radiologically 1 or 2 months after the fracture and is characterized by a relative radiodensity of the ischemic portion of the bone. Treatment should consist of observation and analgesic or anti-inflammatory medications. Revascularization occurs predictably within 2 years of the time of injury.[48, 55]

Nonunion of fractures of the patella is rare, with the incidence ranging from 2.4% to 4.8%.[31, 48] Repeat osteosynthesis is indicated in young active patients. Nonunion is usually well tolerated by inactive patients. Painful nonunions associated with an avascular fragment should be treated by partial patellectomy of the ischemic fragment and reconstruction of the extensor mechanism.

Infection following open reduction and internal fixation of open or closed fractures is a serious complication necessitating immediate surgical debridement and intravenous antibiotics. Nonviable bone fragments should be debrided along with removal of loose hardware. Stable fixation should be retained at least until union of the fracture. Some wounds can be closed loosely over drains if adequate debridement is performed. All attempts should be made to preserve the extensor mechanism. Exposure of articular cartilage to chronic infection leads to progressive articular cartilage destruction, loss of joint space, and poor knee function. Flap coverage of large open wounds is indicated in selected cases.

Failure to regain full knee motion following a fracture of the patella may be secondary to prolonged immobilization, infection, or a poor surgical repair.[7, 48] Studies have demonstrated that cast immobilization for longer than 8 weeks produced only 15%

good results, whereas immobilization for less than 4 weeks produced 83% good results. There was no difference between nonoperative and operative patients.[48] Restriction of motion also can be secondary to arthrofibrosis and infrapatellar contracture syndrome. Closed manipulation is contraindicated and may lead to fracture separation or refracture. Arthroscopic lysis of adhesions or open lysis of adhesions followed by continuous passive motion postoperatively has been shown to be effective in restoring some knee motion.

PROGNOSIS

As with most intraarticular fractures, the prognosis for healing and restoration of function in fractures of the patella is primarily dependent on the amount of articular cartilage damage at the time of injury.[11, 15, 31, 58] Most authors report 70% to 80% good to excellent results following open reduction and internal fixation of fractures of the patella, and approximately 60% good to excellent results following partial patellectomy with repair of the extensor mechanism.[6, 7, 48] Frequent complaints include weakness of the extremity and reduced range of knee motion with difficulty in stair climbing, walking downhill, and kneeling. About 70% of patients will have some complaint following fracture of the patella.[2, 5, 18, 48, 50] Full recovery of knee function after surgery usually requires 6 to 12 months of rehabilitation.[7, 31, 48] Results following total patellectomy are not as favorable, with good to excellent results ranging from 22% to 85%.* The strength of knee extension is diminished following total patellectomy and full extension of the knee requires approximately a 30% increase in quadriceps force.[7, 32, 48]

REFERENCES

1. Anderson LD: Fractures. In Crenshaw AH, (editor): *Campbell's operative orthopaedics,* ed 5, St Louis, 1971, Mosby–Year Book.
2. Andrews JR, Hughston JC: Treatment of patellar fractures by partial patellectomy, *South Med J* 70:809–813, 1977.
3. Ashby ME, Schields CL, Karmy JR: Diagnosis of osteochondral fractures in acute traumatic patellar dislocations using air arthrography, *J Trauma* 15:1032–1033, 1975.
4. Böhler J: Behandlung der Kniescheibenbrüche: Osteosynthese, Teilexstirpation, Extirpation. *Dstch Med Wochenschr,* 86:1209–1212, 1961.

*References 17, 18, 38, 48, 50, 57, 62, 70.

5. Böstman A, Kiviluoto O, Nirhamo J: Comminuted displaced fractures of the patella, *Injury* 13:196–202, 1981.
6. Böstman A, et al: Fractures of the patella treated by operation, *Arch Orthop Trauma Surg,* 102:78–81, 1983.
7. Boström A: Fractures of the patella: A study of 422 patellar fractures, *Acta Orthop Scand* 143(suppl):1–80, 1972.
8. Brooke R: The treatment of fractured patella by excision: A study of morphology and function, *Br J Surg,* 24:733–747, 1936–37.
9. Bruce J, Walmsley R: Excision of the patella—some experimental and anatomic observations. *J Bone Joint Surg* 24:311–375, 1942.
10. Cameron JC: Transverse fracture of the patella, *Glasgow Med J* 10:289–294, 1878.
11. Cargill AO: The long-term effect of the tibiofemoral compartment of the knee joint of comminuted fractures of the patella, *Injury,* 6:309–312, 1975.
12. Del Pizzo W et al: Operative arthroscopy for the treatment of arthrofibrosis of the knee, *Contemp Orthop,* 10:67–72, 1985.
13. Dennis FS: The treatment of fractured patella by the metallic suture, *New York Med J* 43:372–377, 1886.
14. DePalma AF, *The management of fractures and dislocations,* Philadelphia, 1959, WB Saunders.
15. DePalma AF, Flynn JJ: Joint changes following partial and total patellectomy, *J Bone Joint Surg [Am]* 40:395–413, 1958.
16. Dowd GSE: Marginal fractures of the patella, *Injury,* 14:287–291, 1982.
17. Duthie HL, Hutchinson JR: The results of partial and total excision of the patella, *J Bone Joint Surg [Br]* 40:75–81, 1958.
18. Einola S, Aho AJ, Kallio P: Patellectomy after fracture: Long-term follow-up results with special reference to functional disability, *Acta Orthop Scand,* 47:441–447, 1976.
19. Fergusen AB, et al: Relief of patellofemoral contact stress by anterior displacement of the tibial tubercle, *J Bone Joint Surg [Am]* 61:159–166, 1979.
20. Freiberger RH, Kotzen LM: Fracture of the medial margin of the patella: A finding diagnostic of lateral dislocation. *Radiology* 88:902–904, 1967.
21. Garr EL, Moskowitz RW, Davis W: Degenerative changes following experimental patellectomy in the rabbit, *Clin Orthop,* 92:262–304, 1973.
22. Haajanen J: Fractures of the patella: One hundred consecutive cases, *Ann Chir Gyneacol,* 70:32–35, 1980.
23. Hammerle CP, Jocob RP: Chondral and osteochondral fractures after luxation of the patella and their treatment, *Arch Orthop Trauma Surg,* 97:207–211, 1980.
24. Haxton H: The function of the patella and effects of its excision, *Surg Gynecol Obstet* 80:389–395, 1945.
25. Hey Groves EW: A note on the extension apparatus of the knee joint, *Br J Surg* 24:747–748, 1937.

26. Huang LK, et al: Fractured patella: Operative treatment using the tension band principle, *Injury* 16:343–347, 1985.
27. Hughston JC: Subluxation of the patella, *J Bone Joint Surg [Am]* 50:1003–1026, 1968.
28. Jakobsen J, Christensen KS, Rasmussen OS: Patellectomy—a 20-year follow-up, *Acta Orthop Scand* 56:430–432, 1985.
29. Jarvinen A: Über die Kniescheibenbrüche und ihre Behandlung mit besonderer Berücksichtigung der Dauerresultate im Licht der Nachuntersuchungen, *Acta Soc Med Duodecim* 32:81, 1942.
30. Jensenius H: On the results of excision of the fractured patella, *Acta Chir Scand* 102:275–284, 1951.
31. Johnson EE: Fractures of the Patella. In Rockwood C, Green D, Bucholz RW, (editors): *Rockwood and Green's fractures in adults, ed 3,* Philadelphia, 1991, JB Lippincott.
32. Kaufer H: Mechanical function of the patella, *J Bone Joint Surg [Am]* 53:1551–1560, 1971.
33. Kennedy JC, Grainger RW, McGraw RW: Osteochondral fracture of the femoral condyles, *J Bone Joint Surg [Br]* 48:436–440, 1966.
34. Lapidus PW: Longitudinal fractures of the patella, *J Bone Joint Surg* 14:351–379, 1932.
35. Lister J: A new operation for fracture of the patella, *Br Med J* 2:850, 1877.
36. Lotke PA, Ecker ML: Transverse fractures of the patella, *Clin Orthop,* 158:180–184, 1981.
37. Ma Y, et al: Treatment of fractures of the patella with percutaneous suture, *Clin Orthop* 191:241–245, 1984.
38. MacAusland WR: Total excision of the patella for fracture: Report of fourteen cases, *Am J Surg* 72:510–516, 1946.
39. Magnusen PB: *Fractures,* ed 2, Philadelphia, 1936, JB Lippincott.
40. Makin M: Osteochondral fracture of the lateral femoral condyle, *J Bone Joint Surg* 48:436–440, 1966.
41. Malgaigne JF: *Dennis system of surgery,* vol 1, Philadelphia, 1895, Lea Brothers.
42. Maquet PGJ: *Biomechanics of the knee: With application to the pathogenesis and the surgical treatment of osteoarthritis* Berlin, 1976, Springer-Verlag.
43. Maquet PGJ: Considerations on the treatment of patellar fractures, *Acta Orthop Belg* 53:25–33, 1987.
44. McKeever DC: Tibial plateau prosthesis, *Clin Orthop,* 18:86–95, 1955.
45. McMaster PE: Fractures of the patella, *Clin Orthop* 4:24–43, 1954.
46. Milgram JW, Rogers LF, Miller JW: Osteochondral fractures: Mechanisms of injury and fate of fragments, *AJR* 130:651–658, 1978.
47. Müller ME, Allgöwer M, Willinegger H: *Manual of internal fixation: Technique recommended by the AO group,* New York, 1979, Springer-Verlag, pp 249–250.
48. Nummi J: Fracture of the patella: A clinical study of 707 patellar fractures. *Ann Chir Gynaecol, Suppl* 60:179, 1971.
49. Payr E: Zur operativen Behandlung der Kniegelenksteife nach Langdauernder Ruhigstellung, *Zentralbl Chir* 44:809–816, 1917.
50. Peeples RE, Margo MK: Function after patellectomy, *Clin Orthop,* 132:180–186, 1978.
51. Rorabeck CH, Bobechko WP: Acute dislocation of the patella with osteochondral fracture: a review of eighteen cases, *J Bone Joint Surg [Am]* 58:237–240, 1976.
52. Rosenberg NJ: Osteochondral fractures of the lateral femoral condyle, *J Bone Joint Surg [Am]* 46:1013–1026, 1964.
53. Saltzman CL, et al: Results of treatment of displaced patellar fractures by partial patellectomy, *J Bone Joint Surg [Am]* 72 A :1279–1285, 1990.
54. Sanderson MC: The fractured patella: A long-term follow-up study, *Aust N Z J Surg* 45:49–54, 1974.
55. Scapinelli R: Blood supply of the human patella: Its relation to ischaemic necrosis after fracture, *J Bone Joint Surg [Br]* 49:563–570, 1967.
56. Schönbauer HR: Brüche der Kniescheibe, *Chir Orthop* 41:56–79, 1959.
57. Scott JC: Fractures of the patella, *J Bone Joint Surg [Br]* 31:76–81, 1949.
58. Smillie IS: *Injuries of the knee joint,* ed 4, Edinburgh, 1970, E & S Livingstone.
59. Sorensen KH: The late prognosis after fracture of the patella, *Acta Orthop Scand* 34:198–212, 1964.
60. Sprague N, O'Connor RL, Fox JM: Arthoscopic treatment of postoperative knee fibroarthrosis, *Clin Orthop* 166:165–172, 1982.
61. Stimson LA: Treatment of fracture of the patella, *Ann Surg* 28:216–228, 1898.
62. Sutton FS, et al: The effect of patellectomy on knee function, *J Bone Joint Surg [Am]* 48:537–540, 1976.
63. Thiem C: Über die Grösse der Unfallfolgen bei der blutigen und unblutigen Behandlung der einfachen (subcutanen) Querbrüche der Kniescheibe. *Verh Dtsch Ges Chir,* 34:374–383, 1905.
64. Thomson JEM: Comminuted fractures of the patella: Treatment of cases presenting with one large fragment and several small fragments, *J Bone Joint Surg* 17:431–434, 1935.
65. Thomson JEM: Comminuted fractures of the patella: Removal of the loose fragments and plastic repair of the tendon: A study of 554 cases *Surg Gynecol-Obstet* 74:860–866, 1942.
66. Villiger KJ, Behandlungsergebnisse bei Patellafrakturen. *Schweiz Med Wochenschr* 18:595–599, 1965.
67. Watson-Jones R: Excision of the patella (letter), *Br Med J,* 2:195–196, 1945.
68. Weber MJ, et al: Efficacy of various forms of fixation of transverse fractures of the patella, *J Bone Joint Surg [Am]* 62:215–220, 1980.
69. West FE: End results of patellectomy, *J Bone Joint Surg [Am]* 44:1089–1108, 1962.
70. Wilkinson J: Fracture of the patella treated by total excision, *J Bone Joint Surg [Br]* 59:352–354, 1977.

82
Periprosthetic Fractures

MARK L. HARLOW, M.D.
AARON A. HOFMANN, M.D.

Femoral fractures
  Treatment
  Controversies
    Role of cement
    Role of anterior femoral notching

Patellar fractures
  Treatment
Tibial fractures

The management of periprosthetic fractures following total knee arthroplasty poses a difficult challenge to the orthopaedic surgeon. Fractures of the femur, patella, and tibia each present their own particular treatment concerns. The principles for management of these injuries are essentially the same as those for primary knee arthroplasty. Restoration of limb alignment, preservation of bone stock, and maintenance of the integrity of the collateral ligaments and extensor mechanism are the keys to success.

FEMORAL FRACTURES

Fractures of the distal femur following total knee arthroplasty are not an uncommon complication. The incidence in reported series ranged from 0.6% to 2.5%.[11, 42] These injuries commonly occur with minimal trauma and the most frequently implicated risk factor is osteopenia. This may be due to osteoporosis, disuse, rheumatoid arthritis, or prolonged steroid therapy. Other risk factors include notching of the anterior femoral cortex, advanced age, the presence of a revision arthroplasty, and the presence of a neurologic disorder.

Distal femoral fractures following total knee arthroplasty were first reported in the German literature in 1977[31] and in the American literature in 1981.[39] Twenty publications have discussed the treatment of these injuries in a cumulative total of 246 patients.* Of these, 142 patients (58%) were initially managed with closed methods including traction, casting, cast bracing, or combinations of these; 41 patients (29%) failed closed treatment and went on to secondary operative procedures. The remaining 104 patients (42%) were managed initially with operative intervention, including open reduction with internal fixation (ORIF), closed reduction with internal fixation, external fixation, or revision total knee arthroplasty; 14 (13%) of these patients required at least one additional operation to achieve union. The rationale for treatment reflected significant diversity of opinion and was based largely on anecdotal factors. Only 8 of the 19 reports included more than 10 patients. These are discussed below.

Sisto et al.[40] reviewed the results of treatment of 15 supracondylar fractures that were divided into three treatment groups. Group I included four patients treated with closed reduction, cast immobilization, and early weightbearing. Group II included eight patients treated with traction followed by cast or cast-brace immobilization. Group III had three patients treated by immediate ORIF. In group I, three of four patients had knee scores, judged according to the Hospital for Special Surgery (HSS) rating system, that were lower than their preinjury rating, and one patient required a corrective osteotomy. In group II, five of eight had lower HSS scores and one patient had developed a nonunion necessitating surgical treatment. In group III, all three fractures united between 3 and 5 months and all knee scores were unchanged at follow-up. The authors' criteria for success included union of the fracture in proper alignment, maintenance of fixation of the prosthetic com-

*References 2, 3, 6, 9–11, 14, 18, 19, 24, 25, 27, 28, 30, 32, 36, 40, 42.

ponent, and maintenance of 90 degrees of knee motion. The authors recommend gentle closed reduction and skeletal traction for the initial treatment of a displaced supracondylar femur fracture. If satisfactory alignment cannot be maintained in traction they suggest that early open reduction and internal fixation is the treatment of choice.[40]

Merkel and Johnson[25] reviewed 36 fractures including 11 that were undisplaced and 25 that were displaced. The fractures were also categorized retrospectively according to the classification scheme proposed by Neer et al.[26] (Fig 82–1). Twenty-six patients were initially treated using nonoperative means. Nine (35%) of these failed closed treatment due to nonunion (four patients), malunion (two patients), component loosening (two patients), and extensor mechanism dysfunction (one patient). Five fractures were treated with early ORIF and three were treated with early external fixation. In the internal fixation group three of five patients had satisfactory results. One patient died postoperatively and one had an above-knee amputation for sepsis. The three fractures treated with external fixation included one excellent and two good results.

The authors recommend nonoperative treatment for the initial management of these fractures. If a poor functional outcome follows nonoperative treatment they state that the patient can undergo revision arthroplasty with the expectation of a satisfactory outcome. They propose that early operative treatment should be reserved for patients who are not osteopenic, for those who demand a highly functional arthroplasty, and for those in whom adequate closed reduction cannot be maintained. Malalignment of less than 10 degrees in the frontal and sagittal planes was considered acceptable and correlated with a satisfactory clinical outcome. These authors were the first to propose utilization of a fracture classification scheme to direct treatment. They suggested that for Neer grade I fractures the appropriate treatment was immediate casting followed by the implementation of a cast brace at approximately 4 weeks. For grade IIA and IIB fractures, they proposed gentle closed reduction and skeletal traction. If the alignment could not be maintained within 10 degrees of anatomic alignment, then ORIF was recommended. They further recommended that if the femoral component was loose, then the fracture should be allowed to heal with closed treatment followed by late revision arthroplasty.[25]

Cain et al.[6] reported on their series of 14 patients. Ten patients were treated nonoperatively with three resulting in poor outcomes due to nonunion (one patient) and loss of knee motion (two patients). Four

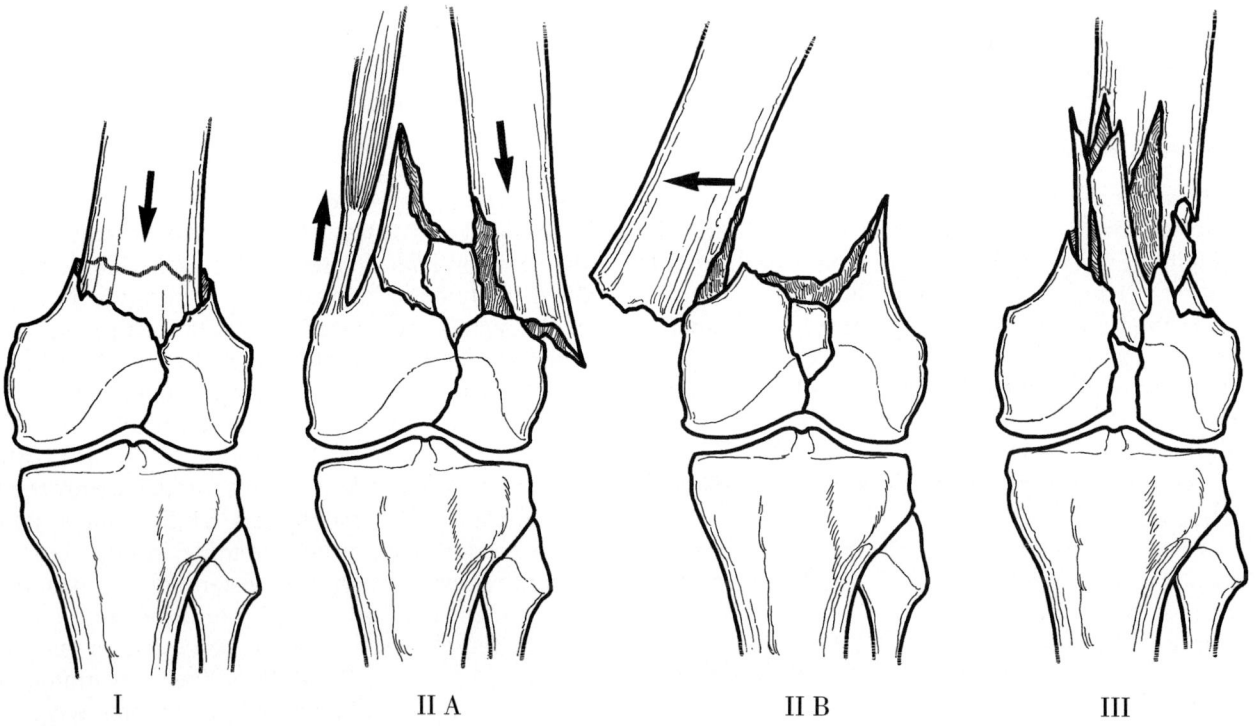

FIG 82–1.
Neer et al.[26] classification of supracondylar femur fractures. (Modified from Neer CS, Grantom S, Shelton M: *J Bone Joint Surg [Am]* 49A:591, 1967. Used by permission.)

patients were treated operatively with three resulting in poor outcomes due to nonunion (two patients) and ligamentous instability (one patient). These authors were the first to propose that translation of the fracture fragments and prosthetic alignment correlated with treatment outcomes. Translations greater than 5 mm were judged more likely to result in a poor clinical result. Furthermore, they proposed that the extent of comminution of the fracture site be considered an important factor for healing. All of their poor results occurred in fractures that were comminuted and translated greater than 5 mm. They concluded that nondisplaced or minimally comminuted fractures could be treated with immediate casting. If the fracture was angulated greater than 10 degrees or translated greater than 5 mm, they recommended closed reduction and skeletal traction. They suggested that failure of closed treatment or a loose femoral component associated with the fracture constituted an indication for early operative intervention.[6]

Culp et al.[10] reported the largest series, which included 61 patients. This is perhaps the only study in which valid comparisons can be made between operative (31 patients) and nonoperative (30 patients) populations. In the nonoperative group, 17 of 30 patients had successful clinical outcomes. Seven malunions and six nonunions were reported in the remainder of this group. Six of these patients required secondary surgical intervention to obtain a satisfactory clinical outcome. In the early operative group, 25 of 31 patients showed satisfactory union. Three malunions and one nonunion were included in this group as were two cases which went on to above-knee amputation for recurrent sepsis. The authors concluded that these injuries are best managed with early secure internal fixation and early motion to minimize the loss of knee motion.[10]

Bogoch et al.[3] reported 12 cases of fracture of the supracondylar femur in patients with rheumatoid arthritis. Eight patients were treated nonoperatively and four were treated with surgical intervention. Eleven fractures healed with the primary treatment and one required a second operative procedure to achieve union. In 10 of the cases the femur was shortened (mean value, 2.8 cm) and in 9 cases the femur was axially malaligned. Two of the patients treated nonoperatively developed subsequent loosening of their femoral components requiring revision arthroplasty. The authors concluded that in the rheumatoid population both treatment modalities are fraught with complications; however, internal fixation is preferred if the patient has good bone stock and has high functional demands.[3]

Nielsen et al.[27] reported their results in 16 patients: 10 patients underwent closed treatment with casting, 4 patients underwent open reduction and plate fixation, and 2 patients underwent closed reduction and internal fixation with Rush pins. In the conservatively treated group of patients and the 2 patients treated with Rush pins, there were no complications and the function of the patients had returned to preinjury status by 1 year. Three of the four cases treated with open reduction and plate fixation developed complications including two deep infections and one loss of fixation resulting in malunion. The authors concluded that patients with stable, undisplaced, or slightly displaced supracondylar fractures may be treated conservatively with a cast and immediate mobilization. The healing time is comparable to that in patients without a knee prosthesis. In patients with unstable or displaced fractures the authors advocate the use of Rush pins as an alternative to conventional plate osteosynthesis in selected cases. They suggest that open reduction and plate fixation may be precarious because of the extensive surgical exposure, the risk of accidental loosening of the prosthesis, and the osteopenia in a bone that has already been mechanically stressed. Plating or revision arthroplasty should be reserved for cases in which the other two modalities have failed.[27]

Figgie et al.[14] reviewed their series of 24 ipsilateral supracondylar fractures above a total knee arthroplasty. The treatment groups included traction followed by cast application (ten patients), ORIF (ten patients), custom total knee arthroplasty with distal femoral allograft (two patients), external fixation (one patient), and primary arthrodesis (one patient). Nine of ten fractures treated conservatively healed primarily. Only five of 10 fractures treated with ORIF healed primarily. Of the remaining five cases, two were salvaged with repeat ORIF and bone grafting and three with a custom total knee arthroplasty. Distal femoral allograft was utilized in two of these cases. The authors further analyzed their results by categorizing the fractures according to the Neer classification. Closed reduction and skeletal traction are recommended for Neer type I or II fractures if the femoral component remains well fixed. If acceptable alignment cannot be maintained, then ORIF with medial and lateral buttress plates is recommended. For Neer type III fractures or Neer type II fractures with poor bone stock, they recommend immediate revision arthroplasty with a custom prosthesis and incorporation of a distal femoral allograft as necessary.[14]

Rand and Franco[30] reported 24 revision total knee arthroplasties for ipsilateral supracondylar fracture above an existing knee arthroplasty. Seventeen of the fractures occurred in patients with primary knee arthroplasties and seven occurred in patients with revision knee arthroplasties. Five patients underwent immediate revision arthroplasty while 19 had surgery between 1 and 12 months postinjury. Six of these 19 underwent revision arthroplasty following failed attempts at ORIF. Sixteen of the cases were revised with a hinged implant while eight utilized a resurfacing implant. Twelve of the 16 (75%) patients receiving hinged implants had postoperative complications in comparison to two of eight (25%) complications in the resurfacing group. Overall, 14 of 24 patients (58%) experienced significant complications. The reported end result was a functioning arthroplasty in 19 of the 24 knees. The authors conclude that these patients present a challenging problem and have an associated high risk of complications. They recommend that modular segmental replacement prostheses should be avoided whenever possible for revisions of supracondylar fractures following total knee arthroplasty.[30]

Treatment

The evaluation of prior treatment outcomes and the establishment of treatment protocols is predicated on the development of a fracture classification system. This assures fair comparison when different treatment modalities are assessed. DiGioia and Rubash[12] have proposed a modified Neer classification that serves this purpose. The classification divides the fractures into three types that are based on the ability to achieve and maintain adequate alignment following closed reduction. The group I fracture is extraarticular (i.e., not involving the bone-implant or bone-cement interface) and nondisplaced as defined by less than 5 mm of translation and less than 5 degrees of angulation in any plane. Group II fractures are extraarticular and defined as those with displacement greater than 5 mm or angulation greater than 5 degrees in any one plane. Grade III fractures are the severely displaced fractures with loss of cortical continuity and are usually associated with greater than 10 degrees of angulation. Grade III fractures may have an intercondylar or total condylar component. The amount of comminution at the fracture site should be graded as minimal or severe based on the amount of potential cortical contact at the fracture site. Minimal comminution requires at least 50% or more contact of opposing cortical bone surfaces, whereas severe comminution is less than 50% cortical contact. In a condensation of the literature values, DiGioia and Rubash have also established guidelines for acceptable alignment of the fracture: less than 5 mm of translation, less than 5 to 10 degrees of angulation, less than 1 cm of shortening, and less than 10 degrees of rotation. The determination of fracture grade and the assessment of alignment criteria can then be useful in choosing the optimal treatment. They have proposed a treatment algorithm based on these parameters (Fig 82–2).

Although traction for management of these fractures may seem an attractive alternative, the effect of prolonged confinement to bed in an elderly person must be considered. From the trauma literature it is known that early fixation of long bone fractures is beneficial to the overall management of the multiple trauma patient, inasmuch as pulmonary complications and decubitus ulcerations are minimized.[4,22] Although this is not a directly analogous situation, the advantages of early mobilization of an elderly patient are apparent. For this reason, one may consider the use of closed reduction and internal fixation using condylar Rush pins as advocated by Ritter and Stiver[34] and Nielsen et al.[27] The use of these percutaneously placed internal splints may facilitate early mobilization of the patient and significantly accelerate the rehabilitative process (Fig 82–3).

Other factors to consider when choosing traction for management include the deforming forces that are brought to bear on the distal fragment by the gastrocnemius (flexion) and adductor magnus (varus). The consensus of authors is that it is difficult to maintain acceptable alignment with tibial pin traction for the type II and III fractures. Union in varus malalignment is common and is associated with a high rate of revision arthroplasty.[14] This leads to overload of the medial compartment and consequent loosening of the tibial component.

If the fracture pattern is not amenable to management with Rush pins, then the principles of rigid internal fixation should be followed. Options for management include a blade plate, a condylar screw and side plate, or an interlocked femoral nail (Fig 82–4). If the fracture is 8 cm or more from the joint line, a Brooker-Wills nail may be used for fixation.[18] A conventional femoral nail may also be used if the distal tip is removed to allow the holes for the interlocking screw to move closer to the joint line. If the bone quality is poor or if there is significant loss of cortical continuity at the time of repair, then the use of autogeneic or allogeneic bone graft may be considered. Also, the use of polymethyl methacrylate (PMMA) may be considered to augment the purchase of the screws in soft bone. There are also occasions when the diminished cortical continuity may require the use of double plating to obtain a stable construct.

If the femoral component is loose, then revision

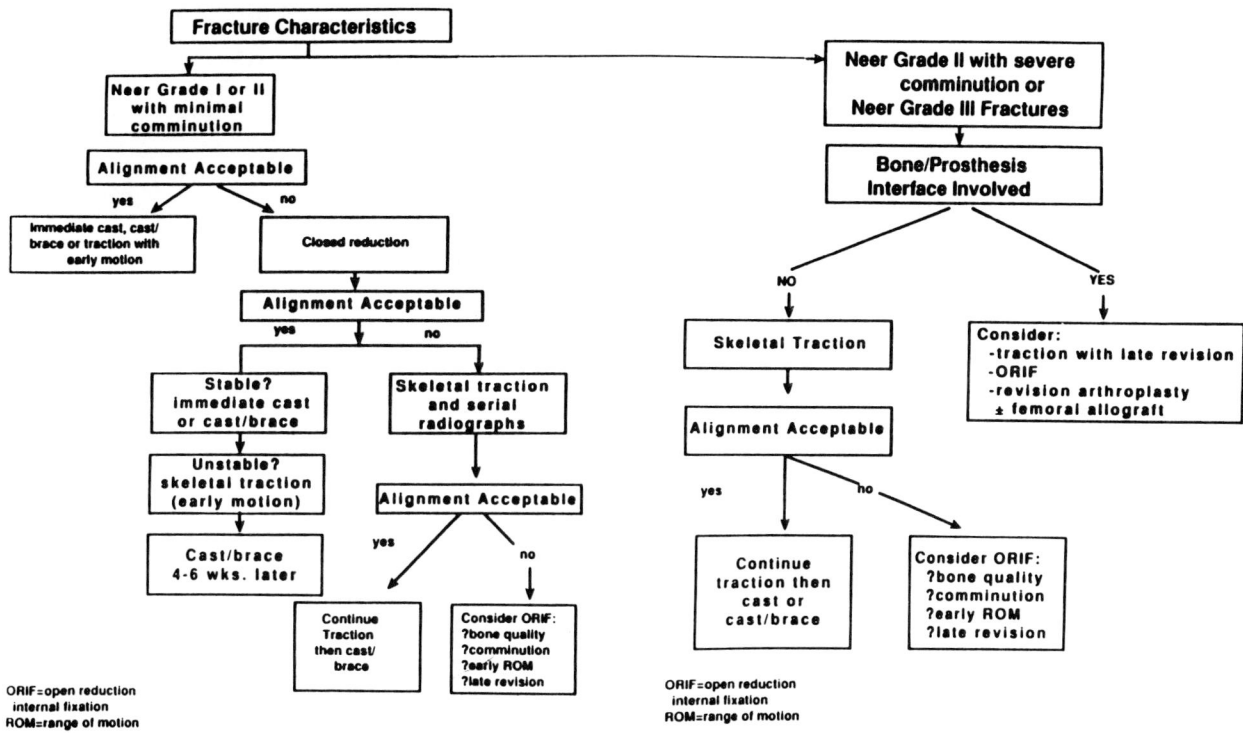

FIG 82–2.
Treatment algorithm for femoral fractures. See text. (From DiGioia A, Rubash H: Clin Orthop 271:135, 1991. Used by permission.)

with a femoral component that includes an intramedullary stem may be the treatment of choice (Fig 82–5). Interlocking screws may be passed through the stem at its proximal extent to enhance rotational control. Augmentation with cortical strut onlay allografts that span the fracture may also prove to be beneficial in minimizing rotational strains. If cement is used to secure the femoral component to the metaphyseal fragment, then care must be taken to avoid extravasation of cement into the fracture planes as this will likely lead to nonunion.

If the supracondylar femur fracture is significantly comminuted and this comminution involves the attachment of the collateral ligaments, then the decision must be made as to whether the fracture will be allowed to heal in situ followed by late revision, or whether early revision with a constrained metaphyseal replacement prosthesis (i.e., a tumor-type prosthesis) would be appropriate.

In general, the patients who present with this complication are of advanced age, have compromised bone quality, and diminished functional expectations. If the fracture is a type I and has inherent stability, then early casting and mobilization would appear to be the appropriate choice. If the fracture is unstable, then the path is less clear. The potential morbidity of prolonged bed rest in skeletal traction must be carefully weighed. If the fracture is amenable to closed reduction and internal fixation, to ORIF, or to revision arthroplasty, then these options should be carefully considered in the context of the patient's overall well-being and his or her functional expectations. These choices must be individualized for each patient.

Controversies

Role of Cement

The role of cement for fixation in revision total knee arthroplasty remains controversial. Cement functions as a grout and has no fundamental adhesive quality. If the distal femur and proximal tibia are thin shells of cortical bone and there is no trabecular bone available for interdigitation of the cement, then the utility of cement must be questioned. The utilization of bone graft, long-stemmed components, and screw fixation of the components to the bone may prove to result in increased longevity.

Role of Anterior Femoral Notching

Numerous authors have cited anterior femoral notching as a significant risk factor for supracondylar femur fracture following total knee arthroplasty.[1, 6, 10, 14, 28] The association of femoral notching with fracture ranged from 21% to 44% in the series that specifically addressed this finding. Culp

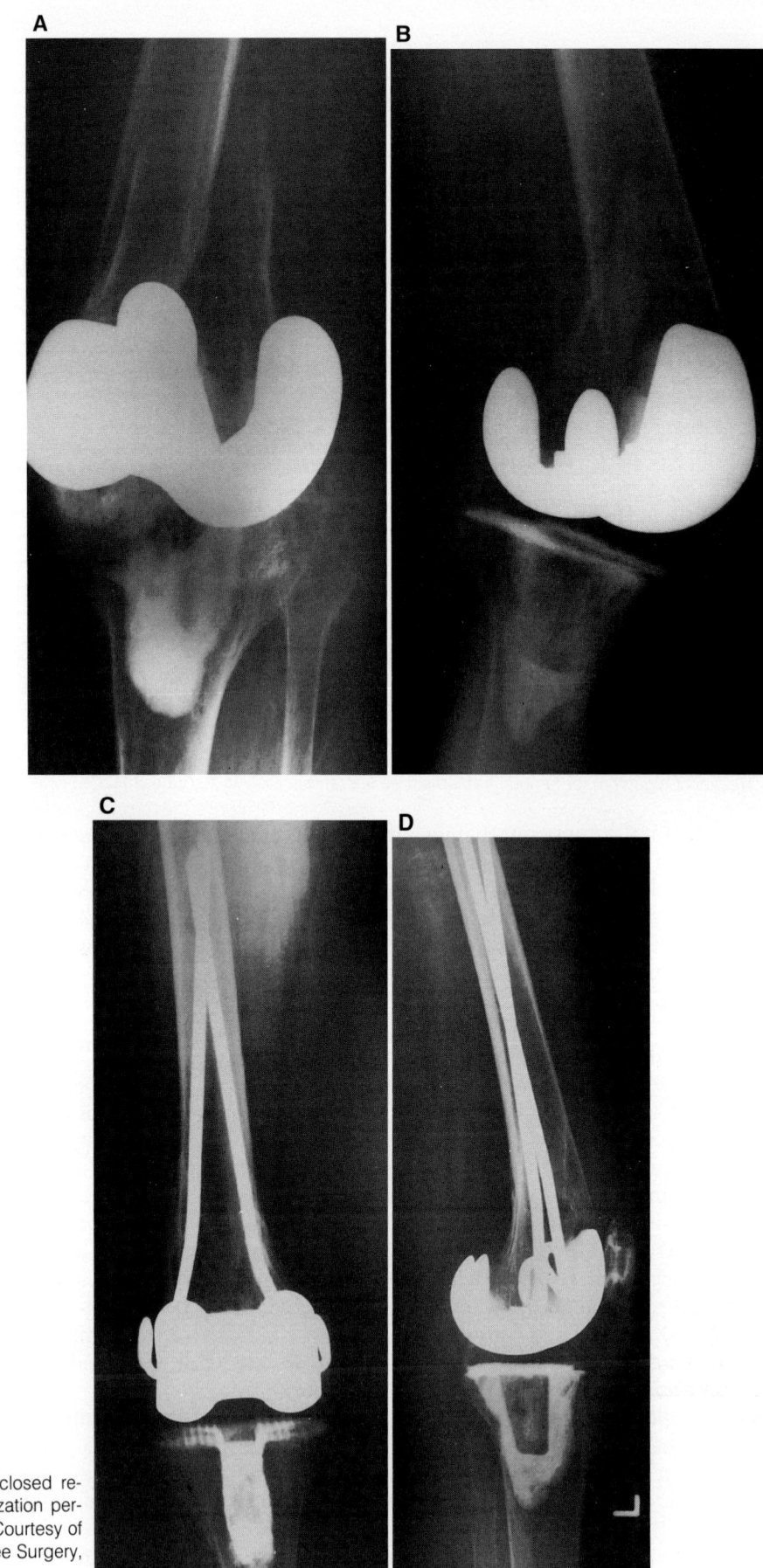

FIG 82-3.
A-D, fracture effectively managed with closed reduction and internal fixation. Early mobilization permitted rapid return to preinjury function. (Courtesy of Merrill Ritter, M.D., Center for Hip and Knee Surgery, Mooresville, Ind.)

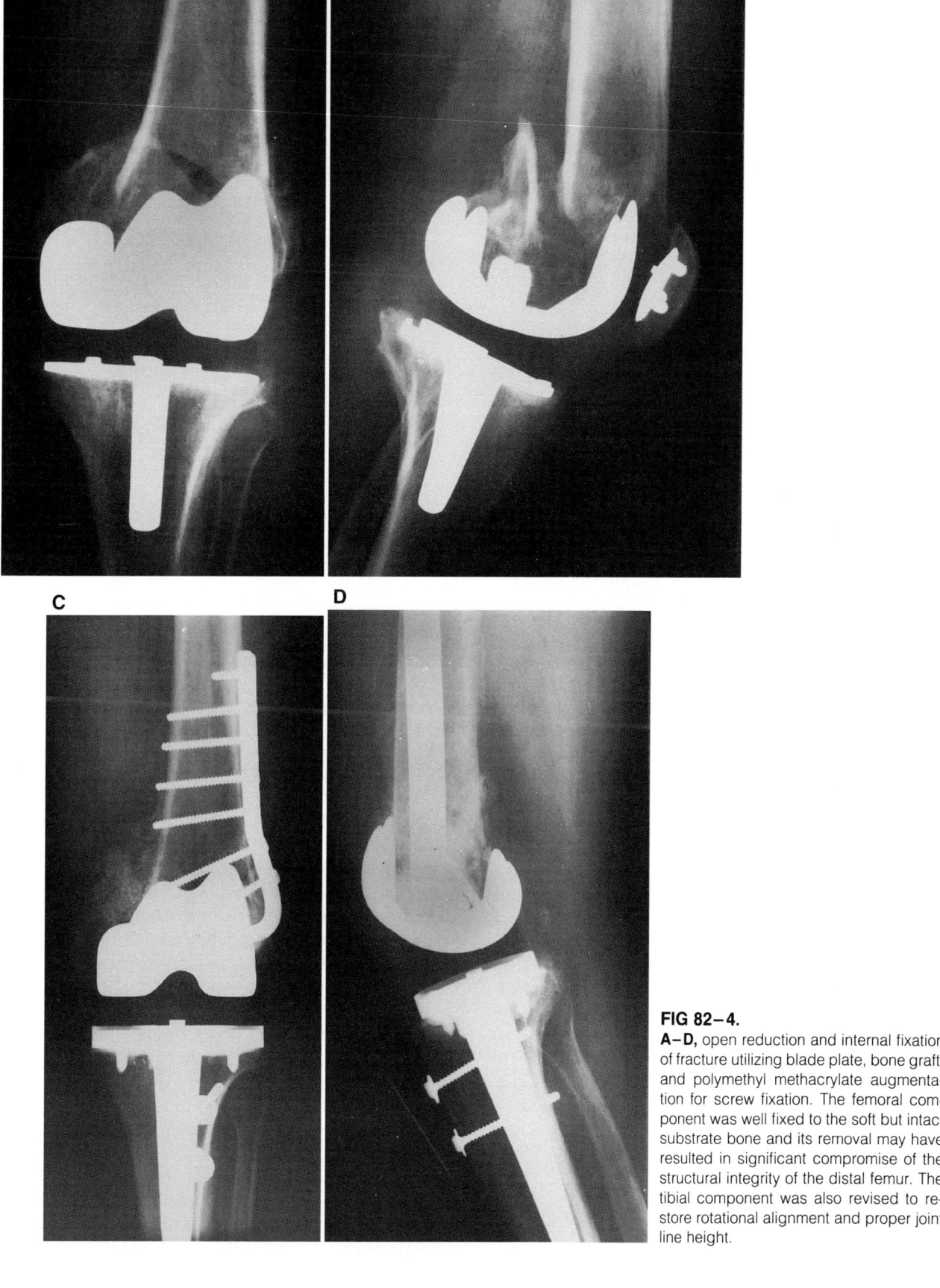

FIG 82–4.
A–D, open reduction and internal fixation of fracture utilizing blade plate, bone graft, and polymethyl methacrylate augmentation for screw fixation. The femoral component was well fixed to the soft but intact substrate bone and its removal may have resulted in significant compromise of the structural integrity of the distal femur. The tibial component was also revised to restore rotational alignment and proper joint line height.

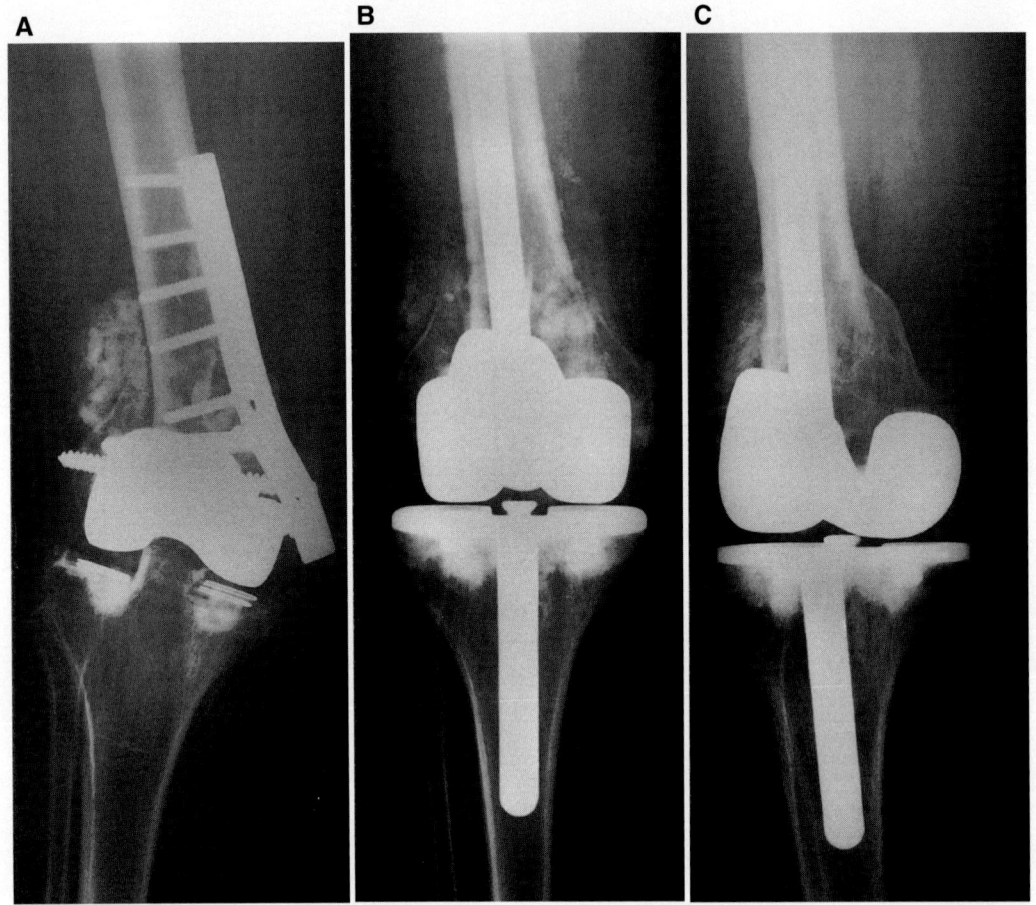

FIG 82–5.
A–C, failed open reduction with internal fixation managed with stemmed revision arthroplasty and bone graft. The patient returned to preinjury functional level. (Courtesy of Kim Bertin, M.D., LDS Hospital, Salt Lake City, Utah.)

et al.[10] in a theoretic model showed that a 3-mm notch in the anterior femur caused a 29% decrease in the polar moment of inertia and thereby decreased the torsional load to failure. This is in contrast to the report by Ritter and colleagues who reviewed 670 cases of which 180 had anterior femoral notching. The notching was reported to be deeper than 3 mm in 138 (20.5%) of these cases. Only two of these 670 cases suffered ipsilateral supracondylar fractures; one with a notched femur and one without. The authors reported that no correlation was found between anterior femoral notching and supracondylar femur fracture, but did state that the cause of these fractures is likely multifactorial in origin and may be attributed to osteopenia, inadequate bone remodeling, stress shielding, or increased use of the extremity following operation.

PATELLAR FRACTURES

As total knee arthroplasty finds greater application in a younger and more active patient population, and as improved implant design leads to increased range of motion, problems pertaining to the patellofemoral articulation are becoming increasingly prevalent. Fractures of resurfaced patellae have a reported incidence from 0.15% to 3.7% in larger series using a total condylar femoral component.[17, 32] The majority of these fractures occur as stress or fatigue fractures and are not associated with a discrete traumatic event. They occur with equal frequency in patients with rheumatoid arthritis or osteoarthritis. They occur with an increased frequency following revision arthroplasty (0.61%) in comparison to primary arthroplasty (0.12%).[17]

The potential etiologic factors are numerous. Compromise of the vascular supply and hence an increased risk of osseous necrosis are associated with a medial parapatellar arthrotomy, lateral retinacular release, and resection of the fat pad. Overresection and excessive excavation of trabecular bone for a cement mantle have also been implicated. Thermal necrosis from the saw and from the polymerization of cement must also be considered. Uneven patellar resection and overthickening of the trochlea may lead to increased contact pressures that may predispose to fracture.

Since 1981, 11 publications have discussed the treatment of these injuries in a cumulative total of 139 patients.* Of these, 73 patients (53%) were managed with nonoperative therapy and 66 patients (47%) were managed with operative intervention. The indications for treatment varied widely among the authors. In the nonoperative group 72 of 73 patients (99%) had satisfactory clinical outcomes. This is in comparison to the operative group, which included 56% (37/66 patients) satisfactory clinical outcomes. It should be noted, however, that these results may reflect the nature of the injuries chosen for the two groups as much as it reflects the effectiveness of the methods. Seven of the 11 reports included more than 10 patients and are discussed below.

Thompson et al.[41] reported 18 patellar fractures in a series of 1,030 total condylar knee arthroplasties. Fifteen fractures were considered to be fatigue or stress fractures, and three were due to trauma. In all cases the treatment was predicated on symptoms and loss of function rather than the radiographic appearance of the fracture. Treatment modalities included partial weightbearing (four fractures), knee immobilizer (four), cylinder cast (two), no treatment (four), and surgery (four). In the operative group, one patient underwent closed reduction, one underwent patellectomy, and two required ORIF. It was noted that secure internal fixation was technically difficult to obtain. The nonoperative group included 10 excellent and four good results, whereas the operative group had three good and one fair result. It was noted that all of the fractures occurred near the central fixation lug and that this may be a predisposing factor for structural weakening of the patella. The authors recommend that careful attention be paid to the accuracy of patellar tracking at the time of soft tissue balancing and that overresection of the patella be avoided.[41]

Ritter and Campbell[32] reported 18 fractures in resurfaced patellae following total knee arthroplasty. Seventeen of these injuries occurred in knees in which a lateral release had not been performed. It has been shown by Scuderi et al.[38] using postoperative technetium bone scans, that there is a higher incidence of vascular compromise in knees with a lateral release compared to those without (56% vs. 15%, respectively). This suggests that disruption of the lateral blood supply to the patella is not the sole factor leading to decreased vascularity that may predispose the patella to fracture. In the Ritter and Campbell series, all patients were asymptomatic at the time the fractures were noted and thus no treatment was rendered. In the 17 fractures noted in patients without a lateral release, all were observed to have lateral patellar bone extending to make contact with the prosthetic lateral femoral condyle. Insofar as lateral release has been positively shown to prevent patellar tilt, it was suggested that these fractures resulted from the increased lateral tension associated with an intact lateral retinaculum and patellar bone lateral to the patellar prosthesis.[32]

Brick and Scott[5] reported 15 patellar fractures following total knee arthroplasty. The average time to fracture presentation was 8.6 months (range, 1–48 months). Seven fractures occurred during normal activities of daily living, and two following postoperative manipulation. Six fractures were asymptomatic. Six knees were treated conservatively using a knee immobilizer and crutches for 6 weeks. Four knees were treated with ORIF, three with partial patellectomy, and two with complete patellectomy. All of the patients treated conservatively had satisfactory clinical outcomes. Three of the four patients treated with ORIF had failures of fixation. These required subsequent complete or partial patellectomy to obtain acceptable clinical outcomes. The results of the patients managed initially by complete or partial patellectomy were suboptimal, owing at least in part to medical infirmity. The authors stated that surgical treatment of patellar fractures can be difficult and that complications are common. Their indications for surgical intervention include a fracture displaced more than 2 cm, a significant extensor lag causing instability, or a loose, displaced patellar prosthesis.[5]

Grace and Sim[17] reviewed 12 patellar fractures in total knee arthroplasties. All patients presented with anterior knee pain and swelling. Treatment was based on the degree of fracture displacement, the amount of comminution, and the fixation of the patellar button. Fractures that had displacement greater than 5 mm, significant comminution, or a loose patellar prosthesis were considered candidates for operative repair. Eight fractures were treated in this fashion. Nonoperative treatment was reserved for those fractures that did not meet the above criteria. Four fractures were treated nonoperatively with 6 weeks of immobilization. Operative procedures included total patellectomy (four fractures), partial pat-

---

*References 5, 7, 16, 17, 20, 23, 32, 35, 37, 41.

ellectomy (two), tension band wiring (one), and circumferential wiring (one). Three of the four patients in the nonoperative group and five of the seven in the operative group had satisfactory clinical outcomes. There were three significant complications in the eight knees managed with operative repair. There was one quadriceps tendon rupture, one refracture, and one deep infection necessitating eventual arthrodesis. The authors recommended that treatment be individualized on the basis of fracture displacement, comminution, and the fixation of the button.[17]

Hozack et al.[20] performed a retrospective multicenter review of 21 patellar fractures. Eleven fractures were related to a traumatic event, whereas nine developed spontaneously. Nineteen fractures were associated with clinical findings, including extensor lag (nine), pain (18), swelling (12), and a palpable quadriceps defect (seven). Nonoperative treatment was selected in five cases. The remainder were treated with operative intervention including ORIF (two), patellectomy (10), and fragment excision with extensor mechanism repair (four). Because the results were drawn from several participating centers, the criteria for decision making were not uniform. Based on their assessment of these cases and on a review of the literature, the authors suggest that nonoperative management is effective for nondisplaced fractures and displaced fractures that do not exhibit an extensor lag. These authors concur with Thompson and colleagues[41] who also suggested that the physical examination was more important than the radiographic appearance when selecting treatment. Hozack et al. state that if nonoperative treatment is not successful, then a patellectomy may be performed for reliably good results. They further state that if a fracture is displaced and associated with an extensor lag, they cannot recommend nonoperative management, but that poor results can be expected with operative treatment. In their series, 12 patients were treated with operative intervention and only 3 (25%) had satisfactory clinical outcomes. When the patellar tendon is avulsed with a segment of the distal pole, these authors advocate excision of this fragment with primary repair of the patellar tendon to the remaining patella.[20]

Goldberg et al.[16] reported on 36 fractures of the resurfaced patella following total knee arthroplasty. These authors were the first to specifically address the effect that fracture type had on clinical outcome. To this end, they suggested a fracture classification including four major types. Type I included fractures that had no involvement of the implant-cement composite or extensor mechanism. Type II fractures do have involvement of the implant-composite or the extensor mechanism or both. Type IIIA are fractures of the inferior pole of the patella associated with a rupture of the patellar tendon. Type IIIB fractures are inferior pole fractures that do not have an associated rupture of the patellar tendon. Type IV includes fracture dislocations of the patella. Fourteen fractures were included in the type I category. All were treated nonoperatively and all had good or excellent results. Six fractures were included in type II. All of these underwent surgical intervention with two good results and four poor results. Eight patients suffered type IIIA fractures. Seven underwent surgical repair (one patient refused) resulting in five poor outcomes. Two patients suffered type IIIB fractures. Both were treated nonoperatively and both had good or excellent results. Six fractures were included in the type IV category. All underwent surgery with four patients subsequently classified as unsatisfactory clinical outcomes. The authors concluded that fractures not associated with loosening of the patellar component, disruption of the extensor mechanism, or major implant malalignment may be successfully managed nonoperatively. The 15 knees in this study treated in this fashion achieved a good or excellent clinical result. Six of the knees undergoing operative repair rated a good or excellent clinical outcome, while nine knees were rated as poor or failed.[16]

Figgie et al.[13] analyzed 36 patellar fractures in total condylar arthroplasties according to the type of fracture and the alignment of the implant. Preinjury radiographs were evaluated using ten criteria established to define neutral alignment. These criteria included factors such as restoration of joint line height, thickness of femoral condyles, mechanical axis, and patellar height, thickness, and coverage. The authors demonstrated that variables of alignment critically affected the rate, severity, and prognosis of patellar fractures. They stated that patellar fractures associated with only minor mismatches between the preoperative and postoperative joint lines and femoral condyle sizes, or those with minor malalignment would, in general, heal well with conservative treatment if the components were firmly fixed and the quadriceps mechanism was intact. Of the 20 knees that demonstrated major malalignment, 19 suffered a more severe patellar fracture and loosening of a component. Surgical management of these injuries should seek to correct the malalignment in addition to addressing the patellar fracture.[13]

Treatment

The decision on how to proceed with management of a fractured patella in total knee arthroplasty is predicated on the answers to two essential questions: Is the extensor mechanism disrupted on physical examination? Is the patellar component loose on radiographic examination? If the answer to both of these questions is no, then nonoperative treatment may be selected with a reasonable expectation of satisfactory clinical outcome. Recommended treatment includes immobilization of the knee for 6 weeks in full extension followed by a graduated program of muscle strengthening and active range-of-motion exercises. In the unlikely event that nonoperative treatment is unsuccessful, or if late symptoms develop, bracing or selective operative intervention may be warranted.

If the answer to either of these questions is yes, then one may consider surgical intervention with the clear understanding that this injury represents a serious complication of total knee arthroplasty and that despite good operative technique, the functional performance of the arthroplasty may be compromised. If operative intervention is selected, the goal is the restoration of the biomechanics of the patellofemoral articulation to its highest possible functional level.

If disruption of the extensor mechanism is associated with an avulsion of the inferior or superior pole of the patella, then resection of the fragment and advancement of the patellar tendon or quadriceps tendon is indicated. Tears of the medial and lateral retinaculum should also be searched for and carefully repaired. If there is a transverse fracture of the body of the patella and the implant is securely fixed to the major fragment, the minor fragment may either be resected or may be secured to the major fragment utilizing cerclage wire fixation. This is one of the few cases where ORIF may be indicated. ORIF with an elaborate construct is to be avoided. If the minor fragment appears thin, dysvascular, or cannot be anatomically reapproximated to the major fragment, then it should be discarded. Postoperatively, a cylinder cast should be employed for approximately 6 weeks followed by appropriate rehabilitation. Straight leg raise exercises and short-arc quadriceps strengthening are preferred along with a program of gentle passive and active assisted range-of-motion (ROM) exercises.

If the fracture is comminuted the initial treatment should be immobilization whether there is an extensor lag present or not. If the fragments are in reasonable approximation they may consolidate to form an acceptable fibrous or osseous union. Function may be assessed following an appropriate period of immobilization and rehabilitation. If symptoms warrant, a partial or total patellectomy may be considered. A total patellectomy with tubulation of the extensor mechanism (sewing of the rolled-under lateral quadriceps tendon to the medial quadriceps tendon and medial retinaculum) has been effective.[8]

If the patellar component is loose and symptomatic, then it should be removed (Fig 82–6). If there is sufficient bone stock remaining, resurfacing may be considered. If bone stock is inadequate, then partial patellectomy may be undertaken, removing only those fragments which cause impingement. Total patellectomy is also an option. Either procedure will result in an approximate 25% decline in quadriceps strength.

If the patellar fracture is associated with significant alteration of joint line height, overthickening of the trochlea, overthickening of the patella, or rotational malposition of the femoral or tibial components, then revision arthroplasty should be strongly considered.

TIBIAL FRACTURES

Tibial fracture is an infrequent complication of total knee arthroplasty. In the only significant series in the literature, Rand and Coventry[29] reported 15 medial tibial plateau fractures in patients who had either the Geometric or Polycentric designs (Howmedica, Rutherford, N.J.). Predisposing factors included limb malalignment, improper component orientation, and osteopenia. Even if fracture union was achieved, all of these fractures were associated with subsequent loosening of the tibial component requiring revision arthroplasty for satisfactory clinical outcome.

When considering treatment, tibial fractures should be subdivided into those that extend into the interface with the implant (i.e., plateau fractures) and those that do not. Fractures that include disruption of the bone-implant interface should be managed with revision of the tibial component combined with stable fixation of the fracture unless the patient is unsuitable for operative intervention for medical reasons. This holds true for both cemented and uncemented implants. If the interface is even partially disrupted it is unlikely that fracture union alone will result in favorable restoration of load distribution, and tibial component loosening will occur. The preferred treatment would be ORIF of the fracture and resurfacing of the tibia with a stemmed base plate. If cement is chosen for fixation, then care must be taken to prevent the extravasation of cement into the fracture planes.

Fractures of the tibial metaphysis and diaphysis that are not associated with loosening of the tibial component may be managed utilizing standard fracture principles. Irrespective of the method chosen, great care must be taken to ensure that proper limb

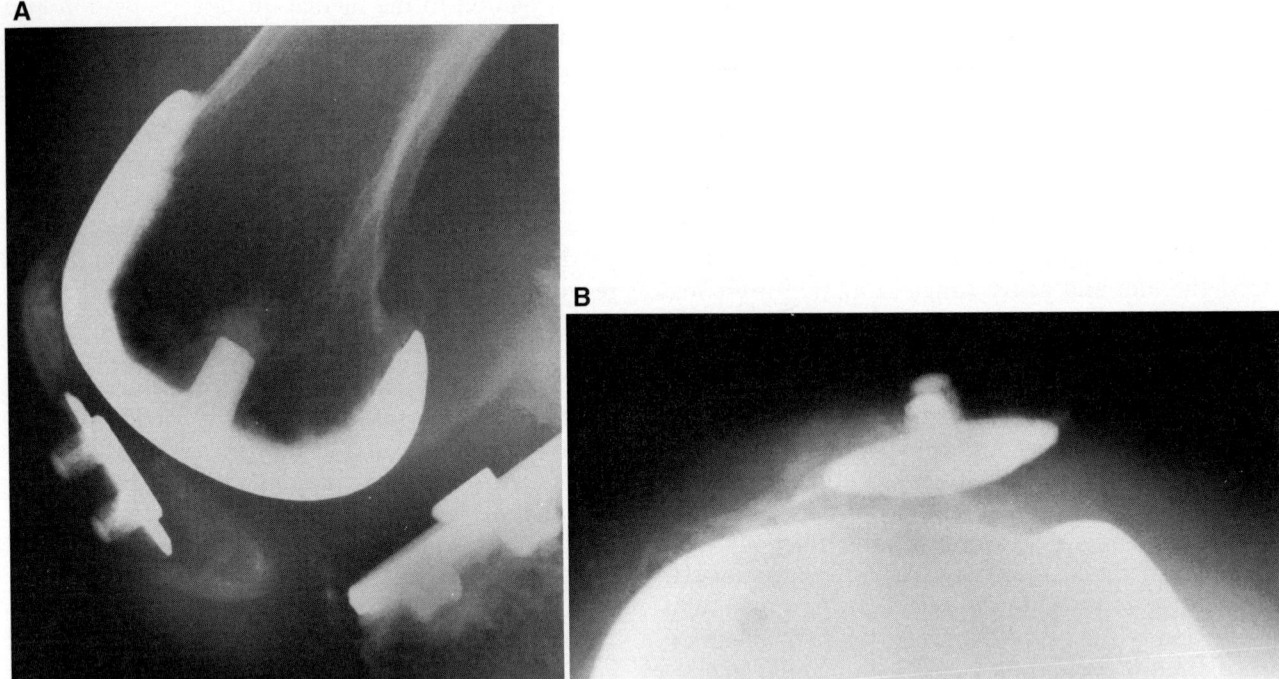

FIG 82-6.
Patellar fracture with dissociation of implant and disruption of extensor mechanism. This was managed successfully with patellectomy and extensor mechanism repair with tubulation.

alignment is maintained. If a nonarticular fracture of the tibia is associated with component loosening, both problems may be successfully addressed utilizing a long-stemmed tibial component that bypasses the fracture by no less than two stem diameters.

REFERENCES

1. Aaron R, Scott R: Supracondylar fracture of the femur after total knee arthroplasty, *Clin Orthop* 219:136, 1987.
2. Anderson SP, Matthews LS, Kaufer H: Treatment of juxtaarticular nonunion fractures at the knee with long stem total knee arthroplasty, *Clin Orthop* 260:104, 1990.
3. Bogoch E, et al: Supracondylar fractures of the femur adjacent to resurfacing and MacIntosh arthroplasties of the knee in patients with rheumatoid arthritis, *Clin Orthop* 229:213, 1988.
4. Bone L, et al: Early vs. delayed stabilization of femoral fractures: A prospective randomized study, *J Bone Joint Surg [Am]* 71:336, 1989.
5. Brick GW, Scott RD: The patellofemoral component of total knee arthroplasty, *Clin Orthop* 231:163, 1988.
6. Cain PR, et al: Periprosthetic femoral fractures following total knee arthroplasty, *Clin Orthop* 208:205, 1986.
7. Clayton ML, Thirupathi R: Patellar complications after total condylar arthroplasty, *Clin Orthop* 170:152, 1982.
8. Coleman SS: Personal communication, 1992.
9. Cordeiro E, et al: Periprosthetic fractures in patients with total knee arthroplasties, *Clin Orthop* 252:182, 1990.
10. Culp RW, et al: Supracondylar fractures of the femur following prosthetic knee arthroplasty, *Clin Orthop* 222:212, 1987.
11. Delport PH, et al: Conservative treatment of ipsilateral supracondylar femoral fracture after total knee arthroplasty, *J Trauma* 24:846, 1984.
12. DiGioia A, Rubash H: Periprosthetic fractures of the femur after total knee arthroplasty, *Clin Orthop* 271:135, 1991.
13. Figgie HE, et al: The effect of alignment of the implant on fractures of the patella after condylar total knee arthroplasty, *J Bone Joint Surg [Am]* 71:1031, 1989.
14. Figgie M, et al: The results of treatment of supracondylar fracture above total knee arthroplasty, *J Arthroplasty* 5:267, 1990.
15. Goldberg VM, et al: The results of revision total knee arthroplasty, *Clin Orthop* 226:86, 1988.
16. Goldberg VM, et al: Patellar fracture type and prognosis in condylar total knee arthroplasty, *Clin Orthop* 236:115, 1988.
17. Grace JN, Sim FH: Fracture of the patella after total knee arthroplasty, *Clin Orthop* 230:168, 1988.
18. Hanks G, et al: Supracondylar fracture of the femur following total knee arthroplasty, *J Arthroplasty* 4:289, 1989.
19. Hirsch D, Bhalla S, Roffman M: Supracondylar fracture of the femur following total knee replacement, *J Bone Joint Surg [Am]* 63:162, 1991.

20. Hozack WJ, et al: The treatment of patellar fractures after total knee arthroplasty, *Clin Orthop* 236:123, 1988.
21. Hungerford DS, Barry M: Biomechanics of the patellofemoral joint, *Clin Orthop* 144:9, 1979.
22. Johnson K, Cadambi A, Seibert G: Incidence of adult respiratory distress syndrome in patients with multiple musculoskeletal injuries: Effect of early operative stabilization of fractures, *J Trauma* 25:375, 1985.
23. Lynch AF, Rorabeck CH, Bourne RB: Extensor mechanism complications following total knee arthroplasty, *J Arthroplasty* 2:135, 1987.
24. Madsen F, et al: A custom-made prosthesis for the treatment of supracondylar femoral fractures after total knee arthroplasty: A report of four cases, *J Orthop Trauma* 3:332, 1989.
25. Merkel K, Johnson E: Supracondylar fracture in the femur after total knee arthroplasty, *J Bone Joint Surg [Am]* 68:29, 1986.
26. Neer C, Grantom S, Shelton M: Supracondylar fracture of the adult femur, *J Bone Joint Surg [Am]* 49:591, 1967.
27. Nielsen BF, Petersen VS, Varmarken JE: Fracture of the femur after knee arthroplasty, *Acta Orthop Scand* 59:155, 1988.
28. Oni OA: Supracondylar fracture of the femur following Attenborough stabilized gliding knee arthroplasty, *Injury* 14:250, 1983.
29. Rand J, Coventry M: Stress fractures after total knee arthroplasty, *J Bone Joint Surg [Am]* 62:226, 1980.
30. Rand J, Franco M: Revision considerations for fractures about the knee. In Goldberg VM, editor: *Controversies of total knee arthroplasty,* New York, 1991, Raven Press.
31. Rinecker H, Haiboeck H: Zur operativen Behandlung periprothetischer Oberschenkelfrakturen nach Kniegelenktotalendoprothesen, *Arch Orthop Unfall* 87:23, 1977.
32. Ritter MA, Campbell ED: Postoperative patellar complications with or without lateral release during total knee arthroplasty, *Clin Orthop* 219:163, 1987.
33. Ritter MA, Faris PM, Keating EM: Anterior femoral notching and ipsilateral supracondylar femur fracture in total knee arthroplasty, *J Arthroplasty* 3:185, 1988.
34. Ritter MA, Stiver P: Supracondylar fracture in a patient with a total knee arthroplasty: A case report, *Clin Orthop* 193:168, 1985.
35. Roffman M, Hirsh DM, Mendes DG: Fracture of the resurfaced patella in total knee replacement, *Clin Orthop* 148:112, 1980.
36. Roscoe MW, Goodman SB, Schatzker J: Supracondylar fracture of the femur after GUEPAR total knee arthroplasty, *Clin Orthop* 241:221, 1989.
37. Scott RD, Turoff N, Ewald FC: Stress fracture of the patella following duopatellar total knee arthroplasty with patellar resurfacing, *Clin Orthop* 170:147, 1982.
38. Scuderi GR, et al: The relationship of lateral release to patella viability in total knee arthroplasty, *J Arthroplasty* 2:209, 1987.
39. Short WH, Hootnick DR, Murry DG: Ipsilateral supracondylar femur fractures following knee arthroplasty, *Clin Orthop* 158:111, 1981.
40. Sisto DJ, Lachiewicz PF, Insall JN: Treatment of supracondylar fractures following prosthetic arthroplasty of the knee, *Clin Orthop* 196:265, 1985.
41. Thompson FM, Wood RW, Insall J: Patellar fractures in total knee arthroplasty, *Orthop Trans* 5:516, 1981.
42. Webster DA, Murray DG: Complications of variable axis total knee arthroplasty, *Clin Orthop* 193:160, 1985.

PART XVII

Tumors About the Knee

83

Tumors and Tumor-Like Lesions of the Knee

VINCENT J. VIGORITA, M.D.
CHARLES GATTO, M.D.
BERNARD GHELMAN, M.D.

Bone tumors of the knee
    Developmental, hamartomatous, and tumor-like lesions
        Cystic lesions of the knee
        Nonossifying fibroma
        Fibrous dysplasia
        Osteochondroma (exostosis)
        Osteoid osteoma
        Eosinophilic granuloma
    Benign tumors
        Chondroblastoma
        Enchondroma
        Periosteal (juxtacortical) chondroma
        Chondromyxoid fibroma
        Osteoblastoma
    Giant cell tumor
    Malignant tumors of the knee
        Osteosarcoma (osteogenic sarcoma)
        Chondrosarcoma
        Malignant fibrous histiocytoma and fibrosarcoma
        Ewing's sarcoma
        Lymphoma
        Multiple myeloma and metastatic carcinoma
            Multiple myeloma
            Metastatic carcinoma
        Secondary malignancies
Synovial tumors
    Benign tumors
        Synovial hemangioma
        Hoffa's disease (synovial lipomatosis)
        Synovial chondromatosis
        Pigmented villonodular synovitis
    Malignant tumors
        Synovial sarcoma
        Epithelioid sarcoma

BONE TUMORS OF THE KNEE

Although bone tumors are relatively rare, the knee is a relatively common site for osseous neoplasms.[16, 24, 33, 40] In fact, one third of bone tumors occur in the region of the knee, approximately half of which occur in the distal femur (Table 83–1). The proximal tibia is the next most common location for intraosseous bone tumors, followed far less commonly by the proximal fibula. Less than 1% of reported bone tumors occur in the patella. Approximately half of the tumors that arise in the bony structures of the knee in general, or distal femur in particular, are malignant (Table 83–2). Bone tumors of the proximal tibia are more commonly benign (60% vs. 40%). Most bone tumors arising in the proximal fibula and patella are benign.

Osteosarcoma is by far the most commonly reported primary knee tumor or tumor-like lesion, making up 32% of all reported cases, followed by osteochondroma (19%), giant cell tumor (15%), nonossifying fibroma (7%), and fibrosarcoma (5%). These tumors in the aggregate constitute over 75% of all primary tumors and tumor-like conditions. At the distal femur, osteosarcoma accounts for approximately 36% of all tumors, followed by osteochondroma (20%), giant cell tumor (13%), nonossifying fibroma (7%), and fibrosarcoma. These tumors and tumor-like lesions account for over 80% of all primary distal femur tumors. In the proximal tibia, the giant cell tumor follows the osteosarcoma (18% vs. 28%), these tumors making up a smaller percentage than tumors at other knee bone sites.

In the proximal fibula, osteosarcoma accounts for 20% of all reported primary bone tumors, followed by osteochondroma (16%), nonossifying fibroma

TABLE 83-1.
Tumor Locations as Percentage of Total Bone Tumors of the Knee

Tumor Location	Percentage of All Bone Tumors	Percentage of Bone Tumors of the Knee
Knee	33.8	100
Distal femur	19.0	56.1
Proximal tibia	12.5	37.0
Proximal fibula	2.2	6.6
Patella	0.1	0.3

TABLE 83-3.
Patellar Bone Tumors in Order of Frequency (%)

Types of Bone Tumor	Percentage of Total Reported Patellar Tumors
Chondroblastoma	32
Osteoblastoma	16
Giant cell tumor	16
Osteochondroma	10
Aneurysmal bone cyst	10
Osteoid osteoma	10
Osteosarcoma	3
Malignant fibrous histiocytoma	3

(14%), giant cell tumor (13%), and Ewing's sarcoma (7%), these five making up 75% of all primary proximal fibula tumors and tumor-like lesions. Fibrosarcoma is a less frequent diagnosis in this bone.

The large majority of tumors occurring in the patella are benign, with chondroblastoma being most frequently reported (32%), followed by giant cell tumor and osteoblastoma, each accounting for approximately 16% (Table 83-3). Kransdorf et al.[15] in 1989 reported 42 proven primary patellar tumors with 90% being benign: chondroblastoma accounted for 38%, giant cell tumor for 19%, and simple bone cyst for 14%.

Developmental, Hamartomatous, and Tumor-Like Lesions

Cystic Lesions of the Knee

The most common cystic-type replacement of bone tissue is that which ensues following the remodeling of bone pursuant to degenerative joint disease. However, there are at least three well-defined primary cystic lesions of the skeleton which may involve bones of the knee joint.

Unicameral Bone Cyst. Unicameral or simple bone cyst is a benign replacement of cancellous bone by a serous fluid, the cause of which is unknown.[7] The lesion occurs most frequently in the proximal femur and proximal humerus. Initiating in the metaphysis, it may be observed progressively down the shaft as the proximal and distal ends of the bone grow away during endochondral ossification. Only 4% of unicameral bone cysts occur at the knee. Unicameral bone cyst is the sixteenth most commonly reported primary osseous knee tumor or tumor-like lesion, with knee locations being most commonly observed in the proximal tibia (56%), followed by the distal femur (32%) and proximal fibula (12%). It has been rarely reported in the patella. Over 80% of unicameral bone cysts present between the ages of 5 and 20 years of age, with the male-to-female ratio being about 2.5:1. Simple bone cysts may cause an expansion of the cortex on the roentgenogram due to the remodeling effect of cortical bone. This may result in fractures, and thus pain, which is not an uncommon presentation of these lesions.

Aneurysmal Bone Cyst. The aneurysmal bone cyst (ABC) is a distinct, benign, pseudotumorous lesion of the bone which is usually differentiated from the simple bone cyst by both its roentgenographic and histopathologic appearance.[47] Its exact cause is not known, but it may be the result of the secondary effects of bone remodeling pursuant to areas of intraosseous vascular disturbances. Twenty-four percent of all ABCs occur at the knee. Classically, the ABC was described as an eccentric, trabeculated lesion in the skeleton, and it may occur at any osseous site. Recent studies have shown that numerous bone lesions may be partly complicated by features of an ABC, and therefore the pathologic diagnosis must be carefully correlated with the roentgenographic appearance to ensure diagnostic accuracy. The ABC is the sixth most common primary osseous knee tumor, constituting 3% of all tumors and tumor-like lesions. Its most common location at the knee is the proximal tibia (48%), followed by the distal femur (38%) and proximal fibula (14%). One percent of these tumors have been reported at the knee in the patella. It is usually metaphyseal in origin, but may extend to the epiphysis in adults. The peak age of the ABC is between 10 and 20 years with 75% of cases occurring

TABLE 83-2.
Ratio of Benign vs. Malignant Bone Tumors in Bones of the Knee*

Tumor Location	Benign Tumors(%)	Malignant Tumors (%)	Ratio
Knee	54	46	1.2:1
Distal femur	49	51	1:1
Proximal tibia	60	40	1.5:1
Proximal fibula	64	36	2:1
Patella	97	3	32:1

*Figures represent reported cases in the literature, not the actual prevalence of these lesions.

under 20 years of age. There is a more equal sex distribution to this lesion than that of the simple bone cyst.

The most common finding clinically is swelling at the lesion which may or may not be painful. In a third of the cases the onset of symptoms may be related to trauma: pathologic fracture may occur. Computed tomography (CT) scanning or magnetic resonance imaging (MRI) may be useful to evaluate the lesion and show mostly a fluid appearance of its contents. Grossly, the periosteum is usually elevated and intact, enveloping a thin rim of reactive bone. The lesion proper may appear bluish owing to acute and chronic bleeding, the cavity itself showing very hemorrhagic-appearing sponge-like cavities filled with blood and other fluid. Although not pulsatile, it is a vascular lesion. Bone tissue walls are thin, often with fibrous septa. The tissue itself is histologically different from that of a simple bone cyst that has a bland membrane as its salient microscopic feature. In an ABC there is a cellular cavity, often with the membranes filled with giant cells (Fig 83–1). The clinical course is variable, but may show progression. Others may spontaneously cease and may slowly ossify, repairing themselves, as is the case with simple bone cysts. ABCs may recur and, as mentioned, may be a complicating feature of a number of other neoplasms such as giant cell tumor, chondroblastoma, chrondomyxoid fibroma, and other lesions.

Ganglion Cysts. These rare benign cysts derive their name from their chemical and pathologic similarity to their far more common soft tissue counterpart.[2] Characteristically, a clear, gelatinous, self-contained lesion is seen in juxtaposition to eroded paraarticular bone.

Nonossifying Fibroma

The nonossifying fibroma (fibrous cortical defect, fibrous metaphyseal defect) is best considered a benign, hamartomatous, or developmental condition of the metaphyseal region of the bone in which there is a mixed fibroblastic, histiocytic, and foam cell proliferation, usually at the incorporation of tendinous or ligamentous insertions of the bone.[39] The anatomic occurrence at certain locations in the distal femur and proximal tibia supports the diagnosis of it occurring as a developmental error, 55% of them occurring at the knee. The nonossifying fibroma is the fourth most common reported tumor-like lesion of the knee, constituting approximately 7% of reported bone tumor cases. The most common location is the distal femur followed by the proximal tibia (54% vs. 33%) and the proximal fibula (13%), with no cases reported in the patella. This lesion occurs predominantly between the ages of 5 and 20 years, with as many as a third of all children aged 4 to 10 years old demonstrating such a lesion, usually a small, asymptomatic, regressing lesion.

Caffey,[8] in a roentgenographic survey of a pediatric population, showed that these lesions are quite common in the developmental group with gradual disappearance as the skeleton reaches maturation. Lesions histologically identical to the nonossifying fibroma in an adult may be seen and are best regarded as a benign fibrous histiocytoma[13] (Fig 83–2). Nonossifying fibromas are most commonly seen in a 1.5:1 male ratio and are most often completely asymptomatic. However, they may be large causing mild pain and pathologic fracture. Multiple nonossifying fibromas with associated pigmented skin lesions and congenital abnormalities have been reported in the literature. Roentgenographically, there is a characteristic lytic lesion located eccentrically, involving the cortex with sclerotic borders. Orientation is along the oblong axis, that is along the length of the bone. These lesions have a gross appearance showing yellowish-brown tissue, which is usually solid in appearance, and histologically are composed of a mixture of cells including giant cells, fibroblasts, histiocytes, and often foam cells. Hemosiderin may be present, as well as areas of collagen production.

Fibrous Dysplasia

Fibrous dysplasia is a slowly growing, developmental defect which replaces cancellous and eventually cortical bone with a fibro-osseous tissue.[18] Numerous

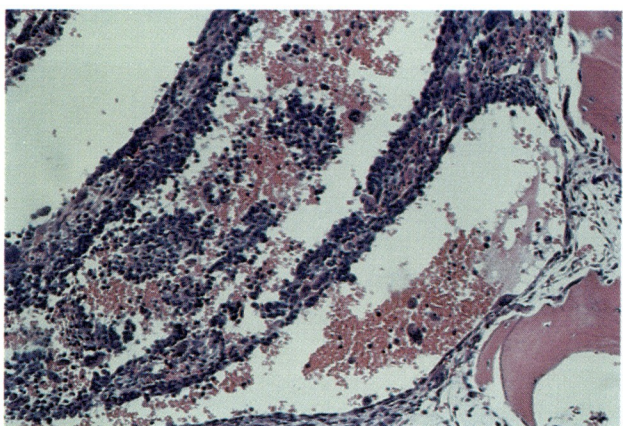

FIG 83–1.
Aneurysmal bone cyst. Photomicrograph of an aneurysmal bone cyst showing large vascular spaces filled with red blood cells. The underlying cancellous bone *(lower right)* is remodeling and is lined by a membrane composed of slender lining cells and multinucleated giant cells. Sinewy membrane extensions filled with mononuclear cells and giant cells course through the open vascular channels.

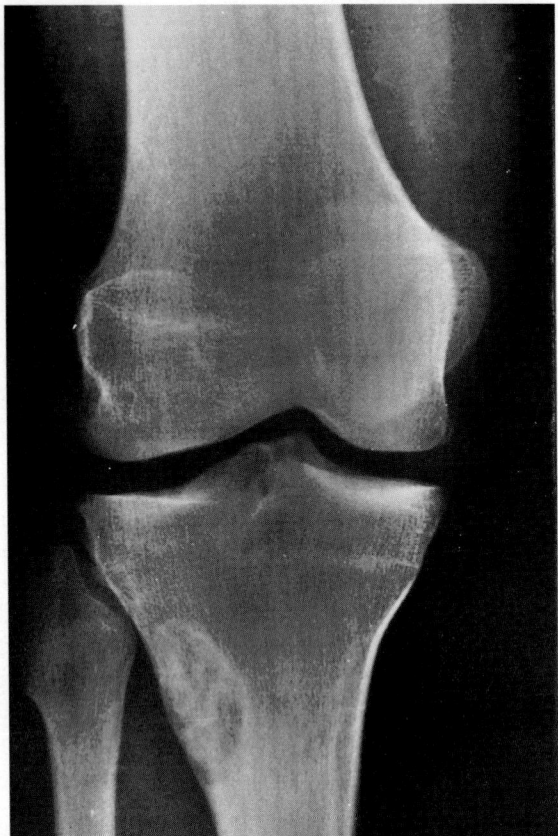

FIG 83–2.
Benign fibrous histiocytoma. Frontal radiograph of a well-defined lucent lesion in the lateral border of the proximal tibial metaphysis. The lesion causes moderate thinning and mild bulging of the adjacent cortex. Areas of increased density are seen in the lesion. This is a healing benign fibrous histiocytoma. The same lesion in a younger patient (note small osteophytes in the medial femoral condyle indicating that this is an adult patient) would be interpreted as a nonossifying fibroma.

sex distribution with symptoms, usually mild, proportional to the extent of the lesion. With lesions involving the proximal fibula or tibia there may be deformation as well as fractures. The radiographic appearance is typical in advanced lesions with replacement of predominantly cancellous, but also cortical bone by a fibrous and osseous stroma leading to relative radiolucency. There is often a fine granularity to the texture of the bone on radiograph, giving a ground-glass appearance. The cortex may be very thin with expansion of the overall diameter of the bone, often with cystic cavities. On gross examination the tumor has a compact, solid appearance with the microscopic appearance showing a replacement of the cancellous tissue by benign-appearing, sparsely cellular fibrous tissue intermixed with irregular spicules of cellular or woven bone (Fig 83–3). Rare foci of cartilage may occur, explaining the very rare complication of malignant tumor such as chondrosarcoma.

The course of fibrous dysplasia begins in childhood but is highly variable and dependent on the extent of the condition. There is eventual skeletal maturation in most cases. In general, there is need for surgical intervention in lower extremity lesions in patients younger than 18 years of age.[45] Sarcomatous transformation is rare, occurring in less than 1% of cases.

More recently, a skeletal lesion with a predilection for the mandible and tibia and initially referred to as an ossifying fibroma owing to prominent osteoblast rimming of bone spicules observed microscopically has been discussed as possibly representing a variant in the spectrum of fibroosseous lesions of the

types of fibrous dysplasia have been described including monostotic and polyostotic variants, polyostotic variants with endocrinopathy and skin lesions (Albright's syndrome), and an unusual type involving the facial bones leading to the appearance of cherubism. Albright's syndrome occurs in less than 5% of fibrous dysplasia cases. In general, fibrous dysplasia in all its variants is seen in the knee in 23% of cases. It is the seventh most common reported tumor or tumor-like lesion of the knee, composing approximately 3% of all cases. It occurs with almost equal distribution in the proximal tibia, distal femur, and proximal fibula, and less frequently in the proximal fibula, with rare occurrences in the patella.

Fibrous dysplasia usually begins in childhood with a peak onset of symptoms between the ages of 5 and 20 years. The more extensive the case, the earlier the onset of symptoms. There is an almost equal

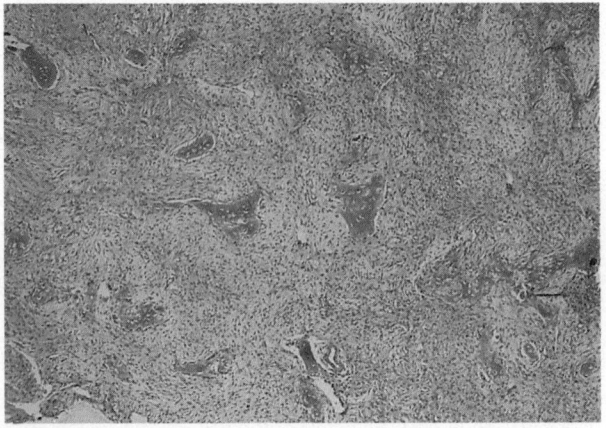

FIG 83–3.
Fibrous dysplasia. Photomicrograph revealing irregularly shaped spicules of cellular woven bone enmeshed in a matrix of bland cellularity producing abundant collagenized matrix, the admixture of irregular woven bone spicules and bland fibrous tissue characteristic of fibrous dysplasia.

skeleton. Campanacci has popularized the term *osteofibrous dysplasia* for this lesion, which is characterized by prominent cortical tibia involvement with anterior bowing[9, 10] (Fig 83–4).

Other fibrous tumors of the bone include periosteal desmoids and desmoplastic fibromas that mimic the abdominal wall desmoid, and are sparsely cellular fibrous lesions. Only 15% of all desmoid-like lesions occur in the knee, accounting for less than 1% of primary osseous tumors. The most common location is the proximal tibia (55%). Ninety percent are found in patients less than 30 years old. There is an equal sex distribution.

Osteochondroma (Exostosis)

Osteochondroma is a benign developmental tumor-like condition which represents an eccentric mass growing away from the joint space, most likely the independent growth of aberrant epiphyseal cartilage during early growth of the skeleton. These eccentric lesions may be sessile or pedunculated, and usually present as a mass. They may or may not be symptomatic depending on pressure effects on nerves or fracture of the stalk. It is the second most common tumor or tumor-like lesion of the knee, making up approximately 19% of all reported cases. Its most common location is the distal femur (61%), followed by the proximal tibia (33%), the proximal fibula (6%), and the patella (less than 1%). Osteochondromas peak in the 10- to 18-year-old age range with growth being greatest during puberty. Osteochondromas usually cease growth after skeletal maturation. Any solitary osteochondroma that continues to grow after skeletal maturation, as well as those changing in size in multiple hereditary exostosis (MHE), should be considered carefully for the diagnosis of chondrosarcomatous transformation. There is a slight male predominance for osteochondroma. The gross pathologic appearance is that of a mature piece of bone capped by a thin cartilaginous cap. Histologically, one sees a band of periosteum covering a proliferating zone of organized columns of chondrocytes which are undergoing endochondral ossification (Fig 83–5). The cap may be variable in thickness and fragments of the cap may fall off after trauma, developing separate growths similar to osseocartilaginous loose bodies seen in synovial loose bodies.

As mentioned, the osteochondroma may be seen as multiple lesions in the condition known as hereditary exostosis,[34] which is ten times less common than a solitary exostosis. In MHE there is often associated skeletal shortening of the involved limb, or deformity, and an increased incidence of malignant trans-

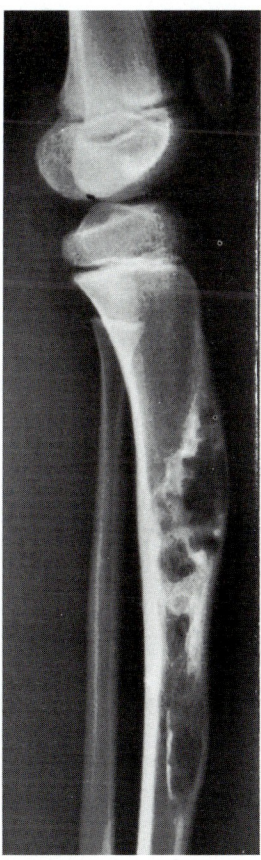

FIG 83–4.
Osteofibrous dysplasia. Lateral radiograph of a well-defined lucent and partially sclerotic lesion involving the anterior cortex of the midtibial shaft. The lesion is located mainly in the diaphyses. There is mild anterior bowing of the tibia with a normal growth plate and epiphysis.

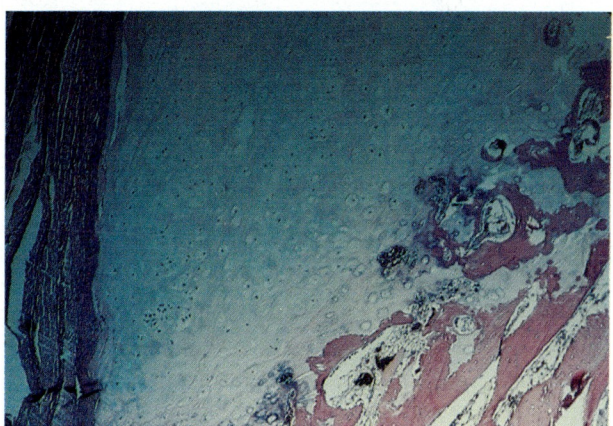

FIG 83–5.
Osteochondroma. Photomicrograph revealing a cartilaginous cap lined by a fibrous periosteum *(top)*. The cartilage cap consists of chondrocytes often lined up in columns which are undergoing endochondral ossification *(central bottom)* similar to that seen at an active epiphysis. The cartilage becomes calcified and then remodels into cancellous bone.

formation, which most likely occurs in 1% to 10% of these cases.

Osteoid Osteoma

Pain, often severe at night, and relieved by aspirin, with a characteristic, hot, well-circumscribed lesion on bone scan, is characteristic of osteoid osteoma, a small, most likely reactive lesion of the skeleton.[26] Osteoid osteoma characteristically occurs as a well-defined nidus of remodeling spicules of cancellous-type bone within the cortex. Less commonly it is seen in the cancellous marrow bone and even less frequently in a subarticular or juxtarticular location. It is the eleventh most common tumor-like lesion in large series, composing approximately 2% of all reported cases, but 13% of all cases occurring in the knee. The most common location in the knee is the cortical bone of the proximal tibia (61%), followed by the distal femur (33%), proximal fibula (5%), and patella (2%).

Osteoid osteoma has a classic roentgenographic appearance and has a peak age of occurrence in the pediatric population, age 11 to 20 years, with 95% of cases occurring between age 5 and 30 years. There is a 2.3:1 male predominance. The lesion is characteristically examined for its associated pain, with the roentgenogram showing a zone of sclerosis. In many cases on the radiograph, and more sensitively on the CT scan, a centralized radiolucent nidus may be detected embedded within the sclerotic cortical bone (Fig 83–6). These lesions may be difficult to localize surgically, but studies with bone scanning agents have indicated that the central lucent nidus is the area of most intense radioactive uptake, a phenomenon which has formed the basis for radioisotope localization techniques to localize this lesion.[48] These lesions may be difficult to see grossly because they may be small, usually less than 1 cm (Fig 83–7). Surgical removal is curative.

Eosinophilic Granuloma

Eosinophilic granuloma is a tumor-like proliferation of chronic inflammatory cells, eosinophils, histiocytes, and Langerhans cells which may involve one or multiple bones, and in rare circumstances may be associated with diabetes insipidus and exophthalmos (Hand-Schüller-Christian disease). Most often the clinical presentation of eosinophilic granuloma to the orthopaedic surgeon is that of a solitary lesion, which not uncommonly presents in the femur or tibia.[21] It often manifests as pain or swelling in the extremity of a child. The lesion may clinically and roentgenographically mimic osteomyelitis, fibrous dysplasia, Ewing's sarcoma, and in some instances even osteo-

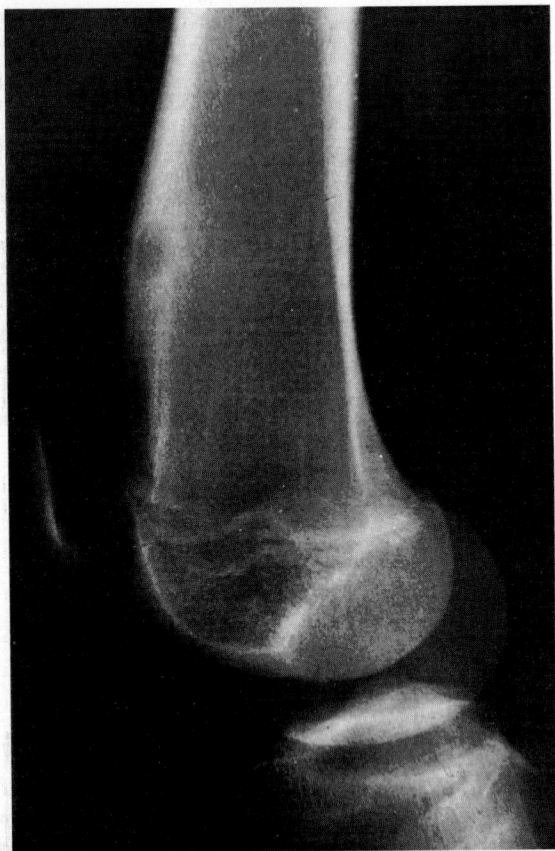

FIG 83–6.
Osteoid osteoma. Lateral radiograph of a small central lucency (the nidus) surrounded by sclerosis in the anterior cortex of the distal femur. At times small central calcifications can be seen in the nidus of an osteoid osteoma.

genic sarcoma. A biopsy is necessary to confirm the diagnosis of eosinophilic granuloma, which is a benign, usually nonprogressive osseous lesion of limited duration. Although lesions have been treated both surgically and with medical intervention, including chemotherapy, the solitary variant may follow a limited course and most likely represents a reactive or transient immunologic abnormality. The diagnosis is confirmed by identifying the diagnostic Langerhans giant cell, a cell which is present normally in numerous anatomic sites, including the skin, but proliferates in rare circumstances. The Langerhans giant cell is identified by the characteristic Birbeck granules, peculiar pentalamellar structures identified by electron microscopy.[49] The Langerhans cells most probably are peripheral antigen-processing cells of bone marrow origin which process various antigens stimulating an immunologic reaction.

Formerly, eosinophilic granuloma was considered part of a spectrum of lesions termed histiocytosis X, which included the solitary eosinophilic granu-

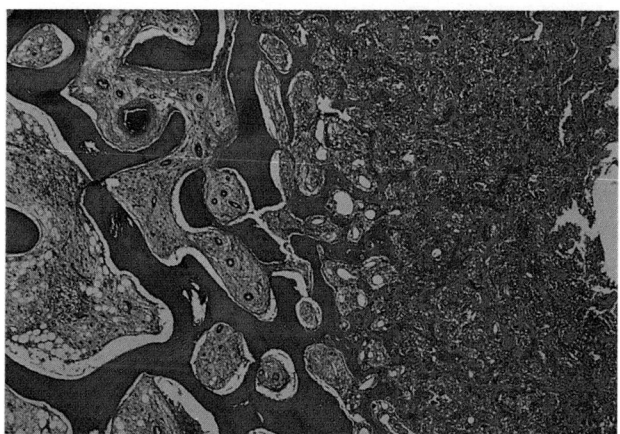

FIG 83-7.
Osteoid osteoma. The well-circumscribed nidus (left) is seen in contradistinction to the surrounding remodeling bone (right) and is characterized by small, interweaving spicules of markedly remodeling bone with osteoblasts forming abundant osteoid in a well-vascularized stroma.

loma, Hand-Schüller-Christian disease and Letterer-Siwe disease. The last disorder, however, is a distinct clinicopathologic entity which carries a poor prognosis and acts clinically more like a progressive lymphoproliferative disorder.

Benign Tumors

Chondroblastoma

Chondroblastoma characteristically occurs as a slowly growing benign lytic lesion over the epiphysis in a skeletally immature person[34] (Fig 83-8). Thirty-six percent of all chondroblastomas occur in the knee. It is the 12th most commonly reported primary osseous tumor of the knee and occurs with almost equal distribution in the proximal tibia (48%) and distal femur (45%). Five percent of knee chondroblastomas occur in the patella with the fibula being the least common site (2%). The peak age of occurrence is between 10 and 20 years of age (85%) with a 1.8:1 male-to-female ratio. The lesion usually presents with pain and may rarely involve the articular cartilage causing symptoms primarily associated with the joint. A fracture into the chondroblastoma may lead to loose bodies, and even mimic osteochondritis dissecans roentgenographically and clinically. The origins of chondroblastoma are not known, but ultrastructural studies have suggested that the major cell in this tumor has some similarities to a primitive cartilaginous cell. Histologically, chondroblastoma is characterized by a polygonal cell population with focal areas of calcification noted in approximately 50% of cases, the calcification often appearing in a linear fashion enveloping individual cells (Fig 83-9). The lesion may be cellu-

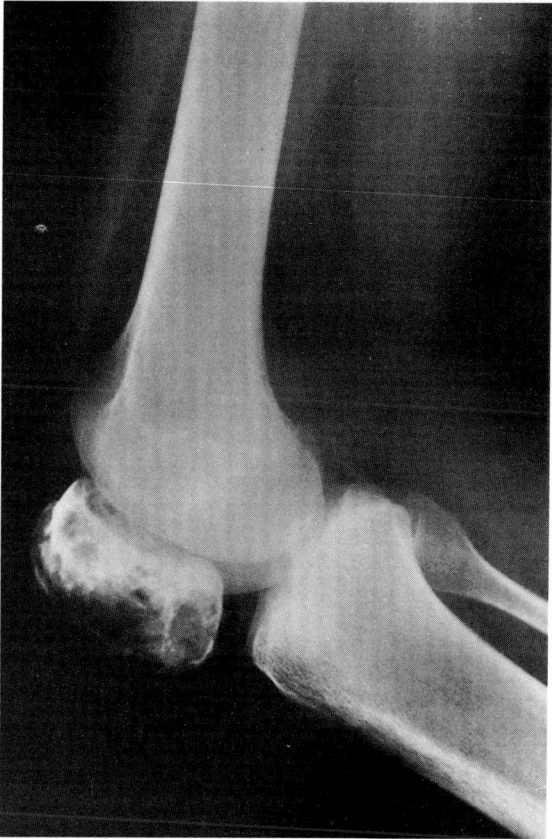

FIG 83-8.
Chondroblastoma. Lateral radiograph of a large, lucent, and partially sclerotic lesion occupying most of the patella in a 17-year-old patient. Plain radiographs and CT scan demonstrated the sclerosis mainly in the periphery of the lesion. There was no evidence for punctate calcifications in the lesion. This is an unusual location for a chondroblastoma (Codman's tumor) which is most often found in the proximal humeral and femoral epiphyses.

lar and may be confused microscopically with a malignant tumor.

Enchondroma

Enchondromas are benign tumors of well-differentiated cartilage. Only 5% of all solitary enchondromas occur in the knee. Enchondromas may occur as a solitary lesion, or as a more developmental problem involving multiple bones. (Ollier's disease). This rare form of enchondromatosis may lead to marked deformities of the involved bone and is associated with development of chondrosarcoma. Solitary enchondroma constitutes approximately 1% of all knee tumors. Its most common location at the knee is the distal femur (41%), followed by the proximal fibula (30%), proximal tibia (29%), and patella (1%). It is most commonly diagnosed in the knee during the first 20 years of life and has no sex predilection.

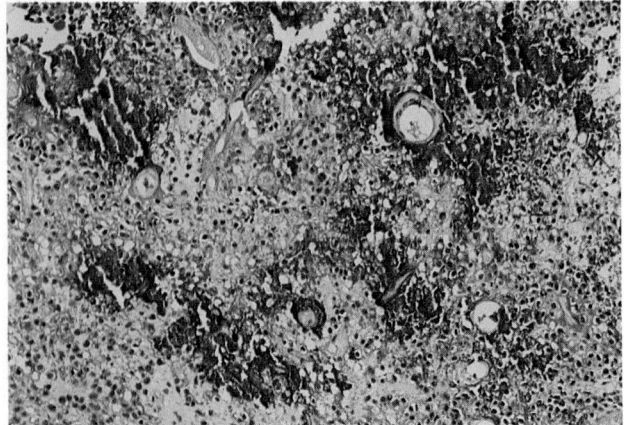

FIG 83-9.
Chondroblastoma. These cellular lesions are characterized by proliferating mononuclear cells producing a grayish-blue chondroid matrix, which focally undergoes calcification, often surrounding individual chondrocytes in a punctate linear fashion. The cell population is polygonal with varying degrees of cytoplasm, chondroid matrix, and calcification.

Enchondromas roentgenographically occur as purely lytic lesions or with a cluster of punctate calcifications. The latter may mimic a chondrosarcoma roentgenographically and histologically (Fig 83–10). Histologically, enchondromas are characterized by well-differentiated cartilage with focal areas of calcification (Fig 83–11). Unlike chondrosarcoma, these lesions are usually not pleomorphic and are usually enveloped by the normal surrounding lamellar bone.

Periosteal (Juxtacortical) Chondroma

Periosteal or juxtacortical chondroma is a benign cartilage tumor usually arising on the surface of cortical bone in the diaphysis or metaphysis.[3] It is most common during adolescence or young adulthood and characteristically has a radiographic appearance of a saucer-shaped indentation of the cortical bone. Because of increased cartilaginous cellularity, it may be misdiagnosed and overtreated. The most common presenting symptoms are pain and swelling. Marginal excision usually suffices.

Chondromyxoid Fibroma

Chondromyxoid fibroma is a benign tumor composed of fibrous tissue, myxoid connective tissue, and tissue differentiating toward cartilage.[19] It almost always arises in regions of fetal metaphyseal cartilage. Forty-five percent of all chondromyxoid fibromas reported in the literature occur in the knee: the proximal tibia accounts for 76%, the distal femur for 15%, and the proximal fibula for 10%. Over 80% of cases in general occur between the ages of 5 and 30 years, with a 1.5:1 male preponderance.

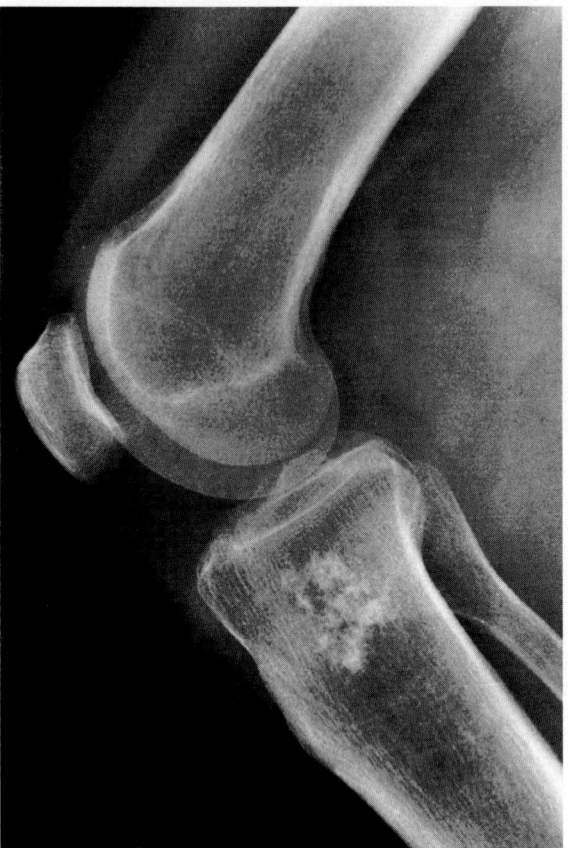

FIG 83-10.
Enchondroma. Lateral radiograph showing punctate calcifications in the proximal metaphyses of the tibia, a lesion which can be confused with a bone infarction.

Osteoblastoma

Osteoblastoma is a benign tumor that is characterized histologically by its similarity to osteoid osteoma in which there is abundant osteoblast cellularity with production of osteoid and bone in an irregular organization.[26] Only 10% of reported osteoblastomas occur in the knee, constituting less than 1% of primary bone tumors of the knee (proximal tibia, 64%; distal femur, 22%). The patella accounts for a surprisingly high percentage of knee cases (14%). Approximately 90% of these tumors occur between age 5 and 30 years, with a 3:1 male predominance. These lesions are usually larger than 2 cm and have a roentgenographic appearance that may vary from one of pure lysis to one in which there is detectable bone formation.

Giant Cell Tumor

Giant cell tumor, or osteoclastoma, occurs at the end of the bones as a well-circumscribed lytic lesion usually abutting the articular cartilage.[11, 27] It derives its

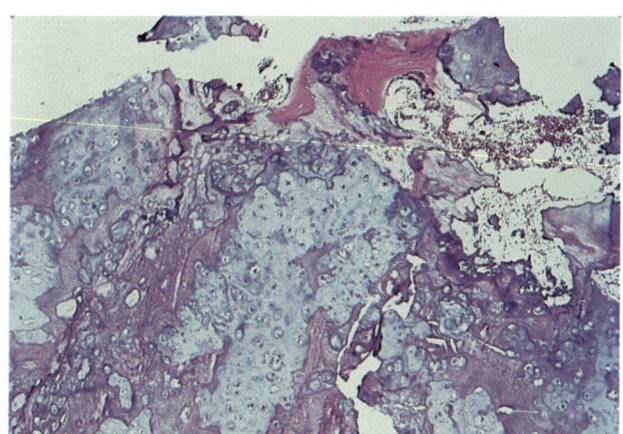

FIG 83-11.
Enchondroma. Proliferative chondrocytes in a grayish-blue matrix are characteristic of enchondromas, which typically calcify *(deep purple)* and remodel into bone *(pink)* in interconnecting islands replacing the underlying normal marrow fat and bone *(upper right).*

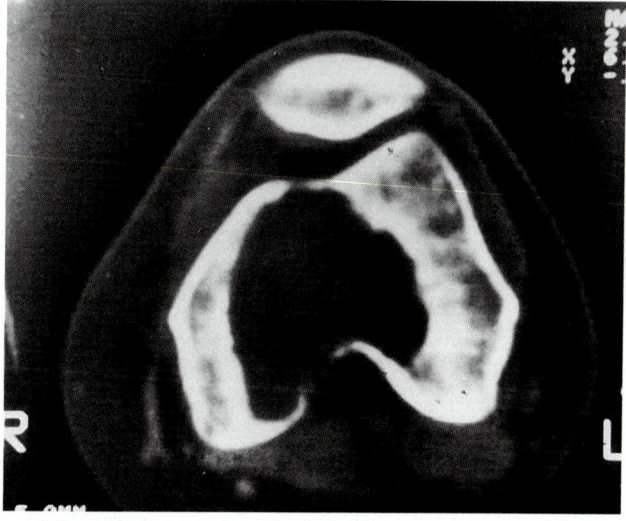

FIG 83-12.
Giant cell tumor of bone. CT scan through the distal femur demonstrating a well-defined lucent lesion replacing most of both femoral condyles. The lucency of the lesion is homogeneous. There is no evidence of calcification in the tumor. Minimal sclerosis surrounds the neoplasm. The posterior cortex of the femur is invaded by the lesion, resulting in a small lucent defect.

name from the microscopic appearance in which there is a sea of multinucleated giant cells enmeshed in a noninflammatory mesodermal mononuclear cell matrix of uncertain histogenesis. Although most giant cell tumors are benign, the lesion may metastasize. Giant cell tumors that are fully malignant from the start and act in a sarcomatous fashion are also well documented in the literature. This is the third most commonly reported primary osseous tumor of the knee, composing 15% of all reported cases, occurring with approximately equal distribution between the distal femur (48%) and proximal tibia (46%); 6% of cases have been reported in the proximal fibula and less than 1% in the patella. The peak age of occurrence for giant cell tumor is the young adult, with 80% of cases occurring between 20 and 40 years of age. It is very rare prior to puberty. Thus lytic lesions at the end of the bone prior to skeletal maturation favor the diagnosis of chondroblastoma, and after skeletal maturation, giant cell tumor. There is a slight female predilection in reported cases.

Clinically, the major symptom is pain, usually in the joint, with decreased range of motion often due to effusion or expansion of the bone. Although the tumor abuts the articular cartilage, it rarely extends into the joint space. There may be swelling, and pathologic fracture is not uncommon. Characteristically, there is a well-defined radiolucent mass on the roentgenogram, with well-defined borders (Fig 83-12). It is usually situated eccentrically at metaphyseal-epiphyseal areas. Classification of giant cell tumors roentgenographically has been proposed and is reputed to be of prognostic value. In the Enneking staging system,[17] stage I "quiescent" lesions appear small and slowly expand with an intact cortex and well-defined borders. Active lesions (stage II) usually show a thinned or missing cortex, but have an intact periosteum. Borders are less clear. This is the most common form encountered. In stage III, or the aggressive giant cell tumor, the cortex is destroyed. The tumor is not confined by the periosteum. Here a large expansive lesion, possibly extending to articular cartilage, suggests rapid growth.

Grossly, giant cell tumors appear as usually solid lesions with a light brown to red color, uniform, without bone or calcification. There may be associated hyperemia and marked bleeding at incision. Histologically, the characteristic uniform and even distribution of giant cells is diagnostic. Histologic study alone and even flow cytometry studies of the DNA content of the nuclei of cells from giant cell tumors are unable to predict which of these lesions will metastasize.

The clinical course of giant cell tumors is highly variable, ranging from local growth over years, to more rapid invasion in brief periods of time. Although malignant transformation has been reported in 5% of cases, one cannot exclude that these malignant giant cell tumors are not sarcomas from the beginning. Malignant giant cell tumors may have fibrosarcomatous, malignant fibrous histiocytomatous, or osteosarcomatous areas, raising the possibility of initial diagnostic accuracy. Radiation treatment is contraindicated because of the potential for sarcomatous stimulation. Local recurrence has been reported in less than 10% with appropriate surgical treatment, and usually occurs within 3 years of surgery. Patients with pulmonary metastases may survive with the appropriate treatment.

Malignant Tumors of the Knee

Osteosarcoma (Osteogenic Sarcoma)

Osteosarcoma, or osteogenic sarcoma, is a highly malignant tumor which, by definition, produces neoplastic osteoid or bone, or both. It characteristically arises within the metaphysis of the long bones and grows circumferentially through the cortex into the soft tissue raising the periosteum. It rarely invades the joint space. Fifty-six percent of all osteogenic sarcomas occur at the knee resulting in it being the most common primary osseous knee tumor reported in the literature (32%). Of osteogenic sarcomas of the knee, 64% occur in the distal femur, 32% in the proximal tibia, 4% in the proximal fibula, and less than 1% in the patella. Osteogenic sarcoma characteristically occurs at the adolescent growth spurt, with the peak age of occurrence between 10 and 20 years of age, 75% of all cases occur between 10 and 30 years of age. There is a male predominance of 1.5:1. In the immature skeleton with an intact growth plate, the epiphysis may act as a relative barrier to its growth. Osteogenic sarcoma typically presents with pain, which is often mild and intermittent initially, but more continuous and exacerbated by deep palpation later. A mass or a swelling may be felt. Rarely one encounters a pathologic fracture. The laboratory hallmark of an osteogenic sarcoma is an elevated alkaline phosphatase, usually in excess of that noted during pediatric growth. The characteristic radiograph reveals a radiodense lesion over the metaphysis with indistinct borders and periosteal elevation (Fig 83–13). The raised periosteum creates a triangle (referred to as Codman's triangle) whose borders are the intact cortex, the tumor, and the periosteum proper. CT scans may be helpful in defining soft tissue or joint penetration, with MRI defining involvement of cancellous and medullary bone.

Grossly, the osteogenic sarcoma is a hard, compact tumor (Fig 83–14). The external layers tend to be softer and more suitable for biopsy. Histologically, osteogenic sarcoma is characterized by the presence of sarcomatous osteoblast cells producing a disorganized maze of calcified tissue including osteoid and bone (Fig 83–15). The lesion may vary from one that is very cellular with little osteoid or bone production to those that are sparsely cellular with abundant calcified matrix being produced. Osteogenic sarcoma, for which there is an animal model in the Great Dane, has a seeming predilection for areas of rapid growth.

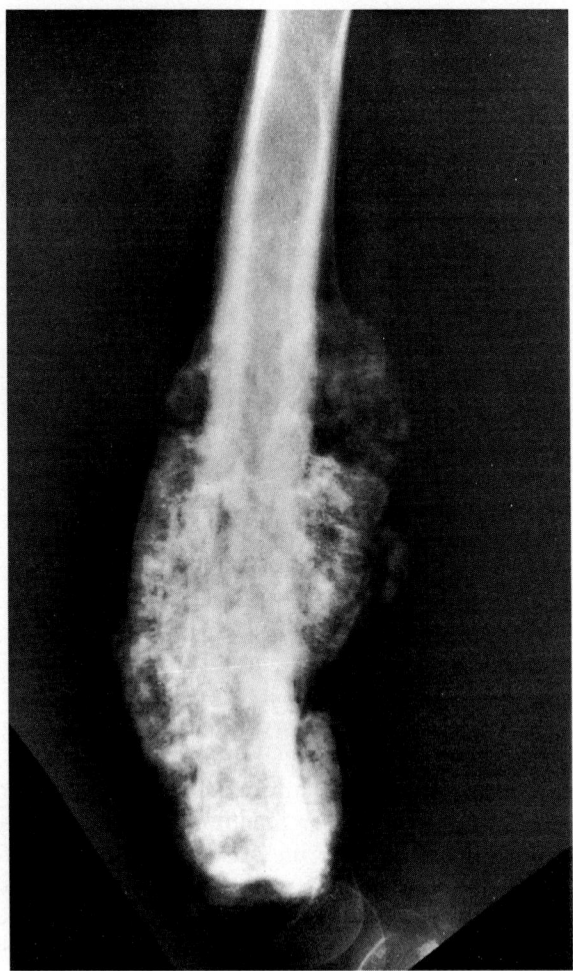

FIG 83–13.
Osteogenic sarcoma. Lateral radiograph showing a large blastic lesion extending from the distal metaphysis to the diaphysis of the femur. Extensive periosteal and tumor bone formation surrounds the distal femur. Periosteal new bone formation tends to be better organized, with areas of density perpendicular or parallel to the involved bone. Tumor bone tends to be disorganized and is usually seen as patches of increased density. The differentiation between periosteal and tumor bone formation is difficult. In this case the epiphysis of the distal femur is not involved by the tumor.

It occurs, as mentioned, in the adolescent growth spurt, and also is seen with increased incidence in bone affected by Paget's disease.[23, 41] Osteogenic sarcoma grows by relatively rapid local expansion and metastases to the lungs. With the advent of adjuvant therapy, including chemotherapy and surgical removal, the 5-year survival of children with osteogenic sarcoma without evidence of disseminated disease, is approximately 60% to 70%.[34, 35] Of prognostic value is the response to preoperative chemotherapy with a favorable outlook when 90% of the tumor is necrosed. Other prognostic indicators include the size and extent of cortical and soft tissue penetration.

Osteosarcoma Variants. Numerous variants of

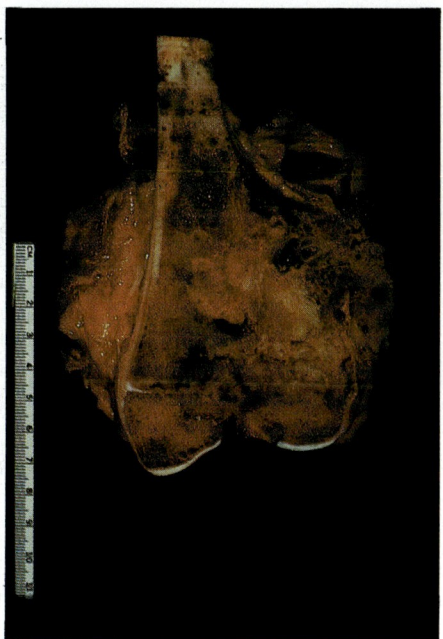

FIG 83–14.
Osteogenic sarcoma. Gross photograph of osteogenic sarcoma at the distal metaphysis of the proximal femur showing a bone-forming lesion expanding into the surrounding soft tissue and lifting up the periosteum *(top right)*. The marrow itself and surrounding soft tissue is replaced by a heterogeneous matrix destroying the bone, the epiphyseal growth plate acting as a relative barrier to spread, with relative sparing of the epiphysis.

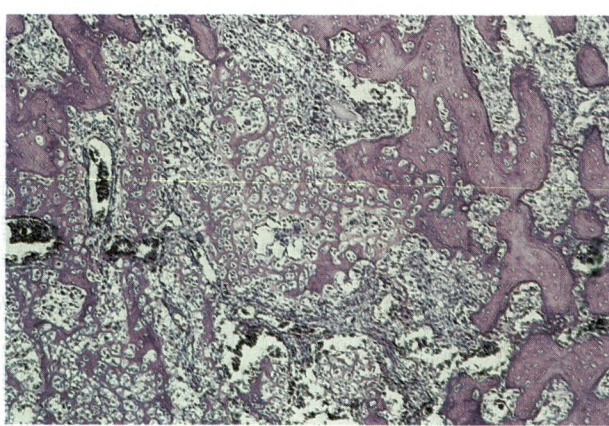

FIG 83–15.
Osteogenic sarcoma. Photomicrograph of osteogenic sarcoma showing the underlying remodeling cancellous bone *(lower left)* being replaced by the juxtaposition of a highly irregular cellular population of cells producing a highly disorganized bone matrix. The replacement of marrow fat and bone by irregular osteoid and bone production is characteristic of osteogenic sarcoma.

osteogenic sarcoma have been described, including a low-grade well-differentiated tumor, a hemorrhagic radiolucent lesion mimicking an aneurysmal bone cyst (telangiectatic osteogenic sarcoma),[36] and one confined to the cortex of bone (intracortical osteogenic sarcoma). Osteogenic sarcomas may also occur on the surface of the bone, and at least three variants have been described: a high-grade osteogenic sarcoma which mimics classic osteogenic sarcoma histologically; a periosteal osteogenic sarcoma that tends toward chondroblastic differentiation, and the most distinctive of the group, the parosteal or juxtacortical osteogenic sarcoma, which is a lesion of fibroblastic differentiation with a predilection for the distal posterior aspect of the distal femur.[38] In addition to the anatomic variants, there are numerous histologic variants, most notably the small cell osteogenic sarcoma which is highly malignant and mimicks an undifferentiated small cell tumor such as Ewing's sarcoma.[31]

Parosteal or juxtacortical osteogenic sarcoma is generally slow-growing. It is the tenth most common primary osseous tumor reported in the literature, accounting for approximately 2% of cases. Sixty-nine percent of all parosteal osteogenic sarcomas occur at the knee, a higher prevalence than classic osteogenic sarcoma. The distal femur is the most common location (86%) occurring posteriorly with growth or swelling into the popliteal space. Ten percent occur in the proximal tibia and 4% percent in the proximal fibula, with no cases reported in the patella. Parosteal or juxtacortical osteogenic sarcoma occurs in an older age group than does classic osteogenic sarcoma, with 95% of all cases occurring between the ages of 15 and 40 years. In contradistinction to classic osteogenic sarcoma, there is a 1.4:1 female predilection. The tumor is characterized by pain and swelling late in the course of the disease with a decreased range of motion.

Roentgenographically, there is a mass at the surface of the bone, which is often radiodense. CT scans and MRI may be useful in ascertaining cortical invasion, a factor which has prognostic significance since the classic juxtacortical surface tumor carries a better prognosis than one involving the medullary cavity. On gross examination the tumor is hard with a pseudocapsule, the tumor itself enveloping the bone. It may be adherent to the soft tissue or the cortex. The clinical course is that of slow progression. Metastases by hematogenous spread may occur more than 5 years after excision. With a wide margin recurrence is rare, but may occur as long as a decade after surgery. Overall, survival is approximately 80%.

Chondrosarcoma

Chondrosarcoma occurs as a malignant lesion within the medullary cavity in a skeletally mature person.[20] Although the classic chondrosarcoma is one which arises de novo in essentially normal bone, chondrosarcoma may develop in preexisting lesions including multiple hereditary exostoses and Ollier's disease.[20] As with osteogenic sarcoma, there are several anatomic and microscopic variants of this tumor. Anatomically, chondrosarcomas may arise either on the surface of the bone—the periosteal chondrosarcoma—or in the soft tissue. They may also complicate, in rare circumstances, benign conditions such as synovial chondromatosis[30] and fibrous dysplasia. Well-described microscopic variants include those which mimic a small cell tumor (mesenchymal chondrosarcoma),[25] those which have a purely lytic appearance and mimic metastatic renal cell carcinoma (clear cell chondrosarcoma),[5] and one in which there is a highly malignant-appearing spindle cell tumor (dedifferentiated chondrosarcoma).[29]

Twelve percent of the classic cases of medullary chondrosarcoma occur at the knee. It is the ninth most commonly reported primary bone tumor, constituting approximately 2% of all bone tumors. Its most common location in the knee is the proximal tibia (54%), followed by the distal femur (40%) and the proximal fibula (6%). In adults, in whom it is most commonly reported, the chondrosarcoma frequently invades the epiphysis and may even involve the joint. Most cases occur between the ages of 30 and 70 years with rare occurrences before age 20 years. There is a 1.6:1 male-to-female ratio. Chondrosarcomas classically show a slow growth often with a nonspecific clinical history, but vague, mild intermittent pain may occur. Epiphyseal involvement, which is common, can cause effusions. Pathologic fractures are rare.

Roentgenographically, there is a slowly growing lytic lesion, which is usually calcified, eroding the inner aspect of the cortical bone leaving a scalloped appearance. It is somewhat eccentric at the metaphyseal area, and unlike osteogenic sarcoma, preferentially grows down the medullary cavity. In general the cortex is thinned and even perforated. Grossly, chondrosarcoma has a bluish-gray appearance with calcifications apparent. There is usually a fine gritty texture present. Microscopically, the tumor is characterized by neoplastic pleomorphic cartilage cells, the degree of differentiation toward cartilage being variable (Fig 83–16). In low-grade lesions there may be only slight cytologic abnormalities making the differential diagnosis from benign enchondromas quite difficult. However, most cases exhibit a degree of variation from cell to cell, and crowding of cells and abnormal mitotic figures, making the diagnosis less difficult. Obviously, large pleomorphic tumors carry a worse prognosis.

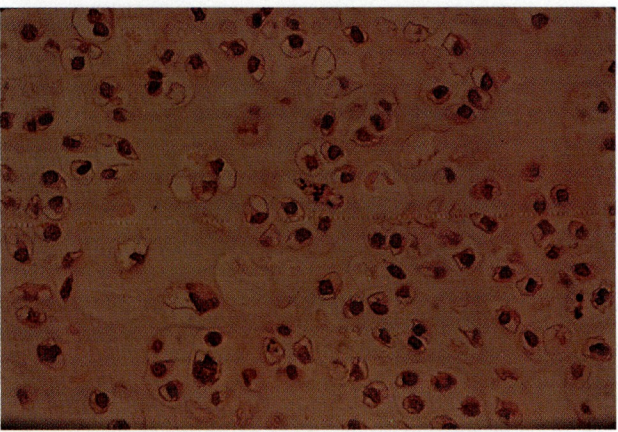

FIG 83–16.
Chondrosarcoma. Photomicrograph of chondrosarcoma revealing pleomorphic chondrocytes with atypical mitoses *(center)* enmeshed in a chondroid matrix. The variation from cell to cell, the highly irregular nuclear configurations, the atypical mitoses, and the often binuclear chondrocytes are typical of a malignant cartilage tumor.

In general, the clinical course is more indolent than that of osteogenic sarcoma. The tumor spreads by the hematogenous route and therefore pulmonary metastases may be encountered.

Dedifferentiated Chondrosarcoma. The dedifferentiated chondrosarcoma is a highly malignant sarcomatous tumor originating in a preexisting chondrosarcoma.[28] It is characterized by the juxtaposition of classic chondrosarcomatous areas with a fully malignant, spindle cell tumor, usually a fibrosarcoma or malignant fibrous histiocytoma. Some believe this tumor to be a pluripotential malignant tumor from its onset. However, the classic roentgenographic appearance showing a typical calcified cartilaginous tumor adjacent to a purely lytic permeating lesion supports a change in an underlying chondrosarcoma. Eighteen percent of all reported dedifferentiated chondrosarcomas occur in the knee, with the tumor accounting for less than 1% of reported knee tumors. The most common location in the knee is the distal femur (76%), followed by the proximal tibia (24%), with no cases reported in the proximal fibula and patella. Its more frequent occurrence in the knee than classic chondrosarcoma suggests a predilection for this site. The tumor usually occurs after age 50 years with the peak between 60 and 70 years of age. There is a slight male predominance. Dedifferentiated chondrosarcoma is a highly malignant tumor with a poor prognosis.

Mesenchymal Chondrosarcoma. Mesenchymal chondrosarcoma is a rare form of chondrosarcoma that is characterized by a population of undifferentiated, mononuclear malignant cells mimicking other small cell malignant tumors such as Ewing's sarcoma and lymphoma.[25] However, admixed with the poorly differentiated small cell population are areas of recognizable chondrosarcoma. The prognosis is poor. Only 8% of cases have been reported in the knee. This rare tumor may occur in the distal femur (50%), proximal fibula (30%), and proximal tibia (20%).

Malignant Fibrous Histiocytoma and Fibrosarcoma

Two predominantly fibroblastic malignancies of the knee are the fibrosarcoma[28] and the malignant fibrous histiocytoma.[12] These highly malignant tumors are more frequently reported in soft tissue, but may occur de novo in bone. They are distinguished by their microscopic appearance, the fibrosarcoma being composed predominantly of spindle cell pleomorphic fibroblasts, often arranged in a herringbone pattern, as opposed to the malignant fibrous histiocytoma (MFH), which is a tumor of heterogeneous cellularity which may include fibroblasts, macrophages, or histiocytes, as well as inflammatory cells. In the MFH the disorganized growth pattern is striking with tumor cells proliferating in a swirling or storiform pattern. Forty-four percent of fibrosarcomas reported in the literature occur at the knee, with fibrosarcoma the fifth most common primary osseous tumor, constituting 5% of all reported tumor cases. Its most common location in the knee is the distal femur (61%), followed by the proximal tibia (34%), and the proximal fibula (5%). Very rare prior to puberty, it is most diffusely distributed between the ages of 15 and 60 years with a relatively equal sex distribution. Pain is the most common feature with frequent occurrence of pathologic fracture. Roentgenographically, the tumor is purely osteolytic, characteristic of most benign and malignant tumors of fibrous origin. The tumor is more indolent than osteogenic sarcoma, particularly those that have a low grade histologically. However, high-grade tumors may spread hematogenously with pulmonary and bone metastases being frequent.

Malignant fibrous histiocytoma has been reported with less frequency than fibrosarcoma (Fig 83-17). Its roentgenographic appearance, clinical symptoms, age, and sex distribution mimic fibrosarcoma. Spindle cell tumors, such as fibrosarcoma and MFH, have been reported as complications of both radiotherapy and bone infarction.

Ewing's Sarcoma

The classic Ewing's sarcoma is a permeating, destructive lesion of the diaphysis of a long bone in a child, with laboratory, clinical, and roentgenographic symptoms often mimicking osteomyelitis.[1] There may be fever, anemia, elevated sedimentation rate, and leukocytosis. The diagnosis is made by the histologic identification of a population of undifferentiated round cells that characteristically have abundant glycogen and therefore are identified with special stains. There are numerous small or round cell tumors that may affect the skeleton either in a primary or secondary fashion, and laboratory expertise is required in differentiating them. These round cell tumors include lymphomas, acute leukemias,[46] and other rarer entities. Thirteen percent of all reported cases of Ewing's sarcoma occur at the knee. It is the eighth most commonly reported primary osseous knee tumor, constituting approximately 3% of all cases. The most common location in the knee is the distal femur (46%), followed by the proximal tibia (35%) and the proximal fibula (19%). Approximately 90% of all cases occur between ages 5 and 25 years with a 1.5:1 male-to-female ratio.

In general Ewing's sarcoma presents with pain,

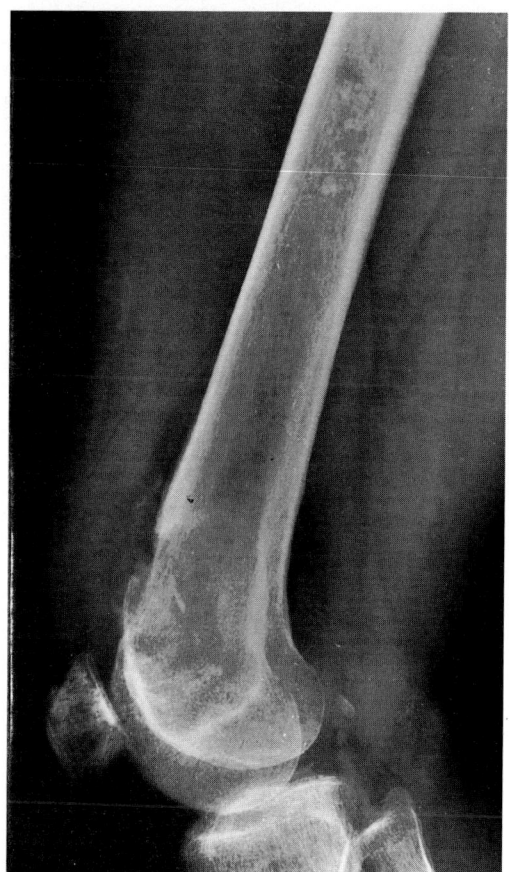

FIG 83-17.
Malignant fibrous histiocytoma. Lateral radiograph demonstrating a poorly defined lucent lesion in the distal metaphysis of the femur. There is destruction of the adjacent cortex in the anterior surface of the distal femur. Faint calcifications are seen in the tumor as well as in the midportion of the femoral shaft. This is a case of bone infarction with superimposed degeneration into a malignant fibrous histiocytoma.

which may be mild and intermittent, but is progressively severe. Swelling occurs early and associated symptoms include weight loss, low-grade fever, anemia, leukocytosis, and increased sedimentation rate. These symptoms may parallel progression of the tumor and indicate a poor prognosis. Radiographic features are variable but the classic Ewing's sarcoma shows a permeating destructive lesion which anatomically invades the cortex and elevates the periosteum, causing a layering or onion-skin appearance of the periosteal tissue (Fig 83–18). The spread of Ewing's sarcoma is more extensive than can be demonstrated by roentgenographic studies. In this regard, CT scans, bone scans, and MRI scans may be helpful.

Grossly, Ewing's sarcoma is a soft, grayish-white tumor with abundant areas of necrosis. The inflammation that accrues with necrosis may lead to misinterpretation of diagnosis. However, in an adequate sample, the diffuse population of homogeneous, small round cells with scant cytoplasm confirms the presence of a malignant tumor. Special stains, which discern the abundance of glycogen within the cytoplasm, can establish the diagnosis and exclude other small cell tumors (Fig 83–19). The histogenesis of Ewing's sarcoma is unknown. The usual clinical course is one of fairly rapid growth and, if left untreated, it will disseminate quickly to other parts of the skeleton and hematogeneously throughout the body, including through lymphatic channels. The prognosis for Ewing's sarcoma has improved dramatically with the advent of adjuvant therapies. Treatment with surgery, chemotherapy, and radiation combined has improved the 5-year survival to the range of 50%.

Lymphoma

Both Hodgkin's and non-Hodgkin's lymphomas can arise de novo in the skeleton although most lymphomas involve the skeleton in secondarily after spread from lymph organs. Most patients with terminal lymphomas from lymph node origin have skeletal involvement at the time of death. However, lymphomas may arise within the skeleton as a primary process. Hodgkin's lymphoma is identified by the recognition histologically of a heterogeneous cell population including eosinophils and plasma cells,

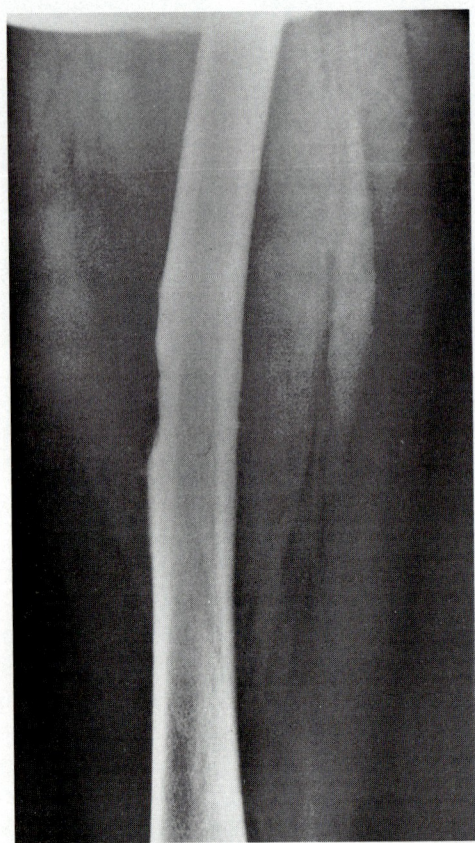

FIG 83–18.
Ewing's sarcoma. Frontal radiographs of the femur showing a shallow defect in the anteromedial cortex of the shaft of the bone. A faint periosteal reaction surrounds this defect. On biopsy this proved to be Ewing's sarcoma. These is a neoplasm that arises from the marrow cavity of the bone. As it grows there is invasion of the cortex and displacement of periosteum. A multilayered periosteal reaction (onion-skin appearance) is typical of Ewing's sarcoma. At times, as in this case, the growth of the neoplasm is not circumferential and results in localized invasion of the cortex and a localized periosteal reaction. The shallow defect (saucer sign) is seen at times in these lesions. The cortical defect is apparently due to pressure by the tumor on the outer surface of the bone.

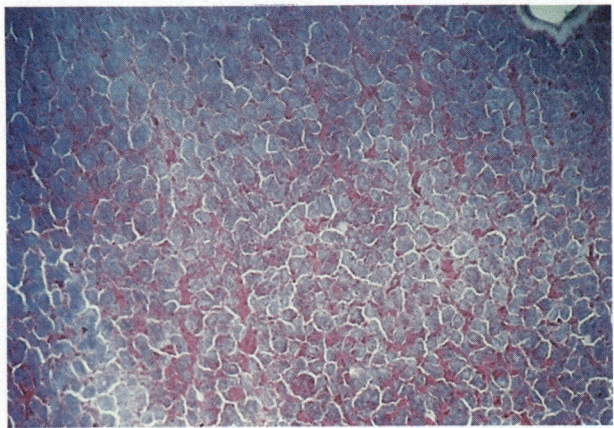

FIG 83–19.
Ewing's sarcoma. Photomicrograph of Ewing's sarcoma revealing a homogeneous cell population characterized by cells with sparse cytoplasm and bland nuclear detail characteristic of this malignant small cell tumor. The pink cytoplasmic glycogen characteristic of Ewing's sarcoma is demonstrated here using a periodic–acid Schiff (PAS) stain, special stains necessitating the differentiation of poorly differentiated round cell and small cell malignant tumors.

but most importantly by the identification of the Reed-Sternberg cell, a cell characterized by its large, mirror-image clear nucleus and red nucleolus. With regard to non-Hodgkin's lymphomas, recent studies utilizing techniques applied to lymphomas arising within lymph nodes have shown that the histologic type, stage, and presence and degree of soft tissue invasion are important indicators of survival potential in non-Hodgkin's lymphoma of the skeleton.[14]

Non-Hodgkin's lymphomas of the skeleton can be classified by the microscopic features of the predominant cell type with the most commonly reported non-Hodgkin's lymphoma of bone being that of a diffusely infiltrative large cell tumor. Those with cleaved nuclei have shown a better prognosis than those which have a noncleaved or immunoblastic appearance. Less commonly described variants of lymphoma include the undifferentiated or Burkitt's type, as well as the well-differentiated or small lymphocytic lymphomas. Long-term survivorship is far more likely in patients who present with osseous lymphomas localized to one bone than those in which the tumor has disseminated in the skeleton. Lymphomas present with a lytic pattern but may have a mixed or primary sclerotic appearance in the skeleton.

Multiple Myeloma and Metastatic Carcinoma

Multiple Myeloma

Multiple myeloma is a malignant tumor of plasma cells which is usually associated with widespread intraosseous proliferation of plasma cells with ensuing destruction and lysis of bone. Multiple myeloma is usually associated clinically with bone pain, with lytic lesions occurring throughout the skeleton, including the extremities, often leading to fracture. The laboratory abnormalities associated with multiple myeloma include hypercalcemia and hypergammaglobulinemia. The plasma cells produce a monoclonal gammopathy, that is, a proliferation of one light chain or one heavy chain, or both, which are identified by immunoelectrophoresis. In screening for multiple myeloma, the hypergammaglobulinemia may be verified by doing serum protein electrophoresis in which a broad band is detected in the gamma globulin range. However, to detect a monoclonal gammopathy, a characteristic of plasma cell malignancies, the diagnostic tests are serum and urine immunoelectrophoresis, which detects the monoclonal production of either a heavy chain (IgM, IgG, IgA, or others) or one light chain (kappa or lambda). Confirmation of the diagnosis can be obtained by bone biopsy, which reveals replacement of the bone marrow space by sheaths of atypical plasma cells. Myeloma is thought to produce a bone resorbing factor (osteoclast activating factor) which explains its destructive lysis of the skeleton. In rare circumstances myeloma may be associated with bone production, a sclerotic variant.

Metastatic Carcinoma

Metastatic cancer to the skeleton is the most common malignant tumor affecting bone, the bone being the third most common site of metastasis, with 60% of cancer patients at autopsy revealing bone metastasis. The most frequently seen tumor sites affecting the skeleton in patients dying of metastatic cancer are the breast, prostate, lung, thyroid, and kidney. Metastatic cancer has a predilection for the marrow space of bone, but in rare circumstances may affect cortical bone, this usually due to metastatic lung cancer. The most commonly affected part of the skeleton is the spine. The lumbar vertebrae are more commonly involved than the thoracic, cervical, and sacral vertebrae, with the exception of prostate cancer, which has a predilection for metastasis to the lumbar and sacral vertebral bodies, and breast and lung cancers, which prefer thoracic vertebrae. Following the spine, the ribs, pelvis, proximal ends of the bones, sternum, and skull are involved by metastatic cancer in decreasing frequency. Factors associated with metastatic spread have, for the most part, been elusive to investigators, but more than likely involve anatomic aspects of the vasculature, perhaps explaining the predilection of prostate cancer for vertebral bodies via Batson's plexus, variability in the susceptibility of different organs, and the different properties of tumor cells themselves.

Metastatic cancer usually causes lysis or destruction, with the most common features of metastatic cancer being radiolucencies and eventual fractures. Thyroid, kidney, lung, and gastrointestinal tumors most commonly cause lysis of the skeleton. Prostate cancer most often causes bone formation and osteoblastic metastases. Breast cancer often gives a mixed picture.

More specifically, in the skeleton it has been estimated that 30% of metastatic osseous lesions are located in the femur, with one third of these occurring below the subtrochanteric region in the shaft or in the supracondylar region.[50] Metastatic lesions may be suspected when a symptomatic lesion is seen on plain films, or abnormal areas are found on bone scan, with either increased or decreased uptake. It should be pointed out that when contemplating biopsy to establish the diagnosis, metastatic renal and thyroid tumors may have a significant increase in vascularity with even palpable pulses or bruits.

The tibia is a relatively infrequent site of involvement by metastatic cancer, and usually tibial metastases occur late in the development of metastatic disease.[4] It should be noted that metastatic bone disease may be the presenting complaint in patients with metastatic cancer, with the primary site not immediately appreciated.[43] In fact, cases in which a primary cancer may be indeterminate after extensive clinical and roentgenographic workup are well known. Even after autopsies in some studies, approximately 1% of patients presenting with metastatic cancer may have an undetectable primary site. More than likely, however, tumors uncovered after a careful search are common tumors, such as breast, lung, thyroid, and kidney tumors, with an increased number of pancreatic cancers evident in this group requiring evaluation.

The reasons for bone-associated changes in metastatic cancer are not clear, but may include a number of factors. Some tumors, such as multiple myeloma, secrete factors such as osteoclast activating factor, which have a direct osteolytic effect. Others secrete parathyroid-like hormones that activate the remodeling cycle, in particular, osteoclastic resorption. Tumors are well known to be associated with both marrow and bone necrosis, processes that may cause definable bone scan and plain film changes. The release of other local bone-mediating factors, as well as the possibility of direct mechanical or pressure effects, may also play a role.

Secondary Malignancies

Malignant bone tumors may occur in rare circumstances as a complication of benign tumors and tumor-like lesions of the skeleton, as well as following infarction and iatrogenic intervention. Chondrosarcomas, for example, may complicate benign cartilaginous conditions, such as MHE and Ollier's disease (enchondromatosis). The incidence varies considerably, but is probably less than 10%. Solitary osteochondromas and solitary enchondromas would be an extremely rare setting for the development of a malignant cartilaginous tumor. Chondrosarcomas have also been described as complicating cases of fibrous dysplasia and synovial chondromatosis,[30] rare phenomena.

Paget's disease, a metabolic disease of bone characterized by a marked increase in osteoblast and osteoclast remodeling of the skeleton, may be a monofocal or multifocal condition. The latter is associated with the development over time of malignant neoplasms, which include osteogenic sarcomas, chondrosarcomas, lymphomas, and even giant cell lesions (Avellino tumor).[23, 41]

Radioactivity may lead to the development of tumors, including leukemias, the classic description being their development in radium watch dial workers following ingestion of radioactive dyes. Postirradiation sarcomas of the skeleton are now well described, and in fact may be predicted in a small percentage of patients treated for a various number of tumors, including lymphomas.[23]

Bone infarction may also be the setting for the development of malignancy in the skeleton. Recently, interest has been generated by a number of reports showing an association between the implantation of orthopaedic devices and the subsequent development of sarcomas at the implant site.[22] However, despite the fact that certain metal components are carcinogenic in laboratory animals, the sporadic and sparse reports of such associations in humans more than likely represents a coincidental occurrence, albeit one of potential serious concern.

In general, malignant transformation may occur in a broad range of lesions. Squamous cell carcinoma may arise in draining sinuses of over many years duration in chronic osteomyelitis. Infarction, of whatever cause, may lead to the development of malignancies, particularly MFH, osteogenic sarcomas, and even, most recently, angiosarcomas. It is of interest that malignancies reported as complications of underlying skeletal disorders are often composed of malignant spindle cell sarcomas, including MFH, which has been reported in chrondromatosis, fibrous dysplasia, radiation disorders, Paget's disease, bone infarction, and even in association, as mentioned, with metallic implants. In general, sarcomas developing in the setting of underlying bone disease are highly malignant and carry a relatively poor prognosis.

SYNOVIAL TUMORS

Benign Tumors

Synovial Hemangioma

Synovial hemangioma usually presents as a solitary benign vascular proliferation, most commonly seen in the knee joints of children and adolescents. Although the patient may be asymptomatic, there may be swelling, mild pain, or limitation of motion, with the pain and swelling in some instances being of several years duration. Radiographic examination reveals a soft tissue mass which may, in severe cases, cause adjacent bone changes such as periosteal reaction or lucent zones. Grossly, the knee joint reveals a soft, doughy, brown mass with proliferating villous synovium, frequently mahogany-stained by hemosiderin deposition. Histologically, there is proliferation of vascular channels of various sizes and shapes with surrounding hyperplastic synovium. Copious hemosiderin may be seen in patients who have had repeated hemarthrosis.

Hoffa's Disease (Synovial Lipomatosis)

In Hoffa's disease there is enlargement of the infrapatellar fat pad on either side of the patellar tendon with resulting pain or aching in the anterior compartment of the knee. Pain may be aggravated by physical activity or extension of the knee, with swelling or recurrent effusion, or both, a consequence. Macroscopically the synovium has a marked papillary proliferative appearance with microscopically evident hyperplasia of the synovial lining cells overlying abundant fat.

Synovial Chondromatosis (Synovial Osteochondromatosis)

The synovium, capable of undergoing metaplasia to cartilage in a broad range of conditions, including trauma and degenerative joint disease, may produce multiple cartilaginous and chondro-osseous loose bodies throughout the joint.[32] Synovial chondromatosis, or synovial osteochondromatosis, is best characterized as a benign tumorous proliferation. Initially embedded in the synovium, the nodules may be dislodged and become free loose bodies ranging in number from a few to several hundred. The characteristic presentation of synovial chondromatosis is a monoarticular condition of the third, fourth, or fifth decades of life with a predilection for the knee. It is usually associated with swelling and may be associated with pain, limitation of motion, and occasionally clicking or locking. Radiographically, the condition is easily recognized if the cartilaginous bodies have undergone calcification or ossification, which they often do. The numerous radiopaque densities range in size from a few millimeters to several centimeters, varying considerably in the extent of calcification and ossification. Arthrography may be useful in diagnosing the noncalcified bodies. Grossly, the synovium shows flaky bodies, or it may have an irregular nodular contour. Whitish, or translucent bluish-gray nodules, ranging greatly in size and shape, may be more obviously attached on the membrane or floating in the joint space (Fig 83–20).

The histopathologic differences of these bodies have supported a distinction between a secondary synovial chondromatosis associated with degenerative joint disease and a primary synovial chondromatosis, not associated with any underlying disorder, the former suggesting a reactive or metaplastic change, and the latter representing a true de novo primary

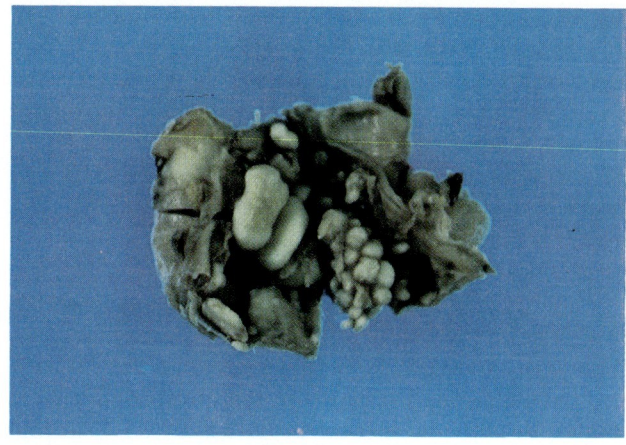

FIG 83–20.
Chondromatosis. Gross photomicrograph of chondromatosis, here seen in a bursa around the knee in which numerous cartilaginous and osseocartilaginous bodies of various shapes and sizes are both freely mobile within the space or focally adherent to the bursal lining membrane.

joint tumor. The loose bodies in the secondary condition classically show more organized cellular growth, such as layers of calcification. However, in primary synovial chondromatosis a more disorganized growth of cartilage cells is often apparent, similar to that seen in the primary cartilaginous disorders such as enchondroma of the bone. Surgical removal of all the nodules is important to prevent recurrence. If the chondro-osseous bodies are entirely free loose bodies within the joint, a fact which may be difficult to ascertain from surgical exposure alone, a thorough cleaning of the joint may suffice. However, the disorder may involve chondro-osseous change within the synovial subintimal connective tissue, a fact that may require total synovectomy to prevent recurrence.

A phenomenon similar to synovial chondromatosis may occur within bursae. In very rare instances, chondrosarcomas may arise in the setting of synovial chondromatosis. This rare condition can be suspected when there is evidence of aggressive growth, such as invasion into adjacent extraarticular tissues. Focal areas of atypical cellularity and increased cellularity in an otherwise unremarkable case of synovial chondromatosis, should not be overdiagnosed. Synovial chondrosarcoma may also arise as a de novo synovial malignancy. The clinical behavior of these neoplasms varies from that of low-grade neoplasms, with a propensity to recur locally, to those that may, in fact, metastasize.

Pigmented Villonodular Synovitis

Although sometimes considered an inflammatory reaction, pigmented villonodular synovitis (PVNS) is a tumorous proliferation of stromal mononuclear and multinucleated giant cells of the fibroblastic histiocytic or fibrohistiocytic cell lineage[37] (Fig 83–21). The nodular growth pattern, the occasionally observed mitotic activity of the stroma, the relative lack of inflammatory cells, and the ability to erode local tissue support the classification of PVNS as a tumor. The name is fitting for only some of the lesions, as PVNS may show little pigmentation, is often a solitary nodular growth with little villous hyperplasia, and in the typical case shows little, if any, inflammation. The joint fluid color is variable, ranging from normal to brownish-red. The synovium may appear diffusely pigmented or, more commonly, focally so. The pigmentation is caused by hemosiderin accumulation from microscopic synovial hemorrhage, giving foci of brown color, as well as by aggregates of lipid-laden macrophages giving a yellow appearance, particularly in the periphery of expanding nodules. Hyperplastic and pigmented changes mimicking those of chronic hemarthrosis in the adjacent synovium are secondary and do not represent the lesion proper.

At least five clinical types of PVNS are identified in the knee: loose body, localized nodule (pedunculated or embedded in the synovium), aggregates of nodules confined to one compartment, truly diffuse involvement of the synovium, and PVNS extending into bursae. The localized nodular and nodular aggregate types are the most common (Fig 83–22). Typically, PVNS is a monoarticular arthritis, usually observed in the early and middle adult period, rarely at the extreme ends of life. Symptoms may be gradual in onset. Clinically, patients may present with discomfort or pain. Swelling, stiffness, locking, or even instability of the knee may occur. Torsion of a pedunculated nodular form of PVNS has been associated with the unusual clinical presentation of acute pain. The most common radiographic finding in the knee is soft tissue swelling. Arthrograms may best demonstrate the nodules as discrete, pitting defects. Bone changes are less frequent, but may include erosions and degenerative changes.

The treatment of PVNS is surgical. If an isolated loose body or nodule is confirmed, arthroscopic surgical excision may be attempted. However, the propensity of the lesions to recur in up to one third of cases requires careful examination of the remainder of the joint to exclude multiple foci. Smaller nodules may be missed, embedded as they are in the subintimal synovial layers. The diffuse form of PVNS is more problematic and requires total synovectomy. If not removed, PVNS will continue to grow and erode into the articular bone. Bursal PVNS also requires adequate surgical excision, and may extend deeply into surrounding soft tissue.

Malignant Tumors

Synovial Sarcoma

Synovial sarcoma is a malignant mesenchymal tumor that usually arises in structures adjacent to the joint, most often in tenosynovial lining anatomic structures.[42] It derives its name from the microscopic appearance which mimics the histologic appearance of the embryonic synovium. It occurs in close association with tendon sheaths, bursae, and joint capsules, and has a propensity to differentiate toward a spindle cell– or fibroblast-like mesodermal cell population, as well as an epithelial population, giving it,

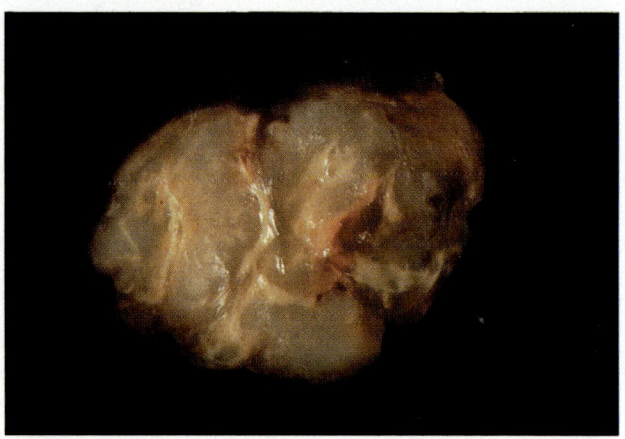

FIG 83–22.
Nodule of pigmented villonodular synovitis. Transected gross nodules of pigmented villonodular synovitis reveal the silk-like nodularity of this tumor-like growth, the nodules themselves matted together and often surrounded by yellowish and tan borders.

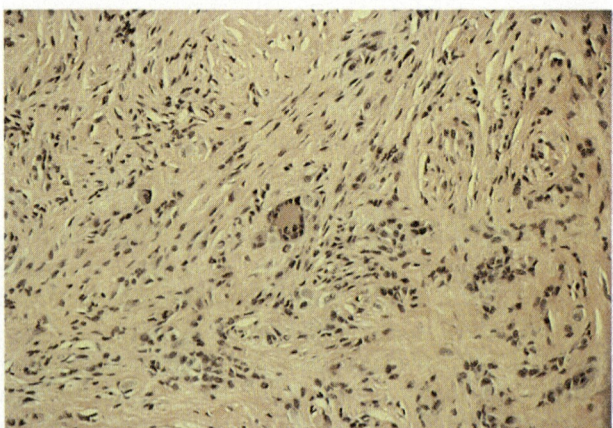

FIG 83–21.
Pigmented villonodular synovitis. Photomicrograph of pigmented villonodular synovitis revealing the characteristic giant cells (center) enmeshed in a matrix of mononuclear cells producing abundant pink collagen. The admixture of mononuclear and giant stromal cells is typical of the group of fibrous histiocytic lesions.

in its classic presentation, a biphasic microscopic appearance. Approximately 70% of the tumors occur in the lower extremity and 15% about the knee. It is the fourth most common soft tissue sarcoma, accounting for approximately 10% of all malignant mesenchymal neoplasms. It is most prevalent between the ages of 15 and 35 years, and the characteristic presentation is that of a painful, palpable soft tissue mass. Roentgenographically, the synovial sarcoma presents as a soft tissue mass with about half the cases demonstrating calcification. There may be local bone changes secondary to a mass effect of an adjacent growing lesion. These malignant lesions recur locally and spread by both regional lymph node and pulmonary metastatic routes. Histologically, the tumor is diagnosed by the identification of a biphasic cell population. Immunocytochemical and immunohistologic staining have demonstrated a mesenchymal tissue in one component and epithelial differentiation in the other (Fig 83–23). Descriptions in the literature of monophasic variants of synovial sarcoma, with a predominance of one of these two cell types, have raised questions about classification.

Prognosis may be related to gross anatomic and histologic findings with a better prognosis in younger patients with tumors less than 5 cm, tumors located in the lower extremity with an epithelial gland cellularity greater than 50%, and a mitotic activity of less than 15 mitoses/10 HPF. A recent multimodality approach involving surgery, radiotherapy, and combined chemotherapy may improve survival in this highly malignant tumor.

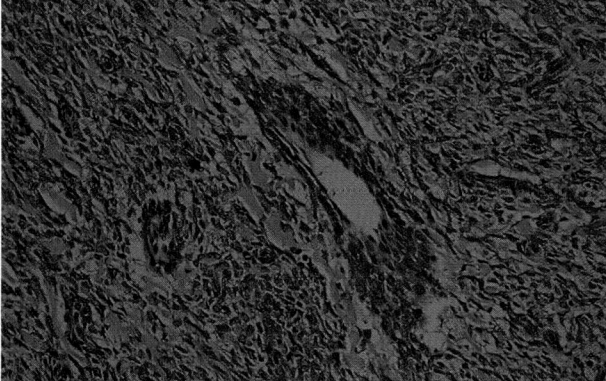

FIG 83–23.
Synovial sarcoma. Photomicrograph revealing the mixed pattern of this tumor recognized histologically by an irregular, often spindle cell pleomorphic cell population, within which are noted glandular elements or gland-like elements *(center)* mimicking the epithelial-like gland formations in epithelial tumors or cancers. The admixture of the epithelial and spindle cell or sarcomatous components is typical of this biphasic, highly malignant neoplasm.

Epithelioid Sarcoma

Epithelioid sarcoma is a malignant soft tissue sarcoma of unknown histogenesis which primarily affects the subcutaneous tissue, fascia, and tendon sheaths of the extremities.[6] It is most commonly seen in the upper extremities as a small, painless, subcutaneous nodule. Because of associated inflammation and even necrotizing granulomatous-like reactions, it may be confused with a benign process. It most often occurs in young males and tends to recur locally after excision. Progression along tendon sheath and lymphatic pathways has been demonstrated. There is a poor prognosis associated with tumors greater than 3 cm and in those that are deeply situated in the soft tissue. Focal necrosis may indicate a worse prognosis. Wide or radical resection may be required.

REFERENCES

1. Bacci G, et al: Long-term results in 144 localized Ewing's sarcoma patients treated with combined therapy, *Cancer* 63:1477–1486, 1989.
2. Bauer TW, Dorfman HD: Intraosseous ganglion: A clinicopathologic study of 11 cases, *Am J Surg Pathol* 6:207–213, 1982.
3. Bauer TW, Dorfman HD, Lathan JT Jr: Periosteal chondroma: A clinicopathologic study of 23 cases, *Am J Surg Pathol* 6:631–637, 1982.
4. Beauchamp CP, Sim FH: Lesions of the tibia. In Sim FH (editor): *Diagnosis and treatment of metastatic bone disease: A multidisciplinary approach to management,* New York, 1987, Raven Press.
5. Bjornsson J, et al: Clear cell chondrosarcoma of bone: Observations in 47 cases, *Am J Surg Pathol* 8:223–230, 1984.
6. Bos GD, et al: Epithelioid sarcoma: An analysis of fifty-one cases, *J Bone Joint Surg [Am]* 70:862–870, 1988.
7. Boseker EH, Bickel WH, Dahlin DC: A clinicopathologic study of simple unicameral bone cysts, *Surg Gynecol Obstet* 127:550–560, 1968.
8. Caffey J: On fibrous defects in cortical walls of growing tubular bones: Their radiologic appearance, structure, prevalence, natural course, and diagnostic significance, *Adv Pediatr* 7:13–51, 1955.
9. Campanacci M: *Bone and soft tissue tumors,* New York, 1991, Springer-Verlag, pp 419–431.
10. Campanacci M, Laus M: Osteofibrous dysplasia of the tibia and fibula, *J Bone Joint Surg [Am]* 63:367–375, 1981.
11. Campanacci M, Baldini N, Boriani S, et al: Giant-cell tumor of bone, *J Bone Joint Surg [Am]* 69:106–114, 1987.
12. Capanna R, et al: Malignant fibrous histiocytoma of bone: The experience at the Rizzoli Institute: report of 90 cases, *Cancer* 54:177–187, 1984.

13. Clarke BE, Xipell JM, Thomas DP: Benign fibrous histiocytoma of bone, *Am J Surg Pathol* 9:806–815, 1985.
14. Clayton F, et al: Non-Hodgkin's lymphoma in bone: Pathologic and radiologic features with clinical correlates, *Cancer* 60:2494–2501, 1987.
15. Kransdorf MJ, Moser RP, Vinh TN, et al: Primary tumors of the patella. A review of 42 cases. *Skeletal Radiol* 18:365–371, 1989.
16. Dahlin DC: *Bone tumors: general aspects and data on 8,542 cases,* edition 2, Springfield, Ill, 1991, Charles C Thomas.
17. Enneking WF: A system of staging musculoskeletal neoplasms, *Clin Orthop* 204:9–24, 1986.
18. Garfin SR, Rothman RH: Case Report 346: Fibrous dysplasia, *Skeletal Radiol* 15:72–76, 1986.
19. Gherlinzoni R, Rock M, Picci P: Chondromyxoid fibroma: The experience at the Istituto Orthopedico Rizzoli, *J Bone Joint Surg [Am]* 65:198–204, 1983.
20. Gitelis S, et al: Chondrosarcoma of bone: The experience at the Istituto Ortopedico Rizzoli, *J Bone Joint Surg [Am]* 63:1248–1257, 1981.
21. Greis PE, Hankin FM: Eosinophiliac granuloma: The management of solitary lesions of bone, *Clin Orthop* 257:204, 1990.
22. Hamblen DL, Carter RL: Sarcoma and joint replacement (editorial), *J Bone Joint Surg [Br]* 66:625–626, 1984.
23. Healey JH, Buss D: Radiation and Pagetic osteosarcoma, *Clin Orthop* 270:128–134, 1991.
24. Huvos AG: *Bone tumors: Diagnosis and prognosis,* ed 2, New York, 1990, WB Saunders.
25. Huvos AG, et al: Mesenchymal chondrosarcoma: A clinicopathologic analysis of 35 patients with emphasis on treatment. *Cancer* 51:1230–1237, 1983.
26. Jackson RP, Reckling FW, Mantz FA: Osteoid osteoma and osteoblastoma: Similar histologic lesions with different natural histories, *Clin Orthop* 128:303–313, 1977.
27. Larsson SE, Lorentzon R, Boquist L: Giant-cell tumor of bone: A demographic, clinical and histopathological study of all cases recorded in the Swedish Cancer Registry for years 1958 through 1968, *J Bone Joint Surg [Am]* 57:167–173, 1975.
28. Larsson SE, Lorentzon R, Boquist L: Fibrosarcoma of bone: A demographic, clinical and histopathological study of all cases recorded in the Swedish Cancer Registry from 1958 to 1968, *J Bone Joint Surg [Am]* 58:412–417, 1976.
29. McCarthy EF, Dorfman HD: Chondrosarcoma of bone with dedifferentiation: A study of eighteen cases, *Hum Pathol* 13:36–40, 1982.
30. Manivel JC, Dehner LP, Thompson R: Case report 460, *Skeletal Radiol* 17:66–71, 1988.
31. Martin SE, et al: Small-cell osteosarcoma, *Cancer* 50:990–996, 1982.
32. Milgram JW: Synovial osteochondromatosis: A histopathological study of thirty cases, *J Bone Joint Surg [Am]* 59:792–793, 1977.
33. Mirra JM, et al, editors: *Bone tumors: Clinical, radiologic and pathologic correlation,* Philadelphia, 1989, Lea & Febiger.
34. Peterson HA: Multiple hereditary osteochondromata, *Clin Orthop* 239:222–230, 1989.
35. Petrilli AS, et al: Increased survival, limb preservation, and prognostic factors for osteosarcoma, *Cancer* 68:733–737, 1991.
36. Pignatti G, et al: Telangiectatic osteogenic sarcoma of the extremities: Results in 17 patients treated with neoadjuvant chemotherapy, *Clin Orthop* 270:99–106, 1991.
37. Rao AS, Vigorita VJ: Pigmented villonodular synovitis (giant-cell tumor of the tendon sheath and synovial membrane), *J Bone Joint Surg [Am]* 66:76–94, 1984.
38. Raymond AK: Surface osteosarcoma, *Clin Orthop* 270:140–148, 1991.
39. Ritschl P, Karnel F, Hajek P: Fibrous metaphyseal defects—determination of their origin and natural history using a radiomorphological study, *Skeletal Radiol* 17:8–15, 1988.
40. Schajowicz F: *Tumors and tumorlike lesions of bone and joints,* New York, 1981, Springer-Verlag.
41. Schajowicz F, Santini Araujo ES, Berenstein M: Sarcoma complicating Paget's disease of bone: A clinicopathological study of 62 cases, *J Bone Joint Surg [Br]* 65:299–307, 1983.
42. Schmidt D, et al: Synovial sarcoma in children and adolescents: A report from the Kiel Pediatric Tumor Registry, *Cancer* 67:1667–1672, 1991.
43. Simon MA, Karluk MB: Skeletal metastases of unknown origin: Diagnostic strategy for orthopedic surgeons, *Clin Orthop* 166:96–103, 1982.
44. Springfield DS, et al: Chondroblastoma: A review of seventy cases, *J Bone Joint Surg [Am]* 67:748, 1985.
45. Stephenson RB, et al: Fibrous dysplasia: An analysis of options for treatment, *J Bone Joint Surg [Am]* 69:400–409, 1987.
46. Thomas LB, et al: The skeletal lesions of acute leukemia, *Cancer* 14:608–620, 1961.
47. Vergel DeDios AM, et al: Aneurysmal bone cyst: A clinicopathologic study of 238 cases, *Cancer* 69:2921–2931, 1992.
48. Vigorita VJ, Ghelman B: Localization of osteoid osteomas—Use of radionuclide scanning and autoimaging in identifying the nidus, *Am J Clin Pathol* 79:223–225, 1983.
49. Wester SM, et al: Langerhans' cell granulomatosis (histiocytosis X) of bone in adults, *Am J Surg Pathol* 6:413–426, 1982.
50. Wilkins RM, Sim FH: Lesions of the femur. In Sim FH (editor): *Diagnosis and treatment of metastatic bone disease: A multidisciplinary approach to management,* New York, 1987, Raven Press.

84

Management of Bone and Soft Tissue Tumors About the Knee

JOHN H. HEALEY, M.D.
RICHARD M. TEREK, M.D.

Bone tumors
   General concepts
   Clinical presentation
   Diagnostic studies
   Biopsy technique
   Staging
   Treatment
      Benign bone tumors
      Malignant bone tumors
      Adjuvant chemotherapy
Surgical technique for malignant bone tumors

Decision making
En bloc excision of the knee
Reconstruction
Endoprostheses
Arthrodesis
Fibular lesions
Metastatic tumors about the knee
Soft tissue tumors
General concepts
Benign soft tissue tumors
Soft tissue sarcomas

Tumors about the knee are relatively common. Bone and soft tissue lesions, both benign and malignant, occur frequently. Metastatic lesions also develop and even present with disease in this location, although less often than in the proximal femur or hip. Tumors must be recognized and treated promptly to optimize oncologic and functional results. General orthopaedists, sports medicine physicians, and knee specialists will encounter many lesions in this region, and must be aware of the types of symptoms that these lesions cause, the workup of the lesions, the spectrum of disease that develops in the knee area, and the therapeutic options for the common diagnostic entities. This chapter presents clinical, epidemiologic, and radiographic information about bone and soft tissue tumors that occur about the knee. It discusses general concepts of staging, biopsy, and treatment. It reviews current data on the function and durability of reconstructions used after tumor excisions. This information is of particular interest to knee surgeons as more salvage knee surgery becomes necessary for nononcologic reasons.

BONE TUMORS

General Concepts

Any bone tumor can occur about the knee. The more common types are discussed below. Caffey[11] reported that 43% of normal children had a developmental or neoplastic bony defect during growth that resolved by adulthood. Among these abnormalities, fibrous cortical defects or metaphyseal conversion defects are the most common (Fig 84–1). An estimated 30% of children will have such a defect in the metaphysis of the distal femur or proximal tibia.[10] The importance of this lesion is to distinguish it from a true neoplasm that requires intervention. The most common benign bone tumor (12% of all tumors, and 50% of benign bone tumors) is the solitary osteochondroma (Fig 84–2). Nearly one half of these develop about the knee. Giant cell tumors frequently (65%) reside in the epiphyseal region of the femur and tibia in young adults.[14] One third of chondroblastomas, the so-called calcifying epiphyseal giant cell tumors,

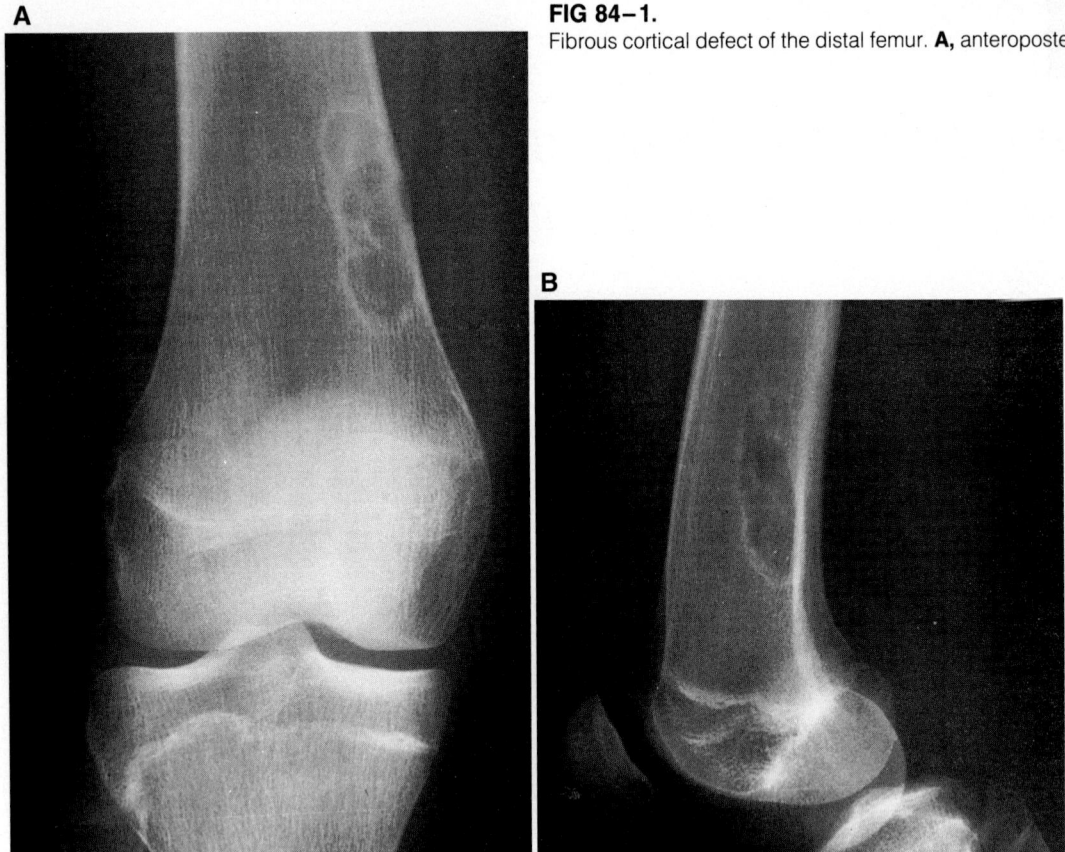

FIG 84–1.
Fibrous cortical defect of the distal femur. **A,** anteroposterior view; **B,** lateral view.

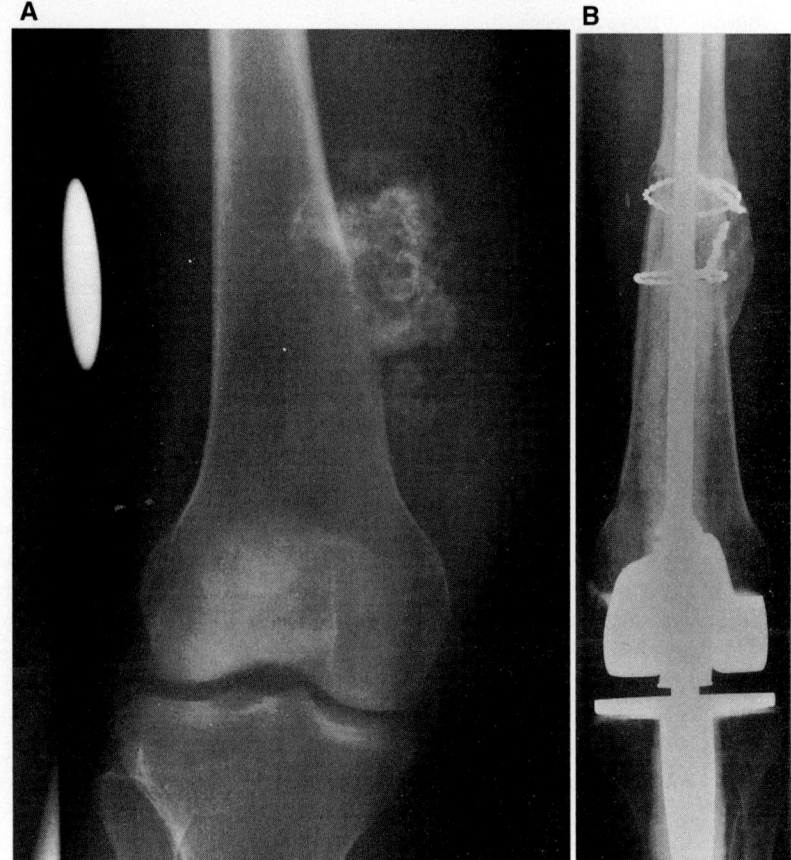

FIG 84–2.
Osteochondroma of the distal femur which developed into a grade II chondrosarcoma. **A,** preoperative; **B,** postoperative after resection and reconstruction with an allograft-prosthesis.

culled from the literature were reported as occurring about the knee, despite their alleged preference for the shoulder tuberosities or the greater trochanter of the hip. The tibial spine and intercondylar notch are typical haunts for this tumor[43] (Fig 84–3). Chondromyxoid fibromas are rare tumors that develop below the knee in 50% of cases, including the proximal tibia and fibula.[19] Curiously, they also have a predilection for the anterior aspect of the femur at the osteocartilaginous junction and are thereby associated with considerable patellofemoral pain. These are but a few of the benign tumors that have an altered anatomic

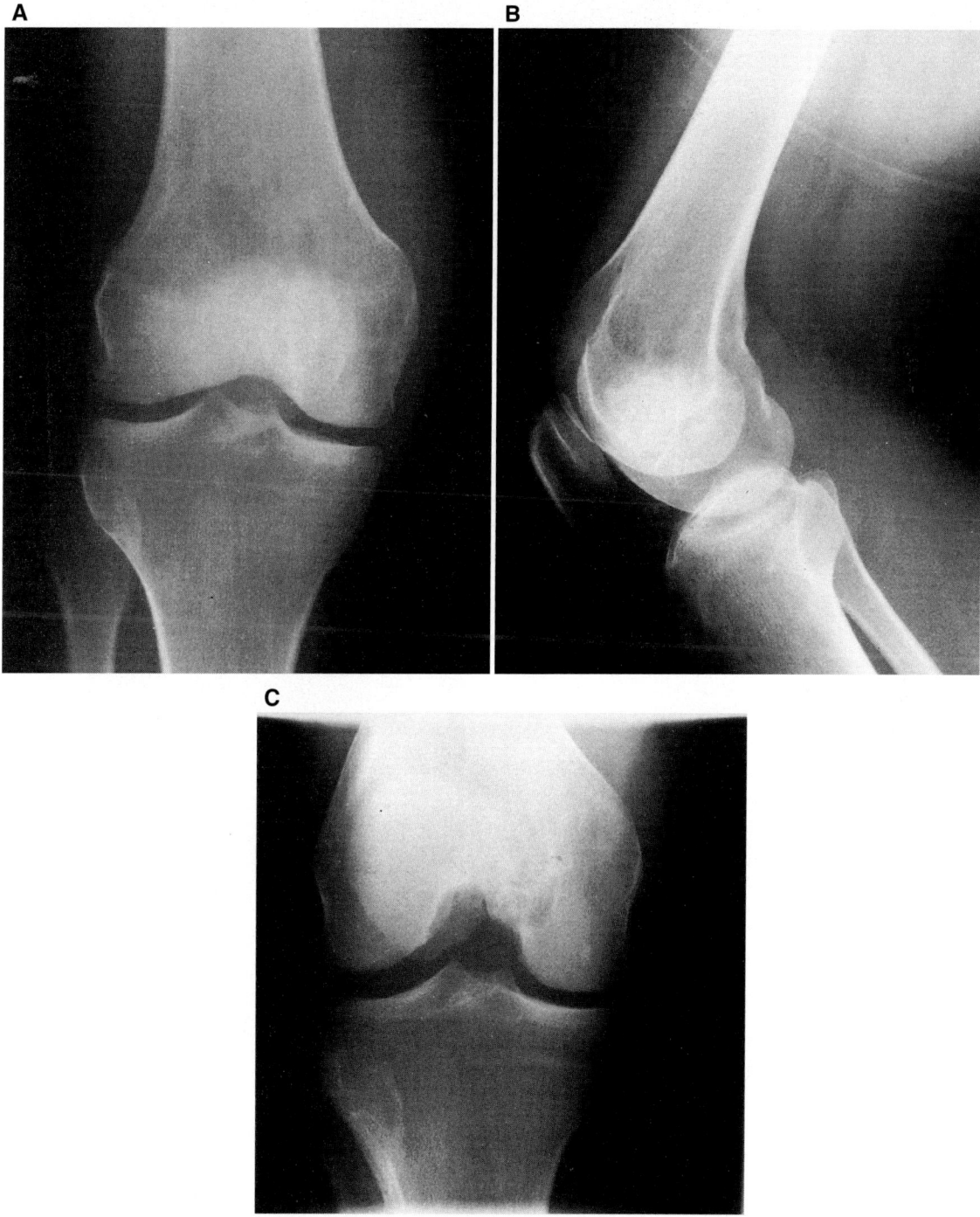

FIG 84–3.
This chondroblastoma of the distal femur is not well visualized on the standard anteroposterior (**A**) and lateral views (**B**), but can be easily seen on the notch view (**C**).

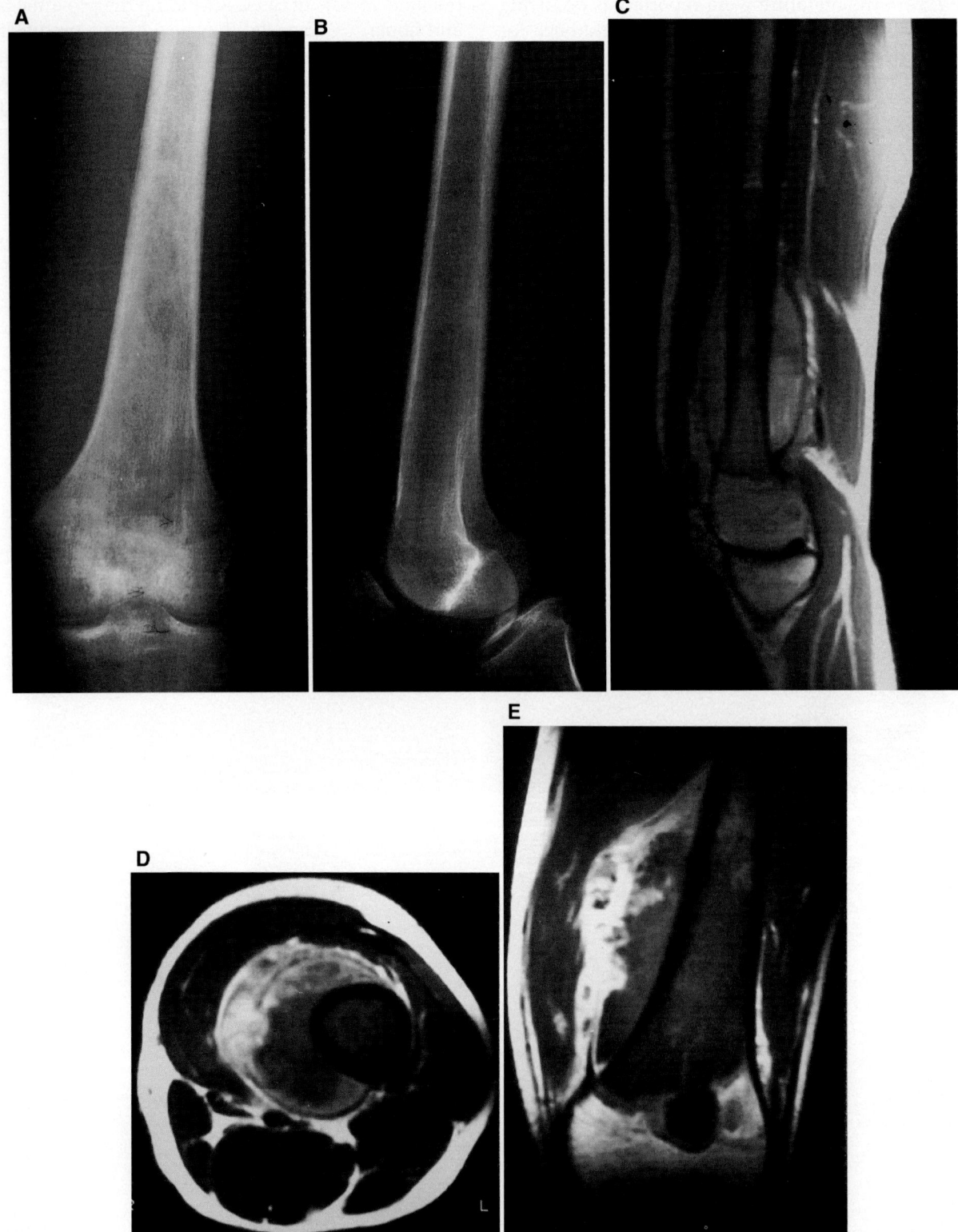

FIG 84-4.
Osteogenic sarcoma of the distal femoral metaphysis. The mixed lytic and blastic pattern is seen, as well as the periosteal reaction, in the anteroposterior **(A)** and lateral **(B)** views. MRI scan demonstrates the soft tissue mass anterior, medial, and posterior to the distal femur as well as the intramedullary extent of the tumor in the sagittal **(C)** and axial **(D)** images. **E,** coronal MRI demonstrates violation of the physis.

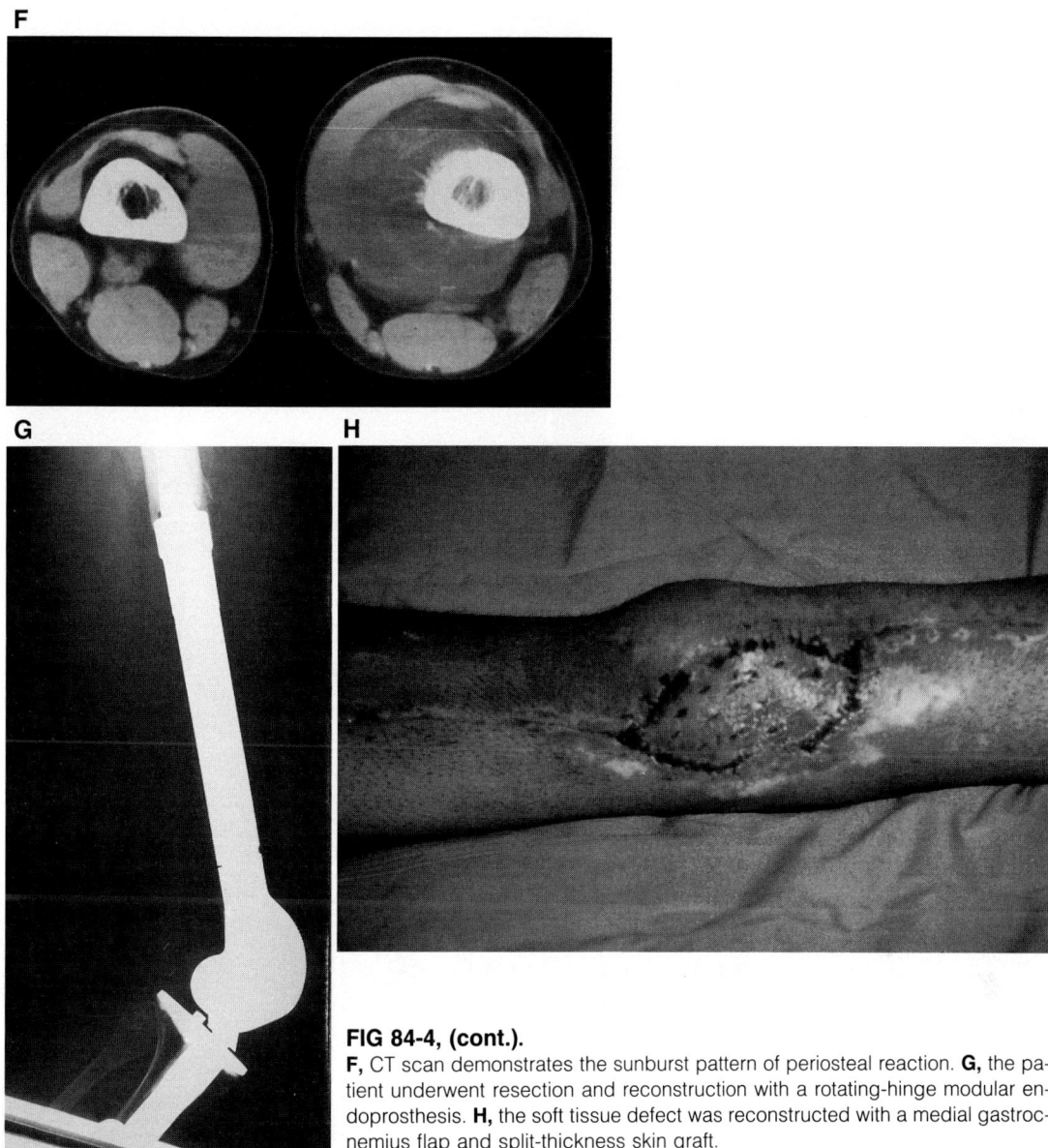

FIG 84-4, (cont.).
F, CT scan demonstrates the sunburst pattern of periosteal reaction. **G,** the patient underwent resection and reconstruction with a rotating-hinge modular endoprosthesis. **H,** the soft tissue defect was reconstructed with a medial gastrocnemius flap and split-thickness skin graft.

distribution or distinctive clinical presentation about the knee.

Malignant tumors occur less often than benign bone tumors, and significantly less often than the developmental lesions that mimic bone tumors. The most common primary bone malignancy is osteogenic sarcoma, and approximately one half of these tumors occur about the knee. The metaphyseal femur is the usual site for fully malignant osteogenic sarcomas (Fig 84-4). Low-grade surface or juxtacortical tumors develop in more diaphyseal locations, and Huvos and Marcove[43] reported that 14 of 24 were on the posterior aspect of the femur (Fig 84-5). In the United States, an estimated 300 osteogenic sarcomas per year occur in the knee region. Chondrosarcomas (Fig 84-6), malignant fibrous histiocytomas, and fibrosarcomas are the other mesenchymal tumors that occur regularly about the knee, approximately one half to two thirds as often as osteogenic sarcomas. These tumors all occur in a somewhat older population. Malignant round cell tumors such as Ewing's sarcoma are classically diaphyseal tumors, yet nearly 50% of them occur in nondiaphyseal locations. Ewing's sarcoma is particularly common in the femur and is the most common malignancy of the fibula. Lymphoma (mixed and histiocytic types) is known to develop as a primary bone tumor in many cases, and seems to have a predilection for the femur in young adults (Fig 84-7). Certainly, metastatic lesions are the most common lesions in older adults with multiple

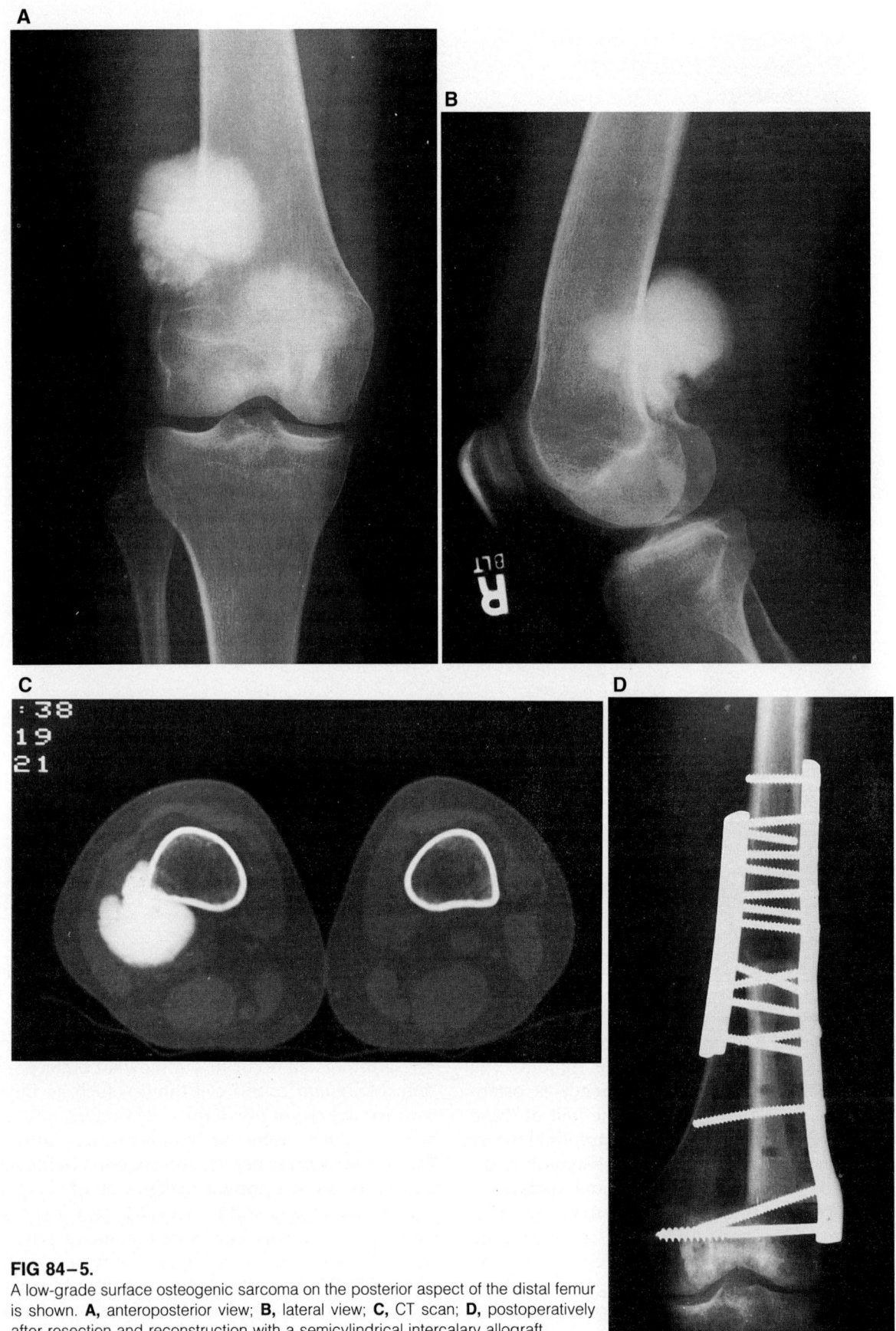

FIG 84–5.
A low-grade surface osteogenic sarcoma on the posterior aspect of the distal femur is shown. **A,** anteroposterior view; **B,** lateral view; **C,** CT scan; **D,** postoperatively after resection and reconstruction with a semicylindrical intercalary allograft.

MANAGEMENT OF BONE AND SOFT TISSUE TUMORS ABOUT THE KNEE 1447

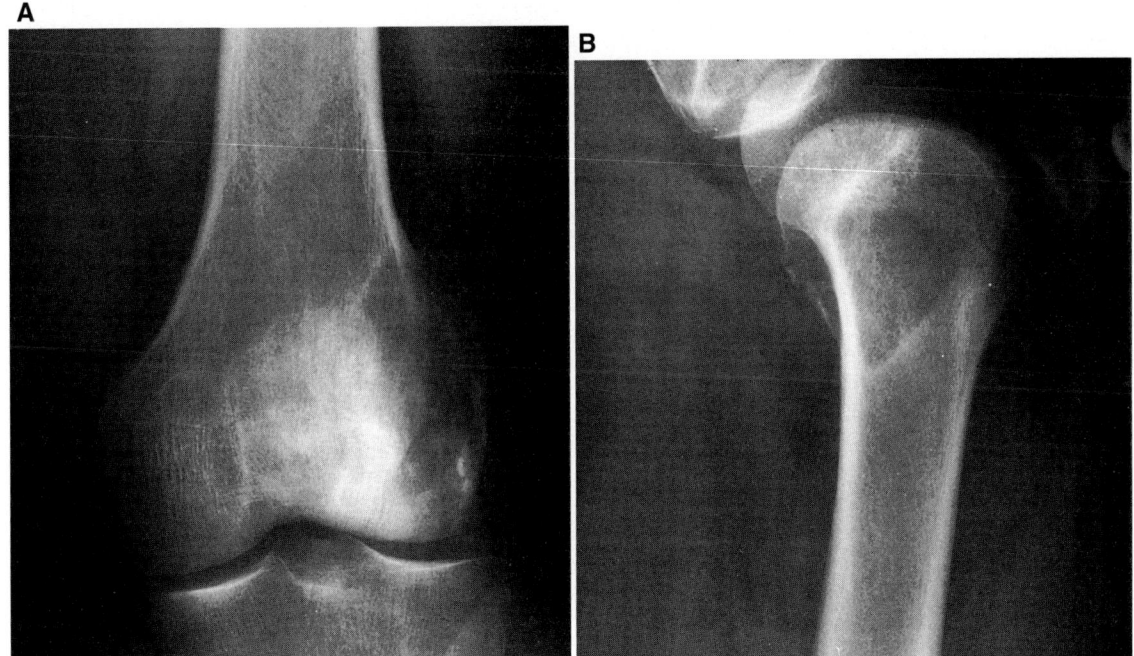

FIG 84–6.
Grade II chondrosarcoma of the lateral femoral condyle. **A,** anteroposterior view; **B,** lateral view.

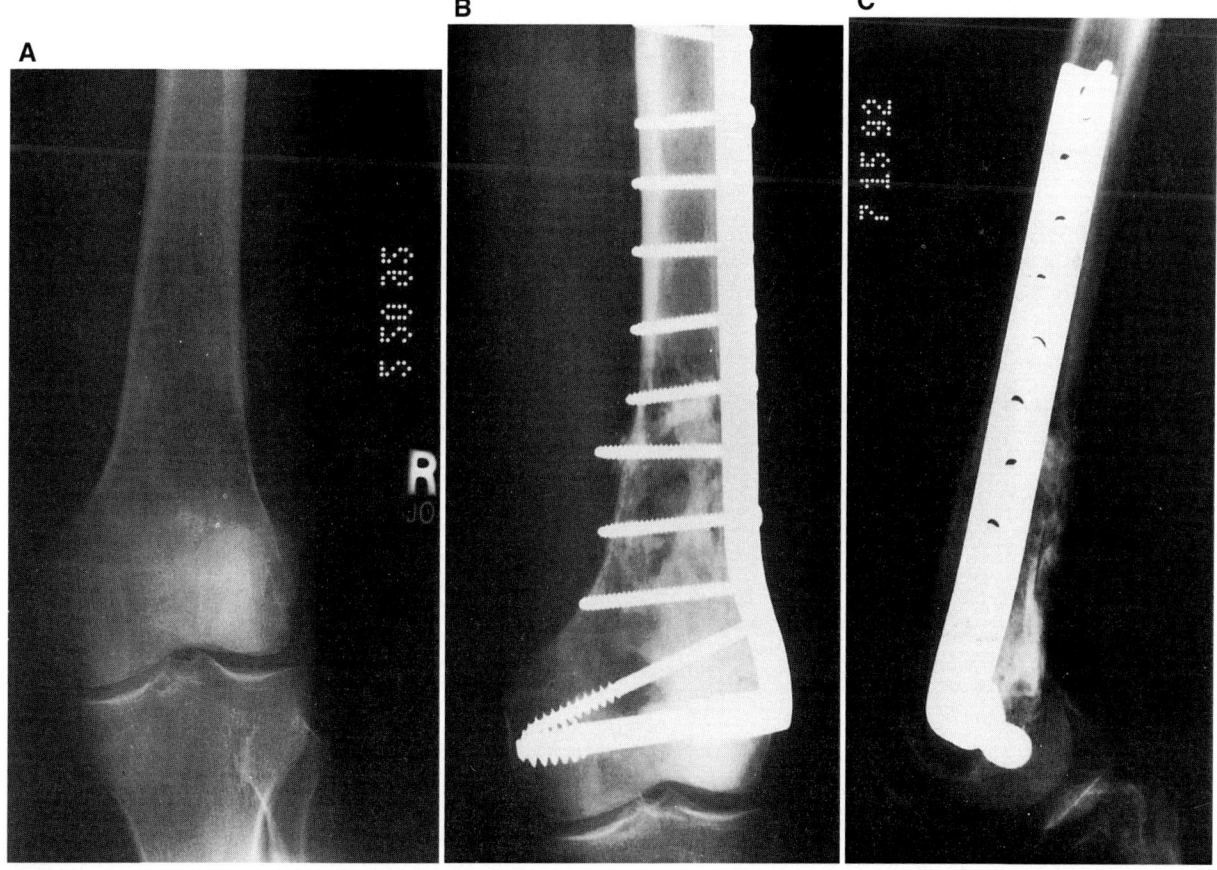

FIG 84–7.
Lymphoma of bone. **A,** a permeating destructive pattern is seen in the anteroposterior view. Healing is seen after internal fixation with a supracondylar screw and side plate and postoperative radiation therapy in anteroposterior **(B)** and lateral **(C)**, views.

myeloma (see Fig 84–26), with breast, renal, and lung cancer the usual suspects in the knee region as elsewhere.

Clinical Presentation

Patients with bone tumors almost always have pain. Slowly growing tumors, however, such as low-grade chondrosarcomas, may be pain-free in as many as one third of patients (Fig 84–8). Patients report that the pain is unresponsive to changes of position, and may even be worse at night or when they are recumbent. A mechanical component is often present as well, heralding structural insufficiency exacerbated by weightbearing. Occasionally lesions may be indolent and symptom-free, only to be diagnosed incidentally. Rarely, a patient sustains a pathologic fracture as the presenting symptom.

The medical history is primarily helpful to exclude infection and congenital conditions. The medical history and focused examination are the investigations most likely to reveal the source of metastatic cancers. It is rare that the family history is contributory. Exceptions include familial osteochondromatosis and newly recognized associations of osteogenic sarcoma with genetic alterations in tumor suppressor genes and familial cancer syndromes.[56]

Coincidental pathologic findings are common in the knee. Thirty percent of patients report that they sustained trauma to the area. Most often the injury merely brings a previously unsuspected lesion to the patient's attention. Rarely is there a significant associated traumatic condition. Patellar pain is ubiquitous. This is particularly true after muscle atrophy and gait abnormalities develop from favoring the affected extremity. The physician must exhibit great restraint and avoid diagnosing the obvious co-morbid condition and miss the offending primary lesion or tumor[44] (Fig 84–9). Therefore, despite the suspicion of a soft tissue injury, malalignment syndrome, or benign intraarticular derangement, all patients should have at least a radiographic examination prior to any operative intervention such as arthroscopy.

Physical examination findings are nonspecific

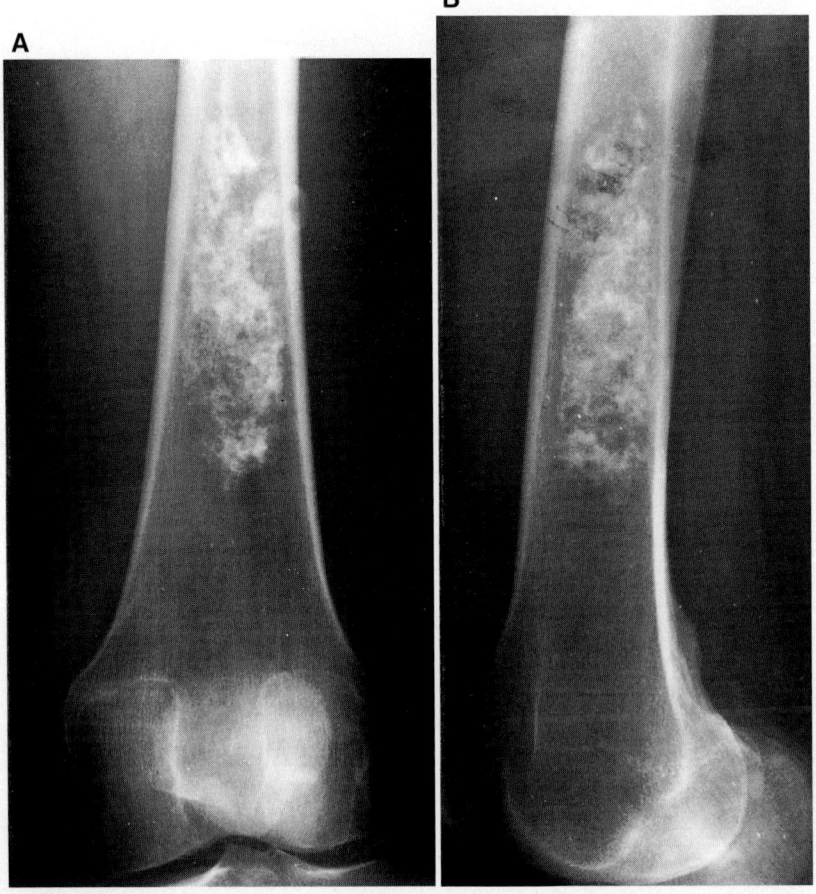

FIG 84–8.
Chondrosarcoma, grade I/II, of the distal femur. **A,** anteroposterior view; **B,** lateral view.

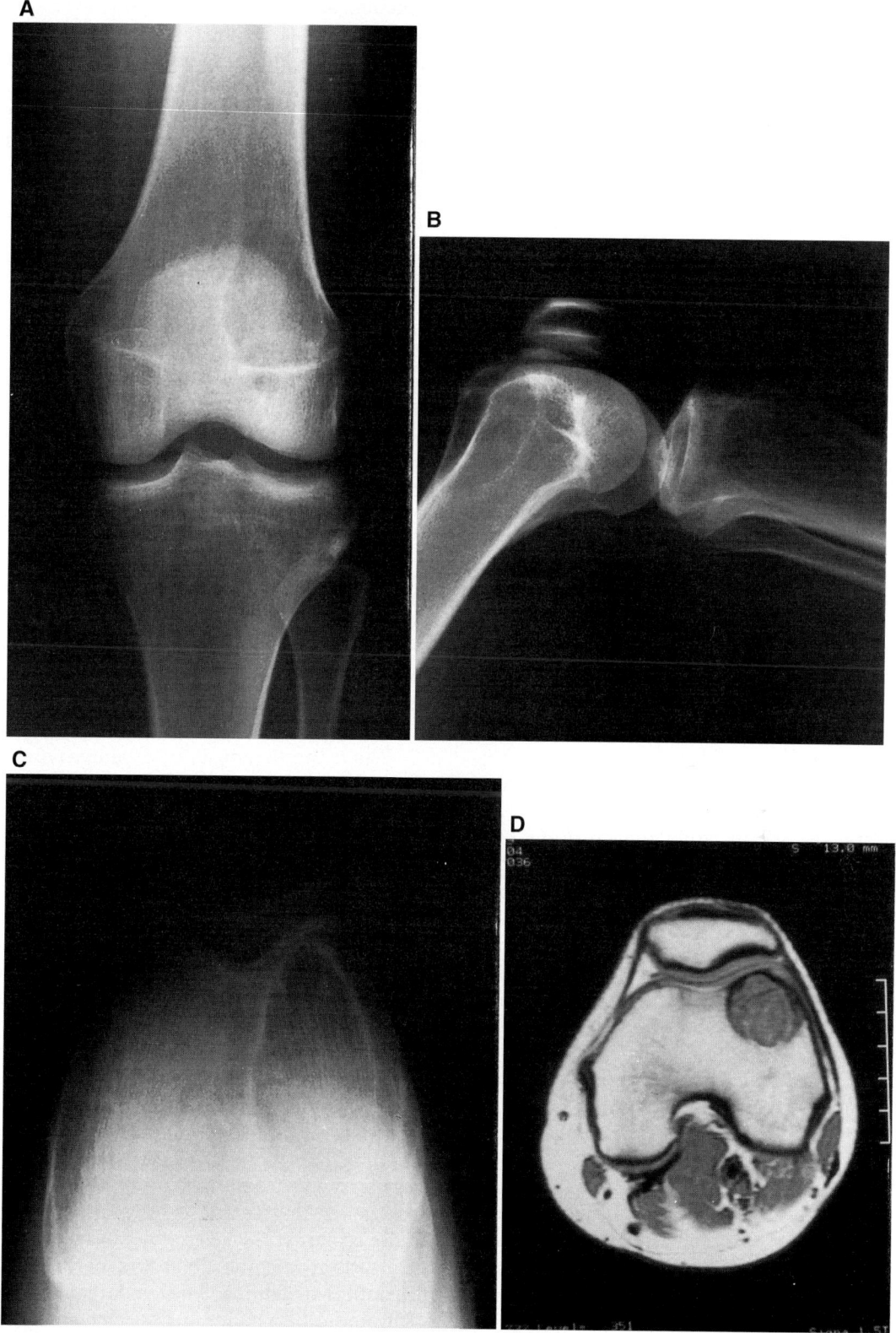

FIG 84–9.
This patient presented with patellofemoral joint pain. Anteroposterior **(A)**, lateral **(B)**, and sunrise **(C)** views, and CT scan **(D)** demonstrate a lytic lesion under the lateral facet of the patellofemoral joint which proved to be a giant cell tumor.

and consist of a palpable mass, painful or limited range of motion, and effusion. Tenderness is variable, and most common in patients with tumors eliciting periosteal reactions. Vascular and neurologic findings are uncommon but do occur. Examination of the hip is important since this may be the source of referred knee pain. Lymphoma is the only primary bone tumor that involves lymph nodes regularly. Lymphadenopathy from tumor involvement occurs in 1% to 2% of spindle cell and round cell sarcomas. General examination of the chest, abdomen, and pelvic organs may reveal the site of the primary cancer in cases of metastatic disease.

Careful physical examination is the most specific indicator of popliteal artery tumor encasement or invasion. If the artery can be palpated and moved over the tumor for the entire length of the lesion, then it can be dissected away safely from a tumor situated in the popliteal space. An effusion is usually only reactive, yet one must suspect tumor involvement of the knee joint. When dealing with malignant tumors an effusion mandates performing a wide tumor excision by removing the joint in an extraarticular fashion.

DIAGNOSTIC STUDIES

Conventional biplane roentgenograms are the most useful and diagnostic tests. They narrow the diagnostic possibilities and suggest whether the tumor is a benign or malignant process. Benign lesions have sharp margins, a narrow zone of transition, and evoke a well-developed host response of bony containment (see Fig 84-9). They may expand the cortical bone, but infrequently destroy it and extend into the soft tissue. Malignant lesions lack a sharp margin, have a wide zone of transition, may permeate cortical and cancellous bone (see Figs 84-7, 84-12, and 84-21), and elicit a primitive host response such as elevating the periosteum (see Figs 84-4, 84-17, and 84-25). The matrix within the lesion can be diagnostic of specific bone tumors. For example, a white cloud of bone is only seen in osteogenic sarcoma.

Osteochondromas and fibrous cortical defects are radiographic diagnoses and need not be biopsied unless tumor growth or symptoms mandate intervention. Virtually all other lesions should be biopsied to confirm the radiographic diagnosis.

Serum tests rarely are specific. The erythrocyte sedimentation rate (ESR) is elevated in most malignant tumors to a mild degree so it does not distinguish them from infections. Multiple myeloma causes significant elevations of the ESR as well as anemia, azotemia, and even hypercalcemia in widespread disease. The alkaline phosphatase level is elevated in 85% of osteogenic sarcomas, and in most patients with Paget's disease of bone. Serum lactate dehydrogenase (LDH) is typically elevated in round cell tumors such as Ewing's sarcoma and lymphoma, with values correlating with tumor burden. Both LDH and alkaline phosphatase have prognostic significance. Patients presenting with elevated levels have lower long-term survival than patients presenting with normal levels.[64] Serum calcium and parathyroid hormone levels are elevated in brown tumors of hyperparathyroidism and these laboratory studies should be checked in all patients with presumed giant cell tumor since these two entities are sometimes impossible to differentiate histologically. Pseudotumors of hemophilia should be suspected by an appropriate history of coagulopathy. Crystalline goutlike deposition disease may demonstrate the diagnostic uric acid or calcium pyrophosphate crystals in synovial fluid. Patients with chondrosarcoma (70%) manifest abnormal glucose tolerance tests[60] and fasting blood sugar values should be determined in these patients. Although a glucose tolerance test is not part of the routine workup of patients with chondrosarcoma, it does suggest that abnormally high levels of circulating insulin levels may stimulate the growth of these tumors.

When the diagnosis of a benign latent lesion is clear, no further imaging is warranted, and one should proceed to biopsy directly. Conversely, if the diagnosis is unclear, or if a more aggressive or possibly malignant lesion is suspected, further imaging will aid in the diagnosis and treatment.

Magnetic resonance imaging (MRI) provides valuable diagnostic information about both benign and malignant lesions, yet still lacks diagnostic precision.[20] The technique excels at defining normal and pathologic anatomy. It is particularly accurate at defining soft tissue, vascular, neural, and marrow space involvement (see Fig 84-4). Conventional spin-echo sequences do not resolve cortical bone involvement as accurately as does computed tomography (CT) scanning. New contrast agents under development show promise for enhancing bone resolution as well as better distinguishing edema and scar from tumor. In the region of the knee, the popliteal artery and its trifurcation, and the tibial and peroneal nerves are the critical structures. Their involvement is a relative contraindication to limb-preserving surgery. Vascular involvement necessitates bypass surgery, and arteriography is useful in preoperative planning (Fig 84-10). Narrowly focused MRI scans taken with only one spin-echo sequence to evaluate intraarticular lesions

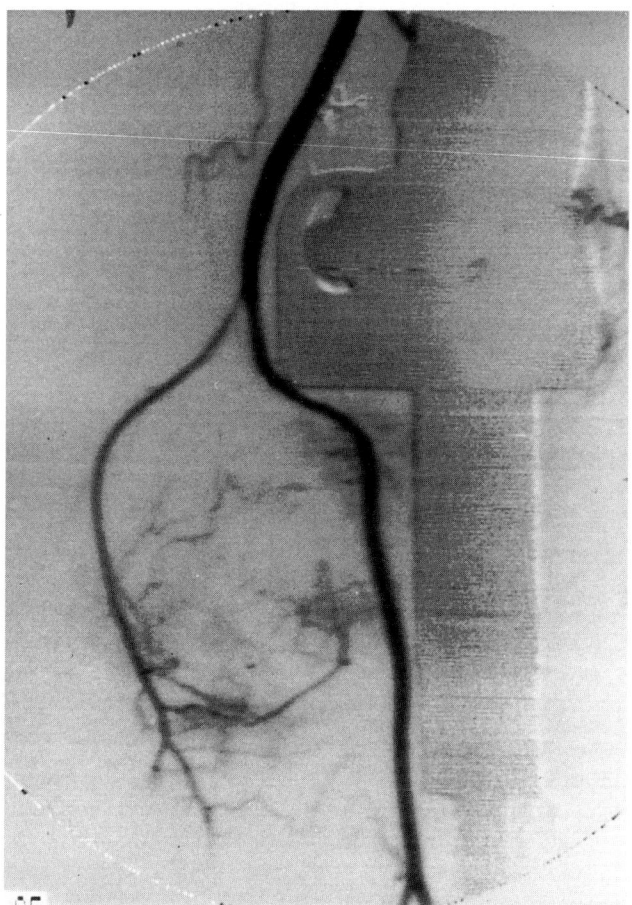

FIG 84–10.
Arteriogram demonstrating involvement of the popliteal artery by a recurrent osteogenic sarcoma.

(meniscal tears) easily miss extraarticular soft tissue and metaphyseal bone tumors. Therefore, a protocol which includes at a minimum a T1-weighted coronal image, a T2-weighted sagittal image, and a gradient echo–weighted axial image should be performed to pick up the unsuspected lesion in the distal femur, proximal tibia, and soft tissues. The evaluation of a tumor requires at least axial T_1 and T_2 imaging in addition to the above sequences.

CT scans are still valuable in imaging bone tumors. This modality remains the best at assessing cortical bone and can detect endosteal cortical erosions not seen on radiographs but caused by tumors, such as low-grade chondrosarcomas that frequent the distal femur and proximal tibia. CT can also detect cortical breakthrough, an important parameter in the Enneking staging system.[24] CT is also sensitive in identifying soft tissue calcification, such as that seen in synovial sarcoma.

Bone tumor staging includes a whole-body technetium 99m pyrophosphate bone scan. If only a localized bone scan has been done (e.g., to evaluate the tibial plateaus or femoral condyles for osteonecrosis), a full-body scan must be repeated since some patients presenting with primary bone tumors will have distant bone metastasis. When metastatic disease is suspected, the bone scan is particularly important since it may identify a better or safer site to biopsy. Gallium scans help to assess soft tissue involvement and distinguish tumor from other conditions that produce a hot bone scan (e.g., regional disuse osteoporosis).[30] Pulmonary metastatic or mediastinal nodal involvement can be ruled out by means of a chest film and CT scan. Chest CT will detect a pulmonary metastasis missed on the plain film and is more sensitive than plain tomography.[16] Table 84–1 summarizes the diagnostic studies we use.

Biopsy Technique

Certain radiologic pictures are diagnostic, as noted above. If classic fibrous cortical defects or osteochondromas are found, particularly as incidental abnormalities, they should not be operated on for diagnostic or treatment purposes. Symptomatic osteochondromas warrant excisional biopsy. The perichondrium and any overlying soft tissue bursae should be completely excised to prevent recurrence. The physician should be careful when ascribing knee pain to the radiographically obvious osteochondroma. The lesions often occur in the medial femoral metaphysis. Since the disease process is developmental and there is uniformly some distortion of the distal femur, patellofemoral malalignment and poor tracking can be seen as well. Patellar pain syndromes in osteochondroma patients may be exacerbated by surgery that weakens the vastus medialis. Excisional biopsy may need to be coupled with lateral retinacular release in such patients, one of the few occasions where

TABLE 84–1.
Recommended Diagnostic Studies of Bone Tumors

Before biopsy	Radiograph (biplanar) of primary site
	Three-dimensional imaging of primary site (MRI or CT)
	Whole-body three-phase bone scan
	Chest radiograph
	Biochemical profile (lactic dehydrogenase, alkaline phosphatase)
	Hematologic profile (complete blood count, erythrocyte sedimentation rate)
Post biopsy	Chest CT (high-grade and low-grade tumors)
	Gallium scan (round cell tumors)
	Bone marrow biopsy (round cell tumors)
Optional	Thallium scan
	Physical examination

it is appropriate to perform incidental reconstructive surgery in tandem with tumor resection. (Incisional biopsy and staged resection are reserved for osteochondromas with large cartilaginous caps, i.e., 1.5 cm as seen on MRI, or growing lesions in adults.) Such lesions either already have, or could convert to, chondrosarcomas and they demand a staged diagnostic and therapeutic approach (see Fig 84-2). Finally, there is little role for prophylactic excision of osteochondroma since the risks of surgery exceed the risk of sarcomatous degeneration of a solitary tumor (estimated at 0.1%). One does not operate simply because a lesion is there and it is abnormal.

Excisional biopsy is good treatment for other lesions where the risk of local recurrence is low and the lesions within the differential diagnosis are all treated similarly. For example, osteoid osteomas should be excised and diagnosed afterward since the diagnostic alternative is Brodie's abscess, a condition which can be treated in the same fashion. Intralesional treatment may be more appropriate for difficult locations.

The most common biopsy technique is the incisional biopsy. Proper technique is necessary to avoid the many complications associated with this procedure.[39, 57, 77] It is the procedure of choice for biopsy of most potentially malignant tumors, particularly when the diagnosis is doubtful, when the tumors are notoriously heterogeneous, or when large amounts of tissue are needed for special tests. The placement of the biopsy incision is crucial since all tissue exposed during the biopsy must be excised in continuity with the tumor mass at the time of the surgical resection. Biopsy incisions about the knee should be over the tumor and in line with extensile exposures that will be used to perform the resection. This typically means that the incision is anteromedial or anterolateral and longitudinal. This minimizes unnecessary extracompartmental contamination and allows for neurovascular exposure during the resection. Posterior and transverse biopsy scars about the knee compromise the extensile exposure needed for an en bloc limb-sparing resection. Biopsy scars should be small to minimize the amount of tissue that must be removed. Large incisions contribute to substantial defects over the knee joint area and serious soft tissue coverage problems. Muscle flaps have improved the options for recouping even large soft tissue defects, permitting limb salvage, and are often used prophylactically when wound healing difficulties are anticipated[40] (see Fig 84-4). Fibular lesions present a particular problem. A longitudinal incision over the anterolateral aspect of the bone is best. The peroneal nerve should not be isolated; otherwise it will have to be sacrificed at the time of subsequent tumor excision if a malignancy is found. Excisional biopsy is a useful option for fibular head lesions, as is discussed later. Intraosseous cartilaginous lesions of the proximal fibula, suspicious of chondrosarcoma, are amenable to primary excision to avoid contaminating the peroneal nerve (Fig 84-11).

Bone biopsies should remove a small amount of bone tissue and preserve the architectural relationship between the lesion and the host bone. A circular or oval hole is the best to minimize stress risers in the bone and reduce the risk of postbiopsy fracture. A trephine works very well, as does the method of connecting multiple drill holes arranged in a circle. If possible, the biopsy should be limited to the soft tissue tumor component to avoid iatrogenic weakening of the bone itself. A frozen section analysis is performed to confirm accurate location and sufficiency of the biopsy. The intraoperative examination may suggest the need for special studies such as electron microscopy, lymphoma typing, and cytogenetics, which require fresh tissue. Multiple cultures are obtained for fungus, acid-fast bacilli, aerobic and anaerobic bacteriologic examination. Prebiopsy antibiotics are avoided since they may prevent the recovery of organisms from the lesion. Tumor spillage should be minimized and meticulous hemostasis obtained. Postoperative ecchymoses and hematoma theoretically contaminate the soft tissues with neoplastic cells and spread the tumor. Absorbable gelatin sponge (Gelfoam), thrombin, hemostatic agents, argon laser, and even cementation of the cortical window in the bone are used as needed to prevent postoperative hemorrhage. If a drain is used, it should be small and placed in line with the incision, and the tract of the drain excised in continuity with the biopsy incision at the time of resection.

Following a bone biopsy it is important to instruct the patient in protective weightbearing to prevent a pathologic fracture. A pathologic fracture does not preclude limb salvage, but it disseminates tumor and makes it more difficult to obtain a wide margin of resection.

A tourniquet is not essential but is an excellent aid when biopsying highly vascular tumors. There is no evidence that a tourniquet avoids, or contributes to tumor dissemination. An elastic bandage should not be used to exsanguinate the limb prior to biopsy.

Percutaneous needle biopsies may work when performed by the surgeon and if the pathologist is comfortable with interpreting small specimens. As for open biopsies, the needle must be placed carefully so that the tract can be excised in continuity with the tumor. Percutaneous biopsies are nondiagnostic or

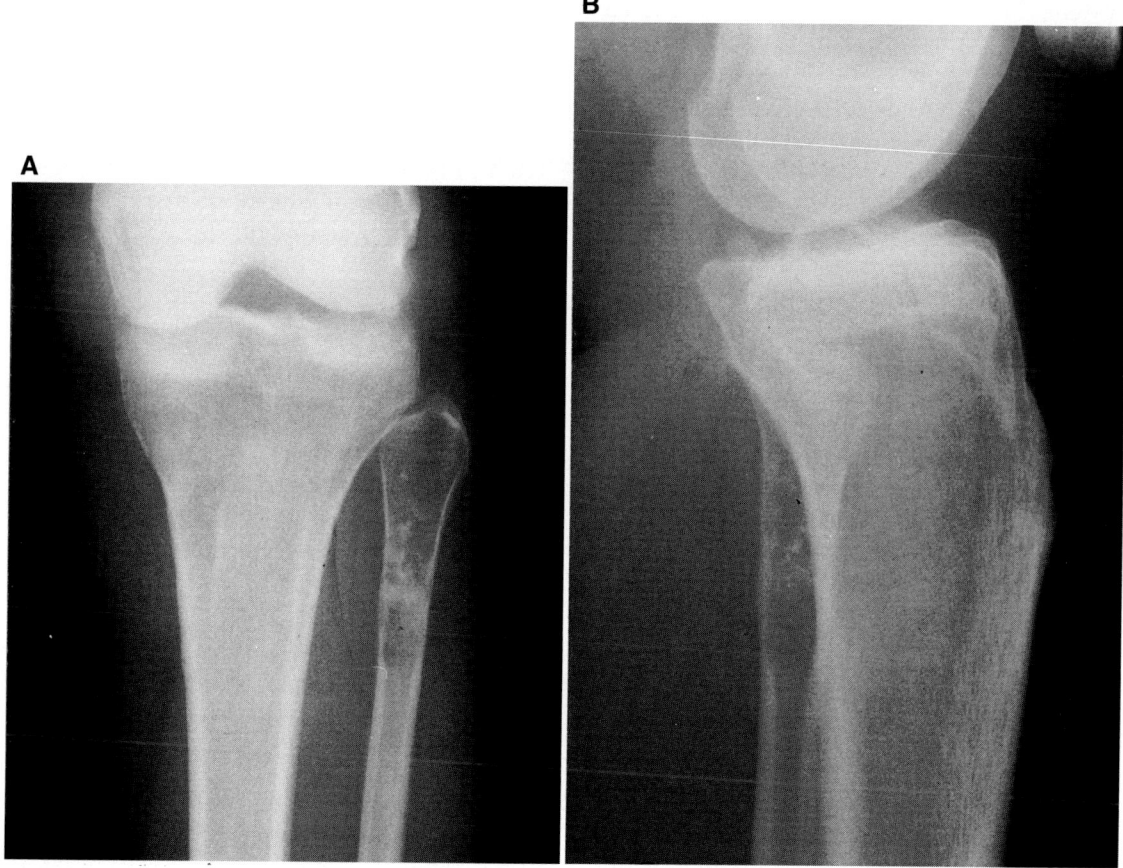

FIG 84–11.
Chondrosarcoma, grade II, of the proximal fibula. **A,** anteroposterior view; **B,** lateral view.

misleading ten times as often as open biopsies. The biopsy technique of preference depends in large part on how much the physician and the patient can live with surprises. Certain lesions, such as a juxtacortical osteogenic sarcoma and myositis ossificans, must be distinguished by a biopsy that preserves the spatial orientation of the tissue, and allows the zonation phenomenon to be seen. A large-core biopsy accomplishes this goal well.

Staging

Staging structures the approach to both benign and malignant tumors. It not only organizes the diagnostic process, but predicts outcome and dictates treatment.

Benign tumors are staged by one of two methods. The Enneking method is more comprehensive but cumbersome.[24] We prefer the simple Campanacci system based solely on the radiograph.[14] Latent lesions (stage A) are contained within bone, without thinning the surrounding cortex. Active lesions (stage B) are within bone, but evoke a cortical reaction: lysis is typical, but sclerosis may occur. Aggressive lesions (stage C) break through the cortex into surrounding soft tissue. Neither system predicts outcome, however. In a recent European-American musculoskeletal tumor society symposium, Campanacci[14] demonstrated that recurrence rates of giant cell tumor treated by intralesional methods did not differ by stage and that the Enneking and Campanacci systems were not statistically different. The value of benign tumor staging seems to be that it forces careful anatomic definition of the tumor which helps plan proper tumor ablation and requisite skeletal reconstruction. Current practice is to treat latent lesions with intralesional methods and usually bone graft. Active lesions may warrant local adjuvants such as cement and cryosurgery. Aggressive lesions may be treated with curettage and an adjuvant or may warrant resection and bone and joint reconstruction if tumor extent and functional considerations dictate.

The staging of malignant bone tumors is much more standardized and prognostically accurate. Multiple systems exist for soft tissue tumors. In the Enneking system,[24] malignant bone tumors are graded based on histologic criteria and metastatic potential as either low grade or high grade. Low-grade lesions are stage I and high-grade lesions are stage II. Substage A or B refers to the anatomic extent of the tumor. *A* denotes that the tumor is confined within the bony compartment, whereas *B* signifies that the tumor extends beyond the compartment into the surrounding joint or soft tissue. Stage III includes metastatic tumors, either high or low grade. Most malignant tumors (both bone and soft tissue) are high grade and extracompartmental, i.e., stage IIB lesions. Round cell tumors such as Ewing's sarcoma are staged differently. About the knee, examples of typical lesions in each stage are shown in the following figures. Figure 84–8—stage IA low-grade intraosseous chondrosarcoma of the distal femoral metadiaphysis; Figure 84–5—stage IB low-grade juxtacortical osteogenic sarcoma (parosteal osteogenic sarcoma); Figure 84–12—stage IIA small classic osteogenic sarcoma; Figure 84–4—stage IIB classic osteogenic sarcoma breaking out into the soft tissue.

Soft tissue extension into the popliteal space poses significant staging problems since the area behind the knee is not bounded by well-developed fascial planes. By definition, the popliteal space is extracompartmental. There is merely loose fat and areolar tissue remaining between a popliteal tumor and the popliteal artery and vein. This has important treatment implications as is demonstrated later. Prognosis has been shown to correlate with these stages, although refinements which take into account the size of the lesion, anatomic site, age, and some measure of biologic aggressiveness will ideally be incorporated into future staging systems. Soft tissue malignancies can be classified by this same system. More informative and predictive are systems that are dealt with later in the chapter.

Surgery is the mainstay for treating all bone and soft tissue malignancies. Wide local excision is the norm, which is defined as the excision of the tumor with a surrounding layer of normal, unreactive tissue on all surfaces. When effective local or systemic adjuvants are available, then a narrower margin of normal tissue resection may suffice. In the absence of an effective adjuvant, very wide or radical compartment excision should be considered to effect a cure. Accurate staging is fundamental to surgical decision making. Functional considerations come into play as well, and clinical judgment is needed. Sometimes it is better to accept a narrow margin to enhance the functional result, particularly in a low-grade tumor where it is still possible to cure most recurrences. Since metastasis is unlikely, this approach is reasonable. On the other hand, high-grade tumors must be treated aggressively from the outset. One should remember that the best chance for cure is from the initial resection. Ablation of all involved structures is the conservative approach that will save lives. Proper staging clarifies biologic potential and anatomic distribution of the tumor, thereby dictating treatment.

Treatment

Benign Bone Tumors

Benign bone tumors that have indisputable radiologic features, such as asymptomatic osteochondromas or metaphyseal cortical defects, do not need to be biopsied or treated. If the diagnosis is in doubt, or known lesions become symptomatic, biopsy and treatment are appropriate. Latent lesions can be treated with curettage and bone grafting. Active and aggressive lesions may require the addition of an adjuvant such as cryosurgery, phenol, bone cement, or a limited en bloc excision. The treatment methods and common technical variations are dealt with in the discussion of the giant cell tumor (GCT), below.

Rare tumors pose interesting specialized problems when they occur about the knee. For example, chondroblastoma has unusual manifestations. It has a predilection for epiphyseal locations that are difficult to see well by conventional radiographic imaging. The subchondral bone in the intercondylar notch and the tibial spine frequently harbors chondroblastoma (see Fig 84–3). Special radiographic views such as the intercondylar notch and tibial plateau views may be helpful to define the lesion and to monitor for possible recurrence.[92] The deep central location limits direct access by conventional routes such as an extraarticular medial or lateral exposure. Intraarticular exposure is sometimes acceptable to limit the amount of normal bone removal that would be needed. The nonweightbearing nature of these special locations makes the transarticular approach feasible. It is critical to protect the remaining joint from tumor implantation. We advocate isolation of the tumor bed with sponges and vigorous joint lavage after tumor removal when approaching a tumor through the joint. Chondroblastomas of the tibia commonly extend along the growth plate and into the tibial tubercle. Coronal and sagittal MRI is often helpful in defining tibial tubercle involvement. Great care must be taken when removing tumors in this location because the remaining shell of cortical bone is subject to avulsion fracture and extensor mechanism disruption. Reinforcement with a screw and washer should be considered and the postoperative rehabili-

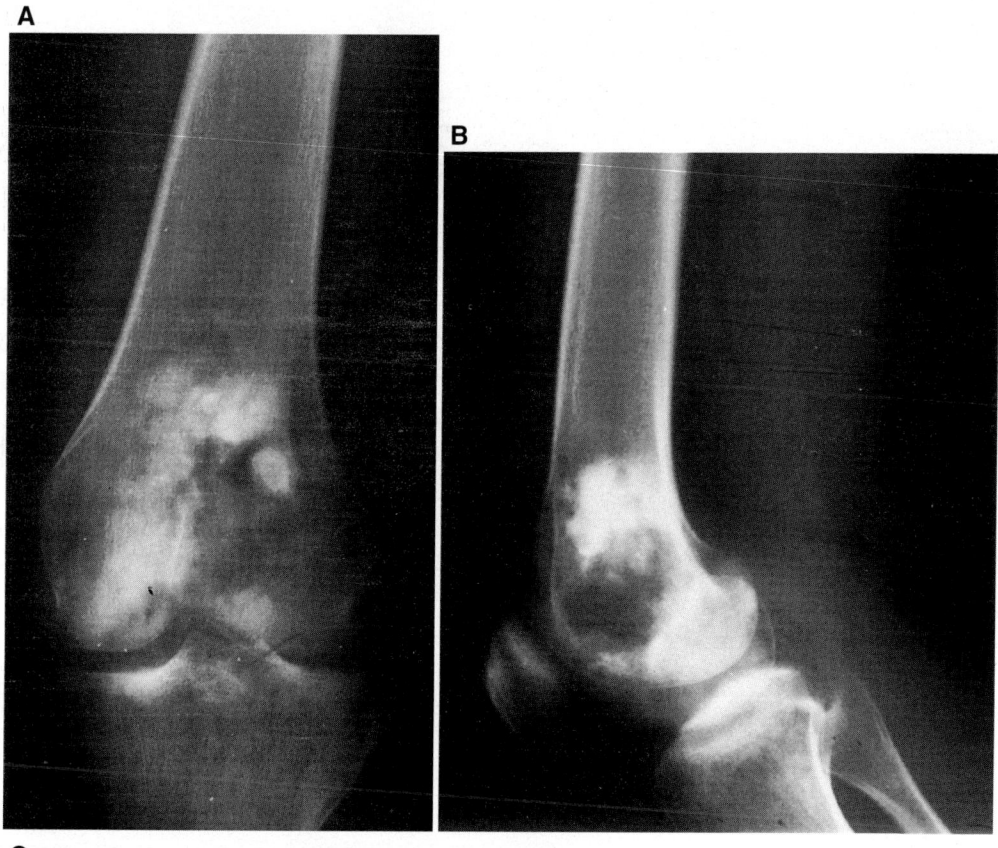

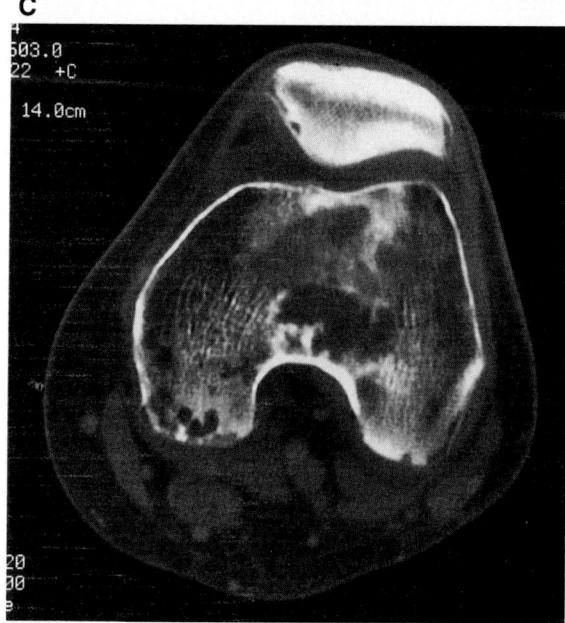

FIG 84-12.
Osteogenic sarcoma of the distal femur, Enneking stage IIA. **A,** anteroposterior view; **B,** lateral view; **C,** CT scan.

tation program suspended when the tubercle is destabilized.

Giant Cell Tumor. Treatment for GCT encompasses the principles previously articulated for benign bone tumors and highlights important variations needed to address the peculiar subchondral location and aggressiveness of this tumor. Most GCTs occur in the epiphyseal distal femur or proximal tibia, and extend to the subchondral bone (see Fig 84-9 and Fig 84-13). Carefully aggressive treatment reduces the historically high recurrence rates to less than 10% and preserves joint function. Simple curet-

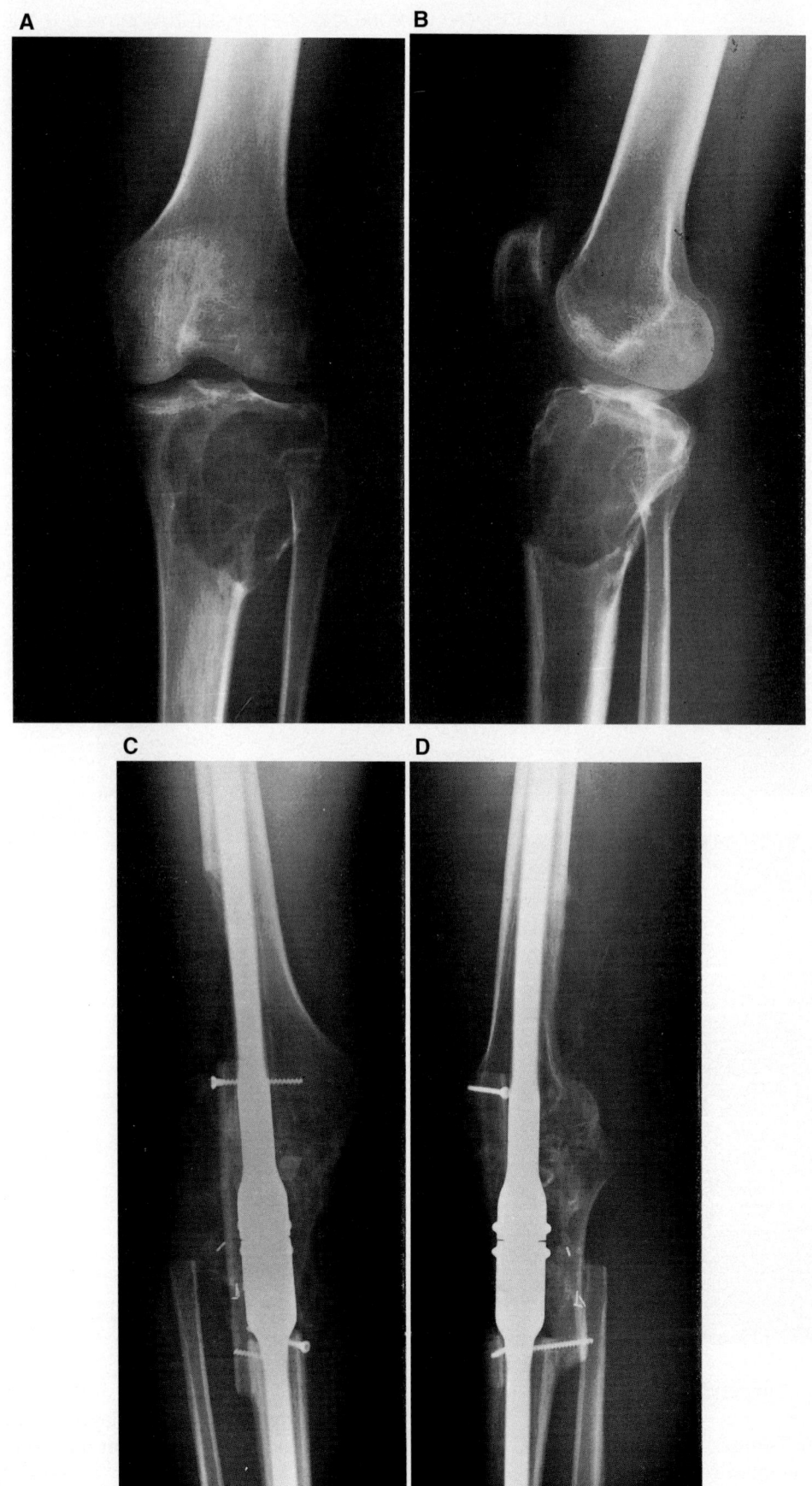

FIG 84–13.
Giant cell tumor of the proximal tibia. **A,** anteroposterior view; **B,** lateral view. The patient wanted a durable reconstruction and an arthrodesis was performed with a Neff nail and femoral turndown graft. Postoperative anteroposterior **(C)** and lateral **(D)** views.

tage has approximately a 50% recurrence rate. At the other extreme, few GCTs relapse after resection, but this treatment has the greatest morbidity and reconstructive difficulty. Prosthetic knee replacement or allografts can salvage cases in which joint destruction or tumor recurrence necessitate joint resection (Fig 84–14). Eccentric tumors may destroy one portion of the knee joint, such as one femoral condyle. Such lesions are well treated by local excision and replacement of a single condyle (or plateau) with an allograft (Fig 84–15). Preservation of joint alignment, stability, and structure contribute to the high success rates reported for this type of "hemi-joint" replacement (see Fig 84–15). The large cancellous surface and interface contribute to more rapid graft healing and incorporation than seen with complete osteochondral allografts. Fortunately, en bloc excision is rarely needed and the intralesional technique is very effective in eradicating the aggressive tumor.

Intralesional surgery is usually best. The tumor is fully exteriorized through a large cortical bone window. The lesion is curetted aggressively and a high-speed burr is used to eliminate fingers of tumor extending though cancellous and subchondral bone. Particular attention is paid to the diaphyseal side of the tumor since most recurrences develop in this often neglected region.

Chemical and physical modalities extend the margin of tumor excision and improve tumor control. Acrylic cement evolves heat and necroses a small rim of surrounding bone. This not only kills tumor but mechanically supports the defect, allowing early weightbearing. Long-term follow-up has shown that the cement functions well and that it need not be replaced electively with bone grafts (Fig 84–16). Supplemental cryosurgery can dramatically extend the volume of bone sterilized, potentially reducing the recurrence rate further.[61] Theoretic objections to cryosurgery include reduced bone healing and a high fracture rate, problems that can be treated preemptively with prophylactic internal fixation. Surface treatments such as phenol application and laser therapy do not penetrate well and have no proven value.

Malignant Bone Tumors

A four-part surgical staging system defines the nature of any tumor excision and specifies the surgical margin that was attained.[24] An intralesional margin occurs when an incision passes through the lesion. Curettage or even translesional amputations are examples of intralesional procedures. Intralesional excision is suitable only for benign lesions. A marginal excision courses through the inflammatory layer around a tumor. The most common example is an excisional biopsy around the tumor pseudocapsule. It usually leaves microscopic disease at the margin of the wound and is associated with routine recurrence of malignant tumors. Reexcision of the tumor and surgical bed with a wide margin is recommended after marginal excision of a malignant bone or soft tissue tumor. A wide excision removes the lesion and a cuff of surrounding normal tissue. Most limb-sparing en bloc excisions for sarcomas are performed by obtaining a wide surgical margin. A radical margin is obtained by removing all of the tumor, the entire soft tissue and bone compartments that contain the tumor, and all structures that course through the compartments. This means removing the entire femur for a distal femoral lesion or the entire quadriceps for a distal vastus lateralis lesion. Amputations are not necessarily more radical than local excisions. For example, an adductor compartment resection is actually more radical than an above-knee amputation for a synovial sarcoma of the distal gracilis.

When an effective adjuvant is available, such as chemotherapy for osteogenic sarcoma or radiotherapy for soft tissue sarcomas, a wide local excision is the current standard of practice. This approach was well articulated in the 1985 NIH Consensus Conference on limb salvage surgery.[67]

Osteogenic Sarcoma. Limb preservation does not compromise survival rates compared to amputation for similar stages and locations of osteogenic sarcomas. Multi-institutional long-term follow-up of patients substantiates the findings of comparable survival rates despite an increase in the local recurrence rate: limb salvage, 11%; above-knee amputation, 8%; hip disarticulation, 0%.[80] These results show that in the era of modern chemotherapy there is no adverse impact on survival when resectable lesions are treated with limb-sparing surgery. Despite chemotherapy, large, poorly responding tumors should be evaluated as if no effective adjuvant exists, and radical resection should be considered the most curative treatment.

Gross survival rates of 80% can be expected for the stage IIA and IIB lower limb lesions. In the Memorial Sloan-Kettering experience, disease-free survivals are durable, with few patients relapsing between the third and tenth year of follow-up.[64] Tibial lesions have significantly better survival than distal femoral tumors,[64] yet limb salvage has less predictable functional results and durability.[42]

Improvement is sorely needed in our ability to retrieve high-risk cases. In contrast to localized stage II lesions, only 15% of patients with distant metastases can be cured. Limb salvage is the humane and onco-

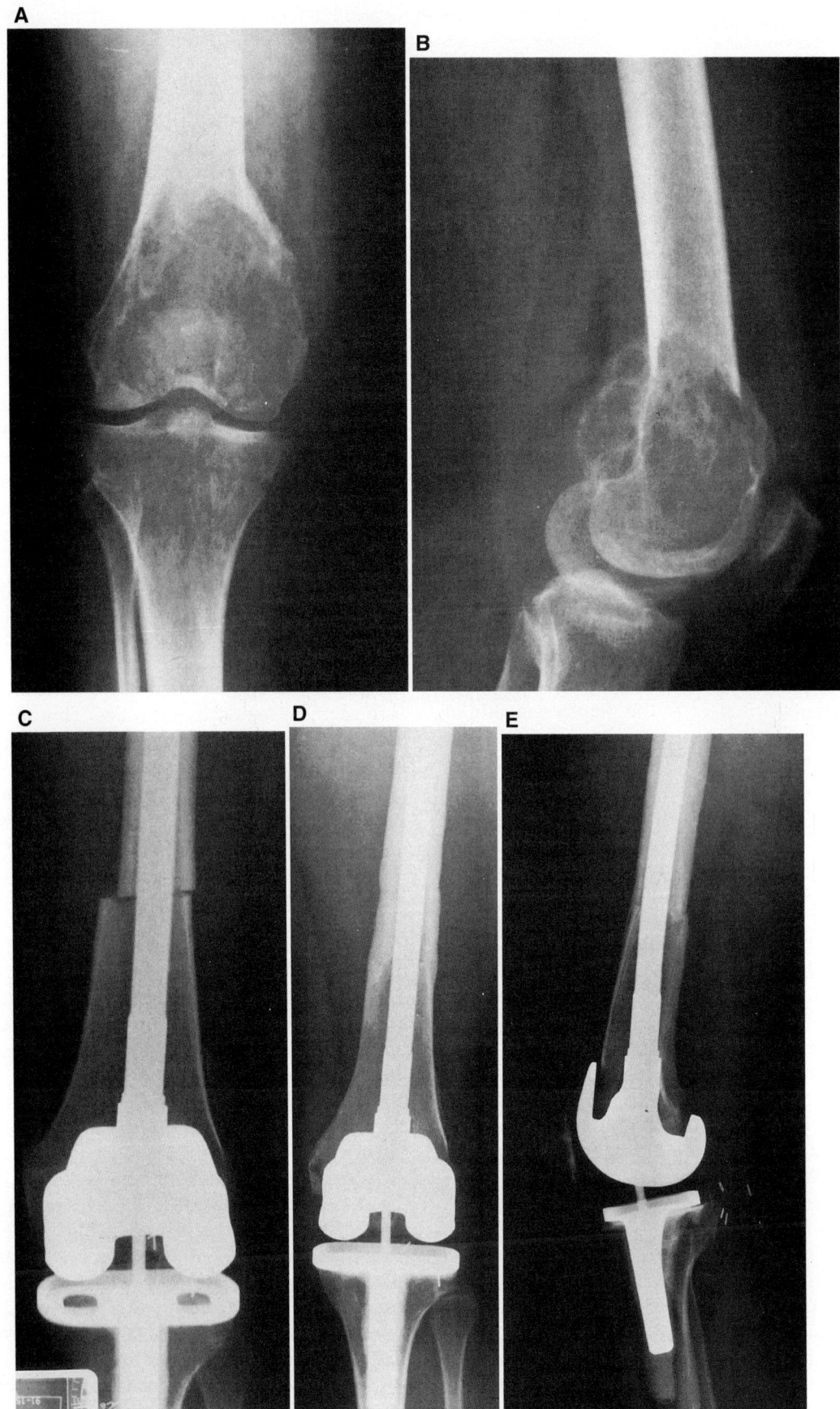

FIG 84-14.
Giant cell tumor of the distal femur. **A,** anteroposterior view; **B,** lateral view. Reconstruction was performed with an allograft-endoprosthesis composite. **C,** Postoperative anteroposterior view. Anteroposterior **(D)** and lateral **(E)** views demonstrate healing of the allograft to the host bone.

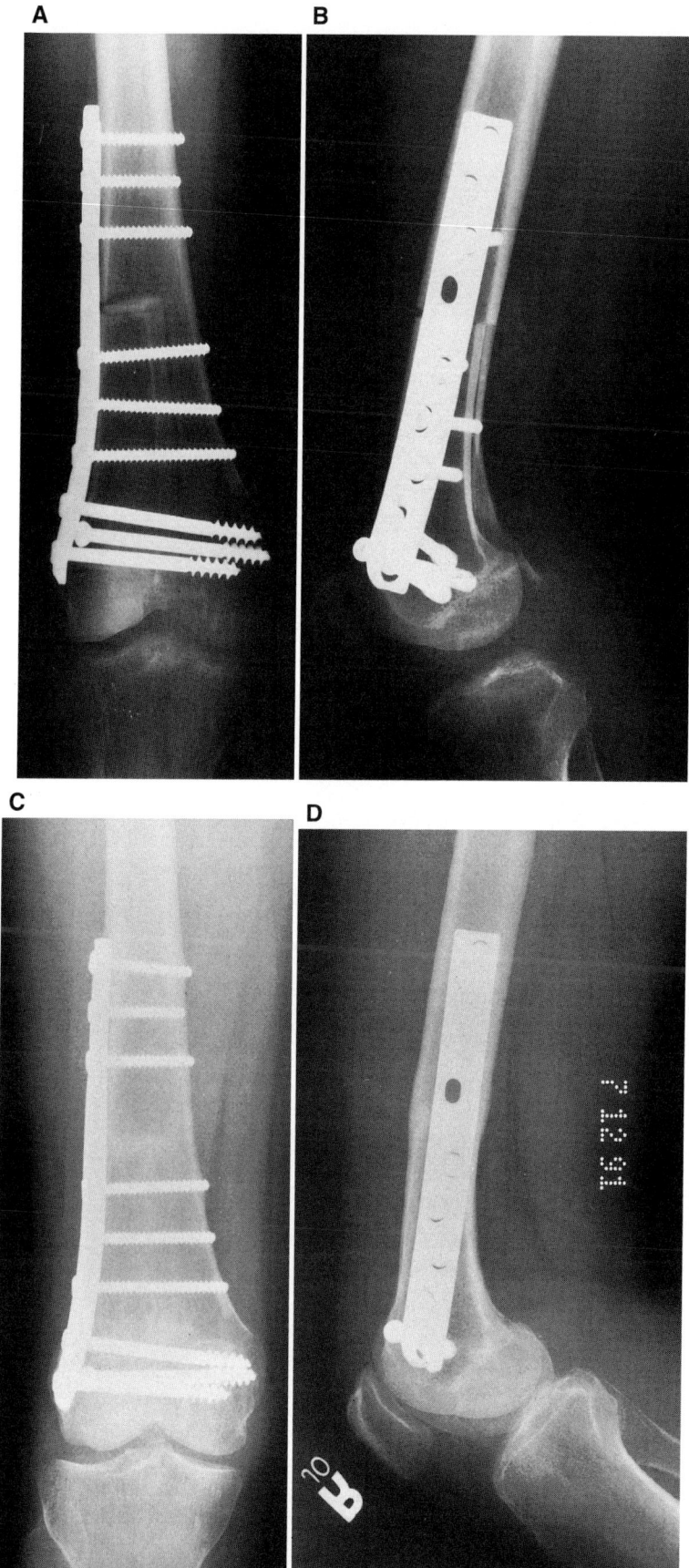

FIG 84–15.
Reconstruction of a lateral femoral condyle which was resected for a giant cell tumor. **A,** anteroposterior view; **B,** lateral view. After healing, anteroposterior **(C)** and lateral **(D)** views.

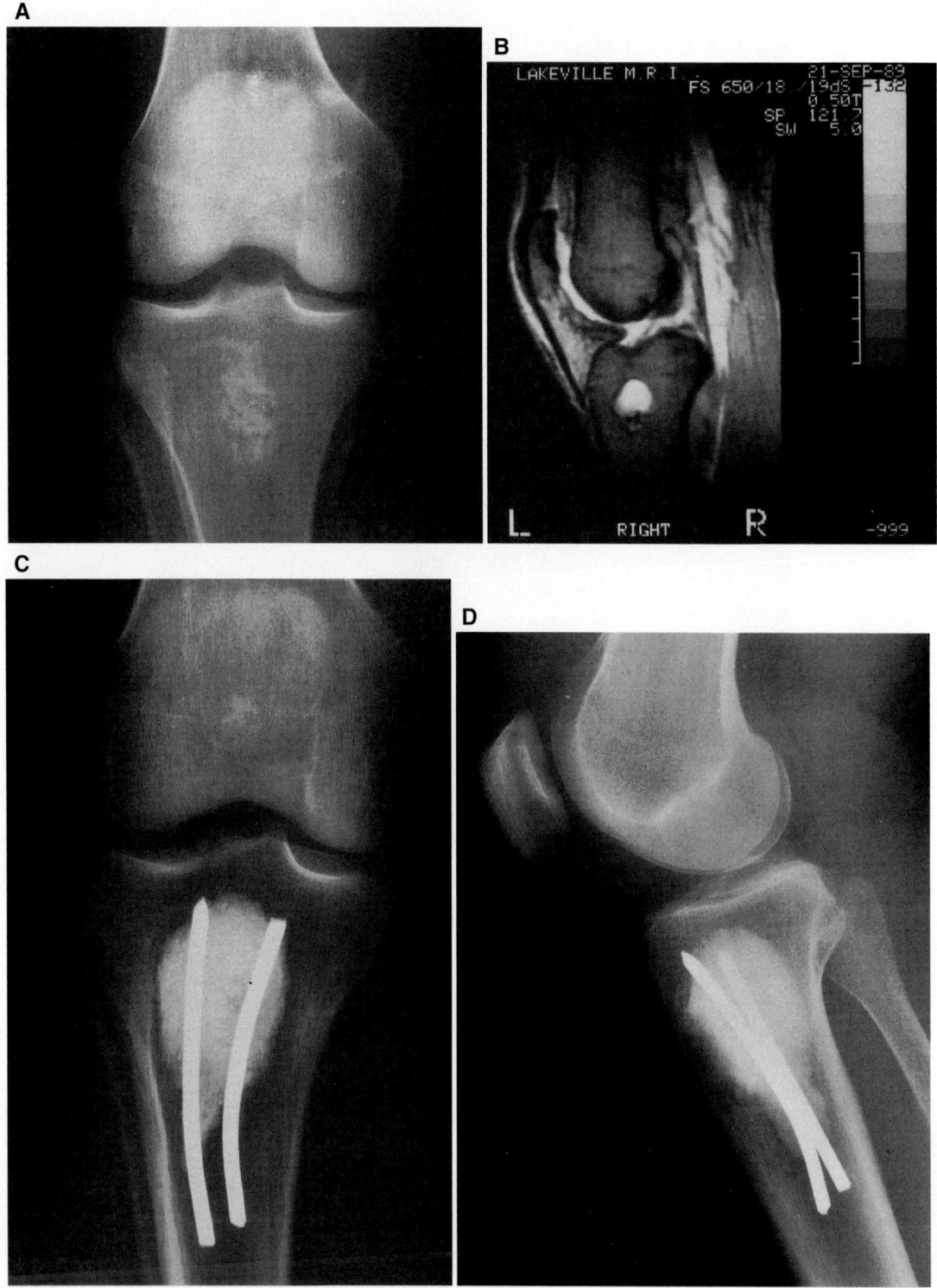

FIG 84–16.
Chondrosarcoma of the proximal tibia, grade I. **A,** anteroposterior view; **B,** CT scan. Lesion was treated with curettage, cryosurgery, and cementation with pins. Postoperative anteroposterior **(A)** and lateral **(D)** views.

logically sound option for these patients. Stage III tumors warrant amputation only when there is a pathologic fracture or uncontrolled symptoms from the primary tumor.

Stage I low-grade osteogenic sarcomas are uncommon, occur in adults, and may spare the knee joint. They develop on the surface (juxtacortical, parosteal) or the intramedullary space.[1, 26, 28, 81, 84–86] Surface tumors involve the marrow space in as many as 20% of cases, an underappreciated fact. Furthermore, just because a tumor is located on the bone surface, it still may harbor high-grade elements. Therefore, biopsy is needed to stage these tumors, which have a predilection for the posterior distal femur. If the tumor is confirmed to be low grade, chemotherapy is contraindicated. Local excision is the preferred treatment, and amputation is only needed for massive tumors involving the neurovascular structures. The reconstruction is based on tumor extent and anatomy. Intercalary or osteoarticular allografts are attractive options since there is no need for chemotherapy that would interfere with wound or bone healing (see Fig 84–5).

Adjuvant Chemotherapy

Adjuvant multiagent chemotherapy is standard treatment for some high-grade malignant bone tumors around the knee. In osteosarcoma, chemotherapy has increased disease-free survival from less than 20% when treatment was by radical surgery alone to approximately 70% when systemic treatment is combined with aggressive local therapy.[10, 64, 74, 75] The data are incontrovertible for osteogenic sarcoma and Ewing's sarcoma. Other histologic tumor types may not be as responsive to existing chemotherapy. Low-grade sarcomas (e.g., "parosteal" osteogenic sarcoma) do not require chemotherapy, and no evidence exists for recommending routine adjuvant chemotherapy for high-grade soft tissue sarcomas or chondrosarcoma.

Because of the low tumor incidence, it is difficult to accrue sufficient cases to test all potential combinations of chemotherapeutic agents and establish which is the best option. Furthermore, the small number of cases prevents us from demonstrating a statistically significant improvement in cure rates above the current 70% for osteosarcoma. We use osteosarcoma and Ewing's sarcoma as paradigms to show the current approach to high-grade malignant tumors.

When an osteogenic sarcoma is diagnosed, most patients will already have microscopic foci of metastatic disease. Systemic treatment is needed to eliminate micrometastases. Preoperative chemotherapy rapidly shrinks bulky primary and metastatic tumor. In the estimated 85% of patients who have responsive tumors, the distance, or margin, increases between the sarcoma and the popliteal vessels—the rate-limiting distance that determines tumor resectability. Preoperative chemotherapy increases the rate at which limbs can be saved. The extent of necrosis induced in the primary tumor determines the effectiveness of chemotherapy. Long-term results of chemotherapy based on high-dose methotrexate administration show that the extent of necrosis in the resected specimen predicts the disease-free survival.[64] Coupled with measurement of the surgical margin, necrosis also predicts the likelihood of local tumor control (or conversely, the recurrence rate.) Unfortunately, the idea that the response to preoperative chemotherapy should govern the choice of postoperative chemotherapy and allow tailoring of effective postoperative chemotherapy has not worked.[64, 76] New regimens, based on ifosfamide and cisplatinum may induce greater primary tumor necrosis than that seen with methotrexate, but they have not yet demonstrated cure rates superior to more traditional regimens. It is presumed that agents which give higher rates of necrosis result in higher rates of long-term survival, but, long-term follow-up is needed to determine if the predictive value of tumor necrosis obtained with one type of chemotherapy can be extrapolated to new chemotherapy protocols.

Another advantage of preoperative chemotherapy is that it provides time for the manufacture of custom endoprostheses for reconstruction of the salvaged limb.[74, 75] It also provides time for the patient and surgeon to establish a therapeutic relationship prior to surgical intervention.[79] This pays great dividends when supervising the postoperative rehabilitation or dealing with surgical complications.

Many centers give adjuvant chemotherapy to all patients with high-grade spindle cell sarcomas similar to osteogenic sarcoma, certain high-grade chondrosarcomas, high-grade fibrosarcomas, and malignant fibrous histiocytoma. Evidence is sparse to support this practice, however. Exciting new biologic agents may produce further improvement in survival of human osteogenic sarcomas, as they have done in naturally occurring canine osteogenic sarcoma. We are currently testing muramyl tripeptide phosphoenthanolamine (MTP-PE), a modulator of macrophage function, as a salvage agent for high-risk and relapsed cases of osteogenic sarcoma.

Combination chemotherapy is also mandatory in treating small cell malignancies such as Ewing's sarcoma. Initial aggressive chemotherapy not only clears micrometastatic disease but dramatically shrinks, or even obliterates, the primary tumor. Local control depends on sterilization of the primary tumor site. Radiation often succeeds in this regard, but it has a very high short- and long-term complication rate. Local recurrence is reported in as many as 28% of irradiated cases. About the knee, radiation of the growth plates will predictably produce a severe limb length inequality. Knee joint contractures are common as well.[53] Pathologic fracture and delayed union or nonunion are common sequelae of the high doses of radiation used (50 Gy). Finally, a startlingly high rate of secondary radiation-associated malignancy has been reported (1% per year).[37] Therefore, most oncologists now recommend resection of the primary bone as the best way to achieve local control and avoid long-term complications. When the bone is "dispensable," such as the fibula, there is little controversy. When the femur is the primary site, however, the best method for local control is not always clear. We recommend wide local excision and prosthetic replacement of the knee or diaphyseal replacement of the femur as dictated by the tumor location (Fig 84–17). Supplemental radiation is still occasionally needed if a wide margin is not obtained.

SURGICAL TECHNIQUE FOR MALIGNANT BONE TUMORS

Decision Making

Surgical decision making for malignant lesions about the knee is complex. It depends on many factors. Accurate surgical staging and pathologic diagnosis are of major importance. Imaging studies after preliminary chemotherapy should be repeated before making a final decision about which surgical procedure to recommend. The extent of bone and joint and soft tissue and neurovascular involvement are evaluated as well. The chemotherapeutic response based on tumor shrinkage, pain relief, biochemical changes (decreased alkaline phosphatase and LDH) and improvement in the imaging characteristics are assessed. If all of the tests are favorable, limb sparing is proper. If there is no improvement, amputation is safer. Decision analysis of amputation vs. limb salvage has been modeled and favors limb salvage for tumors about the knee.[65] Oncologic principles must not be compromised just to preserve a limb because local recurrence and death will be the outcome.

The patient's age plays a major role in determining the type of surgical procedure that should be employed. Major limb length inequality will occur in young children who lose their distal femoral and proximal tibial physes. The expandable prostheses touted for these patients are too small and biomechanically inadequate for the demands placed on the knee joint[47, 48, 52] (Fig 84–18). Furthermore, they must be expanded every 6 months to keep pace with growth. Children recovering from cancer and chemotherapy should not be subjected to additional repetitive surgeries. If the transection level is within 7 cm of the lesser trochanter, stump-extending alternatives such as turnplasty or rotationplasty may be considered[12, 29, 35, 63, 87] (Fig 84–19). If a longer stump is feasible and the patient does not want a rotationplasty, then amputation remains the most suitable surgical option.

MRI provides accurate documentation of the proximal and distal margins of tumor, and particularly the extent of intramedullary involvement[83] (see Fig 84–4). The presence of "skip" metastases are excluded by MRI and bone scan. Whether limb salvage or amputation is chosen, the bone is transected approximately 3 to 5 cm away from the bony limit of disease, although even these margins may be difficult to obtain in small children.

En Bloc Excision of the Knee

Limb-sparing wide excision of the knee joint is an oncologically valid option to amputation.[59] The surgical techniques of resection and reconstruction continue to evolve. These procedures should be performed in centers with extensive experience in the methods and with access to multidisciplinary oncologic care for the patients.

A tourniquet is applied to obtain a dry field during cementation of an endoprosthesis or if bleeding is a problem. The incision is placed longitudinally as dictated by the medial or lateral biopsy scar, with care taken not to compromise a potential site of proximal amputation with unnecessary incisions. The "no-touch" technique is adhered to assiduously. The saphenous vein and nerve are preserved if possible. Flaps are created either above the fascia or below the fascia, as required. Retaining the fascia improves and facilitates wound closure and healing, but should not be done at the expense of a wide margin. The semimembranosus, pes, and medial gastrocnemius are detached as necessary to allow exposure of the popliteal vessels. The popliteal areolar tissue is retained with the tumor. The vascular adventitia is split and the artery and vein are shelled out separately, ligating all branches. The vessels are mobilized distally past the popliteal trifurcation. The muscles are incised at the predetermined level down to the femur. The femur is transected and frozen sections are ob-

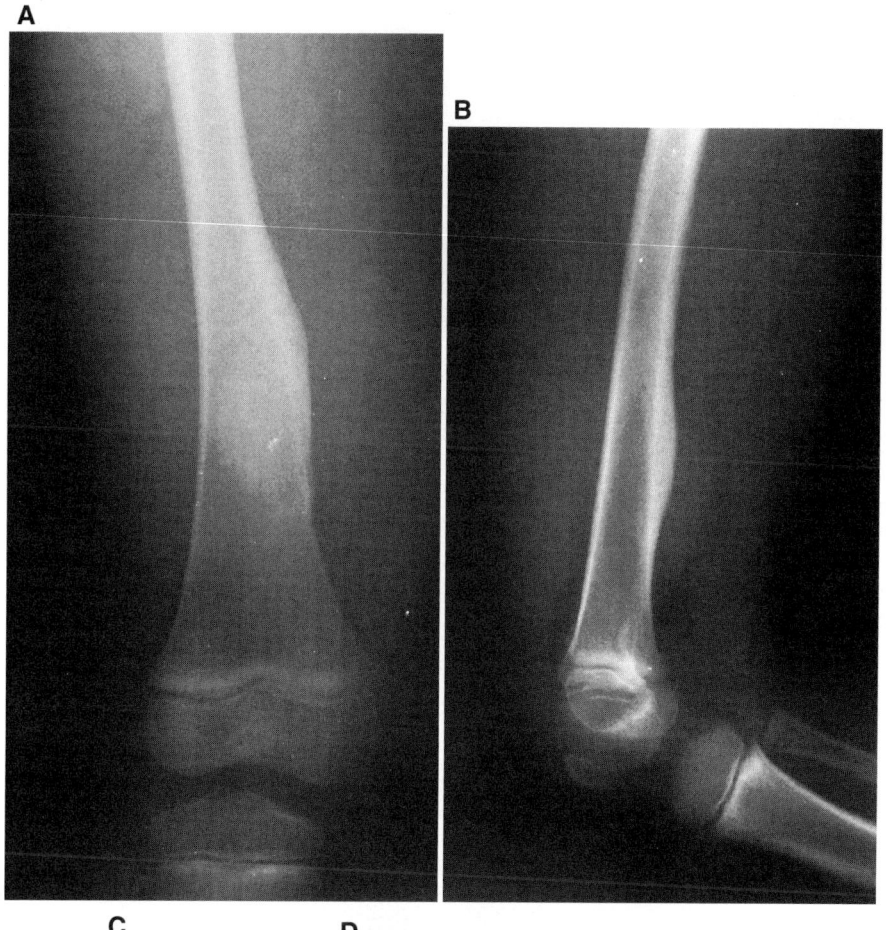
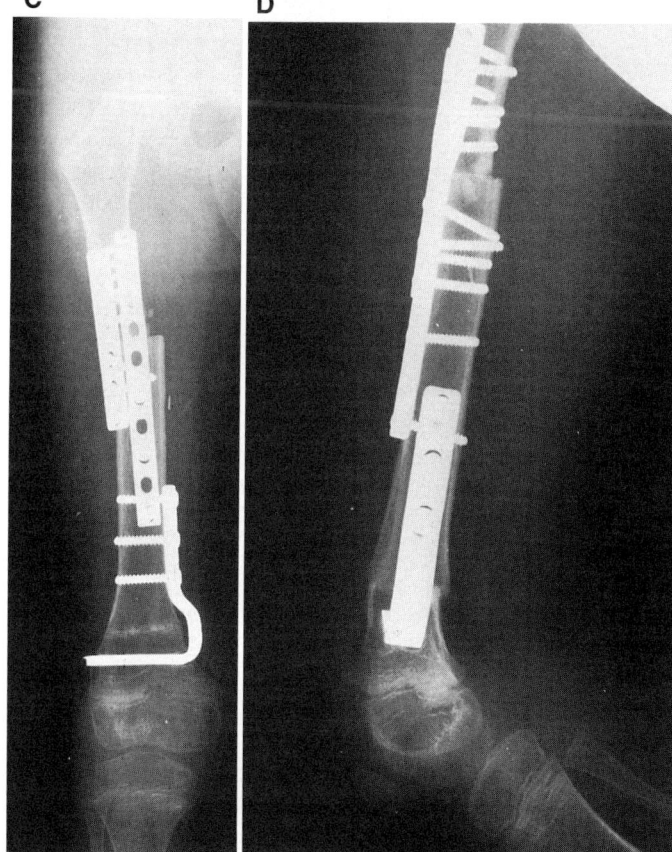

FIG 84-17.
Ewing's sarcoma affecting the diaphysis of the femur. **A,** anteroposterior view; **B,** lateral view. The patient underwent resection and reconstruction with an intercalary allograft. Postoperative anteroposterior **(A)** and lateral **(D)** views.

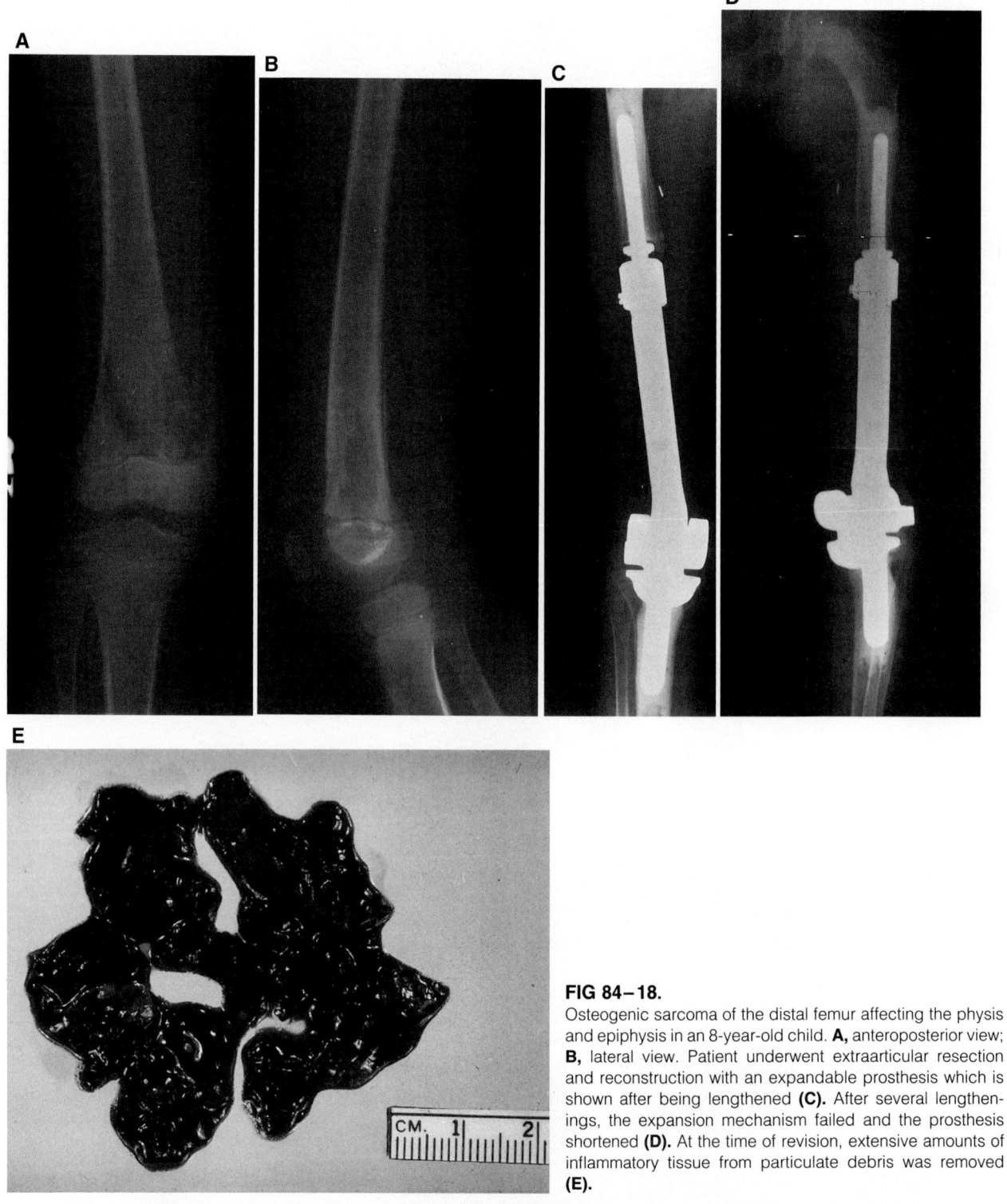

FIG 84–18.
Osteogenic sarcoma of the distal femur affecting the physis and epiphysis in an 8-year-old child. **A,** anteroposterior view; **B,** lateral view. Patient underwent extraarticular resection and reconstruction with an expandable prosthesis which is shown after being lengthened **(C).** After several lengthenings, the expansion mechanism failed and the prosthesis shortened **(D).** At the time of revision, extensive amounts of inflammatory tissue from particulate debris was removed **(E).**

tained of the retained host bone and soft tissue proximal margin of the resection.

Tumor location and invasiveness determine the required extent of resection. Traditionally, distal femoral and proximal tibial sarcomas should be excised widely by removing the entire joint. Extraarticular excision is necessary for tumors invading the joint (anterior lesions associated with an effusion) and those tracking along the capsule (posterior tumors involving the posterior cruciate ligament). When per-

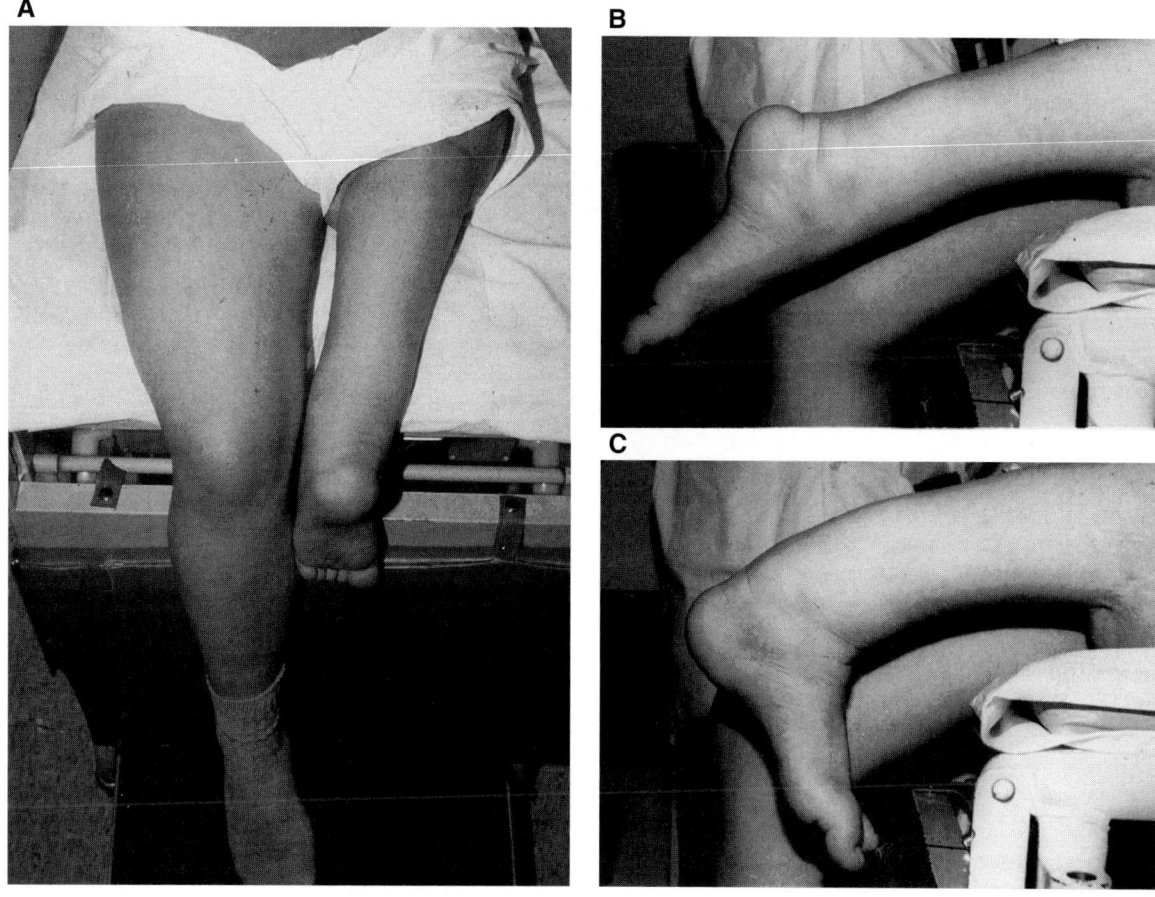

FIG 84–19.
This patient had an osteogenic sarcoma of the distal femur and underwent resection and reconstruction with a rotationplasty (**A**). **B,** full extension; **C,** flexion of the "knee."

forming an extraarticular excision it is difficult to preserve any extensor mechanism. Nevertheless, the rectus femoris is rarely involved with tumor and can usually be saved. In some cases a useful extensor mechanism can be maintained by staying out of the joint, preserving the anterior portion of the quadriceps tendon and the patella (cutting the patella coronally and leaving the cartilage and subchondral bone and synovium with the knee joint) (Fig 84–20).

Intraarticular excisions conserve one side of the joint and are technically easier to perform. Care must be exercised to avoid tumor in the capsular and periarticular tissues. More reconstructive options exist after intraarticular excisions (e.g., osteoarticular allografts), and functional results are theoretically superior to extraarticular excision. Improvements in preoperative imaging and adjuvant therapies foster this more conservative surgical approach. Performed selectively, intraarticular excision is appropriate for approximately 75% of patients treated by limb-sparing surgical resection without compromising local recurrence or survival rates.

If the extraarticular technique is chosen, the popliteal trifurcation vessels behind the tibia are protected. The tibia is cut 10 to 15 mm below the joint line, keeping the popliteus in continuity with the joint and tumor mass. If the intraarticular technique is chosen, the ligaments are cut well away from the tumor, ideally at their tibial insertions.

The technique for proximal tibial resection is similar.[55] Care must be taken to preserve vascularity to local structures such as the medial gastrocnemius that must be used for the soft tissue reconstruction. Since soft tissue coverage is particularly problematic after tibial resections, plans are made for not only local muscle flap coverage (see Fig 84–4) but for possible free tissue transfers such as latissimus dorsi microvascular transfers[40] (Fig 84–21).

RECONSTRUCTION

Reconstructive options about the knee include prosthetic arthroplasty, arthrodesis, and osteoarticular allografts. Each alternative must be adapted to the na-

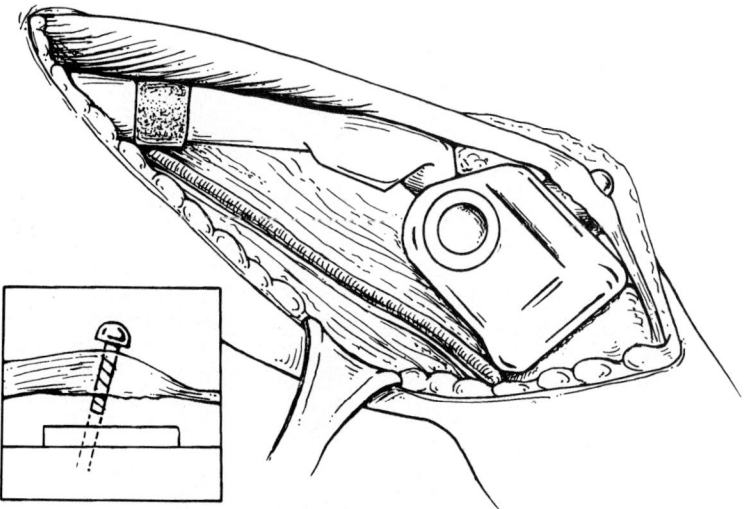

FIG 84-20.
Illustration of an extraarticular resection of the knee maintaining the anterior half of the patella and rectus femoris as an extensor mechanism. If the insertion of the patellar tendon is sacrificed, the patella can be attached to the tibial component with a screw.

ture of the tumor resection and the magnitude and quality of the structural defect. Although intimately related, the resection must be performed independently of the reconstruction to avoid compromising the oncologic success of the procedure. No tumor was ever cured by an allograft.

Endoprostheses

Prosthetic knee replacement is the preferred method of reconstruction in patients who have high-grade malignancies resected, and those in whom both sides of the joint were removed. The potentially short life expectancy of the patient, the need to resume chemotherapy promptly, and the compromise of bone healing during chemotherapy make segmental joint replacement the logical choice. Since soft tissues and ligamentous supports are lacking, a constrained prosthesis is needed. Segmental defects averaging 24 cm in our series require coupled replacement of the bone shaft. There is significant difficulty in making the level of resection exact since there is limited exposure of the bony shaft. Resection lengths are typically off by 1 cm or more. Custom prostheses do not allow for the clinical reality of variable resection lengths. Modular systems provide greater flexibility, and currently available models have interchangeable segments every 2 to 3 cm in length. The long lever arms on constrained prostheses create huge forces on the components, bone, and interface.

Efforts to reduce mechanical failure have centered around improving prosthetic design, metallurgy, and prosthetic fixation. Prosthetic designs have varied to reduce and dampen loads applied to the prosthesis (cement)-bone interface.

The most commonly used components employ a rotating-hinge design and reconstruct an anatomic joint line. The Kinematic, (Howmedica, Rutherford, N.J.),[70] Stanmore (Royal National Orthopaedic Hospital, England), and Finn (Biomet, Warsaw, Ind.)[72] designs are most popular. They are well adapted to situations where a significant amount of the extensor mechanism is preserved. When the extensors are absent, as after classic extraarticular excision, a novel ball-and-socket design is appropriate. The Burstein-Lane prosthesis allows 3.5 degrees of knee hyperextension and 2.5 degrees of internal-external rotation, and operates through a "sloppy hinge" mechanism[66] (Fig 84-22). There has also been interest in reducing the prosthetic constraint needed by combining the joint replacement with a segmental allograft. Gitelis and Piasecki[34] refer to these reconstructions as "alloprostheses." About the knee, an alloprosthesis can provide ligamentous and capsular tissue as well as replace the deficient segment. Arguably, one could then use a partially constrained component, resurfacing the articular surface of the allograft and repairing the allograft soft tissues to the remaining host structures.

Most prostheses are made of titanium to reduce weight and maximize strength. Particulate debris is a significant problem with all existing designs, especially in light of the young age of so many tumor patients. Differences in long-term effects of titanium, cobalt-chromium, and stainless steel will no doubt influence the selection of prostheses in the future. These issues are particularly important in devices that have metal-on-metal gear mechanisms like the existing expandable prostheses. The worst metal wear problems we have encountered have been in such

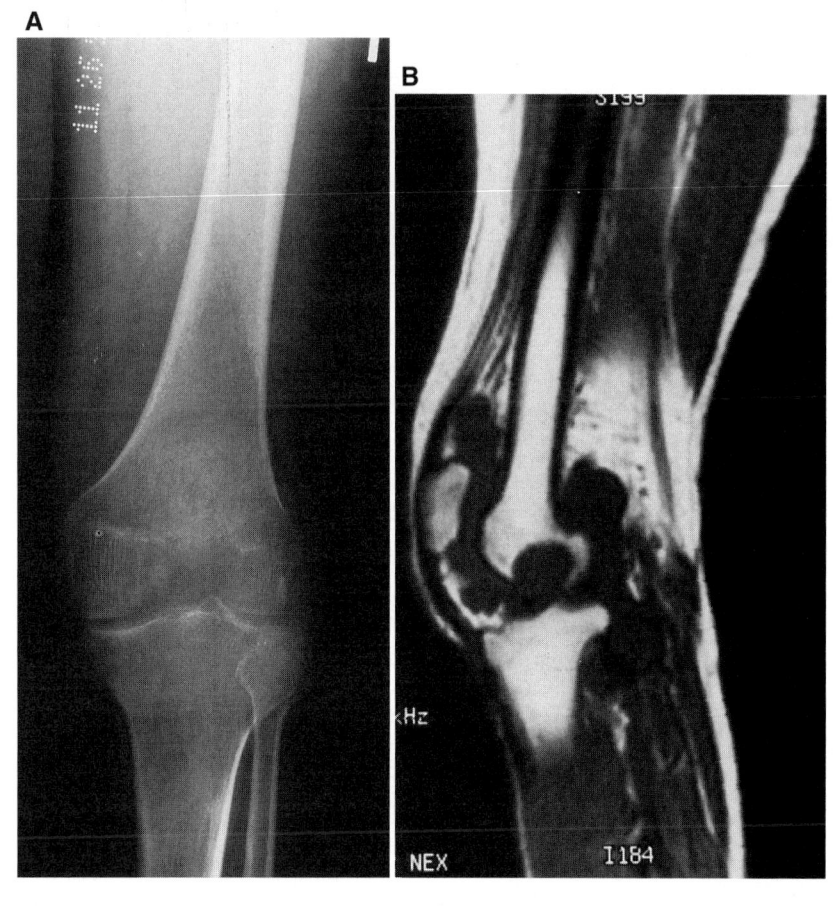

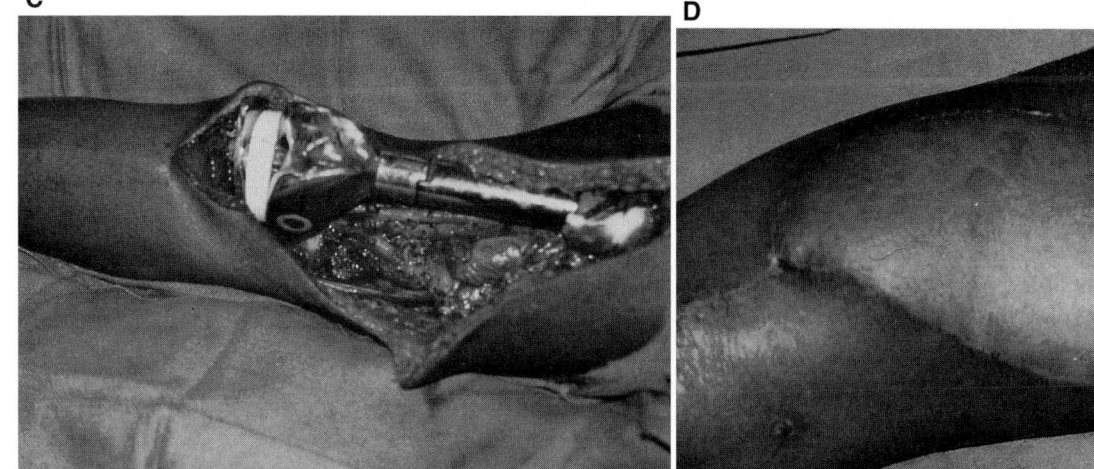

FIG 84–21.
This patient had undergone multiple arthroscopic procedures for a presumed intraarticular lesion. Anteroposterior radiograph **(A)** shows a destructive lesion in the distal femur and sagittal MRI **(B)** demonstrates an intraarticular and extraarticular soft tissue mass, which was a synovial sarcoma. Curative resection was attempted which necessitated an extraarticular resection and removal of contaminated anterior soft tissues. **C,** endoprosthetic reconstruction and soft tissue defect. **D,** soft tissue defect was reconstructed with a latissimus dorsi free flap.

prostheses (see Fig 84–18). Polyethylene wear has not been reported to be a problem in oncologic reconstructions. Now that more patients and limbs are being saved, this problem will undoubtedly surface in the near future.

Interface problems have been addressed by moving away from cementation of prostheses. It is prudent to remember, however, that cement may be the best solution for very ill patients on chemotherapy who may not be able to integrate bone into prosthe-

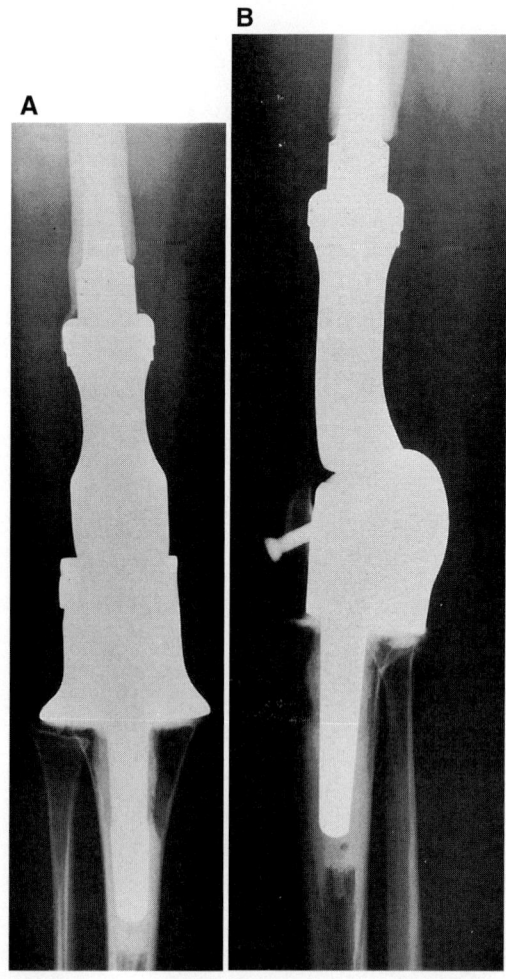

FIG 84-22.
Radiographs of the Burstein-Lane prosthesis. The extensor mechanism can be reconstructed by attaching the patella or patellar tendon to the tibial component. Extramedullary bridging is seen at the junction of the prosthesis with the femur. **A,** anteroposterior view; **B,** lateral view.

sis dependably. The role of biologic fixation remains to be defined in tumor reconstructive surgery. Various uncemented fixation strategies are popular. Unfortunately, no comparative studies have been done to evaluate the relative merits of the techniques. Fluted stems give excellent cortical bone purchase, but the radius of prosthetic curvature rarely matches that of the host bone. It is not surprising then that such prostheses are apt to split the host shaft. Intramedullary porous ingrowth is an attractive concept with which most reconstructive surgeons are familiar. Data on the effectiveness and durability of such prostheses are lacking. Chao and colleagues[17, 36] and others[18] advocated extramedullary porous fixation to take advantage of the periosteal-periprosthetic sleeve of bone that reliably forms at the junction of bone and component. Animal models support the use of this fixation method and early clinical results from several centers have been favorable. Unfortunately, the large cuff of bone that develops during the first postoperative year seems to attenuate over time as stresses bypass the newly formed bone. Finally, extramedullary plates, with or without interlocking screws, are very popular in Europe. They provide excellent torsional stability and may facilitate porous ingrowth. Unfortunately, they are very rigid and contribute to extensive bone loss attributed to the stress bypass effect, and may be subject to greater metal debris problems. Only careful clinical and radiographic evaluation will determine which prostheses produce the most functional and long-lived reconstructions.

A final issue is the uncertain role for custom prostheses. Satisfactory options exist using standard modular components for distal femoral reconstructions. Unusual anatomic situations in the femur may require unique, customized solutions. For example, when long resections leave the femoral isthmus insufficient to secure a stem, interlocking screws matching the intrinsic femoral neck anteversion give excellent fixation (Fig 84-23). This custom design feature allows limb salvage and hip joint preservation. Total femur replacement and most proximal tibial replacements are ideal candidates for custom-designed prostheses.

Segmental knee replacement yields good to excellent results in most cases. Pain-free, unassisted, and unlimited ambulation are the usual outcome. Function is inversely proportional to the magnitude of the bone and soft tissue resection required to remove the tumors. Functionally, knee replacement cancer patients have better velocity, endurance, and oxygen utilization than amputees.[69] Endoprosthetic reconstruction is chosen most often by patients and surgeons alike.

Complications are routine both early and late after major joint resection and reconstruction. Acutely, the most frequent complication is marginal wound necrosis seen in as many as 25% of cases of large femoral tumor and in most tibial resections. Wound healing problems are treated aggressively since they can delay the resumption of chemotherapy and compromise patient survival. Local muscle (gastrocnemius) or free tissue transfers (latissimus dorsi) are required to achieve a tension-free closure with muscle coverage over all prostheses and allografts. If a wound slough still occurs, prompt wound revision and muscle coverage are performed. Attentive wound management saves most tenuous limbs. Aseptic loosening occurs in as many as 25% of patients at 5 years follow-up.[41] Revision surgery successfully salvages most cases of prosthetic failure

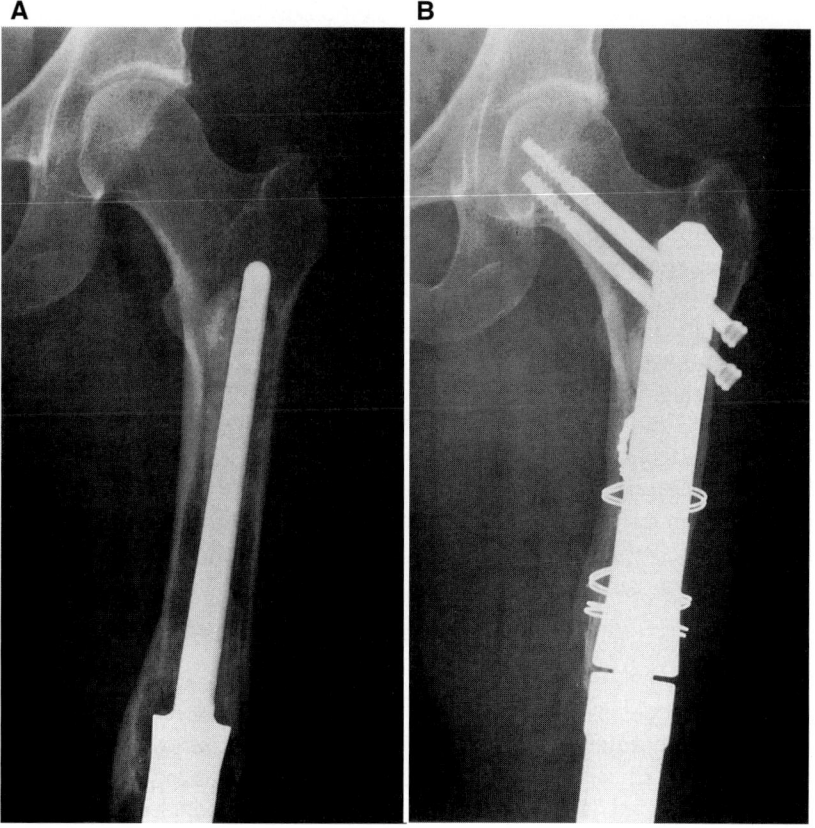

FIG 84–23.
A, anteroposterior radiograph of the proximal femur demonstrating a loose femoral component in a patient who had a resection of the distal femur. **B,** endoprosthetic reconstruction was performed utilizing a custom implant with proximal interlocking screws into the femoral neck.

from aseptic loosening. Wound healing problems and infection plague attempted revisions and careful soft tissue management is critical. Tibial failures are often converted to above-knee amputations when complicated by infection since there is a reasonable functional level after amputation. Femoral lesions warrant more aggressive attempts at revision since even a poor salvage is usually better than a high above-knee amputation or hip disarticulation.

Good results require proper postoperative management. Suction drains are kept in place until drainage is minimal. Antibiotic prophylaxis is used until the wound healing is secure. Physical therapy and continuous passive motion of the knee begin when the wound is dry and healing well. Knee flexors are often stronger than the residual knee extensors. Knee flexion contractures are avoided by splinting the knee in extension at night. This is critical in patients with absent quadriceps because a flexion contracture prevents them from keeping their weightbearing axis anterior to the knee flexion axis and precludes a stable stance phase during gait.

Arthrodesis

Arthrodesis is an alternative to endoprosthesis after resecting a malignant or recurrent benign tumor about the knee[6, 13, 19] (see Fig 84–13). Various combinations of autologous or allogeneic grafts and intramedullary devices span the skeletal defect. Many surgeons prefer arthrodesis whenever the entire extensor mechanism is absent. Campanacci and Costa[13] use an anterior hemicylindrical sliding graft taken from either the tibia or femur, whereas Enneking and Shirley[25] use a hemidiaphyseal graft sagittally turned down (up) from the remaining unaffected host bone. The method usually uses an intramedullary rod inserted antegrade from the greater trochanter-femoral neck. Since the diameter of the femur and tibia rarely match, Neff (personal communication) modifies the technique. He joins a larger-diameter femoral rod inserted retrograde to an appropriately sized tibial fluted rod inserted antegrade. The rods lock at the knee and supplemental grafts are placed around the rods. Improved fixation results and avoids a second incision at the hip, but can lead to insurmountable difficulty in extracting the rods if necessitated by infection or other complication. Campanacci and Costa achieved union in 92% of cases eventually, using repeated bone grafting in 15% of cases. Full weight-bearing was regained within 2 years in all patients with solid fusions. Infection occurred in 19% of cases, half of which were salvageable while half contributed to nonunion.[13] These problems are serious and often prompt patients to request secondary amputation.

Simon et al.[80] compared the functional outcome and gait performance of patients with successful knee fusions, arthroplasty, and amputation after tumor resections. There was no difference between the three groups. Some contend that the durability of the fusion makes it the preferred reconstruction. The slow healing and difficulty with sitting that limit patients may be a worthwhile long-term investment for patients who survive their cancer, but are an unnecessary cost to patients who still succumb to their disease.

Intercalary defects in the femoral or tibial shafts behave similarly owing to the defect length, deficient soft tissue, and presence of two osteosynthesis sites. Vascularized[9,45,91] and nonvascularized fibular grafts have been used to span arthrodeses and diaphyseal defects.[23] Enneking[23] noted that the likelihood of graft fracture increases dramatically whenever the graft length exceeds 12 cm. Vascularized fibulae seem to heal faster and hypertrophy faster than nonvascularized fibular grafts.[21] Unfortunately, the fibula substitutes poorly for the mechanical properties of a normal femur. Fractures typically occur during the time it takes the fibula to hypertrophy sufficiently. The fibular strengthening process takes about 2 or more years. Allografts solve the mechanical problem dependably, but leave a biologic problem of being slow to unite to host bone. Furthermore, although allografts have been used successfully to span arthrodesis defects, approximately 25% will not unite at one junction and will require secondary bone grafting. This encourages the search for a mechanically sound alternative method that promotes bone healing. Some surgeons now combine allografts for structural support and vascularized fibulae for enhanced healing potential.

As demonstrated, many options for reconstruction exist after limb salvage and the treatment should be individualized. We believe that it is most functional and compassionate to keep all patients functioning, walking, and bending their knees during their remaining lifetimes by means of endoprostheses. Selected tumors have diaphyseal defects reconstructible by intercalary allografts. When used in patients requiring chemotherapy, all allografts have unacceptably high infection, fracture, and nonunion rates. These complications seem to be less salvageable than similar problems encountered in prostheses. Whichever reconstruction option is chosen, patients should be selected carefully and educated before and after limb preservation. This is particularly true for patients treated with segmental knee replacements.

All of these reconstructive alternatives restrict patient function. Altered muscle balance, stability, and proprioception affect function of salvaged limbs and may contribute to falls. These problems are compounded in patients who suffer peripheral neuropathies from chemotherapy (cisplatinum, vincristine, and others). Patients should be counseled that despite undergoing limb salvage surgery, they will be permanently disabled.[78]

FIBULAR LESIONS

Fibular lesions encompass a broad spectrum of diagnoses. Benign conditions include a disproportionate prevalence of aneurysmal bone cysts (Fig 84–24), enchondromas, unicameral bone cysts, and GCTs. Malignant lesions include Ewing's sarcoma (the most common malignant tumor of the fibula), and chondrosarcoma (see Fig 84–11), as well as the rare spindle cell sarcoma. Benign lesions are approached through a longitudinal lateral incision, with care taken to isolate the peroneal nerve. Primary resection[54,58] or excisional biopsy is the most suitable technique for benign-aggressive, and questionably malignant lesions. This solves the diagnostic and therapeutic problems expeditiously. It also minimizes the risk of peroneal nerve neuropraxia or tumor recurrence that is inherent in staged biopsy-excision procedures. There is a limited role for surgical adjuvants in treating benign-aggressive or low-grade malignant tumors of this bone. Tumors that are probably high-grade sarcomas, suitable for chemotherapy, should have an incisional biopsy rather than primary resection. Since peroneal nerve sacrifice is essential to obtain a satisfactory margin around a proximal fibular malignancy, biopsy contamination does not compromise the ability to save the nerve at the time of definitive tumor resection (Fig 84–25). Appropriate systemic therapy should be selected for such tumors, as for tibial and femoral lesions. As long as one major arterial supply to the limb remains, en bloc wide excision may be considered. Arteriography is helpful in preoperatively planning resection of the proximal fibula. On the other hand, sarcomas frequently extend across

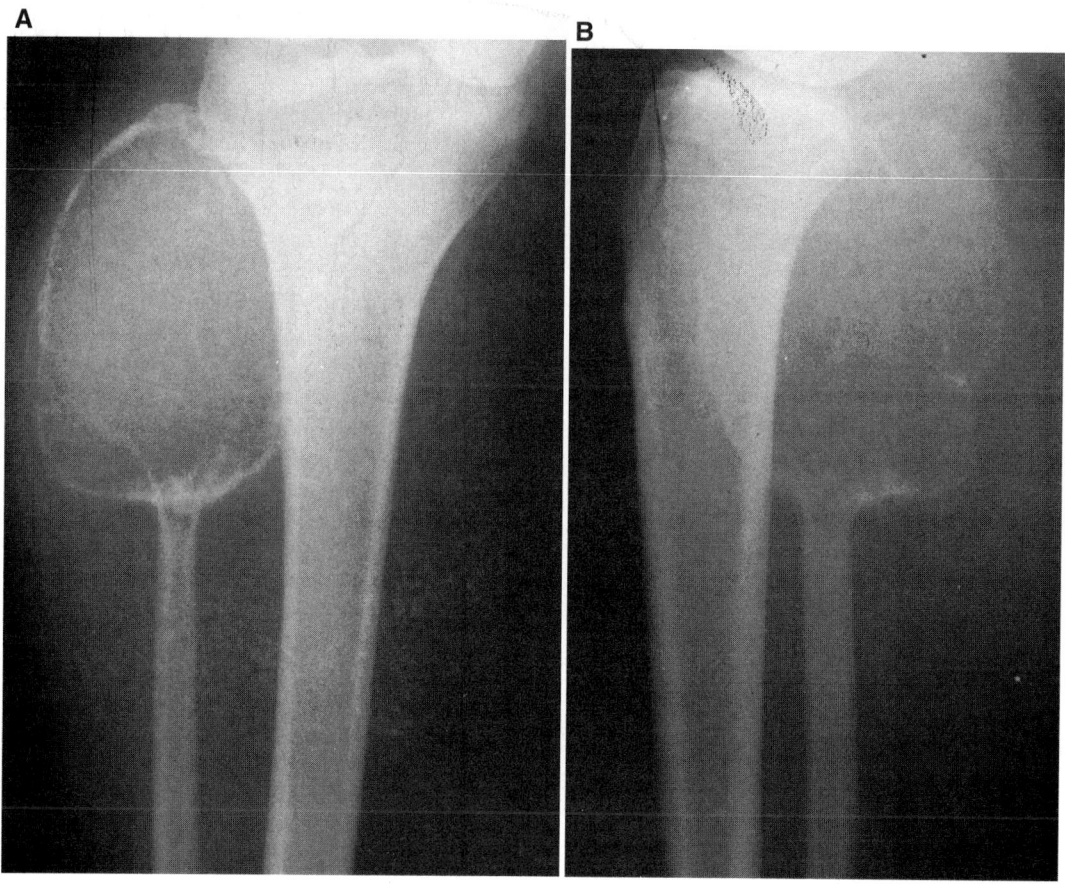

FIG 84-24.
Aneurysmal bone cyst of the proximal fibula. **A**, anteroposterior view; **B**, lateral view.

the tibial fibular joint or involve the popliteal artery trifurcation, precluding safe limb salvage. Amputation still has a role in fibular sarcomas. When excision is performed, lateral ligament reconstruction can be performed with the use of suture anchors in the lateral tibia.

METASTATIC TUMORS ABOUT THE KNEE

Metastatic lesions about the knee cause pain, swelling, and pathologic fracture. They are usually identified because of symptoms in a patient with a known cancer, but occasionally are the initial manifestation of a cancer. Breast, kidney, and prostate cancer, along with multiple myeloma, are the most common primary cancers. Typically, there are many lesions, so the entire femur (or tibia) must be evaluated to exclude the presence of a significant lesion in the proximal femur causing referred knee pain. Small deposits that are mechanically stable should be treated with protected weightbearing and radiotherapy. If pain does not relent promptly, surgery is needed. Poor surgical candidates with less than 3 months to live may get relief from a cast brace that allows weightbearing. Pathologic fracture of the supracondylar femur requires surgery in most instances. Good to excellent results are obtained in 70% of patients after fixing the fracture with a 95-degree blade plate or Zickel supracondylar nails reinforced with polymethyl methacrylate.[38] Rigid fixation palliates symptoms and improves the quality of life (see Fig 83–7). Postoperative radiotherapy is usually indicated to stop tumor progression. Destructive epiphyseal disease of the proximal tibia or distal femur is best treated by local resection and total knee replacement. When the joint is involved or a stable construct cannot be achieved with internal fixation, a resection arthroplasty and knee replacement meet the goal of palliation (Fig 84–26). Tissue such as the extensor mechanism is preserved, even if it is involved with tumor. In these circumstances, function is a priority. A more constrained prosthesis than is apparently necessary is used since tumors tend to progress and destabilize the components. Palliative amputation

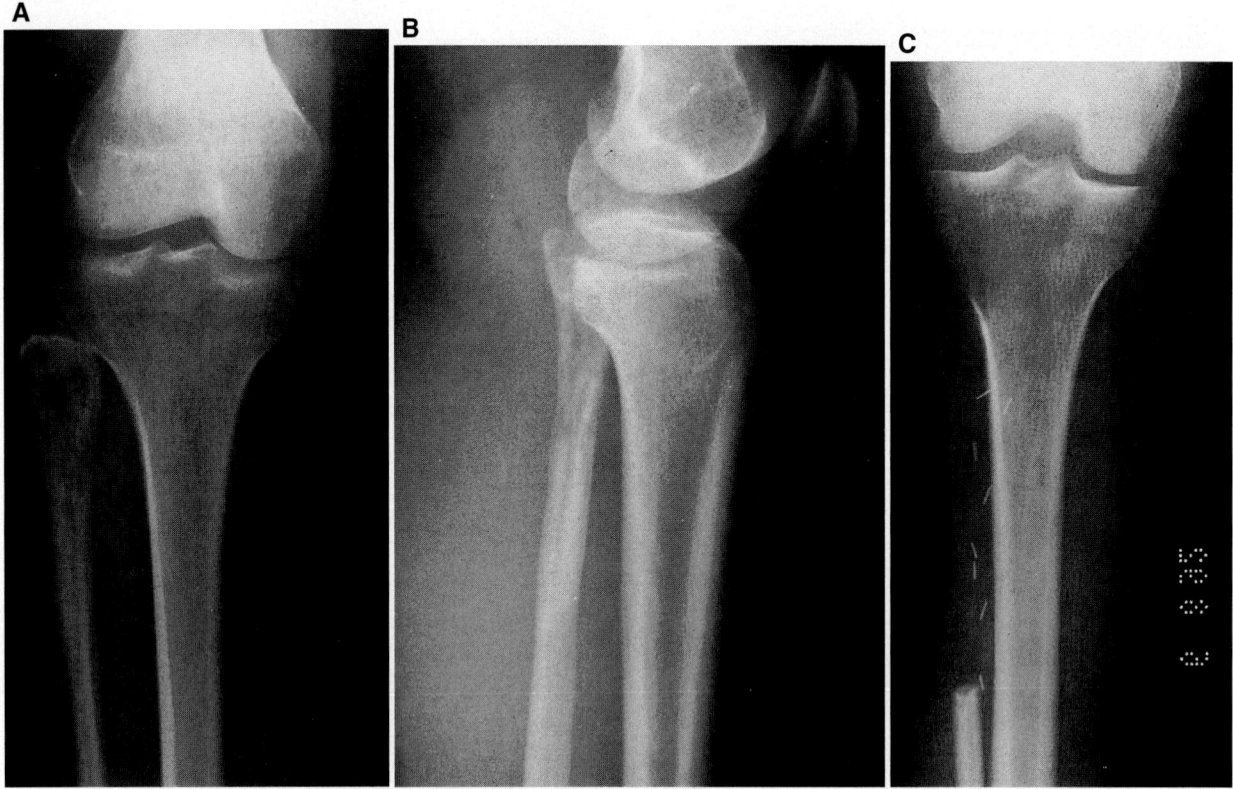

FIG 84-25.
Osteogenic sarcoma of the proximal fibula. **A,** anteroposterior view; **B,** lateral view. **C,** the resection includes the peroneal nerve and lateral cortex of the proximal tibia.

may be the fastest, most dependable treatment for uncontrollable lesions (Fig 84-27).

SOFT TISSUE TUMORS

General Concepts

Soft tissue tumors are approximately ten times more frequent than bone tumors. This applies to both benign and malignant tumors. The tumors are noted to be painless masses by most patients, although pain may be present. Rapid growth is often reported in cases that turn out to be malignancies. It reflects not only the cell proliferation rate but hemorrhage and necrosis within the tumor. Physical examination is fundamental to identifying unrecognized masses about the knee and thigh. The relationship of tumors to the knee joint and important neurovascular structures is defined.

The diagnostic imaging workup should be focused. Plain films and MRI or CT with contrast are the only relevant tests. Other studies waste time and resources and rarely provide information that alters diagnosis or treatment. Exceptions are arthrography (with or without CT) to best demonstrate extension of a mass into or out of the joint and sonography, which helps to define cystic lesions. These studies are warranted to distinguish tumors from popliteal or meniscal cysts when the clinical picture is not clear. Complete staging studies such as chest CT scans can be performed selectively in patients who have an established malignant tumor.

Biopsy is the definitive diagnostic test. As for bone tumors, the physician must make a determination at this time if the local experience and facilities are suitable to treat the most involved tumor that is within the differential diagnosis. If not, the patient should be referred to a specialty center.

Biopsy technique varies with the clinical situation, tumor size, and location. It can be asked why soft tissue tumors should be biopsied since the only effective treatment is surgical. While surgery is the treatment of choice for all soft tissue tumors, from the most benign to the most malignant, the magnitude of the resection, extent of surgical margins, possibilities for preoperative radiation therapy or investigational chemotherapy, or intraoperative placement of brachytherapy catheters, and appropriate patient counseling justify a discrete biopsy procedure.

The simplest, least expensive procedure is needle

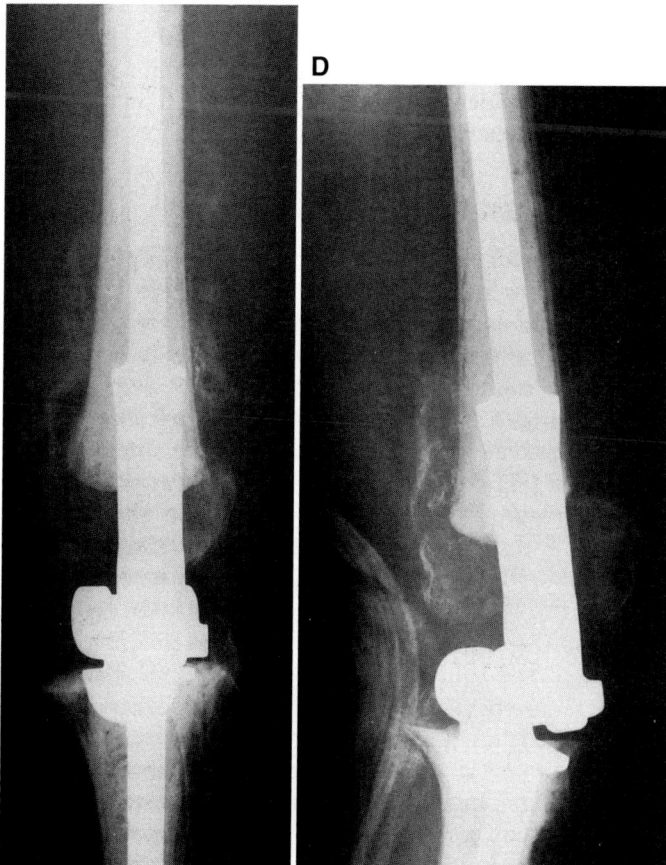

FIG 84–26.
An unreconstructable pathologic fracture through a distal femur extensively involved with multiple myeloma was treated with resection and endoprosthetic reconstruction. **A** and **C,** anteroposterior views; **B** and **D,** lateral views.

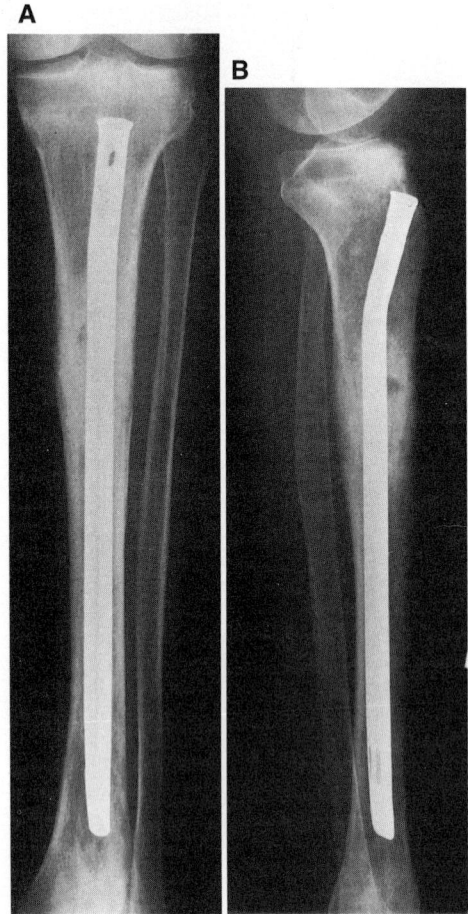

FIG 84–27.
Metastatic colon cancer to the tibia was initially treated with internal fixation followed by radiation therapy. **A,** anteroposterior view; **B,** lateral view. Intractable pain recurred and the patient elected to undergo an above-knee amputation.

aspiration. This office procedure gives immediate diagnostic information about cystic lesions. If typical joint or ganglion fluid is not obtained, then more expensive imaging or more invasive diagnostic tests should be done. Aspiration biopsy cytology can be diagnostic. Prior to performing any major tumor resection we recommend that the diagnosis be more firmly established by histologic means.

Needle biopsy is often sufficient. The track must be noted for inclusion in the resection specimen and care should be taken to avoid straying into new compartments. A common error is to plunge through the tumor and strike the underlying bone, or extend through a restraining fascial compartment.

When the diagnosis is fairly certain, superficial tumors can be excised marginally, staying above the fascia. This approach is most suitable for lipomas. Since fatty tumors are notoriously difficult to evaluate by frozen section histologic analysis, primary excision is permissible. Other superficial small (<3 cm) lesions should also be removed by this technique. Superficial large lesions should be biopsied before removal since malignant tumors necessitate removal of greater amounts of normal tissue.

Although deep lesions are much more often malignant than superficial lesions, most deep lesions are still benign. Deep large tumors must always be biopsied to assure both the adequacy of their subsequent resection and to avoid overtreatment of benign lesions. Deep small tumors are uncommon and present an unusual set of clinical compromises for the surgeon to deal with. Excisional biopsy will prove satisfactory for most tumors, but is inadequate for a higher percentage of deep than superficial tumors. Incisional biopsy necessitates a second procedure to remove both benign and malignant tumors. Both incisional and excisional biopsy contaminate, and necessitate removal, of much more tissue than would have been required had primary wide excision been done. Thus there is a rationale for incisional biopsy, excisional biopsy, and primary wide excision in dealing with deep small lesions. The final decision depends on the extent of additional disability that would be anticipated from a potential secondary wide excision. If the extra disability is minimal, then a preliminary biopsy procedure is warranted. Conversely, if the only opportunity to obtain a wide surgical margin without undue sacrifice of important structures is at the time of the initial procedure, then a primary wide excision should be chosen.

Benign Soft Tissue Tumors

Most benign lesions are treated by simple excision and have low recurrence rates. Lipomas are among the most common of all lesions. Most are superficial, but intramuscular lipomas are frequently seen in the distal thigh. When deep, painful, or demonstrably growing, they are excised by local enucleation. Atypical lipomas are common in the deep intramuscular tissue (Fig 84–28). They have a propensity to grow and recur. Excision of atypical lipomas should be en bloc and careful follow-up must be sustained.

Popliteal cysts may be primary or secondary and are the most common soft tissue masses found behind the knee. The workup includes imaging studies when the tumor lacks typical characteristics. If the presumed cyst is not in the typical location adjacent to the semimembranosus or medial gastrocnemius, or if fluid cannot be aspirated, then ultrasound and other imaging studies should be performed. Soft tissue sarcomas may simulate popliteal cysts. Another solid tumor is suspected if the arthrogram does not

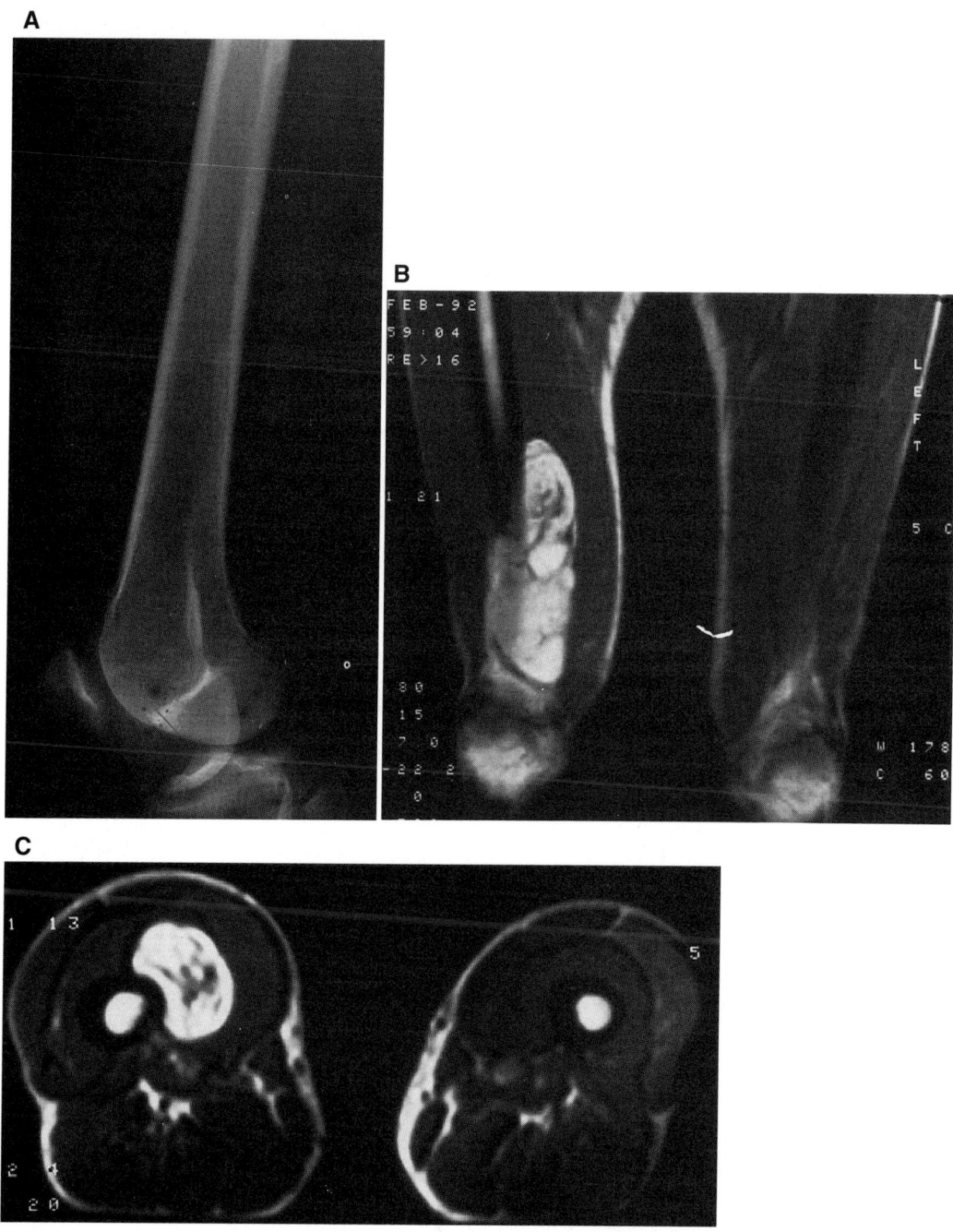

FIG 84-28.
A, lateral radiograph demonstrates a mass on the anterior surface of the femur. Coronal **(B)** and axial **(C)** MRI scans demonstrate a soft tissue mass with the density of fat surrounding the anterior and medial aspects of the distal femur. Results of a biopsy showed an atypical lipoma which was enucleated.

show communication between the joint and the lesion, or if the sonogram shows echogenic solid areas. MRI and a biopsy should be performed in such circumstances. If there is preoperative diagnostic uncertainty, care must be taken to avoid contaminating popliteal neurovascular structures with tumor. Needle biopsy of the mass maximizes the opportunity to cure the potential malignancy with less than an amputation. Symptomatic cysts refractory to conservative treatment are excised. Popliteal cysts in children are usually painless and most regress spontaneously.[22]

Extraabdominal desmoid tumors are aggressive, infiltrating tumors that may develop following trauma. They recur multiply, grow extensively, and may develop in multiple sites within the extremity.

Surgery is the only effective treatment,[73] yet surgery may trigger tumor growth if the excision is incomplete. Imaging these tumors is extremely difficult, even with MRI, since the density of the tumor is the same as the surrounding tissue. Therefore, imaging should be done with contrast agents: gadolinium for MRI and intravenous contrast for CT, since desmoids are enhancing lesions.[2] Wide excision is preferred. Adjuvant radiotherapy is reported to reduce local recurrence, but compromises follow-up examination of the radiated tissue and may rarely contribute to secondary sarcomatous degeneration. We use radiation selectively for recurrent cases or situations in which recurrence is both a high probability and of high consequence if it does occur[3, 62] (Fig 84–29). Some oncologists suggest chemotherapy for these tumors, using agents such as methotrexate, vincristine, and actinomycin D.[71, 89] Despite encouraging literature reports, response rates and magnitudes do not justify routine chemotherapy. Occasionally, significant responses to estrogen antagonists and nonsteroidal anti-inflammatory drugs are obtained.[15, 50, 88]

Synovial chondromatosis is an uncommon cause of painful knee swelling and effusion. Metaplastic foci of cartilage develop in the synovium and are diagnostic. These foci become calcified or even ossified and are usually visible radiographically. They may detach and appear as loose bodies in the joint, but usually remain fixed in the joint capsule or synovium. Double contrast arthrography demonstrates these deposits particularly well. Histologically, the tissue appears very active and even pseudomalignant on occasion. Complete synovectomy and removal of the loose bodies are the indicated treatment. Arthroscopic treatment will often suffice. Isolated loose bodies rarely recur, whereas extensive multifocal synovial involvement is difficult to eradicate.

Pigmented villonodular synovitis (PVNS) is a monoarthritis, most commonly seen around the knee. It occurs in young and middle-aged adults. Similar to synovial chondromatosis, it is an inflammatory condition and is associated with a substantial amount of joint pain and sensitivity and recurrent hemarthrosis. Roentgenograms usually show only nonspecific synovitis, but erosions on both sides of the joint may result. Various inflammatory arthropathies and chronic infections such as tuberculosis can have this same appearance, clinically and radiographically. Asymmetric cysts on one side of the joint have been mistaken for giant cell tumors and malignant neoplasms. Histologically, nonspecific synovitis with focal hemorrhage, and rheumatoid arthritis must be distinguished from PVNS. Mild diffuse synovial disease can be treated by arthroscopic synovectomy. Extensive, erosive, and recurrent synovial disease is best treated by open total synovectomy, usually through two incisions (Fig 84–30). Localized nodular disease requires wide local excision to eradicate the tumor. Recurrent disease may require en bloc excision of the joint or even amputation to effect a cure. Radiation synovectomy using intraarticular dysprosium may be effective in selected cases, but one must always weigh the risks of potentially malignant radiation therapy to treat what is entirely a benign condition.

Periarticular muscle is the most common site for intramuscular hemangiomas. The knee capsule occasionally and the distal vastus muscles frequently are the sites for this developmental, neoplastic condition (Fig 84–31). Symptomatic masses usually arise in the third and fourth decades. They typically have a dull aching pain that becomes severe and throbbing after exercise. Adolescents seem to be particularly prone to this activity-related pain from hemangiomas. Smaller lesions may be exquisitely sensitive to percussion despite lacking tenderness to deep palpation. Intramuscular hemangiomas are multifocal in at least 25% of cases. Therefore, although excision may be very effective in eliminating pain, recurrence is frequent. Excision must be done judiciously to remove all the identifiable tumor, yet preserve important joint and muscle tissue. Inadequate tumor excision merely spreads the disease in the periarticular tissue, contributes to tumor recurrence, and is associated with chronic pain and disability in many instances.

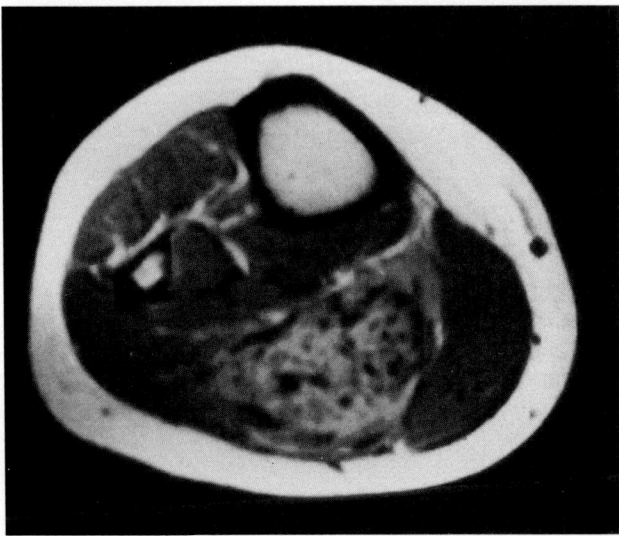

FIG 84–29.
MRI scan of the leg demonstrating a recurrent desmoid tumor in the posterior compartment. Because of its proximity to neurovascular structures, a marginal resection was performed and radiation therapy with brachytherapy catheters was administered.

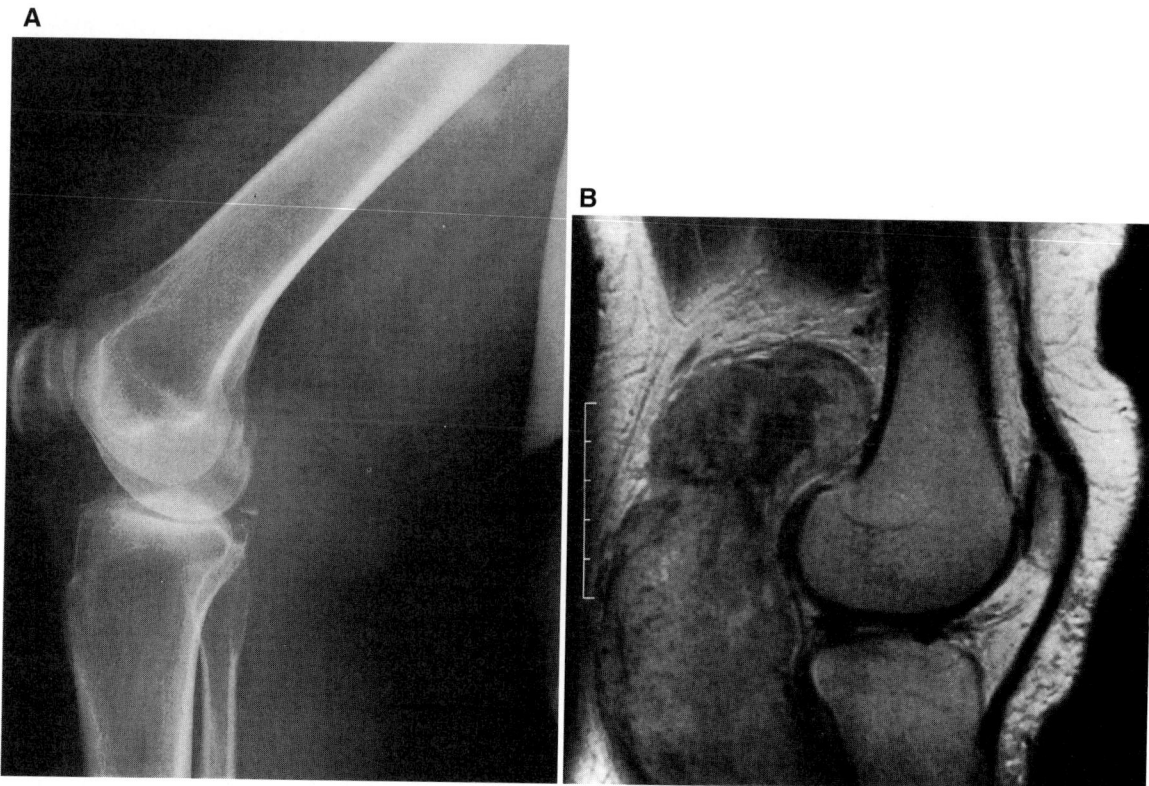

FIG 84-30.
Extensive pigmented villonodular synovitis in the popliteal fossa was treated with open synovectomy. **A,** lateral radiograph; **B,** sagittal MRI scan.

Experimental techniques such as interferon-α administration[27] and intravascular sclerosis by embolization or injection hold promise for improved treatment of this disorder.

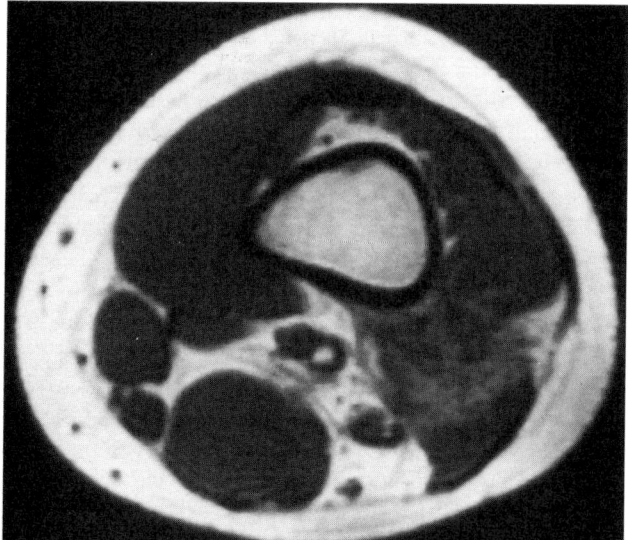

FIG 84-31.
MRI scan demonstrating an intramuscular hemangioma involving the long head of the biceps femoris.

Soft Tissue Sarcomas

Approximately one third of soft tissue sarcomas occur in the thigh or knee region. All histologic subtypes are found in tumors in this region. As yet, there is no prognostic significance to the different tumor diagnoses. Malignant fibrous histiocytoma and liposarcoma are the most common. Around the knee, synovial sarcoma is also common, and soft tissue "bone" malignancies such as mesenchymal and myxoid chondrosarcoma occur despite the overall rarity of these lesions. Perhaps the tumors that are most important to distinguish are embryonal rhabdomyosarcoma (ERMS) in children and young adults since chemotherapy plays an important role in their cure. Malignant peripheral nerve sheath tumors are among the most difficult to image accurately due to common intraneural spread and they are refractory to adjuvant therapies. Some authors question whether these facts preclude successful limb salvage surgery for such tumors. At this time there is little diagnostic or therapeutic value to subclassification of soft tissue sarcomas.

There are no reliable physical examination signs that distinguish between benign and malignant soft tissue lesions. Clinical symptoms and signs are important, however, in providing the information needed to decide which lesions warrant biopsy. Several general principles govern decision making. All persistent or growing deep masses should be biopsied. Painful masses require biopsy, even though soft tissue sarcomas are usually pain-free. Physical examination reveals the approximate size of the mass and its attachment to superficial or deep structures. Tumors fixed to skin or deep structures also must be biopsied. Lymphadenopathy can be incidental or related to infection or neoplastic spread. Most sarcomas metastasize via the hematogenous route and lymphatic involvement is uncommon (1%–5%). Several sarcomas such as epithelioid sarcoma, ERMS, clear cell sarcoma, and to a lesser extent, synovial sarcoma have a propensity to spread via the lymphatic system. The presence of enlarged regional lymph nodes raises the possibility of a mass being a high-grade malignancy and makes biopsy mandatory. Transillumination is a useful technique to evaluate superficial lesions. Meniscal or ganglion cysts will often transmit light because of their fluid-filled nature. These simple tests can obviate the need for formal biopsy of trivial lesions, as well as highlight those tumors that must be biopsied.

As noted previously, one should be parsimonious in ordering tests. Plain films are very important for identifying soft tissue calcifications commonly seen in such tumors as hemangiomas and synovial sarcomas. MRI or contrast-enhanced CT is needed for three-dimensional imaging of the lesion. They may show important diagnostic information such as central necrosis or fluid-fluid levels, but are nonspecific diagnostically. Bone scans have poor accuracy and poor positive predictive value in soft tissue sarcomas. Gallium scans may be helpful for certain round cell tumors such as Ewing's sarcoma, but are insensitive for mesenchymal tumors, failing to image primary and recurrent lesions under 5 cm reliably. Important staging studies such as chest CT can be performed selectively after malignancy is confirmed histologically.

The most important prognostic factor in patients with soft tissue sarcomas is the histologic grade of the tumor.[32] Survival is inversely proportional to grade. Broder I and II, well-differentiated, Musculoskeletal Tumor Society (MSTS) stage I tumors have the best prognosis, and the Broder III and IV, poorly differentiated, MSTS stage II tumors have the worst prognosis. In addition, size (greater or less than 5 cm) and location (superficial or deep to the fascia) of the lesion are important. Invasiveness may be an important additional factor. Karakousis et al.[46] found the lowest survival rates in patients with nerve, artery, or bone involvement. LaQuaglia et al.[51] found this to be true even in children with chemotherapy-responsive tumors such as ERMS. Most of the large deep tumors are extracompartmental (Enneking stage IIB). The Hadju system, which is based on tumor grade, size, and depth relative to the deep fascia, is more predictive of survival and local control than the MSTS staging system.[32] Several investigators have reported independent prognostic value for tumor DNA ploidy (diploid, good prognosis; aneuploid, bad prognosis).[4]

Because of the locally invasive nature of these lesions, local recurrence rates of 30% are seen with local excision alone of high-grade sarcomas greater than 5 cm. Radical compartment resection or wide excision plus radiation therapy (50–60 Gy) reduce local recurrence rates to approximately 10%.[7] Preoperative radiotherapy and marginal excision work as effectively in selected cases. Patients should undergo wide repeat excision of lesions "totally" removed by an excisional biopsy. In such cases, gross tumor remains in one third of patients, microscopic tumor in one third, and most of the others have undetectable cancer that would inevitably recur without the reexcision. However, despite reexcision of incompletely excised tumors, the results are not as good as when the tumor is adequately excised initially.[5] This approach of aggressive local excision plus adjuvant radiotherapy for high-grade sarcomas effectively controls local disease, preserves functional limbs, and does not compromise survival. The role of radiation therapy in large, low-grade sarcomas remains to be determined. Brachytherapy does not improve the results, but external beam radiation may.[7] Small sarcomas (<5 cm), whether high or low grade, superficial or deep, can be treated with excision alone and no radiation therapy. Local recurrence with this technique is 10%, 5-year survival is 94%, and neither outcome is improved with chemotherapy or radiation therapy.[33] Primary amputation continues to have a role for bulky, invasive tumors where vascular, bone or joint, and soft tissue reconstruction cannot restore reasonable function in the extremity[90] (Fig 84–32). Amputation for extensive recurrent disease remains the procedure of choice.

Radiation oncologists use various methods to deliver adjuvant radiotherapy. At Memorial Sloan-Kettering brachytherapy is used whenever possible to administer the equivalent of 60 Gy via iridium or iodine beads.[7, 8] Intraoperatively placed catheters are loaded 5 days postoperatively to allow for early wound healing.[68] Treatment is completed after 5 days of radiation rather than the 6 weeks required for conventional cobalt external beam radiotherapy. Several

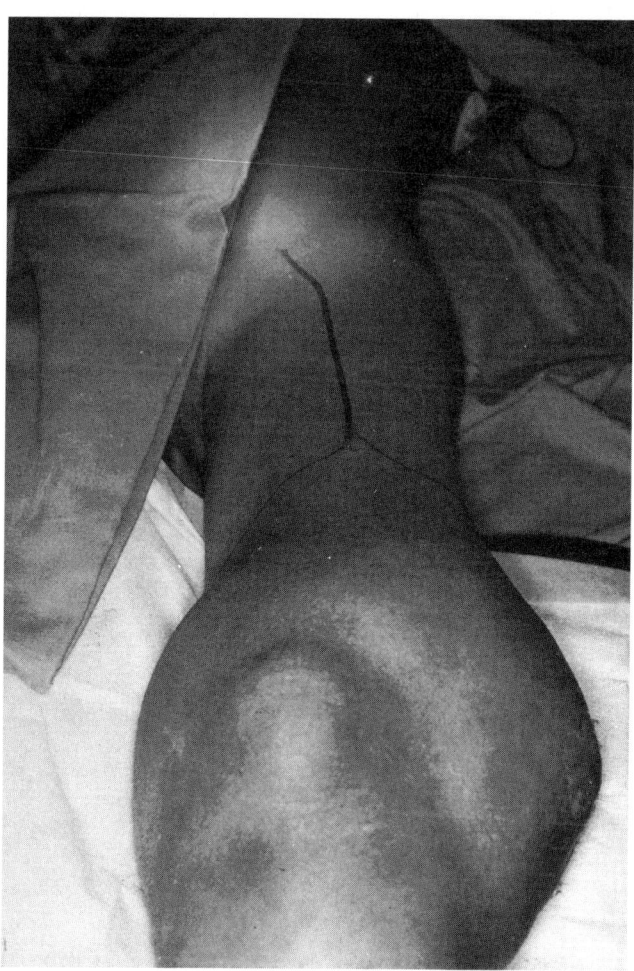

FIG 84–32.
A large soft tissue sarcoma which was eroding through the skin laterally and involved all compartments of the thigh was treated with a primary amputation.

centers are experimenting with intraoperative radiotherapy in combination with either pre- or postoperative radiotherapy. Early results have shown this to be an effective technique, although at the expense of toxicity to neural structures.[49, 82]

Since there is a 40% to 80% mortality of high-grade soft tissue sarcoma, the need for systemic therapy is obvious. Adjuvant chemotherapy remains a tantalizing prospect to improve the outcome in soft tissue sarcoma patients. Doxorubicin-containing protocols appear to be the most effective for metastatic disease. However, promising reports of effective single- and multiagent chemotherapy regimens have not been corroborated in most randomized trials of adjuvant treatment. Chemotherapy for localized soft tissue sarcomas is still investigational.

Soft tissue tumors are within the orthopaedist's purview. Careful workup, staging, limb-sparing surgery, and adjuvant radiation therapy for large high-grade sarcomas are the standards of care. The orthopaedist is in the best position to reconstruct the patient's limb to optimize functional results.

REFERENCES

1. Ahuja SC, et al: Juxtacortical (parosteal) osteogenic sarcoma. Histological grading and prognosis, *J Bone Joint Surg [Am]* 59:632, 1977.
2. Alman BA, et al: Aggressive fibromatosis, *J Pediatr Orthop* 12:1, 1992.
3. Assad WA, et al: Role of brachytherapy in the management of desmoid tumors, *Int J Radiat Oncol Biol Phys* 12:901, 1986.
4. Bauer HCF, Kreicbergs A, Tribukait B: DNA content prognostic in soft tissue sarcoma, *Acta Orthop Scand* 62:187, 1991.
5. Bell RS, et al: The surgical margin in soft-tissue sarcoma, *J Bone Joint Surg [Am]* 71:370, 1989.
6. Benevenia J, et al: Resection arthrodesis of the knee for tumor: Large intercalary allograft and long intramedullary nail technique. In Brown KLB, editor: *Complications of limb salvage. Prevention, management and outcome,* International Symposium on Limb Salvage, Montreal, 1991, p 69.
7. Brennan MF, et al: The role of multimodality therapy in soft-tissue sarcoma, *Ann Surg* 214:328, 1991.
8. Brennan MF, et al: Local recurrence in adult soft-tissue sarcoma. A randomized trial of brachytherapy, *Arch Surg* 122:1289, 1987.
9. Brown KL: Limb reconstruction with vascularized fibular grafts after bone tumor resection, *Clin Orthop* 262:64, 1991.
10. Caffey J: On fibrous defects in cortical walls of growing tubular bones. Their radiologic appearance, structure, prevalence, natural course, and diagnostic significance, *Adv Pediatr* 7:13, 1955.
11. Caffey J: *Pediatric x-ray diagnosis: A textbook for students and practitioners of pediatrics, surgery, and radiology,* ed 5, St Louis, 1967, Mosby–Year Book.
12. Cammisa FP, et al: The Van Ness tibial rotationplasty. A functionally viable reconstructive procedure in children who have a tumor of the distal end of the femur, *J Bone Joint Surg* 72:1541, 1990.
13. Campanacci M, Costa P: Total resection of distal femur or proximal tibia for bone tumors. Autogenous bone grafts and arthrodesis in twenty-six cases, *J Bone Joint Surg [Br]* 61:455, 1979.
14. Campanacci M, et al: Giant cell tumor of bone, *J Bone Joint Surg [Am]* 69:106, 1987.
15. Case records of the Massachusetts General Hospital. Case 5–1989, *N Engl J Med* 320:301, 1989.
16. Chang AE, Schaner EG, Conkle DM: Evaluation of computed tomography in the detection of pulmonary metastases, *Cancer* 43:913, 1979.
17. Chao EY, Sim FH: Modular prosthetic system for segmental bone and joint replacement after tumor resection, *Orthopedics* 8:641, 1985.

18. Cobb JP, et al: Extracortical bone bridging to enhance fixation. In Brown KLB, editor: *Complications of limb salvage. Prevention, management and outcome,* International Symposium on Limb Salvage, Montreal, 1991, p 409.
19. Dahlin DC: Chondromyxoid fibroma of bone with emphasis on its morphological relationship to benign chondroblastoma, *Cancer* 9:195, 1956.
20. Dalinka MK, et al: The use of magnetic resonance imaging in the evaluation of bone and soft tissue tumors, *Radiol Clin North Am* 28:461, 1990.
21. Dell C, Burchardt H, Glowczewskie FP Jr: A roentgenographic, biomechanical, and histologic evaluation of vascularized and non-vascularized segmental fibular canine autografts, *J Bone Joint Surg [Am]* 67:105, 1985.
22. Dinham JM: Popliteal cysts in children, *J Bone Joint Surg [Br]* 57:69, 1975.
23. Enneking WF: Autogenous cortical bone graft in the reconstruction of segmental skeletal defects, *J Bone Joint Surg* 62-A:1039, 1980.
24. Enneking WF: A system of staging musculoskeletal neoplasms, *Clin Orthop* 204:9, 1986.
25. Enneking WF, Shirley PD: Resection-arthrodesis for malignant and potentially malignant lesions about the knee using an intramedullary rod and local bone grafts, *J Bone Joint Surg [Am]* 62:1039, 1977.
26. Enneking WF, Springfield D, Gross M: The surgical treatment of parosteal osteosarcomas in long bones, *J Bone Joint Surg [Am]* 67:125, 1985.
27. Ezekowitz RA, Mullikan JB, Folkman J: Interferon alpha-2a therapy for life-threatening hemangiomas of infancy. *N Engl J Med* 326:1456, 1992.
28. Farr GH, Huvos AG: Juxtacortical osteogenic sarcoma. An analysis of fourteen cases, *J Bone Joint Surg [Am]* 54:1205, 1972.
29. Finn HA, Simon MA: Limb-salvage surgery in the treatment of osteosarcoma in skeletally immature individuals, *Clin Orthop* 262:108, 1991.
30. Finn HA, et al: Scintigraphy with gallium-67 citrate in staging of soft-tissue sarcomas of the extremity, *J Bone Joint Surg [Am]* 69:886, 1987.
31. Finn HA, et al: The Finn knee: Rotating hinge replacement of the knee. Preliminary report of new design. In Brown K, editor: *Complications of limb salvage. Prevention, management and outcome,* International Symposium on Limb Salvage, Montreal, 1991, p 413.
32. Gaynor JJ, et al: Refinement of clinicopathologic staging for localized soft tissue sarcoma of the extremity: A study of 423 adults, *J Clin Oncol* 10:1317, 1992.
33. Geer RJ, et al: Management of small soft-tissue sarcoma of the extremity in adults, *Arch Surg* 127:1285, 1992.
34. Gitelis S, Piasecki P: Allograft prosthetic composite arthroplasty for osteosarcoma and other aggressive bone tumors, *Clin Orthop* 270:197, 1991.
35. Gottsauner-Wolf F, et al: Rotationplasty for limb salvage in the treatment of malignant tumors at the knee. A follow-up study for seventy patients, *J Bone Joint Surg [Am]* 73:1365, 1991.
36. Gottsauner-Wolf F, et al: Extracortical bone bridging for endoprosthetic shaft anchorage in segmental bone/joint defect replacement. In Brown KLB, editor: *Complications of limb salvage. Prevention, management and outcome,* International Symposium on Limb Salvage, Montreal, 1991, p 439.
37. Greene MH, et al: Subsequent cancer in patients with Ewing's sarcoma, *Cancer Treat Rep* 63:2043, 1979.
38. Healey JH, Lane JM: Treatment of pathologic fractures of the distal femur with the Zickel supracondylar nail, *Clin Orthop* 250:216, 1990.
39. Heare TC, Enneking WF, Heare MM: Staging techniques and biopsy of bone tumors, *Orthop Clin North Am* 20:273, 1989.
40. Horowitz SM, Lane JM, Healey JH: Soft-tissue management with prosthetic replacement for sarcomas around the knee, *Clin Orthop* 275:226, 1992.
41. Horowitz SM, et al: Prosthetic, extremity, and patient survival in limb salvage. In Brown KLB, editor: *Complications of limb salvage. Prevention, management and outcome,* International Symposium on Limb Salvage, Montreal, 1991, p 139.
42. Horowitz SM, et al: Prosthetic arthroplasty of the knee after resection of a sarcoma in the proxiaml end of the tibia, *J Bone Joint Surg [Am]* 73:286, 1991.
43. Huvos AG, Marcove RC: Chondroblastoma of bone: A critical review, *Clin Orthop* 95:300, 1973.
44. Joyce MJ, Mankin HJ: Caveat arthroscopy: Extra-articular lesions of bone simulating intra-articular pathology of the knee, *J Bone Joint Surg [Am]* 65:289, 1983.
45. Jupiter JB, Bour CJ, May JW: The reconstruction of defects in the femoral shaft with vascularized transfers of fibula bone, *J Bone Joint Surg [Am]* 69:365, 1987.
46. Karakousis CP, et al: Feasibility of limb salvage and survival in soft tissue sarcomas, *Cancer* 57:484, 1986.
47. Kenan S, Bloom N, Lewis MM: Limb-sparing surgery in skeletally immature patients with osteosarcoma. The use of an expandable prosthesis, *Clin Orthop* 270:223, 1991.
48. Kenan S, Lewis MM: Limb salvage in pediatric surgery: The use of the expandable prosthesis, *Orthop Clin North Am* 22:121, 1991.
49. Kinsella TJ, et al: Preliminary results of a randomized study of adjuvant radiation therapy in resectable adult retroperitoneal soft tissue sarcoma, *J Clin Oncol* 6:18, 1988.
50. Klein WA, et al: The use of indomethacin, sulindac, and tamoxifen for the treatment of desmoid tumors associated with familial polyposis, *Cancer* 60:2863, 1987.
51. LaQuaglia MP, et al: Factors predictive of mortality in pediatric extremity rhabdomyosarcoma, *J Pediatr Surg* 25:238, 1990.
52. Lewis MM: The use of an expandable and adjustable prosthesis in the treatment of childhood malignant bone tumors of the extremity, *Cancer* 57:499, 1986.
53. Lewis RJ, Marcove RC, Rosen G: Ewing's sarcoma: Functional effects of radiation therapy, *J Bone Joint Surg [Am]* 59:325–331, 1977.
54. Malawar MM: Surgical management of aggressive and

malignant tumors of the proximal fibula, *Clin Orthop* 186:172, 1984.
55. Malawer MM, McHale KA: Limb-sparing surgery for high grade malignant tumors of the proximal tibia: Surgical technique and a method of extensor mechanism reconstruction, *Clin Orthop* 239:231, 1989.
56. Malkin D, et al: Germ line p53 mutations in a familial syndrome of breast cancer, sarcomas, and other neoplasms, *Science* 250:1233, 1990.
57. Mankin HJ, Lange TA, Spanier SS: The hazards of biopsy in patients with malignant primary bone and soft-tissue tumors, *J Bone Joint Surg [Am]* 64:1121–1127, 1982.
58. Marcove RC, Jensen MJ: Radical resection for osteogenic sarcoma of fibula with preservation of limb, *Clin Orthop* 125:173, 1977.
59. Marcove RC, Rosen G: En bloc resections for osteogenic sarcoma, *Cancer* 45:3040, 1980.
60. Marcove RC, Shoji H, Harlen M: Altered carbohydrate metabolism in cartilaginous tumors, *Contemp Surg* 5:53, 1974.
61. Marcove RC, Weis LD, Vaghaiwalla MR: Cryosurgery in the treatment of giant cell tumors of bone: A report of 52 consecutive cases, *Cancer* 41:957, 1978.
62. McCollough WB, et al: Radiation therapy for aggressive fibromatosis, *J Bone Joint Surg [Am]* 73:717, 1991.
63. Merkel KD, Gebhardt M, Springfield DS: Rotationplasty as a reconstructive operation after tumor resection, *Clin Orthop* 270:231, 1991.
64. Meyers PA, et al: Chemotherapy for nonmetastatic osteogenic sarcoma: The Memorial Sloan-Kettering experience, *J Clin Oncol* 10:5, 1992.
65. Moskowitz AJ, Pauker SG: A decision analytic approach to limb-sparing treatment for adult soft-tissue and osteogenic sarcoma, *Cancer Treat Symp* 3:11, 1985.
66. Muschler GF, et al: A custom femoral prosthesis for reconstruction of large defects following wide excision for sarcoma. Results and prognostic factors, *Orthopedics* 1993 (in press).
67. NIH Consensus Conference: Limb-sparing treatment of adult soft-tissue sarcomas and osteosarcomas, *JAMA* 254:1791, 1985.
68. Ormsby MV, et al: Wound complications of adjuvant radiation therapy in patients with soft-tissue sarcoma, *Ann Surg* 210:93, 1991.
69. Otis JC, Lane JM, Krol MA: Energy cost during gait in osteosarcoma patients after resection and knee replacement and after above the knee amputation, *J Bone Joint Surg [Am]* 67:606, 1985.
70. Rand JA, Chao EYS, Stauffer RN: Kinematic rotating hinge total knee arthroplasty, *J Bone Joint Surg [Am]* 69:489, 1987.
71. Raney B, et al: Nonsurgical management of children with recurrent or unresectable fibromatosis, *Pediatrics* 79:394, 1987.
72. Roberts P, et al: Prosthetic replacement of the distal femur for primary bone tumors, *J Bone Joint Surg [Br]* 73:762, 1991.
73. Rock MG, et al: Extra-abdominal desmoid tumors, *J Bone Joint Surg [Am]* 66:1369, 1984.
74. Rosen G, Marcove RC, Caparros B: Primary osteogenic sarcoma. The rationale for preoperative chemotherapy and delayed surgery, *Cancer* 43:2163, 1979.
75. Rosen G, Murphy ML, Huvos AG: Chemotherapy, en bloc resection and prosthetic bone replacement in the treatment of osteogenic sarcoma, *Cancer* 37:1, 1976.
76. Rosen G, et al: Preoperative chemotherapy for osteogenic sarcoma: Selection of postoperative chemotherapy based on the response of the primary tumor to preoperative chemotherapy, *Cancer* 49:1221, 1982.
77. Simon MA: Biopsy of musculoskeletal tumors, *J Bone Joint Surg [Am]* 64:1253, 1982.
78. Simon MA: Limb salvage for osteosarcoma, *J Bone Joint Surg [Am]* 70:307, 1988.
79. Simon MA, Nachman J: The clinical utility of preoperative therapy for sarcomas, *J Bone Joint Surg [Am]* 68:1458, 1986.
80. Simon MA, et al: Limb-salvage treatment versus amputation for osteosarcoma of the distal end of the femur, *J Bone Joint Surg [Am]* 68:1331–1337, 1986.
81. Smith J, et al: Parosteal (juxtacortical) osteogenic sarcoma. A roentgenological study of 30 patients, *J Can Assoc Radiol* 29:167, 1978.
82. Suit HD, et al: Treatment of the patient with M0 soft tissue sarcoma, *J Clin Oncol* 6:854, 1988.
83. Sundaram M, et al: Magnetic resonance imaging in planning limb-salvage surgery for primary malignant tumors of bone, *J Bone Joint Surg [Am]* 68:809, 1986.
84. Unni KK, et al: Parosteal osteogenic sarcoma, *Cancer* 37:2466, 1976.
85. Unni KK, Dahlin DC, Beabout JW: Periosteal osteogenic sarcoma, *Cancer* 37:2476, 1976.
86. van der Heul RO, von Ronnen JR: Juxtacortical osteosarcoma. Diagnosis, differential diagnosis, treatment, and an analysis of eighty cases, *J Bone Joint Surg [Am]* 49:415, 1967.
87. Van Nes CP: Rotationplasty for congenital defects of the femur, *J Bone Joint Surg [Br]* 32:12, 1950.
88. Waddell WR, Kirsch WM: Testolactone, sulindac, warfarin, and vitamin K for unresectable desmoid tumors, *Am J Surg* 161:416, 1991.
89. Weiss AJ, Lackman RD: Low dose chemotherapy of desmoid tumors, *Cancer* 64:1192, 1989.
90. Williard WC, et al: Comparison of amputation with limb-sparing operations for adult soft tissue sarcoma of the extremity, *Ann Surg* 215:269, 1992.
91. Wood MB: Free vascularized bone transfers for nonunions, segmental gaps, and following tumor resection, *Orthopedics* 9:810, 1986.
92. Zucchi V, Odella F, Mapelli S: Benign epiphyseal chondroblastoma adjacent to the femoral intercondylar fossa, *Ital J Orthop Traumatol* 10:369, 1984.

Index

A

Abrasion arthroplasty
　for chondromalacia, 613
　for degenerative arthritis, 585–591
　upper tibial osteotomy and, 591–592
Acceleration, definition, 96
Achilles tendon graft
　in patellar tendon rupture repair, 477
　in PCL reconstruction, 880–881
Acquired immunodeficiency syndrome (AIDS)
　case definition, 351
　epidemiology, 348–349
　HIV infection in (see Human immunodeficiency virus infection)
　transfusions and, 1212
Acromegaly, 127
Acrylic interpositional arthroplasties, 1051, 1053
Active movement testing, for patellofemoral rehabilitation, 923–924
Activities
　in pediatric knee disorders, continuing care, 292–293
　return to, after rehabilitation, 950–951
Activities of daily living, coactivation in, 116, 117–118
Activity level, osteotomy and, 1024, 1026
Acufex Knee Signature System, 678–679
Adduction-abduction, normal moment patterns in walking, 99–100
Adductor magnus, 43

ADL (activities of daily living), coactivation in, 116, 117–118
Adolescents
　chondromalacia patellae, 396
　developmental considerations, 279–280
　pain, 285
　psychosocial needs, 289
　teaching, 291
AGC prosthesis, modular system characteristics, 1300
AIDS (see Acquired immunodeficiency syndrome)
Albright's syndrome, 1424
Alfentanil, in arthroscopic surgery, 301
Alkaline phosphatase, in bone tumors, 1450
Allografts
　freeze-dried soft tissue, 575
　meniscal (see Meniscal allotransplantation)
Allografts in ligament surgery, 653, 654, 751, 865–893
　anterior cruciate ligament, 871–873
　intraarticular repair, 751
　postoperative management, 879
　technique, 873–879
　two-incision rear-entry guide technique, 878, 880
　biomechanics, 870–871
　cruciate ligaments, 642, 653, 654
　donor screening and prevention of disease transmission, 866–867
　frontiers, 889
　histology, 869–870

human allograft reconstruction results, 885–889
immunogenicity, 869
indications, 871
posterior cruciate ligament postoperative management, 884–885
　technique, 879–884
procurement and storage, 867–868
secondary sterilization, 868–869
α-adrenergic antagonists, for reflex sympathetic dystrophy, 374
Aminocaproic acid, in hemophilia, 335–336
Aminoglycoside, in total knee arthroplasty, 1269
Amoxicillin, in total knee arthroplasty, 1266
Ampicillin, in total knee arthroplasty, 1269
Amputation
　dislocations and, 1002–1003
　for infected total knee arthroplasty, 1276
Amyloidomas, radiography, 129
Analgesia (see also Anesthesia; Pain management)
　epidural, in total knee arthroplasty, 1232–1233
　patient-controlled (see Patient-controlled analgesia)
　pediatric, 286–287
Anametric total knee replacement, 1070
Anatomically Graduated Components prosthesis, modular system characteristics, 1300

Anatomy, 15–54
　anterior aspect of knee, 45, 46–47
　arthroscopic (see Arthroscopic anatomy)
　blood supply, 51–52
　capsule, 24
　failed knee replacement and, 1279–1281
　hyaline or articular cartilage, 32–33
　innervation, 47–51
　lateral aspect of knee, 39–43, 1200, 1203–1204
　ligaments, 26–32
　medial aspect of knee, 35–39, 1200, 1201–1202
　menisci, 33–35, 527–528, 529
　normal skeletal structures, 15
　bone, 16–18, 20
　bony architecture, 17, 18–19, 20–22
　magnetic resonance imaging, 161–163
　patella, 22–24
　tibiofibular joint, 24
　patellofemoral joint, 381–382, 416–419
　posterior aspect of knee, 42–46, 1200, 1205
　proximal tibia, 1369–1370
　synovium, 24–26
Anderson Knee Stabler, 957–959, 961
Anderson splint, 260
Andrews (ACL) procedure, 806–807, 809
Anemia, roentgenographic evaluation, 139
Anesthesia for knee surgery, 299–314
　arthroscopic surgery, 300–301, 493
　general anesthesia, 301–302

xxv

Anesthesia for knee
surgery (cont.)
general vs. local
anesthesia, 301
local anesthesia, 302
postoperative local
analgesia, 302–303
local anesthetics,
306–308
complications of
regional anesthesia,
309–310
toxicity, 308–309
monitoring standards,
299–300
postoperative pain
management, 310
nonsteroidal
anti-inflammatory
drugs, 310–311
opioid analgesia,
311–312
total knee arthroplasty,
303
preoperative
assessment,
303–305
regional anesthesia,
305–309
Anesthesia for stress
examination,
664–665
Anesthetic sympathetic
blockade, in reflex
sympathetic
dystrophy,
372–373, 375
Aneurysmal bone cysts,
1422–1423, 1471
Anger, pediatric, 280
Angiography of pulmonary
embolism, 1221
Angulatory deformities
arthroscopic debridement
and, 593
bone loss in, 1333–1334
femoral, 1338
tibial, 1334–1338,
1339–1340
osteotomy and,
1020–1021, 1024,
1026, 1028 (see
also Osteotomy for
arthritic knee)
pediatric, 262
posttraumatic,
262–263
tibia vara (Blount's
disease), 263–264
treatment, 262
Antacids
for children, 294
NSAIDs interacting with,
326–327

Anterior approaches to
knee, 55–59
anterolateral (Kocher),
57, 58–59
anteromedial, 56–57
subvastus, 57, 58
Insall approach, 57
midline, 55, 57
with osteotomy of tibial
tubercle, 66–67
Anterior aspect of knee,
anatomy, 45, 46–47
Anterior cruciate ligament
congenital absence, 212
development, 9, 11, 12
examination, 667–670
in knee stability, 85–86,
87, 114
magnetic resonance
imaging, 172,
174–177
Anterior cruciate ligament
anatomy, 26–32
arthroscopic view, 28,
503, 510–511
attachment sites, 27, 29
blood supply, 31, 32
diagram, 28
flexion and extension, 30
magnetic resonance
imaging, 29, 34,
174–177
mechanoreceptors and
motion, 27
Anterior cruciate
ligament-deficient
knees
degenerative changes,
725
laxity testing (see
KT-1000 arthrometer)
meniscal injuries in,
minimal intervention
surgery, 727
meniscal repairs in, 561
sidestep cut in, 102–103
Anterior cruciate ligament
injuries, 723–735
distribution of
disruptions, 658
functional knee bracing,
963–967
with lateral ligamentous
injuries, 717–718
laxity, 660
with medial collateral
ligament injuries,
710–711
minimal intervention
surgery, 727
natural history
complete injury,
723–726
partial injury, 726

nonoperative treatment
and rehabilitation,
723–735
atrophy, 728
biomechanics,
727–728
bracing, 730–731
complete Injury,
731–732
hamstring
rehabilitation,
729–730
knee strengthening,
728–729
partial injury, 732
patient selection,
726–727
nursing care (see
Nursing care of
ligament injuries)
pediatric, 252
midsubstance tears,
254–255, 256, 257
tibial spine fractures,
252–254
prophylactic knee
bracing, 958–962
surgery (see Anterior
cruciate ligament
reconstruction)
Anterior cruciate ligament
reconstruction
with allografts, 871–873
biomechanics,
870–871
postoperative
management, 879
technique, 873–879
two-incision rear-entry
technique, 878, 880
arthroscopic (see
Arthroscopic ACL
reconstruction)
candidates, 747–748
developments, 865
extraarticular, 800–803
Andrews procedure,
806–807, 809
Arnold-Coker
procedure, 805, 807
biomechanics, 801,
802–803
complications, 802,
807–808
Ellison procedure, 803,
805, 806
indications, 802
intraarticular vs., 640
James procedure, 805,
808
Losee procedure, 803,
805
MacIntosh procedure,
803, 804–805

pes anserinus transfer,
807, 809
results, 801–802
historical perspective,
638, 639, 640–642,
747
with iliotibial band (see
Iliotibial myofascial
transfer)
indications and surgical
philosophy for
management,
747–755
intraarticular, 749,
791–792
conventional
two-incision
technique, 792–796
extraarticular vs., 640
graft strength
considerations, 749
graft types, 750–752
graft vascularity, 749
isometric
considerations,
749–750
single-incision
endoscopic
reconstruction,
796–800
intraarticular
semitendinosus,
813–827
Hendler procedure,
821–824, 825
patellar tendon graft
vs., 824–825
semitendinosus as
ACL substitute,
813–817
technical
considerations,
817–821
with Kennedy LAD,
829–837
clinical results,
831–832
procedure, 832–836
for knee dislocation,
1003, 1004, 1005
operative repair,
748–749
with patellar tendon
grafts (see Patellar
tendon grafts in ACL
reconstruction)
prosthetic (see
Prosthetic cruciate
ligament
reconstruction)
Anterior cruciate ligament
rehabilitation
protocol, 951
forms, 972–977

return to activities and sports, 950
Anterior drawer test, 666, 668
Anterior femoral notching, in total knee replacement, 1409, 1412
Anterior tibial artery, recurrent branch, supplying blood to knee soft tissue, 1280
Antibiotics in total knee arthroplasty
  adverse effects, 1270
  antibiotic-loaded cement, 1271–1272
  aspiration and, 1272
  doses, 1268
  long-term suppression of infection, 1270–1271
  perioperative, 1264–1266
  therapy, 1268
Anticoagulants, total knee arthroplasty and, 1211
Antifibrinolytic agents, in hemophilia, 335–336
Anti-inflammatory medications
  nonsteroidal (see Nonsteroidal anti-inflammatory drugs)
  in wound healing, 1282–1283
Antimalarials
  for osteoarthritis, 327
  for rheumatoid arthritis, 328
Antirheumatic drugs, 321–322
  clinical evaluation
    aspirin and other salicylates, 322–324
    other NSAIDs, 324–326
    second- and third-line drugs, 327–329
  individualizing dosage, 322
  principles of adjusting dose, 322
  slow-acting, for children, 286
AO classification of supracondylar and intercondylar distal femoral fractures, 1358, 1359

Apical ectodermal ridge, 7
Apprehension sign of Fairbanks, 393, 423, 424
Arcuate ligaments, anatomy, 39–40
Arginine vasopressin, in hemophilia, 335
Argon lasers, in arthroscopy, 522
Arnold-Coker (ACL) procedure, 805, 807
Arteria genus suprema, supplying blood to knee soft tissue, 1280
Arthralgia, HIV infection and, 357
Arthritic knees
  arthroscopy (see Arthroscopic treatment of degenerative arthritis)
  gait analysis, 103
  ligament releases (see Ligament releases in arthritic knee)
  osteotomy (see Osteotomy for arthritic knee)
Arthritis (see also specific types)
  HIV-associated, 357
  infection-associated, 131–132
  Lyme, pediatric, 268
  after patellar fracture, 1401
  roentgenographic evaluation, 126–130, 131–132
  septic, pediatric, 267–268
Arthrodesis
  in bone tumor reconstruction, 1469–1470
  for infected total knee arthroplasty, 1274–1275
Arthrodesis
  for failed knee replacement
    external fixation, 1346–1347
    general principles, 1346
    internal fixation, 1347–1348
    intramedullary nail fixation, 1348, 1349
    union and nonunion rates, 1345

Arthrography, 149–150
  computed tomography with, 149–150, 152–154
Arthropathy and hemophilia, 331–345
  pathogenesis, 336–338
  radiographic changes, 338, 339
  treatment of knee
    acute hemarthrosis, 338–339
    chronic hemophilic arthropathy, 340–344
    subacute hemarthrosis, 339–340
Arthroscope, 488, 489
Arthroscopic ACL reconstruction with patellar tendon graft, 757–771
  allografts, 758, 759
  anterior exposure, 764
  equipment, 758, 759
  femoral notch preparation, 761–762
  femoral site selection, 762–763
  fixation of graft, 767–769
  harvesting autograft, 765–767
  historical perspective, 757–758
  initial diagnostic arthroscopy, 760–761
  isometry testing, 764–765
  lateral incision, 761
  passage of graft, 767
  passage of rear-entry drill guide, 763
  portal selection, 759
  postoperative care, 769
  setup, 759, 760
  tibial guide placement, 764
  tibial hole preparation, 765, 766
  with semitendinosus graft, 816–817
  Hendler procedure, 821–824, 825
Arthroscopic anatomy, 497
  femoral condyles and tibial plateaus, 501–502

intercondylar notch and cruciate ligaments, 502–503
menisci, 503–505
patellofemoral joint, 500–501
suprapatellar pouch and plicae, 497–500
Arthroscopic debridement
  for degenerative arthritis, 585, 591, 592–593, 594
  for osteonecrosis, 610
Arthroscopic equipment
  arthroscope, 488, 489
  camera systems, 488
  historical perspective, 483–484, 487–488
  instrument guides and fixation techniques, 491–492
  instruments, 488
    mechanical, 489, 490
    nonmechanical, 489
  lasers, 492–493
  lighting systems, 488, 489, 490
  motorized equipment, 490–491
Arthroscopic laser surgery, 492–493, 515–524
  carbon dioxide laser, 521
  contact Nd:YAG laser, 517–521
  delivery systems, 517–522
  excimer laser, 521–522
  future directions, 522–523
  Ho:YAG laser, 522
  KTP and argon lasers, 522
  meniscal resection, 517–522, 545
Arthroscopic lavage, 594
Arthroscopic meniscal repair, 559–571
  classification of tears, 560
  complications, 568–569
  diagnostic arthroscopy and instrumentation, 561–562
  future directions, 569
  indications, 560–561
  inside-out technique
    lateral tears, 565–566
    medial tears, 563–565
  intraarticular, posterior incision combined with, 69–71
  outside-in technique for anteromedial and anterolateral tears, 566–567

Arthroscopic meniscal
  repair *(cont.)*
  rehabilitation, 567–568
  results, 568
Arthroscopic
  meniscectomy,
  527–557
  anatomy, 527–529
  complex and
    degenerative tears,
    552–553
    discoid meniscus,
      553–554
    perimeniscal cysts,
      553
  indications and goals,
    538, 540
  with lasers, 517–522,
    545
  pediatric, 250, 251
  posterior rim, 545
  postoperative
    management, 554
  primary cleavage tears
    cleavage flap tears,
      551–552
    pure cleavage tear,
      550–551
  principles, 540–542
    anterior exposure,
      542–543
    instrumentation,
      544–545
    posterior visualization,
      543
    two-portal technique,
      541, 543–544
  results, 554–555
  tear patterns and
    pathogenesis,
    528–538
  vertical longitudinal
    tears, 546–548
  vertical radial tears,
    548–550
Arthroscopic PCL
  reconstruction with
  patellar tendon graft,
  surgical technique,
  897–906
Arthroscopic portal sites
  accessory anteromedial
    and anterolateral,
    513
  anterolateral, 505, 506
  anteromedial, 505–506
  central ("Swedish"), 506
  midpatellar lateral, 508
  posteromedial and
    posterolateral,
    507–508
  superomedial and
    superolateral, 506
  sweep of knee, 508–513

Arthroscopic synovectomy,
  625–626
  technique, 626, 627
Arthroscopic treatment of
  degenerative
  arthritis, 583–596
  abrasion arthroplasty
    and upper tibial
    osteotomy,
    591–592
  alignment and
    debridement,
    592–593
  arthroscopic and
    radiographic
    findings, 593–594
  cartilage repair problem,
    584
  debridement, 592–593
  diagnostic arthroscopy,
    592
  early arthroscopy,
    583–584
  lavage, 594
  Pridie procedure and
    abrasion
    arthroplasty,
    584–591
Arthroscopy
  anesthesia, 300–301,
    493
    general, 301–302
    general vs. local, 301
    local, 302
    postoperative local
      analgesia, 302–303
  chondral lesions,
    616–617
  chondromalacia
    diagnosis, 611–612
    treatment, 612–614
  historical perspective,
    482–483
  ligament injuries,
    641–642
  osteochondral fractures,
    615–616
  osteochondritis
    dissecans
    adult lesions,
      601–602
    juvenile form, 600
  before osteotomy, 1029
  past, present, and future,
    481–485
  in patellofemoral
    malalignment
    diagnosis, 447–448
  pediatric, 3, 231
  physical therapy after,
    935–937
  portals, 67–69
  surgical approaches,
    493–494

  tibial plateau fracture
    fixation, 1386
Arthrotomy incisions,
  patellar circulation
  and, 55, 56
Articular cartilage
  anatomy, 32–33, 382
  arthroscopic removal,
    612–613
  lesion classification,
    611–612 *(see also*
    Cartilage lesion
    rehabilitation)
Articular nerve
  anatomy
    lateral articular nerve,
      51
    posterior articular
      nerve, 48–49
  innervated tissues, 109
Articular surface design
  in artificial knee
    congruent joint
      surfaces, 1144
    incongruent joint
      surfaces,
      1144–1145
    justification for
      unconforming
      designs, 1145–1146
    kinematics and
      mechanics of knee,
      1146–1148
    Oxford knee,
      1148–1155
  in human knee,
    1143–1144
Articular surfaces of knee,
  injuries and
  diseases
  chondromalacia,
    611–614
  osteochondritis
    dissecans,
    597–606
  osteonecrosis, 606–611
  traumatic lesions,
    614–617
Articulating surfaces in
  total knee
  replacement,
  retrieval analysis,
  1252–1256
Artificial cruciate ligament
  reconstruction (*see*
  Prosthetic cruciate
  ligament
  reconstruction)
ASIF classification of tibial
  plateau fractures,
  1372–1374
Aspirin
  in pediatric pain
    management, 294

  as prophylaxis for
    thromboembolic
    disease, 1222
  for rheumatolgic
    disorders
    clinical evaluation,
      322–324
    side effects and
      toxicity, 324
Athletic injuries
  bracing, 957–969
  history of ligament
    reconstruction,
    638–639
Athletics, return to, after
  rehabilitation,
  950–951
Atropine, 310
Autogenous grafts
  bone grafting for tibial
    deficiency,
    1336–1338,
    1339–1340
  ligament repair, 652–653
  intraarticular ACL
    reconstruction,
    750–751
Avascular necrosis
  of patella, after patellar
    fracture, 1401
  subchondral,
    radiography,
    142–143
Avulsion fractures, lateral
  tibial plateau, 713,
  717
Avulsion fragments, 1001,
  1002
Axial loading of knee, 82,
  83
Axial rotation of tibia, 79
Azathioprine, for
  rheumatoid arthritis,
  328

B

Baker's cysts, imaging, 124
Bare nerve endings,
  107–108
Basket forceps, for
  arthroscopic
  meniscectomy, 544
Beath pin, in ACL
  reconstruction, 799
β-adrenergic antagonists,
  for reflex
  sympathetic
  dystrophy, 374
Biceps tendon
  anatomy, 42–43
  transfer in ACL
    reconstruction, 803,
    806

Bicompartmental knee replacement/bicondylar knees
evolution, 1059–1062
with mobile meniscal bearings, 1169
Biofeedback
electromyographic, in cartilage lesion rehabilitation, 932–933
pediatric, 285
Biomechanics, 75–94
allograft reconstruction, 870–871
anterior cruciate ligament injuries, 727–728
contact area and role of menisci, 80–81
cruciate ligaments, 1146
functional activities analysis for rehabilitation, 922–924
gait (see Gait analysis)
Kennedy LAD, 829–831
knee replacement
cementless, 1107–1109
designs (see Total knee replacement design biomechanics)
meniscal bearing, 1158–1166
retrieval analysis, 1251–1260
lateral capsuloligamentous complex, 714–715
medial capsuloligamentous complex, 704–706
muscles, 1146
osteotomy, 1020–1021
patellofemoral joint (see Patellofemoral joint, biomechanics)
stability, 81
joint surface, 81
ligamentous, 82–87
loading and, 82, 83
menisci, 81–82
stability and motion, 107–120
surface motion at knee
axial rotation, 79
instantaneous center of motion, 75–78
rolling, sliding, and crossed four-bar linkage, 78–79
tibial plateau fractures, 1371

Biopsy technique for bone tumors, 1451–1453
Bipartite patellae, 215, 399
anteroposterior radiograph, 124
in patellofemoral pain differential diagnosis, 427–428
pediatric, 241
Blood clotting, biochemical basis, 331–332
Blood coagulation, 331–332
Blood loss, in total knee arthroplasty, 1213, 1214
Blood supply
to cruciate ligaments, 31, 32
to knee, 51–52
soft tissues, 1279–1281
to medial meniscus, 35
to patella, 23–24
Blount disease, 219–223, 263–264
classification, 219
clinical features, 219, 220
etiology and incidence, 219
infantile vs. late-onset, 263–264
roentgenographic evaluation, 145, 219–220, 264
treatment, 220–223
osteotomies, 221–223
Rab technique for correction, 264, 265
Bone
biopsy technique, 1451–1453
cortical vs. cancellous, 16
normal anatomy, 16–18, 20
Bone contusion, magnetic resonance imaging, 188, 189
Bone cysts
aneurysmal, 1422–1423, 1471
unicameral, 1422
Bone grafting in internal fixation of distal femoral fractures, 1364, 1365
Bone grafting in total knee arthroplasty, 1333–1344
femoral bone loss, 1338

revision arthroplasty, 1301, 1338, 1340
central medullary deficiency, 1341, 1342
cystic deficiencies, 1340, 1342
peripheral tibial plateau or condylar bone loss, 1342–1344
tibial bone loss
defects greater than 12 mm deep, 1334–1338, 1339–1340
defects 6 to 12 mm deep, 1334
Bone infarction, malignancies and, 1436
Bone infection, radionuclide imaging, 197–199
Bone metastasis, 1435–1436
Bone-patellar tendon-bone grafts (see Patellar tendon grafts in ACL reconstruction; Patellar tendon grafts in PCL reconstruction)
Bone scans (see also Nuclear scans)
bone tumors, 1451
patellofemoral pain, 425
reflex sympathetic dystrophy, 366–367
Bone tumors, 1421–1422, 1441–1448
benign, 1427–1428
benign vs. malignant by location, 1422
clinical presentation, 1448–1450
developmental, hamartomatous, and tumor-like lesions, 1422–1427
diagnostic studies, 1450–1451
biopsy technique, 1451–1453
staging, 1453–1454
fibular lesions, treatment, 1470–1471
giant cell tumor, 1428–1429
treatment, 1455–1457, 1458–1459
locations by percentage, 1422

malignant, 1429–1435
metastatic tumors, treatment, 1471–1472, 1473–1474
multiple myeloma and metastatic carcinoma, 1435–1436
reconstruction, 1465–1466
arthrodesis, 1469–1470
endoprostheses, 1466–1469
secondary malignancies, 1436
surgical technique for malignant tumors
decision making, 1462
en bloc excision of knee, 1462, 1464–1465, 1466
treatment
benign tumors, 1454–1457, 1458–1460
malignant tumors, 1457, 1461–1462, 1463
Bony architecture, normal anatomy, 17, 18–19, 20–22
anteroposterior and lateral roentgenogram, 21
anteroposterior view, 17
knee motion, 17
landmarks, 18–19
"screw-home mechanism," 22
Borrelia burgdorferi, Lyme arthritis from, 268
Boston and Brigham unicompartmental arthroplasty, 1059
Bowleg, 217–218 (see also Blount disease)
Bracing
for anterior cruciate ligament-deficient knee, 730–731
for athletic injuries, 957–969
functional knee braces, 963–967
prophylactic knee braces, 957–962
rehabilitative knee braces, 962–963
after iliotibial band transfer, 783, 789
instrumented testing, 697

Bracing (cont.)
  after ligament reconstruction, 984–985
  patellar, 434–435
  for posterior cruciate ligament injuries, 742, 743
  rehabilitative, 948, 949
  for tibial plateau fractures, 1379
Breaststroker's knee, pediatric, 239–240
Bretylium, 309
Brief's ACL reconstruction technique, 254, 255
Bruises, magnetic resonance imaging, 189
Bruser approach, 59
Bupivacaine, 308
  in arthroscopic surgery, 302–303
  cardiotoxicity, 308
  in postoperative pain management, 311–312
Bursae around knee, 428
  anatomy, 25, 428
  pathology, 25–26
Bursitis, 399
  magnetic resonance imaging, 184, 187
  in patellofemoral pain differential diagnosis, 426–427
  prepatellar, with total knee prosthesis, 150
Burstein-Lane prosthesis, 1466, 1468

C

Calcium, in bone tumors, 1450
Calcium channel blockers, for reflex sympathetic dystrophy, 374
Calcium pyrophosphate deposition disease (CPDD), radiography, 128, 138
Camelback sign, 423, 424
Camera systems for arthroscopy, 488
Campanacci method of bone tumor staging, 1453
Can-Am brace, 963
Cancellous bone, anatomy, 16
Capnography, 300

Capsaicin, for reflex sympathetic dystrophy, 374
Capsular anatomy, 24
Capsular dehiscence, in total knee replacement, 1263
Capsular tears, physical examination, 665–667
Carbamazepine, for reflex sympathetic dystrophy, 373
Carbon dioxide, end-tidal, monitoring, 300
Carbon dioxide lasers, in arthroscopy, 521
Carbon fiber implants
  in ACL reconstruction, 840
  for polyethylene joint components, 1181, 1254–1255
Cardiac arrest, from spinal anesthesia, 309
Cardiac morbidity, perioperative, total knee replacement and, 303–304
Cardiac toxicity, from bupivacaine, 309
Cartilage
  arthrography, 150
  arthroscopic removal, 612–613
  CT/arthrography, 150–151
  in degenerative arthritis, 584, 593
Cartilage lesion rehabilitation, 921–941
  assessment, 924
  chondromalacia patellae (see Chondromalacia patellae rehabilitation)
  meniscal repairs, 939
  osteochondritis dissecans, 937–939
  patellofemoral pain (see Patellofemoral pain, rehabilitation)
  physical therapy after arthroscopic procedures, 935–937
  physical therapy after patellar realignment, 937
  prehabilitation evaluation, 921–922
  assessment, 924

biomechanical analysis of functional activities, 922–924
subjective and objective information, 922
Cartilage lesions
  classification, 611–612
  laser debridement, 613
Cast bracing, for tibial plateau fractures, 1379
Cast immobilization, for tibial plateau fractures, 1378
Casting, pediatric, 281–282
  teaching needs, 291–292
Cat-scratch bacillus, 357
Causalgia (see also Reflex sympathetic dystrophy), pathophysiology, 368–371
Cave approach, 60, 61
CD4 counts, in HIV infection, 350–351
Cefazolin, in total knee arthroplasty
  prophylactic, 1264, 1265
  treatment dose, 1269
Cefuroxime, in total knee arthroplasty, 1264
Cement, in total knee replacement, 1409
Central medullary deficiency, bone grafting in revision total knee arthroplasty, 1341, 1342
Central nervous system, local anesthetic toxicity, 308
Cephalosporins, in total knee arthroplasty, 1264, 1270
Cephalothin, in total knee arthroplasty, 1269
Cephapirin, in total knee arthroplasty, 1265, 1269
Ceramic biomaterials, future directions, 1174
Cerebral palsy, radiography, 133
Chemical synovectomy, 626
Chemotherapy for bone tumors, 1461–1462
Children (see Pediatric knee)

Chloroprocaine, 307–308
  in arthroscopic surgery, 303
Chloroquine
  for osteoarthritis, 327
  for rheumatoid arthritis, 328
Chondral fractures, rehabilitation, 937–939
Chondral lesions, 616–617
Chondrification, development, 7, 8, 9
Chondroblastomas, 1427, 1428
  of distal femur, 1441, 1443
  frequency, 1422
  pediatric, 266
Chondromalacia, primary, 184
Chondromalacia fabellae, 240
Chondromalacia patellae, 393–397, 611
  arthroscopic treatment, 612–614
  CT/arthrography, 152, 153
  diagnosis, 611
  arthroscopic, 611–612
  historical perspective, 404, 415
  magnetic resonance imaging, 183, 184
  pediatric, 232–233
Chondromalacia patellae rehabilitation, 924
  and biomechanical rationale for treatment, 924–935
  electromyographic biofeedback, 932–933
  flexibility and, 925
  inflammation and, 924–925
  isokinetic exercise, 930–931
  open-chain and closed-chain activities, 931–932
  patient education, 934–935
  proprioceptive training, 930, 931, 932
  resistive closed-chain exercise, 933, 935
  stair climbing vs. stairs, 933–934, 936
  stationary bicycle, 929

strengthening and, 925–927
  isometric quadriceps sets, 927
  manual resistance exercises, 929
  neuromuscular electrical stimulation, 928–929
  terminal knee extension, 927–928
  vastus medius obliquus exercise, 927
 taping, 929, 930
 therapeutic plan, 924
Chondromatosis, synovial, 1437, 1476
Chondromyxoid fibromas, 1428, 1443
Chondrosarcomas, 1431–1432, 1447
 biopsy technique, 1452, 1453
 complicating other conditions, 1436
 dedifferentiated, 1432
 glucose tolerance and, 1450
 mesenchymal, 1432–1433
 treatment, 1454–1455, 1460
Cho semitendinosus procedure, 816
Chronic dislocation of patella (CDP), 406–407, 408
 pediatric, 236
Chronic subluxation of patella (CSP), 406, 407
 pediatric, 234–235
Ciprofloxacin, in total knee arthroplasty, 1269
Cisplatinum, for bone tumors, 1461
Clindamycin, in total knee arthroplasty, 1264, 1265, 1266
 treatment dose, 1269
Clonidine, for reflex sympathetic dystrophy, 374
Closed-chain kinetic exercises, 433
Closed reduction and internal fixation, of periprosthetic distal femoral fractures, 1408, 1410
Cloutier nonconstrained knee arthroplasty, 1060, 1062

Cloutier prosthesis, 1129–1132
Coagulation, 331–332
Codeine, 992
Codivilla tendon lengthening and repair, 473
CO_2 lasers, in arthroscopy, 521
Cold compressive therapy, 783, 790
Cold treatment
 for patellofemoral pain, 429
 pediatric, 285
Collagen
 in bone anatomy, 16–17
 in ligaments, 26, 27
 in menisci, 33
Collateral ligaments
 arthrography, 150, 152
 lateral (see Lateral collateral ligament)
 laxity, 661, 662, 665
 magnetic resonance imaging, 170, 179–183
 medial (see Medial collateral ligament)
 physical examination, 664, 665
Compliance index determination, definition, 674
Compression boots, in thromboembolic disease, 1223
Compression plates, in arthrodesis for failed knee replacement, 1347–1348
Compression ultrasonography, in deep venous thrombosis, 1219
Computed tomography
 with arthrography, 150, 152–154
 bone tumors, 1450, 1451
 extensor mechanism injuries, 413
 indications, 148–149
 patellofemoral pain, 424–425, 446–447, 463
 tibial plateau fractures, 1375–1376
Condylar buttress plate, 1362, 1363–1364
Condylar prostheses
 conforming, 1314–1315
 constrained, 1065, 1069, 1309–1316

Condyles (see also Femoral condyles; Tibial condyles), magnetic resonance imaging, 34
Congenital deformities, 209–227
 absence of anterior cruciate ligament, 212
 bipartite patellae, 215
 Blount disease (see Blount disease)
 discoid meniscus, 215–216, 250–251
 dislocation and subluxation, 209–210
  classification, 210, 211
  clinical examination, 210, 212
  pathologic findings, 210–211
  treatment, 211–212, 213–214
 dislocation of patella, 213–214, 215
 genu varum and genu valgum, 217–218, 262
 malalignments, 258–259
 nail-patella syndrome, 136, 214
 popliteal cysts, 216, 267
Congenital diseases, roentgenographic evaluation, 134–136
Congruent meniscal bearings in knee arthroplasty (see Meniscal bearing knee replacement)
Connective tissue disease, radiography, 129–130
Constrained knee arthroplasty, 1305–1323
 clinical review, 1318–1320
 historical aspects, 1305–1308
 indications, 1308
  conforming condylar prostheses, 1314–1315
  constrained condylar prostheses, 1065, 1069, 1309–1316
  PCL-retaining prostheses, 1315–1316
  posterior stabilized prostheses, 1314

  rigid-hinge prostheses, 1309
  rotating-hinge prostheses, 1309, 1311–1312
 revision algorithm, 1317
 surgical techniques, 1316
  bone stock assessment, 1317
  closure, 1318
  debridement of bone and soft tissue, 1317
  exposure, 1316
  implantation, 1318
  ligamentous and musculotendinous assessment, 1317, 1318
  postoperative management, 1318
  preparation of bone stock for prosthesis implantation, 1317–1318
  prosthesis removal, 1316–1317
  trial reduction, 1318
Continuing care, pediatric (see Pediatric knee, continuing care)
Continuous passive motion, 946
 after ligament reconstruction, 985–986
 in PCL rehabilitation, 906
 after total knee arthroplasty, 1235
Coonse-Adams quadriceps turndown, 66
Coping, pediatric, 288–289
Cortical bone, anatomy, 16
Corticosteroids
 for children, 286
 for osteoarthritis, 327
 for rheumatoid arthritis, 328
 in wound healing, 1283
Cortisone, in wound healing, 1283
Coumadin, total knee arthroplasty and, 1211
Crossed four-bar linkage, 78–79
Cruciate condylar prosthesis, 1065, 1067, 1069
Cruciate ligaments
 anatomy, 26–32
  arthroscopic, 502–503
  insertion into bone, 26, 27

Cruciate ligaments (cont.)
  arthrography, 150
  examination, 667–671
  history of reconstruction, 638, 639, 640–642
  kinematics and biomechanics, 1146
  in knee stability, 85–87, 641
  magnetic resonance imaging, 172, 174–178
  preserved in total knee arthroplasty
    historical development, 1060, 1063
    total condylar knee prostheses, 1125–1126, 1128
  prosthetic reconstruction (see Prosthetic cruciate ligament reconstruction)
  repair in knee dislocation, 1003, 1004–1006
  sacrifice in total knee arthroplasty, 1170–1171
Cruciate-substituting knee arthroplasty
  history of knee arthroplasty at Hospital for Special Surgery, 1179–1182
  Insall-Burstein Posterior Stabilized prosthesis, clinical results, 1187–1192
  posterior cruciate ligament sacrifice or substitution
    advantages, 1182–1183
    clinical function, 1192–1193
    clinical results at Mayo Clinic, 1193–1194
    complications of PCL substitution, 1194–1196
    survivorship analysis, 1194, 1195
  Posterior Stabilized prosthesis, 1185–1186
    design rationale, 1186–1187
  Total Condylar prosthesis, 1183
    design, 1183–1184
    long-term results, 1184–1185

Crutch walking, after ligament reconstruction, 986–987, 988, 989
Cryo/Cuff Aircast, 742
Cryopreservation of meniscal allografts, 575
CT (see Computed tomography)
CTi brace, 963, 965
Cutting forceps, for arthroscopic meniscectomy, 544
Cyclophosphamide, for rheumatoid arthritis, 328
Cystic deficiencies, bone grafting in revision total knee arthroplasty, 1340, 1342
Cystic lesions, 1422–1423
Cystic rheumatoid arthritis, 128
Cysts
  ganglion, 1423
  imaging, 124, 128, 129
    arthrography, 149
    magnetic resonance imaging, 149
  meniscal, 149, 172
  perimeniscal, arthroscopic meniscectomy for, 553
  popliteal, 216, 1474–1475
    imaging, 124, 128
    pediatric, 267
Cytomegalovirus, transfusion-transmitted, 1211–1212

D

DDAVP, in hemophilia, 335
Debridement
  arthroscopic
    for degenerative arthritis, 585, 591, 592–593, 594
    for osteonecrosis, 610
  in constrained knee arthroplasty, 1317
  in infected total knee arthroplasty, 1272–1273
  by laser, 613
  before osteotomy, 1029
Dedifferentiated chondrosarcomas, 1432

Deep peroneal nerve, assessment after ligament reconstruction, 984
Deep venous thrombosis in knee arthroplasty, 1218 (see also Thromboembolic disease in knee arthroplasty)
  detection methods, 1218–1220
  incidence, 1220–1221
  after osteotomy, 1034–1035
  radiography, 148, 150
  regional anesthesia and, 305
Delayed exchange of prosthesis, in infected total knee arthroplasty, 1273–1274
Demerol, 992
Dermatomyositis, radiography, 130
Desmoid tumors, 1475–1476
Developmental horizons, 3–11
Developmental stages, 277
  adolescents, 279–280
  infants, 277–278
  preschool children, 278–279
  school-age children, 279
Diabetes mellitus, wound healing and, 1284
Diaphyseal dysplasia, radiography, 140–141
Diazepam, 308
  in pediatric pain management, 286
Didanosine, 356
Diet, pediatric, 287, 294
Diflunisal, 325
  in postoperative pain management, 310
Dilaudid, 992
Discoid lateral meniscus, arthroscopic analysis, 505
Discoid meniscus, 215–216
  pediatric, 250–251
  torn, arthroscopic meniscectomy for, 553–554
Dislocation
  femorotibial joint, imaging, 146, 147

proximal tibiofibular joint (see Proximal tibiofibular joint, dislocation)
traumatic (see Traumatic dislocation of knee)
Dislocation and subluxation of knee, congenital, 209–210, 259
  classification, 210, 211
  clinical examination, 210, 212
  pathologic findings, 210–211
  treatment, 211–212, 213–214, 259
Displacement, definitions, 96
Distal femoral extension osteotomy, 1033, 1034
Distal femoral varus osteotomy, 1033–1034, 1035
  results, 1037
Distal femur
  bone tumors, types and percentages, 1421
  fractures (see also Supracondylar and intercondylar distal femoral fractures)
    epiphyseal and physeal, 243–246
    periprosthetic fractures, internal fixation, 1408–1419
    plate and screw assemblies, 1360–1362, 1363, 1364
  lateral approach, 65–66
  osteochondromas, 1441, 1442
Disuse, effects on musculoskeletal tissue, 945–946
Dolophine, 992
DonJoy custom ACL orthosis, 965
DonJoy Gold Point, 963
Duocondylar total knee arthroplasty, 1122–1125
Duopatellar total knee arthroplasty, 1123–1125
Dynamic condylar screw, 1362, 1363
  insertion technique, 1364, 1366
Dyonics Dynamic Cruciate Tester, 678–679

Dysplasia
  diaphyseal, 140–141
  epiphyseal, 135
  fibrous, 140, 1423–1425
  radiography, 135, 136, 140–141

E

Early exchange of prosthesis, in infected total knee arthroplasty, 1273
Ectoderm, development, 7
Edema reduction, in cartilage lesion rehabilitation, 925
Education, in patellar rehabilitation, 428–429
Effusions of knee, examination and grading, 663
Ehlers-Danlos syndrome, radiography, 134
Eicosapentaenoic acid, for osteoarthritis, 327
Electrical muscle stimulation
  after ligament reconstruction, 986, 987
  in patellofemoral pain, 421
Electromyographic biofeedback, in cartilage lesion rehabilitation, 932–933
Electromyographic coactivation, in activities of daily living, 117–118
ELISA diagnosis of HIV infection, 352
Ellison (ACL) procedure, 803, 805, 806
Ely test, 424
Embryology
  developmental horizons, 3–11
  evolution of knee, 3
Emotional reactions, pediatric, 280
Enchondromas, 1427–1428, 1429
  roentgenographic evaluation, 137
Endoprosthetic reconstruction for bone tumors, 1466–1469

Enneking method of bone tumor staging, 1453–1454
Enzyme-linked immunosorbent assay, in diagnosis of HIV infection, 352
Eosinophilic granulomas, 1426–1427
Ephaptic conduction, in reflex sympathetic dystrophy, 369–371
Epidural analgesia, postoperative, 311–312
Epidural anesthesia
  in arthroscopic surgery, 301
  complications, 309–310
  in reflex sympathetic dystrophy, 373
Epiphyseal and physeal fractures, 242–243
  distal femoral, 243–244
  prognosis, 245–246
  treatment, 244–245
  proximal tibial, 246–247
  tibial tubercle, 247–248
Epiphyseal dysplasias, radiography, 135
Epiphyseal-metaphyseal osteotomy, for Blount disease, 222–223
Epiphysiodesis, in Blount disease, 221
Epithelioid sarcomas, 1439
Equilibrium, definitions, 97–98
Erdheim-Chester disease, radiography, 138–139
Eryops, 3, 4, 5
Erythrocyte sedimentation rate, in bone tumors, 1450
Erythromycin, in total knee arthroplasty, 1266
Erythropoietin, recombinant human, in total knee arthroplasty, 1212–1213
Ewing's sarcoma, 1433–1434, 1445, 1463
  adjuvant chemotherapy, 1461–1462
Excessive lateral pressure syndrome (ELPS), 398
Excimer lasers, in arthroscopy, 522

Exercise *(see also specific types)*
  effect on knee laxity, 697
  functional, 949–950
  pediatric, 287, 294
  static vs. dynamic, 420–421
Exostoses *(see also Osteochondromas),* roentgenographic evaluation, 136–137
Extension
  patellofemoral joint and, 90
  tibial motion and, 79
Extension contractures, pediatric, 260–262
Extensor disruptions, in total knee arthroplasty, 1328–1330
Extensor mechanism *(see also Patellofemoral joint)*
  anatomy, 469
  in chronic hemophilic arthropathy, 341–342
  patellofemoral disease and, magnetic resonance imaging, 183–187
Extensor mechanism injuries, 403–414
  classification, 404, 405
  historical perspective, 403–404
  patellofemoral dysplasia, 404–405
    chronic dislocation of patella, 406–407, 408
    chronic subluxation of patella, 406, 407
    lateral patellar compression syndrome, 405–406
    recurrent dislocation of patella, 406, 408
  pathomechanical basis, 407, 409, 410, 411
  radiologic evaluation, 409–413
    CT and MRI, 413
External fixation
  for failed knee replacement, 1346–1347
  pediatric, 282
Extremities, developmental horizons, 3–11

F

Fabella syndrome, 240
Fabellofibular ligaments, anatomy, 39–40
Factor replacement, in hemophilia, 334–335
Failure to progress, 951–952
Fairbanks apprehension sign, 393, 423, 424
Fascia anatomy
  lateral aspect, 39, 40
  medial aspect, 35, 36
Fat embolism syndrome, 1221
Fat pad syndrome, in patellofemoral pain differential diagnosis, 428
FDA approval process for prosthetic ligaments, 842–843
Feaney brace, 963
Fear, pediatric, 280, 285
Femoral axis, in patellofemoral joint biomechanics, 87, 88
Femoral condyles
  anatomy, 20
  arthroscopic visualization, 501–502, 510
  design principles in meniscal bearing arthroplasty, 1148, 1149
  embryology, 8–9, 11
  peripheral bone loss, bone grafting in revision total knee arthroplasty, 1342, 1343
  wear patterns, arthroscopic analysis, 497, 498
Femoral fractures
  distal *(see Distal femur, fractures)*
  periprosthetic, 1405–1408
    role of anterior femoral notching, 1409
    role of cement, 1409
    treatment, 1408–1409, 1410–1412
    treatment algorithm, 1409
  radiography, 125

Femoral metaphyseal displacement osteotomy, 1032–1033
Femoral nerve anatomy, 50–51
Femoral tunnel, in intraarticular ACL reconstruction
  conventional two-incision technique, 794–796
  single-incision endoscopic reconstruction, 798–799
Femorotibial joint, dislocation at, imaging, 146, 147
Femur
  bone loss, bone grafting for, 1338
  chondrification, 7, 8
  development, 7–9, 11
  distal (see Distal femur)
  knee replacement design
    biomechanics fixation, 1090–1092
    kinematics, 1080–1081
  surface motion between tibia and, 77, 78–79
  in total knee arthroplasty, 1244–1245
Fenamic acid, 326
Fenoprofen, 326
Fentanyl, in arthroscopic surgery, 301
Fibrosarcomas, frequency, 1421
Fibrous cortical defects, 1441, 1442 (see also Nonossifying fibromas)
  pediatric, 266
Fibrous dysplasia, 1423–1425
  roentgenographic evaluation, 140
Fibrous histiocytomas
  benign, 1424
  malignant, 1433
Fibula
  anatomy and development, 24
  proximal, bone tumors, types and percentages, 1421–1422
Fibular lesions, treatment, 1470–1471
Ficat technique, 412

Financial concerns of parents, 281
Fish oil, for osteoarthritis, 327
Fitness, hemophilia and, 333–334
Fixation (see External fixation; Internal fixation)
Fixation of knee replacements, retrieval analysis, 1257–1259
Flaps, for wound closure in failed knee replacement, 1288–1291
Flexibility
  in cartilage lesion rehabilitation, 923, 925
  of patellofemoral joint, testing, 445
Flexion
  cruciate ligaments and, 86–87
  patellofemoral joint and, 90
    biomechanics, 87–89
  sliding and rolling of femur on tibia with, 77, 78
  tibial motion and, 79
Flexion contractures
  ligament release, 1207–1209
  pediatric, 259–260, 261
Flexion-extension
  angle, in gait cycle, 99
  normal moment patterns in walking, 99, 100
Flexion reflex, 111–112
Flexion-rotation drawer test, 667–668
Fluorescein monitoring of wound healing, 1285–1286
Fluorosis, radiography, 141
Food and Drug Administration approval process for prosthetic ligaments, 842–843
Football, history of ligament reconstruction, 638–639
Forceps for arthroscopic meniscectomy
  cutting, 544
  grasping, 545

Fractures (see also specific anatomic locations)
  computed tomography, 151
  magnetic resonance imaging, 185, 189, 190
  osteochondral, 614–616
  pediatric, 242–248
  around prosthesis (see Periprosthetic fractures)
  radiography, 124, 125, 143–146
Freeman-Swanson prosthesis, 1063–1064
Free tissue transfer, for wound closure in failed knee replacement, 1291
Freeze-dried soft tissue allografts, 575
Fulkerson anteromedialization technique, 457, 458, 459–461
Fulkerson-Schutzer classification of patellofemoral pain, 425, 426
Functional activities, biomechanical analysis for rehabilitation, 922–924
Functional exercises, 949–950
Functional knee braces, 963–967
  for ACL-deficient knee, 730–731
  comparison, 963

G

Gait
  crutch walking after ligament reconstruction, 986–987, 988, 989
  definition, 95
  normal, 99
  osteotomy and, 1027
Gait analysis, 95–105
  in anterior knee pain, 422
  in arthritic knees, 103
  definitions, 95–98
  equilibrium between internal and external forces acting on bodies, 97–98

  high tibial osteotomy and, 103
  human locomotion, 98–99
    adaptation to sidestep cut in ACL-deficient knee, 102–103
    angular motion at knee joint, 99
    magnitude of moment during walking, 100
    maximum moment amplitudes and walking speed, 100
    normal gait, 99
    normal moment patterns during walking, 99–100
    running and sidestep cut, 101–102
  kinematics of motion, 95–97
  kinetics, 97
  after total knee replacement, 103–104
Galeazzi-Baker technique for patellofemoral realignment, 234, 235
Galeazzi tenodesis, 452, 454
Gallium 67 citrate scintigraphy, 197
Ganglion cysts, 1423
Gastrocnemius
  anatomy, 43, 46
  stretching, 430, 432
Gastrocnemius muscle flap, for wound closure in failed knee replacement, 1288–1290
Gastrocnemius-soleus, stretching, 925
Gate control theory of pain transmission, 368–369
Gaucher's disease, radiography, 138, 139
General anesthesia
  for knee arthroscopy, 301–302
  local vs., 301
Genesis prosthesis, modular system characteristics, 1300
Genetics, hemophilia, 332–333
Genicular arteries circulation, 31, 51–52

supplying blood to knee soft tissue, 1279–1280
Gentamicin, in total knee arthroplasty, 1269, 1270
  added to cement, 1271–1272
Genucom Knee Analysis System, 678, 688–689
Genu valgum, 217, 218, 262
Genu varum, 217–218, 262 (see also Blount disease)
Geometric prosthesis, 1059, 1060
Geometric total knee arthroplasty, 1119–1121
Giant cell tumors of bone (osteoclastomas), 1428–1430, 1449
  frequency, 1421, 1422
  treatment, 1455–1457, 1458–1459
Gliding motion between femur and tibia, 77, 78–79
Glucocorticoids, in wound healing, 1283
Glucose tolerance, chondrosarcomas and, 1450
Gold, for rheumatoid arthritis, 327
Golgi receptors, 108
Gore-Tex ligament, 752
  biomechanical testing results, 843
  concept, 843–844
  indications, 849–850
  new developments, 850
  results, 846–849
  technique, 844–846
Gore-Tex II ligament, 850, 851
Gout, 126–127
Gracilis tendon anatomy, 43
Gracilis tendon grafts
  in ACL reconstruction, 750–751
    semitendinosus grafts with, 823 (see also Semitendinosus tendon grafts)
  healing and, 947
  in PCL reconstruction
    clinical results, 916
    discussion, 916–917
    technique, 913–916

Grafts (see Allografts; Autogenous grafts; and specific types)
Grasping forceps, for arthroscopic mensicectomy, 545
Groves cruciate ligament reconstruction, 638
GUEPAR hinge, 1048, 1064
Guilt
  parental, 281
  pediatric, 280
Gunston polycentric prosthesis, 1055, 1057, 1058

H

Haemophilus influenzae, pediatric knee infections from, 267, 268
Hamstrings
  rehabilitation in ACL-deficient knee, 729–730
  stretching, 430, 431, 925, 926
  tightness assessment, 423–424, 425
Hauser procedure, 452–454
Headache, from spinal anesthesia, 309
Heat polishing, for polyethylene joint components, 1255
Heat treatment
  for patellofemoral pain, 429
  pediatric, 285
Heavy metal poisoning, roentgenographic evaluation, 139
Hemangiomas
  intramuscular, 1476–1477
  synovial, 1436–1437
Hemarthrosis (see also Hemophilia)
  acute, treatment, 338–339
  after ligament reconstruction, 993
  pediatric, 230–231
  subacute, treatment, 339–340
  synovium of, 622
  in total knee replacement, 1263

Hematologic considerations in total knee arthroplasty, 1211–1216
  intraoperative period, 1213
  postoperative period, 1213–1214
  preoperative period, 1211–1213
Hemodynamics, regional anesthesia and, 305–306
Hemoglobinopathies, roentgenographic evaluation, 139
Hemophilia (see also Hemarthrosis)
  arthropathy in pathogenesis, 336–338
  radiographic changes, 338, 339, 341–343
  biochemical basis of coagulation, 331–332
  classification, 629
  clinical course, 333–334
  diagnosis, 333, 335
  genetics, 332–333
  knee treatment
    acute hemarthrosis, 338–339
    chronic hemophilic arthropathy, 340–344
    subacute hemarthrosis, 339–340
  pediatric, 231
  radiography, 129
  synovectomy and, 629–630
  treatment, 334, 335
    complications of transfusion therapy, 336
    doses of factor for replacement, 334–335
    nonblood products, 335–336
Hemophilus influenzae, pediatric knee infections from, 267, 268
Hemorrhage, in hemophilia, 333, 336–337
Hendler procedure, 821
  surgical technique, 821–824, 825

wound closure and postoperative care, 824
Henning retractor, 564
Heparin, in thromboembolic disease, 1223, 1224
Hepatitis, transfusion-transmitted, 1212
Hepatitis B, hemophilia transfusion therapy and, 336
Hepatitis C, hemophilia transfusion therapy and, 336
Herbert prosthesis, 1048
Hereditary osteo-onychodysplasia (HOOD), radiography, 136
High tibial osteotomy
  abrasion arthroplasty and, for degenerative arthritis, 591–592
  gait analysis and, 103
  for osteonecrosis, 610–611
Hinge arthroplasties, 1046, 1146
  concept and history, 1306, 1307
  early failures, 1047–1048
  later experiences with conventional hinges, 1048–1049
  lessons from, 1046–1047
  rigid hinges, 1306, 1307, 1309
    results, 1319
  rotating hinges, 1306, 1307, 1309
    indications, 1309, 1310–1311
    results, 1319
  rotationally nonconstrained hinges, 1049, 1050–1051, 1052
Hip abductors, strengthening, 434
Hip adductors, strengthening, 433–434
Histiocytomas, fibrous
  benign, 1424
  malignant, 1433
Histology of allografts, 869–870
HIV (see Human immunodeficiency virus infection)

Hodgkin's lymphoma, 1434–1435
Hoffa's disease/syndrome, 399, 1437
Hoppenfeld medial approach, 60
Hospital for Special Surgery, total knee arthroplasty, 1064
  duocondylar prosthesis, 1064
  duopatellar prosthesis, 1064–1065
  history, 1179–1180
  Insall-Burstein Posterior Stabilized prosthesis results, 1187–1191
  posterior-stabilized prosthesis, 1065
  stabilocondylar prosthesis, 1065
  Total Condylar prosthesis, 1065
  unicondylar replacement, 1057, 1059
Housemaid's knee, 399
Ho:YAG lasers, in arthroscopy, 522
Human immunodeficiency virus infection, 347–363
  arthritis related to, radiography, 131–132
  clinical syndromes
    acute retroviral syndrome, 350
    asymptomatic infection, 350–351
    pediatrics, 351–352
    symptomatic infection, 351
  diagnosis, 352–353
  epidemiology, 348–349
  hemophilia transfusion therapy and, 336
  musculoskeletal disease and, complications, 356–357
  prophylaxis and treatment of pathogens, 356
  total knee replacement and, 342
  transfusions and, 1212
  transmission, 353
    in allotransplantation, 574–575, 746–747, 748
    parenteral, 354–355
    perinatal, 353–354
    sexual, 353
    surgery issues, 355
  treatment, 355–356

virology, 349
Humphry's ligament, 34
Hyaline cartilage anatomy, 32–33
Hyaline cartilage injury, healing, 946
Hydromorphone, 992
Hydroxyapatite-coated implants, 1106, 1107
Hydroxychloroquine
  for osteoarthritis, 327
  for rheumatoid arthritis, 328
Hydroxypyridinoline cross-linking, 523
Hyperextension, congenital, 258
Hypermobility syndrome, pediatric, 258
Hyperostoses, roentgenographic evaluation, 140–141
Hyperparathyroidism, roentgenographic evaluation, 138
Hyperphosphatasia, radiography, 141
Hypophosphatasia, 138

I

Ibuprofen, 326
  for children, 286
Ifosfamide, for bone tumors, 1461
Iliotibial band
  in ACL reconstruction, 751, 797, 803–806, 808
  history, 640
  anatomy, 39, 43, 418, 419, 713–714, 773–774
  magnetic resonance imaging, 41, 43
  in knee stability, 85
  stretching, 429, 430, 925
  transection in lateral valgus release, 1207
Iliotibial (friction) band syndrome, 39, 399, 428
Iliotibial myofascial transfer, 773–790
  anatomy, 773–774
  contraindications, 775
  history, 773
  postoperative care, 782–783, 786, 790
  results, 789–790
  surgical modification, 786

surgical technique, 775–789
theoretical considerations, 774–775
Imagery, for children, 285
Imaging (see Roentgenographic evaluation and other modalities)
Immediate exchange of prosthesis, in infected total knee arthroplasty, 1273
Immobilization
  effects on musculoskeletal tissue, 945–946
  pediatric, 281–283, 293
  as rehabilitation phase, 948
Immunogenicity of allografts, 879
Immunology of meniscal allotransplantation, 576
Implants (see Prostheses)
Incisional massage, after ligament reconstruction, 994–995
Incisions (see Surgical approaches)
Independence, pediatric, 288–289
Indium 111-labeled leukocyte scintigraphy, 197–198
  case reports, 203–204
Indium 111-labeled polyclonal antibodies, 199
Indomethacin, 325
  for children, 286
  in postoperative pain management, 310
Inertia, definition, 97
Infants
  developmental considerations, 277–278
  pain in, 284
  teaching, 291
Infected total knee arthroplasty, 1172, 1261–1278
  definition, 1261–1262
  diagnosis
    causative organisms, 1267–1269
    clinical findings, 1266
    laboratory findings, 1266–1267

factors associated with, 1262
  choice of prosthesis, 1262–1263
  wound problems, 1263–1264
prevention
  controlled surgical environment, 1265
  long-term, 1265–1266
  perioperative antibiotics, 1264–1265
  postoperative management, 1265
  preoperative planning, 1264
treatment and results
  amputation, 1276
  antibiotic-loaded cement, 1271–1272
  antibiotic therapy, 1269
  arthrodesis, 1274–1275
  aspiration and antibiotics, 1272
  delayed exchange, 1273–1274
  early exchange, 1273
  immediate exchange, 1273
  long-term suppression with antibiotics, 1270–1271
  open debridement, 1272–1273
  resection arthroplasty, 1275
  specific regimens, 1269–1270
  surgical options, 1272
Infection
  bone, radionuclide imaging, 197–199
  computed tomography, 148
  with Kennedy ligament augmentation device, 831
  after osteotomy, 1036
  after patellar fracture, 1401
  pediatric knee, 267–268
  from regional anesthesia, 310
  roentgenographic evaluation, 130–133
Infectious complications, orthopedic, of HIV infection, 356–357
Inflammation, in cartilage lesion rehabilitation, 924–925

Inflammatory musculoskeletal complications of HIV infection, 356–357
Infrapatellar bursitis, magnetic resonance imaging, 184, 187
Infrapatellar contracture syndrome, rehabilitation and, 952
Infrapatellar plicae, arthroscopic anatomy, 499–500
Inhibitors, hemophilia transfusion therapy and, 336
Innervation of knee joint, 47–51, 109–110
　lateral aspect, 49
　ligaments, 108
　medial aspect, 48
　popliteal space, 50
Insall anterior approach to knee, 57
Insall-Burstein Posterior Stabilized prosthesis, 1314
　clinical results
　　Hospital for Special Surgery, 1187–1191
　　other institutions, 1191–1192
　design modifications, 1181
　dislocations with, 1195–1196
　patellofemoral complications, 1188, 1191
Insall-Burstein II Posterior Stabilized prosthesis
　design concept, 1181–1182
　dislocations with, 1195–1196
　modular system characteristics, 1300
Instability (see Stability)
Instantaneous center of motion, 75–78
Integraft stent, 840–841
Intercondylar distal femoral fractures (see Supracondylar and intercondylar distal femoral fractures)
Intercondylar notch, arthroscopic anatomy, 502
Intermittent compression boots, in thromboembolic disease, 1223

Internal-external rotation, normal moment patterns in walking, 99–100
Internal fixation
　for failed knee replacement, 1347–1348
　for periprosthetic distal femoral fractures, 1408–1409
　proximal tibial osteotomy and, 1036
Interpositional arthroplasties, 1051, 1053
Intraarticular ACL reconstruction (see Anterior cruciate ligament reconstruction, intraarticular)
Intraarticular fractures, osteotomy and, 1036
Intraarticular loose bodies, CT/arthrography, 152, 153
Intramedullary fixation
　for distal femoral fractures, 1361–1362, 1363
　for failed knee replacement, 1348, 1349
Intramuscular nerves, 109
Intravenous regional sympathetic blockade, in reflex sympathetic dystrophy, 373
Involved-uninvolved differences, definition, 674
Iodine 131-labeled fibrinogen scan, in deep venous thrombosis, 1220
Ischemia, perioperative, 312
Isokinetic exercise, 421, 950
　in cartilage lesion rehabilitation, 930–931
Isometric exercise, 420–421, 949
Isotonic exercise, 421, 949

J

James (ACL) procedure, 805, 808
Jaroschy technique, 412

Jerk test, 669
Joint debridement before osteotomy, 1029
J sign, 410
Jumper's knee, 399
Juvenile osteochondritis, 598, 600–601
Juvenile rheumatoid arthritis
　diagnosis, 268–269
　prognosis, 269
　radiography, 128, 129
　synovectomy, 625
　treatment, 269
Juxtacortical chondromas, 1428
Juxtacortical osteogenic sarcomas, 1431

K

Kennedy ligament augmentation device (LAD), 749, 752
　ACL reconstruction with, 829–837
　　clinical results, 831–832
　　procedure, 832–836
　biomechanics, 829–830
　　load-sharing concept, 830–831
　infection and synovitis, 831
Ketoprofen, 326
Ketorolac, in postoperative pain management, 310–311
Kinematic conflict, total knee replacement and, 1059, 1062–1064
Kinematic (Howmedica) total knee, 1126–1129
Kinematic prosthesis, 1069
Kinematic rotating hinge, 1049, 1052
Kinematics, 95–97
　cruciate ligaments, 1146
　knee replacement designs, 1080–1087
　muscles, 1146
　patellofemoral, 384, 385, 1147
　sagittal, 1146–1147
Kinematic Stabilizer prosthesis, 1193–1194
　dislocations with, 1195
Kinemax prosthesis, modular system characteristics, 1300
Kinetics, 97

Kirschner wires, in knee dislocation management, 1005, 1006
Kissing osteophytes, 1100
Klippel-Trenaunay-Weber syndrome, radiography, 135–136
Knee joint development, 9
Knee laxity (see Laxity)
Knee motion (see also Gait analysis)
　ligaments and, 83–85
　limitation after ligament reconstruction, 993
　musculature in, 113–118
　after patellar fracture, 1401–1402
　regulation, 113
　six degrees of freedom, 17, 20
　surface
　　axial rotation, 79
　　instantaneous center of motion, 75–78
　　rolling, sliding, and crossed four-bar linkage, 78–79
Knee replacement (see Total knee replacement)
Knives, for arthroscopic mensicectomy, 544
Knock-knee, 217, 218, 262
Kocher anterolateral approach to knee, 57, 58–59
KT-1000 arthrometer
　application to surgical results, 690–695
　comparison examination of patients awake and under anesthesia, 686–690
　components, 674
　definition, 673
　description and positioning, 677
　illustration, 674
　in vitro testing, 679–680
　normal and ACL-deficient knees, 680–686
　in PCL insufficiency, 695–697
　technical pitfalls, 677–678
　testing reproducibility and device comparison, 678–679

KTP lasers, in arthroscopy, 522
K-wires, in knee dislocation management, 1005, 1006

L

Labelle technique, 412
Lachman test, 667, 723
　for lateral capsuloligamentous complex injuries, 716
　for medial capsuloligamentous complex injuries, 707
　passive 15-lb, definition, 673
　passive 20-lb, definition, 673
　passive 30-lb, definition, 673
　posterior, 670
Lactate dehydrogenase, in bone tumors, 1450
LAD (see Kennedy ligament augmentation device)
Langenskiöld classification for Blount disease, 219
Langerhans giant cell, 1426
Lasers
　in arthroscopy (see Arthroscopic laser surgery)
　components, 516
　for debridement of cartilage lesions, 613
　modes, 516, 517
　principles, 515–517
Laskin unicondylar and unicompartmental replacement experience, 1057
Lateral approaches to knee, 59–60
Lateral articular nerve, 51, 109
Lateral aspect of knee, anatomy, 39–42, 1200, 1203–1204
　innervation, 49
Lateral capsuloligamentous complex injuries, 712
　anatomy, 712–714
　biomechanical factors, 714–715

clinical approach, 715–716
distribution of disruptions, 660
management, 716–720
pediatric, 258
Lateral collateral ligament
　anatomy, 40, 41, 43, 181
　elevation in lateral valgus release, 1208
　in knee stability, 85
　laxity, 661, 662
　magnetic resonance imaging, 41, 179, 181–183
　physical examination, 664, 665
　in proximal tibiofibular joint dislocation, 1011–1012
Lateral genicular artery, supplying blood to knee soft tissue, 1279–1280
Lateral instability, surgical repair, 719–720
Lateral meniscus
　anatomy, 33–35
　arthrogram, 152
　arthroscopic visualization, 35, 509, 511, 513
　discoid, arthroscopic analysis, 505
　posterolateral incision for arthroscopic repair, 70–71
Lateral patellar compression syndrome, 405–406
　pediatric, 233
　conservative treatment, 233–234
　surgical correction, 234–235
Lateral retinaculum, stretching, 925, 926
Lateral thrust, osteotomy and, 1027
Lateral tibial plateau, avulsion fracture, 713, 717
Lateral tibiofemoral osteoarthritis with valgus deformity, osteotomy for, 1032–1033
Laurin patellar tilt angle, 424, 446
Lavage, arthroscopic, for degenerative arthritis, 594

Laxity
　effect of exercise on, 697
　generalized ligamentous, 697–698
　knee replacement design kinematics, 1080
Laxity testing devices, 673–700 (see also KT-1000 arthrometer)
　definitions and terminology, 673–675
　for knee braces, 697
　normal and ACL-deficient knees, 680–686
　testing reproducibility and device comparison, 678–679
LCS total knee system (see New Jersey Low-Contact-Stress total knee system)
Leeds-Keio ligament, 752
　biomechanical testing results, 843
　concept, 854–855
　results, 857–858
　technique, 855–857
Lenox Hill brace, 730, 731, 963, 964
　studies, 965
Letterer-Siwe disease, 1427
Levine brace, 435
Levo-Dromoran, 992
Levorphanol, 992
Lidocaine, 308
　in arthroscopic surgery, 302, 303
Ligament augmentation device (see Kennedy ligament augmentation device)
Ligament healing, 947–948
　physiology, 649
　biologic replacement grafts, 651–653
　phase I: inflammation, 649
　phase II: matrix and cellular proliferation, 649–650
　phase III: remodeling, 650
　phase IV: maturation, 650–651
Ligament injuries
　diagnosis and classification, 657–672

history of surgical treatment, 637–644
　continuing debate, 640–641
　development of current treatment rationale, 641
　football and knee trauma, 638–639
　Hey Groves and reconstruction, 638
　past decade, 641–642
　rotatory instability, 639–640
mechanisms, 647–649, 657–659
medical history, 657
nursing care (see Nursing care of ligament injuries)
observation, 659–663
pediatric (see Pediatric knee, ligament injuries)
physical examination
　anterior cruciate ligament, 667–669
　capsular tears, 666–667
　collateral ligaments, 664, 665
　palpation, 663–665
　posterior, 670–671
postoperative rehabilitation, 653–654
Ligamentomuscular protective reflex, 110–111
Ligament releases in arthritic knee, 1199–1210
　anatomy, 1199–1205
　balancing
　　flexion contracture, 1207–1209
　　valgus deformity, 1206–1207, 1208
　　varus deformity, 1205–1206
Ligament-spindle reflex, 112
Ligaments (see also specific ligaments)
　anatomy, 26–32
　development, 9, 10, 11, 12
　hypermobility, signs, 230
　innervation, 108
　insertion into bone, 26, 27
　knee replacement design biomechanics, 1079–1081

in knee stability, 82–87, 107 (*see also* Reflexes active about knee)
material properties, 646–647
morphology, 645–646
transplants
allografts (*see* Allografts in ligament surgery)
autografts, 652–653
Ligastic ligament
biomechanical testing results, 843
concept, 858–859
results, 860–861
technique, 859–860
Lighting systems for arthroscopy, 488, 489, 490
Limbs, developmental horizons, 3–11
Lipidoses, roentgenographic evaluation, 138–139
Lipomas, treatment, 1474, 1475
Lipomatosis, synovial, 1437
Lipscomb and Anderson's ACL reconstruction technique, 255, 257
Livingston's vicious cycle, 368
Loading
in running and sidestep cut, 101–102
stability and, 82, 83
Load-sharing, with Kennedy LAD, 830–831
Local anesthesia, 306–308
general anesthesia vs., 301
for knee arthroscopy, 302
nerve fiber types and, 309
postoperative, 302–303
sites of action, 307
toxicity, 308–309
Locomotion (*see* Gait analysis)
Losee (ACL) procedure, 803, 805
Losee test, 669–670
Low-Contact-Stress (LCS) total knee system (*see* New Jersey Low-Contact-Stress total knee system)
Low-contact stress prosthesis, 1136–1137, 1138

Lumbar sympathetic blockade, in reflex sympathetic dystrophy, 372–373
Lupus erythematosus, systemic, radiography, 129
Lyme arthritis
pediatric, 268
radiography, 132–133
synovectomy, 631
Lymphomas of bone, 1434–1435, 1445, 1447

M

MacAusland hinge, 1047–1048
MacIntosh (ACL) procedure, 803, 804–805
MacIntosh arthroplasty, 1051, 1053
Macrodystrophia lipomatosa, radiography, 136
Magnetic resonance imaging, 159–193
bone tumors, 1450–1451
collateral ligaments
lateral, 179, 181–183
medial, 179, 180
cruciate ligaments
anterior, 172, 174–177
posterior, 177–178
extensor mechanism injuries, 413
hemophilic arthropathy, 338
meniscal lesions
diagnosis, 540
horizontal cleavage-based tears, 537
menisci, 161, 163–172, 173
lateral, 34, 35
normal anatomy, 29, 30, 34, 35, 37, 41, 43, 161–163
osseocartilaginous structures, 187–193
osteochondritis dissecans, 598, 599
osteonecrosis, 609
patellofemoral pain, 425
physics, 159–160
posterior cruciate ligament injuries, 739, 740, 741

quadriceps tendon rupture, 470
technique, 160–161
tibial plateau fractures, 1376–1377
Malacia, definition, 393
Mammals, evolution of knee, 3, 4, 5
Manual resistance exercise, in cartilage lesion rehabilitation, 929
Maquet dome osteotomy, 1030
Maquet technique for anterior and medial displacement of tibial tuberosity, 456
Marfan syndrome, radiography, 134
Marmor modular knee, 1057
Marrow hyperplasia, magnetic resonance imaging, 191–192
Marshall-MacIntosh graft, LAD-augmented, 831–832
Maximum manual test, 675
definition, 673–674
Mayo Clinic, PCL-substitution arthroplasty, 1193–1194
McConnell taping, 929, 930
McDavid lateral hinge prophylactic brace, 958, 961
McKeever implant, 1051, 1053
MDP (methylene disphosphonate) scans, 196
case reports, 200–201
Mechanoreceptors, 107–109
Medial approaches to knee, 60–61, 62
Medial articular nerve, 109
Medial aspect of knee, anatomy, 35–39, 1200, 1201–1202
innervation, 48
Medial capsuloligamentous complex injuries
anatomy, 703–704, 705
associated injuries, 709–712
biomechanical factors and histologic studies, 704–706

clinical approach, 706–707
distribution of disruptions, 658
nonoperative management, 708–709
operative management, 709, 710, 711
pediatric, 257–258
physical examination, 707–708
prophylactic knee bracing, 958–962
Medial collateral ligament
anatomy, 37–39, 179, 703–704
arthrogram, 152
flexion and extension, 39
in knee stability, 84–85
laxity, 661, 662
magnetic resonance imaging, 37–39, 170, 179, 180
physical examination, 664, 665
stability in total knee arthroplasty, 1245
Medial genicular artery, supplying blood to knee soft tissue, 1279–1280
Medial meniscus
anatomy, 33–35
cross section, 33
magnetic resonance imaging, 34
peripheral blood supply, 35
arthroscopic visualization, 34, 510–513
posteromedial incision for arthroscopic repair, 69–70
Medial patellofemoral ligament anatomy, 418
Medial patellotibial ligament anatomy, 418
Medial tibiofemoral osteoarthritis with varus deformity, osteotomy for, 1029–1030
Medications, in pediatric pain management, 286–287, 294
Melorheostosis, radiography, 141
Membrane interpositional arthroplasty, 1046

Meniscal
	allotransplantation, 573–581
		biology, 574
		graft selection, 575–576
		immunologic response, 576
		meniscus procurement, sterilization, and storage, 574–575
		surgical techniques, 576
	clinical experience (failed allograft), 576–580
	evolution, 573–574
	future directions, 578
	rationale, 574
Meniscal bearing knee replacement, 1136–1137, 1138, 1157–1177
	articular surface design in artificial knee
		congruent joint surfaces, 1144
		femoral condyle, 1148
		incongruent joint surfaces, 1144–1145
		justification for unconforming designs, 1144–1146
		kinematics and mechanics of knee, 1146–1148
		meniscal bearing, 1149
		Oxford Knee, 1149–1155
		tibial plateau, 1148–1149
	articular surface design in human knee, 1143–1144
	clinical application of mobile meniscal bearings
		bicompartmental knee replacement, 1169
		cruciate-sacrificing rotating platform, 1170–1171
		isolated patellofemoral replacement, 1171–1172
		tricompartmental knee replacement, 1169–1170
		unicompartmental knee replacement, 1168–1169
	congruent, 1143–1156
	contact stress analysis of mobile and fixed bearings, 1163–1164, 1165
	design principles of meniscal bearing, 1148–1149
	failure modes of rotating bearing patella replacements, 1164
	fixation of mobile meniscal bearings, 1164, 1167–1168
	future directions, 1173–1175
	history and development of mobile bearings, 1157
	Oxford knee (see Oxford meniscal bearing prosthesis)
	retrieval and simulator specimens, 1158, 1166
	revision total knee replacement, 1172–1173
	surface geometry, 1158–1163
	survivorship analysis of cemented and cementless replacements, 1173, 1174
	wear properties of mobile and fixed bearings, 1164
Meniscal cysts
	arthrography, 149
	magnetic resonance imaging, 172
Meniscal tears
	in ACL-deficient knee, 724
	arthroscopic repair (see Arthroscopic meniscal repair)
	classification, 560
	open repair, 567
	patterns and pathogenesis, 528, 530
		complex degenerative tear, 538
		horizontal tear, 530, 532–537
		vertical longitudinal tear, 530, 531–532
		vertical transverse tear, 538, 539
	pediatric, 250
Meniscectomy
	arthroscopic (see Arthroscopic meniscectomy)
	degenerative changes after, 34
	effect on knee stability, 81, 82
	historical perspective, 559
Menisci
	anatomy, 33–35, 527–528, 529
	arthroscopic, 503–505
	arthrography, 149, 152
	arthroscopy (see Arthroscopic meniscal repair; Arthroscopic meniscectomy)
	development, 10, 11, 249–250
	discoid, 215–216
		lateral, arthroscopic analysis, 505
		pediatric, 250–251
		torn, arthroscopic meniscectomy for, 553–554
	function, 34–35
	healing, 947
	joint surface contact area and, 80–81
	in knee stability, 81–82
	lateral (see Lateral meniscus)
	load bearing and, 80–81
	magnetic resonance imaging, 161, 163–172, 173
	medial (see Medial meniscus)
	optical tissue properties, 522–523
	rehabilitation after repair, 939
Meniscofemoral ligaments, 34
	in discoid meniscus, 216
	pseudotear, magnetic resonance imaging, 171
Meperidine, 992
	for pediatric pain, 286
Mepivacaine, in arthroscopic surgery, 303
Merchant technique/view, 412, 424
Mesenchymal chondrosarcomas, 1432–1433
Mesoderm development, 7
Metal-backed knee replacements, retrieval analysis, 1256–1257
Metallic interpositional arthroplasties, 1051, 1053
Metastatic tumors, 1435–1436
	treatment, 1471–1472, 1473–1474
Methadone, 992
Methotrexate
	for bone tumors, 1461
	for rheumatoid arthritis, 328
Methylene disphosphonate scans, 196
	case reports, 200–201
Methylprednisolone, for rheumatoid arthritis, 328
Metronidazole, in total knee arthroplasty, 1269
Micheli's ACL reconstruction technique, 254, 256
Microfractures (stress fractures)
	magnetic resonance imaging, 189
	patellar
		in patellofemoral pain differential diagnosis, 428
		pediatric, 240–241
	radiography, 145, 146
Miller-Galante prosthesis, 1114, 1132–1133, 1135
Miller-Galante II prosthesis, 1114, 1115
	modular system characteristics, 1300
MKS II brace, 966
Mobility, in total knee arthroplasty, 1233–1234
Mold arthroplasty, 1053
Moment of force, definition, 97
Morphine, 992
	for pediatric pain, 286
	in postoperative pain management, 311–312
Morphology, developmental chronology, 5
Motion about knee (see Knee motion)

Movement testing, for patellofemoral rehabilitation, 923–924
MRI (see Magnetic resonance imaging)
Mueller classification of tibial plateau fractures, 1372–1374
Multicentric reticulohistiocytosis, radiography, 138
Multiple myeloma, 1435
Muscle nerves, 109
Muscle receptors, innervation, 109
Muscles
 anterior, anatomy, 45, 46
 atrophy in ACL-deficient knee, 728
 electrical stimulation after ligament reconstruction, 986, 987
 inhibition from edema in cartilage lesions, 925
 kinematics and biomechanics, 1146
 posterior, anatomy, 42–46
 slow vs. fast twitch fibers, 420
 strengthening (see Strengthening)
Muscle spindle, 108, 112
Muscular coactivation, 113–118
Muscular control of knee stability and motion, 107, 113–118 (see also Reflexes active about knee)
Muscular strength, biomechanical assessment for patellofemoral rehabilitation, 923
Musculoskeletal disease, HIV infection and, 356–357
Musculoskeletal tissue disuse and immobilization, 945–946
 healing, 946–947
Myeloma, multiple, 1435
Myocardial infarction, perioperative reinfarction, 304

N

Nafcillin, in total knee arthroplasty, 1269
Nail-patella syndrome, 214
 radiography, 136
Nalbuphine, 992
Naloxone, 311
 in pediatric pain management, 286
Naproxen, 326
 in postoperative pain management, 310
Narcotics
 for pediatric pain, 286–287
 in postoperative pain management, 311
 dosage and contraindications, 992
Nd:YAG lasers, in arthroscopy, 517–521
Neer classification of supracondylar femur fractures, 1406
 modified, 1408
Negative predictive accuracy of laxity testing, definition, 675
Neoplasms about knee (see also Tumors), pediatric, 264–267
Neoplastic complications of HIV infection, 357–358
Nerve anatomy, 47–51, 109–110
 lateral aspect, 49
 ligament innervation, 108
 medial aspect, 48
 popliteal space, 50
Neural reflex arcs, 107–113
Neurologic complications
 after reduction of proximal tibiofibular joint dislocation, 1014
 of regional anesthesia, 310
Neuromuscular disease, roentgenographic evaluation, 133–134
Neuromuscular electrical stimulation, in cartilage lesion rehabilitation, 928–929
Neuromuscular stimulators, 945–946

Neurons, wide dynamic range, in reflex sympathetic dystrophy, 369
Neuropathic joint disease, roentgenographic evaluation, 132, 133
Neurovascular assessment of lower extremity, after ligament reconstruction, 984
New Jersey Low-Contact-Stress (LCS) total knee system, 1157
 components, 1159
 development, 1168–1169
 fixation elements, 1167
 rotating platform, 1170, 1172
 tibial component, 1162
 surface geometry, 1158–1159, 1160
 survivorship, 1173
Newtonian (inertial) frame of reference, 96
Nicotinic acid, wound healing and, 1283–1284
Noiles hinge, 1049, 1051
Non-Hodgkin's lymphomas, 1435
Nonossifying fibromas, 1423 (see also Fibrous cortical defects)
 frequency, 1421–1422
 pediatric, 266
Nonsteroidal anti-inflammatory drugs (NSAIDs)
 classification, 325
 effect of food or antacids, 326–327
 for patellofemoral pain, 429
 for pediatric pain, 286, 294
 in postoperative pain management, 310–311
 for reflex sympathetic dystrophy, 373
 for rheumatologic disorders, 321, 322
 clinical evaluation, 322–327
 side effects and toxicity, 324
 total knee arthroplasty and, 1211
 in wound healing, 1282–1283

Notchplasty, in intraarticular ACL reconstruction
 conventional two-incision technique, 794
 single-incision endoscopic reconstruction, 797
Noyes flexion rotation drawer test, 707
Noyes-Stabler classification of articular cartilage lesions, 612
NSAIDs (see Nonsteroidal anti-inflammatory drugs)
Nubain, 992
Nuclear scans, 195–205
 bone infection, 197–199
 case reports, 199–205
 image production, 195–196
 knee, 199
 principles, 195–197
 radiopharmaceuticals, 195
Numorphan, 992
Nursing care for total knee arthroplasty, 1229–1238
 postoperative care
 clinical monitoring, 1236–1237
 continuous passive motion, 1235
 discharge planning, 1237–1238
 occupational therapy, 1237
 pain management, 1235–1236
 preoperative program, 1229–1231
 mobility, 1233–1234
 pain management, 1231–1233
 patient education, 1231
 preparation for surgery, 1234–1235
Nursing care of ligament injuries, 983–996
 postoperative
 continuous passive motion, 985–986
 crutch walking, 986–987, 988, 989
 electrical muscle stimulation, 986
 leg bracing, 984–985
 neurovascular assessment of lower extremity, 984
 pain assessment, 987–990

Nursing care of ligament injuries *(cont.)*
  patient-controlled analgesia, 990, 991, 992
  psychosocial aspects, 990–991
  wound drainage, 984, 985
  postoperative complications, 991, 993
    hemarthrosis, 993
    incisional binding, 994–995
    motion limitation, 993
    patellar immobilization, 993–994
    sepsis, 993
    thrombophlebitis, 993
  preparation for discharge, 995
  treatment decisions, 983
Nursing care of pediatric patient, 277–295
Nutrition, pediatric, 287, 294

O

Ober test, modified, 424
Obesity
  morbid, total knee replacement and, 304–305
  pediatric, 287
Oblique anteromedial incision, 60, 61
Oblique popliteal ligament, semimembranosus muscle and, 45
Obturator nerve anatomy, 49
Occupational therapy for total knee arthroplasty, 1237
Ochronosis, 127
Omnifit prosthesis, modular system characteristics, 1300
OMNI Scientific lateral hinge prophylactic brace, 958
Omni-TS7 brace, 963, 964
Onychoosteodysplasia, hereditary, 214
Open reduction and internal fixation
  distal femoral fractures, 1360–1364, 1365
  periprosthetic, 1407–1408, 1411–1412

patellar fractures, 1397, 1399
tibial plateau fractures, 1381–1386
Opiates, sites of action, 307
Opioids
  for arthroscopy anesthesia, 301
  for pediatric pain, 286
  for reflex sympathetic dystrophy, 373–374
Opium tincture, 992
Ortholoc I total knee replacement, 1088
Ortholoc II total knee replacement, 1089
Orthopedic Specialty Hospital, rehabilitation protocols, forms, 971–981
Orthotics, patellar, 435
Osgood-Schlatter disease, 399, 403
  in patellofemoral pain differential diagnosis, 426
  pediatric, 238–239
  radiography, 143, 144
Osseocartilaginous structures, magnetic resonance imaging, 187–193
Osteitis deformans (Paget disease), 436
  juvenile, 141
  radiography, 139–140
Osteoarthritis, 127
  arthroscopy *(see* Arthroscopic treatment of degenerative arthritis*)*
  aspirin and other salicylates for, 323
  contractures in, 1199
  diagnosis, 315–316
  experimental treatment, 322, 327
  knee pain in, 1018
  osteotomy *(see* Osteotomy for arthritic knee*)*
  of patellofemoral joint, 397
  posterior cruciate ligament in, 1072
  radiography, 127
  unicompartmental knee replacement in, 1098, 1099–1100, 1102
    Oxford knee, 1152–1154

Osteoblastomas, 1428
Osteoblasts, in bone formation, 17–18
Osteochondral fractures, 614–616
Osteochondritis dissecans
  epidemiology, 598
  etiology, 597–598
  magnetic resonance imaging, 184, 186, 189–190
  management of adult lesions, 601–606, 607
  management of juvenile form, 598, 600–601
  of patella, 397, 427
  pediatric, 248–249
  presentation, 598
  radiology, 142, 598, 599
  rehabilitation, 937–939
  treatment algorithm, 608
Osteochondromas, 1425–1426
  biopsy technique, 1451–1452
  of distal femur, 1441, 1442
  frequency, 1421, 1422
  pediatric, 266
  radiography, 136
Osteochondromatosis, synovial, 1437
Osteoclastomas *(see* Giant cell tumors of bone*)*
Osteoclasts, 19–20
Osteogenesis imperfecta, radiography, 134–135
Osteogenic sarcomas *(see* Osteosarcomas*)*
Osteoid osteomas, 1426, 1427
  biopsy technique, 1452
  pediatric, 266
Osteomalacia, roentgenographic evaluation, 137, 138
Osteomyelitis
  in AIDS patients, 356–357
  in children and adolescents, 268
  in neonates, 268
  radiography, 130–131
Osteonecrosis, 606–608
  magnetic resonance imaging, 190–191, 609
  pathology, 609–610
  roentgenographic evaluation, 141–143, 608–609
  treatment, 610–611

Osteopenia, with cemented total knee replacements, 1091
Osteopetrosis, radiography, 141
Osteoporosis, radiography, 133
Osteosarcomas, 1430–1431, 1444–1445, 1446
  Enneking stage II, 1455
  frequency, 1421, 1422
  magnetic resonance imaging, 192
  pediatric, 266–267
  treatment, 1457, 1461, 1464–1465, 1472
    adjuvant chemotherapy, 1461
Osteotomy
  for Blount disease, 221–223
  Fulkerson anteromedialization technique, 457, 458, 459–461
  high tibial, 103, 591–592, 610–611
  patellar, 462
  tibial tubercle, anterior approaches to knee with, 66–67
Osteotomy for arthritic knee, 1019–1043
  choice of osteotomy
    distal femoral varus osteotomy, 1033–1034, 1035
    lateral tibiofemoral osteoarthritis with valgus deformity, 1032–1033
    medial tibiofemoral osteoarthritis with varus deformity, 1029–1030
    proximal tibial valgus osteotomy, 1030–1032
  complications
    infection, 1036
    internal fixation, 1036
    intraarticular fracture, 1036
    nonunion, 1036
    peroneal palsy, 1035
    thromboembolic disease, 1034–1035
    undercorrection, 1034
    vascular injury, 1036
  patient selection, 1021
    activity level, 1024, 1026
    age, 1021

angular deformity,
1020–1021, 1024,
1026, 1028
bone loss, 1026
cosmesis, 1027
lateral thrust, 1027
patellofemoral pain,
1027
personality, 1021
range of motion, 1024
rheumatoid arthritis,
1026
stability, 1026
tibiofemoral
subluxation, 1027
weight, 1026
pre- and postoperative
radiographs,
1022–1025
preoperative evaluation
arthroscopy and joint
debridement, 1029
patient education,
1029
physical examination,
1027–1028
physical therapy,
1028–1029
radiographic
examination, 1028
surgical planning,
1029
rationale, 1019–1020
results
distal femoral varus
osteotomy, 1037
proximal tibial valgus
osteotomy,
1036–1037
proximal tibial varus
osteotomy, 1037
rheumatoid arthritis,
1026
total knee arthroplasty
after, 1037–1041
failed osteotomy, 1041
radiographs,
1038–1040
OTI Performer brace, 963
Outerbridge classification
of chondromalacia,
611–612
Overuse injuries, pediatric
(see Pediatric knee,
overuse injuries)
Oxacillin, in total knee
arthroplasty, 1269
Oxford meniscal bearing
prosthesis, 1136,
1168, 1170
clinical experience, 1152
components, 1149, 1151
design concept,
1149–1150, 1158

function of meniscal
bearings,
1154–1155
illustration, 1137
unicompartmental
arthroplasty for
osteoarthritis,
1152–1154
in vitro studies,
1150–1152
Oxidative degradation of
polyethylene joint
components, 1255
Oxymorphone, 992

P

Pacinian corpuscles, 108
Paddu ACL reconstruction,
816, 817
Paget disease, 1436
juvenile
(hyperphosphatasia),
141
roentgenographic
evaluation, 139–140
Pain
patellofemoral (see
Patellofemoral pain)
pediatric
functional knee pain,
269
misconceptions, 284
in reflex sympathetic
dystrophy
management,
372–374
mechanisms, 368–371
in total knee arthroplasty,
1298
Pain intensity assessment
scales, 1231–1232
Pain management (see
also Analgesia;
Anesthesia)
assessment after
ligament
reconstruction,
987–990
pediatric, 283–287
assessment, 283–285
interventions,
285–287
postoperative, 310
nonsteroidal
anti-inflammatory
drugs, 310–311
opioid analgesia,
311–312
reflex sympathetic
dystrophy, 368–371
total knee arthroplasty
postoperative care,
1235–1236

preoperative
assessment,
1231–1233
treatment modalities,
429
Pantapon, 992
Parathyroid hormone, in
bone tumors, 1450
Parents
effect of pediatric
disorders on,
280–281
presence needed by
children, 286
Parosteal osteogenic
sarcomas, 1431
Passive patellar tilt test,
393, 423, 444, 445
Passive physiologic
movement testing,
for patellofemoral
rehabilitation, 924
Patella
anatomy, 381–382,
416–420
arthroscopic, 500–501
magnetic resonance
imaging, 34
normal, 22–24
anomalies, 399
arthroscopic
visualization, 510
bipartite, 215, 399
anteroposterior
radiograph, 124
in patellofemoral pain
differential
diagnosis, 427–428
pediatric, 241
blood supply, 23–24
bone tumors, types and
percentages, 1422
chondrification, 9, 11
chondromalacia (see
Chondromalacia
patellae)
circulation, arthrotomy
incisions and, 55, 56
classification of types, 23
contact areas, in knee
flexion, 89, 419
entrapment, rehabilitation
and, 952
functions, 23, 391
immobilization after
ligament
reconstruction,
993–994
knee replacement design
biomechanics,
1083–1087,
1089–1090
medial and lateral glide,
410

metal-backed
components,
1108–1109
failure, 1113–1114
nail-patella syndrome,
214
osteochondritis
dissecans, 397
osteochondrosis
(Sinding-Larsen-
Johansson
syndrome), 399
in patellofemoral pain
differential
diagnosis, 426
pediatric, 239
physical examination,
392–393
realignment, physical
therapy after, 937
replacement, rotating
bearing, 10, 1164
resurfacing,
tricompartmental
knee replacement
and, 1062
static and dynamic
orientation, 922
taping, 929, 930
tendinitis
diagnosis, 462
in patellofemoral pain
differential
diagnosis, 426
surgery, 462
tilt, 398
trauma, 397
Patella alta, 409, 411
lateral radiograph, 124,
143
Patella downturn
approaches, 66
Patella infera, 409, 411
Patellar complications in
total knee
replacement, 1297,
1325-1332
clunk syndrome,
1326–1327
component failure,
1326
extensor disruptions,
1328–1330
Insall-Burstein
prosthesis, 1188,
1191
instability, 1327–1328
loosening, 1325–1326
surgical technique and,
1330
Patellar dislocation, 398,
442–443
acute, pediatric,
241–242

Patellar dislocation (cont.)
  chronic, 406–407, 408
    pediatric, 236
  congenital, 213–214, 215
  recurrent, 406, 408
    pediatric, 235–236
Patellar fractures, 1393–1403
  classification, 1394
  complications, 1401–1402
  diagnosis, 1394–1395
  historical perspective, 1393
  magnetic resonance imaging, 184, 185
  mechanisms of injury, 1393–1394
  pediatric, 242
  periprosthetic, 1412–1414
    treatment, 1414–1415, 1416
  prognosis, 1402
  stress fracture
    in patellofemoral pain differential diagnosis, 428
    pediatric, 240–241
  in total knee arthroplasty, 1329
  treatment, 1395–1400
    marginal and osteochondral fractures, 1401
    open fractures, 1401
    open reduction and internal fixation, 1397, 1399
    operative vs. nonoperative, 1395
    partial patellectomy, 1399
    surgical options, 1395, 1397
    total patellectomy, 1399–1400
Patellar glide testing, 423, 444, 445
Patellar osteotomy, 462
Patellar plica, medial, arthroscopic anatomy, 499
Patellar sleeve, pediatric fractures, 242
Patellar subluxation, 397–398
  chronic, 406, 407
    pediatric, 234–235
Patellar tendon
  anatomy, 382, 469
    arthroscopic, 503, 504
  bone grafting technique, 1170
  magnetic resonance imaging, 34
  in patellofemoral joint biomechanics, 90
  reconstruction, history, 639, 640–641
  rupture, 469–470, 473–474
    radiography, 143
    repair, 474–477
  in total knee arthroplasty, 1329
Patellar tendon grafts in ACL reconstruction, 641, 652–653
  arthroscopy (see Arthroscopic ACL reconstruction, with patellar tendon graft)
  bone-tendon-bone grafts, 641, 751, 837, 850–851
  conventional two-incision technique, 792–794, 796
  semitendinosus grafts vs., 824–825
  single-incision endoscopic reconstruction, 796–797, 799–800
Patellar tendon grafts in PCL reconstruction, 895–911
  clinical experience, 907–908
  historical perspective, 895–896
  indications, 896–897
  postoperative rehabilitation, 906–907
  protocol forms, 909–910
  surgical technique
    equipment, 898
    examination under anesthesia, 897–898
    graft harvest, 898–899
    graft passage and fixation, 904–906
    graft preparation, 899
    tunnel placement, 899–904
Patellectomy, 461–462
  for patellar fractures, 1393
    partial, 1399
    periprosthetic fractures, 1415, 1416
    total, 1399–1400
Patellofemoral congruence, radiographic measurement, 411, 412–413
Patellofemoral disease and extensor mechanism, magnetic resonance imaging, 183–187
Patellofemoral dysplasia, 404–405
  chronic dislocation of patella, 406–407, 408
  chronic subluxation of patella, 406, 407
  classification, 405
  lateral patellar compression syndrome, 405–406
  pediatric (see Pediatric knee, patellofemoral dysplasia)
  recurrent dislocation of patella, 406, 408
Patellofemoral hemiarthroplasty, 462
Patellofemoral joint
  anatomy, 381–382, 416–419
    arthroscopic, 500–501
  arthritis after patellar fracture, 1401
  arthroscopic visualization, 510
  biomechanics, 383, 419–420, 1147
    closed-chain and open-chain loading, 387, 388
    contact area and pressures, 88–89, 384, 386–387
    forces and force transmission, 89–90
    functions, 87
    kinematics, 384, 385, 1147
    loading with activity, 387–388
    motion, 87–88
    Q angle, 383, 385
    stability, 90–91
  classification of disorders, 404, 405
  complications with Insall-Burstein prosthesis, 1188, 1191
  contact areas, 22
  injuries (see Extensor mechanism injuries)
  overuse, pediatric, 237–238
  reaction force, 419–420
  replacement, isolated, 1171–1172
Patellofemoral joint surgery, 441–468
  articular degeneration without malalignment, 461–462
    author's approach, 464
  classification for approach, 447
  patellofemoral malalignment
    anteriorization, 455–457
    anteromedialization, 457–458, 459–461
    arthroscopic diagnosis, 447–448
    author's approach, 463–464
    distal realignment, 451–455, 458–459
    factors involved, 231
    lateral release and medial imbrication, 450–451, 452, 453
    procedures, 448–449
    proximal realignment by lateral release, 449–450, 451
  soft tissue disorders without malalignment, 462–463
Patellofemoral pain, 391–402
  anatomy and biomechanics, 416–420
  classification, 393
    presence of cartilage damage, 393–397
    usually normal cartilage, 399
    variable cartilage damage, 397–399
  diagnosis, 441–442
    differential, 426–428
    history, 391–392, 442–443
    physical examination, 392–393, 421–424, 443–445
    principles, 442
    radiologic evaluation, 424–426, 446–447

electrical stimulation, 421
Fulkerson-Schutzer classification, 425, 426
malalignment in, 415–416
mechanisms, 416
muscle physiology, 420
muscle strengthening, 420–421
osteotomy and, 1027
rehabilitation, 428 (*see also* Chondromalacia patellae rehabilitation)
extrinsic support, 434–435
modalities, 429
patient education, 428–429
regimen, 435
strengthening, 430–434
stretching, 429–433
surgery (*see* Patellofemoral joint surgery)
treatment, 399–400
nonoperative, 415–439, 447
Patellofemoral plicae
diagnosis and treatment, 462–463
pain, 398–399
Pathologic fractures, radiography, 145–146
Patient-controlled analgesia (PCA)
after ligament reconstruction, 990, 991, 992
pediatric, 286
in postoperative pain management, 311
in total knee arthroplasty, 1232
Patient education, in patellar rehabilitation, 428–429
PCA implants, 1133–1136
clinical results, 1111–1112
tibial component damage, 1253
PCA total knee, 1133–1136
Pediatric HIV infection, 351–352

Pediatric knee, 229–275 (*see also* Adolescents; Congenital deformities; Developmental stages)
acute trauma
acute patellar dislocation, 241–242
late effects, 248
patellar fractures, 242
patellar sleeve fractures, 242
physeal and epiphyseal fractures, 242–248
angulatory deformities, 262
posttraumatic, 262–263
tibia vara (Blount's disease), 263–264
treatment, 262
arthroscopy, 3, 231
congenital malalignments, 258–259
continuing care, 290
activity, 292–293
cast care, 291–292
health promotion, 293–294
medication regimen, 294
nursing and ancillary care, 290
school, 290
self-care, 293
teaching needs, 290–294
developmental considerations, 277
adolescents, 279–280
infants, 277–278
preschool children, 278–279
reactions to illness and hospitalization, 280
school-age children, 279
evaluation, 230–231
extension contractures, 260–261
treatment, 261–262
flexion contractures, 259–260, 261
functional knee pain, 269
hemarthrosis, 230–231
infections, 267–268

ligament injuries, 251–252
anterior cruciate ligament, 252–255, 256, 257
hypermobility syndrome, 258
lateral collateral ligament, 258
medial collateral ligament, 257–258
posterior cruciate ligament, 255–257
meniscal anatomy and development, 249
meniscal injuries
discoid meniscus, 250–251
tears, 250
neoplasms
chondroblastoma, 266
fibrous cortical defect and nonossifying fibroma, 266
incidence and evaluation, 264–266
miscellaneous, 267
osteochondroma, 266
osteoid osteoma, 266
osteosarcoma, 266–267
popliteal cyst, 267
nursing care, 277–295
osteochondritis dissecans, 248–249
overuse injuries, 236–237
bipartite patellae, 241
breaststroker's knee, 239–240
chondromalacia fabellae, 240
Osgood-Schlatter disease, 238–239
patellar stress fractures, 240–241
patellofemoral overuse, 237–238
risk factors, 237
Sinding-Larsen-Johansson syndrome, 239
synovial plicae, 240
parental considerations, 280–281
patellofemoral dysplasia, 231
chondromalacia, 232–233
chronic patellar dislocation, 236
chronic subluxating patella, 234–235
clinical features, 232

etiology, biomechanics, and risk factors, 231–232
lateral patellar compression syndrome, 233–234
radiographic evaluation, 232
recurrent patellar dislocation, 235–236
physical care
immobilization, 281–283
misconceptions about pain, 284
nutrition and weight management, 287
pain management, 283–287
psychosocial care
coping, 288–289
independence, 289
social interaction, 289–290
resources, 295
rheumatoid arthritis (*see* Juvenile rheumatoid arthritis)
slow-acting antirheumatic drugs for, 286
Pelligrini-Stieda disease, radiography, 126
Penicillamine, for rheumatoid arthritis, 327–328
Penicillin G, in total knee arthroplasty, 1269
Penicillins, in total knee arthroplasty, 1264, 1269, 1270
Perimeniscal cysts, arthroscopic meniscectomy for, 553
Periosteal chondromas, 1428
Peripatellar causes of knee pain, 399
Peripheral nerve block, in arthroscopic surgery, 301
Peripheral tibial plateau or condylar bone loss, bone grafting in revision total knee arthroplasty, 1341, 1342
Periprosthetic fractures, 1298, 1302, 1405–1417
femoral, 1405–1408
role of anterior femoral notching, 1409

Periprosthetic fractures (cont.)
  role of cement, 1409
  treatment, 1408–1409, 1410–1412
  treatment algorithm, 1409
  patellar, 1412–1414
    treatment, 1414–1415, 1416
  tibial, 1415–1416
Peroneal nerve
  assessment after ligament reconstruction, 984
  recurrent, anatomy, 51
Peroneal nerve palsy
  dislocations and, 1003
  after osteotomy, 1035
  in tibial plateau fracture, 1387, 1388
Pes anserinus tendons
  anatomy, 43
  transfer in ACL reconstruction, 807, 809
Pes muscles, saphenous nerve and, 36
PFC total knee arthroplasties, clinical results, 1112
Pharmacologic interventions in pediatric pain management, 286–287, 294
Phenylbutazone, 326
Phenytoin, for reflex sympathetic dystrophy, 373
Physeal and epiphyseal fractures, 242–243
  distal femoral, 243–244
  prognosis, 245–246
  treatment, 244–245
  proximal tibial, 246–247
  tibial tubercle, 247–248
Physical care of children
  immobilization, 281–283
  nutrition and weight management, 287
  pain management, 283–287
    assessment, 283–285
    interventions, 285–287
Physical therapy
  after arthroscopy, 935–937
  before osteotomy, 1028–1029
  after patellar realignment, 937
  for reflex sympathetic dystrophy, 372
  for total knee arthroplasty, 1233–1234, 1235–1237
Pigmented villonodular synovitis (PVNS), 1437–1438
  management, 1476, 1477
  synovectomy, 622, 628–629
Pin care, pediatric, 282–283
Pinch test, of graft isometry, 767
Pin tract complications, in arthrodesis for failed knee replacement, 1347
Piroxicam, 326
Pivot shift test, 669, 707, 723
Plantaris tendon anatomy, 46
Plate and screw assemblies, for distal femoral fractures, 1362–1364, 1365, 1366
Play therapy, 288–289
Plethysmography, in deep venous thrombosis, 1220
Plicae, 26
  arthroscopic anatomy, 498, 499–500
  CT/arthrography, 153–154
  magnetic resonance imaging, 184, 185
  patellofemoral diagnosis and treatment, 462–463
  pain, 398–399
  pediatric, 240
Plica syndrome, in patellofemoral pain differential diagnosis, 426
Pneumocystis carinii pneumonia (PCP), 356
Pogrund approach, 59
Poliomyelitis, radiography, 133
Polycentric knee arthroplasty, 1117–1119, 1121
Polyethylene joint components
  carbon-reinforced, 1181, 1254–1255
  modifications, 1254–1255
  resins for, 1254
  retrieval analysis, 1254–1258
  wear
    failure from, 1246–1247
    in Oxford Knee, 1154–1155
Polyflex ligament, 840
Polymethyl methacrylate, blood loss and, 1213
Polymyositis, radiography, 130
Popliteal angle, in hamstring tightness assessment, 423–424, 425
Popliteal artery
  supplying blood to knee soft tissue, 1279, 1280
  tibial fractures and, 246
Popliteal cysts, 216, 1474–1475
  imaging, 124, 128
  pediatric, 267
Popliteal fossa
  anatomy, 42, 44
  surgical anatomy, 64, 65
Popliteal space, innervation, 50
Popliteus muscle, function, 40, 42
Popliteus tendon
  elevation in lateral valgus release, 1208
  magnetic resonance imaging, 35, 171
Porous Coated Anatomic (PCA) implants, 1133–1136
  clinical results, 1111–1112
  tibial component damage, 1253
Porous-coated implants
  biology and surgical considerations, 1105–1107
  clinical results, 1111–1112
  complications, 1112–1114
  design, 1107–1109
  retrieval studies, 1109–1111
Townley's development, 1055
Positive predictive accuracy of laxity testing, definition, 675
Posterior approaches to knee, 63–65
Posterior articular nerve, 109
  anatomy, 48–49
Posterior aspect of knee, anatomy, 42–46
Posterior cruciate condylar knee, 1125–1126, 1128
Posterior cruciate ligament
  arthroscopic visualization, 511–512
  development, 10, 11, 12
  examination, 670–671
  knee replacement design biomechanics, 1080, 1081
  in knee stability, 76, 85, 86
  magnetic resonance imaging, 177–178
  in total knee replacement
    gait analysis and, 103–104
    new arguments and data, 1071–1072
    retention vs. sacrifice, 1063, 1069
Posterior cruciate ligament
  anatomy, 26–32
  arthroscopic, 502
  attachment sites, 29, 30
  blood supply, 32
  diagram, 28
  flexion and extension, 30
  magnetic resonance imaging, 30, 34, 177
  stabilizing function, 30–32
Posterior cruciate ligament-deficient knees
  grading system, 897
  instability, 742
  KT-1000 arthrometer and, 695–697
Posterior cruciate ligament injuries, 737–744
  distribution of disruptions, 659
  magnetic resonance imaging, 739, 740, 741
  mechanism, 737–738

with medial collateral
 ligament injuries,
 711–712
medical history,
 738–739
natural history, 739–741
nonoperative
 management,
 741–742, 743
pediatric, 255–257
Posterior cruciate ligament
 reconstruction
 with allografts
 postoperative
 management,
 884–885
 technique, 879–884
 with bone-patellar
 tendon-bone
 autografts (see
 Patellar tendon
 grafts in PCL
 reconstruction)
 historical perspective,
 638, 641
 for knee dislocation,
 1003, 1004, 1005
 with Ligastic ligament,
 860, 861
 with semitendinosus and
 gracilis tendons,
 913–917
 clinical results, 916
 discussion, 916–917
 technique, 913–916
Posterior cruciate ligament
 rehabilitation
 protocol, 951
 forms, 978–981
 return to activities and
 sports, 950
Posterior cruciate
 ligament-retaining
 prostheses,
 1315–1316
Posterior drawer test, 670,
 671
 for lateral
 capsuloligamentous
 complex injuries,
 716
 for medial
 capsuloligamentous
 complex injuries,
 707
Posterior incision combined
 with arthroscopic
 intraarticular
 meniscal repair,
 69–71
Posterior Lachman test,
 670
Posterior oblique ligament
 anatomy, 703, 704

Posterior portion of knee,
 anatomy, 1200,
 1205
Posterior Stabilized
 prosthesis, 1065,
 1067, 1185–1186
 biomechanics,
 1081–1083
 clinical function,
 1192–1193
 design rationale,
 1186–1187
 Insall-Burstein (see
 Insall-Burstein
 Posterior Stabilized
 Prosthesis)
 modifications, 1181
 original design,
 1180–1181
 survivorship analysis,
 1194, 1195
Posterior tibial nerve,
 assessment after
 ligament
 reconstruction, 984
Posterolateral approach to
 knee, 63
Posterolateral capsule,
 examination, 664,
 666–667
Posterolateral rotatory
 instability, surgical
 repair, 718–719
Posteromedial approach to
 knee, 61–63
Posteromedial capsule,
 examination, 664,
 665, 666
Prednisone, for reflex
 sympathetic
 dystrophy, 373
Prepatellar bursitis,
 magnetic resonance
 imaging, 187
Preschool children
 developmental
 considerations,
 278–279
 pain in, 284–285
 teaching, 291
Press Fit Condylar
 prosthesis,
 1137–1139
 clinical results, 1112
 modular system
 characteristics, 1300
Pridie procedure
 for chondromalacia, 613
 for degenerative arthritis,
 584–585
Prilocaine, in arthroscopic
 surgery, 303
Procaine, in arthroscopic
 surgery, 303

Pro-Col xenograft
 bioprosthesis, 841
Profunda femoris artery,
 supplying blood to
 knee soft tissue,
 1280
Progressive resistive
 exercises, 949
Prophylactic knee braces
 Anderson Knee Stabler,
 947, 957–959
 studies, 957–962
 types, 957
Proplast ligament, 840
Propofol, in arthroscopic
 surgery, 301–302
Proprioceptive training, in
 cartilage lesion
 rehabilitation, 930,
 931, 932
Prostheses (see also
 specific types)
 knee replacement (see
 Total knee
 replacement)
 ligaments, 642 (see also
 Kennedy ligament
 augmentation
 device)
 roentgenographic
 evaluation,
 147–148, 149,
 150
Prosthetic cruciate
 ligament
 reconstruction, 642,
 839–864
 advantages, 839–840
 classification of
 prosthetic ligaments,
 841–842
 FDA approval process,
 842–843
 future, 861–862
 Gore-Tex ligament
 biomechanical testing
 results, 843
 concept, 843–844
 indications, 849–850
 new developments,
 850
 results, 846–849
 technique, 844–846
 historical perspective,
 840–841
 intraarticular ACL
 reconstruction,
 751–752
 Leeds-Keio ligament
 biomechanical testing
 results, 843
 concept, 854–855
 results, 857–858
 technique, 855–857

Ligastic ligament
 biomechanical testing
 results, 843
 concept, 858–859
 results, 860–861
 technique, 859–860
 Stryker Dacron ligament
 biomechanical testing
 results, 843
 concept, 850–851
 results, 852–854
 technique, 851–852
Prosthetic reconstruction
 for bone tumors,
 1466–1469
Proximal fibula bone
 tumors, types and
 percentages,
 1421–1422
Proximal tibia
 anatomy, 1369–1370
 fractures, epiphyseal and
 physeal, 246–248
 transverse lateral
 approach, 67, 68
Proximal tibial metaphyseal
 osteotomy, 1030,
 1031
Proximal tibial valgus
 osteotomy,
 1030–1032
 results, 1036–1037
 total knee replacement
 after, 1037–1041
 failed osteotomy, 1041
 radiographs,
 1038–1040
Proximal tibial varus
 osteotomy, 1032
 results, 1037
Proximal tibiofibular joint
 dislocation, 1009–1015
 classification,
 1010–1011
 historical perspective,
 1009–1010
 mechanism,
 1011–1012
 prognosis and
 complications, 1014
 roentgenographic
 findings, 1012
 signs and symptoms,
 1012
 surgical anatomy,
 1009–1010
 treatment, 1012–1014
 oblique and horizontal
 types, 1010
 subluxation, 1010, 1011,
 1012
Pseudogout, 127
 calcium pyrophosphate
 crystals in, 622

Pseudogout *(cont.)*
  radiography, 127
Psychosocial aspects of ligament injury rehabilitation, 990–991
Psychosocial care of children
  coping, 288–289
  independence, 289
  social interaction, 289–290
Pulmonary capillary wedge pressure, 300
Pulmonary embolism
  asymptomatic, 1222
  in knee arthroplasty, 1221–1222 *(see also* Thromboembolic disease in knee arthroplasty)
  regional anesthesia and, 305
Pulmonary osteoarthropathy, hypertrophic, 127
Pulse oximetry, 300
PVNS (pigmented villonodular synovitis), 1437–1438
  management, 1476, 1477
  synovectomy, 622, 628–629
Pyknodysostosis, radiography, 141
Pyle's disease, radiography, 135

Q

Q angle *(see* Quadriceps angle)
Quadriceps
  anatomy, 45, 46, 382
  loading
    tibial anterior displacement and, 115
    tibial internal rotation and, 115–116
  strengthening in PCL rehabilitation, 906–907
  stretching, 430, 433
  tear, magnetic resonance imaging, 184, 186
  tendinitis, 399
Quadriceps active test, 662, 668
  definition, 674

Quadriceps angle, 46–47, 90, 91, 383, 385, 417–418
  measurement, 409, 417, 443
  in patellofemoral examination, 392–393, 443
Quadriceps force, 420
Quadriceps neutral angle, 675, 676
  definition, 674
Quadricepsplasty, for pediatric extension contractures, 261–262
Quadriceps setting exercises, 927
Quadriceps snip of Insall, 67
Quadriceps tendon
  anatomy, 469
  in patellofemoral joint biomechanics, 87–91
  rupture, 469–470
  radiography, 143
  repair, 470–473
  in total knee arthroplasty, 1328–1329
Quadriceps turndown, 66
Quinolones, in total knee arthroplasty, 1269

R

Rab technique for correction of Blount's disease, 264, 265
Radiation synovectomy, 626–628
Radical flexor release for flexion contracture, 260, 261
Radioactivity, tumors from, 1436
Radiologic analysis *(see* Roentgenographic evaluation *and other modalities)*
Radionuclide orthopedic imaging *(see* Bone scans; Nuclear scans)
Radiopharmaceuticals, 195
Range of motion
  mobilization for tibial plateau fractures, 1378
  observation and recording, 660–661, 662

osteotomy and, 1024
  as rehabilitation goal, 945
  as rehabilitation phase, 948–949
  in stress examination, 663–664
  in total knee arthroplasty, 1298
Rectus femoris anatomy, 46, 418
Recurrent dislocation of patella (RDP), 406, 408
  pediatric, 235–236
Recurrent peroneal nerve anatomy, 51
Recurvatum, congenital, 258
Reflexes active about knee
  flexion reflex, 111–112
  ligamentomuscular protective reflex, 110–111
  ligament-spindle reflex, 112
  sensorimotor acquired reflex, 112–113
Reflex sympathetic dystrophy, 365–377
  clinical presentation, 365–366
  diagnosis, 371
  investigative studies, 366–367
  patellofemoral pain from, 399
  pathophysiology, 367–371
  pediatric, 248
  terminology, 365
  treatment, 371
    algorithm, 374–375
    pain management, 372–374
    physical therapy, 372
Regional anesthesia
  complications, 309–310
  physiology, 306, 307, 308
  for total knee arthroplasty, 305–306
Regression, pediatric, 280
Rehabilitation after knee ligament injury or surgery, 943–955
  ACL reconstruction, 951
  failure to progress, 951–952
  forms, 971–981
  functional exercises, 949–950

general protocol, 948–951
goals and principles, 945
immobilization and bracing, 948
isokinetic exercises, 950
isometric exercises, 949
isotonic or progressive resistive exercises, 949
musculoskeletal tissues
  characteristic changes, 946
  effects of disuse and immobilization, 945–946
  healing, 946–948
patient differentiation and, 943–944
PCL reconstruction, 906, 910–911, 951
procedure selection and, 944
progressive weightbearing, 949
range-of-motion phase, 948–949
return to activities and sports, 950–951
surgical techniques and, 944–945
Rehabilitation of cartilage lesions *(see* Cartilage lesion rehabilitation)
Rehabilitative knee braces, 962–963
Reiter's syndrome, in HIV infection, 357
Relaxation, pediatric, 285
Resection arthroplasty
  for failed knee replacement, 1348–1350
  for infected total knee arthroplasty, 1275
Resins, for polyethylene joint components, 1254
Resistive closed-chain exercise, in cartilage lesion rehabilitation, 933, 935
Respiratory depression, from epidural narcotics, 311
Retinaculum
  anatomy, 382, 418
  median patellar, tear, magnetic resonance imaging, 184

Retrieval analysis of knee replacements, 1251–1260
factors affecting performance
articulating surfaces, 1252–1256
fixation, 1257–1259
metal backing, 1256–1257
methods, 1251–1252
Retroviruses, 349
Reverse pivot shift test, 667
Revision total knee replacement (*see* Total knee replacement revision)
Rheumatoid arthritis, 127, 128 (*see also* Rheumatologic disorders affecting knee)
Arthritis Foundation classification, 623
aspirin and other salicylates for, 323
cystic, 128
diagnosis, 315–316
imaging, 127–128
juvenile (*see* Juvenile rheumatoid arthritis)
osteotomy, 1026
synovectomy, 621–622
contraindications, 623
indications, 622–623
results, 624–625
technique, 623–624
total knee replacement and, 304, 1262
wound healing in, 1283
Rheumatoid nodules, radiography, 128
Rheumatologic disorders affecting knee, 315–329 (*see also* Ligament releases in arthritic knee)
diagnostic considerations, 315–316
NSAIDs, 322
synovial fluid
abnormal, 316–319
normal, 316
synovianalysis, 315, 316
characteristics of abnormal synovial fluid, 318, 319–321
technique, 319
treatment, 321–322
clinical evaluation of antirheumatic drugs, 322–327

experimental osteoarthritis treatment, 327
individualizing drug dosage, 322
principles of adjusting drug dose, 322
second- and third-line drugs in rhemumatoid arthritis, 321-322, 327–329
Rickets, roentgenographic evaluation, 137–138
Rigid-hinge prostheses, 1306, 1307, 1309
Roentgenographic evaluation, 123–148
angular deformity in osteotomy, 1028
arthritides, 126–130
Blount disease, 219–220
bone tumors, 1450–1451
congenital diseases, 134–136
enchondromas, 137
exostoses, 136–137
extensor mechanism injuries, 409–413
fibrous dysplasia, 140
heavy metal poisoning, 139
hemoglobinopathies and anemia, 139
hemophilic arthropathy, 338, 339, 341–343
hyperostoses, 140–141
hyperparathyroidism, 138
infection, 130–133
lipidoses, 138–139
neuromuscular disease, 133–134
neuropathic joint disease, 132, 133
normal bony architecture, 21
osteonecrosis, 141–143, 608–609
Paget disease, 139–140
patellofemoral pain, 424, 446–447
pediatric patellofemoral dysplasia, 232, 233
prostheses, 147–148, 149, 150
proximal tibiofibular joint dislocation, 1012
pulmonary embolism, 1221
reflex sympathetic dystrophy, 366, 367

rickets and osteomalacia, 137–138
scurvy, 138
soft tissue, 124–126
tibial plateau fractures, 1375
trauma, 143–147
views, 123–124
Roentgen stereophotogrammetric analysis, 1108
Rolling motion between femur and tibia, 77, 78–79
Rosenberg semitendinosus procedure, 817, 819
Rotating bearing patella replacement, 10, 1164
Rotating-hinge prostheses, 1306, 1307, 1309
indications, 1309, 1310–1311
Rotatory instability, history, 639
Roux-Elmslie-Trilat procedure, 455
Roux-Goldthwait procedure, 452, 454
RSA (roentgen stereophotogrammetric analysis), 1108
Ruffini endings, 108
Running
biomechanical analysis for patellofemoral rehabilitation, 923
gait analysis, 101

S

Sagittal kinematics of knee, 1146–1147
Sagittal plane diagrams of knee, congruent and incongruent joint surfaces, 1144–1145
Salicylates
in pediatric pain management, 294
for rheumatolgic disorders
clinical evaluation, 322–324
side effects and toxicity, 324
Salter-Harris type I fracture, fixation technique, 244–245

Salter-Harris type II fracture
fixation technique, 244–245
magnetic resonance imaging, 244
Salter-Harris type III fracture, fixation technique, 245
Salter-Harris type IV fracture, fixation technique, 245
Salter III injury, radiography, 143, 144
Saphenous nerve
anatomy, 51
pes muscles and, 36
Sarcomas (*see also specific types* and Bone tumors)
epithelioid, 1439
osteogenic
magnetic resonance imaging, 192
pediatric, 266–267
soft tissue, 1477–1479
synovial, 1438–1439
radiography, 125, 126
Sartorius anatomy, 43
Scaffold device, in cruciate ligament reconstruction, 842
Schatzker classification of tibial plateau fractures, 1372, 1373
School-age children
developmental considerations, 279
pain in, 285
teaching, 291
School concerns, 290
Scintigraphy, 197–198
Screw fixation for osteochondritis dissecans, 603–606
Screw-home mechanism, 22, 79, 418
Screw plate devices, for distal femoral fractures, 1362–1364, 1365, 1366
Scuderi technique, 472–473
Scurvy, roentgenographic evaluation, 138
Sedatives, in pediatric pain management, 286
Segond fracture, 717
radiography, 145
Semimembranosus tendon anatomy, 43, 45

INDEX

Semitendinosus tendon anatomy, 43
Semitendinosus tendon grafts
  in ACL reconstruction, 750–751, 813–817
    Hendler procedure, 821–824, 825
    with Kennedy LAD, 832–836
    patellar tendon grafts vs., 824–825
    technical considerations, 817–821
  healing and, 947
  in PCL reconstruction
    clinical results, 916
    discussion, 916–917
    technique, 913–916
Sensitivity of laxity testing, definition, 674–675
Sensorimotor acquired reflex, 112–113
Sensory receptors of knee, 107–109
Sepsis, after ligament reconstruction, 993
Septic arthritis
  in children and adolescents, 267–268
  in neonates, 267
Settegast technique, 412
Shiers hinge, 1047
Sidestep cut, gait analysis, 101–103
Sinding-Larsen-Johansson syndrome, 399
  in patellofemoral pain differential diagnosis, 426
  pediatric, 239
Skeletal traction and early mobilization, for tibial plateau fractures, 1379
Skill development, in muscular coactivation, 114
Skin grafting, for wound closure in failed knee replacement, 1288
Skin necrosis, in total knee replacement, 1263–1264
Skin slough, in total knee replacement, 1263
Sliding motion between femur and tibia, 77, 78–79
Sling and reef procedure, 803, 805

Slocum test, 665, 666
Smoking, wound healing and, 1283–1284
Social interaction, pediatric, 289–290
Soft tissues
  anatomy
    anterior aspect, 45, 46–47
    lateral aspect, 39–42
    medial aspect, 35–39
    posterior aspect, 42–46
  contractures (*see* Ligament releases in arthritic knee)
  in failed knee replacement
    anatomy, 1279–1281
    coverage options, 1286–1291
    wound healing, 1281–1286
  roentgenographic evaluation, 124–126
  tumors, 1472, 1474
    benign, treatment, 1474–1477
    sarcomas, treatment, 1477–1479
Soleus muscle anatomy, 46
Soleus muscle flap, for wound closure in failed knee replacement, 1290
Specificity of laxity testing, definition, 675
Spherocentric prosthesis, 1049, 1050, 1257
Spinal anesthesia
  in arthroscopic surgery, 301
  complications, 309
  differential spinal blockade, in reflex sympathetic dystrophy, 372
Sports
  history of ligament reconstruction, 638–639
  return to, after rehabilitation, 950–951
Sports injuries, bracing, 957–969
Squamous cell carcinoma, radiography, 131, 132
Squats, biomechanical analysis for patellofemoral rehabilitation, 923

Stability, 81
  history of rotatory instability treatment, 639–640
  joint surface, 81
  knee replacement failures and, 1244–1245
    revision arthroplasty, 1297–1298
  ligamentous, 82–87
  ligament-spindle reflex in, 112
  loading and, 82, 83
  menisci and, 81–82
  musculature in, 107, 113–118
  osteotomy and, 1026
  patellofemoral, 90–91
    testing, 444–445
  in total knee arthroplasty, 1327–1328
  after PCL reconstruction, 907
Stabilocondylar prosthesis, 1065, 1068
Stair climbing
  biomechanical analysis for patellofemoral rehabilitation, 923
  in cartilage lesion rehabilitation, 933–934, 936
Staphylococcus aureus
  pediatric knee infection from, 267, 268
  total knee arthroplasty infection from, 1267, 1268
Staphylococcus epidermidis
  radionuclide imaging of infection, 203, 205
  total knee arthroplasty infection from, 1267
Staphylococcus osteomyelitis, radiography, 130
Static observation of knee, 922
Stationary bicycle, in cartilage lesion rehabilitation, 929
Steinmann pin, in knee dislocation management, 1004
Stents, in cruciate ligament reconstruction, 842
Sterilization of allografts, secondary, 868–869
Steroids (*see* Corticosteroids)

Strength, biomechanical assessment for patellofemoral rehabilitation, 923
Strengthening
  of ACL-deficient knee, 728–729
  in cartilage lesion rehabilitation, 925–929
  exercise types, 420–421
  in patellofemoral rehabilitation, 430–434
Strengthening exercises, 949, 950
Streptococci, total knee arthroplasty infection from, 1267
Stress, parental, 281
Stress examination
  anesthesia, 664–665
  range of motion, 663–664
Stress fractures
  magnetic resonance imaging, 189
  patellar
    in patellofemoral pain differential diagnosis, 428
    pediatric, 240–241
  radiography, 145, 146
Stretching, in patellofemoral rehabilitation, 429–433
Stryker Dacron ligament
  biomechanical testing results, 843
  concept, 850–851
  results, 852–854
  technique, 851–852
Stryker knee laxity tester, 678–679, 688–689, 697
Subchondral avascular necrosis, radiography, 142–143
Subchondral bone, healing, 946
Subluxation
  congenital (*see* Dislocation and subluxation of knee, congenital)
  patellar, 397–398
    chronic, 234–235, 406, 407
    pediatric, 234–235
  proximal tibiofibular joint, 1010, 1011, 1012

Sufentanil, in arthroscopic surgery, 301
Sulfasalazine, for rheumatoid arthritis, 328
Sulindac, 325–326
Superficial peroneal nerve, assessment after ligament reconstruction, 984
Supracondylar and intercondylar distal femoral fractures, 1357–1368
  classification, 1358, 1359
  clinical evaluation, 1357–1358
  nonoperative management, 1358, 1360
  open reduction and internal fixaton, 1360
    bone grafting, 1364, 1365
    insertion of dynamic condylar screw, 1364, 1366
    surgical implants, 1361–1364
    surgical planning, 1360
    unicondylar fractures, 1360–1361
  operative management, 1358
  operative vs. nonoperative management, 1357, 1358
  results and complications, 1367
  periprosthetic supracondylar fractures, 1405–1412
  after total knee replacement, 1364, 1366–1367
Suprapatellar pouch, arthroscopic anatomy, 497, 499
Surgery (see also specific types), HIV transmission and, 355
Surgical approaches, 55–71
  anterior, 55–59
  anterior approach to knee with osteotomy of tibial tubercle, 66–67
  arthroscopic, 67–69

arthrotomy incisions and patellar circulation, 55, 56
combined posterior incision and arthroscopic intraarticular meniscal repair, 69–71
lateral, 59–60
lateral approach to distal femur, 65–66
medial, 60–61, 62
patella downturn approaches, 66
posterior, 63–65
posterolateral, 63
posteromedial, 61–63
transverse lateral approach to proximal tibia, 67, 68
Sympathectomy, surgical, for reflex sympathetic dystrophy, 373
Sympathetic blockade, in reflex sympathetic dystrophy, 372–373, 375
Synovectomy, 621–633
  arthroscopic, 625–626
    technique, 626, 627
  chemical and radioisotope, 626–628
  contraindications, 623
  in hemophilia, 629–630
  historical perspective, 621
  indications, 622–623
  for juvenile rheumatoid arthritis, 625
  for Lyme disease, 631
  for pigmented villonodular synovitis, 628–629
  results, 624–625
  for rheumatoid arthritis, 621–625
  for subacute hemarthrosis, 340
  for synovial chondromatosis, 630
  technique, 623–624
Synovial chondromatosis, 1437, 1476
  radiography, 125
  synovectomy, 630
Synovial fluid
  abnormal, 316–317
    characteristics, 318, 319–321
    classification, 317, 319
  normal, 316

Synovial folds, anatomy, 426, 427
Synovial hemangiomas, 1436–1437
Synovial lipomatosis (Hoffa's syndrome), 399, 1437
Synovial plicae (see Plicae)
Synovial sarcomas, 1438–1439
  radiography, 125, 126
Synovial tumors
  benign, 1436–1438
  malignant, 1438–1439
Synovianalysis, 315, 316
  characteristics of abnormal synovial fluid, 318, 319–321
  technique, 319
Synovitis (see also Pigmented villonodular synovitis; Rheumatoid arthritis; Synovectomy), with Kennedy LAD, 831
Synovium anatomy, 24–26
Systemic lupus erythematosus, radiography, 129

T

Tamoxifen, for osteoarthritis, 327
Taping
  in cartilage lesion rehabilitation, 929, 930
  patellar, 435
Technetium 99m HMPAO, 198–199
Technetium 99m methylene disphosphonate scans, 196
  case reports, 200–201
Teenagers (see Adolescents)
Tendinitis, peripatellar, 399
Tendon anatomy, 22
  insertion into bone, 26, 27
  posterior, 42–44, 46
Tendon grafts (see also specific tendons), in patellar tendon rupture repair, 477
TENS (transcutaneous electrical nerve stimulation)
  for patellofemoral pain, 429

pediatric, 285
Terminal knee extension, 927–928
Thermography, in reflex sympathetic dystrophy evaluation, 367
Thigh muscle atrophy, in ACL-deficient knee, 728
Thromboembolic disease in knee arthroplasty, 1217–1225, 1284
  deep venous thrombosis, 1218
  detection methods, 1218–1220
  incidence, 1220–1221
  pathophysiology, 1217–1218
  prophylaxis, 1222–1223
  pulmonary embolism, 1221–1222
  treatment, 1222–1223
Thrombophlebitis, after ligament reconstruction, 993
Thrombosis, deep venous (see Deep venous thrombosis)
Tibia
  anterior displacement, quadriceps loading and, 115
  axial rotation, 79
  congenital anterior subluxation, 258–259
  development, 7, 8, 9, 11, 24
  internal rotation, quadriceps loading and, 115–116
  knee replacement design biomechanics
    fixation, 1092–1093
    kinematics, 1080–1082
  periprosthetic fractures, 1415–1416
  proximal (see Proximal tibia)
  surface motion between femur and, 77, 78–79
  in total knee arthroplasty, 1244–1245
Tibial artery, anterior, recurrent branch, supplying blood to knee soft tissue, 1280

Tibial axis, in patellofemoral joint biomechanics, 87, 88
Tibial bone loss, bone grafting for
  defects greater than 12 mm deep, 1334–1338, 1339–1340
  defects 6 to 12 mm deep, 1334
Tibial condyles
  anatomy, 21
  embryology, 9, 11
Tibial nerve, posterior, assessment after ligament reconstruction, 984
Tibial osteochondrosis (see Osgood-Schlatter disease)
Tibial osteotomy, high
  abrasion arthroplasty and, for degenerative arthritis, 591–592
  gait analysis and, 103
  for osteonecrosis, 610–611
Tibial plateau
  anatomy, 20, 21
  arthroscopic, 502
  bone loss, osteotomy and, 1026
  design principles in meniscal bearing arthroplasty, 1148–1149
  peripheral bone loss, bone grafting in revision total knee arthroplasty, 1341, 1342
  surgical approaches, 1379–1381
Tibial plateau fractures, 1369–1392
  anatomy, 1369–1370
  classification, 1372–1374
  clinical findings, 1374–1375
  complications, 1386–1388
  computed tomography, 151
  conservative management, 1377
  cast bracing, 1379
  cast immobilization, 1378
  early range-of-motion mobilization, 1378
  skeletal traction and early mobilization, 1379
  lateral tibial plateau avulsion fracture, 713, 717
  mechanism of injury, 1370–1372
  open reduction and internal fixation, 1381
  bicondylar fracture, 1383, 1385
  cleavage fracture, 1381–1382
  cleavage with depression fracture, 1382–1383, 1384
  complex fracture, 1383, 1385–1386
  depression fracture, 1382
  fracture fixation and arthroscopy, 1386
  medial condyle fracture, 1383
  postoperative care, 1388–1389
  radiographic evaluation, 1375–1377
  surgical approaches to tibial plateau, 1379–1381
  surgical goals and principles, 1389
Tibial rotation, Q angle and, 418
Tibial spine fractures, pediatric, 252–253
  prognosis, 253–254
  treatment, 253
Tibial tubercle
  anteriorization, 455–457, 461
  fractures, 247–248
  osteotomy, anterior approaches to knee with, 66–67
Tibial tunnel, in intraarticular ACL reconstruction
  conventional two-incision technique, 794–796
  single-incision endoscopic reconstruction, 797–798
Tibia vara, 263–264
  infantile vs. late-onset, 263
  Rab technique for correction, 264, 265
  roentgenographic diagnosis, 264
Tibiofemoral joint
  contact area, 80–81
  subluxation, osteotomy and, 1027
Tibiofibular joint
  normal anatomy, 24
  proximal, dislocation (see Proximal tibiofibular joint, dislocation)
Tobramycin, in total knee arthroplasty, 1269
  added to cement, 1271–1272
Toddlers
  pain in, 284
  teaching, 291
Toddler's fracture, radiography, 143, 144
Tolmetin, 326
Tomography, tibial plateau fractures, 1375, 1376
Total Condylar prosthesis, 1125, 1126
  clinical results, 1183, 1192–1193
  Hospital for Special Surgery, 1184–1185
  other institutions, 1185
  development, 1065, 1066
  original design, 1179–1180, 1183–1184
  failure mechanism, 1239
  rotating platform, 1171
  survivorship analysis, 1194, 1195
  tibial component damage, 1253
Total Condylar II prosthesis, 1180
  retrieval analysis, 1258
  stability with, 1244–1245
Total Condylar III prosthesis, 1301
  results, 1319–1320
Total knee replacement
  anesthesia, 303
  preoperative assessment, 303–305
  regional, 305–309
  bone grafting (see Bone grafting in total knee arthroplasty)
  categories of knee prostheses, 1307
  cementless, 1105–1116
    biologic and surgical considerations of porous ingrowth fixation, 1105–1107
    clinical results, 1111–1112
    complications, 1112–1114
    components, 1239
    failure, 1242–1243
    implant design, 1107–1109
    implant retrieval studies, 1109–1111
    University Hospitals of Cleveland results, 1114–1115
  in chronic hemophilic arthropathy, 341, 342, 343
  condylar system, 1320
  conforming condylar device, illustration, 1308
  constrained condylar device (see also Constrained knee arthroplasty), illustration, 1308
  distal femoral fractures after, 1364, 1366–1367
  failed
    arthrodesis for, 1345–1348
    resection arthroplasty for, 1348–1349
    soft tissue considerations, 1279–1295
  fractures after (see Periprosthetic fractures)
  gait analysis after, 103–104
  infection (see Infected total knee arthroplasty)
  loosening of prosthetic components, 147–148, 149
  meniscal bearing (see Meniscal bearing knee replacement)
  motion and posterior cruciate ligament, 1071
  nursing care (see Nursing care for total knee arthroplasty)
  occupational therapy, 1237

overload of bone and ligaments, 1239
patellar complications (see Patellar complications in total knee replacement)
posterior cruciate ligament in
  new arguments and data, 1071–1072
  retention vs. sacrifice, 1063, 1069
posterior cruciate ligament-retaining device, illustration, 1308
posterior cruciate ligament retention
  cruciate-sparing total condylar knee, 1125–1126, 1128
  Duocondylar and Duopatellar, 1122–1125
  early controversy, 1063
  Geometric, 1119–1121
  Kinematic, 1126–1129
  meniscal bearing prostheses, 1136–1137, 1138
  Miller-Galante, 1132–1133, 1135
  Polycentric, 1117–1119, 1121
  Porous Coated Anatomic, 1133–1136
  Press Fit Condylar, 1137–1139
  stability and, 1245
  Townley and Cloutier, 1129–1132
posterior cruciate ligament sacrifice or substitution
  advantages, 1182–1183
  clinical function, 1192–1193
  clinical results of posterior stabilization at Mayo Clinic, 1193–1194
  complications of PCL substitution, 1194–1196
  survivorship analysis, 1194, 1195
posterior-stabilized device, illustration, 1308

principles and design problems, 1070–1071
prosthetic modular systems, 1300
after proximal tibial valgus osteotomy, 1037–1041
  failed osteotomy, 1041
  radiographs, 1038–1040
retrieval analysis, 1251–1260
  articulating surfaces, 1252–1256
  fixation, 1257–1259
  metal backing, 1256–1257
  methods, 1251–1252
rigid-hinge device, illustration, 1307
rotating-hinge device, illustration, 1307
soft tissue considerations in failed knee replacement, 1279-1295
  anatomy, 1279–1281
  coverage options, 1286–1291
  postoperative monitoring, 1285–1286
  wound healing, 1281–1284
survivorship at 15 years, 1139
transfusion considerations, 1211–1216
  intraoperative period, 1213
  postoperative period, 1213–1214
  preoperative period, 1211–1213
Total knee replacement design
  biomechanics, 1079–1096
  design of revision components, 1094
  fixation
    femoral component, 1090–1092
    tibial component, 1092–1093
  kinematics
    patella, 1083–1087
    posterior-stabilized total knee replacement, 1081–1083

tibia-femur, 1080–1081
strength of components, 1093–1094
wear, 1087–1090
Total knee replacement evolution, 1045–1078, 1305–1308
  acrylic and metallic interpositional arthroplasties, 1051, 1053
  bicondylar knees, 1059–1062
  future, 1069–1072
  hinges, 1046–1051, 1052
  Hospital for Special Surgery pedigree, 1064–1069, 1070
  membrane interpositional arthroplasty, 1046
  mold arthroplasty, 1053
  Townley's development, 1053–1055, 1056
  tricompartmental arthroplasty, 1062–1064
  unicondylar knee prosthesis, 1055, 1057–1059
Total knee replacement failure mechanisms, 1239–1249
  cement-bone interface failure, 1240–1244
  cementless knees, 1242–1244
  initial fixation, 1242
  instability, 1244–1245, 1297–1298
  stiff total knee replacement, 1245–1246
  wear, 1246–1247
Total knee replacement revision
  bone grafting in, 1338–1344
  final implant selection and fixation, 1301–1302
  general considerations, 1298
  implant removal, 1301
  indications, 1297–1298
  modular systems, 1300
  preoperative assessment and planning, 1298–1299
  prosthesis selection, 1299

surgical approach, 1299
Tourniquet, in total knee arthroplasty, 1213
Townley prosthesis, 1129, 1131, 1132
Townley's development of knee arthroplasty, 1053–1055, 1056
Townsend brace, 963
Traction
  pediatric, 282
  for periprosthetic distal femoral fractures, 1408
Tranexamic acid, in hemophilia, 335–336
Transcutaneous electrical nerve stimulation (TENS)
  for patellofemoral pain, 429
  pediatric, 285
Transfusion considerations in total knee arthroplasty, 1211–1216
  intraoperative period, 1213
  postoperative period, 1213–1214
  preoperative period, 1211–1213
Transfusion therapy for hemophilia, complications, 336
Transverse ligament, pseudotear, magnetic resonance imaging, 170
Trauma
  acute pediatric
    acute patellar dislocation, 241–242
    late effects, 248
    patellar fractures, 242
    patellar sleeve fractures, 242
    physeal and epiphyseal fractures, 242–248
  articular surface
    chondral lesions, 616–617
    osteochondral fractures, 614–616
    computed tomography, 148
    magnetic resonance imaging, 188, 189

Trauma *(cont.)*
  patellofemoral joint (extensor mechanism), 397, 403
    classification, 405
    roentgenographic evaluation, 143–147
Traumatic dislocation of knee, 999–1008
  classification and diagnosis, 999–1000
  evaluation, 1000–1002
  rehabilitation, 1007–1008
  structures involved on posterolateral and lateral side, 1007
  treatment
    historical results, 1002–1003
    nonoperative management, 1003–1004
    operative techniques, 1004–1007
    timing, 1003
Trevor's disease, imaging, 134, 135
Tricompartmental knee replacement
  evolution, 1062–1064
  with mobile meniscal bearings, 1169–1170
Tricyclic antidepressants, for reflex sympathetic dystrophy, 373
Tripartite patella, 399
Tuberculosis, HIV infection and, 357
Tuberculous osteomyelitis, radiography, 131
Tuberous sclerosis, radiography, 136
Tumors *(see also specific types)*
  magnetic resonance imaging, 192
  pediatric neoplasms, 264–267

U

UCI prosthesis, 1059–1060, 1061
Ultrasonography, deep venous thrombosis, 1219–1220
Unicameral bone cysts, 1422
Unicompartmental gonarthrosis, arthroscopy *(see Arthroscopic treatment of degenerative arthritis)*
Unicompartmental knee replacement, 1097–1103
  advantages, 1097–1098
  evolution, 1055, 1057–1059
  future developments, 1102
  historical perspective, 1097
  implant design, 1101–1102
  with mobile meniscal bearings, 1168–1169
  operative procedure, 1099–1100
    component positioning, 1100
    component sizing, 1100–1101
  for osteoarthritis, 1098, 1099–1100, 1102
  Oxford knee, 1152–1154
  patient selection, 1098–1099
  rehabilitation, 1102
  surgical options, 1097–1098
  survivorship curve, 1098
Unicondylar knee prosthesis, 1055, 1057–1059 *(see also Unicompartmental knee replacement)*
University Hospitals of Cleveland, cementless total knee replacement results, 1114–1115
University of California at Irvine (UCI) prosthesis, 1059–1060, 1061
Uphill principle, 81

V

Valgus deformity of knee
  arthroscopic debridement and, 593
  ligament release, 1206–1207, 1208
  osteotomy and, 1020–1021, 1024, 1026, 1028 *(see also Osteotomy for arthritic knee)*
  roentgenogram, 1200
  type II, reconstruction options, 1311–1315
Valgus stress test, for medial collateral ligament injury, 707
Vancomycin, in total knee arthroplasty
  prophylactic, 1264, 1265
  therapy, 1269, 1270
  treatment dose, 1269
Variable resistance exercise, 421
Varus deformity of knee
  arthroscopic debridement and, 593
  ligament release, 1205–1206
  osteotomy and, 1020–1021, 1026, 1028 *(see also Osteotomy for arthritic knee)*
  roentgenogram, 1200
Vascular disease, wound healing and, 1283, 1284
Vascular injury, after osteotomy, 1036
Vascular supply *(see Blood supply)*
Vastus lateralis anatomy, 419
Vastus medialis anatomy, 46
Vastus medialis muscle flap, for wound closure in failed knee replacement, 1290
Vastus medialis obliquus
  anatomy, 418–419, 703
  in cartilage lesion rehabilitation exercise, 927, 928
  functional closed-chain activities, 932
  evaluation of deficiency, 410
  in medial collateral ligament injury, 707
Velocity, definition, 96
Vena cava filters, in thromboembolic disease, 1223
Venography, ascending, in deep venous thrombosis, 1218
Venous thrombosis, deep *(see Deep venous thrombosis)*
Ventilation perfusion (V/Q) scans, for pulmonary embolism, 1221

W

Wagner oblique metaphyseal osteotomy, 1030
Walking *(see also Gait analysis)*
  biomechanical analysis for patellofemoral rehabilitation, 922–923
  moment patterns, 99–100
Walldius hinge, 1047
Warfarin
  in thromboembolic disease, 1222, 1224
  total knee arthroplasty and, 1211
Weight, osteotomy and, 1026
Weightbearing, progressive, 949
Weight management, pediatric, 287
Wiberg classification of patellar morphology, 416, 417
Withdrawal (flexion) reflex, 111–112
Wound complications, infected total knee arthroplasty from, 1263–1264
Wound drainage, after ligament reconstruction, 984, 985
Wound healing, in failed knee replacement, 1281–1284
  postoperative monitoring, 1285–1286
Wrisberg's ligament, 34
Wrisberg-type discoid meniscus, 216

Y

Young hinge, 1048

Z

Zalcitabine, 356
Zarins procedure, modified, 816, 817
Zidovudine, 356